EXPERTddx™

PEDIATRICS

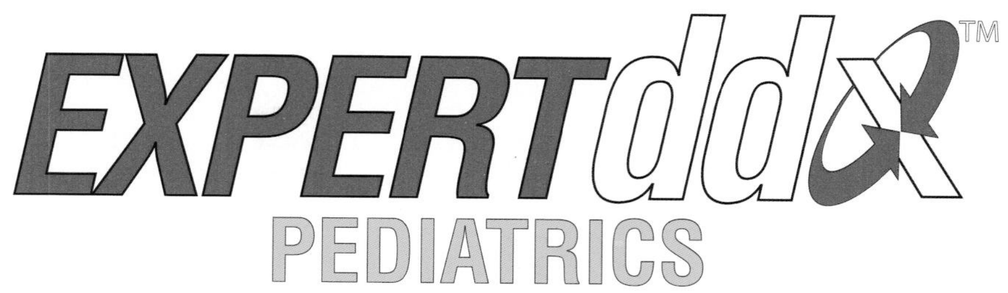

Christopher G. Anton, MD
Assistant Professor of Radiology and Pediatrics
Associate Director of Radiology Residency Program
University of Cincinnati College of Medicine
Cincinnati Children's Hospital Medical Center
Cincinnati, Ohio

Alexander J. Towbin, MD
Assistant Professor of Radiology and Pediatrics
University of Cincinnati College of Medicine
Director of Radiology Informatics
Associate Director of Thoracoabdominal Imaging
Cincinnati Children's Hospital Medical Center
Cincinnati, Ohio

Bernadette L. Koch, MD
Associate Professor of Radiology and Pediatrics
University of Cincinnati College of Medicine
Associate Director of Physician Services and Education
Cincinnati Children's Hospital Medical Center
Cincinnati, Ohio

Eva Ilse Rubio, MD
Assistant Professor of Radiology and Pediatrics
University of Cincinnati College of Medicine
Cincinnati Children's Hospital Medical Center
Cincinnati, Ohio

Daniel J. Podberesky, MD
Assistant Professor of Radiology and Pediatrics
University of Cincinnati College of Medicine
Chief, Division of Thoracoabdominal Imaging
Cincinnati Children's Hospital Medical Center
Cincinnati, Ohio

B.J. Manaster, MD, PhD, FACR
Professor of Radiology
University of Utah School of Medicine
Salt Lake City, Utah

Susan I. Blaser, MD, FRCPC
Associate Professor of Neuroradiology
University of Toronto
Staff Neuroradiologist
The Hospital for Sick Children
Ontario, Canada

Sara M. O'Hara, MD, FAAP
Associate Professor of Radiology and Pediatrics
University of Cincinnati College of Medicine
Chief, Division of Ultrasound
Cincinnati Children's Hospital Medical Center
Cincinnati, Ohio

Lane F. Donnelly, MD
Professor of Radiology and Pediatrics
University of Cincinnati College of Medicine
Radiologist-in-Chief
Cincinnati Children's Hospital Medical Center
Cincinnati, Ohio

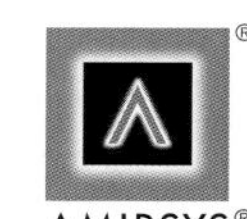

AMIRSYS®
Names you know. Content you trust.®

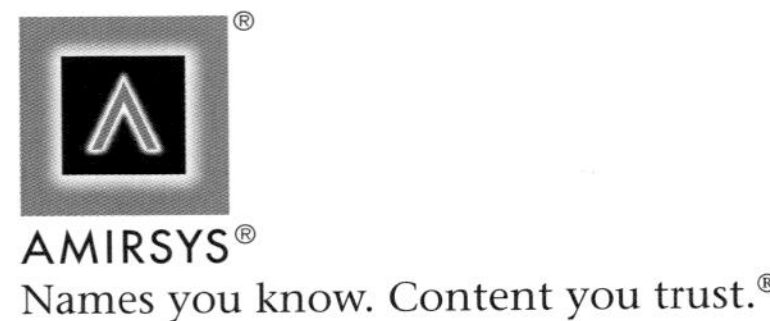

AMIRSYS®
Names you know. Content you trust.®

First Edition

Composition by Amirsys, Inc., Salt Lake City, Utah

Printed in Canada by Friesens, Altona, Manitoba, Canada

ISBN: 978-1-931884-13-6

Notice and Disclaimer

The information in this product ("Product") is provided as a reference for use by licensed medical professionals and no others. It does not and should not be construed as any form of medical diagnosis or professional medical advice on any matter. Receipt or use of this Product, in whole or in part, does not constitute or create a doctor-patient, therapist-patient, or other healthcare professional relationship between Amirsys Inc. ("Amirsys") and any recipient. This Product may not reflect the most current medical developments, and Amirsys makes no claims, promises, or guarantees about accuracy, completeness, or adequacy of the information contained in or linked to the Product. The Product is not a substitute for or replacement of professional medical judgment. Amirsys and its affiliates, authors, contributors, partners, and sponsors disclaim all liability or responsibility for any injury and/or damage to persons or property in respect to actions taken or not taken based on any and all Product information.

In the cases where drugs or other chemicals are prescribed, readers are advised to check the Product information currently provided by the manufacturer of each drug to be administered to verify the recommended dose, the method and duration of administration, and contraindications. It is the responsibility of the treating physician relying on experience and knowledge of the patient to determine dosages and the best treatment for the patient.

To the maximum extent permitted by applicable law, Amirsys provides the Product AS IS AND WITH ALL FAULTS, AND HEREBY DISCLAIMS ALL WARRANTIES AND CONDITIONS, WHETHER EXPRESS, IMPLIED OR STATUTORY, INCLUDING BUT NOT LIMITED TO, ANY (IF ANY) IMPLIED WARRANTIES OR CONDITIONS OF MERCHANTABILITY, OF FITNESS FOR A PARTICULAR PURPOSE, OF LACK OF VIRUSES, OR ACCURACY OR COMPLETENESS OF RESPONSES, OR RESULTS, AND OF LACK OF NEGLIGENCE OR LACK OF WORKMANLIKE EFFORT. ALSO, THERE IS NO WARRANTY OR CONDITION OF TITLE, QUIET ENJOYMENT, QUIET POSSESSION, CORRESPONDENCE TO DESCRIPTION OR NON-INFRINGEMENT, WITH REGARD TO THE PRODUCT. THE ENTIRE RISK AS TO THE QUALITY OF OR ARISING OUT OF USE OR PERFORMANCE OF THE PRODUCT REMAINS WITH THE READER.

Amirsys disclaims all warranties of any kind if the Product was customized, repackaged or altered in any way by any third party.

Library of Congress Cataloging-in-Publication Data

Expertddx. Pediatrics / [edited by] Christopher G. Anton. -- 1st ed.
p. ; cm.
Includes index.
ISBN 978-1-931884-13-6
1. Children--Diseases--Diagnosis--Atlases. 2. Diagnosis, Differential--Atlases. I. Anton, Christopher G. II. Title: Pediatrics.
[DNLM: 1. Pediatrics--methods--Handbooks. 2. Diagnosis, Differential--Handbooks. WS 39 E96 2009]
RJ51.D53E97 2010
618.92--dc22

2009037206

To my wife, my best friend and three children: Mackenzie, Lily, and Joshua. They have sacrificed many hours in allowing me to complete this book. It is also dedicated to my father, who I attempt to emulate as a dad and a radiologist.

"To me, there are three things we all should do every day. We should do this every day of our lives. Number one is laugh. You should laugh every day. Number two is think. You should spend some time in thought. And number three is, you should have your emotions moved to tears, could be happiness or joy. But think about it. If you laugh, you think, and you cry, that's a full day. That's a heck of a day. You do that seven days a week, you're going to have something special."

Excerpt from a speech given by
Jimmy Valvano at ESPY Awards on March 3, 1993.

CGA

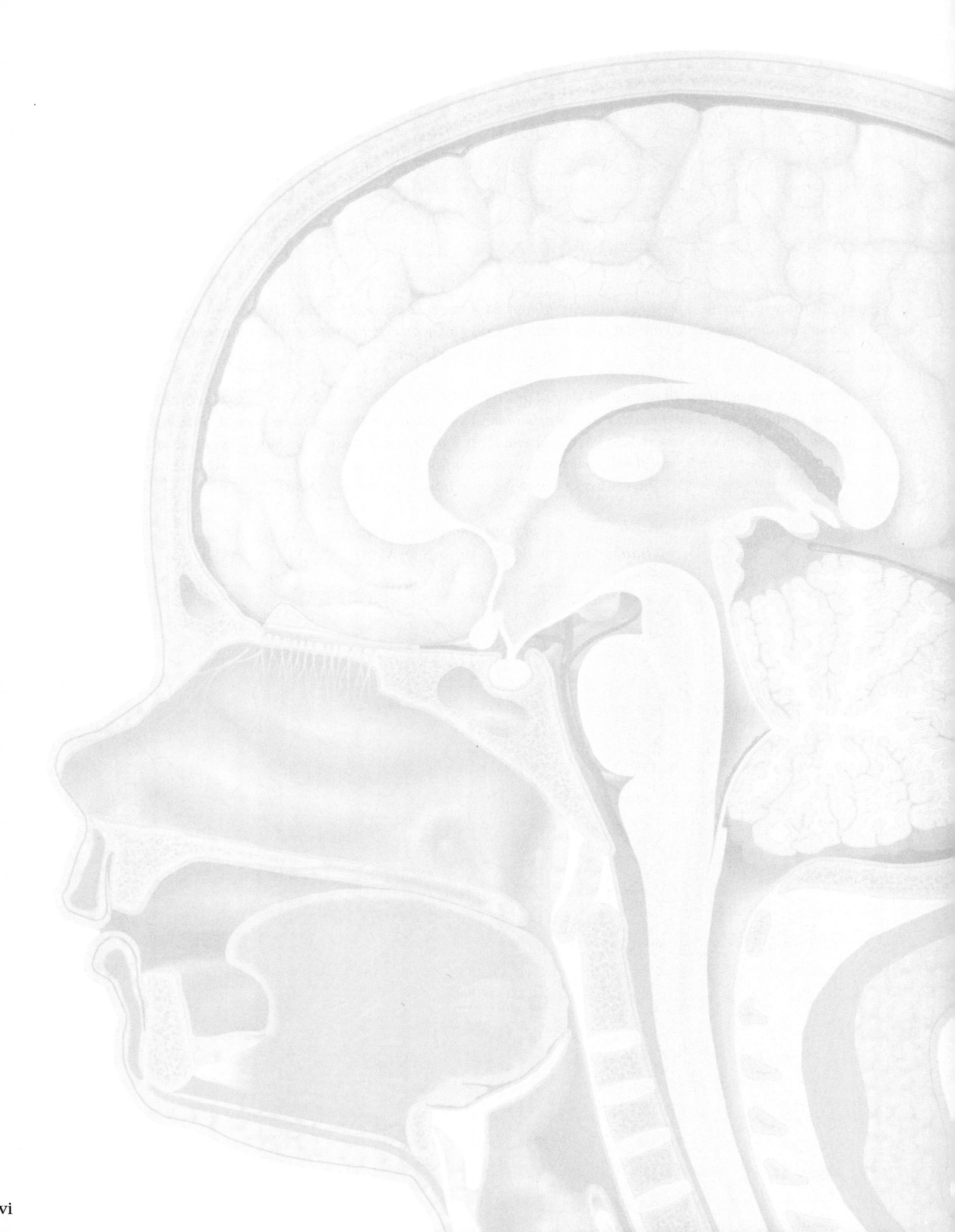

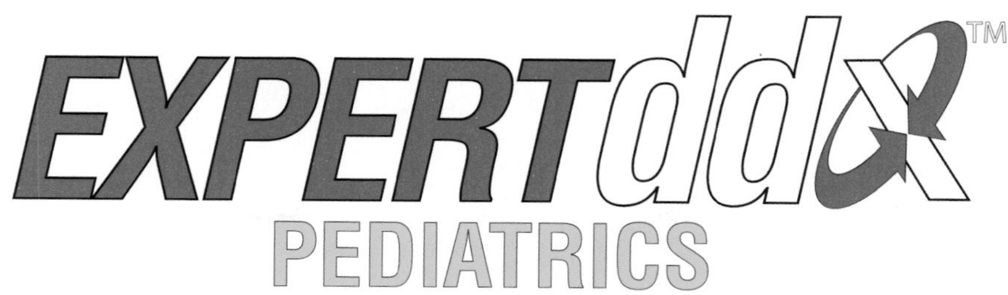

Once the appropriate technical protocols have been delineated, the best quality images obtained, and the cases queued up on PACS, the diagnostic responsibility reaches the radiology reading room. The radiologist must do more than simply "lay words on" but reach a real conclusion. If we cannot reach a definitive diagnosis, we must offer a reasonable differential diagnosis. A list that's too long is useless; a list that's too short may be misleading. To be useful, a differential must be more than a rote recitation from some dusty book or a mnemonic from a lecture way back when. Instead, we must take into account key imaging findings and relevant clinical information.

With these considerations in mind, we at Amirsys designed our Expert Differential Diagnoses series—EXPERTddx for short. Leading experts in every subspecialty of radiology identified the top differential diagnoses in their respective fields, encompassing specific anatomic locations, generic imaging findings, modality-specific findings, and clinically based indications. Our experts gathered multiple images, both typical and variant, for each EXPERTddx. Each features at least eight beautiful images that illustrate the possible diagnoses, accompanied by captions that highlight the pertinent imaging findings. Hundreds more are available in the eBook feature that accompanies every book. In classic Amirsys fashion, each EXPERTddx includes bulleted text that distills the available information to the essentials. You'll find helpful clues for diagnoses, ranked by prevalence as Common, Less Common, and Rare but Important.

Our EXPERTddx series is designed to help radiologists reach reliable—indeed, expert—conclusions. Whether you are a practicing radiologist or a resident/fellow in training, we think the EXPERTddx series will quickly become your practical "go-to" reference.

Anne G. Osborn, MD
Executive Vice President and Editor-in-Chief, Amirsys, Inc.

Paula J. Woodward, MD
Executive Vice President and Medical Director, Amirsys, Inc.

H. Ric Harnsberger, MD
CEO, Amirsys, Inc.

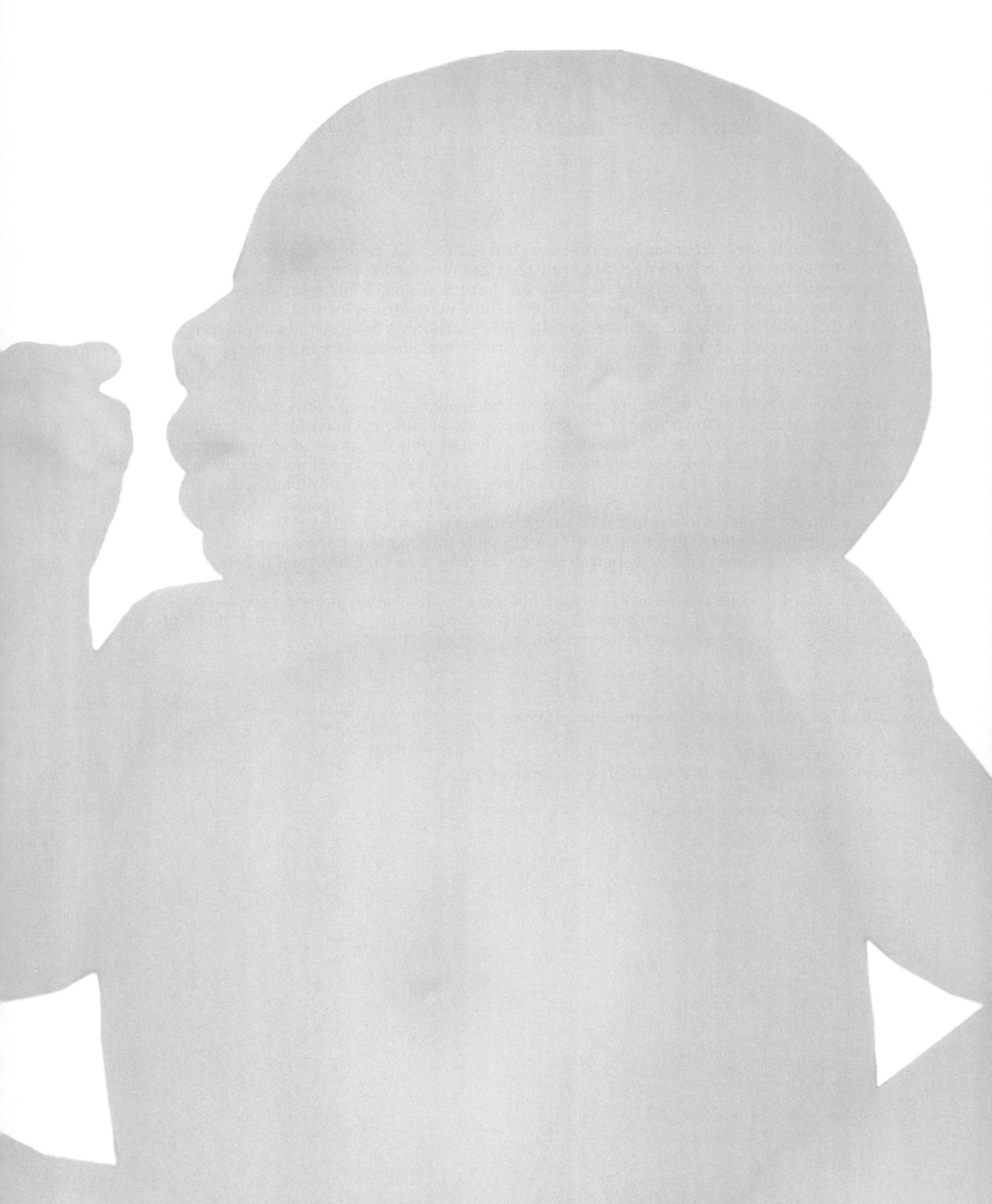

PREFACE

Many radiologists are uncomfortable interpreting pediatric imaging studies; some may even be tempted to return the study to the bottom of a stack of films or leave it in the PACS system for someone else to read. We hope that using *EXPERTddx: Pediatrics* will reduce the hesitation and remove much of the stress of reading that "pediatric" case. This book was written to provide useful information for radiologists at all levels of experience and expertise.

Our goal was to create a comprehensive ddx textbook as a resource for pediatric imaging interpretation. *EXPERTddx: Pediatrics* is not meant to be an all inclusive source for pediatric imaging, although the book provides an extensive insight to the most common to the more complex pediatric disease processes that one encounters. For example, a neonate with a liver mass, what could it be? What are the important clinical and imaging findings in formulating this ddx? What are uncommon or rare possibilities?

The format of this book is similar to others in the EXPERTddx series. We have divided *EXPERTddx: Pediatrics* into anatomical sections: Cardiac, Chest, Gastrointestinal, Genitourinary, Musculoskeletal, Brain, Head and Neck, and Spine. Each chapter begins with a list of the different diagnoses for either the clinical or imaging scenario. This is followed by helpful clues on imaging as well as clinical pearls that can aid in unlocking each ddx. Each chapter ends with a large image gallery showing representative examples of each ddx.

I am grateful to Dr. Lane Donnelly and Amirsys for giving me the opportunity to work on this book. I am deeply grateful to my co-authors for their significant time dedication and contributions to *EPERRTddx: Pediatrics*. I hope this has been as an enjoyable and rewarding process for them as it has been for me. I would also like to acknowledge Dr. Alan Brody for his guidance over the years and contributing author Dr. Daniel Podberesky for his patience while I bounced many a questions off him.

In addition, I would also like to acknowledge Melissa Hoopes, Ashley Renlund, and Dr. Tony Zarka for their editorial expertise. I could not have completed the book without their support.

We have poured a great deal of ourselves with time and hard work into this book. We hope that this book will be a valuable resource for daily radiology practices.

Christopher G. Anton, MD
Assistant Professor of Radiology and Pediatrics
University of Cincinnati College of Medicine
Associate Director of Radiology Residency Program
Cincinnati Children's Hospital Medical Center
Cincinnati, Ohio

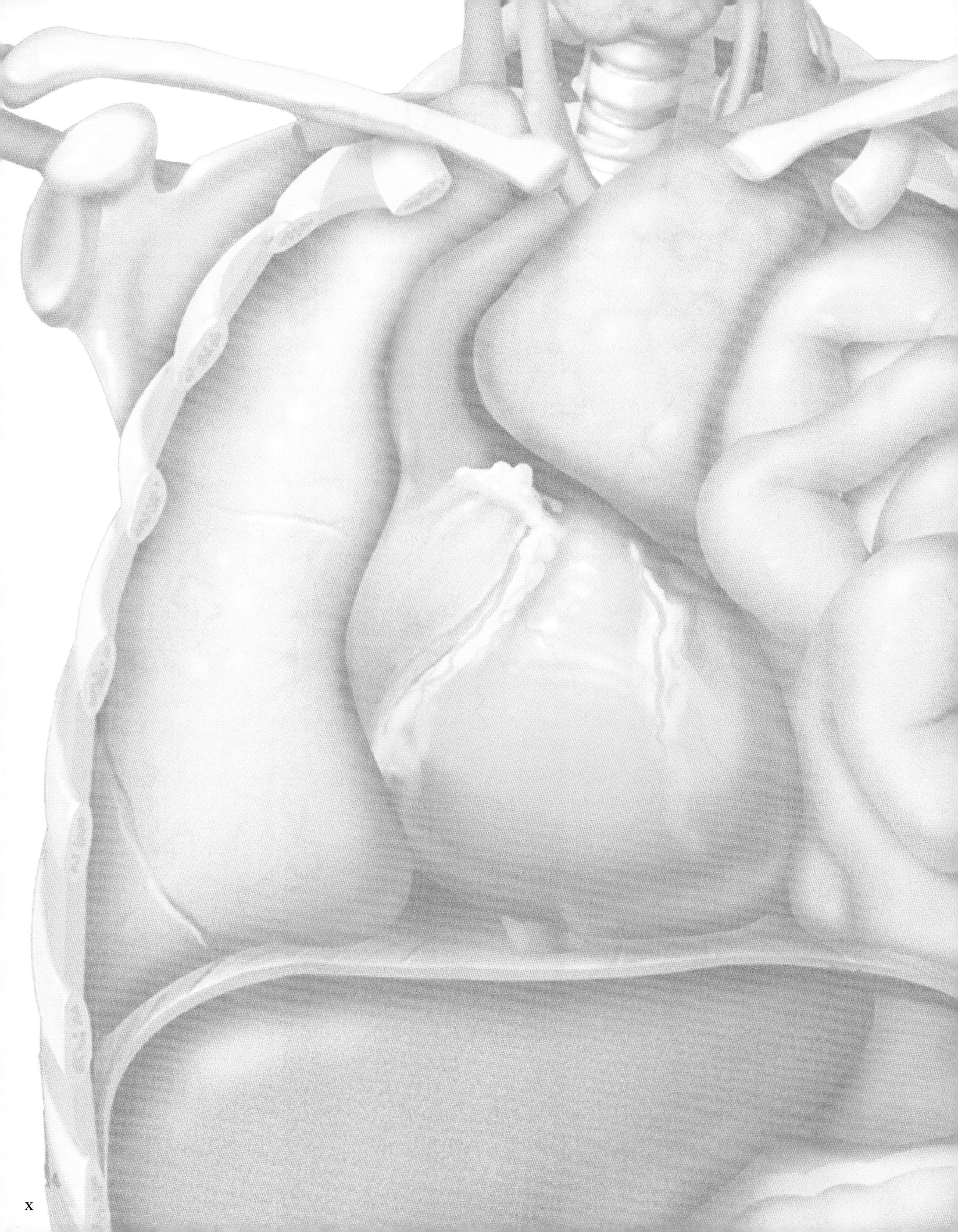

ACKNOWLEDGMENTS

Text Editing
Kellie J. Heap
Arthur G. Gelsinger, MA
Katherine Riser, MA
Dave L. Chance, MA

Image Editing
Jeffrey J. Marmorstone
Danny C. La

Medical Text Editing
Anthony I. Zarka, MD

Art Direction and Design
Lane R. Bennion, MS
Richard Coombs, MS
Laura C. Sesto, MA

Associate Editor
Ashley R. Renlund, MA

Production Lead
Melissa A. Hoopes

Some images were previously published in Manaster BJ, May DA, Disler DG. Musculoskeletal Imaging: The Requisites. 2nd edition. Philadelphia, PA: Mosby, Elsevier; 2002. Each of these images is identified by "MSK Req" in the caption.

These images appear as follows: section.page.image; 5.4.2; 5.23.6; 5.57.2; 5.67.1; 5.83.2; 5.85.3; 5.111.5; 5.114.1; and 5.114.2.

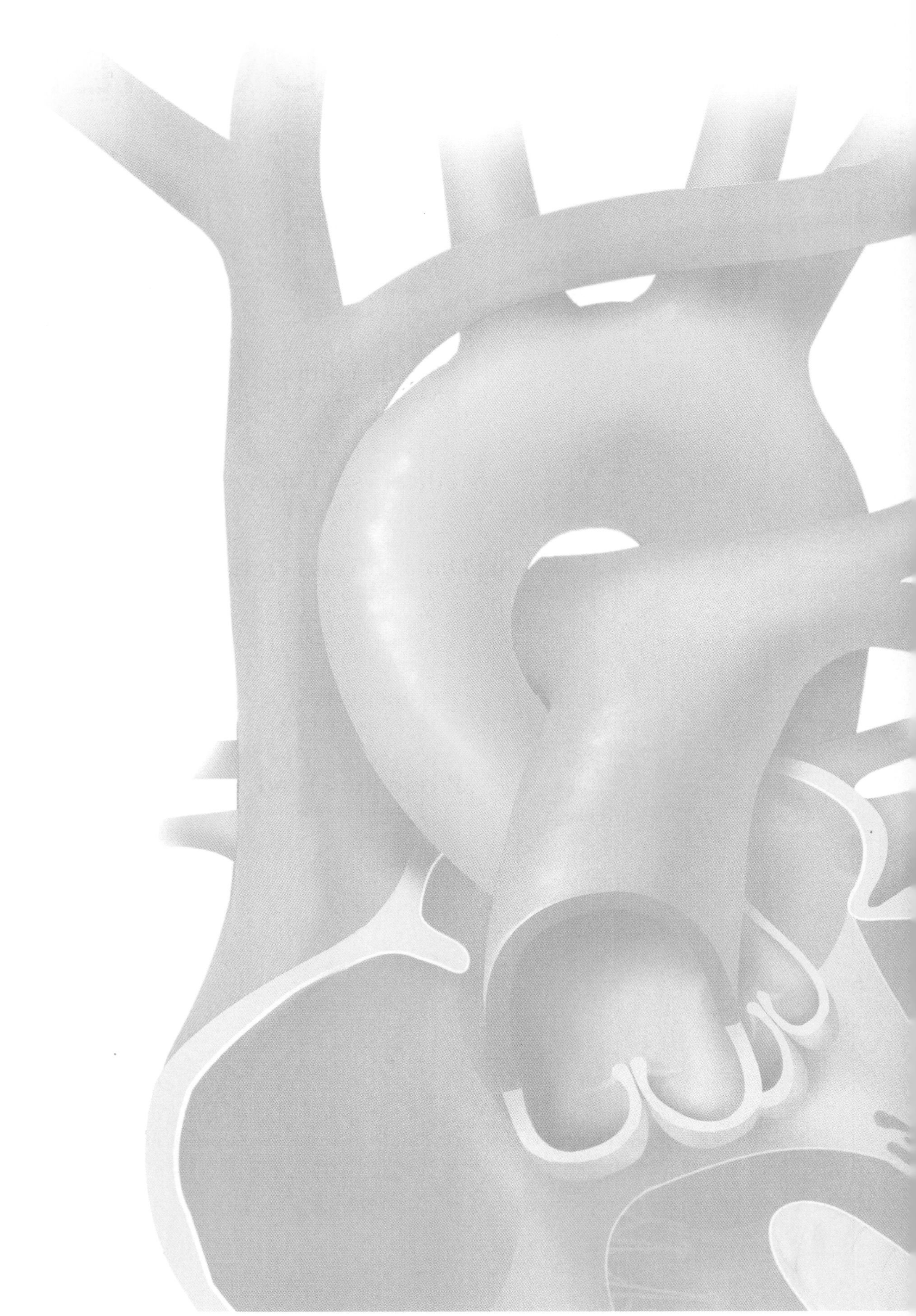

SECTIONS

TABLE OF CONTENTS

SECTION 1
Cardiac

SECTION 2
Chest

SECTION 3
Gastrointestinal

SECTION 4
Genitourinary

SECTION 5
Musculoskeletal

SECTION 6
Brain, Head and Neck

SECTION 7
Spine

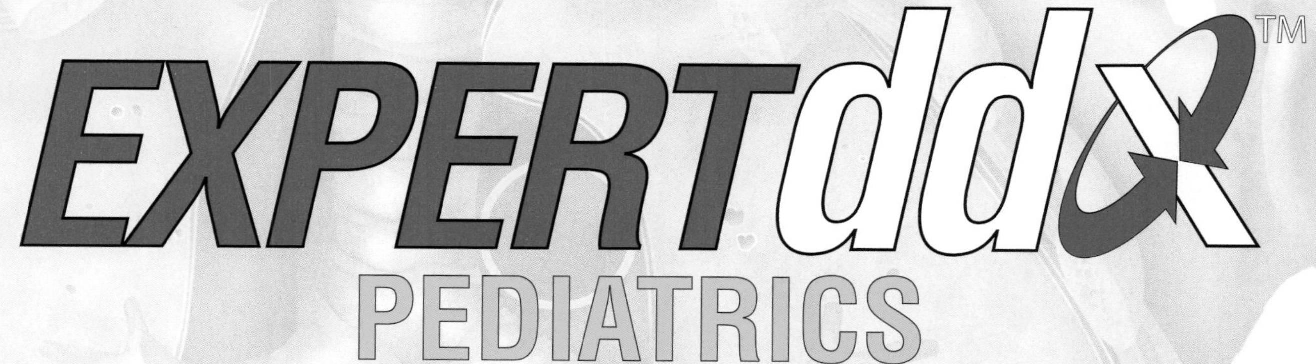
EXPERTddx™
PEDIATRICS

SECTION 1
Cardiac

HIGH OUTPUT HEART FAILURE

DIFFERENTIAL DIAGNOSIS

Common
- Intracardiac Shunt
- Vein of Galen Aneurysmal Malformation
- Anemias

Less Common
- Vascular Malformations
- Hemangioendothelioma
- Teratoma

Rare but Important
- Parkes-Weber
- Chorioangioma

ESSENTIAL INFORMATION

Key Differential Diagnosis Issues
- Age of patient: Newborn, toddler, child, or adolescent?
- Prior medical history
  - Underlying congenital heart defect or aortic anomaly
  - Infectious history or postinfectious syndrome
  - Chronic medical conditions or therapy
- Intracardiac vs. extracardiac cause?

Helpful Clues for Common Diagnoses
- **Intracardiac Shunt**
  - Ventricular septal defect
    - Most common cardiac anomaly in general population
    - Radiograph findings: Hyperexpanded lungs, large round heart, plump pulmonary vessels most conspicuous at hila
  - Atrioventricular septal defect
    - Commonly associated with Down syndrome
    - Radiograph findings: Hyperexpanded lungs, large round heart, plump pulmonary vessels most conspicuous at hila
  - Anomalous coronary artery
    - Most commonly, left coronary artery arises from pulmonary artery origin
    - Preferential flow away from myocardial muscular bed into pulmonary circulation results in ventricular ischemia
    - Imaging features: Marked cardiomegaly (CM); left ventricular and atrial enlargement conspicuous on lateral view
- **Vein of Galen Aneurysmal Malformation**
  - Congenital arteriovenous fistulous communicate between midline intracranial arteries and vein of Galen or other fetal venous structures
  - Poor prognosis
    - Choroidal type
    - Fetal hydropic changes
    - Congestive heart failure with intracranial bruit
  - Intracranial findings
    - Large midline vascular anomaly
    - Hydrocephalus
    - Encephalomalacia
- **Anemias**
  - Sickle cell disease
    - Longstanding anemia leads to global CM
    - Physiologic contributions: High output of anemia, poor oxygen delivery to coronary arteries, pulmonary arterial hypertension
    - More common in older children, adolescents
  - β-thalassemia
    - Severe anemia leads to global CM
    - Physiologic contributions: High output anemia, elevated iron levels/deposition from transfusions
    - May manifest earlier in childhood

Helpful Clues for Less Common Diagnoses
- **Vascular Malformations**
  - Typical locations: Head, neck, extremities, liver
  - Classification of vascular anomalies (these lesions grow commensurate with child)
    - High-flow vascular lesions (arteriovenous malformations and arteriovenous fistulae)
    - Low-flow vascular lesions (venous, lymphatic, venolymphatic)
- **Hemangioendothelioma**
  - a.k.a. infantile hepatic hemangioma
    - Hypervascular liver mass seen in infants
    - May have cutaneous hemangiomas, especially multiple
  - Imaging
    - May be multiple rounded lesions or single dominant lesion

- US: Hypoechoic
- CT: Round, enhancing lesions; may enhance from periphery to center
- MR: Bright on T2, isointense/dark on T1

- ○ Cardiovascular sequelae/manifestations
  - Significant arteriovenous shunting may lead to high output failure
  - Aorta may be diminutive distal to lesion
  - Disseminated intravascular coagulopathy may occur

- **Teratoma**
  - ○ Germ cell tumor presumably arising from multipotential cells
  - ○ Typical locations
    - Sacrococcygeal region, arising from Hensen node
    - Neck
    - Oropharynx
    - Abdomen
    - Retroperitoneum
  - ○ More common in females
  - ○ Findings associated with increased risk for congestive heart failure
    - Larger lesions
    - Significant solid tissue component
    - Large feeding vessels/robust internal vascularity
    - Intralesional hemorrhage
    - Placentomegaly
    - Hydropic changes in fetus
  - ○ Sacrococcygeal teratoma (SCGT)
    - Classified into types 1-4 based on extrapelvic vs. intrapelvic components
    - SCGT findings associated with heart failure: Aortic velocity > 60 cm/sec; IVC diameter > 4.1 mm (21-28 weeks gestation); reversed hypogastric flow
  - ○ Cervical teratomas
    - Differential consideration is lymphatic malformation if multicystic
    - Other considerations: Airway management, intracranial involvement

Helpful Clues for Rare Diagnoses

- **Parkes-Weber**
  - ○ Rare extremity soft tissue overgrowth syndrome due to vascular anomaly
    - Limb overgrowth
  - ○ Combined vascular malformation; capillary malformation, high-flow AVMs ± lymphatic malformation
  - ○ May result in high output heart failure
- **Chorioangioma**
  - ○ Benign, rare placental tumor
  - ○ Consists of small caliber vascular structures and stroma
  - ○ Often seen at base of umbilical cord, with vascular supply arising near or from umbilical vessels
  - ○ Potential fetal sequelae
    - Hydropic changes
    - Growth restriction

Intracardiac Shunt

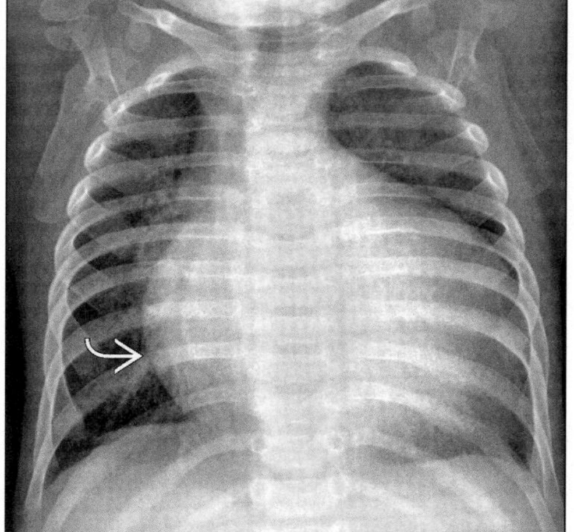

AP radiograph in this 8-month-old child who presented with wheezing and grunting shows new and significant enlargement of the cardiac silhouette ➔. An anomalous coronary artery was discovered.

Intracardiac Shunt

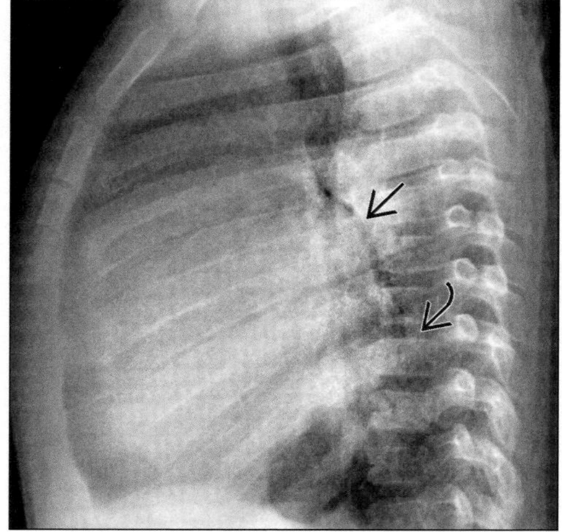

Lateral radiograph of the same child demonstrates left atrial and ventricular enlargement with the posterior border of the heart ➔ overlapping with the spine and causing airway compression ➔.

HIGH OUTPUT HEART FAILURE

(**Left**) *AP radiograph shows mild cardiac enlargement and increased caliber of the pulmonary vessels in a child with a ventricular septal defect.* (**Right**) *AP radiograph shows marked cardiomegaly and florid pulmonary vascular congestion in a 3-month-old child with diabetic embryopathy and an unbalanced atrioventricular septal defect.*

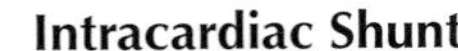

Intracardiac Shunt

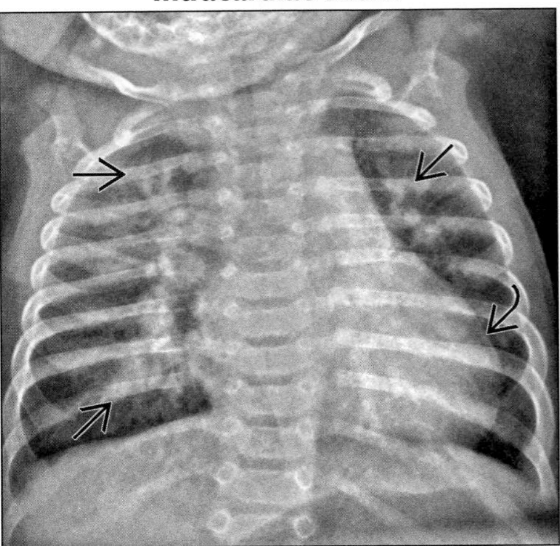

Intracardiac Shunt

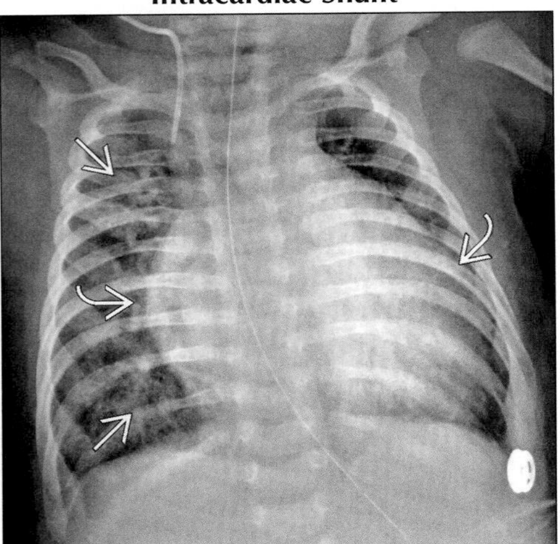

(**Left**) *AP radiograph shows a patient with cardiomegaly due to severe complex congenital heart disease, including situs inversus, transposition of the great vessels, and large atrial/ventricular septal defects.* (**Right**) *Axial T2WI MR of the same patient shows global enlargement of all 4 chambers of the heart. The large ventricular septal defect is depicted. Cine imaging demonstrated globally depressed ventricular systolic function.*

Intracardiac Shunt

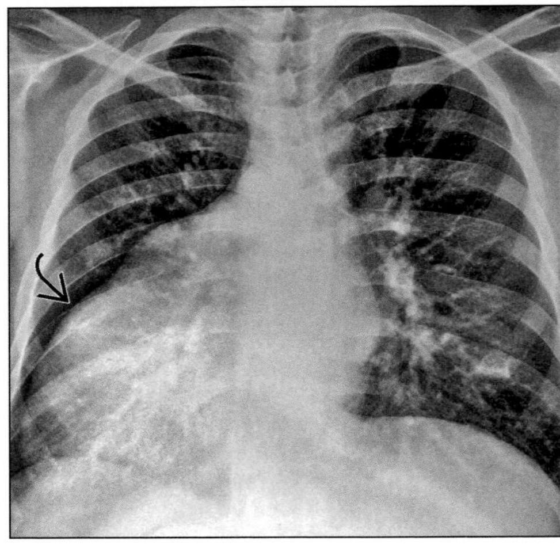

Intracardiac Shunt

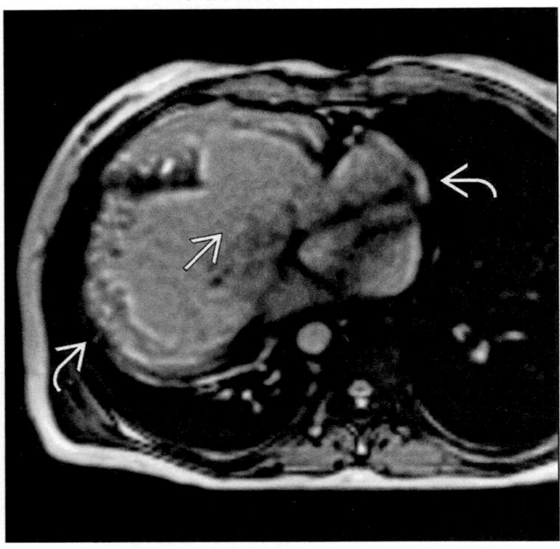

(**Left**) *AP radiograph shows severe cardiac enlargement in a newborn with intractable heart failure and a prenatally diagnosed intracranial lesion.* (**Right**) *Coronal ultrasound in the same child shows the very large caliber interhemispheric vascular abnormality and profound hydrocephalus.*

Vein of Galen Aneurysmal Malformation

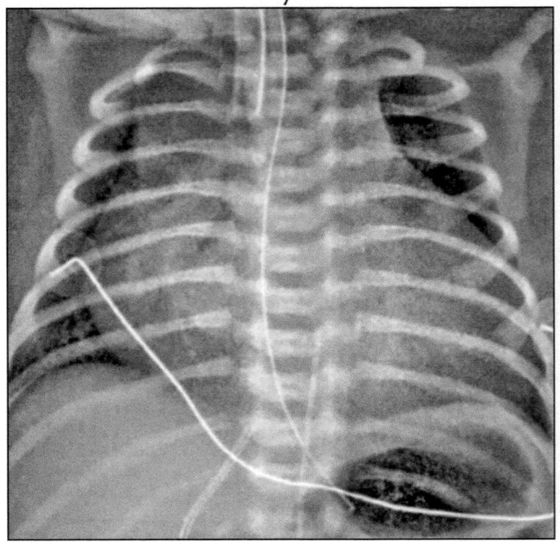

Vein of Galen Aneurysmal Malformation

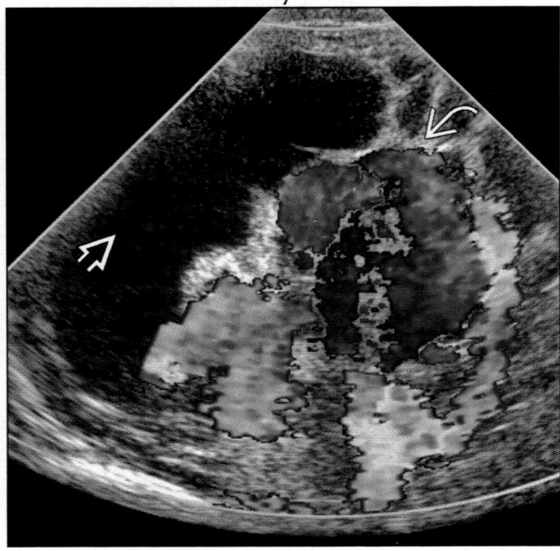

HIGH OUTPUT HEART FAILURE

Vein of Galen Aneurysmal Malformation

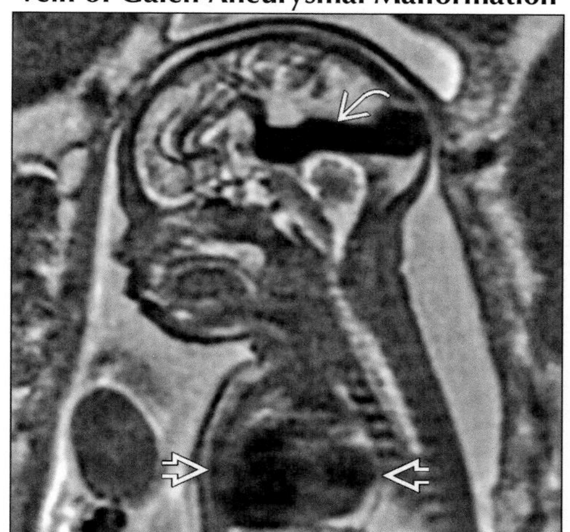

Vein of Galen Aneurysmal Malformation

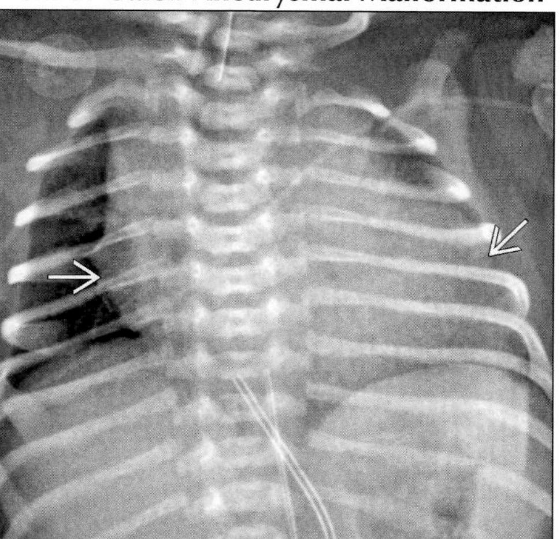

(Left) *Sagittal T2WI MR in a 33-week-old fetus shows a large supratentorial midline vascular anomaly consistent with a choroidal vein of Galen malformation. Note the cardiomegaly; the enlarged left ventricle extends nearly to the spine.* ***(Right)*** *AP radiograph of the same female at birth shows persistent cardiac enlargement. The heart assumed a more normal appearance after several embolizations of the intracranial lesion.*

Anemias

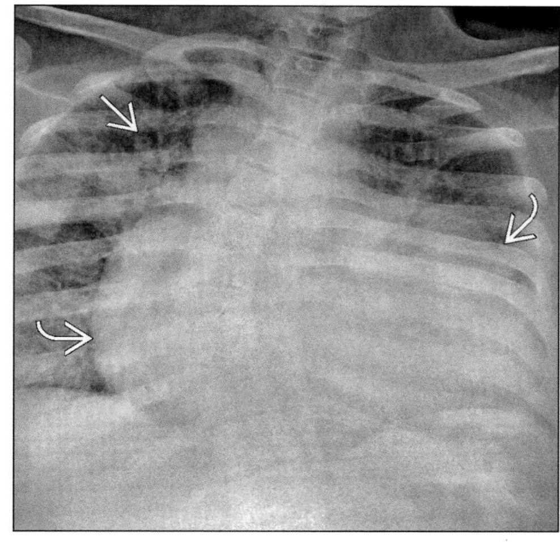

Anemias

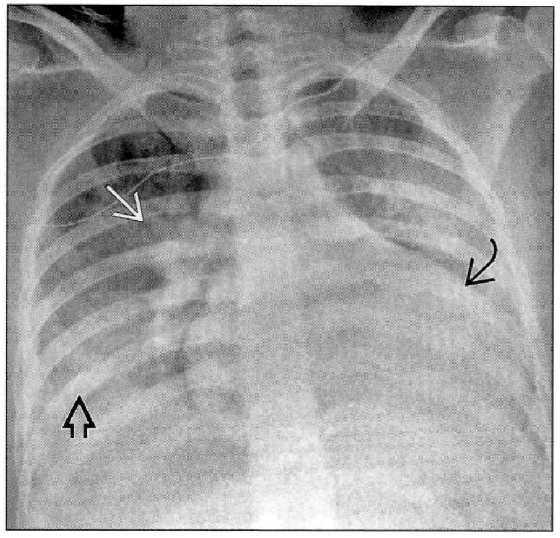

(Left) *AP radiograph shows marked cardiomegaly and pulmonary edema in this teenage female with advanced sickle cell disease. She died from complications of the disease 1 month after this radiograph.* ***(Right)*** *AP radiograph in a patient with hemoglobin S-β-thalassemia disease demonstrates cardiomegaly, pulmonary vasculature congestion, and bibasilar haziness of pleural effusions.*

Vascular Malformations

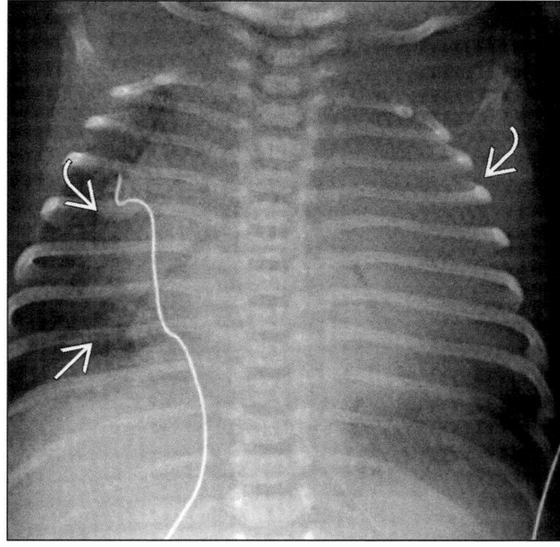

Vascular Malformations

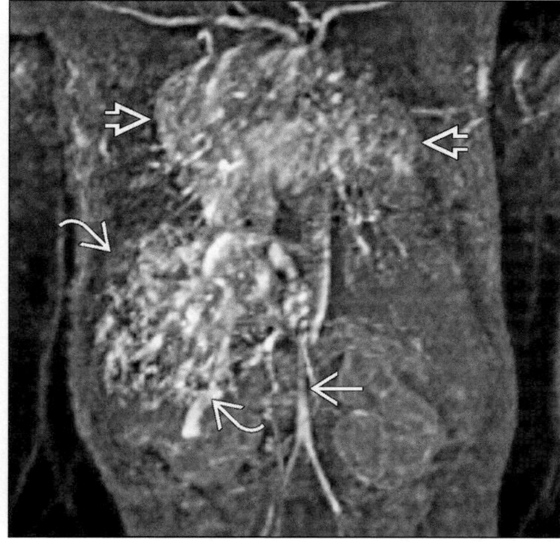

(Left) *AP radiograph shows massive cardiac enlargement and pulmonary edema in this newborn with a prenatally diagnosed liver lesion.* ***(Right)*** *Coronal T1 C+ SPGR MIP MR in the same child shows the large tangled vascular malformation in the right lobe of the liver with marked cardiac enlargement, particularly right atrial enlargement. Note the bulging right heart border. Caliber of the aorta below the lesion is narrowed.*

HIGH OUTPUT HEART FAILURE

*(**Left**) AP radiograph shows only mild cardiomegaly in this 3 year old with a parotid gland arteriovenous malformation (AVM) who nonetheless showed clinical signs of congestive heart failure. (**Right**) AP catheter angiography in the same child shows the large right parotid gland AVM served primarily by the right external carotid artery and drained by the internal jugular vein and retromandibular vein. It was successfully embolized.*

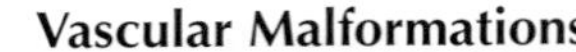

Vascular Malformations

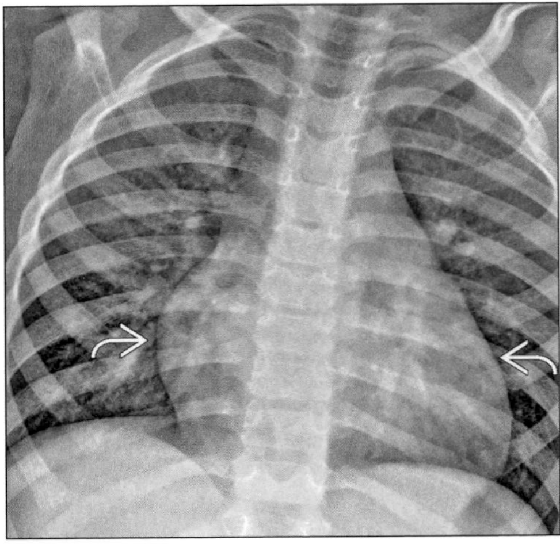

Vascular Malformations

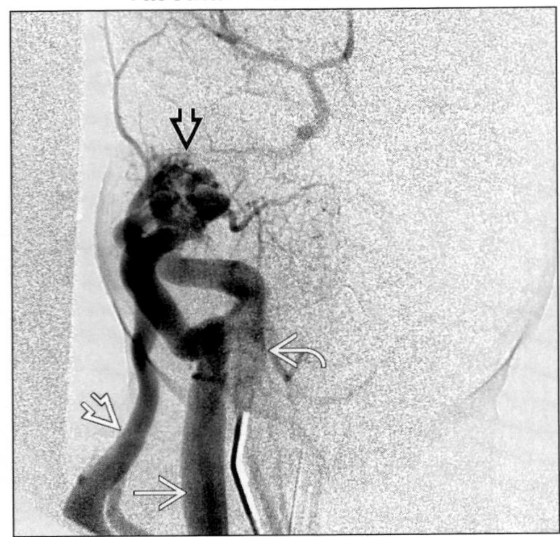

*(**Left**) AP radiograph obtained on the day of birth shows nonspecific cardiomegaly and prominent soft tissue contour of the upper abdomen, presumably the liver. (**Right**) Axial CECT of the same infant shows a large vascular lesion occupying the left lobe of the liver. The hepatic artery is dilated; the aorta is not well seen due to the indwelling umbilical catheter but appears diminutive in caliber.*

Hemangioendothelioma

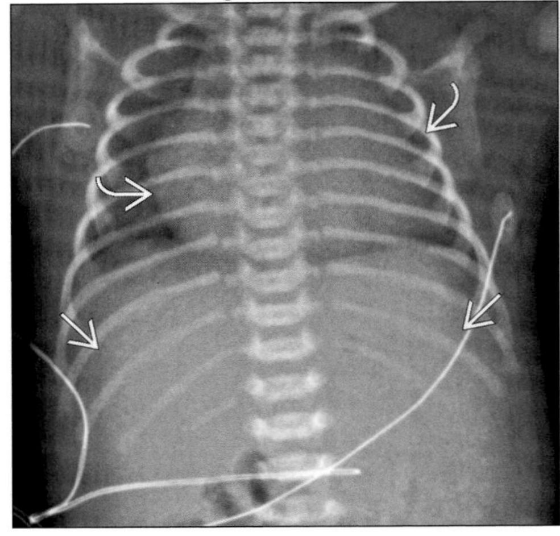

Hemangioendothelioma

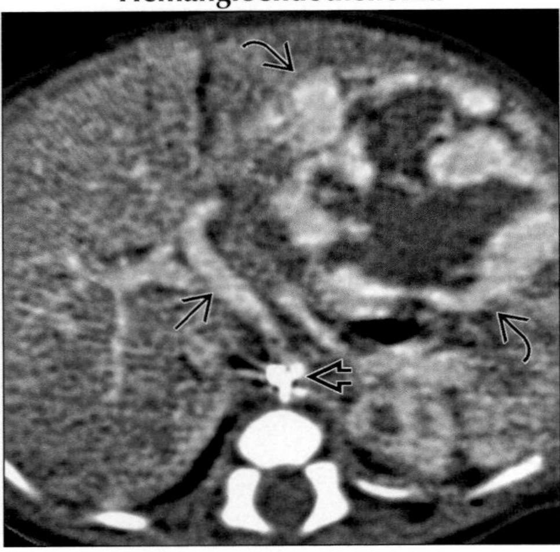

*(**Left**) Coronal T2WI MR in a 31-week-old fetus shows a moderately enlarged heart and massive intra-/extrapelvic mass. The placenta was also thickened. There was concern for mirror syndrome, in which maternal fluid accumulation and pre-eclampsia occur in the setting of developing fetal hydrops. (**Right**) Lateral radiograph shows the infant at birth. A portion of the mass is seen. The heart is still enlarged here but improved after resection.*

Teratoma

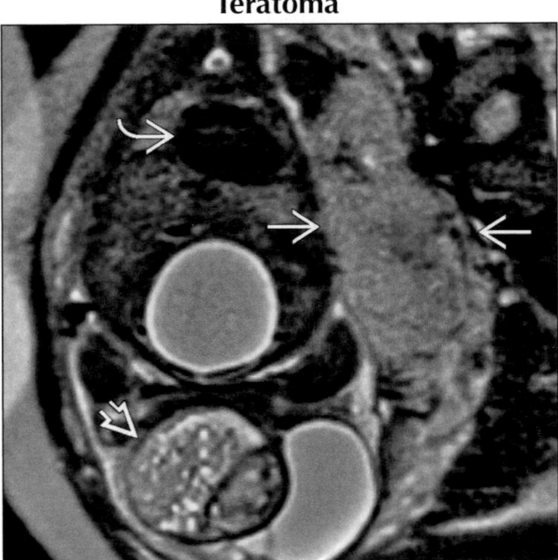

Teratoma

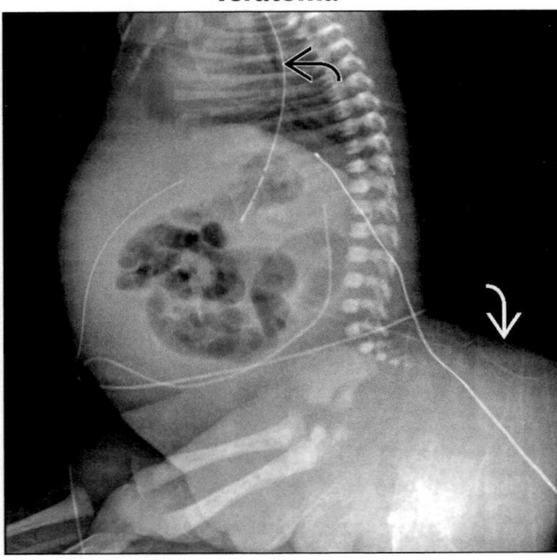

HIGH OUTPUT HEART FAILURE

Teratoma

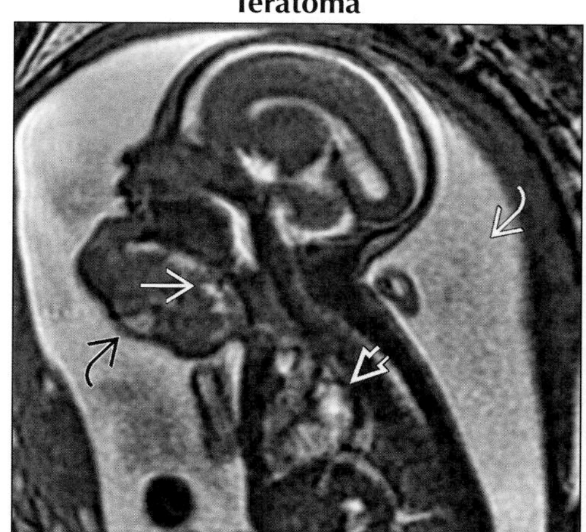

Teratoma

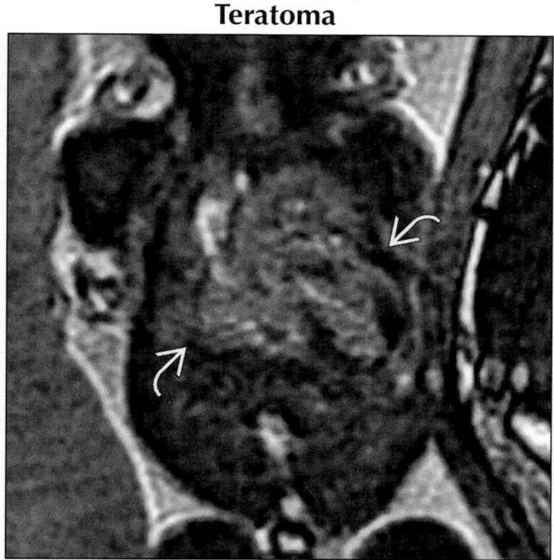

(Left) *Sagittal T2WI MR in a 23-week-old fetus shows a cervical teratoma with prominent internal vessels. Cardiac chambers are globally enlarged. Note the mild polyhydramnios, likely from mass effect on the esophagus.* ***(Right)*** *Coronal T2WI MR shows the full extent of the cardiomegaly in the same infant. Internal hemorrhage of the teratoma at birth resulted in disseminated intravascular coagulopathy and death.*

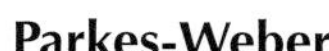

Parkes-Weber

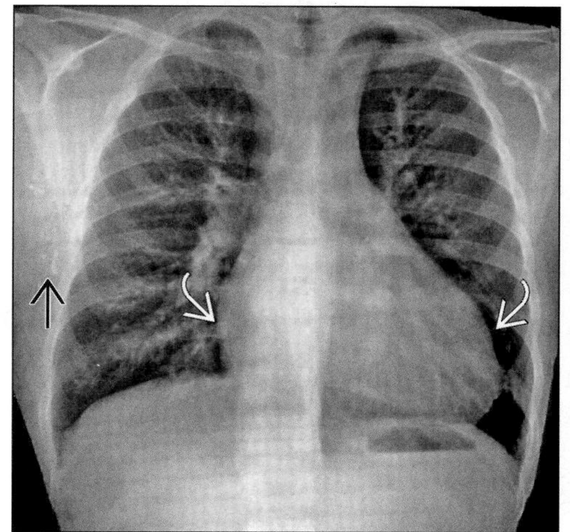

Parkes-Weber

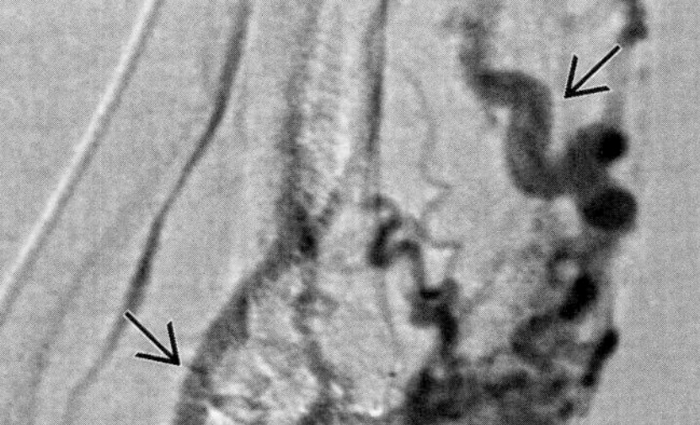

(Left) *AP radiograph shows moderate cardiomegaly in this teenager with an extensive arteriovenous malformation involving the right chest wall, shoulder, and extremity to the elbow. Note the prominence of the soft tissues around the axilla and prior embolization coils.* ***(Right)*** *Lateral catheter angiography of the same child obtained during embolization shows a tangle of engorged high-flow vessels around the right elbow.*

Chorioangioma

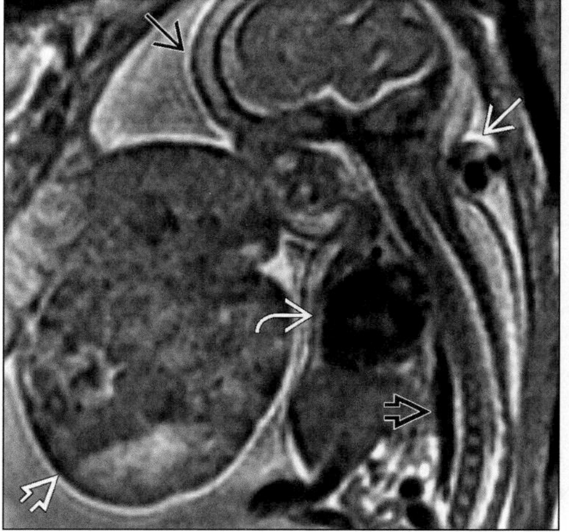

Chorioangioma

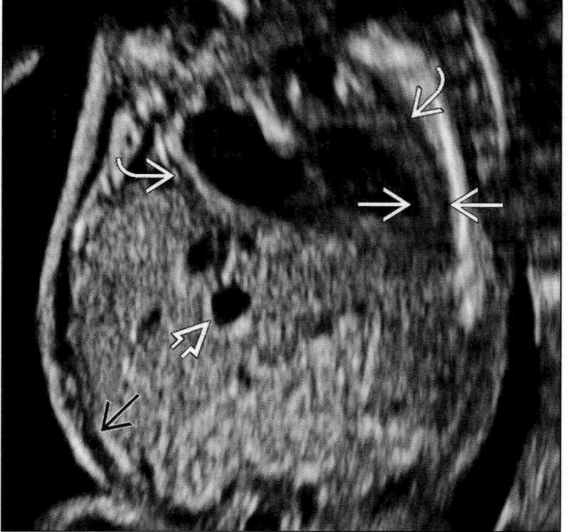

(Left) *Sagittal T2WI MR shows a large, heterogeneous placental mass affecting this 26-week-old fetus. Note the skin edema, cord edema, cardiomegaly, and engorged aorta.* ***(Right)*** *Coronal prenatal ultrasound shows the same fetus with global cardiomegaly and thickened ventricular walls. The umbilical vein is dilated. Skin edema is observed. Fetal echocardiography showed global ventricular dysfunction.*

MASSIVE CARDIOMEGALY

DIFFERENTIAL DIAGNOSIS

Common
- Ebstein Anomaly
- Infectious Cardiomyopathy
- Idiopathic Cardiomyopathy
- Pericardial Effusion

Less Common
- High Output Failure
- Ventricular Septal Defect (VSD)
- Atrioventricular Septal Defect (AVSD)
- Aortic Coarctation
- Anomalous Coronary Artery

Rare but Important
- Pulmonary Artery Atresia with Intact Ventricular Septum
- Glycogen Storage Disease
- Cardiac Tumors

ESSENTIAL INFORMATION

Key Differential Diagnosis Issues
- Age of onset and duration of symptoms
  - Cardiomegaly present at birth or new diagnosis in a previously healthy child?
- Cyanotic vs. noncyanotic patient presentation?

Helpful Clues for Common Diagnoses
- **Ebstein Anomaly**
  - Abnormally formed right-sided heart structures
    - Inferiorly displaced and fixed position of tricuspid valve leaflets
    - "Atrialization of right ventricle" refers to incorporation of right ventricular muscle into right atrium
  - Earlier diagnosis/presentation associated with poorer prognosis
  - Patients are often cyanotic
  - Imaging appearance
    - Often described as "wall-to-wall" heart
    - Contour of heart may be box-like
- **Infectious Cardiomyopathy**
  - Patients noncyanotic
  - Often acute/subacute onset of dyspnea, wheezing
  - Etiologies
    - Viral (enterovirus, parvovirus, adenovirus, coxsackie virus)
    - Diphtheria
    - Lyme disease
- **Idiopathic Cardiomyopathy**
  - May represent prior episode of infection
  - Biopsies may be nonspecific & unrevealing
- **Pericardial Effusion**
  - Patients are noncyanotic; may demonstrate pulsus paradoxus
  - Imaging appearance described as "water bottle" heart
  - Etiologies
    - Viral cardiomyopathy
    - Systemic lupus erythematosus
    - Sarcoidosis
    - Trauma

Helpful Clues for Less Common Diagnoses
- **High Output Failure**
  - Noncyanotic heart disease
  - Often seen with vascular malformations or soft tissue neoplasms
    - Vein of Galen malformation
    - Hemangioendotheliomas when seen extensively throughout liver
    - Parkes-Weber syndrome: Soft tissue vascular malformation with arteriovenous malformation; associated with extremity hemihypertrophy
  - Anemias
    - Sickle cell in advanced stages
- **Ventricular Septal Defect (VSD)**
  - Patients are noncyanotic
  - Degree of cardiac enlargement depends upon size of defect
  - Imaging appearance
    - Increased pulmonary arterial and venous flow
    - Hyperexpanded lungs
- **Atrioventricular Septal Defect (AVSD)**
  - Patients are noncyanotic
  - Strong association with Down syndrome
  - Features of AVSD
    - Deficient atrial, ventricular septa
    - Abnormal mitral and tricuspid valves
    - Associated with hepatomegaly, failure to thrive
  - Imaging appearance
    - Markedly enlarged heart
    - Increased pulmonary arterial and venous flow
    - Hyperexpanded lungs
- **Aortic Coarctation**
  - Localized type

- Focal ring-like narrowing in region of ductus
  - Diffuse type
    - Long segment of narrowing
  - Associations
    - Turner syndrome, trisomy 21, maternal diabetes
    - Intracardiac abnormalities: Bicuspid aortic valve, mitral/tricuspid valve abnormalities, VSD, PDA, AVSD
  - Imaging associations
    - "3" sign, formed by pre-/post stenosis aortic dilation with "waist" of stenosis
    - Notching/erosion of underside of 4th-9th posterior ribs in later childhood
- **Anomalous Coronary Artery**
  - Patients are noncyanotic
  - Most commonly, left coronary artery arises from pulmonary artery
  - Preferential flow away from myocardial muscular bed into pulmonary circulation, results in ischemia
  - Imaging features
    - Severe cardiac enlargement
    - Left ventricular and atrial enlargement conspicuous on lateral view

Helpful Clues for Rare Diagnoses

- **Pulmonary Artery Atresia with Intact Ventricular Septum**
  - Infants develop rapid cyanosis
  - Degree of right ventricular development variable
    - Cardiomegaly may be mild, moderate, or severe
  - Patients are ductal dependent and interatrial flow dependent
- **Glycogen Storage Disease**
  - Noncyanotic cardiomyopathy
  - Types 2, 3, 4 may involve cardiac muscle
  - Type 2 (Pompe disease) classically results in profound cardiomyopathy
    - Severe myocardial hypertrophy
    - Smooth muscle involvement
    - Skeletal muscle involvement, including diaphragm
    - Macroglossia
    - Hepatomegaly
- **Cardiac Tumors**
  - Rhabdomyomas (most common)
    - Associated with tuberous sclerosis
    - May be solitary or multiple
    - Echogenic on ultrasound
    - Benign but may cause symptoms due to mass effect
    - Usually spontaneously resolve
    - No calcifications expected
  - Teratoma
    - Often mixed cystic/solid with fat components with calcification
    - May demonstrate prominent vessels internally
  - Fibroma
    - Inhomogeneous on all modalities
    - Calcifications common

Ebstein Anomaly

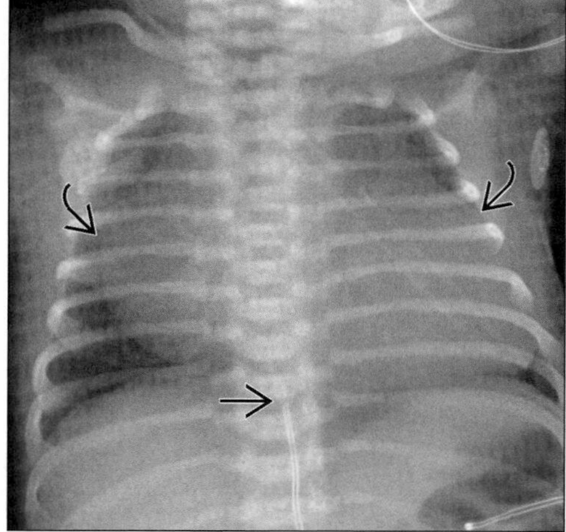

Frontal radiograph in this newborn shows a severely enlarged heart ⇾, which occupies nearly the entire thorax. An umbilical venous catheter projects over the inferior vena cava →.

Ebstein Anomaly

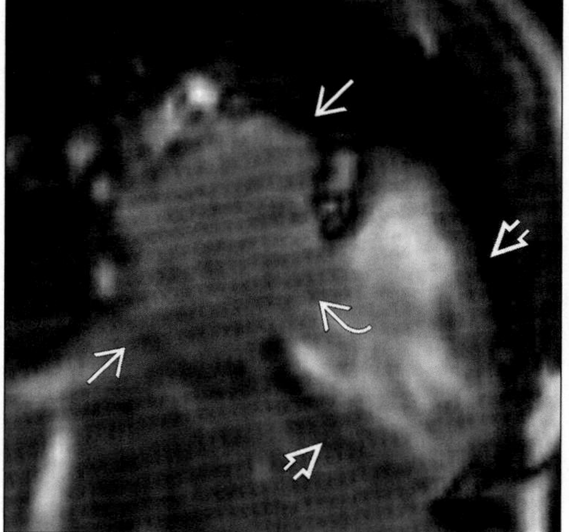

Coronal oblique MR cine in the same child 2 years later shows marked enlargement of the right ventricle ➡ and right atrium ➡, with florid tricuspid valve regurgitation ➡.

MASSIVE CARDIOMEGALY

Ebstein Anomaly

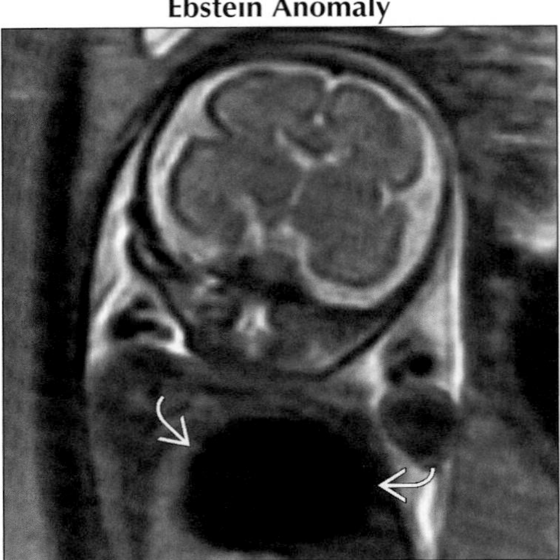

Infectious Cardiomyopathy

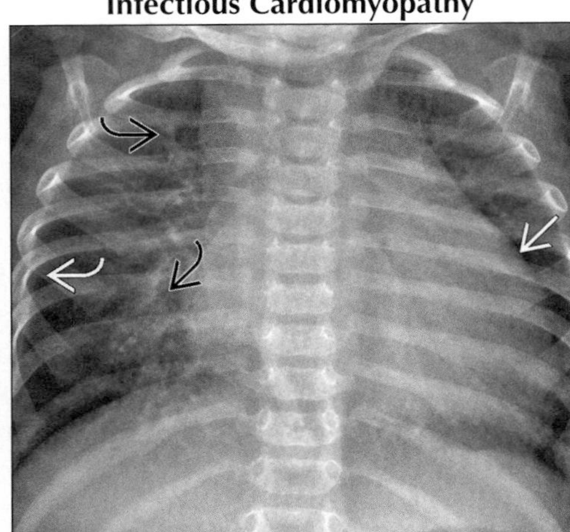

(Left) *Coronal T2WI MR shows a large, globular heart ➔ in a 27-week fetus with Ebstein anomaly confirmed with echocardiography. In these patients, total lung volumes are calculated due to the risk of pulmonary hypoplasia.* ***(Right)*** *Frontal radiograph shows cardiomegaly ➔, mild pulmonary vasculature congestion ➔, and a small pleural effusion ➔ in this 2 year old who presented with respiratory distress. Blood cultures grew parvovirus.*

Idiopathic Cardiomyopathy

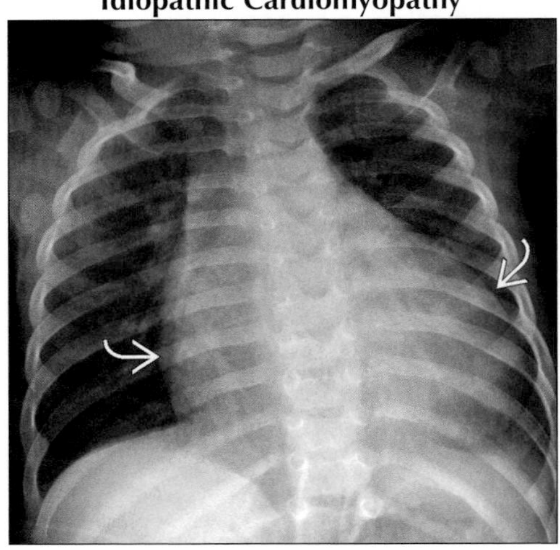

High Output Failure

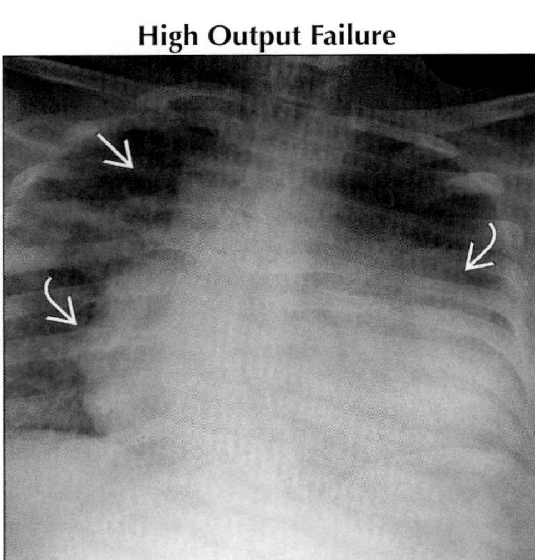

(Left) *Frontal radiograph unexpectedly reveals dilated cardiomyopathy ➔ in this 1 year old who presented with wheezing and dyspnea. Blood cultures were negative, and the heart muscle biopsy was nonspecific.* ***(Right)*** *Frontal radiograph shows increased heart size ➔ in this teenager with end-stage sickle cell disease. Mild pulmonary edema is present ➔.*

High Output Failure

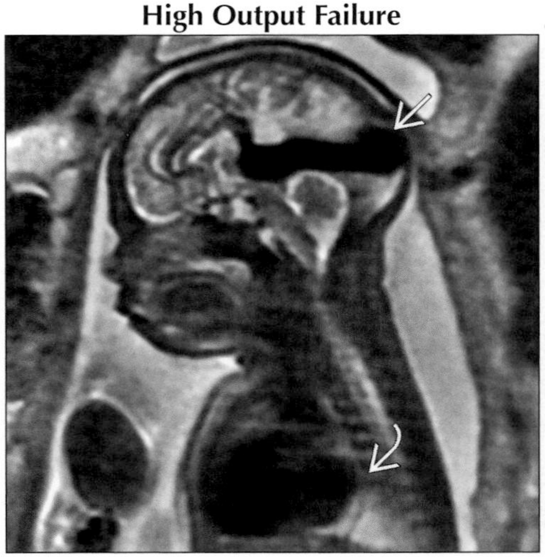

High Output Failure

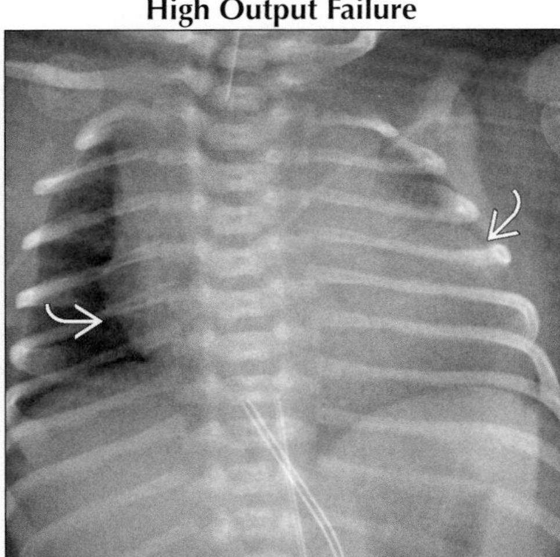

(Left) *Sagittal T2WI MR shows a 33-week fetus with posterior expansion of a dilated heart ➔ and a massive intracranial flow void corresponding to a vein of Galen aneurysm ➔.* ***(Right)*** *Frontal radiograph shows the same baby in the immediate postnatal period. The markedly increased heart size ➔ reflects a high output state from the intracranial vascular malformation (not shown).*

MASSIVE CARDIOMEGALY

Anomalous Coronary Artery

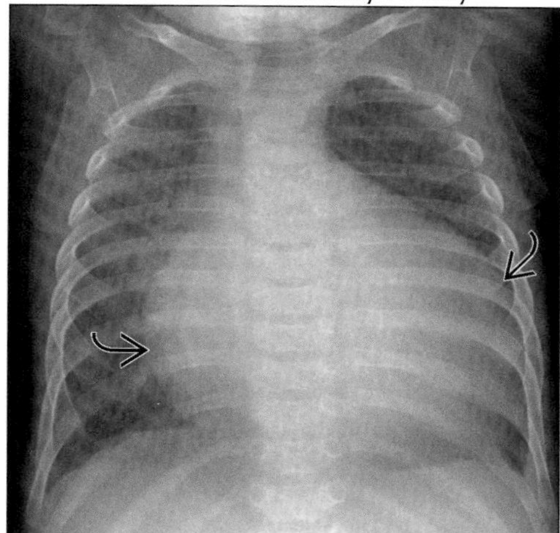

Anomalous Coronary Artery

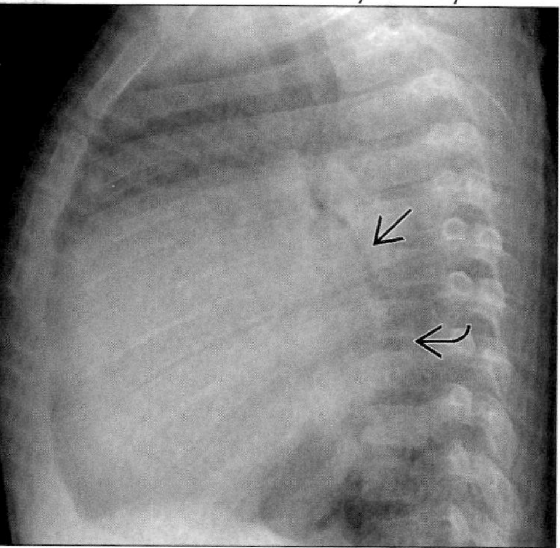

(Left) *Frontal radiograph shows moderate to severe enlargement of the heart → in this 8 month old who presented with dyspnea and poor feeding. Echocardiography demonstrated anomalous origin of the left coronary artery from the main pulmonary artery.* ***(Right)*** *Lateral radiograph obtained at the same time shows left ventricular and left atrial enlargement projecting as a soft tissue density extending posteriorly →, compressing the left main bronchus →.*

Glycogen Storage Disease

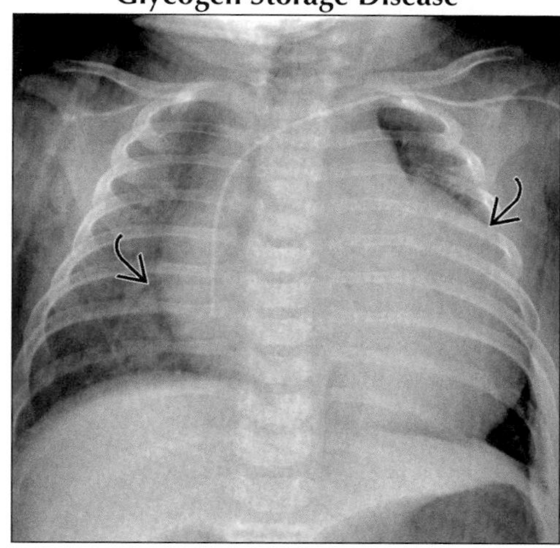

Glycogen Storage Disease

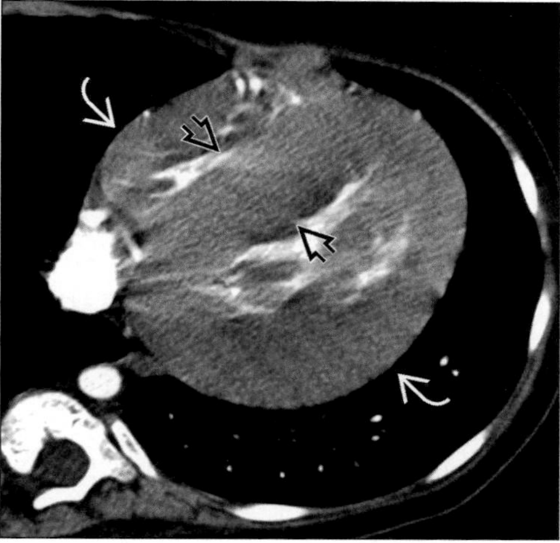

(Left) *Frontal radiograph shows significant cardiac enlargement → in this 3 month old with Pompe disease, a lysosomal storage disorder resulting in accumulation of glycogen in skeletal and cardiac muscles, hepatomegaly, and macroglossia.* ***(Right)*** *Axial CECT shows profound thickening of the right and left ventricular walls → and interventricular septum → in a 12 year old with Pompe disease presenting with chest pain. The cardiac chambers are nearly slit-like.*

Cardiac Tumors

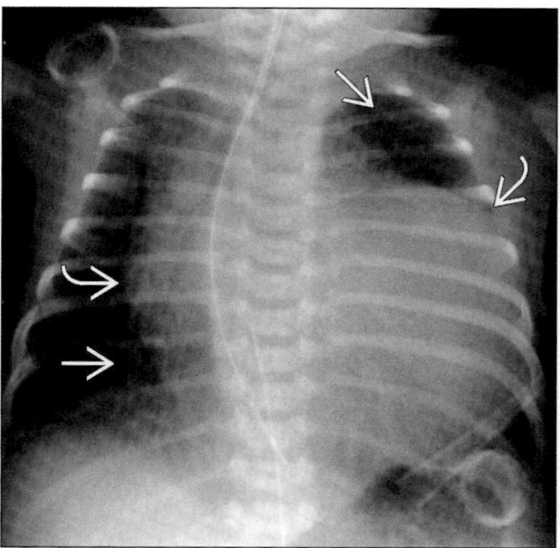

Cardiac Tumors

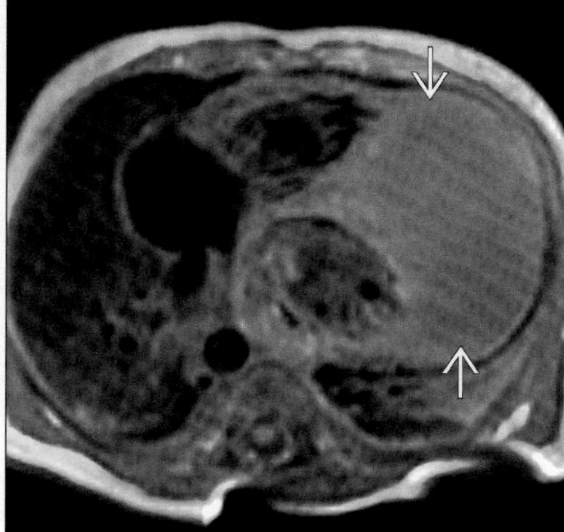

(Left) *Frontal radiograph shows severe cardiomegaly → in this infant with tuberous sclerosis and a massive left ventricular rhabdomyoma. Note that the pulmonary vessels are normal in caliber →.* ***(Right)*** *Axial T1WI MR in the same child shows the homogeneous intermediate signal intensity myocardial rhabdomyoma →. This child's symptoms were treated with inotropic agents and the lesion resolved spontaneously over time.*

ACYANOTIC HEART DISEASE WITH NORMAL VASCULARITY

DIFFERENTIAL DIAGNOSIS

Common
- Aortic Coarctation
- Aortic Stenosis

Less Common
- Interrupted Aortic Arch
- Pulmonary Stenosis

ESSENTIAL INFORMATION

Key Differential Diagnosis Issues
- Obstructive lesions cause acyanotic heart disease with normal pulmonary vascularity
- Patients with small, left-to-right shunts have normal vascularity
- In neonates, increased pulmonary vascular resistance causes left-to-right shunt to have normal vascularity

Helpful Clues for Common Diagnoses
- **Aortic Coarctation**
  - Stenosis in proximal descending aorta
    - Usually just beyond origin of left subclavian artery
  - 5-8% of congenital heart defects (CHD)
  - 2x more common in males
  - Associations: Turner syndrome, bicuspid aortic valve, ventricular septal defect
  - Severe coarct presents when ductus closes
  - Mild coarct presents with upper extremity hypertension and ↓ lower extremity pulses
  - Rib notching not usually seen on chest x-ray (CXR) until after age 6
  - Treatment options: Surgical repair, angioplasty, stent placement
- **Aortic Stenosis**
  - Types: Supravalvular, valvular, or subaortic
  - Valvular aortic stenosis is most common
    - Accounts for 3-6% of CHD
    - 4x more common in males
    - ~ 20% have associated cardiac anomaly
    - Severity related to degree of obstruction
    - CXR: Normal or with cardiomegaly, vascular congestion, and poststenotic dilation of ascending aorta
  - Subaortic stenosis can be discrete or diffuse
  - Supravalvular is least common

Helpful Clues for Less Common Diagnoses
- **Interrupted Aortic Arch**
  - Discontinuity of aorta (1% of all CHD)
  - Associations: DiGeorge syndrome and 22q11 deletion
  - 3 types: Isolated, simple, and complex
    - Isolated: No other cardiac anomalies
    - Simple: Associated with ventricular septal defect and patent ductus arteriosus
    - Complex: Associated with complex CHD
- **Pulmonary Stenosis**
  - Types: Valvular, subvalvular, supravalvular, or in branch pulmonary arteries
  - Valvular stenosis is most common
    - 7-9% of all CHD
    - Presents with asymptomatic murmur
    - CXR: Dilated main pulmonary artery
    - Treatment: Balloon valvuloplasty

Aortic Coarctation

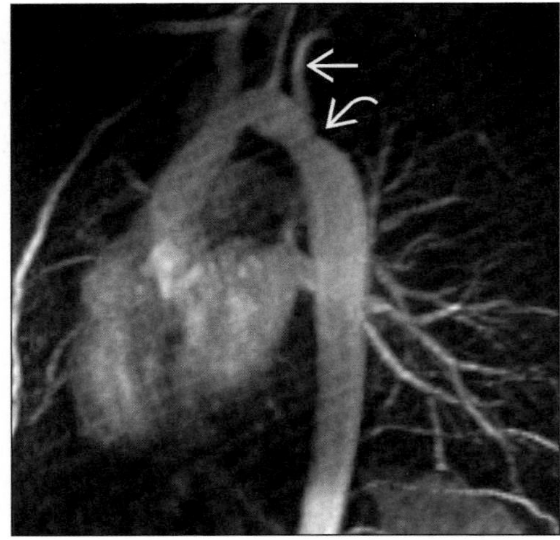

Sagittal MIP of T1 C+ subtraction MR shows a focal area of stenosis in the proximal descending aorta ➡ just distal to the origin of the left subclavian artery ➡.

Aortic Coarctation

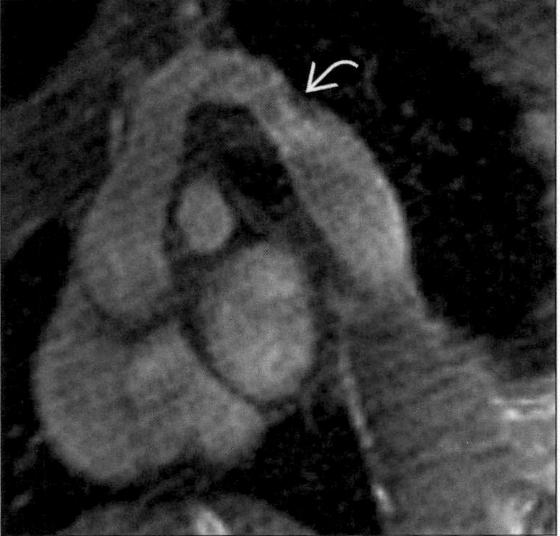

Oblique view from a cardiac MR shows a focal area of narrowing in the proximal descending aorta ➡. Coarctation of the aorta is associated with Turner syndrome and a bicuspid aortic valve.

Aortic Stenosis

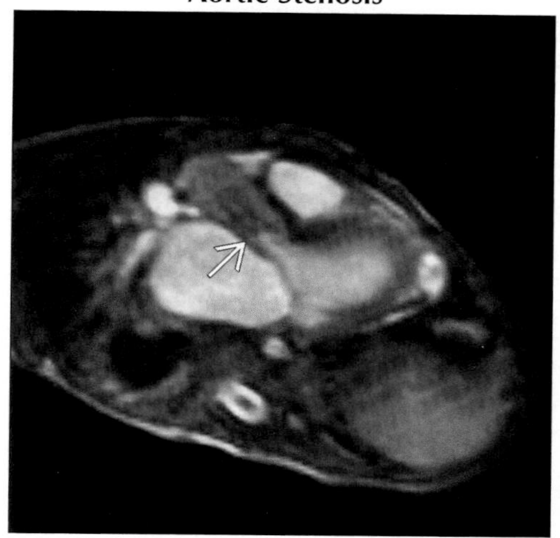

Aortic Stenosis

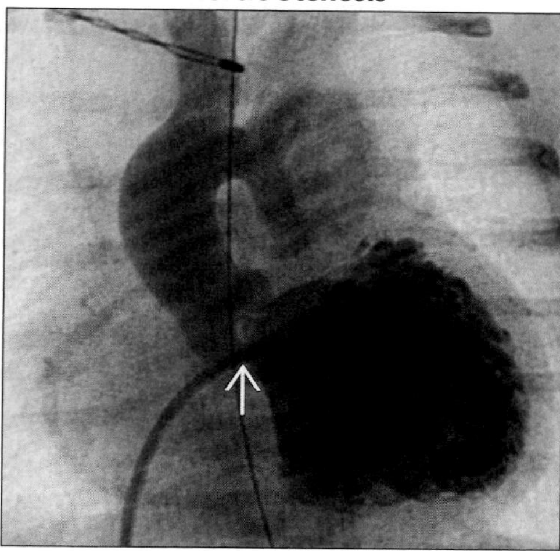

(Left) *Oblique view of the left ventricular outflow tract on a cardiac MR shows a focal jet of turbulent blood just distal to the aortic valve ➔. Valvular aortic stenosis is the most common type of aortic stenosis.* ***(Right)*** *AP view from a cardiac catheterization shows narrowing of the left ventricular outflow tract at the level of the aortic valve ➔. Aortic stenosis is associated with other cardiac anomalies in approximately 20% of patients.*

Interrupted Aortic Arch

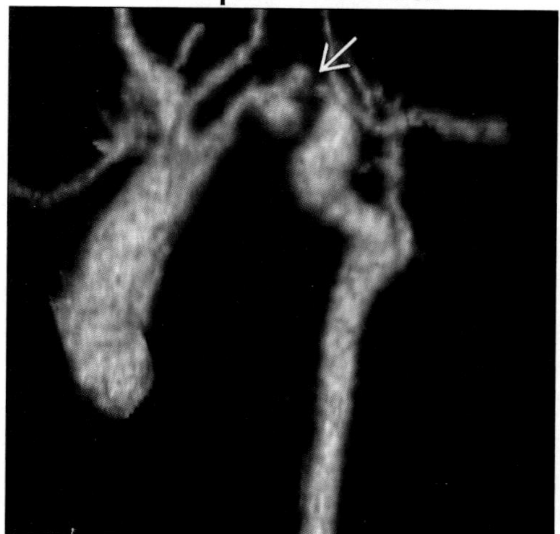

Interrupted Aortic Arch

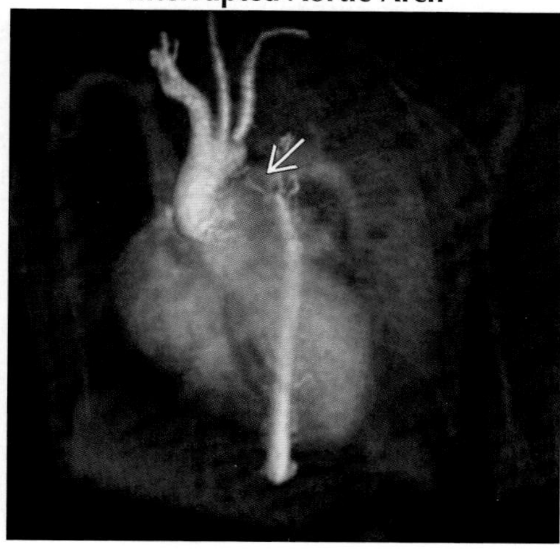

(Left) *Oblique 3D reconstruction shows a focal interruption of the aortic arch ➔. The remainder of the aortic arch is narrowed and tortuous. An interrupted aortic arch is associated with DiGeorge syndrome and 22q11 deletion.* ***(Right)*** *Oblique 3D reconstruction in a different patient shows a simple interruption of the aortic arch ➔. Interrupted aortic arches can be isolated, simple, or complex.*

Pulmonary Stenosis

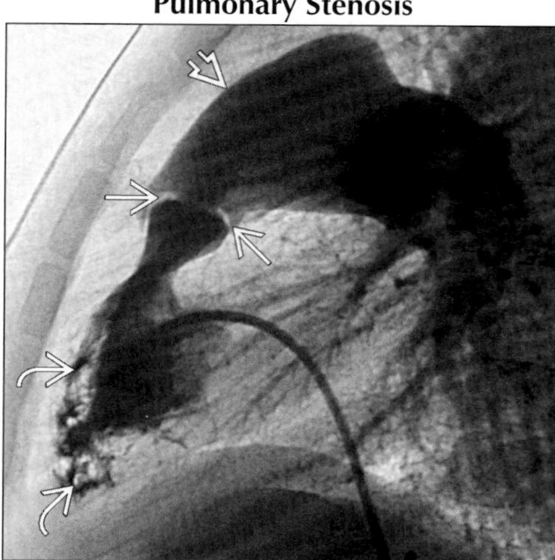

Pulmonary Stenosis

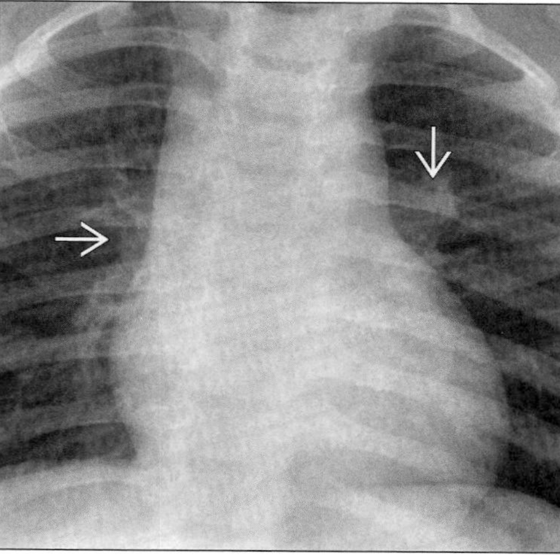

(Left) *Lateral cardiac catheterization shows thickening and stenosis of the pulmonary valve ➔, as well as trabeculation of the right ventricle ➔. The main pulmonary artery is dilated ➔. Poststenotic dilation of the main and left main pulmonary arteries often accompanies valvular pulmonary stenosis.* ***(Right)*** *AP radiograph of the chest shows prominence of the central pulmonary arteries ➔. The peripheral pulmonary arteries are normal and not well seen.*

ACYANOTIC HEART DISEASE WITH INCREASED VASCULARITY

DIFFERENTIAL DIAGNOSIS

Common
- Atrial Septal Defect (ASD)
- Ventricular Septal Defect (VSD)
- Patent Ductus Arteriosus (PDA)

Less Common
- Atrioventricular Septal Defect (AVSD)
- Partial Anomalous Pulmonary Venous Return

Rare but Important
- Hemangioendothelioma
- Vein of Galen Aneurysmal Malformation

ESSENTIAL INFORMATION

Key Differential Diagnosis Issues
- Increased vascularity seen with left-to-right shunts
  - Shunt causes volume overload of right heart, which leads to increased blood flow to pulmonary arteries
- Left-to-right shunts can have cardiac and extracardiac causes
- Small left-to-right shunts are often asymptomatic
- Eisenmenger syndrome results from long-term left-to-right shunt
  - Elevated pulmonary artery pressure → reversal of shunt, oxygen desaturation, and cyanosis

Helpful Clues for Common Diagnoses
- **Atrial Septal Defect (ASD)**
  - 2nd most common isolated congenital heart defect (CHD) after bicuspid aortic valve
    - Accounts for up to 30% of CHD
    - More common in females
  - 3 types: Secundum, primum, and sinus venosus
    - Secundum is most common (92.5%)
  - Secundum ASDs < 3 mm close spontaneously by 18 months
  - Secundum ASDs > 6-7 mm require follow-up echocardiography until age 4-5
    - If not closing, then surgical or interventional closure needed
    - On MR, secundum ASD can be differentiated from normal wall thinning by thickening at edge of defect
  - Primum ASDs are associated with atrioventricular valve abnormalities
  - Sinus venosus ASD is associated with anomalous pulmonary venous connection
  - ASDs have fixed and split-second heart sound
- **Ventricular Septal Defect (VSD)**
  - Most common CHD in children
    - VSD occurs in 50% of children with CHD
    - VSD is isolated defect in 20% of children with CHD
  - 2 main locations: Membranous or muscular septum
    - Membranous defects account for 70% of VSDs
    - Multiple defects can be present
  - Associated with Down syndrome, DiGeorge syndrome, Turner syndrome
  - Holosystolic murmur on auscultation
  - Small VSDs often close spontaneously
    - Large VSDs can be closed surgically or with catheter intervention
- **Patent Ductus Arteriosus (PDA)**
  - Ductus arteriosus connects proximal descending aorta to main pulmonary artery
    - Essential for fetal circulation
  - Normally closes spontaneously after birth
    - Prostaglandins can help keep ductus arteriosus open
    - Indomethacin helps to close duct
  - Risks for PDA: Prematurity, prenatal infection
    - 65% of infants born < 28 weeks of fetal gestation have PDA
  - Accounts for 5-10% of all CHD
  - 2x more common in females
  - Most cases are sporadic
    - Increased risk with Down syndrome, Holt-Oram syndrome, and Carpenter syndrome
  - Continuous machinery murmur at upper left sternal border
  - For some types of CHD, survival is dependent on PDA
    - Ductal dependent lesions for systemic flow: Hypoplastic left heart, critical aortic stenosis, interrupted aortic arch
    - Ductal dependent cyanotic lesions: Pulmonary atresia, transposition of great arteries

Helpful Clues for Less Common Diagnoses

- **Atrioventricular Septal Defect (AVSD)**
  - a.k.a. endocardial cushion defect
  - Deficiency of atrioventricular septum
    - Associated with common atrioventricular valve and abnormal arrangement of valve leaflets
  - Most severe form allows all chambers of heart to communicate
  - Pulmonary hypertension develops in infancy or childhood
  - Associated with Down syndrome
- **Partial Anomalous Pulmonary Venous Return**
  - Uncommon to be seen as isolated CHD
    - Usually associated with ASD (80%)
  - Most common location for anomalous pulmonary venous drainage is from right lung
    - Anomalous drainage is usually to superior vena cava or right atrium

Helpful Clues for Rare Diagnoses

- **Hemangioendothelioma**
  - a.k.a. infantile hepatic hemangioma
  - Most common benign liver tumor in children
    - Accounts for ~ 60% of neonatal liver tumors
    - 85% diagnosed in 1st 6 months of life
  - Symptoms include abdominal distension, hepatomegaly, congestive heart failure, and respiratory distress
    - Other symptoms: Consumptive coagulopathy (Kasabach-Merritt syndrome) and rupture with intraperitoneal hemorrhage
    - Can be associated with hypothyroidism
  - ~ 50% have cutaneous hemangiomas
  - Multiple lesions may be present
  - Celiac and hepatic arteries often enlarged
  - Lesions should regress with age
    - Symptomatic lesions treated with medical or surgical therapy
  - On radiograph, see increased pulmonary vascularity and hepatomegaly
- **Vein of Galen Aneurysmal Malformation**
  - Account for 1% of all intracranial vascular malformations
    - 30% of vascular intracranial malformations in children
  - Ectatic vascular structure is median prosencephalic vein, not vein of Galen
  - Occurs due to direct communication between arterial network and median prosencephalic vein
  - After birth, there is increase in blood flow through malformation
    - Up to 80% of left ventricular output may supply brain
    - Leads to increased cardiac output and heart failure
  - Usually associated with other intracranial venous anomalies

Atrial Septal Defect (ASD)

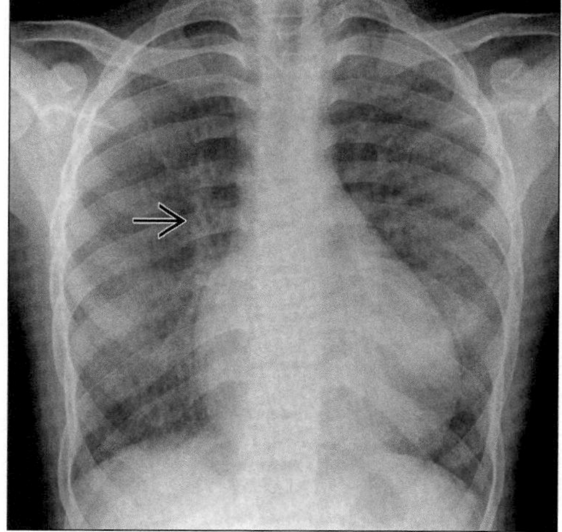

AP radiograph of the chest shows cardiomegaly and increased pulmonary vascularity ⇒. Atrial septal defects are the 2nd most common isolated congenital heart defect.

Atrial Septal Defect (ASD)

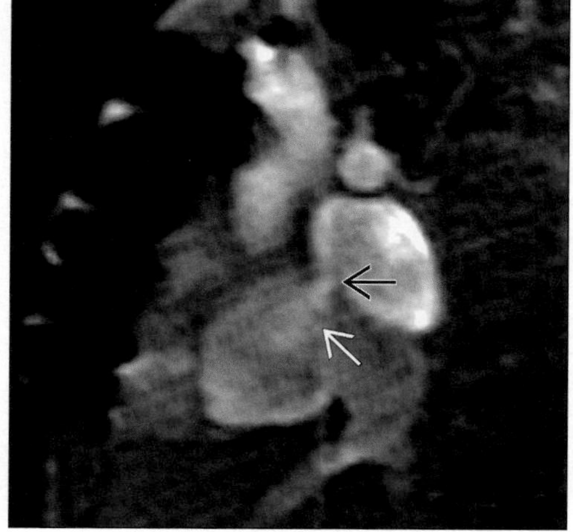

Oblique sagittal image from a cardiac MR shows a jet of turbulent flow ➡ through a small atrial septal defect ⇒. Small atrial septal defects often close spontaneously.

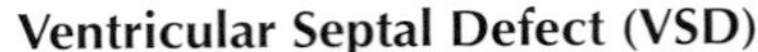

(**Left**) *Four chamber view from a cardiac MR shows a moderate ventricular septal defect →. Ventricular septal defects are the most common congenital heart defect in children.* (**Right**) *Short axis view of a cardiac MR shows a small ventricular septal defect →. Ventricular septal defects are associated with Down syndrome, DiGeorge syndrome, and Turner syndrome. Small defects usually close spontaneously.*

Ventricular Septal Defect (VSD)

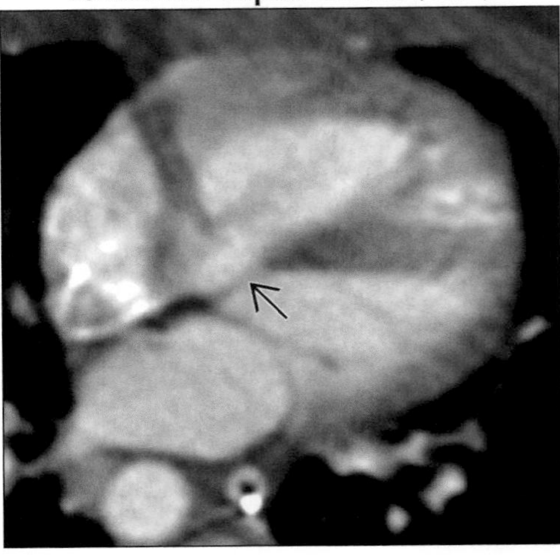

Ventricular Septal Defect (VSD)

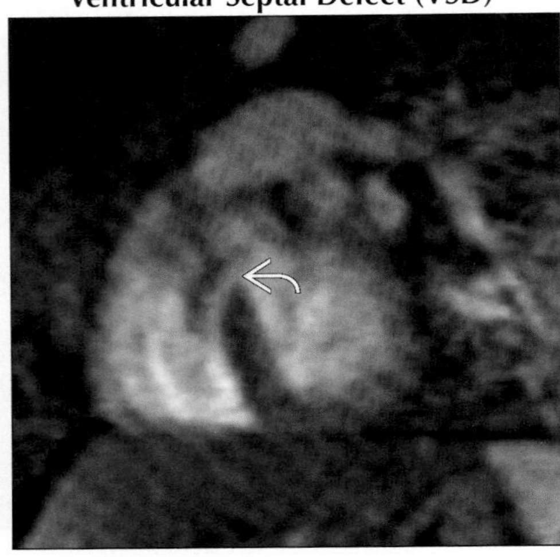

(**Left**) *Axial CECT shows a vascular connection → between the main pulmonary artery → and the descending aorta →. A patent ductus arteriosus is essential for fetal circulation but should close spontaneously after birth.* (**Right**) *Sagittal CECT shows a vascular communication → between the main pulmonary artery → and the proximal descending aorta →. Prematurity and prenatal infection are risks for a patent ductus arteriosus.*

Patent Ductus Arteriosus (PDA)

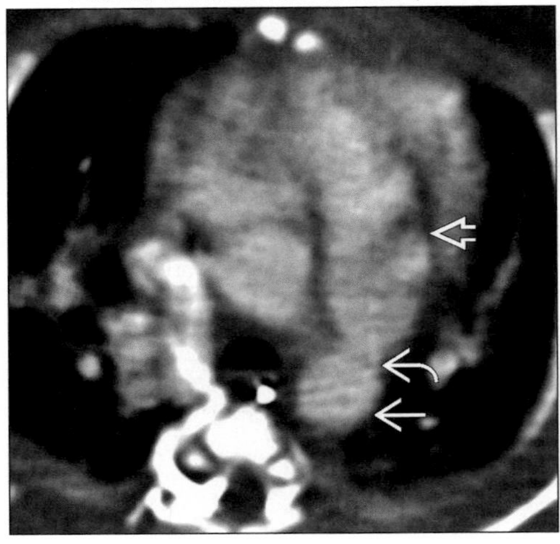

Patent Ductus Arteriosus (PDA)

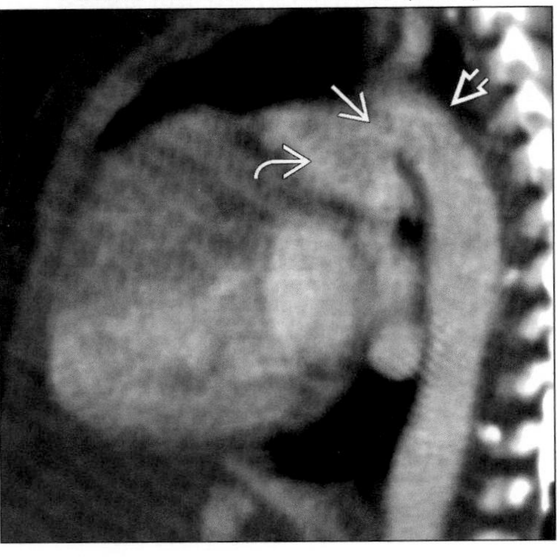

(**Left**) *Coronal MIP of T1 C+ subtraction MR shows anomalous connection at the right upper lobe pulmonary vein → and the superior vena cava →. Partial anomalous pulmonary venous return is usually associated with an atrial septal defect (not shown).* (**Right**) *Oblique 3D reconstruction of the pulmonary veins shows an anomalous right upper lobe pulmonary vein →. The anomalous vein usually drains to the superior vena cava or right atrium.*

Partial Anomalous Pulmonary Venous Return

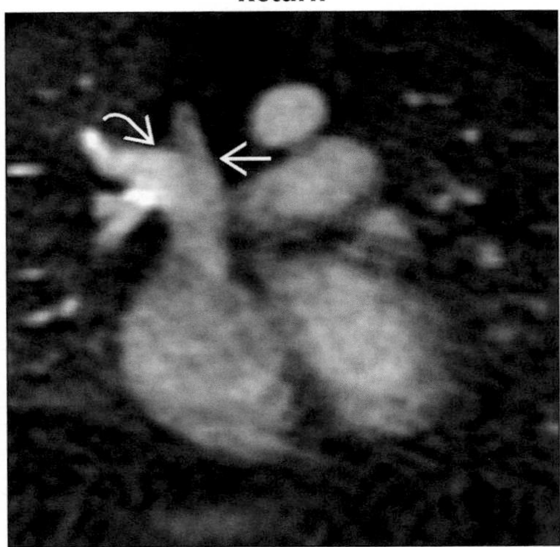

Partial Anomalous Pulmonary Venous Return

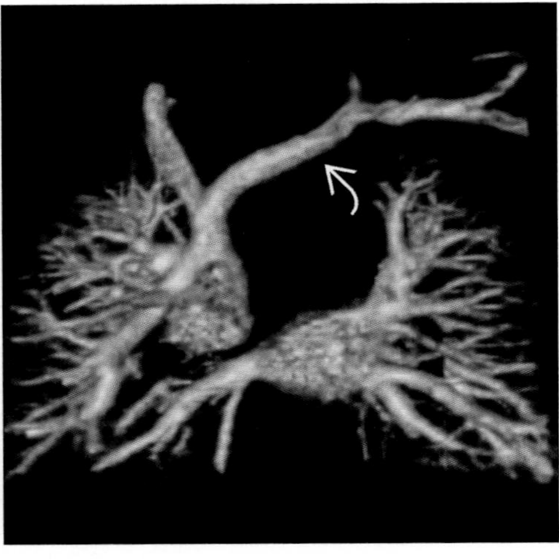

Hemangioendothelioma

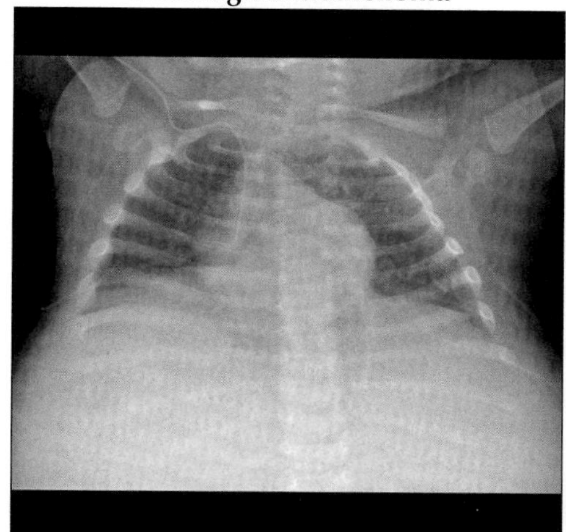

Hemangioendothelioma

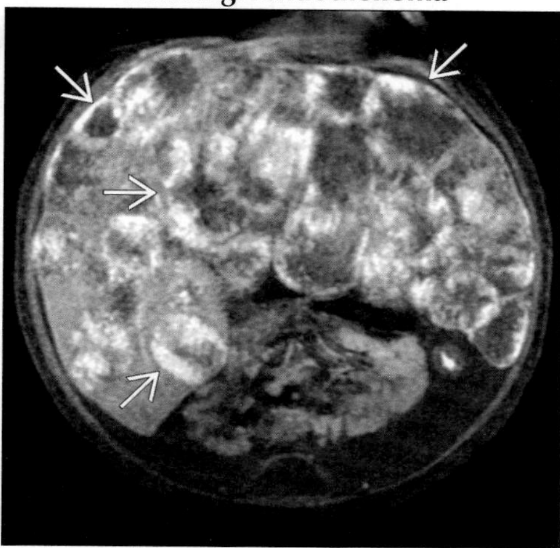

(Left) *AP radiograph of the chest shows mild increased pulmonary vascularity and bulging of the upper abdomen. Hepatic hemangioendotheliomas are the most common benign liver tumor in children.* ***(Right)*** *Coronal T1WI C+ FS MR shows peripheral nodular enhancement of innumerable liver lesions ➡, which nearly replace the liver. Patients with hemangioendothelioma can present with hypothyroidism, congestive heart failure, and abdominal distension.*

Vein of Galen Aneurysmal Malformation

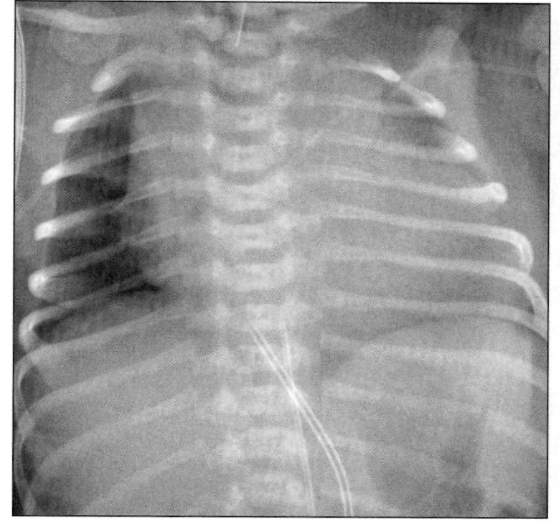

Vein of Galen Aneurysmal Malformation

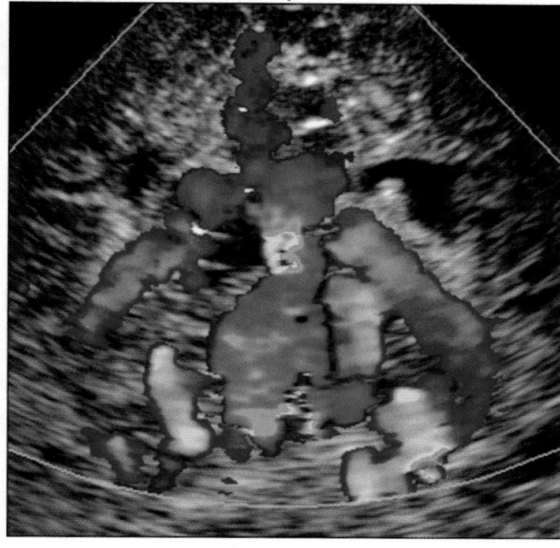

(Left) *AP radiograph of the chest shows cardiomegaly. The pulmonary vascularity is not well seen because of the large heart. Vein of Galen malformations occur due to a direct communication between the arterial network and the median prosencephalic vein.* ***(Right)*** *Coronal ultrasound of the head shows increased color Doppler flow. A vein of Galen malformation accounts for 1% of all intracranial vascular malformations but 30% of malformations in children.*

Vein of Galen Aneurysmal Malformation

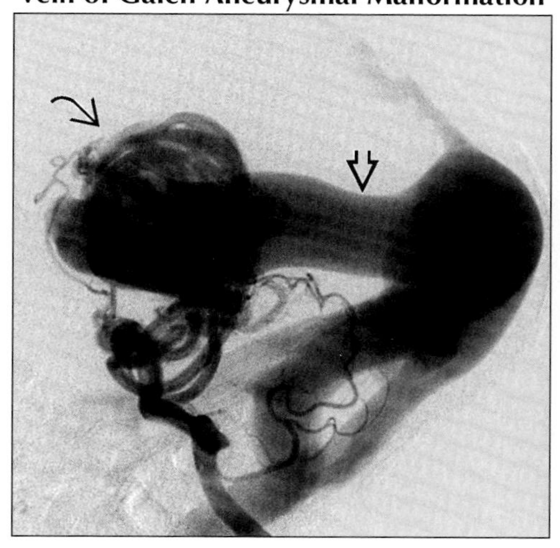

Vein of Galen Aneurysmal Malformation

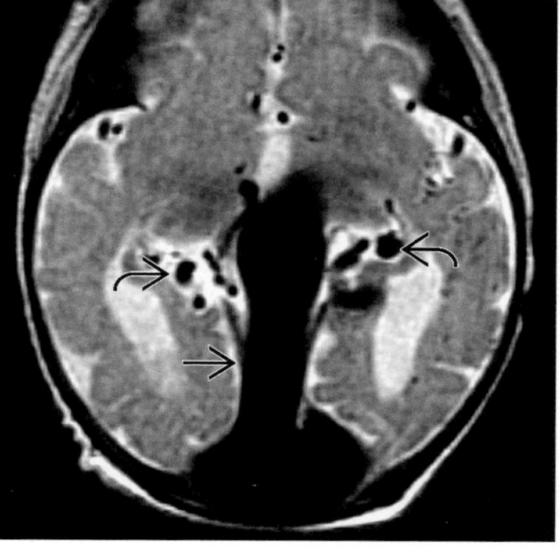

(Left) *Lateral catheter angiography with injection in a vertebral artery shows multiple abnormal vessels centrally ➚ with abnormal early draining into a markedly enlarged vein of Galen malformation ⇨.* ***(Right)*** *Axial T2WI MR shows a massively dilated vein of Galen malformation ➡ and multiple abnormal arterial collaterals bilaterally ➚. Up to 80% of cardiac output in these patients supplies the brain. This can cause high output heart failure.*

CYANOTIC HEART DISEASE WITH DECREASED VASCULARITY

DIFFERENTIAL DIAGNOSIS

Common
- Tetralogy of Fallot (TOF)
- Pulmonary Atresia (PA)
- Tricuspid Atresia

Less Common
- Tricuspid Stenosis
- Ebstein Anomaly
- Transposition Complexes

Rare but Important
- Truncus Arteriosus
- Severe Pulmonary Artery Stenosis with R to L Shunt
- Total Anomalous Pulmonary Venous Return (TAPVR)
- Single Ventricle
- DORV with Pulmonic Stenosis
- Uhl Disease (Parchment RV)
- Isolated RV Hypoplasia

ESSENTIAL INFORMATION

Helpful Clues for Common Diagnoses
- **Tetralogy of Fallot (TOF)**
  - Most common cyanotic CHD in childhood
  - Tetrad includes
    - RV outflow obstruction
    - RV hypertrophy
    - VSD
    - Aorta overriding VSD/interventricular septum
  - Variants
    - Trilogy: PA stenosis with RV hypertrophy
    - Pentalogy: Tetrad plus ASD
    - Pink tetralogy: Tetralogy with mild pulmonic stenosis
  - Radiographic appearance
    - Boot-shaped heart with upturned apex
    - Concave PA segment
    - Right arch (25%)
  - Treatment
    - Reconstruction of RV outflow tract by muscle resection and enlargement
    - Closure of VSD
- **Pulmonary Atresia (PA)**
  - Radiographically similar to TOF
  - Reticular pulmonary vascularity
- **Tricuspid Atresia**
  - No direct communication between RA and RV
    - ASD or patent foramen ovale are always present
    - Transposition of great arteries in 30% has different appearance
    - VSD is common
  - Radiographic appearance
    - Convex left cardiac border, upturned apex
    - Concave PA segment
    - Straight right heart border
    - ↑ vascularity if TGA in (30%)

Helpful Clues for Less Common Diagnoses
- **Tricuspid Stenosis**
  - Isolated tricuspid stenosis is usually congenital, but carcinoid can cause stenosis
  - Rheumatic heart disease
- **Ebstein Anomaly**
  - Displacement of tricuspid leaflets into RV inflow
    - Effectively "atrializes" portion of RV
    - Mostly regurgitant lesion but can be obstructive
    - Associated with right bundle branch block and arrhythmias
  - Radiographic appearance
    - Convex right heart border
    - Cardiomegaly (box-shaped heart)
  - Treatment includes valve reconstruction and pacemaker placement
- **Transposition Complexes**
  - Most common CHD with early cyanosis
  - Narrow superior mediastinum
  - If PS or PA, then decreased vascularity
  - Aorta is at right of MPA
    - Anterior and to right in d-TGA
    - More to right and less anterior in DORV
    - Superimposed, parallel great vessels give rise to narrow mediastinum "string"
    - RA and RV enlargement has "egg-on-side" appearance
    - Thus "egg-on-a-string"
  - Pulmonary vascularity increases as pulmonary resistance decreases
    - Increased pulmonary blood flow is "classic" pattern
    - Decreased pulmonary blood flow is normal early in life
    - Decreased pulmonary blood flow when pulmonic stenosis is present
  - Treatment

- Early treatment is aimed at providing mixing of blood and involves atrial balloon septostomy
- Jatene arterial switch procedure is current standard of care

Helpful Clues for Rare Diagnoses

- **Truncus Arteriosus**
  - Always large VSD present
    - Type 1: Single main PA originates from truncus as common artery
    - Type 2: Right and left PA arise separately from truncus
    - Type 3: Right and left PA arise from clearly separate origins on truncus
    - Type 4: "Pseudotruncus," arteries supplying lungs arise from descending aorta
  - Radiographic appearance
    - Right aortic arch in 35%
    - Cardiomegaly often at birth
    - Pulmonary vascularity can be increased, normal, or decreased
    - Enlarged aorta (truncus)
- **Severe Pulmonary Artery Stenosis with R to L Shunt**
  - Radiographically similar to TOF
- **Total Anomalous Pulmonary Venous Return (TAPVR)**
  - Typically described as variable or increased vascularity but can be initially decreased due to elevated pulmonary resistance in newborn period
- **Single Ventricle**
  - Variable radiographic appearance
    - Pulmonic stenosis: Normal heart size, decreased vascularity
    - No pulmonic stenosis: Cardiomegaly, large MPA, ↑ pulmonary vascularity, and congestive heart failure
  - Usually, RV is underdeveloped
  - Treatment is staged repair
    - Ultimately leads to Fontan
- **DORV with Pulmonic Stenosis**
  - Both great arteries arise from RV
  - Radiographic appearance depends on degree of pulmonic stenosis
    - No pulmonic stenosis: Cardiomegaly and ↑ pulmonary vascularity
    - Pulmonic stenosis: Small heart and decreased vascularity
- **Uhl Disease (Parchment RV)**
  - Congenitally, near complete absence of RV myocardium
    - Normal tricuspid valve
    - Preserved septum and left ventricle
  - Physiologically, forward flow through RV is impeded
- **Isolated RV Hypoplasia**
  - Very rare
  - Trabeculated sinus portion of RV fails to form
  - Physiologically, forward flow through RV is impeded

Tetralogy of Fallot (TOF)

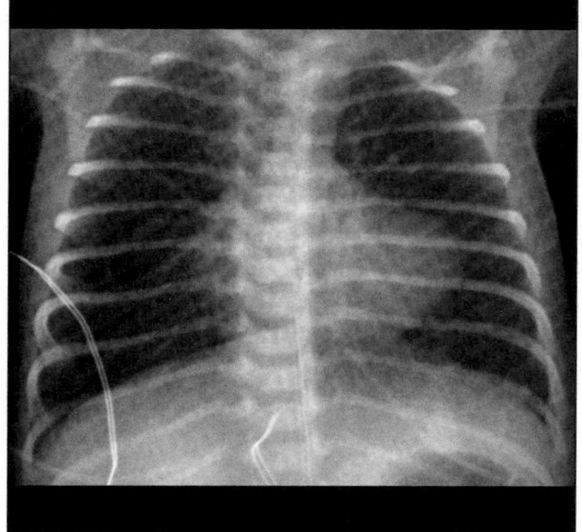

Anteroposterior radiograph shows upturned cardiac apex, hypoplastic pulmonary artery segment, and decreased vascularity. Many chest radiographs in newborns of tetralogy of Fallot are not as classic as this.

Tetralogy of Fallot (TOF)

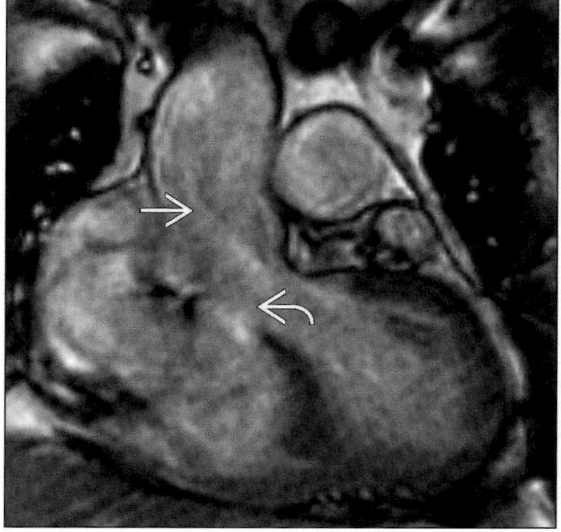

Coronal GRE MR shows the aorta ➔ overriding the VSD ➔ & the thickened right ventricular myocardium in this older patient who did not have repair early in life and now has pulmonary hypertension.

CYANOTIC HEART DISEASE WITH DECREASED VASCULARITY

(Left) *Anteroposterior radiograph shows decreased pulmonary vascularity, a right arch, a hypoplastic pulmonary artery segment, and an upturned cardiac apex in tetralogy of Fallot with pulmonary atresia. This patient had 5 major aortopulmonary collaterals from the descending aorta.* **(Right)** *Axial CTA shows RPA ➙ and LPA ➡ supplied by a large collateral from the ventral surface of the aorta ↷. Showing continuity and size of the PAs is an important role of CT/MR.*

Pulmonary Atresia (PA)

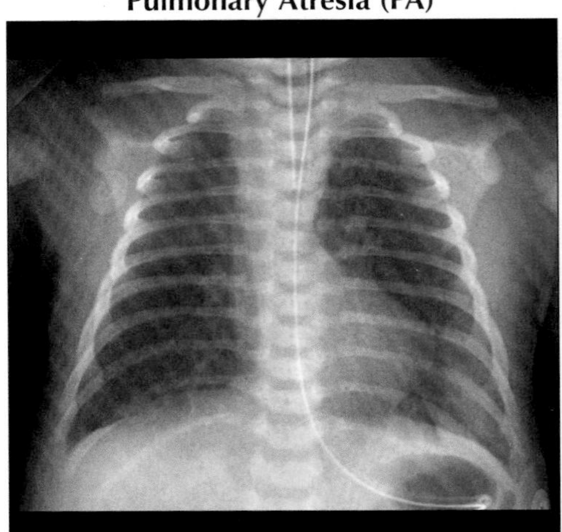

Pulmonary Atresia (PA)

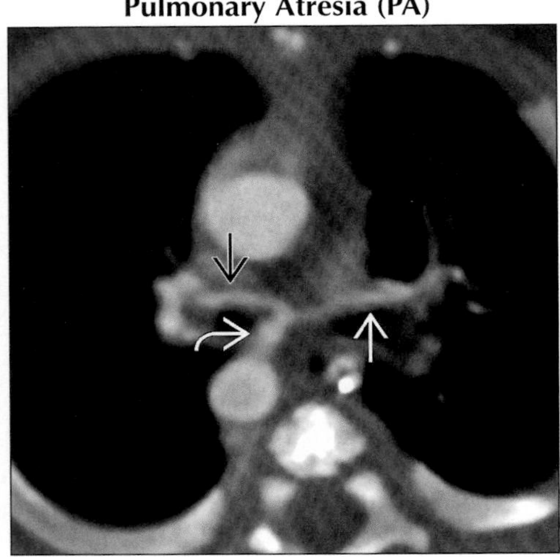

(Left) *Anteroposterior radiograph shows mildly decreased pulmonary vascularity, a straight right heart border, and a convex left heart border.* **(Right)** *Axial CECT shows plate-like atresia of the tricuspid valve ➙ and a hypoplastic RV ➡. Blood flow can only get to the RV via a VSD; therefore, development of the right heart and pulmonary artery depends on the size of the VSD. Atrial mixing of the blood in a right to left shunt causes the cyanosis.*

Tricuspid Atresia

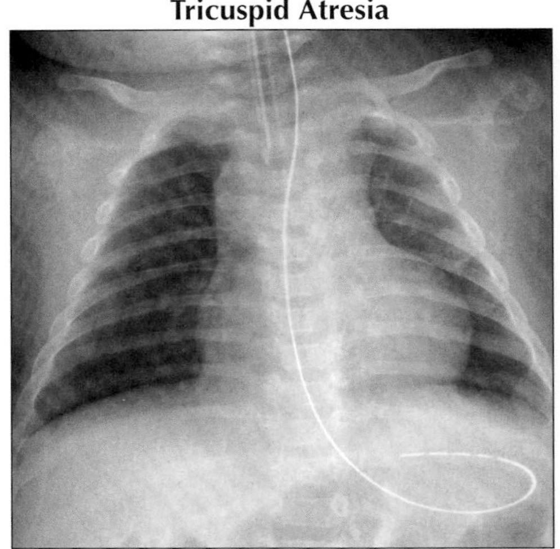

Tricuspid Atresia

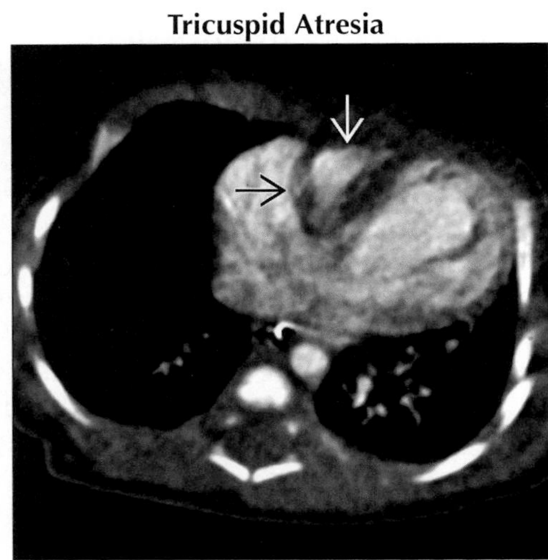

(Left) *Anteroposterior radiograph shows an enlarged cardiac silhouette and decreased pulmonary vascularity in this cyanotic newborn. The right atrium was enlarged.* **(Right)** *Four chamber view GRE MR shows a stenotic tricuspid valve with a plate-like appearance of the atresia ➡, a small RV ➡, and a large VSD ↷. Flow through the tricuspid valve was confirmed by echo. Severity of stenosis and hypoplasia of the RV prevented 2 ventricle repairs.*

Tricuspid Stenosis

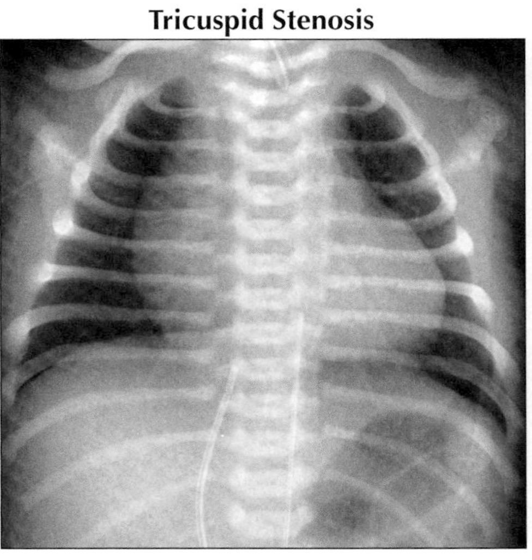

Tricuspid Stenosis

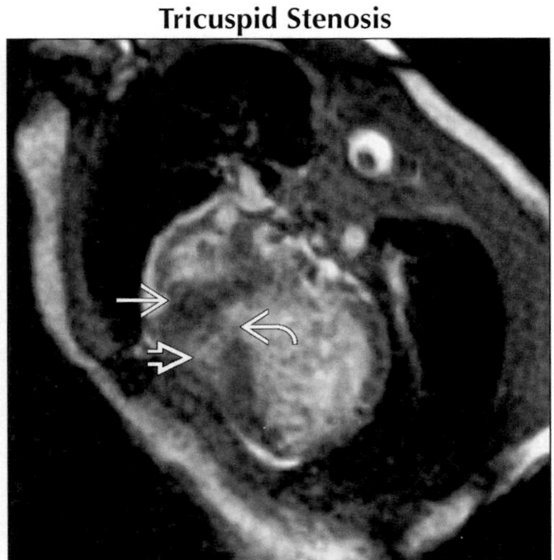

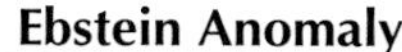

Ebstein Anomaly

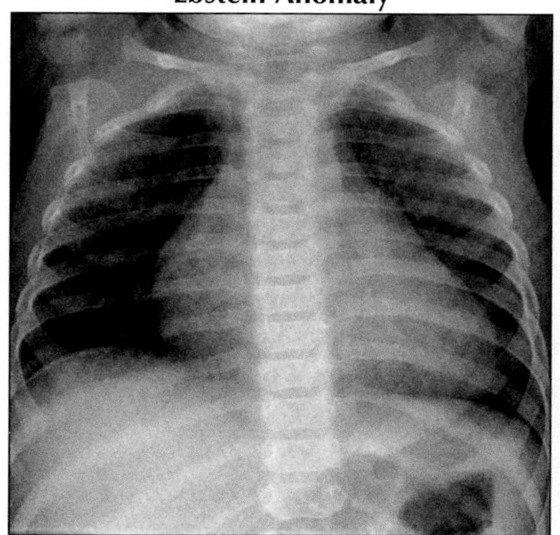

Ebstein Anomaly

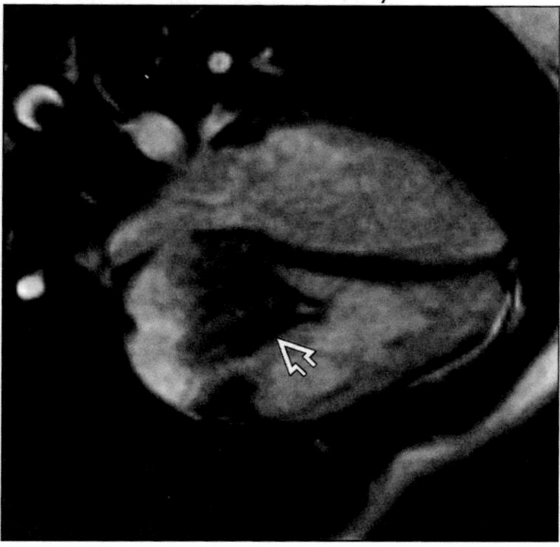

(Left) *Anteroposterior radiograph shows prominent convexity to the right heart border and a large heart. Later in life the patient's heart became box-shaped.* ***(Right)*** *Four chamber view GRE MR shows a large amount of dephasing (dark signal) in the regurgitant blood flow through the tricuspid valve, causing enlargement of the right atrium. A portion of the RV is atrialized by the tricuspid valve in this relatively mild case of Ebstein anomaly.*

Transposition Complexes

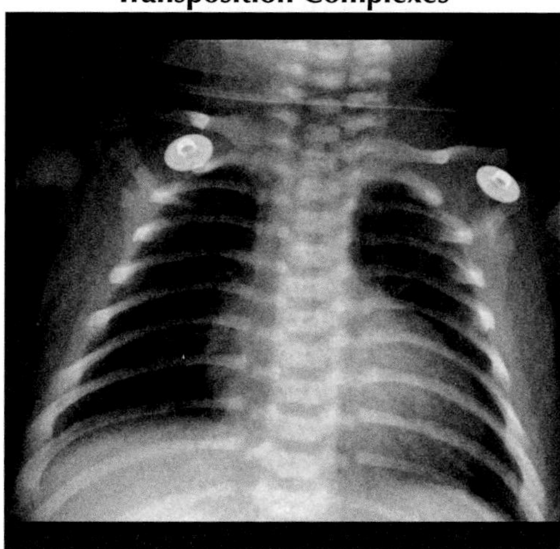

Truncus Arteriosus

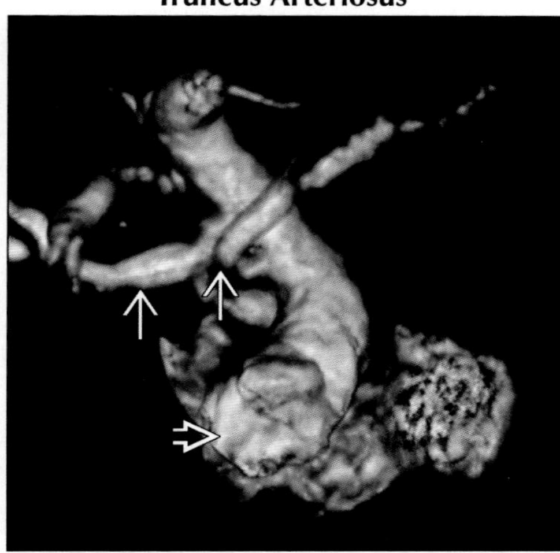

(Left) *AP radiograph shows a large heart with a narrow mediastinum and decreased vascularity due to pulmonic stenosis. The presence of decreased pulmonary vascularity in transposition complexes depends on the pulmonary vascular resistance and degree of pulmonary stenosis.* ***(Right)*** *Right posterior oblique 3D reconstruction shows the large ascending truncus with 2 separate origins for the PAs from the undersurface of the truncus arch.*

Severe Pulmonary Artery Stenosis with R to L Shunt

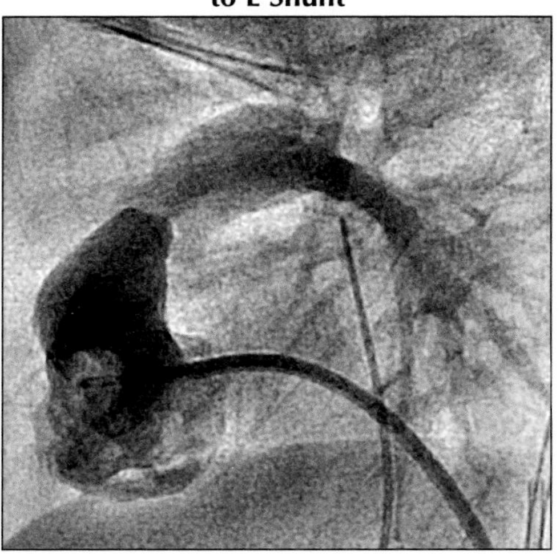

DORV with Pulmonic Stenosis

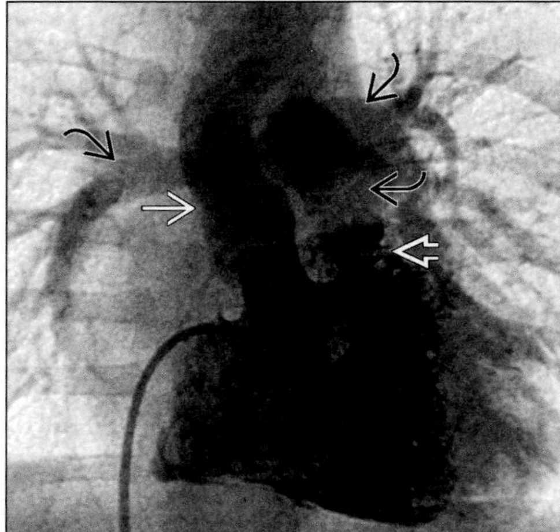

(Left) *Lateral catheter angiography shows a RV injection and tight stenosis of PV. Right to left shunting at the atrial level resulted in cyanosis.* ***(Right)*** *Anteroposterior catheter angiography shows a typical case of double outlet right ventricle (DORV). Most DORV have increased pulmonary flow. This patient has moderate PS. Frontal projection during a right ventricular injection shows filling of the aorta and pulmonary arteries with PV stenosis.*

CYANOTIC HEART DISEASE WITH VARIABLE OR INCREASED VASCULARITY

DIFFERENTIAL DIAGNOSIS

Common
- Transposition of Great Arteries (d-TGA)

Less Common
- Total Anomalous Pulmonary Venous Return (TAPVR)
- Atrioventricular Septal Defect (AVSD)
- Truncus Arteriosus

Rare but Important
- Single Ventricle
- Tricuspid Atresia
- Eisenmenger Physiology
- Double Outlet Right Ventricle (DORV)

ESSENTIAL INFORMATION

Key Differential Diagnosis Issues
- Normal chest radiograph does not exclude congenital heart disease (CHD)
- Pulmonary vascularity is variable
- Many lesions are known prenatally or evaluated soon after birth due to cyanosis

Helpful Clues for Common Diagnoses
- **Transposition of Great Arteries (d-TGA)**
  - Most common CHD with early cyanosis
  - Aorta is anterior and right of main pulmonary artery (MPA)
    - Superimposed, parallel great vessels give rise to narrow mediastinum ("string")
    - Right atrium (RA) and right ventricle (RV) enlargement has "egg-on-side" appearance
    - Thus, creates "egg-on-a-string"
  - Pulmonary vascularity increases as pulmonary resistance decreases
    - Increased pulmonary blood flow is "classic" pattern
    - Decreased pulmonary blood flow in pulmonic stenosis
  - Early treatment tries to provide mixing of right and left blood
    - Rashkind procedure is atrial septostomy with balloon catheter
    - Prostaglandin E1 to keep patent ductus arteriosus (PDA)
  - Later treatment is related to correcting blood flow
    - Jatene arterial switch procedure is current standard of care
    - Atrial switch (baffles) used in past include Mustard or Senning procedures

Helpful Clues for Less Common Diagnoses
- **Total Anomalous Pulmonary Venous Return (TAPVR)**
  - Supracardiac type (50%); infrequently obstructed
  - Cardiac type (30%)
  - Infracardiac type (15%); most obstructed
  - Mixed type (5%)
  - Appearance depends on degree of obstruction to pulmonary venous return
    - Obstructed: Small or normal heart size with severe pulmonary edema
    - Unobstructed: Increased pulmonary vascularity and "snowman" silhouette or pretracheal density (newborn)
    - MR or CT to define anatomy
  - Improved pre- and perioperative care along with better surgical techniques has resulted in low mortality
    - Infracardiac and those with complex cardiac lesion have increased mortality
  - Postoperative course is complicated by obstruction of venous return
- **Atrioventricular Septal Defect (AVSD)**
  - 40% have Down syndrome
  - Radiographic appearance
    - Cardiomegaly: Moderate to marked
    - Prominent pulmonary artery segment
    - Increased pulmonary vascularity
    - Skeletal findings of Down syndrome
  - Frequently present in asplenia and polysplenia
  - Angiographically shows "goose neck" deformity of left ventricular outflow
  - Patch closure of ASD/VSD with reconstruction of left AV valve
- **Truncus Arteriosus**
  - Failure of division of truncus to form aorta and PA
    - Always large VSD
    - Type 1: Single main PA originates from truncus
    - Type 2: Right and left PA arise separately from truncus
    - Type 3: Right and left PA arise from clearly separate origin on truncus
    - Type 4: "Pseudotruncus," arteries supplying lungs arise from descending aorta

- Radiographic appearance
  - Right aortic arch (35%)
  - Cardiomegaly: Often at birth
  - Pulmonary vascularity increases as pulmonary resistance decreases
  - Enlarged aorta (truncus)
- Treatment
  - Usually early with small valved allographs for RV to PA reconstruction

Helpful Clues for Rare Diagnoses

- **Single Ventricle**
  - Variable radiographic appearance
    - Pulmonic stenosis: Normal heart size, decreased vascularity
    - No pulmonic stenosis: Cardiomegaly, large MPA, ↑ pulmonary vascularity, congestive heart failure
  - Imaging is important in identifying single ventricle as left or right ventricle
  - Usually RV is underdeveloped
  - Treatment is staged repair
    - Ultimately leads to Fontan
- **Tricuspid Atresia**
  - TGA is common (30%)
  - Radiographic appearance with TGA
    - Cardiomegaly
    - Increased pulmonary vascularity
    - Narrow pedicle if TGA
  - Radiographic appearance with normally related great vessels
    - Normal to small heart
    - Elevated apex
    - Concave PA segment and ↓ vascularity
    - Straight right heart border
  - Treatment is initially aimed at keeping PDA open
    - Initial surgical procedure may be Blalock-Taussig shunt or Glenn procedure
    - Final pathway results in Fontan
- **Eisenmenger Physiology**
  - Chronic left to right shunt resulting in increased pulmonary vascular resistance
    - Becomes right to left shunt
    - Causes cyanosis
  - Rare today due to early treatment of ASD, VSD, PDA
  - Radiographic appearance
    - Enlarged PA with distal pruning
- **Double Outlet Right Ventricle (DORV)**
  - Both great arteries arise from RV
  - Radiographic appearance depends on degree of pulmonic stenosis
    - No pulmonic stenosis: Cardiomegaly and ↑ pulmonary vascularity
    - Pulmonic stenosis: Small heart and decreased vascularity
  - Taussig-Bing anomaly: Incomplete form of TGA
    - Aorta is anterior and to right of PA
    - PA straddles ventricular septum
    - Subaortic stenosis and coarctation is usually present, causing blood to shunt to PA and resulting in ↑ vascularity

Transposition of Great Arteries (d-TGA)

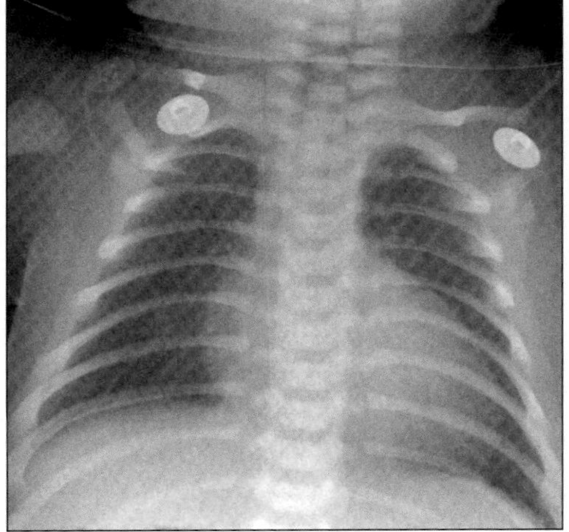

Anteroposterior radiograph shows cardiomegaly, narrow mediastinum, and ↑ pulmonary vascularity in a cyanotic newborn. The mediastinum is narrow due to superimposition of aorta and pulmonary arteries.

Transposition of Great Arteries (d-TGA)

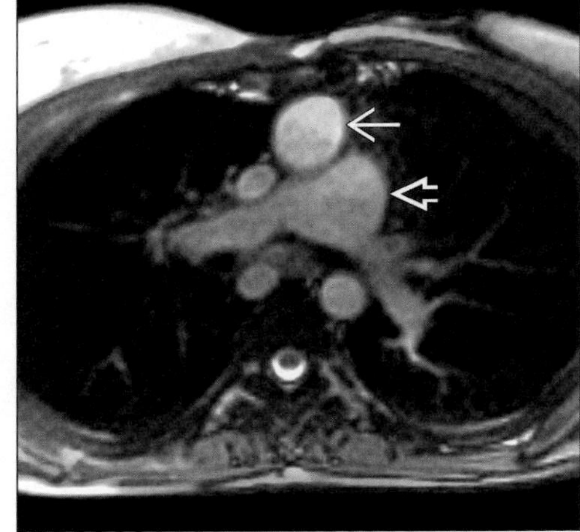

Axial GRE MR shows the aortic root ➔ anterior and slightly to the right of the main pulmonary artery ➔, which is subsequently aligned with the aorta on the plain film, and a narrow mediastinum.

CYANOTIC HEART DISEASE WITH VARIABLE OR INCREASED VASCULARITY

Total Anomalous Pulmonary Venous Return (TAPVR)

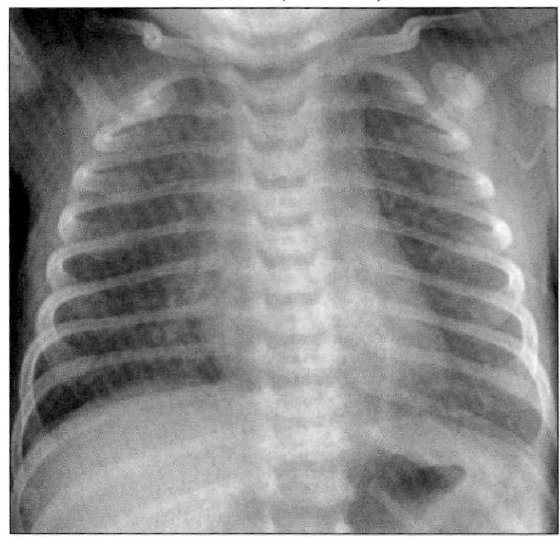

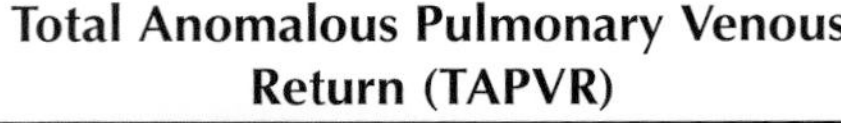

Total Anomalous Pulmonary Venous Return (TAPVR)

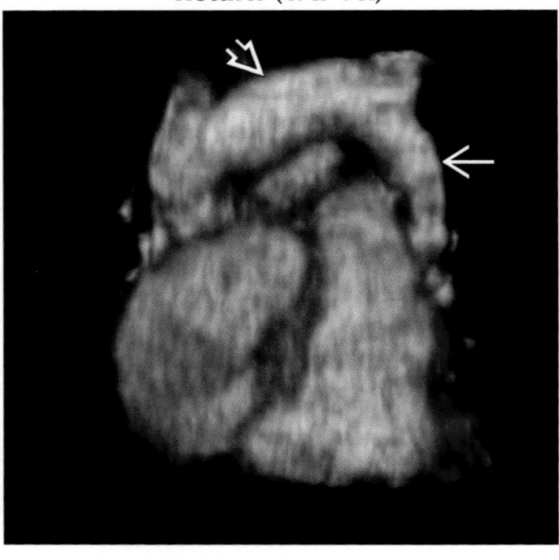

(Left) *Anteroposterior radiograph shows a newborn with supracardiac TAPVR. The lungs are hyperinflated and pulmonary vascularity is increased. The cardiomediastinal silhouette is normal.* ***(Right)*** *Coronal cardiac CT shows a 3D surface rendering of the vertical vein returning the pulmonary venous blood to a dilated left brachiocephalic vein and then into the superior vena cava. Later in life, this forms the "snowman" appearance in supracardiac TAPVR.*

Total Anomalous Pulmonary Venous Return (TAPVR)

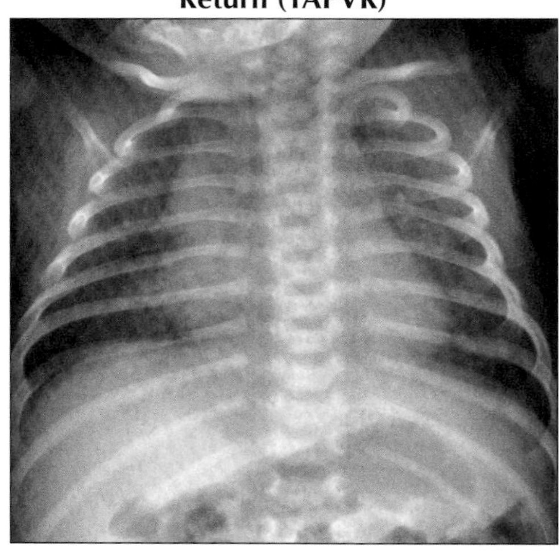

Total Anomalous Pulmonary Venous Return (TAPVR)

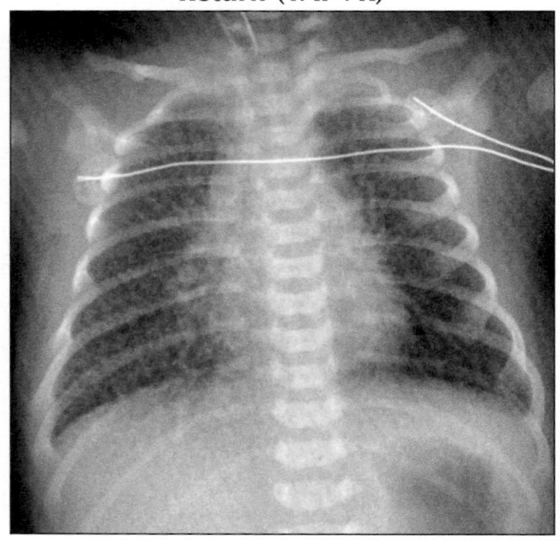

(Left) *Anteroposterior radiograph shows increased pulmonary vascularity and a wide superior mediastinum, giving this case a somewhat "snowman" appearance, which is uncommonly seen in an early diagnosis.* ***(Right)*** *AP radiograph shows hyperinflation of the lungs with increased vascularity, with interstitial pulmonary edema indicated by Kerley-B lines and normal heart size. This is a newborn with infracardiac TAPVR.*

Atrioventricular Septal Defect (AVSD)

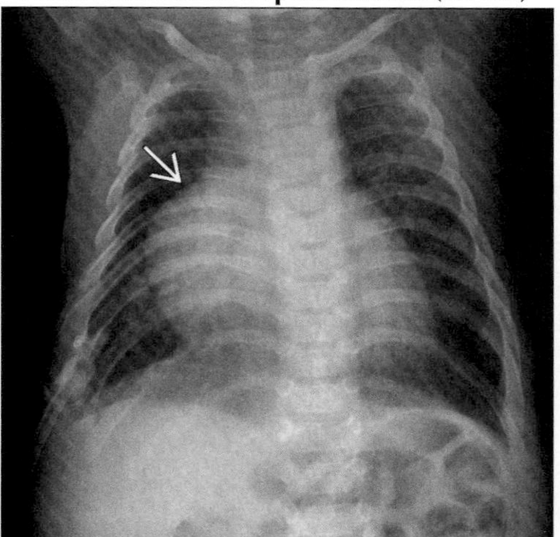

Atrioventricular Septal Defect (AVSD)

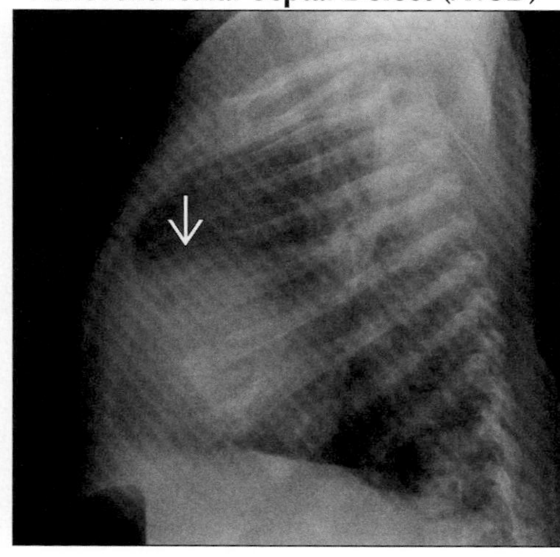

(Left) *Anteroposterior radiograph shows a very large right atrium (RA) creating a shelf with the right upper lobe. Due to the variable appearance of the RA on chest radiographs, RAs must be at least moderately enlarged to appear abnormal.* ***(Right)*** *Lateral radiograph shows the hyperinflation with flattening of the diaphragms and shelf-like interface of the enlarged right atrium with the lung. Only the RA interfaces with the lung in this way.*

CYANOTIC HEART DISEASE WITH VARIABLE OR INCREASED VASCULARITY

Truncus Arteriosus

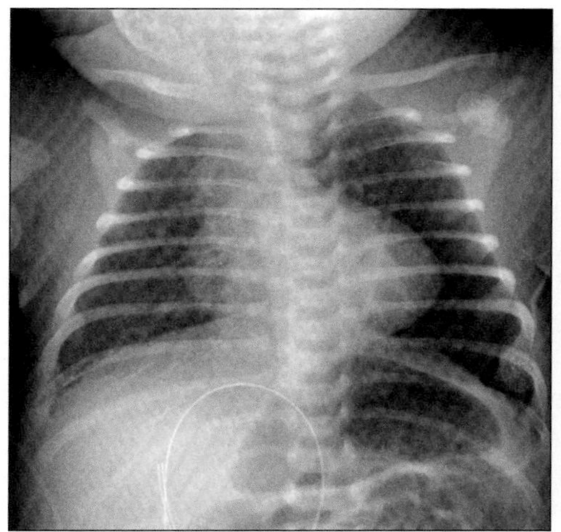

Truncus Arteriosus

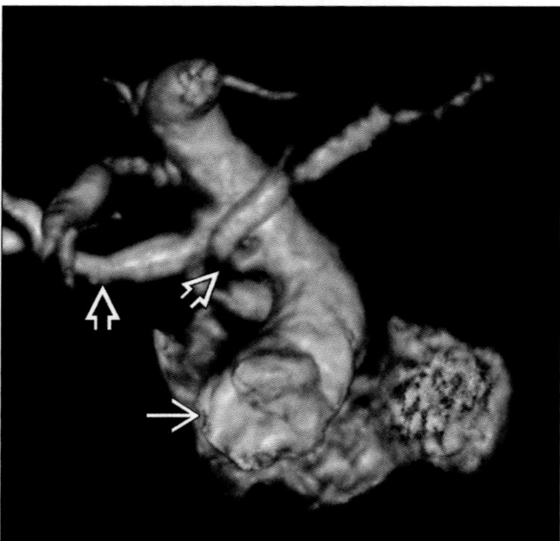

*(**Left**) AP radiograph shows cardiomegaly with decreased pulmonary vascularity and a large right aortic arch in a newborn with cyanosis. The apex of the heart is upturned due to RV hypertrophy, similar to tetralogy of Fallot.* *(**Right**) Right posterior oblique 3D reconstruction shows the large ascending truncus ➔ with 2 separate origins for the pulmonary arteries from the undersurface of the truncus arch ➔.*

Single Ventricle

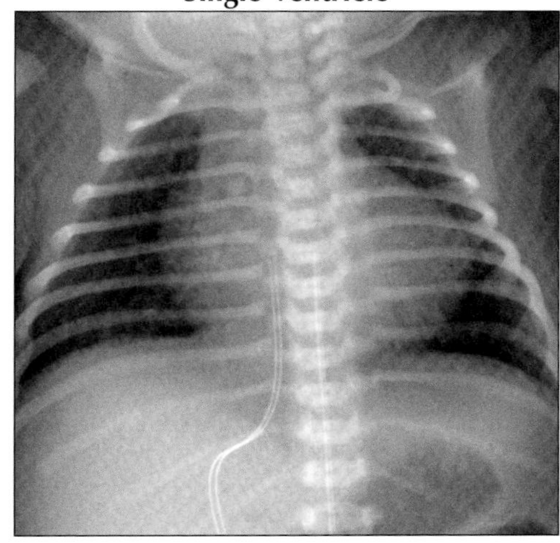

Single Ventricle

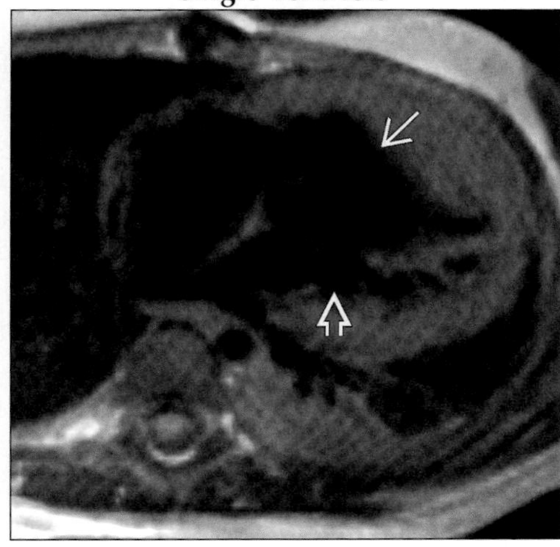

*(**Left**) AP radiograph shows cardiomegaly with decreased pulmonary vascularity in this newborn with single ventricle morphology and double inlet left ventricle with pulmonic stenosis. The aorta arises from the anterior chamber, which is a morphological left ventricle.* *(**Right**) Axial T1WI MR shows the same patient with an anterior, large left ventricle ➔ and a small right ventricle ➔, which give rise to a stenotic pulmonary artery.*

Eisenmenger Physiology

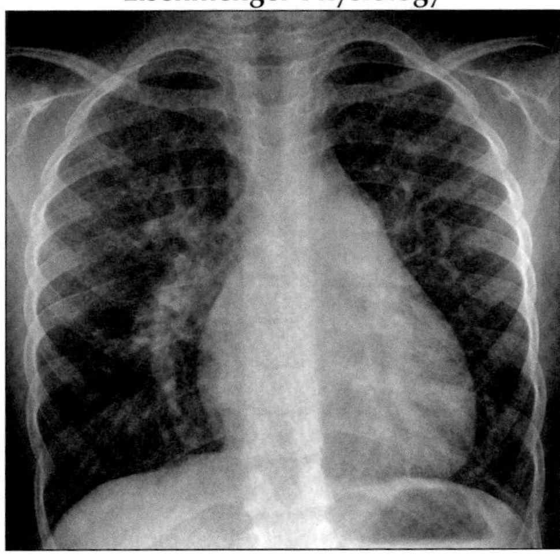

Double Outlet Right Ventricle (DORV)

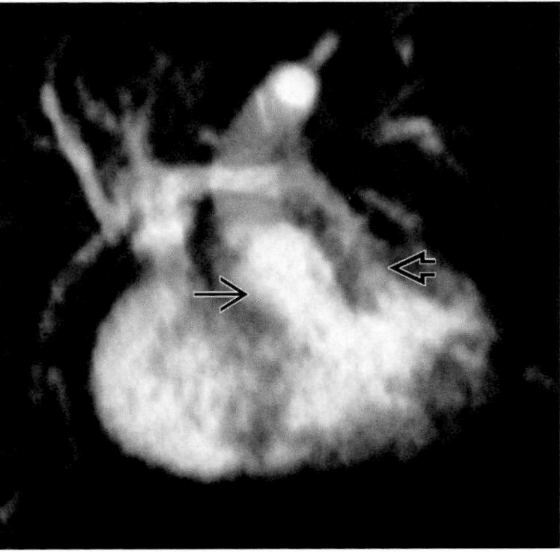

*(**Left**) Posteroanterior radiograph shows a large cardiac silhouette with large pulmonary arteries in a patient with an ASD that was undiagnosed until the intracardiac reversed shunt began to cause cyanosis.* *(**Right**) Oblique MIP of T1 C+ subtraction MR shows the aorta ➔ and pulmonary artery ➔ both arising from the right ventricle. The PV is stenotic, resulting in decreased pulmonary vascularity on the chest radiograph. The RV (not shown) was small.*

RIGHT ATRIAL ENLARGEMENT

DIFFERENTIAL DIAGNOSIS

Common
- Atrial Septal Defect (ASD)
- Tetralogy of Fallot
- Pulmonary Embolus

Less Common
- Atrioventricular Septal Defect (AVSD)
- Dilated Cardiomyopathy

Rare but Important
- Scimitar Syndrome
- Ebstein Anomaly
- Tricuspid Atresia

ESSENTIAL INFORMATION

Key Differential Diagnosis Issues
- Difficult to diagnose on chest x-ray (CXR)
- Look for prominent right heart border
- Need echocardiogram to identify cause

Helpful Clues for Common Diagnoses
- **Atrial Septal Defect (ASD)**
  - 2nd most common congenital heart defect (CHD) after bicuspid aortic valve
    - Accounts for up to 30% of CHD
    - More common in females
  - 3 types: Secundum (92.5%), primum, and sinus venosus
  - Left-to-right shunt causes volume overload of right heart and chamber enlargement
  - Secundum ASDs < 3 mm close spontaneously by 18 months
  - Secundum ASDs > 6-7 mm require follow-up echocardiography until age 4-5
    - If not closing on its own, surgical or interventional closure required
  - On MR, secundum ASD can be differentiated from normal wall thinning by thickening at edge of defect
  - Primum ASDs are associated with atrioventricular valve abnormalities
  - Sinus venosus ASDs are associated with anomalous pulmonary venous connection
- **Tetralogy of Fallot**
  - Combination of 4 cardiac malformations
    - Ventricular septal defect, overriding aorta, subpulmonic stenosis, and right ventricular hypertrophy
  - Most common cyanotic heart disease
  - Accounts for 10% of all CHD
  - Can be associated with other CHD
    - e.g., pulmonary atresia, absent pulmonary valve, double outlet right ventricle, AVSD, ASD, and right aortic arch
  - Classic CXR of "boot"-shaped heart
    - Due to upward displacement of cardiac apex and narrowed mediastinum from hypoplastic pulmonary outflow tract
  - Hypercyanotic "tet spells" begin at several months of age when agitated
    - Can be resolved by placing knees to chest
    - Increases systemic vascular resistance and promotes systemic venous return
  - Associated with trisomy 21, 18, or 13, and DiGeorge syndrome
  - Surgical options include complete repair or palliative surgery followed by complete repair
    - Blalock-Taussig shunt for palliation
  - Now have good long-term prognosis
- **Pulmonary Embolus**
  - Pulmonary artery obstruction caused by embolism or thrombus
  - Uncommon in children
  - ~ 17% of all childhood thromboembolism
  - Seen in up to 4% of pediatric autopsies
  - Thrombosis associated with underlying risk
    - Risk factors include malignancy, CHD, central venous line, lupus, vascular malformations, or renal disease
    - Idiopathic thrombosis is uncommon in children (4%)
    - Congenital thrombophilia leads to thrombus with trauma, burns, or surgery
  - 30-60% have associated deep vein thrombosis
  - Central venous lines are most common risk factor for thrombus in children
  - Chronic pulmonary embolism → right heart failure

Helpful Clues for Less Common Diagnoses
- **Atrioventricular Septal Defect (AVSD)**
  - a.k.a. endocardial cushion defect
  - Has common atrioventricular valve with abnormal arrangement of valve leaflets and deficiency of septum
  - Most severe form allows all chambers of heart to communicate

- Pulmonary hypertension develops in infancy or early childhood
- Associated with Down syndrome

- **Dilated Cardiomyopathy**
  - Characterized by ventricular dilation and decreased contractility
  - Often presents with heart failure
  - Multiple etiologies: Viral myocarditis, CHD, Takayasu arteritis, metabolic disorders, and nutritional deficiencies
  - Most often thought to be idiopathic
  - CXR with cardiomegaly and pulmonary congestion

Helpful Clues for Rare Diagnoses

- **Scimitar Syndrome**
  - a.k.a. hypnogenetic right lung
  - Partial anomalous pulmonary venous return from right lung to inferior vena cava (IVC)
  - Associations: Right lung hypoplasia, pulmonary sequestration, left superior vena cava, and cardiac dextroposition
    - Other associations: ASD, hypoplastic right pulmonary artery, "horseshoe" lung, and right diaphragmatic hernia
  - "Scimitar" sign is large pulmonary vein that courses anteriorly and inferiorly from hilum to diaphragm
    - In 66% of cases, scimitar vein drains entire right lung
    - In 10-20% of cases, scimitar vein is stenotic just distal to junction of IVC
    - Scimitar vein can insert in IVC or right atrium
  - Scimitar syndrome: Scimitar vein with right-sided pulmonary hypoplasia and systemic collateral vessels to right lung
  - 2 types: Infantile and pediatric/adult
    - Infantile form presents with failure to thrive, tachypnea, and heart failure
    - High incidence of other CHD in infantile form
    - Infantile form has 45% mortality
    - Pediatric/adult form is often found incidentally on CXR
- **Ebstein Anomaly**
  - Inferior displacement of tricuspid valve
    - Displacement results in atrialization of proximal right ventricle and tricuspid regurgitation
  - Accounts for < 1% of CHD
  - Associated with ASD and pulmonary atresia
  - Maternal lithium therapy is risk factor
  - CXR shows massive cardiomegaly and increased vascularity
    - Cyanotic lesion
- **Tricuspid Atresia**
  - Rare congenital cardiac malformation
  - Cyanotic heart lesion
  - Associated with ASD, ventricular septal defect, right ventricular hypoplasia, and pulmonary outflow obstruction
  - Can be treated with Fontan procedure

Atrial Septal Defect (ASD)

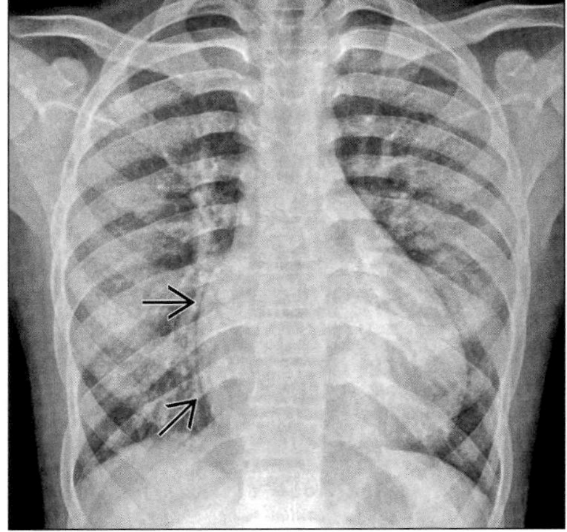

AP radiograph of the chest shows a prominent right heart border ➔ and increased vascularity. An atrial septal defect is the 2nd most common congenital heart defect after a bicuspid aortic valve.

Atrial Septal Defect (ASD)

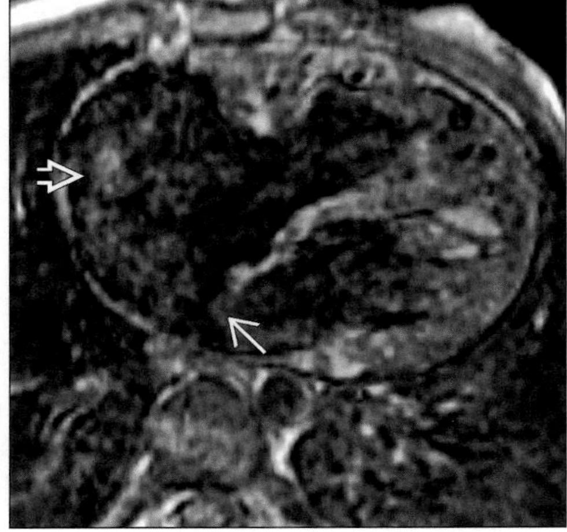

Four chamber view T1WI MR shows a large atrial septal defect ➔. The right atrium is enlarged ➔. Atrial septal defects account for 30% of all congenital heart defects.

RIGHT ATRIAL ENLARGEMENT

*(**Left**) Four chamber view from a cardiac MR shows an atrial septal defect ➡. A faint jet of flow passing through the defect is present ➡. The right atrium is enlarged ➡. Secundum defects are the most common type of defect and occur in more than 90% of patients. (**Right**) Three chamber view from a cardiac MR shows a small atrial septal defect with a jet of blood ➡ crossing from the left atrium to the right atrium. The right atrium is enlarged.*

Atrial Septal Defect (ASD)

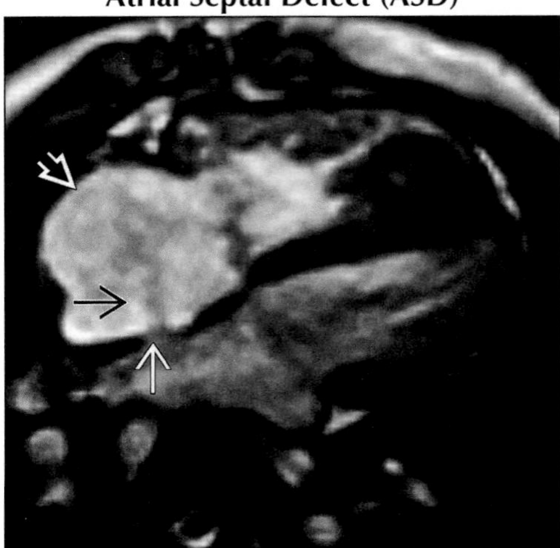

Atrial Septal Defect (ASD)

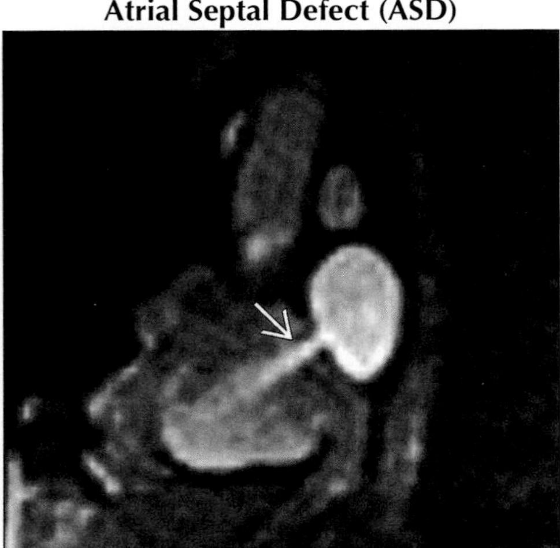

*(**Left**) AP radiograph of the chest shows an enlarged heart with an upturned apex ➡, which gives the heart its typical boot-shaped appearance. Tetralogy of Fallot is a combination of 4 cardiac defects: Ventricular septal defect, overriding aorta, subpulmonic stenosis, and right ventricular hypertrophy. (**Right**) Three chamber view from a cardiac MR shows an overriding aorta ➡ and a ventricular septal defect ➡.*

Tetralogy of Fallot

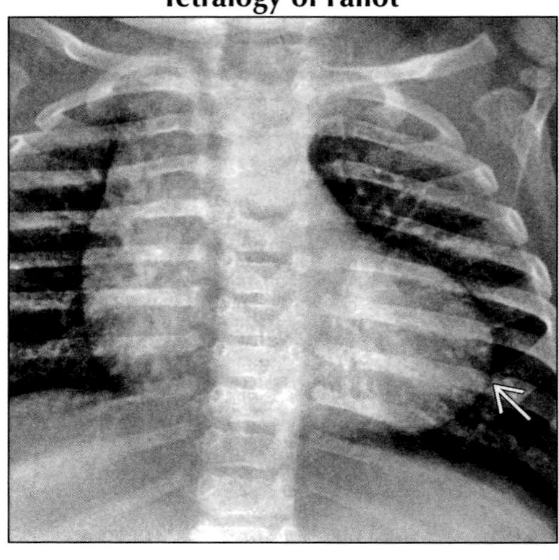

Tetralogy of Fallot

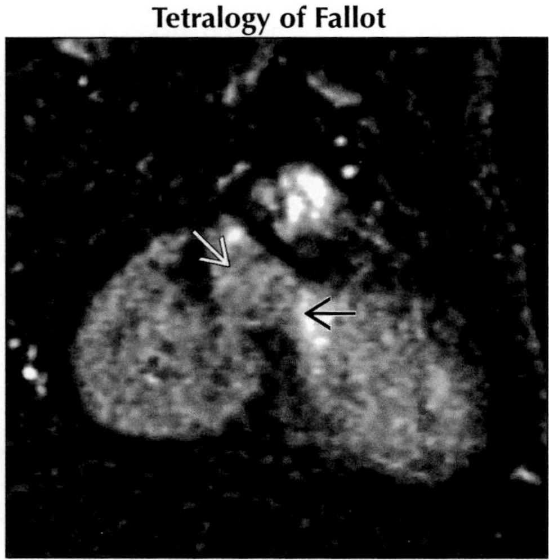

*(**Left**) Axial CECT in the same patient shows a filling defect in the left lower lobe pulmonary artery ➡. Pulmonary embolism is uncommon in children. The most common risk factors in children include malignancy, central venous lines, and congenital heart disease. (**Right**) Anterior V/Q scan shows multiple, large, mismatched defects ➡. The findings are consistent with a high probability for pulmonary embolism.*

Pulmonary Embolus

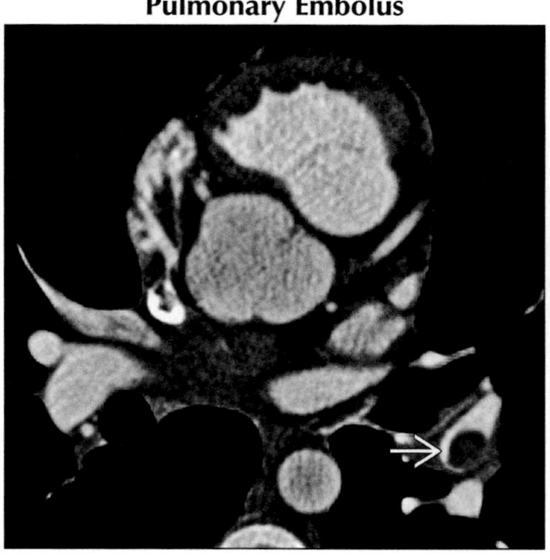

Pulmonary Embolus

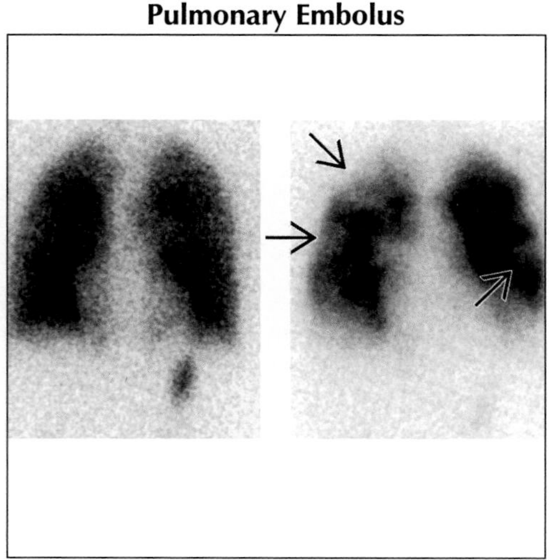

Dilated Cardiomyopathy

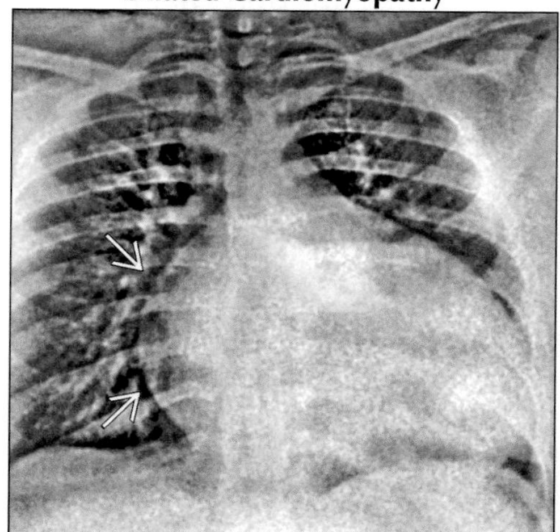

Dilated Cardiomyopathy

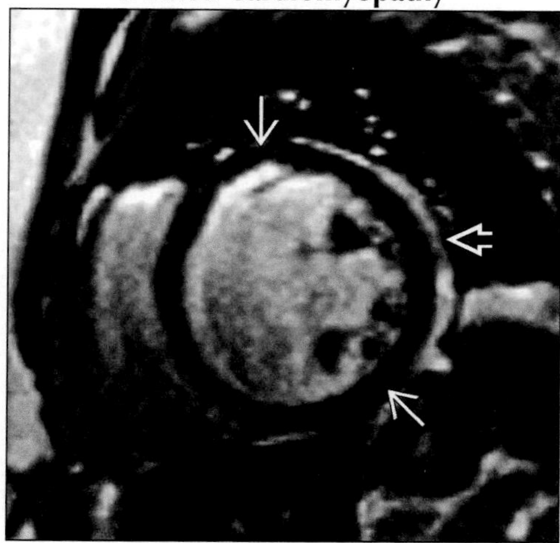

(Left) *AP radiograph of the chest shows an enlarged cardiac silhouette and pulmonary vascular congestion. The right heart border is prominent ➡. Dilated cardiomyopathy is characterized by ventricular enlargement and decreased contractility.* ***(Right)*** *Short axis 2 chamber view from a cardiac MR shows a dilated left ventricle with a thinned wall ➡. There is a small pericardial effusion ➡. Patients often present in heart failure.*

Scimitar Syndrome

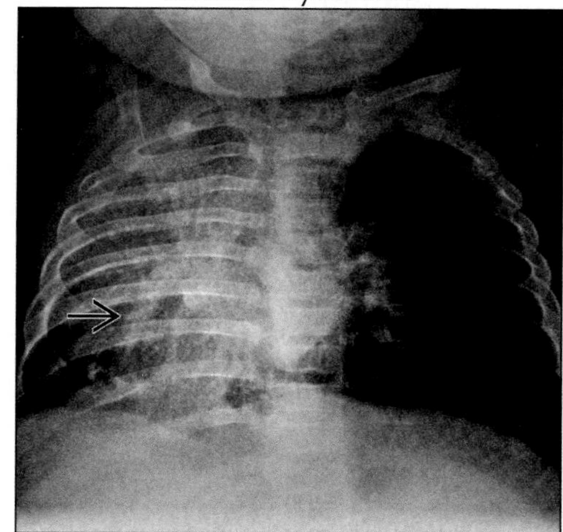

Scimitar Syndrome

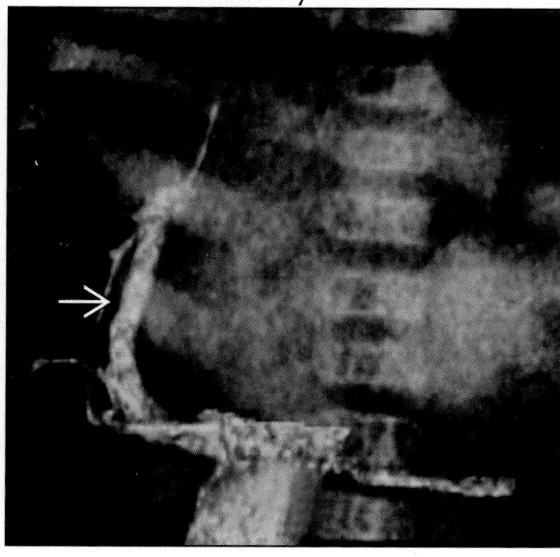

(Left) *AP radiograph of the chest shows an enlarged scimitar vein in the right lower lung ➡. The heart and mediastinum are shifted to the right due to the right-sided pulmonary hypoplasia. The scimitar vein is a large pulmonary vein that drains the right lung.* ***(Right)*** *Oblique 3D volumetric reconstruction from a CECT shows the large scimitar vein ➡ draining to the inferior vena cava at its junction with the right atrium.*

Ebstein Anomaly

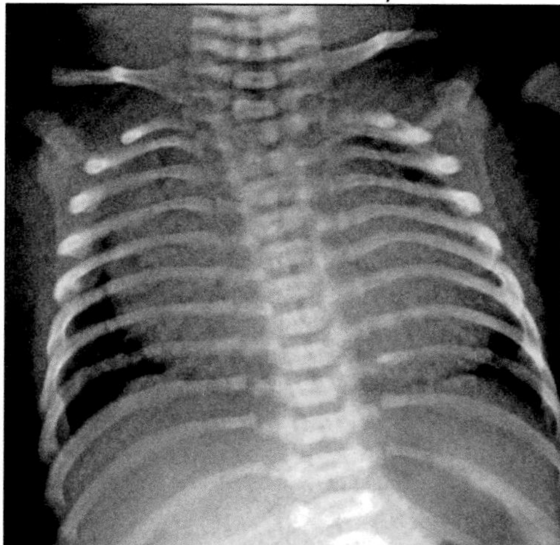

Ebstein Anomaly

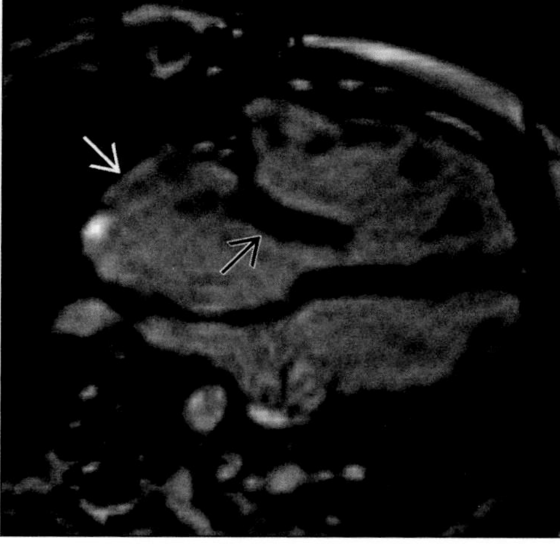

(Left) *AP radiograph of the chest shows massive cardiomegaly. Ebstein anomaly is due to inferior displacement of the tricuspid valve, leading to atrialization of the proximal right ventricle and tricuspid regurgitation. Massive cardiomegaly is characteristic.* ***(Right)*** *Four chamber view from a cardiac MR in the same patient several years after the repair shows continued enlargement of the right atrium ➡. A tricuspid regurgitant jet is present ➡.*

RIGHT VENTRICLE ENLARGEMENT

DIFFERENTIAL DIAGNOSIS

Common
- Pulmonary Hypertension (PH)
- Atrial Septal Defect (ASD)

Less Common
- Dilated Cardiomyopathy
- Pulmonary Stenosis
- Pulmonary Thromboembolism (PTE)

Rare but Important
- Tricuspid Regurgitation

ESSENTIAL INFORMATION

Key Differential Diagnosis Issues
- Causes: ↑ pulmonary vascular resistance, ↑ right heart blood volume

Helpful Clues for Common Diagnoses
- **Pulmonary Hypertension (PH)**
  - In neonatal period, persistent PH of newborn is most common cause of PH
    - Association: Neonatal lung disorders → increased pulmonary vascular resistance
  - Causes of PH in children: Congenital heart defect (CHD) and pulmonary disease
  - Occurs in CHD when pulmonary blood flow or vascular resistance is ↑
  - Main pulmonary artery is larger than aorta
- **Atrial Septal Defect (ASD)**
  - 2nd most common isolated CHD
  - 3 types: Secundum (92.5%), primum, and sinus venosus
  - MR: Differentiated from normal wall thinning by thickening at edge of defect

Helpful Clues for Less Common Diagnoses
- **Dilated Cardiomyopathy**
  - Typical dilated ventricles & ↓ contractility
  - Often presents with heart failure
  - Multiple etiologies: Viral myocarditis, CHD, Takayasu arteritis, metabolic disorders, and nutritional deficiencies
  - Most often thought to be idiopathic
  - CXR: Cardiomegaly and pulmonary congestion
- **Pulmonary Stenosis**
  - Types: Valvular, subvalvular, supravalvular, or in branch pulmonary arteries
  - Valvular most common (7-9% of all CHD)
    - CXR: Dilated main pulmonary artery
- **Pulmonary Thromboembolism (PTE)**
  - Uncommon in children
  - Risk factors: Central venous lines, malignancy, CHD, lupus, vascular malformations, or renal disease
  - 30-60% have deep vein thrombosis
  - Chronic PTE → right heart failure and PH

Helpful Clues for Rare Diagnoses
- **Tricuspid Regurgitation**
  - Can be seen as part of Ebstein anomaly or as isolated anomaly
  - Isolated tricuspid regurgitation can be caused by papillary muscle rupture
    - Rare cause in children
    - Papillary rupture can occur in utero

Pulmonary Hypertension (PH)

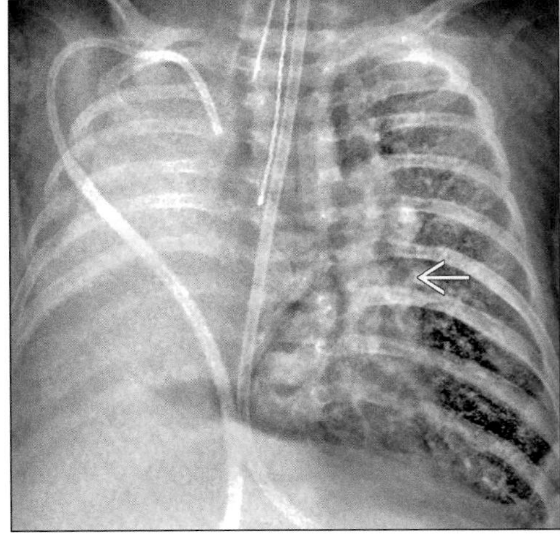

AP radiograph of the chest shows complete consolidation of the right hemithorax with a rightward shift of the heart and mediastinum due to pulmonary hypoplasia. The left hilum is enlarged ➡.

Pulmonary Hypertension (PH)

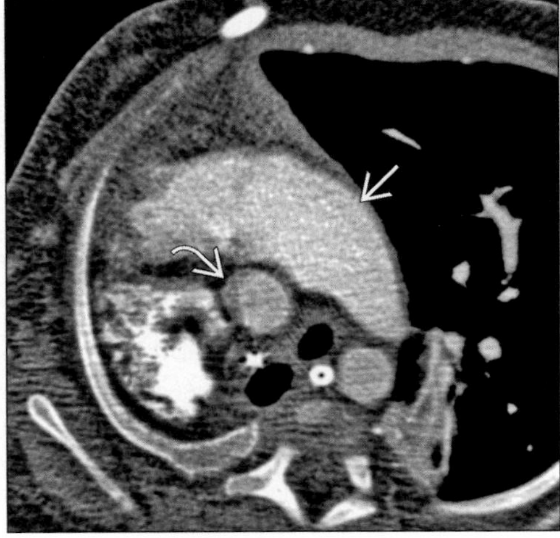

Axial CECT in the same patient shows massive enlargement of the main pulmonary artery ➡, which is larger than the aorta ➡. This is a sign of pulmonary hypertension.

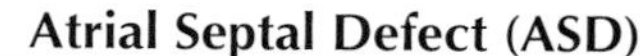

Atrial Septal Defect (ASD)

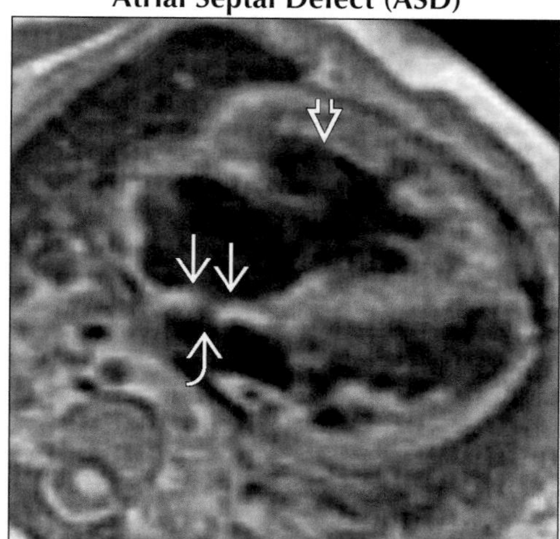

Atrial Septal Defect (ASD)

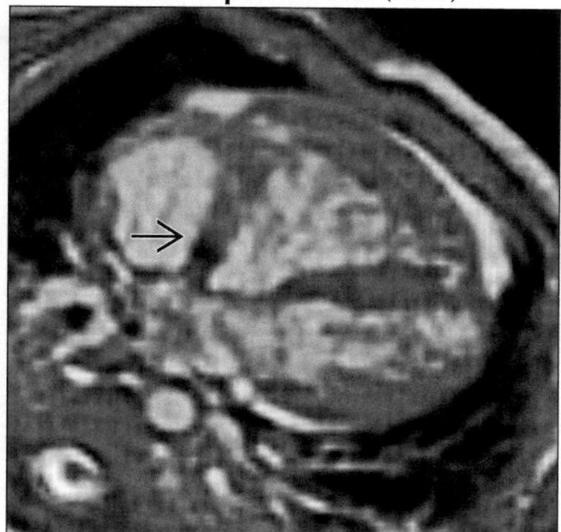

(Left) *Four chamber view from a cardiac MR shows a small atrial septal defect ➔. The right ventricle is also enlarged ➔. Atrial septal defects can be distinguished from normal thinning of the atrial wall by thickening at the edge of the defect ➔.* ***(Right)*** *Four chamber view from a cardiac MR in the same patient shows a jet of blood ➔ passing through the atrial septal defect. Atrial septal defects are the 2nd most common isolated heart defect.*

Dilated Cardiomyopathy

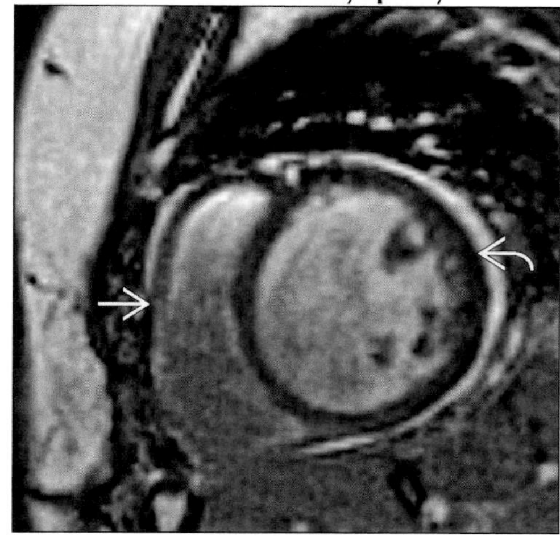

Pulmonary Stenosis

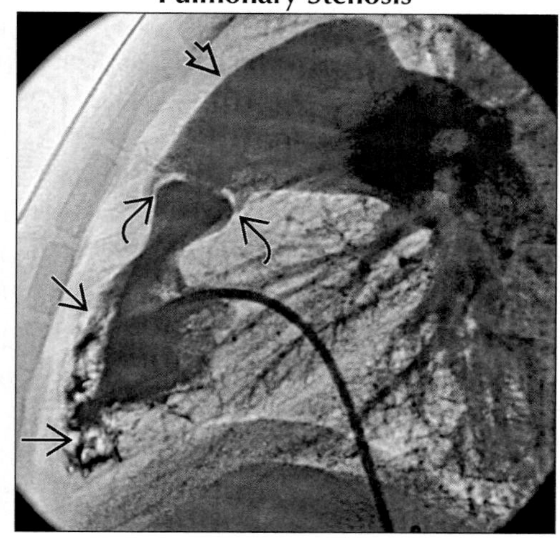

(Left) *Short axis view from a cardiac MR shows a dilated left ➔ and right ➔ ventricle. Dilated cardiomyopathy often presents with heart failure.* ***(Right)*** *Lateral catheter angiography of the right ventricular outflow tract shows considerable trabeculation and hypertrophy of the right ventricle ➔. The pulmonary valve is thickened and stenotic ➔. There is poststenotic dilation of the main pulmonary artery ➔.*

Pulmonary Thromboembolism (PTE)

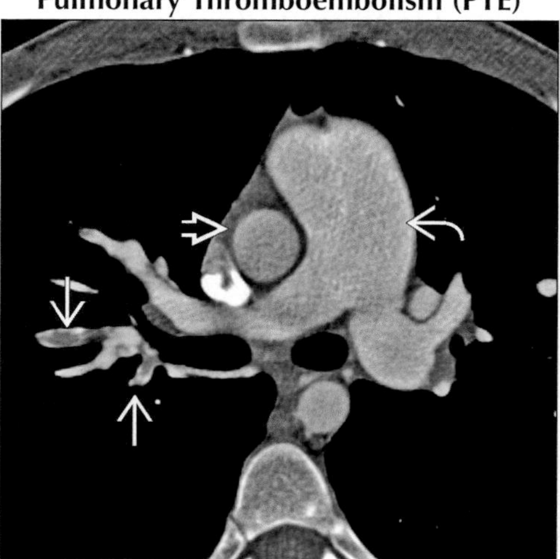

Tricuspid Regurgitation

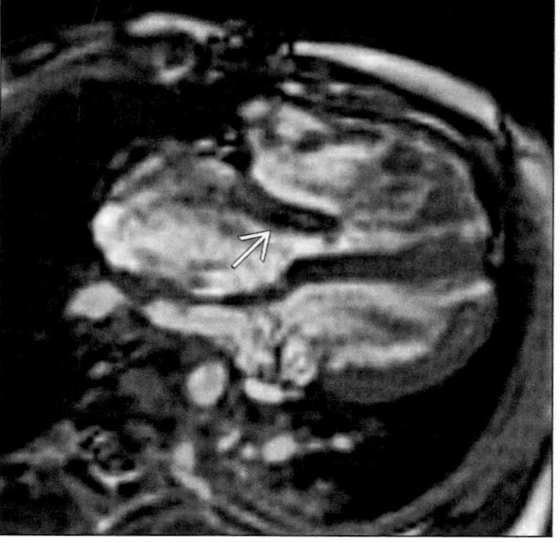

(Left) *Axial CECT shows multiple filling defects in the branch vessel of the right pulmonary artery ➔. The main pulmonary artery ➔ is enlarged compared to the aorta ➔. Although pulmonary embolism is uncommon in children, chronic pulmonary embolism can lead to right heart failure.* ***(Right)*** *Four chamber view of a cardiac MR shows a regurgitant jet arising from the tricuspid valve ➔. This patient's tricuspid regurgitation is due to an Ebstein anomaly.*

SMALL PULMONARY ARTERY

DIFFERENTIAL DIAGNOSIS

Common
- Congenital Venolobar Syndrome
  - Scimitar Syndrome
  - Pulmonary Hypoplasia
- Tetralogy of Fallot

Less Common
- Pulmonary Stenosis
- Supravalvular Aortic Stenosis

Rare but Important
- Takayasu Arteritis
- Alagille Syndrome
- Rubella
- Ehlers-Danlos Syndrome
- Cutis Laxa

ESSENTIAL INFORMATION

Key Differential Diagnosis Issues
- 2 broad categories: Congenital venolobar syndrome and pulmonary stenosis

Helpful Clues for Common Diagnoses
- **Congenital Venolobar Syndrome**
  - Heterogeneous group of pulmonary developmental anomalies
    - Most consistent components are hypogenetic lung and partial anomalous pulmonary venous return
    - Includes scimitar syndrome, partial anomalous pulmonary venous return, congenital absence of pulmonary artery, and pulmonary sequestration
  - Pulmonary sequestration is most common
  - Patients are usually asymptomatic
  - Associations: Cardiac and spinal anomalies
- **Scimitar Syndrome**
  - a.k.a hypogenetic right lung
  - Specific type of congenital venolobar syndrome
    - Definition: Scimitar vein with right-sided pulmonary hypoplasia and systemic collaterals vessels to right lung
  - Scimitar vein: Partial anomalous pulmonary venous return from right lung to inferior vena cava
    - Courses anterior and inferior from hilum to diaphragm
    - Can insert in inferior vena cava or right atrium
  - 2 types: Infantile and pediatric/adult
    - Infantile form presents with failure to thrive, tachypnea, and heart failure; 45% mortality
    - High incidence of other congenital heart defects (CHD) in infantile form
    - Pediatric/adult form is usually incidental finding on chest x-ray (CXR)
- **Pulmonary Hypoplasia**
  - Small lung with alveoli and bronchi present
  - CXR: Small hemithorax, small hilum, and ipsilateral mediastinal shift: Ipsilateral ↓ pulmonary vascularity
  - More common on right
- **Tetralogy of Fallot**
  - Combination of 4 cardiac defects
    - Ventricular septal defect, overriding aorta, subpulmonic stenosis, and right ventricular hypertrophy
  - Most common cyanotic heart disease
  - Accounts for 10% of CHD
  - Classic CXR with boot-shaped heart
    - Due to upward displacement of cardiac apex and narrowed mediastinum from hypoplastic pulmonary outflow tract
  - Associated with trisomy 21, 18, or 13 and DiGeorge syndrome

Helpful Clues for Less Common Diagnoses
- **Pulmonary Stenosis**
  - Types: Valvular, subvalvular, supravalvular, or in branch pulmonary arteries
  - Valvular stenosis is most common
    - 7-9% of all CHD
    - Present with asymptomatic murmur
    - CXR: Dilated main pulmonary artery, small peripheral vessels
    - Treatment: Balloon valvuloplasty
- **Supravalvular Aortic Stenosis**
  - Supravalvular is least common type of aortic stenosis
    - Narrowing of aortic root at or above sinotubular ridge
    - Accounts for < 10%
    - Frequently seen in Williams syndrome
    - Association: Pulmonary artery stenosis

Helpful Clues for Rare Diagnoses
- **Takayasu Arteritis**
  - Chronic vasculitis of unknown etiology

- Large vessel vasculitis affects aorta, its main branches, and pulmonary arteries
- 3rd most common vasculitis of childhood
  - Most commonly presents between 10-20 years of age
  - 8.5x more common in females
- Associated with tuberculosis infection
- Pulseless arteritis is characteristic of chronic disease
- Pulmonary arteries involved in ~ 85%
- Often leads to hypertension, congestive heart failure, or aortic regurgitation
- CXR aorta: Undulating border, segmental calcification
- CXR pulmonary arteries: Oligemia
- CT or MR shows thickened arterial wall with enhancement
- Treated with steroids

- **Alagille Syndrome**
  - Genetic disorder
  - Characterized by 5 major features
    - Paucity of bile ducts, peripheral pulmonary stenosis, "butterfly" vertebral bodies, posterior embryotoxon, and abnormal facies
    - Also associated with complex CHD
  - 20-25% require liver transplant
- **Rubella**
  - a.k.a. German measles
  - > 80% risk of congenital defects if acquired in 1st 12 weeks of pregnancy
  - Now rare due to vaccination
  - Outcome depends on gestational age at time of infection
    - Classic abnormalities: Cataracts, heart defects, and sensorineural deafness
    - Cardiac defects: Patent ductus arteriosus, pulmonary artery stenosis, pulmonary artery hypoplasia
- **Ehlers-Danlos Syndrome**
  - Multiple types
  - Ehlers-Danlos type 4 is vascular type
  - Features: Acrogeria; thin, translucent skin; ecchymoses and hematomas; arterial, digestive, and obstetric complications
  - Arterial complications are leading cause of death
    - Complications most common in medium and large vessels
    - Complications include arterial rupture, aneurysm, and dissection
    - Complications uncommon in childhood
  - Association: Peripheral pulmonary stenosis
- **Cutis Laxa**
  - Characterized by loose sagging skin with decreased elasticity and resilience
  - Multiple modes of inheritance
  - Autosomal recessive form is associated with severe internal organ complications
    - Gastrointestinal and genitourinary diverticula, diaphragmatic hernia, and emphysema
  - Peripheral pulmonary stenosis is most common cardiovascular anomaly
    - Occurs in 90%
    - Other cardiovascular anomalies: Aortic coarctation and aortic aneurysm

Congenital Venolobar Syndrome

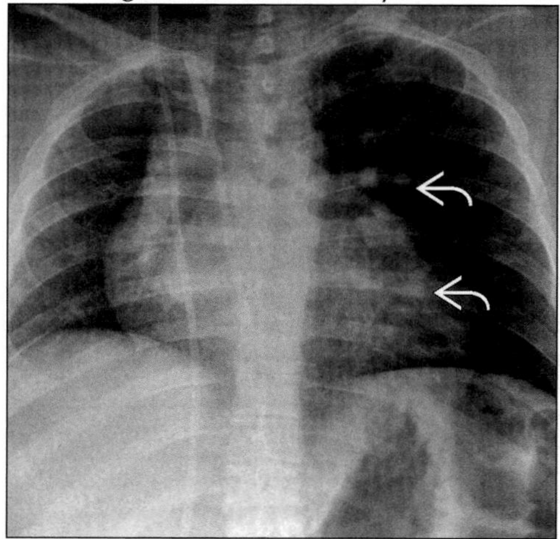

AP radiograph of the chest shows a small right hemithorax and enlarged left-sided pulmonary arteries ➔. Patients with congenital venolobar syndrome are often asymptomatic.

Congenital Venolobar Syndrome

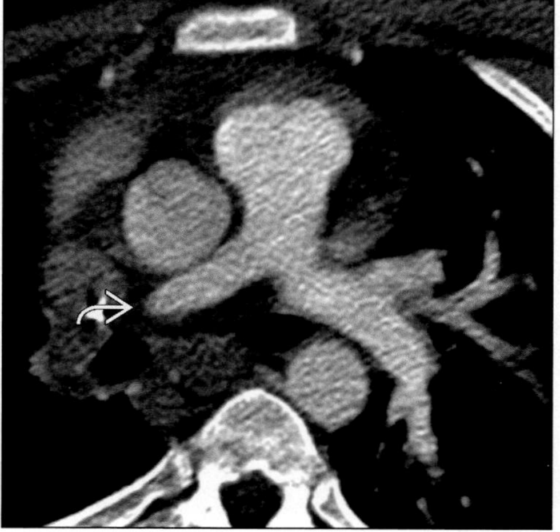

Axial CECT shows abrupt termination of the right pulmonary artery ➔. Congenital venolobar syndrome is a heterogeneous group of developmental anomalies and includes absence of the pulmonary artery.

SMALL PULMONARY ARTERY

(Left) *AP radiograph of the chest shows a small right hemithorax and a curvilinear scimitar vein* ➔ *extending to the right hemidiaphragm. Scimitar syndrome is a specific type of congenital venolobar syndrome.* **(Right)** *Coronal MIP of T1 C+ subtraction MR in the same patient shows the scimitar vein* ➔ *draining into the inferior vena cava at the level of the diaphragm. The scimitar vein is a partial anomalous pulmonary venous connection to the inferior vena cava.*

Scimitar Syndrome

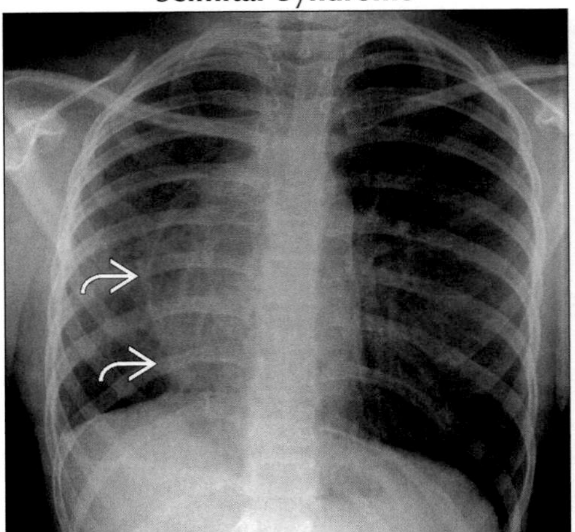

Scimitar Syndrome

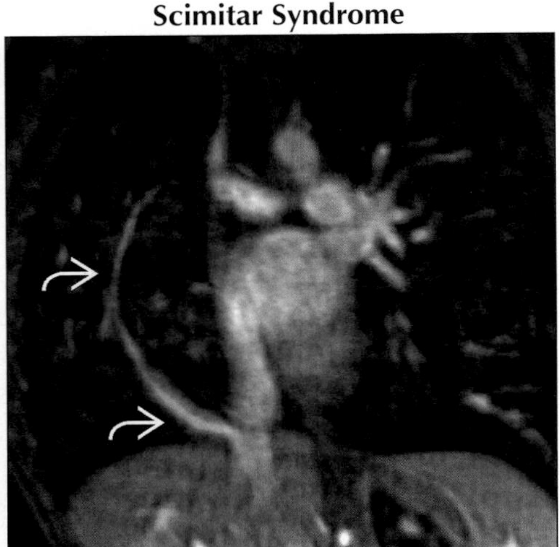

(Left) *AP radiograph of the chest shows a small right hemithorax with rib crowding and absent pulmonary markings. The heart and mediastinum are shifted to the right. Pulmonary hypoplasia or agenesis is more common on the right.* **(Right)** *Axial CECT shows congenital absence of the right lung and hyperinflation of the left lung. The left lung crosses midline anteriorly* ➔*. The heart and mediastinum occupy the right chest* ➔*.*

Pulmonary Hypoplasia

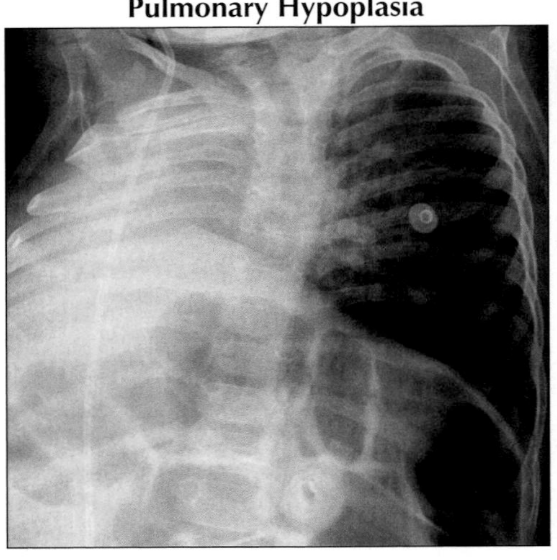

Pulmonary Hypoplasia

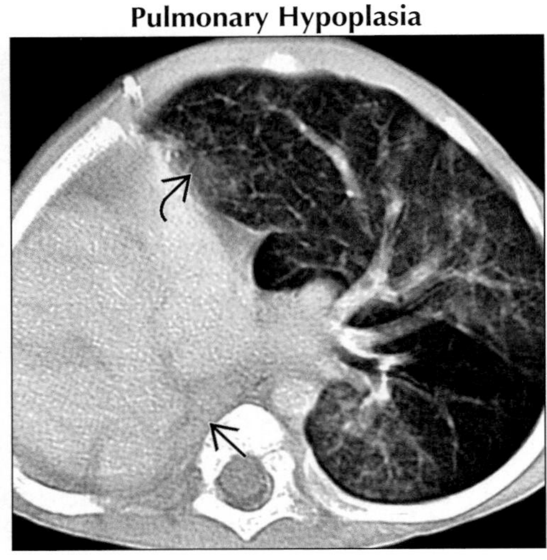

(Left) *AP radiograph of the chest shows a normal-sized heart with an upturned cardiac apex* ➔*. The peripheral pulmonary arteries are not seen. Tetralogy of Fallot is the most common cyanotic heart disease accounting for 10% of all congenital heart defects.* **(Right)** *Axial CECT shows a ventricular septal defect at the level of the overriding aorta* ➔*. The right ventricular wall is thickened and trabeculated* ➔*. Subpulmonic stenosis is not shown.*

Tetralogy of Fallot

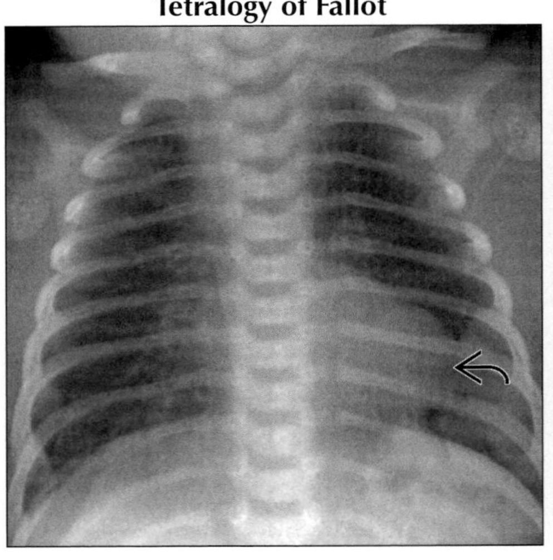

Tetralogy of Fallot

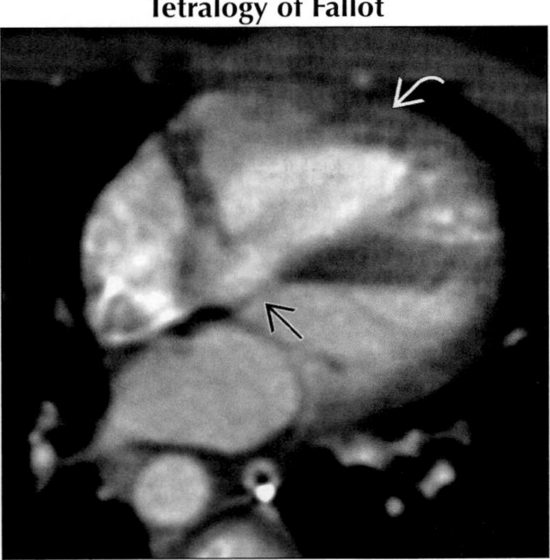

Pulmonary Stenosis

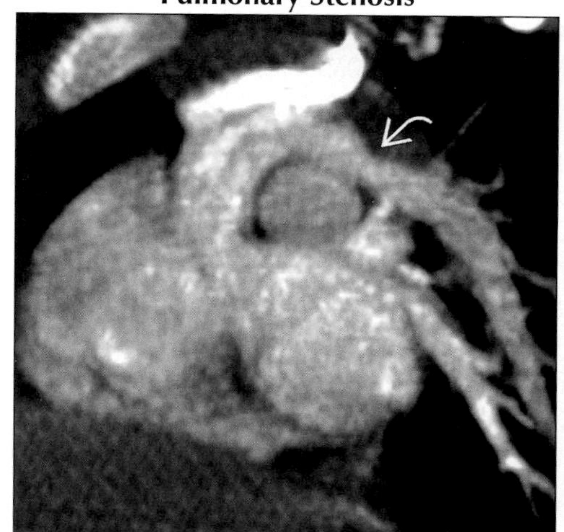

Supravalvular Aortic Stenosis

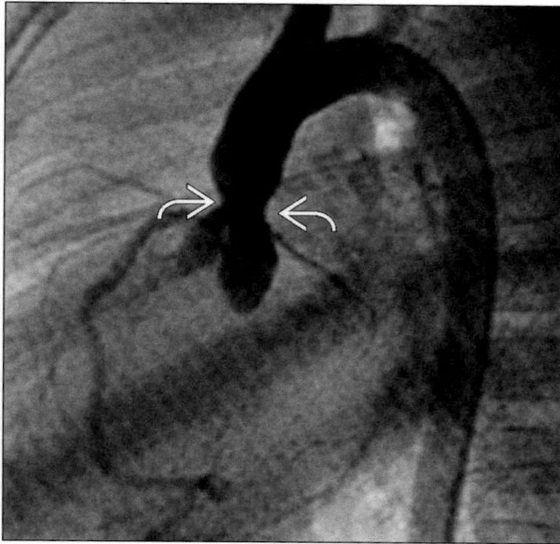

*(**Left**) Oblique CECT shows focal narrowing at the origin of the left pulmonary artery ➔. Pulmonary stenosis can be valvular, subvalvular, supravalvular, and at the level of the branch pulmonary arteries. (**Right**) Lateral catheter angiography shows focal narrowing of the ascending aorta just above the level of the aortic valve ➔. Supravalvular aortic stenosis is associated with Williams syndrome. It accounts for less than 10% of aortic stenosis cases.*

Takayasu Arteritis

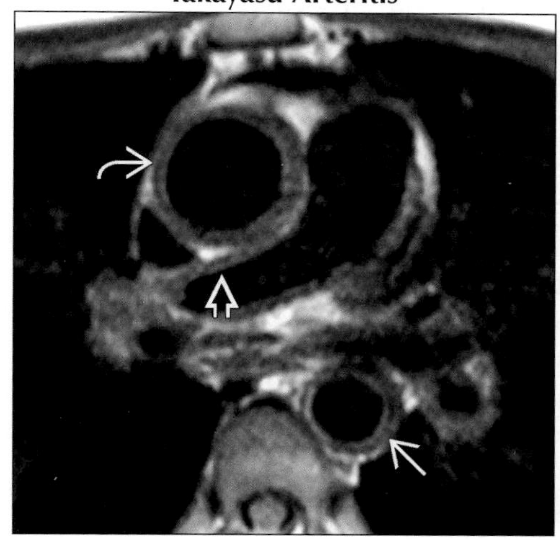

Takayasu Arteritis

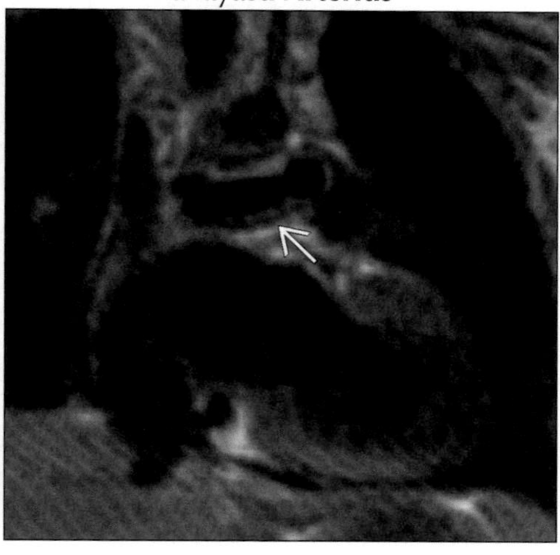

*(**Left**) Axial T1WI MR shows thickening of the wall of the ascending aorta ➔, descending aorta ➔, and right pulmonary artery ➔. Takayasu arteritis is a chronic vasculitis of unknown etiology. (**Right**) Coronal T1WI MR in a different patient shows thickening of the wall of the right pulmonary artery ➔. Takayasu arteritis commonly affects the aorta, its branches, and the pulmonary artery. It is the 3rd most common vasculitis in children.*

Alagille Syndrome

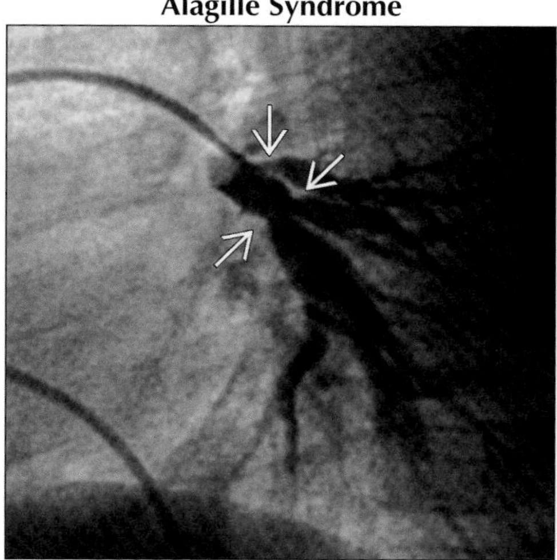

Alagille Syndrome

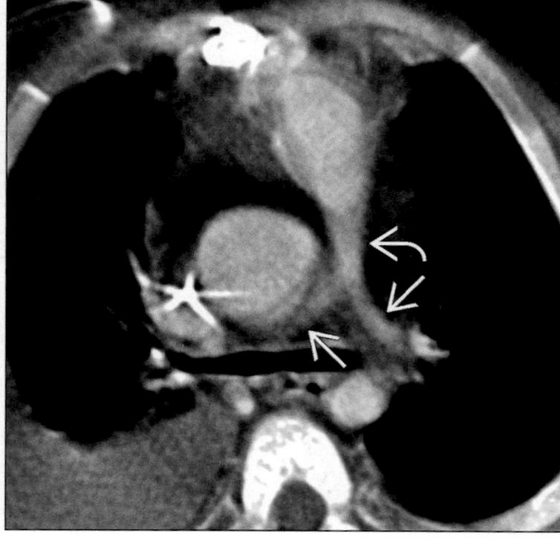

*(**Left**) Lateral catheter angiography of the left pulmonary artery shows multiple areas of branch pulmonary stenosis ➔. Alagille syndrome is characterized by paucity of bile ducts, peripheral pulmonary stenosis, "butterfly" vertebral bodies, posterior embryotoxon, and abnormal facies. (**Right**) Axial CECT shows focal stenosis of the distal main pulmonary artery ➔ and the right and left pulmonary artery ➔.*

PROMINENT PULMONARY ARTERY

DIFFERENTIAL DIAGNOSIS

Common
- Pulmonary Hypertension (PH)
- Left-to-Right Shunts

Less Common
- Pulmonary Thromboembolism
- Pulmonary Stenosis

Rare but Important
- Absent Pulmonary Valve

ESSENTIAL INFORMATION

Key Differential Diagnosis Issues
- Underlying causes: Pulmonary hypertension or ↑ pulmonary blood flow

Helpful Clues for Common Diagnoses
- **Pulmonary Hypertension (PH)**
  - In neonatal period, persistent PH of newborn is most common cause of PH
    - Associated with neonatal respiratory conditions that result in elevated pulmonary vascular resistance
  - Causes of PH in children: Congenital heart defects (CHD) and pulmonary disease
    - Occurs in CHD when pulmonary blood flow or vascular resistance is increased
  - Main pulmonary artery is larger than aorta
- **Left-to-Right Shunts**
  - Any CHD with significant shunt → PH
  - ↑ blood flow to pulmonary bed
    - Over time, smooth muscle hypertrophy of vascular wall
    - PH eventually progressive, irreversible
  - Eisenmenger syndrome: When pulmonary pressure is greater than systemic vascular resistance and shunt reverses
  - Cyanosis in Eisenmenger syndrome

Helpful Clues for Less Common Diagnoses
- **Pulmonary Thromboembolism**
  - Pulmonary artery obstruction caused by embolism or thrombus
  - Uncommon in children
  - Risk factors: Malignancy, CHD, central venous line, lupus, vascular malformations, or renal disease
    - Central venous lines are most common risk factor for thrombus in children
  - 30-60% have deep vein thrombosis
  - Chronic pulmonary embolism → right heart failure and PH
- **Pulmonary Stenosis**
  - Types: Valvular, subvalvular, supravalvular, or in branch pulmonary arteries
  - Valvular stenosis is most common
    - 7-9% of all CHD
    - CXR: Dilated main pulmonary artery

Helpful Clues for Rare Diagnoses
- **Absent Pulmonary Valve**
  - Characterized by narrowed pulmonic annulus and rudimentary cusps, pulmonary artery dilation, and VSD
    - Constellation of findings, i.e., tetralogy of Fallot with absent pulmonary valve
  - Often associated with VSD

Pulmonary Hypertension (PH)

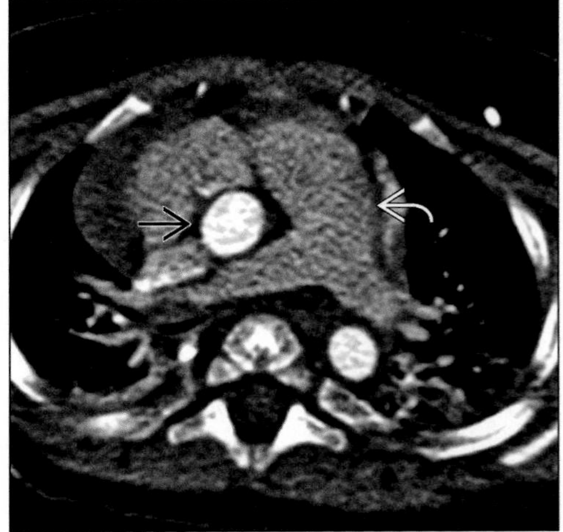

Axial CECT in a patient with a history of a congenital diaphragmatic hernia shows a dilated main pulmonary artery ➡ with a transverse diameter greater than the transverse diameter of the aorta ➡.

Pulmonary Hypertension (PH)

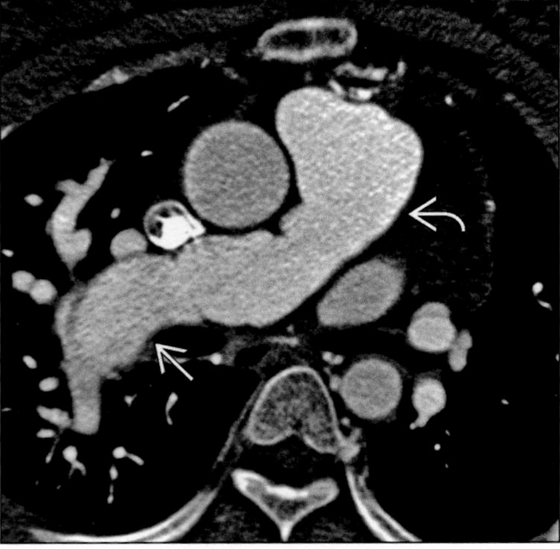

Axial CECT shows a dilated and ectatic main ➡ and right main pulmonary arteries ➡. Common causes of pulmonary hypertension in children include pulmonary disease and congenital heart defects.

PROMINENT PULMONARY ARTERY

Pulmonary Thromboembolism

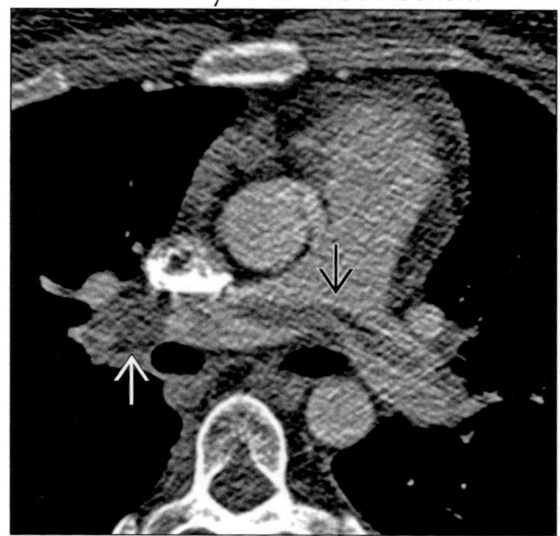

Pulmonary Thromboembolism

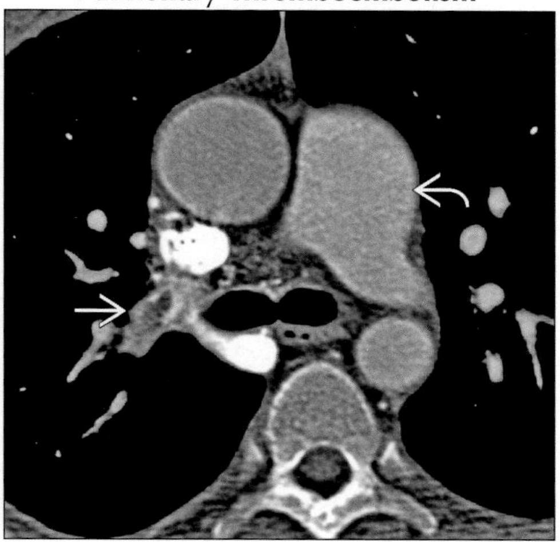

(Left) *Axial CECT shows a saddle pulmonary embolism at the bifurcation of the pulmonary artery* →. *A large thrombus is also present in the right main pulmonary artery* ➡. *Pulmonary embolism is uncommon in children.* ***(Right)*** *Axial CECT shows thrombus in the right main pulmonary artery* ➡ *and a dilated main pulmonary artery* ↪. *The most common risk factor for pulmonary embolism in children is the presence of a central venous line.*

Pulmonary Stenosis

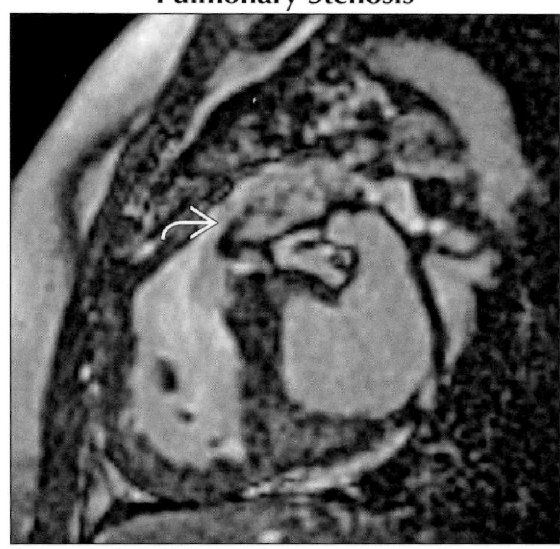

Pulmonary Stenosis

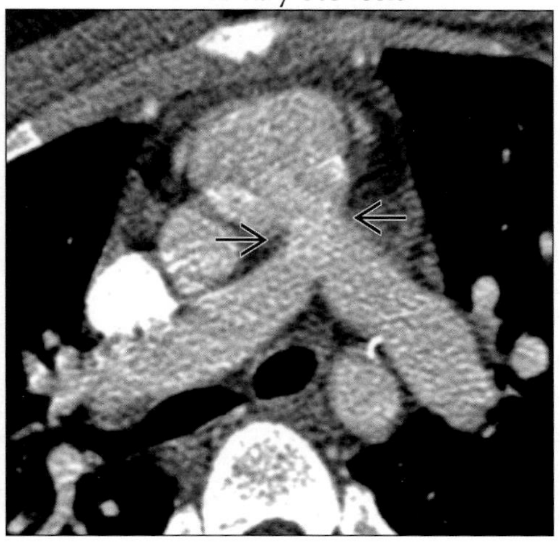

(Left) *RVOT view from a cardiac MR shows a turbulent jet in the proximal main pulmonary artery* ↪ *due to valvular pulmonary stenosis, which is the most common type of pulmonary stenosis.* ***(Right)*** *Axial CECT shows focal narrowing of the main pulmonary artery at the origin of the left and right pulmonary arteries* →. *Supravalvular pulmonary stenosis, as seen in this patient, is associated with Williams syndrome.*

Absent Pulmonary Valve

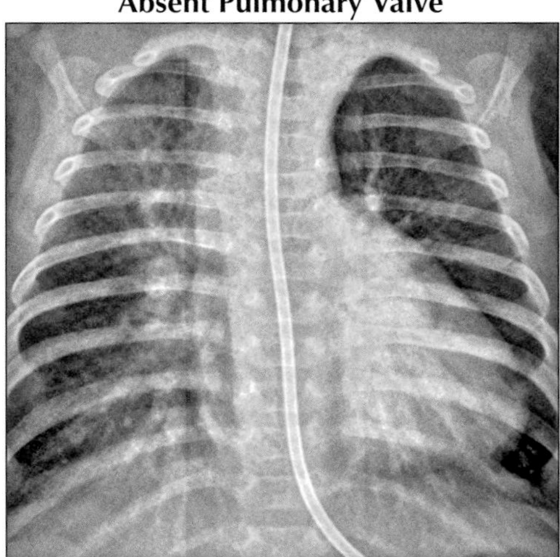

Absent Pulmonary Valve

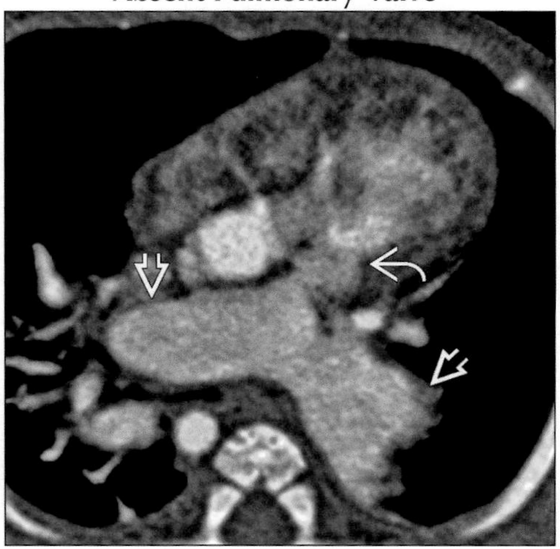

(Left) *Anteroposterior radiograph of the chest shows markedly enlarged central and peripheral pulmonary arteries.* ***(Right)*** *Axial CECT shows focal narrowing at the pulmonary valve annulus* ↪. *The left and right pulmonary arteries are dilated* ⇨. *Absent pulmonary valves are characterized by a narrowed pulmonic annulus, rudimentary valve cusps, dilated pulmonary arteries, and a ventricular septal defect.*

LEFT ATRIAL ENLARGEMENT

DIFFERENTIAL DIAGNOSIS

Common
- Ventricular Septal Defect (VSD)
- Patent Ductus Arteriosus (PDA)

Less Common
- Heart Failure
  - Dilated Cardiomyopathy
- Hypertrophic Obstructive Cardiomyopathy
- Hypertension

Rare but Important
- Mitral Valve Stenosis
- Mitral Valve Regurgitation
- Left Atrial Myxoma

ESSENTIAL INFORMATION

Key Differential Diagnosis Issues
- Left atrial enlargement can be caused by left-to-right shunts, mitral valve disease, or left ventricular dysfunction
- Chest radiograph findings
  - Double density of heart, splaying of carina, and posterior displacement of esophagus

Helpful Clues for Common Diagnoses
- **Ventricular Septal Defect (VSD)**
  - Most common congenital heart defect in children
    - Occurs in 50% of children with congenital heart defect
    - Isolated defect in 20% of children with congenital heart defect
  - 2 main locations: Membranous or muscular septum
    - Membranous defects account for 70% of VSDs
    - Multiple defects can be present
  - Associated with Down syndrome, DiGeorge syndrome, Turner syndrome
  - Holosystolic murmur on auscultation
  - Small VSDs often close spontaneously
    - Large VSDs can be closed surgically or with catheter intervention
- **Patent Ductus Arteriosus (PDA)**
  - Ductus arteriosus connects proximal descending aorta to main pulmonary artery
    - Essential for fetal circulation
  - Normally closes spontaneously after birth
    - Prostaglandins can help keep ductus arteriosus open
    - Indomethacin helps to close duct
  - Risks for PDA: Prematurity, prenatal infection
    - 65% of infants born < 28 weeks of fetal gestation have PDA
  - Accounts for 5-10% of all congenital heart defects
  - 2x more common in females
  - Most cases are sporadic
    - Increased risk with Down syndrome, Holt-Oram syndrome, and Carpenter syndrome
  - Continuous machinery murmur at upper left sternal border
  - For some types of congenital heart defect, survival is dependent on PDA
    - Ductal dependent lesions for systemic flow: Hypoplastic left heart, critical aortic stenosis, interrupted aortic arch
    - Ductal dependent cyanotic lesions: Pulmonary atresia, transposition of great arteries

Helpful Clues for Less Common Diagnoses
- **Heart Failure**
  - Inability of heart to pump sufficient blood to meet metabolic needs of body
    - Heart failure leads to decreased cardiac output
  - Common causes: Congenital heart defect, viral myocarditis, dilated cardiomyopathy, and occult arrhythmias
  - Congenital heart defect is most common cause of heart failure in children < age 1
  - Other causes are also known as heart muscle disease
    - Muscular disease is most common cause of heart failure and transplant in children older than 1 year old
    - 1/3 of patients with muscular disease die or require transplant within 1 year of presentation
  - **Dilated Cardiomyopathy**
    - Characterized by ventricular dilation and decreased contractility
    - Often presents with heart failure
    - Multiple etiologies: Viral myocarditis, congenital heart defect, Takayasu arteritis, metabolic disorders, and nutritional deficiencies

- Most often thought to be idiopathic
- Chest radiograph shows cardiomegaly and pulmonary congestion

- **Hypertrophic Obstructive Cardiomyopathy**
  - Most common hereditary cardiac disorder
    - Autosomal dominant disorder
  - Usually presents in adolescence or later
  - Asymmetric septal hypertrophy leads to left ventricular outflow tract obstruction
  - Can present with sudden death
- **Hypertension**
  - Increasing prevalence in children and adolescents
    - Association of hypertension and obesity
  - Left ventricular hypertrophy is finding of end-organ damage
    - Can be seen in up to 41% of children with hypertension
  - Hypertension is often due to underlying disorder
    - Renal parenchymal disease is most common cause
    - Other causes: Endocrine disorders, aortic coarctation, renal vascular disease, and pheochromocytoma
  - Secondary hypertension is more common in children than adults
  - Echocardiogram to evaluate for left ventricular hypertrophy

Helpful Clues for Rare Diagnoses

- **Mitral Valve Stenosis**
  - If acquired, due to rheumatic heart disease
    - Mitral valve affected in 65-70% of rheumatic fever
    - Rheumatic fever is uncommon in developing countries
  - Echocardiogram is used to determine severity and identify left atrial thrombus
- **Mitral Valve Regurgitation**
  - Systolic retrograde flow from left ventricle to left atrium
  - Most common valvular disease in United States
  - Prevalence increases with age
  - Cause in young adults: Rheumatic fever
  - Endocarditis can cause mitral regurgitation
  - Volume overload with increased preload leads to left atrial and left ventricular enlargement
- **Left Atrial Myxoma**
  - Myxomas are 3rd most common cardiac tumor after rhabdomyomas and fibromas
  - Can occur in all regions of heart
    - Can cause compression of cardiac structures
    - Valvular insufficiency
    - Outflow obstruction
    - Sudden death
    - Mitral regurgitation can occur with left atrial myxoma

Ventricular Septal Defect (VSD)

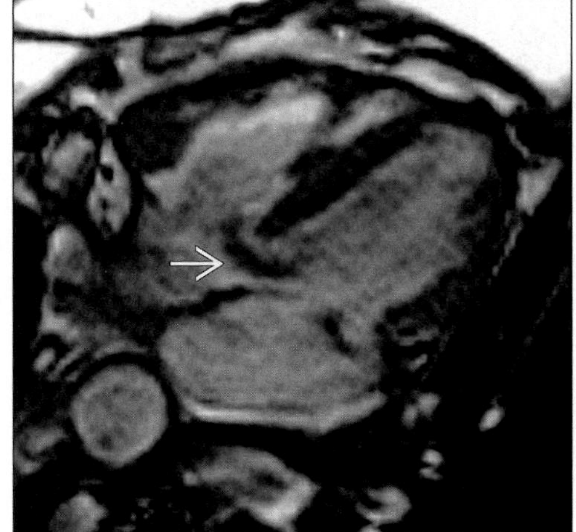

Four chamber view from a cardiac MR shows a ventricular septal defect with a jet of turbulent blood flow ➡. Ventricular septal defects are the most common congenital heart defects.

Ventricular Septal Defect (VSD)

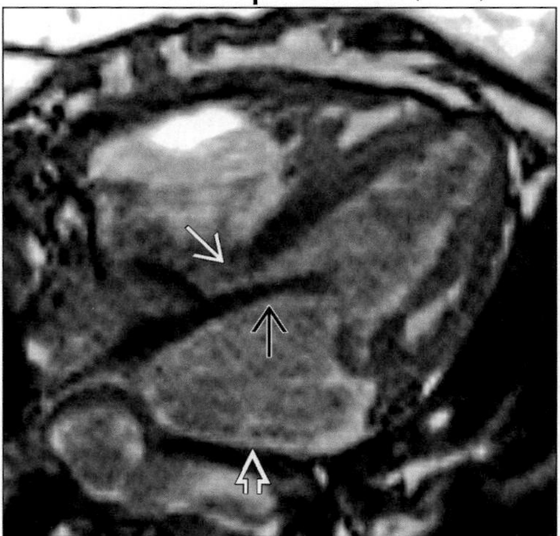

Four chamber view from a cardiac MR shows the mitral valve ➡ next to a ventricular septal defect ➡. The left atrium is enlarged ➡. Ventricular septal defects can close spontaneously.

LEFT ATRIAL ENLARGEMENT

*(**Left**) Short axis 2 chamber view from a cardiac MR shows a ventricular septal defect near the pulmonary outflow tract. Ventricular septal defects are associated with Down syndrome, DiGeorge syndrome, and Turner syndrome. (**Right**) Left anterior oblique catheter angiography with the catheter tip in the aortic arch shows a large patent ductus arteriosus. Risk factors for a PDA include prematurity and prenatal infection.*

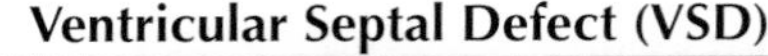

Ventricular Septal Defect (VSD)

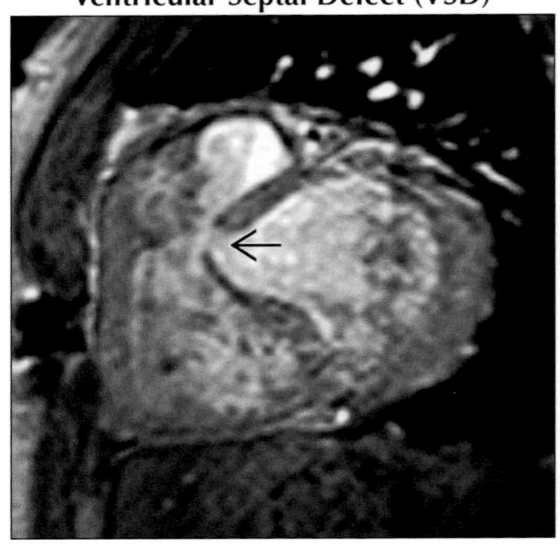

Patent Ductus Arteriosus (PDA)

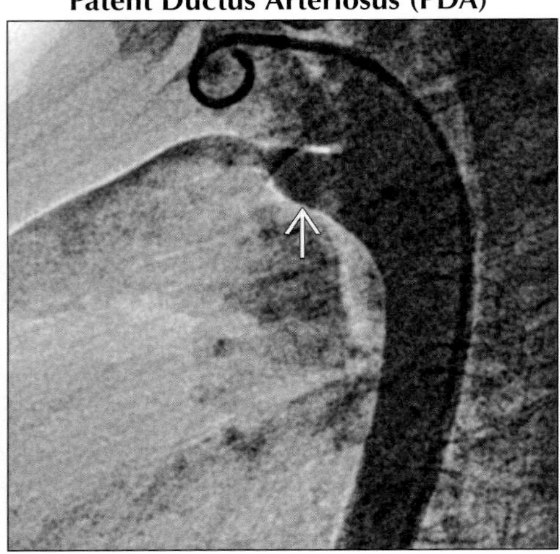

*(**Left**) Axial CECT shows a vascular connection between the main pulmonary artery and the descending aorta. A PDA is essential for normal fetal circulation but normally closes spontaneously after birth. (**Right**) Coronal CECT shows a patent ductus arteriosus between the main pulmonary artery and the descending aorta. Although most PDAs are sporadic, they can be associated with Down, Holt-Oram, and Carpenter syndromes.*

Patent Ductus Arteriosus (PDA)

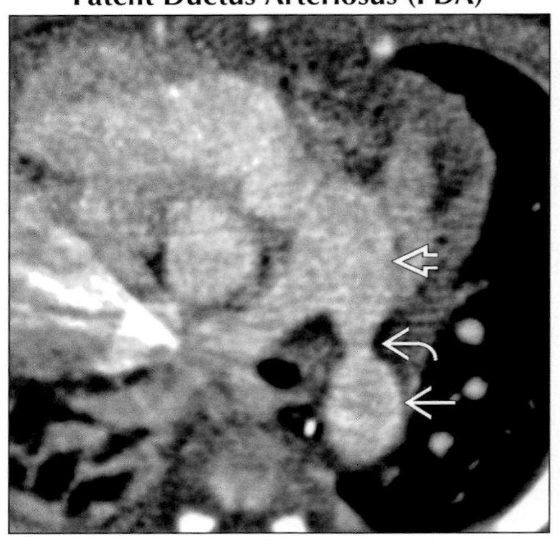

Patent Ductus Arteriosus (PDA)

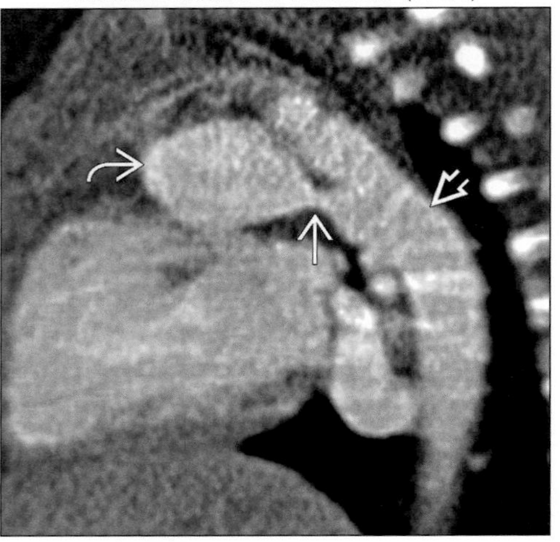

*(**Left**) AP radiograph shows cardiomegaly and pulmonary edema. Heart failure is the inability of the heart to pump sufficient blood to the organs. Congenital heart defects are the most common cause of heart failure in children younger than 1 year. (**Right**) AP radiograph shows marked enlargement of the heart. The bronchi are splayed, a sign of left atrial enlargement. Patients with dilated cardiomyopathy often present with heart failure.*

Heart Failure

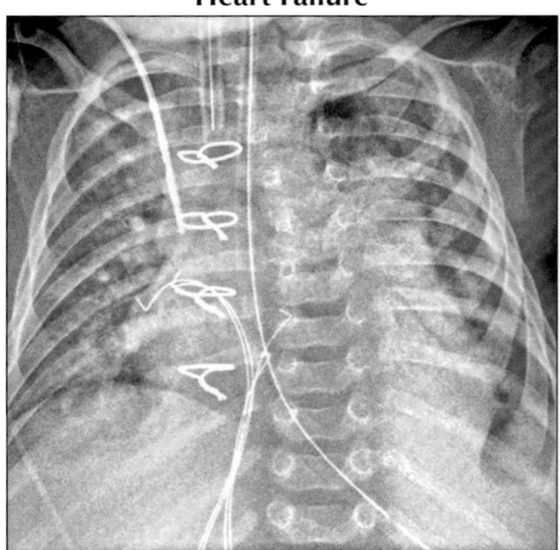

Dilated Cardiomyopathy

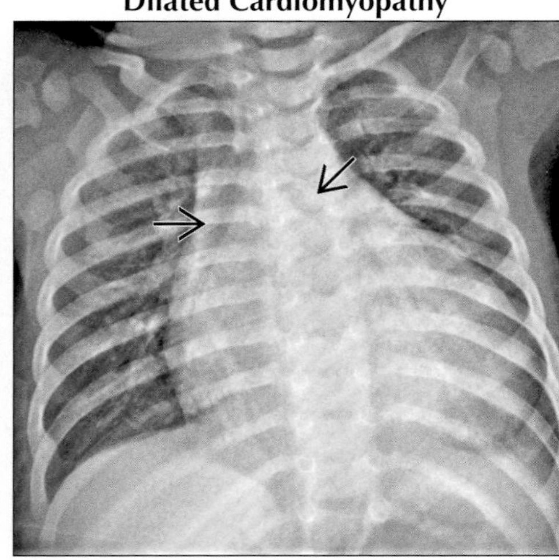

Dilated Cardiomyopathy

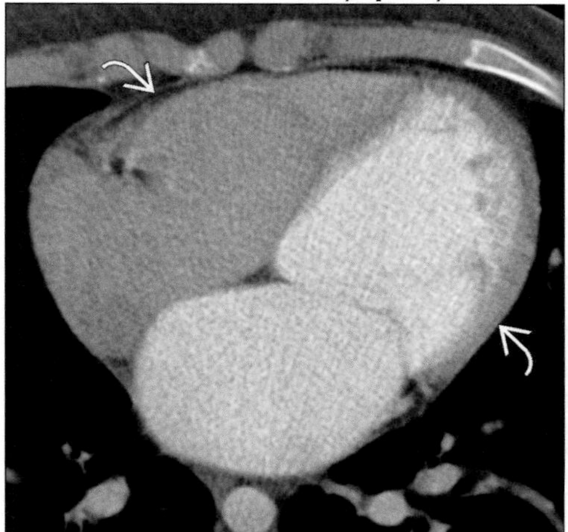

Dilated Cardiomyopathy

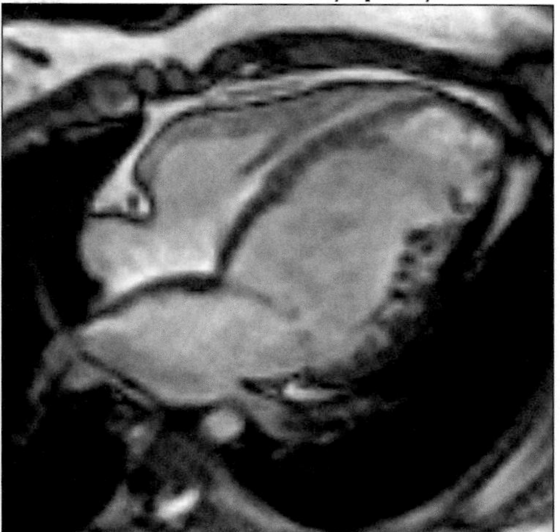

(Left) *Axial CECT shows marked enlargement of all 4 chambers. The cardiac walls are thinned ➡. Dilated cardiomyopathy is characterized by enlarged ventricles and decreased contractility.* ***(Right)*** *Four chamber view from a cardiac MR shows enlargement of all 4 chambers of the heart. While dilated cardiomyopathy is usually idiopathic, potential etiologies include viral myocarditis, congenital heart defects, and metabolic disorders.*

Hypertrophic Obstructive Cardiomyopathy

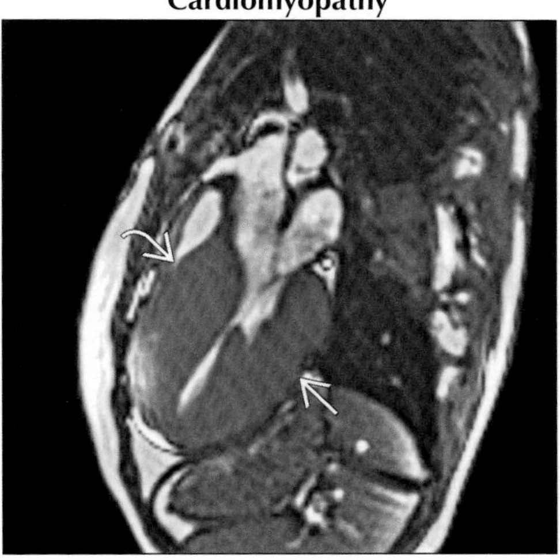

Hypertrophic Obstructive Cardiomyopathy

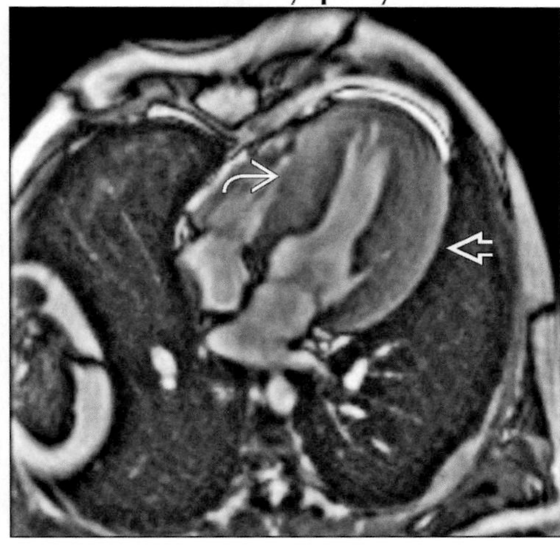

(Left) *LVOT view of a cardiac MR shows marked thickening of the left ventricular wall ➡ and intraventricular septum ➡. This is the most common hereditary cardiac disorder.* ***(Right)*** *Four chamber view from a cardiac MR shows thickening of the left ventricular wall ➡ with asymmetric septal hypertrophy ➡. Asymmetric septal hypertrophy can lead to left ventricular outflow tract obstruction and sudden death.*

Mitral Valve Stenosis

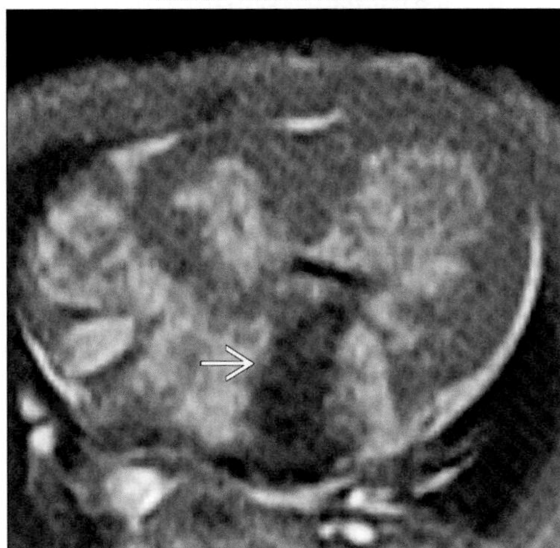

Mitral Valve Regurgitation

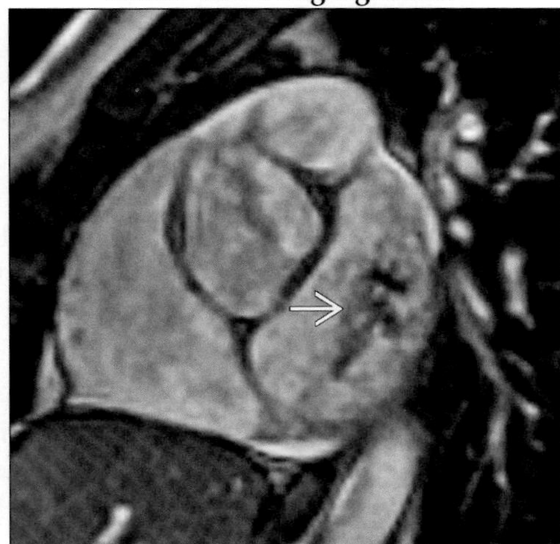

(Left) *Four chamber view from a cardiac MR in a patient with a complex congenital heart defect shows a large regurgitant jet ➡ in an enlarged left atrium.* ***(Right)*** *Oblique short axis view from a cardiac MR shows a regurgitant jet of turbulent flow ➡ in an enlarged left atrium. Mitral regurgitation is the most common valvular disease in the USA, and its prevalence increases with age.*

DIFFERENTIAL DIAGNOSIS

Common
- Marfan Syndrome
- Turner Syndrome
- Aortic Stenosis

Less Common
- Takayasu Arteritis
- Neurofibromatosis Type 1 (NF1)
- Ehlers-Danlos Syndrome

Rare but Important
- Trauma
- Loeys-Dietz Syndrome
- Tuberous Sclerosis
- Mycotic Aneurysm

ESSENTIAL INFORMATION

Key Differential Diagnosis Issues
- Dilated aorta often caused by aortic aneurysm
  - Causes of aortic aneurysm: Connective tissue disorders, vasculitis, trauma, or infection

Helpful Clues for Common Diagnoses
- **Marfan Syndrome**
  - Autosomal dominant connective tissue disorder
  - Characteristic features: Dural ectasia, bullae and pneumothorax, arachnodactyly, ectopia lentis, and retinal detachment
  - Affects multiple systems, including cardiovascular, musculoskeletal, central nervous, pulmonary, and ocular
    - Cardiovascular manifestations: Aortic annulus ectasia, aortic aneurysm, aortic valve insufficiency, aortic dissection
    - Death caused by aortic dissection, congestive heart failure, or valvular disease in > 90%
  - Dilated aortic root seen in 60-80% of adults and leads to aortic insufficiency
    - Prophylactic surgery: When diameter of sinus of Valsalva is > 5 cm
  - Musculoskeletal deformities include pectus excavatum, pectus carinatum, or scoliosis
- **Turner Syndrome**
  - Monosomy of X chromosome (45 XO)
  - Characteristic features include short stature, webbed neck, lymphedema, short 4th metacarpals, and gonadal insufficiency
  - Lymphatic malformation on prenatal ultrasound
  - Congenital heart defects (CHD): Bicuspid aortic valve, aortic coarctation, partial anomalous pulmonary venous return
    - Generalized dilation of aorta can occur
  - Potential complication: Aortic dissection
    - Risks for dissection: Hypertension, bicuspid aortic valve, and coarctation
- **Aortic Stenosis**
  - Can be valvular, subaortic, or supravalvular
  - Valvular aortic stenosis is most common
    - Accounts for 3-6% of CHD
    - 4x more common in males
    - ~ 20% have associated cardiac anomaly
    - Chest x-ray (CXR) can show cardiomegaly, vascular congestion, or poststenotic dilation of ascending aorta
  - Subaortic stenosis can be discrete or diffuse
    - Discrete form is caused by thin fibromuscular membrane
    - In diffuse form, stenosis extends along ventricular septum
  - Supravalvular is least common
    - Narrowing of aortic root at or above sinotubular ridge
    - Association: Pulmonary artery stenosis

Helpful Clues for Less Common Diagnoses
- **Takayasu Arteritis**
  - Chronic vasculitis of unknown etiology
  - Large vessel vasculitis affects aorta, its main branches, and pulmonary arteries
  - 3rd most common vasculitis of childhood
    - Most commonly presents between 10-20 years of age
    - 8.5x more common in females
  - Associated with tuberculosis infection
  - Pulseless arteritis is characteristic of chronic disease
  - Often leads to hypertension, congestive heart failure, or aortic regurgitation
  - CXR aorta: Undulating border, segmental calcification
    - Aortic aneurysms can occur
  - CXR pulmonary arteries: Oligemia
  - CT or MR shows thickened arterial wall with enhancement

- **Neurofibromatosis Type 1 (NF1)**
  - Autosomal dominant disorder
  - Affects 1:3,000 individuals
  - Characteristic features: Café au lait macules, benign neurofibromas, plexiform neurofibromas, and iris hamartomas
  - NF1 vasculopathy is uncommon component of NF1
    - Affects medium and large vessels
    - Aneurysms, stenoses, and arteriovenous malformations occur
    - Renal artery is most commonly affected
    - Aortic aneurysms and stenoses are common
- **Ehlers-Danlos Syndrome**
  - Ehlers-Danlos type 4 is vascular
  - Features: Acrogeria; thin, translucent skin; ecchymoses and hematoma; and arterial, digestive, and obstetric ruptures
  - Arterial complications are leading cause of death
    - Complications most common in medium and large vessels
    - Complications include arterial rupture, aneurysm, and dissection
    - Complications uncommon in childhood
  - Association: Peripheral pulmonary stenosis

Helpful Clues for Rare Diagnoses

- **Trauma**
  - Most common cause of death in children
  - Traumatic aortic injuries are uncommon
    - Iatrogenic trauma is most common cause of aortic injury in children
  - More common in teenage years
  - Associated traumatic injuries are common
- **Loeys-Dietz Syndrome**
  - Syndrome with craniofacial and vascular manifestations
  - Vascular features include arterial aneurysms and tortuosity
    - Aneurysms → rupture or dissection
  - Features of Marfan syndrome
  - 2 types distinguished by phenotype
    - Type 1: Hypertelorism, broad or bifid uvula, cleft palate, craniosynostosis
    - Type 2: No cleft palate, craniosynostosis, or hypertelorism
  - Aortic root aneurysm are common
    - Dissection occurs at smaller size and earlier age than Marfan syndrome
- **Tuberous Sclerosis**
  - Autosomal dominant disorder
  - Classic triad: Epilepsy, mental retardation, and adenoma sebaceum
  - Characterized by hamartomas of multiple organ systems
    - Cardiac rhabdomyomas and renal angiomyolipomas are most common
  - Brain findings include subcortical tubers, subependymal nodules, and segmental giant cell astrocytomas
  - Aortic aneurysms have been reported
    - Aortic aneurysms develop at early age
- **Mycotic Aneurysm**
  - Uncommon in children
  - Can occur in infants secondary to umbilical arterial line placement

Marfan Syndrome

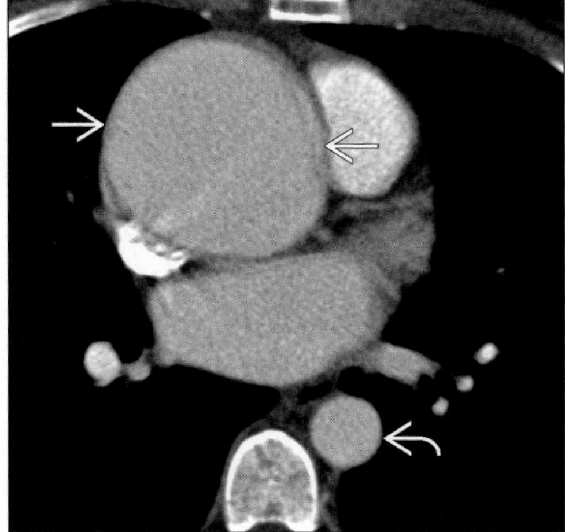

Axial CECT shows a markedly dilated aortic root ➡. The descending aortic arch has a normal caliber ↩. Marfan syndrome is characterized by arachnodactyly and ocular lens dislocation.

Marfan Syndrome

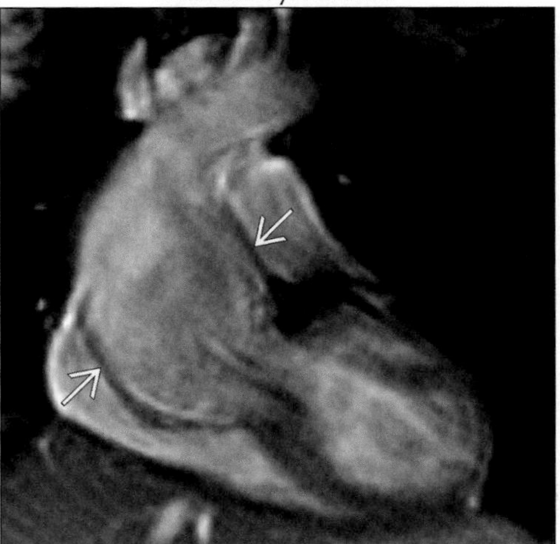

Oblique sagittal from a cardiac MR shows marked dilation of the aortic root ➡. Marfan syndrome is an autosomal dominant disorder. The most common cause of death is aortic dissection.

DILATED AORTA

Turner Syndrome

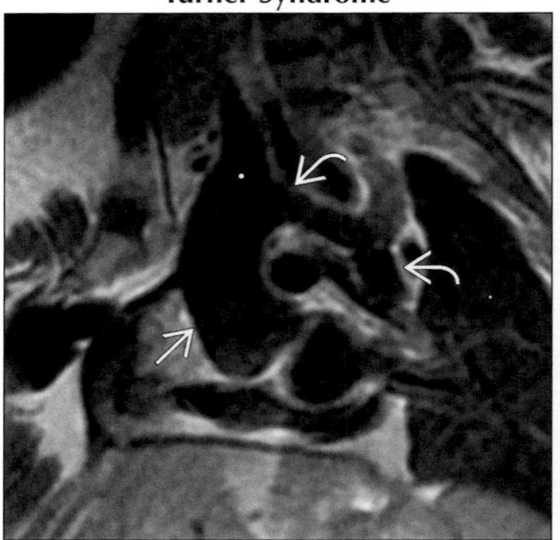

Turner Syndrome

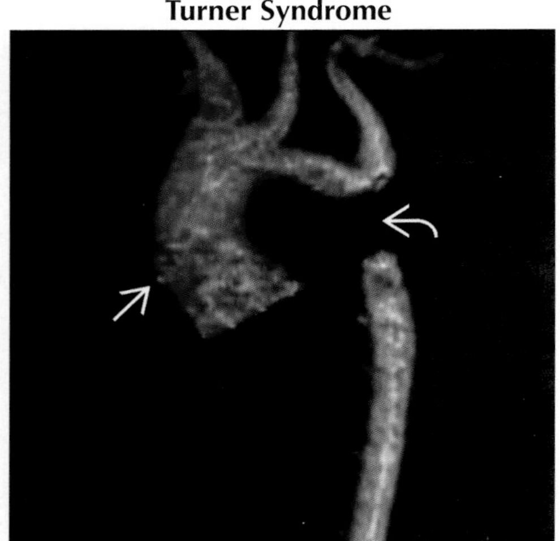

*(**Left**) Oblique sagittal from a cardiac MR shows mild dilation of the ascending aorta ➡ and stenosis of a long segment of the aortic arch ➡. Bicuspid aortic valve, aortic coarctation, and aortic dissection are the most common cardiovascular anomalies in Turner syndrome. (**Right**) 3D reconstruction shows mild dilation of the ascending aorta ➡ and a focal defect ➡ (stent repair for coarctation) in the descending aorta.*

Turner Syndrome

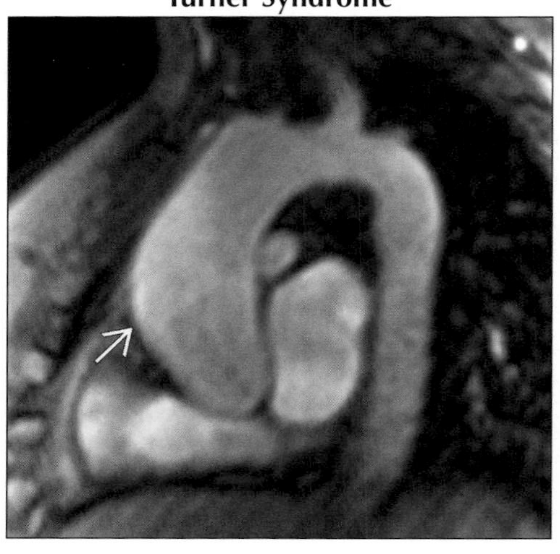

Aortic Stenosis

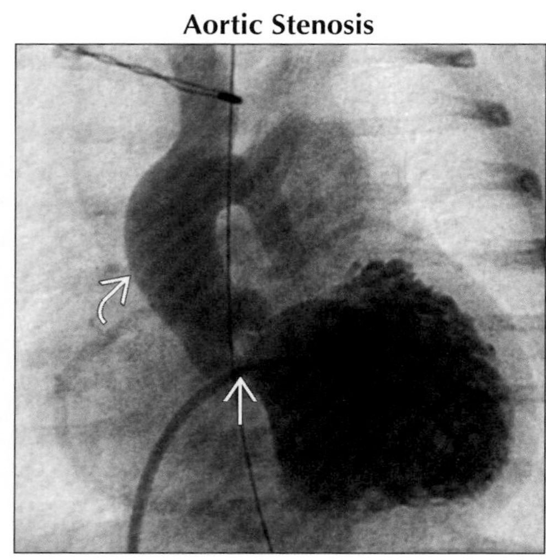

*(**Left**) Oblique sagittal cardiac MR shows moderate dilation of the ascending aorta ➡. Aortic dissection is a major risk in Turner syndrome due to hypertension, bicuspid aortic valve, and coarctation. (**Right**) Left anterior oblique view of a cardiac catheterization shows narrowing of the aortic valve ➡ and mild to moderate poststenotic dilation of the ascending aorta ➡. Valvular aortic stenosis is the most common type of aortic stenosis.*

Takayasu Arteritis

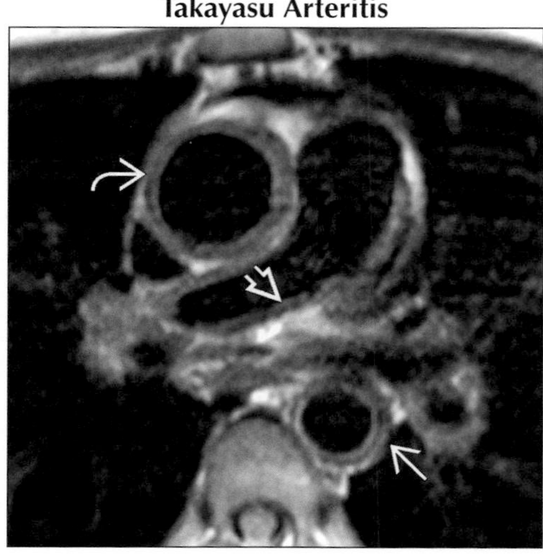

Takayasu Arteritis

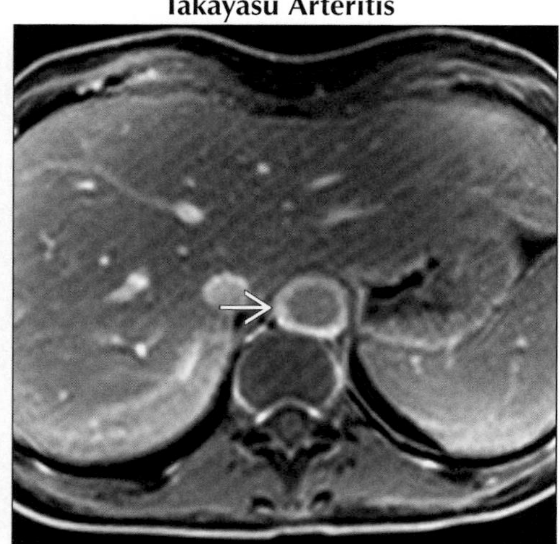

*(**Left**) Axial T1WI MR shows a thickened wall of the ascending ➡ and descending ➡ aorta as well as of the right main pulmonary artery ➡. The ascending aorta is moderately dilated. Takayasu arteritis is a chronic vasculitis of unknown etiology. (**Right**) Axial T1WI C+ FS MR shows an enhancing, thickened wall of the descending aorta ➡. Takayasu arteritis is a vasculitis of large vessels, such as the aorta, its branches, and the pulmonary arteries.*

Ehlers-Danlos Syndrome

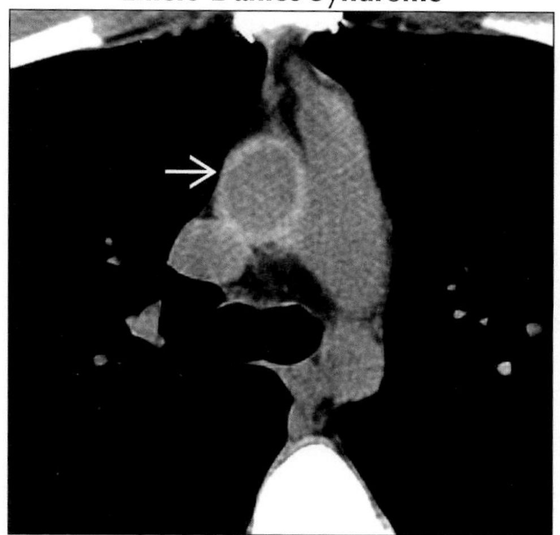

Trauma

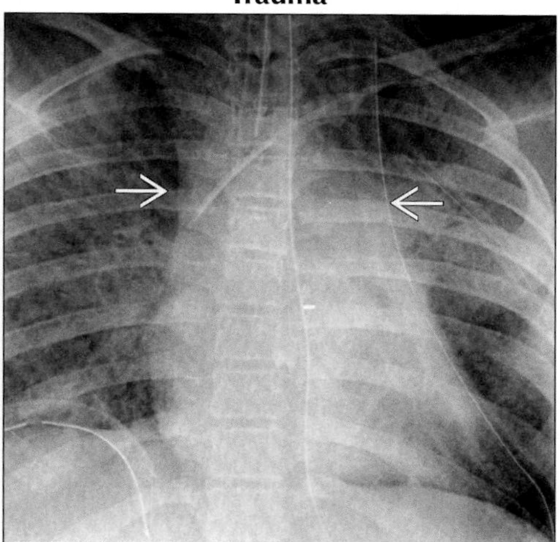

(Left) *Axial NECT shows hyperdensity and thickening of the wall of the ascending aorta ➡. The hyperdensity was thought to be due to mural thrombus in this patient with Ehlers-Danlos. Type 4 Ehlers-Danlos is the vascular type and is associated with aneurysm, dissection, and arterial rupture.* ***(Right)*** *AP radiograph of the chest shows a widened mediastinum ➡ along with pulmonary edema. Trauma is the most common cause of death in children.*

Trauma

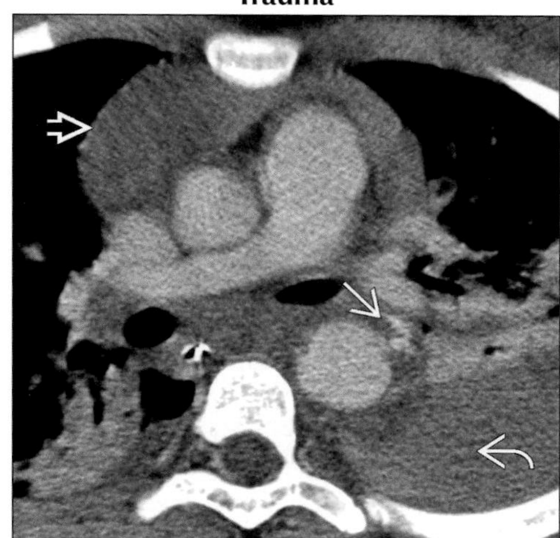

Trauma

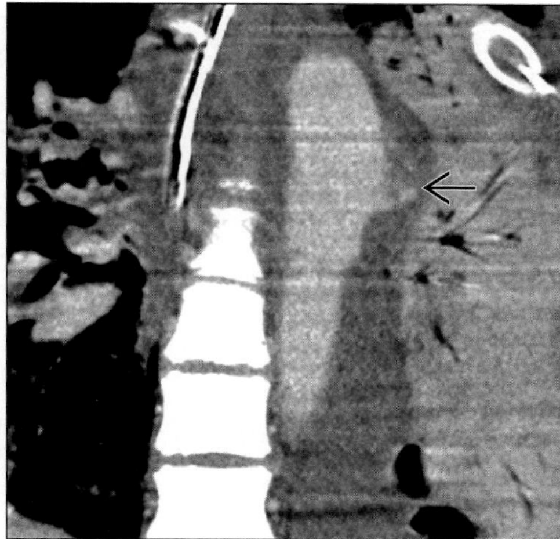

(Left) *Axial CECT shows a focal aortic transection with active extravasation of contrast ➡. Additional findings include a mediastinal hematoma ➡ and left hemothorax ➡. Traumatic aortic injuries are uncommon in children. When they do occur, they are more common in the teenage years.* ***(Right)*** *Coronal CECT in the same patient shows irregularity and extravasation ➡ from the descending aorta.*

Loeys-Dietz Syndrome

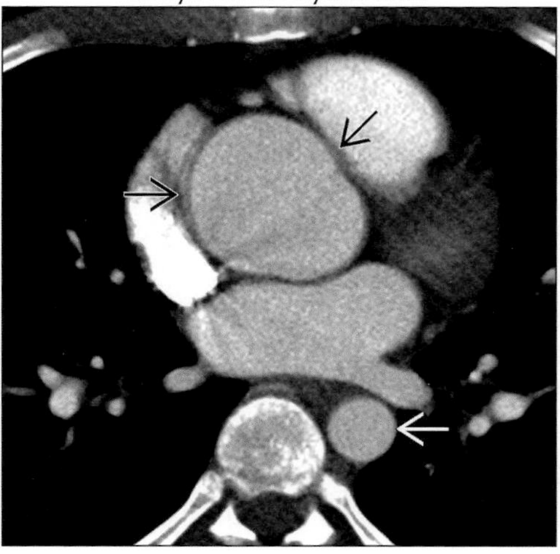

Loeys-Dietz Syndrome

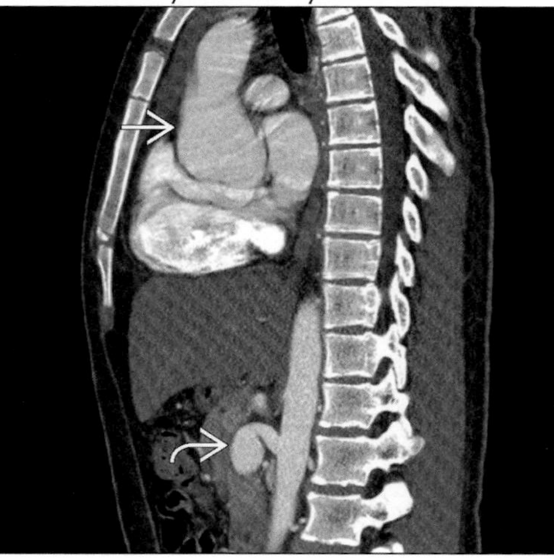

(Left) *Axial CECT shows marked dilation of the ascending aorta ➡. The descending aorta has a normal caliber ➡. Loeys-Dietz syndrome has craniofacial and vascular anomalies. Characteristic vascular malformations include arterial aneurysms and tortuosity.* ***(Right)*** *Sagittal CECT shows a markedly dilated ascending aorta ➡ and aneurysm and tortuosity of the superior mesenteric artery ➡.*

CONGENITAL AORTIC ANOMALIES

DIFFERENTIAL DIAGNOSIS

Common
- Left Aortic Arch with Aberrant Right Subclavian Artery
- Aortic Coarctation
- Double Aortic Arch

Less Common
- Right Aortic Arch with Aberrant Left Subclavian Artery
- Right Aortic Arch with Mirror-Image Branching

Rare but Important
- Interrupted Aortic Arch
- Cervical Aortic Arch
- Persistent 5th Aortic Arch
- Pulmonary Sling

ESSENTIAL INFORMATION

Helpful Clues for Common Diagnoses
- **Left Aortic Arch with Aberrant Right Subclavian Artery**
  - Right subclavian artery has separate origin as last vessel from arch or proximal descending aorta
  - No diverticulum at origin of aberrant right subclavian artery
  - Patients usually asymptomatic as no vascular ring is present
  - Radiograph may show left aortic arch and impression on posterior wall of trachea
  - Esophagram, AP view
    - Impression on left side of barium column, which continues obliquely superiorly and to right
  - Esophagram, lateral view
    - Posterior indentation on barium column on lateral view
  - CT and MR will show aberrant right subclavian artery coursing posterior to esophagus and superiorly to right
- **Aortic Coarctation**
  - Focal narrowing of upper thoracic aorta at level of insertion of ductus arteriosus
    - Less commonly long segment or may be associated with diffuse tubular hypoplasia of aortic arch and isthmus
  - Cardiomegaly and increased pulmonary vascularity with edema may be present in infants
  - "3" sign may be present
  - Notching of undersurface of ribs may develop in longstanding severe cases
  - Collateral flow best identified by CTA and MRA; can be quantified by MR
- **Double Aortic Arch**
  - Both limbs usually complete, but 1 side may be atretic (30%)
    - Atretic limb remains in fibrous continuity with descending aorta
  - Although variable, right limb is usually larger (dominant) and higher in position than left
  - Most commonly: Left arch anterior and left of trachea, right arch posterior and right of esophagus
    - Limbs join posteriorly to form left-sided descending aorta
  - Symptoms usually present early
  - Radiograph may show dominant arch and compression on both sides of trachea
  - Esophagram, AP view
    - Compression on both sides of esophagus
  - Esophagram, lateral view
    - Posterior impression
  - CT and MR demonstrate relative sizes of limbs and degree of associated tracheal narrowing
  - Rarely associated with intracardiac defects

Helpful Clues for Less Common Diagnoses
- **Right Aortic Arch and Aberrant Left Subclavian Artery**
  - Left subclavian artery has separate origin
    - Last vessel from arch or proximal descending aorta
  - May be associated with diverticulum of Kommerell
  - Radiograph may show right aortic arch and impression on posterior wall of trachea
  - Esophagram, AP view
    - Impression on right side of barium column which continues obliquely superiorly to left
  - Esophagram, lateral view
    - Posterior indentation on esophagus
  - CT and MR will show aberrant left subclavian artery coursing posterior to esophagus and superiorly to left

- Vascular ring completed by left ligamentum arteriosum to left pulmonary artery
- Low association (10%) with intracardiac defects

- **Right Aortic Arch with Mirror-Image Branching**
  - 3 vessels arise from right aortic arch in following order
    - Left innominate artery coursing anterior to trachea
    - Right carotid artery
    - Right subclavian artery
  - Impression on right side of trachea and right arch are visible on frontal chest radiograph
  - Lateral chest radiograph does not show impression on posterior wall of trachea
  - Esophagram, AP view
    - Shows corresponding impression on right wall of esophagus
  - Esophagram, lateral view
    - No impression on posterior wall of esophagus
  - High association (90%) with intracardiac defects
    - Tetralogy of Fallot, truncus arteriosus, and double-outlet right ventricle most common defects

Helpful Clues for Rare Diagnoses

- **Interrupted Aortic Arch**
  - Interruption may occur at different sites along arch
    - Most common site is between origins of left carotid artery and left subclavian artery (2/3 of cases)
  - Postnatally, blood supply to lower half of body requires patent ductus arteriosus
- **Cervical Aortic Arch**
  - Arch found above level of clavicle
    - May reach level of C2 vertebra
  - Usually right arch
  - May have associated symptomatic vascular ring
- **Persistent 5th Aortic Arch**
  - Both arches appear on same side of trachea with superior-inferior relationship
  - Both arches may be patent or superior arch may be interrupted with patent inferior arch
- **Pulmonary Sling**
  - Origin of left pulmonary artery has distal origin from main pulmonary artery and courses sharply to left
  - Passes between trachea and esophagus
  - Associated with long-segment tracheal narrowing
    - Narrowing due to complete tracheal rings and anomalous tracheal branching

Left Aortic Arch with Aberrant Right Subclavian Artery

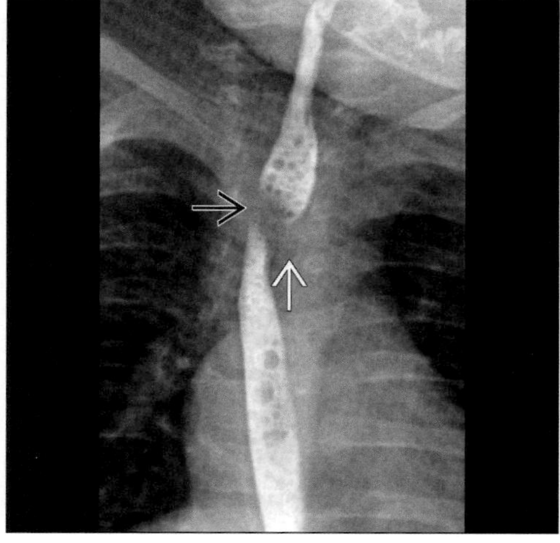

Anteroposterior esophagram shows a left aortic arch displacing the esophagus to the right ➔. There is a filling defect in the contrast column running obliquely and superiorly to the right ➔.

Left Aortic Arch with Aberrant Right Subclavian Artery

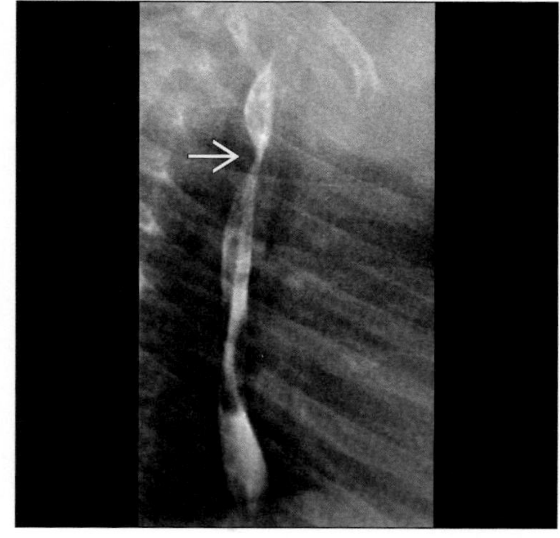

Lateral esophagram shows a posterior impression on the esophagus ➔. The findings on the AP and lateral views are consistent with a left aortic arch with an aberrant right subclavian artery.

CONGENITAL AORTIC ANOMALIES

*(**Left**) Coronal T1WI MR shows a left-sided aortic arch ➡ with an aberrant right subclavian artery ➡. Because the ligamentum arteriosum is on the left side, there is no vascular ring, and the patients are often asymptomatic. Pressure on the esophagus may cause dysphagia. (**Right**) Posterior 3D reconstruction shows the aberrant subclavian artery ➡ as the last vessel from the arch. CT and MR are replacing UGI studies for investigating vascular rings.*

Left Aortic Arch with Aberrant Right Subclavian Artery

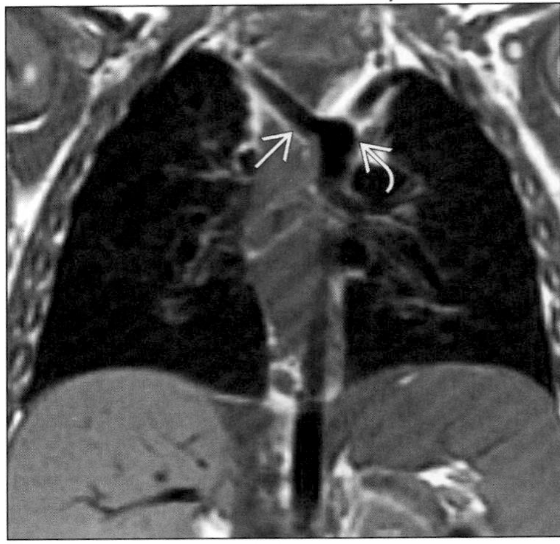

Left Aortic Arch with Aberrant Right Subclavian Artery

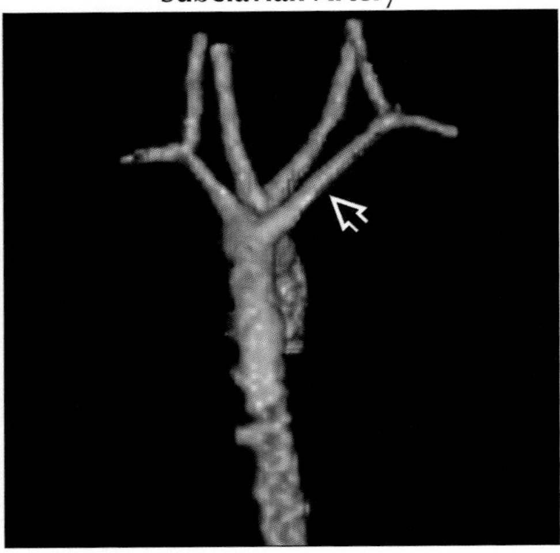

*(**Left**) PA radiograph shows the "3" sign. A superior convexity ➡ of the aortic arch is followed by the concavity of the coarctation ➡ and a lower convexity caused by poststenotic dilatation ➡. Most coarctations are corrected before radiographic signs have time to develop. (**Right**) Oblique MRA in the same patient shows the coarctation ➡ with poststenotic dilatation ➡ of the proximal descending aorta.*

Aortic Coarctation

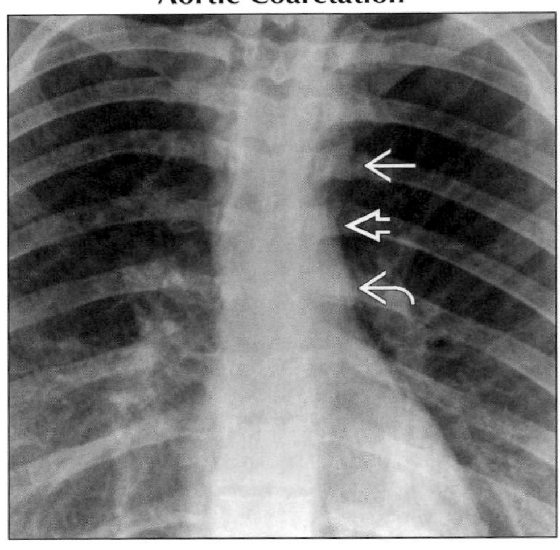

Aortic Coarctation

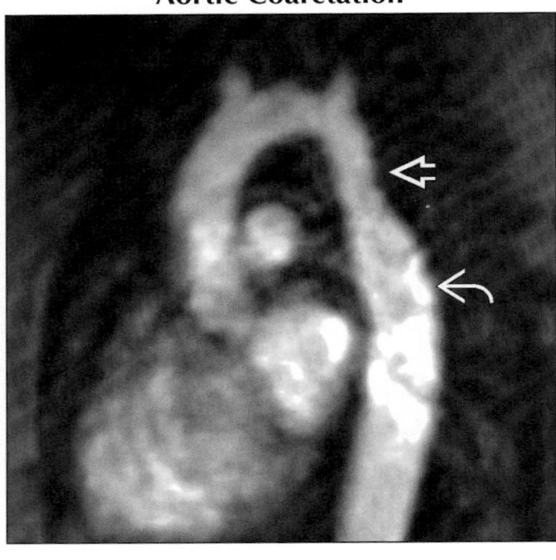

*(**Left**) Sagittal T1WI MR shows focal narrowing of the aorta ➡ with mild poststenotic dilatation ➡. The left subclavian artery is dilated ➡ as it contains collateral blood. (**Right**) Sagittal MRA shows the focal narrowing ➡ of the proximal descending aorta. Multiple prominent intercostal arteries ➡ are seen returning collateral blood flow. Phase-contrast MR imaging can be used to quantify the amount of flow that is diverted around the obstruction.*

Aortic Coarctation

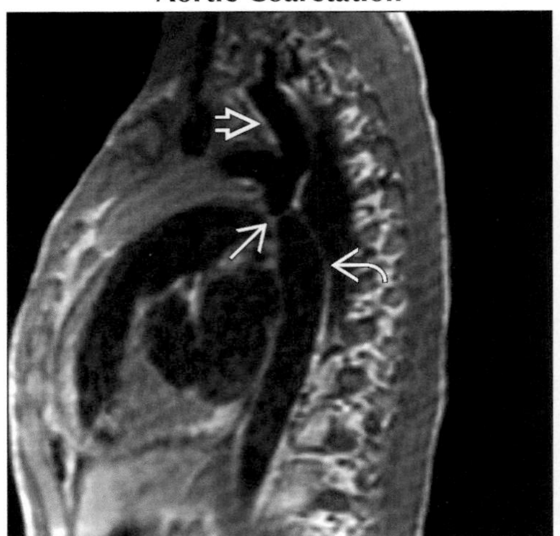

Aortic Coarctation

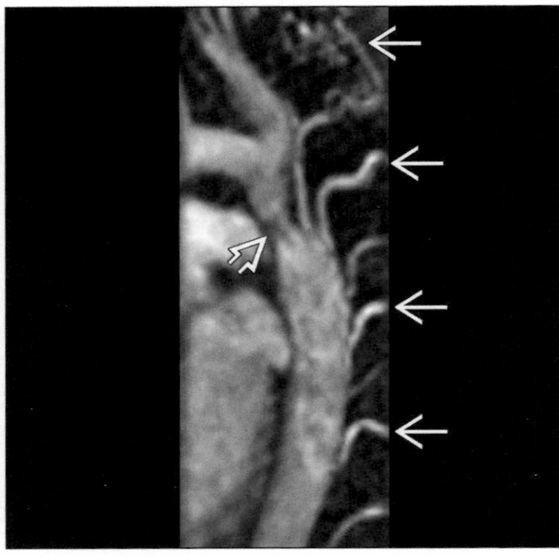

Double Aortic Arch

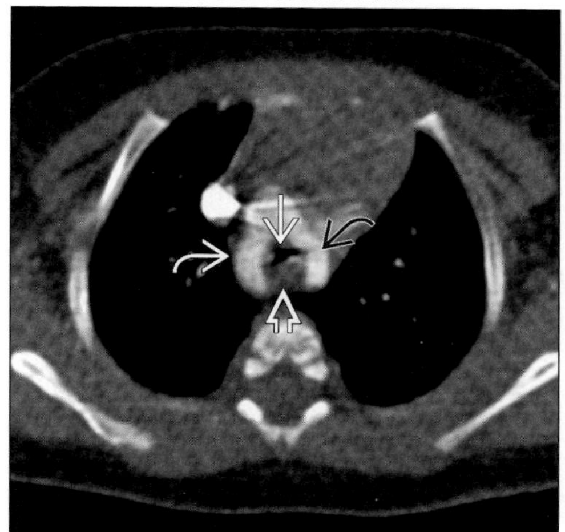

Double Aortic Arch

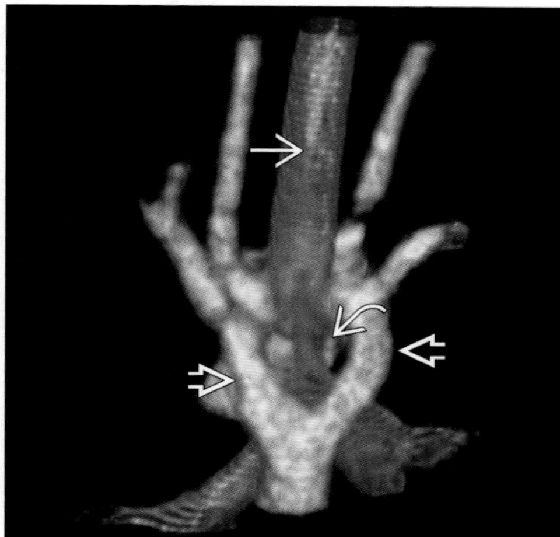

(Left) *Axial CECT shows the larger (dominant) right aortic arch and a smaller left arch encircling a narrowed trachea and esophagus.* ***(Right)*** *Coronal 3D reconstruction shows the double aortic arch encircling the trachea. Note the caliber change of the trachea as it passes through the vascular ring. The tightness of this ring determines the severity of symptoms and how early in life these symptoms appear.*

Double Aortic Arch

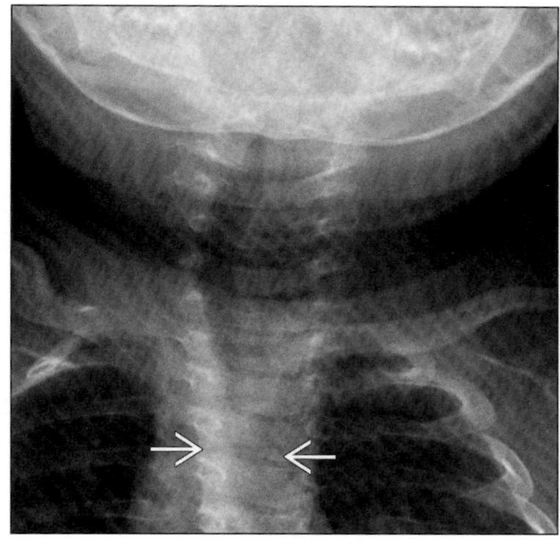

Double Aortic Arch

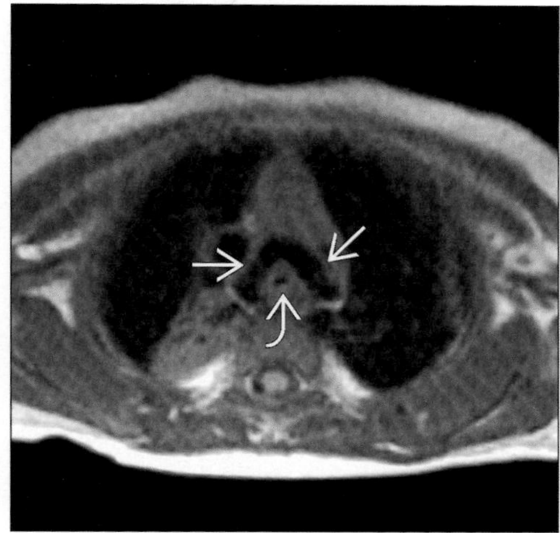

(Left) *Anteroposterior radiograph shows a straight distal trachea with loss of definition of the tracheal walls. The walls of the trachea should be well defined, and the distal trachea deviated slightly to the right side. An aortic anomaly should be excluded in any young child with recurrent respiratory symptoms.* ***(Right)*** *Axial T1WI MR in the same patient shows the dual limbs of the double aortic arch as it encircles a narrowed trachea.*

Right Aortic Arch with Aberrant Left Subclavian Artery

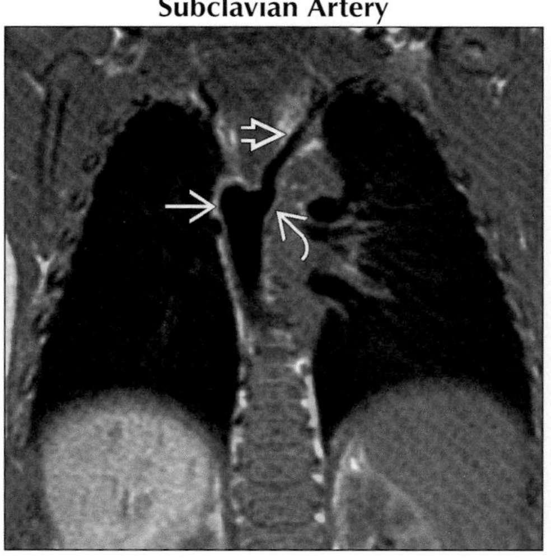

Right Aortic Arch with Aberrant Left Subclavian Artery

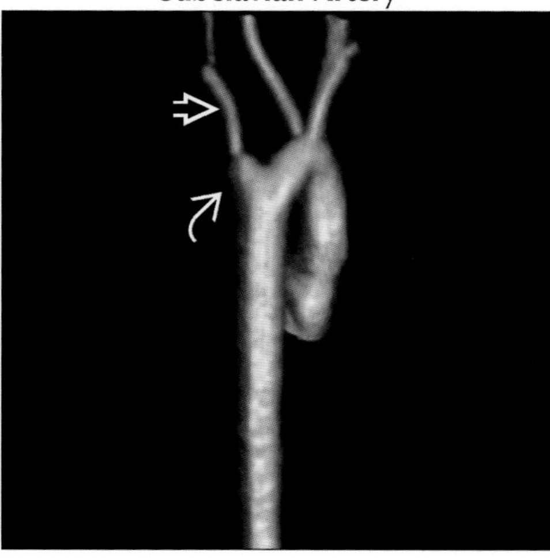

(Left) *Coronal T1WI MR shows a right-sided aortic arch with an aberrant left subclavian artery arising from the diverticulum of Kommerell.* ***(Right)*** *Posterior 3D reconstruction shows the prominent diverticulum giving rise to the aberrant left subclavian artery. A vascular ring is completed by a ligamentum arteriosum. The diverticulum itself also contributes to the symptoms.*

CONGENITAL AORTIC ANOMALIES

(Left) Axial T1WI MR shows a right-sided aortic arch ➡ and a prominent diverticulum of Kommerell ➡, which passes posterior to the trachea ➡. (Right) Sagittal T1WI MR shows a prominent diverticulum of Kommerell ➡ passing posterior to the trachea ➡. In this instance, there is a significant change in the caliber of the trachea as it passes anterior to the diverticulum.

Right Aortic Arch with Aberrant Left Subclavian Artery

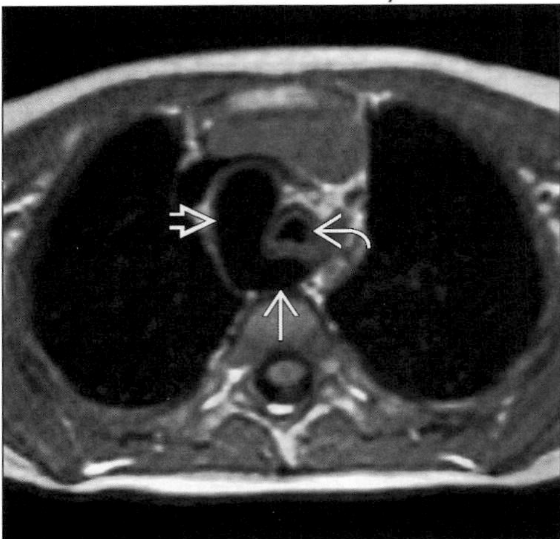

Right Aortic Arch with Aberrant Left Subclavian Artery

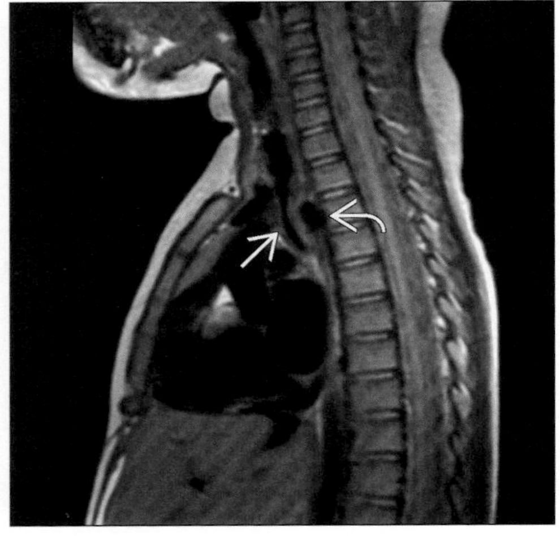

(Left) Posteroanterior radiograph shows a right arch ➡ displacing the trachea ➡ to the left. Note the evidence of prior surgery. There is a high correlation of mirror-image branching with congenital heart disease. (Right) Frontal 3D reconstruction shows the arch ➡ passing to the right of the trachea ➡ with the branches from the aorta arising as follows: Left innominate artery ➡, right common carotid artery ➡, and right subclavian artery ➡.

Right Aortic Arch with Mirror-Image Branching

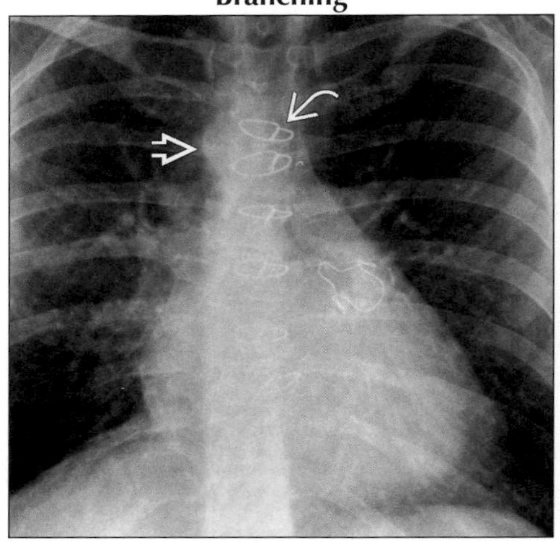

Right Aortic Arch with Mirror-Image Branching

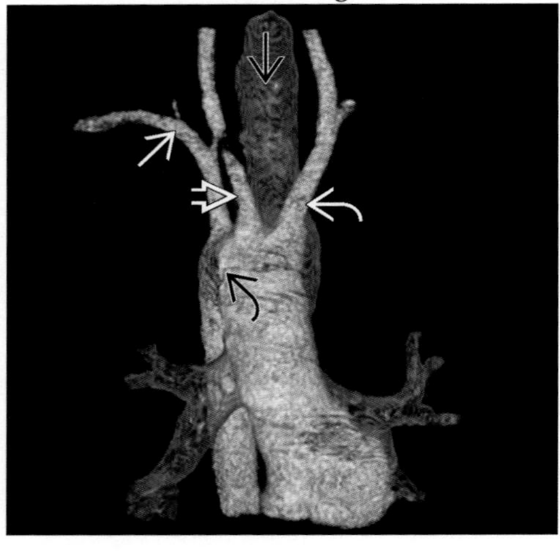

(Left) Oblique 3D reconstruction shows interruption of the aortic arch distal to the origin of the left carotid artery ➡, the most common site of an interruption. There is a large ductus arteriosus ➡ connecting the main pulmonary artery ➡ to the descending aorta ➡. (Right) Oblique 3D reconstruction shows the right and left pulmonary arteries ➡ arising from the main PA ➡ and the left subclavian artery ➡ arising from the residual distal arch.

Interrupted Aortic Arch

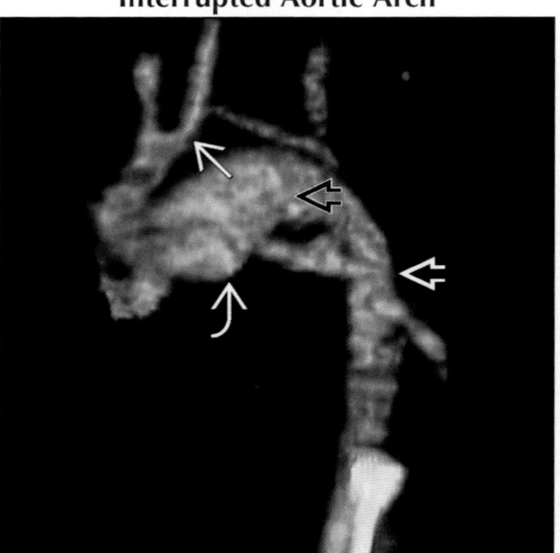

Interrupted Aortic Arch

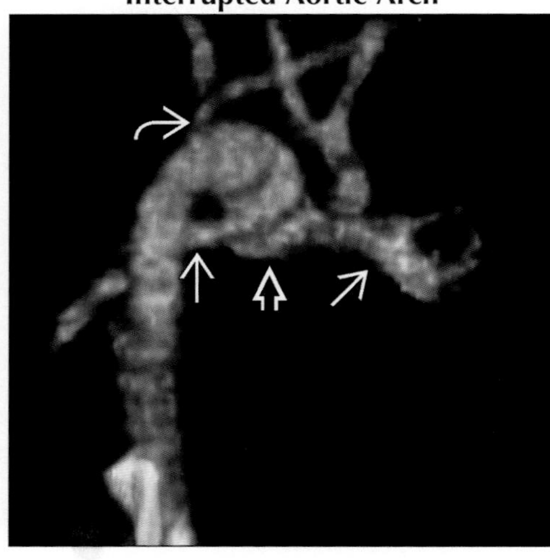

CONGENITAL AORTIC ANOMALIES

Cervical Aortic Arch

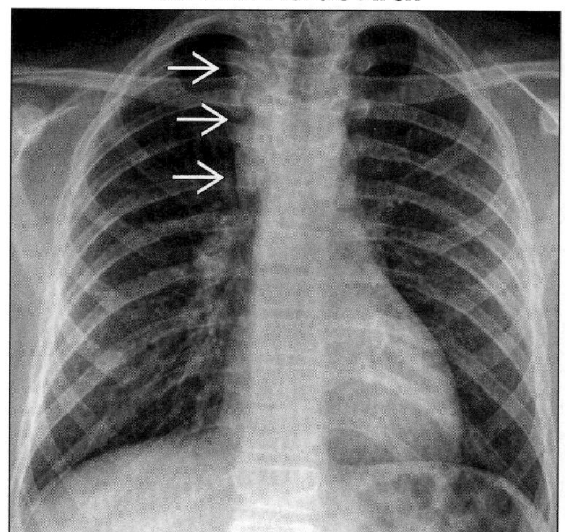

Cervical Aortic Arch

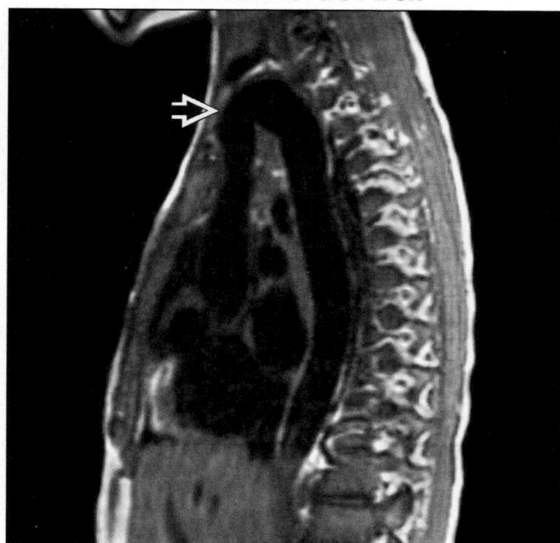

(Left) *Posteroanterior radiograph shows a soft tissue density extending above the level of the clavicle into the superior mediastinum ➔ on the right. A cervical arch is more often right-sided and is then usually associated with a contralateral descending aorta.* ***(Right)*** *Sagittal T1WI MR shows the arch ➔ extending superiorly into the base of the neck. Although a vascular ring may be present, only approximately 50% of such patients are symptomatic.*

Persistent 5th Aortic Arch

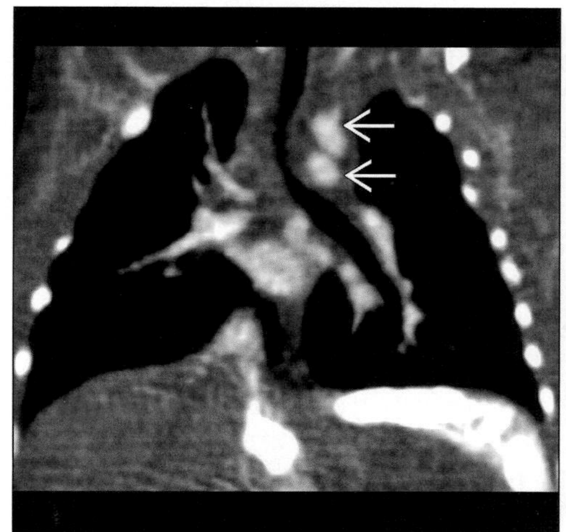

Persistent 5th Aortic Arch

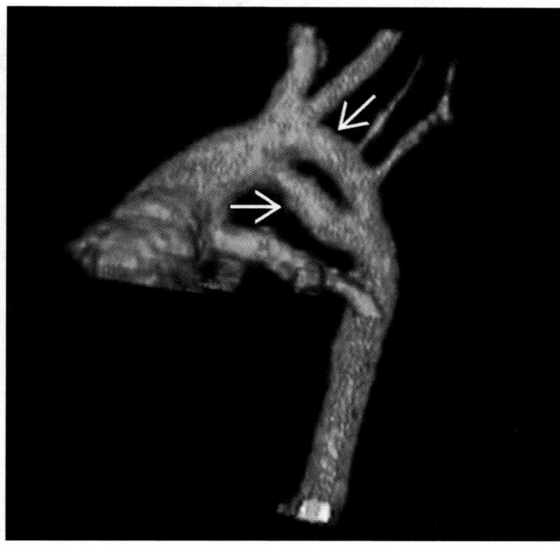

(Left) *Coronal CECT shows 2 arches to the left of the trachea, which have a superior-inferior relationship ➔.* ***(Right)*** *Oblique 3D reconstruction shows 2 patent arches ➔. Less commonly the superior arch may be interrupted, in which case a common trunk gives rise to the origin of all 4 brachiocephalic vessels. Although it can be an incidental finding, a persistent 5th arch is frequently associated with intracardiac anomalies.*

Pulmonary Sling

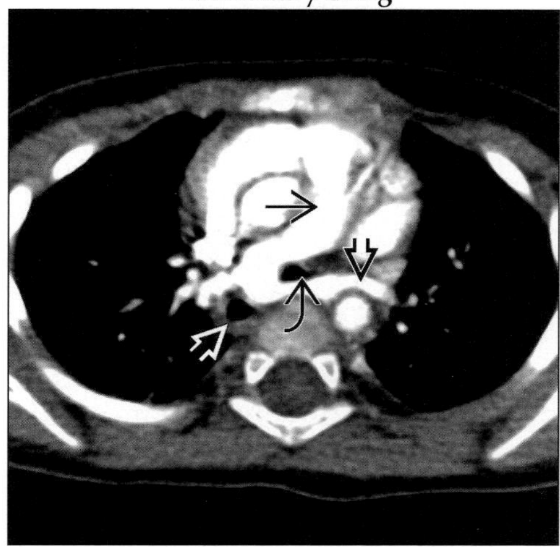

Pulmonary Sling

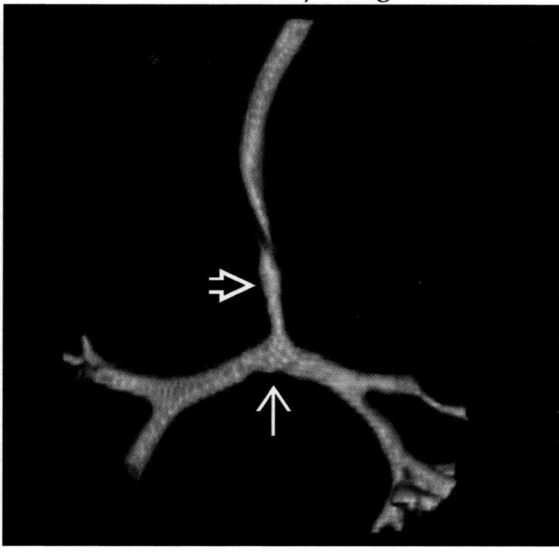

(Left) *Axial CECT shows the left main pulmonary artery ➔ arising from the distal portion of the main pulmonary artery ➔, looping to pass between the trachea ➔ and the displaced esophagus ➔.* ***(Right)*** *Frontal 3D reconstruction shows long-segment narrowing of the trachea ➔, which also appears round, suggesting complete tracheal rings. The carina has an inverted "T" appearance ➔, a common finding in patients with a pulmonary arterial sling.*

LEFT HEART OBSTRUCTIVE LESION

DIFFERENTIAL DIAGNOSIS

Common
- Aortic Coarctation
- Hypoplastic Left Heart
- Aortic Stenosis

Less Common
- Interrupted Aortic Arch
- Hypertropic Obstructive Cardiomyopathy
- Mitral Valve Stenosis

Rare but Important
- Cardiac Rhabdomyomas
- Pseudocoarctation
- Shone Complex
- Cor Triatriatum

ESSENTIAL INFORMATION

Key Differential Diagnosis Issues
- Left ventricular outflow tract obstruction (LVOTO) is common congenital abnormality
  - Multiple anomalies can cause LVOTO
- Causative lesion often at level of aortic valve, mitral valve, aorta, or left ventricle
- Presentation depends on severity of lesion
  - Critical LVOTO presents as ductus arteriosus begins to close
    - ↓ systemic and coronary perfusion, acidosis, end-organ injury, and shock
    - Prostaglandins help keep ductus open
  - Less severe LVOTO presents later
    - Failure to thrive, tachypnea, pulmonary vascular congestion

Helpful Clues for Common Diagnoses
- **Aortic Coarctation**
  - Stenosis in proximal descending aorta
    - Usually just beyond origin of left subclavian artery
    - Stenosis may be discrete or long
  - 5-8% of congenital heart defects (CHD)
  - 2x more common in males
  - Associations: Turner syndrome, bicuspid aortic valve, ventricular septal defect (VSD)
  - Severe coarct presents when ductus closes
  - Mild coarct presents with upper extremity hypertension and ↓ lower extremity pulses
  - Hypertension is major cause of long-term morbidity
    - If uncorrected, ~ 90% die by age 60
  - Rib notching not usually seen on chest x-ray (CXR) until after age 6
  - Treatment options: Surgical repair, angioplasty, or stent placement
- **Hypoplastic Left Heart**
  - Abnormal development of left heart leading to LVOTO
    - Usually includes hypoplasia of left ventricle (LV), aorta, and aortic arch, as well as atresia of aortic and mitral valves
    - LV does not extend to cardiac apex
  - Accounts for up to 3.8% of CHD
    - 70% occur in males
  - Systemic blood flow is dependent on patent ductus arteriosus (PDA)
  - Atrial septal defect (ASD) is required
    - Left-to-right shunt decompresses pulmonary circulation
  - CXR with cardiomegaly and ↑ vascularity
  - Can be diagnosed in utero
  - 2 major surgical treatment options: Transplant or staged palliation
    - Staged palliation: Norwood procedure (near birth), bidirectional Glenn (6-8 months), and Fontan (18-48 months)
- **Aortic Stenosis**
  - Can be valvular, subaortic, or supravalvular
  - Valvular aortic stenosis is most common
    - Accounts for 3-6% of CHD
    - 4x more common in males
    - ~ 20% have associated cardiac anomaly
    - Severity related to degree of obstruction
    - 10-15% present before age 1
    - Infants can present with congestive heart failure and cardiogenic shock
    - Patients > 1 year are often asymptomatic
    - Older children can present with early fatigue, chest pain, syncope, or systolic ejection murmur
    - CXR can be normal or show cardiomegaly, vascular congestion, and poststenotic dilation of ascending aorta
    - Treatment: Surgery or catheterization
  - Subaortic stenosis can be discrete or diffuse
    - Discrete form is caused by thin fibromuscular membrane
    - Membrane arises from ventricular septum and extends to mitral valve
    - Other cardiac anomalies in ~ 30% of patients

- Discrete form is due to abnormal shear forces during contraction
- Diffuse form is less frequent
- In diffuse form, stenosis extends along ventricular septum
  - Supravalvular is least common (< 10%)
    - Narrowing of aortic root at or above sinotubular ridge
    - Frequently seen in Williams syndrome
    - Association: Pulmonary artery stenosis

Helpful Clues for Less Common Diagnoses

- **Interrupted Aortic Arch**
  - Discontinuity of aorta
  - Accounts for 1% of CHD
  - Associations: DiGeorge syndrome and 22q11 deletion
  - 3 types: Isolated, simple, and complex
    - Isolated: No other cardiac anomalies
    - Simple: Associated with VSD and PDA
    - Complex: Associated with complex CHD
- **Hypertropic Obstructive Cardiomyopathy**
  - Most common hereditary cardiac disorder
  - Asymmetric septal hypertrophy → LVOTO
  - Can present with sudden death
- **Mitral Valve Stenosis**
  - If acquired, due to rheumatic heart disease
    - Mitral valve affected in 65-70% of rheumatic fever
    - Rheumatic fever is uncommon in developing countries
  - Echocardiogram used to determine severity and identify left atrial thrombus

Helpful Clues for Rare Diagnoses

- **Cardiac Rhabdomyomas**
  - Most common pediatric heart tumor
  - Most common cardiac tumor diagnosed prenatally
  - 80% of patients have tuberous sclerosis
  - Usually intraventricular
  - Echogenic on echocardiogram
  - Natural history of spontaneous regression
- **Pseudocoarctation**
  - Elongation and kinking of aortic arch and narrowing of aortic isthmus
  - Elongation leads to ↑ distance between left common carotid and left subclavian
  - CXR with superior mediastinal mass
- **Shone Complex**
  - Multiple levels of left heart obstruction
  - Initial description had 4 anomalies
    - Supraannular mitral ring, subaortic stenosis, parachute mitral valve, and aortic coarctation
    - Other anomalies include valvular mitral or aortic stenosis, supravalvular aortic stenosis, or interrupted aortic arch
  - Presentation reflects level of dominant obstructive lesion
- **Cor Triatriatum**
  - Accounts for 0.1-0.4% of CHD
  - Left atrium divided by fibromuscular membrane
  - Associated with ASD
  - Can cause pulmonary venous congestion

Aortic Coarctation

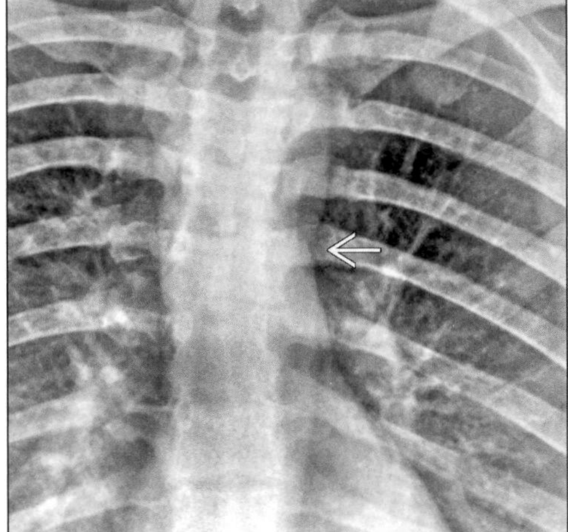

PA radiograph of the chest shows the undulating contour of the proximal descending aorta ➡. The coarctation is usually in the proximal descending aorta just distal to the left subclavian artery.

Aortic Coarctation

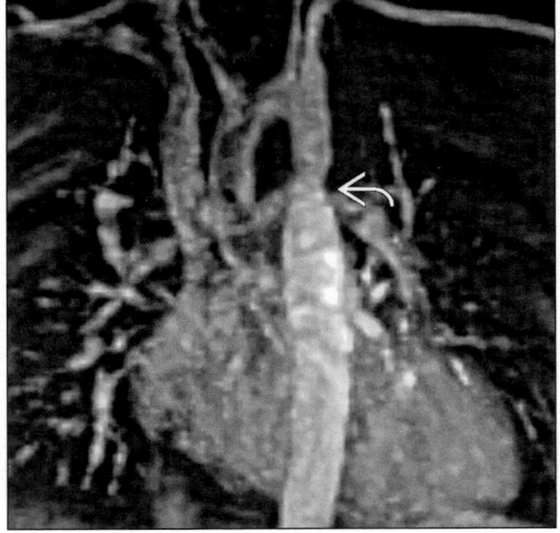

Coronal MIP of T1 C+ subtraction MR in the same patient shows coarctation in the proximal descending aorta ➡. The length of stenosis in coarctation can be focal or long.

LEFT HEART OBSTRUCTIVE LESION

*(**Left**) PA radiograph of the chest shows notching in the 3rd-5th ribs on the left ➔. Rib notching, not seen until at least age 6, is caused by dilated intercostal arteries that act as collateral vessels to bypass a coarctation. (**Right**) Oblique MIP of T1 C+ subtraction MR shows severe coarctation of the aorta with a "string" sign of the severely stenotic segment ➔. Severe coarctations present when the ductus arteriosus closes.*

Aortic Coarctation

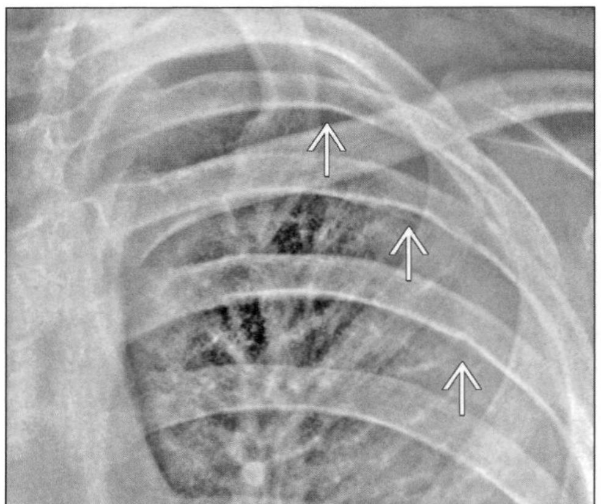

Aortic Coarctation

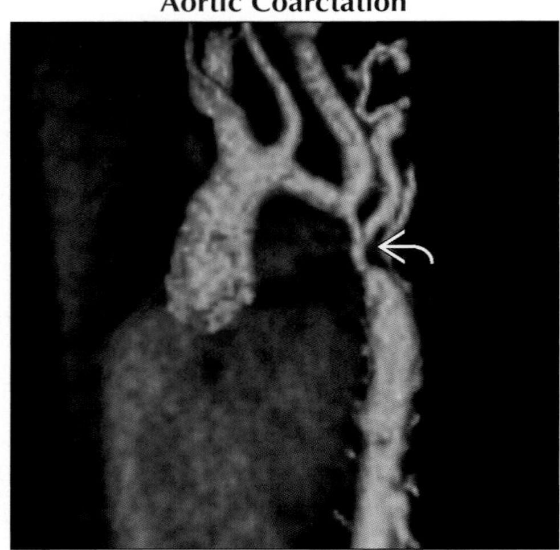

*(**Left**) AP radiograph of the chest shows a normal-sized heart and a diffuse hazy opacity of the lungs representing pulmonary vascular congestion. A hypoplastic left heart can appear on a chest x-ray with cardiomegaly or as a normal-sized heart. (**Right**) Axial CECT shows significant hypoplasia of the left ventricle ➔ and an atrial septal defect ➔. The atrial septal defect is required to decompress the pulmonary circulation.*

Hypoplastic Left Heart

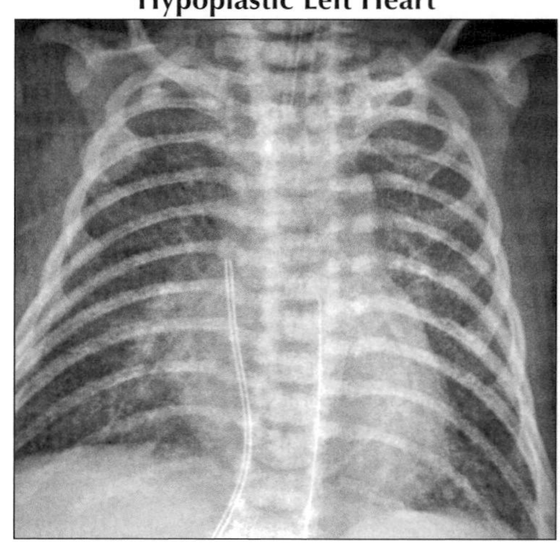

Hypoplastic Left Heart

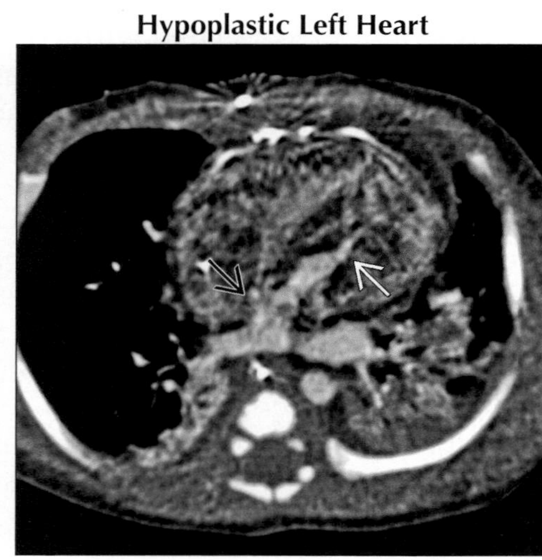

*(**Left**) Left anterior oblique angiography shows valvular aortic stenosis ➔ in this poststenotic dilation of the ascending aorta ➔. Valvular aortic stenosis is the most common type of aortic stenosis. The age of presentation is dependent on the severity of the stenosis. (**Right**) Oblique 3-chamber cardiac MR shows a hypointense jet ➔ due to valvular aortic stenosis. Valvular aortic stenosis can be treated with surgery or catheterization.*

Aortic Stenosis

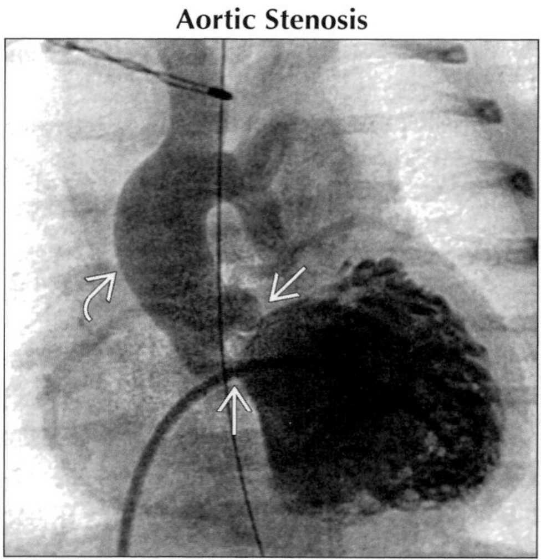

Aortic Stenosis

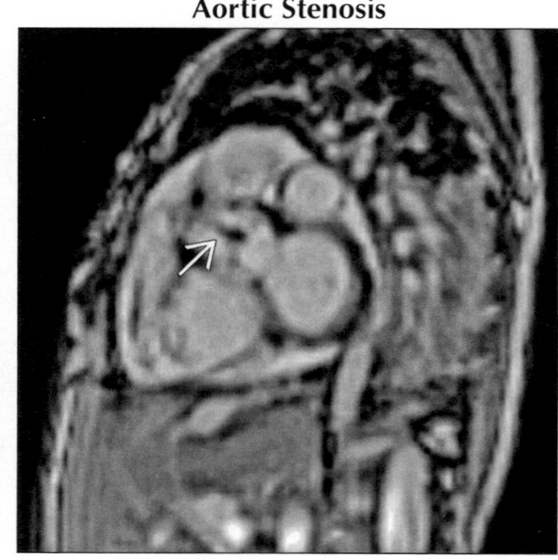

Interrupted Aortic Arch

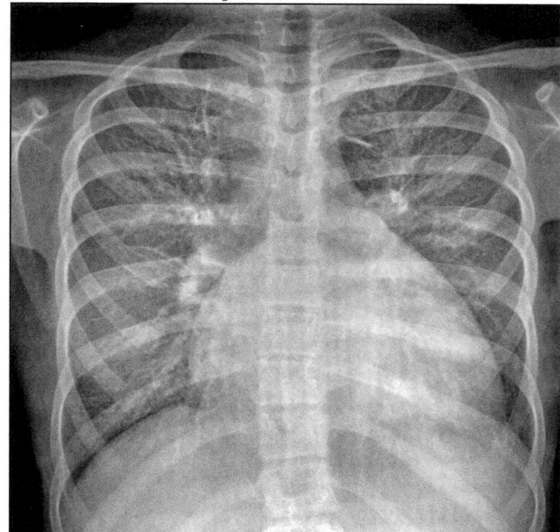

Interrupted Aortic Arch

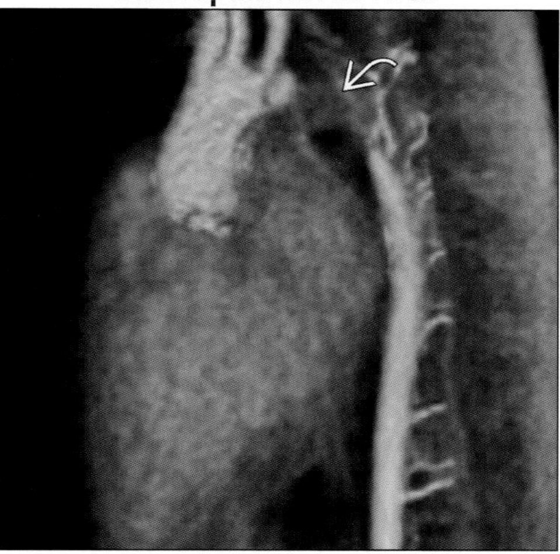

(Left) *AP radiograph of the chest shows cardiomegaly and an absent aortic arch shadow. An interrupted aortic arch is uncommon and accounts for 1% of congenital heart defects.* ***(Right)*** *Oblique MIP of T1 C+ subtraction MR shows interruption of the aortic arch ➡. There are 3 types of an interrupted arch: Isolated, simple, or complex. Interrupted aortic arch is associated with DiGeorge syndrome and 22q11 deletion.*

Hypertropic Obstructive Cardiomyopathy

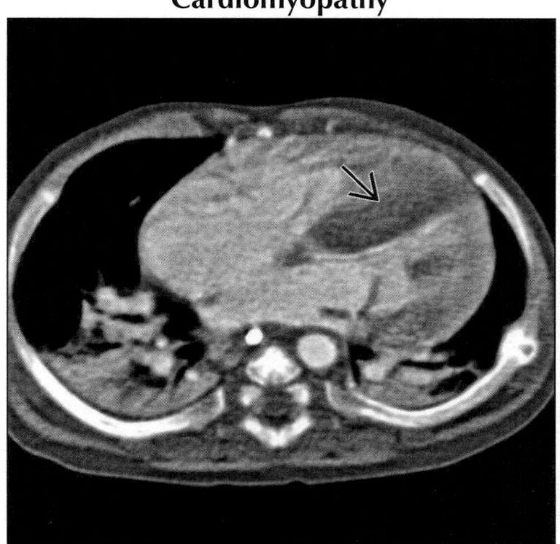

Hypertropic Obstructive Cardiomyopathy

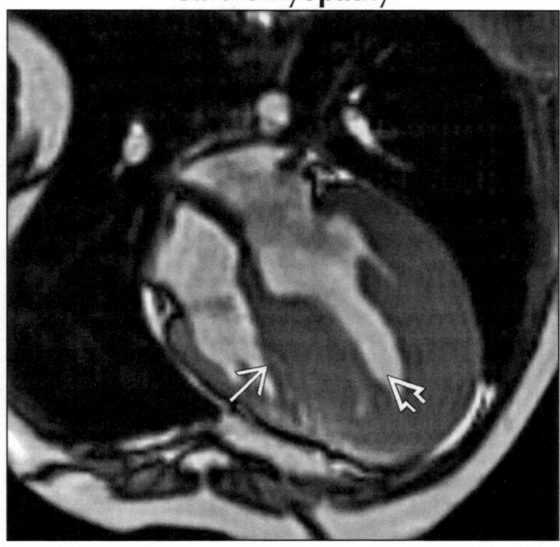

(Left) *Axial CECT shows cardiomegaly and hypertrophy of the intraventricular septum ➡. Hypertrophic obstructive cardiomyopathy is the most common hereditary cardiovascular disorder.* ***(Right)*** *Oblique 4-chamber view from a cardiac MR shows asymmetric septal hypertrophy ➡. The septal hypertrophy narrows the left ventricle ➡. Hypertrophic obstructive cardiomyopathy can present with sudden death.*

Cardiac Rhabdomyomas

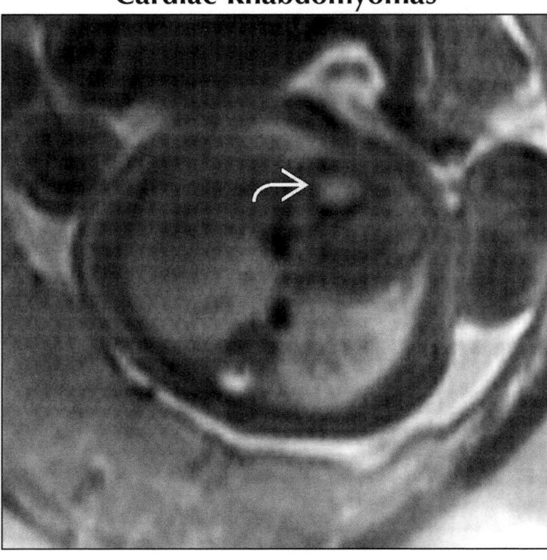

Pseudocoarctation

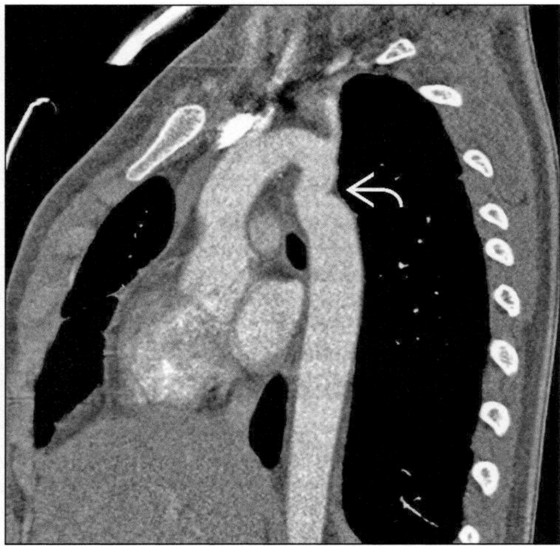

(Left) *Oblique fetal MR shows a hyperintense lesion in the fetal heart ➡. Cardiac rhabdomyomas are the most common cardiac tumor diagnosed prenatally. Nearly 80% of patients with a cardiac rhabdomyoma have tuberous sclerosis, as was the case with this patient.* ***(Right)*** *Oblique CECT shows elongation and kinking of the proximal descending aorta ➡. On chest x-ray, there is often a superior mediastinal mass due to the tortuous aorta.*

HETEROTAXIA SYNDROMES

DIFFERENTIAL DIAGNOSIS

Common
- Total Situs Inversus

Less Common
- Left-Sided Isomerism
- Right-Sided Isomerism

ESSENTIAL INFORMATION

Helpful Clues for Common Diagnoses
- **Total Situs Inversus**
  - All nonsymmetric organs (cardiac structures, lungs, liver, spleen, stomach) are exactly reversed from normal
  - Estimated occurrence = .01% of general population
    - Risk of congenital heart disease slightly more common than general population
  - May be seen in Kartagener syndrome

Helpful Clues for Less Common Diagnoses
- **Left-Sided Isomerism**
  - Slightly more common in females
  - Significantly better prognosis
  - Cardiac findings
    - Less severe cardiac disease with normal to increased pulmonary vascularity; usually noncyanotic
    - Common: Interrupted inferior vena cava, bilateral functional left atria, septal defects
    - May have bilateral superior vena cavae
  - Pulmonary findings
    - Bilateral bi-lobed lungs
    - Both main bronchi lie under pulmonary arteries
  - Intraabdominal findings
    - Midline or left-sided liver; may have absent gallbladder
    - Indeterminate/variable stomach position, may be in right upper quadrant
    - Multiple spleens (which may be located right, left, or centrally within abdomen)
    - Malrotation may be present
- **Right-Sided Isomerism**
  - Slightly more common in males
  - More dire prognosis
  - Cardiac findings
    - More severe cardiac disease with normal to decreased pulmonary vascularity; often cyanotic
    - Common: Anomalous pulmonary venous return, bilateral functional right atria, atrioventricular canal defects, pulmonary outflow tract obstruction, single ventricle
    - May have bilateral superior vena cavae
  - Pulmonary findings
    - Bilateral tri-lobed lungs
    - Both main bronchi course over pulmonary arteries
  - Intraabdominal findings
    - Midline liver
    - Indeterminate/variable stomach position
    - Absent spleen
    - Malrotation common

Total Situs Inversus

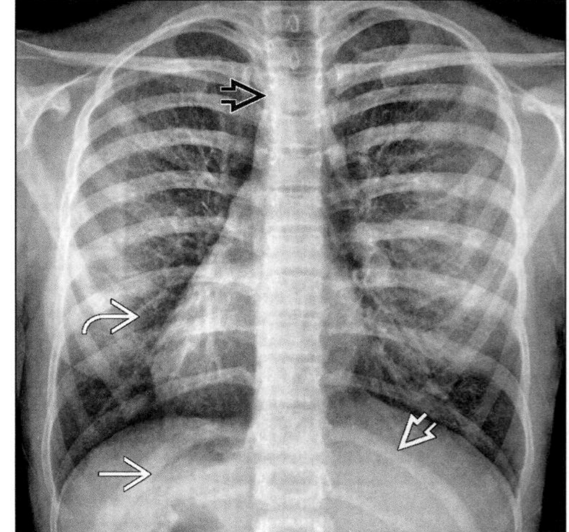

AP radiograph shows dextrocardia ➨, the stomach in the right upper quadrant ➨, the liver in the left upper quadrant ➨, and a right aortic arch displacing the trachea leftward ➨.

Left-Sided Isomerism

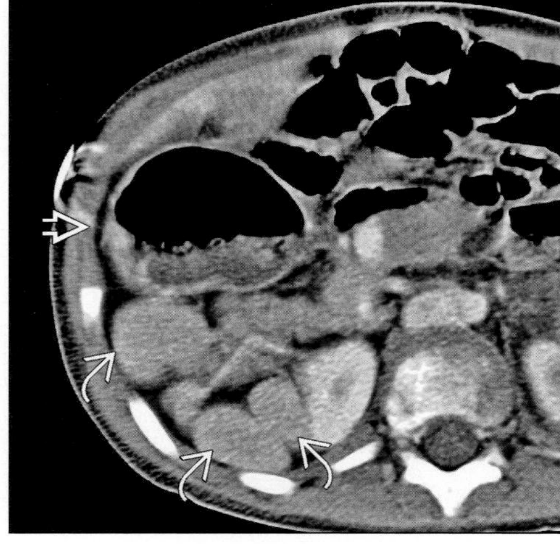

Axial CECT shows an incidentally noted right-sided stomach ➨ and multiple splenules ➨ in a 2 year old imaged for trauma. Abnormal bowel distribution was also noted, consistent with malrotation.

Left-Sided Isomerism

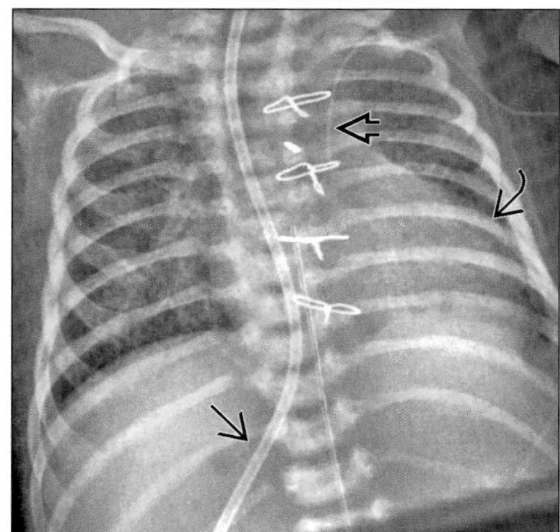

Left-Sided Isomerism

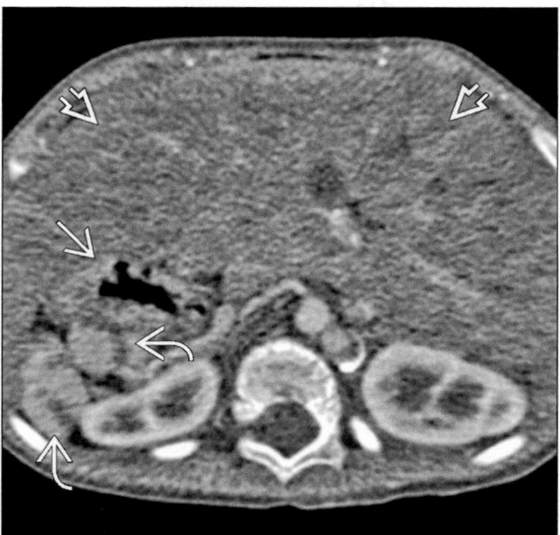

*(**Left**) AP radiograph shows leftward orientation of the cardiac apex, a feeding tube coursing into a right upper quadrant stomach, and a central line coursing into a left superior vena cava. (**Right**) Axial CECT of the same child shows the liver extending across the midline, a right upper quadrant stomach, and a cluster of splenic tissue in the right upper quadrant.*

Right-Sided Isomerism

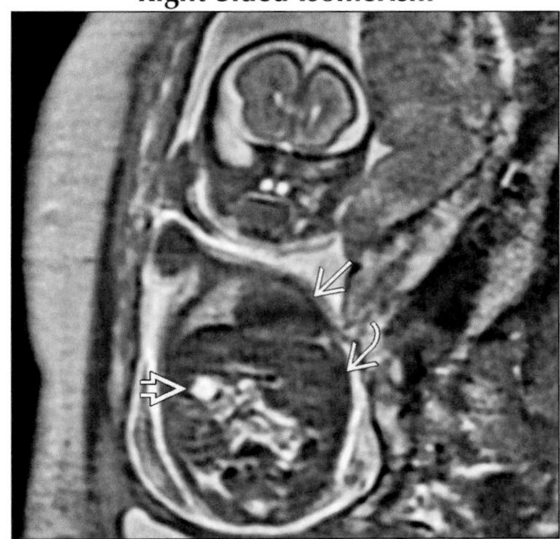

Right-Sided Isomerism

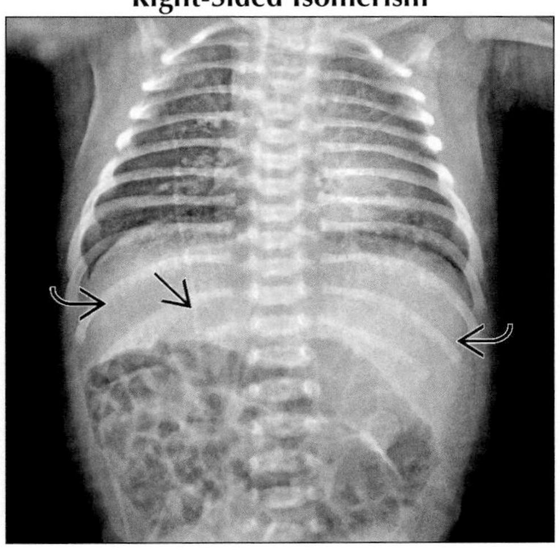

*(**Left**) Coronal T2WI MR shows a fetus with the liver and heart on the left and the stomach on the right. Determining situs in a fetus can be tricky; if the baby is in breech position, facing the maternal left, then the baby's left is by the maternal spine, as depicted here. (**Right**) Frontal radiograph shows the same baby at birth. The liver is predominantly left-sided. The stomach is faintly seen. A sulfur colloid study confirmed asplenia.*

Right-Sided Isomerism

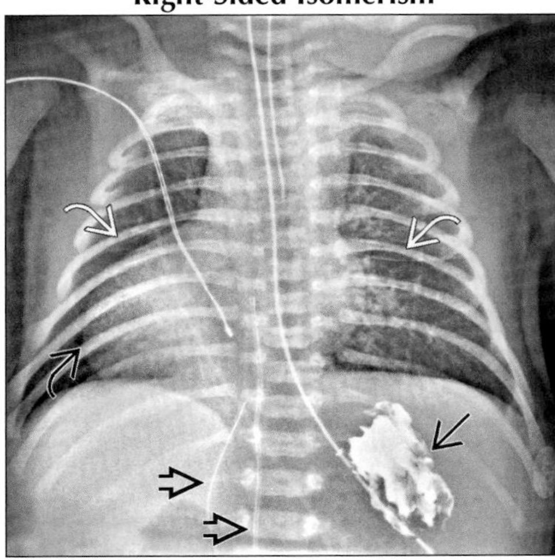

Right-Sided Isomerism

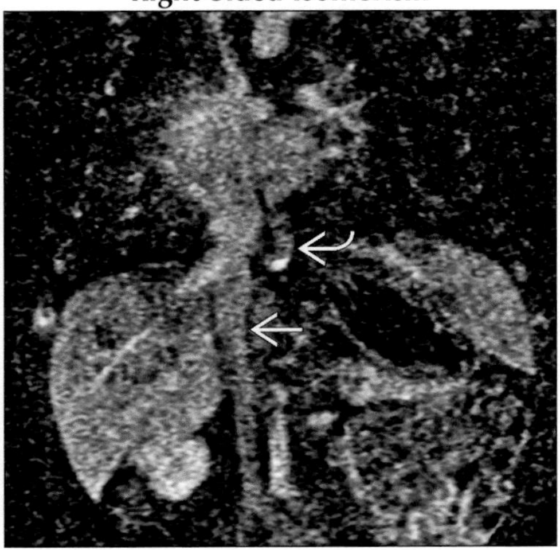

*(**Left**) AP radiograph shows dextrocardia and a left-sided stomach. Note the umbilical catheters in the aorta and inferior vena cava, both positioned to the right of the midline. Faintly seen are bilateral minor fissures. (**Right**) Coronal T1 C+ subtraction MR in the same child shows total anomalous pulmonary venous return, with infradiaphragmatic drainage of the pulmonary veins into the inferior vena cava.*

Enlarged Lingual Tonsils

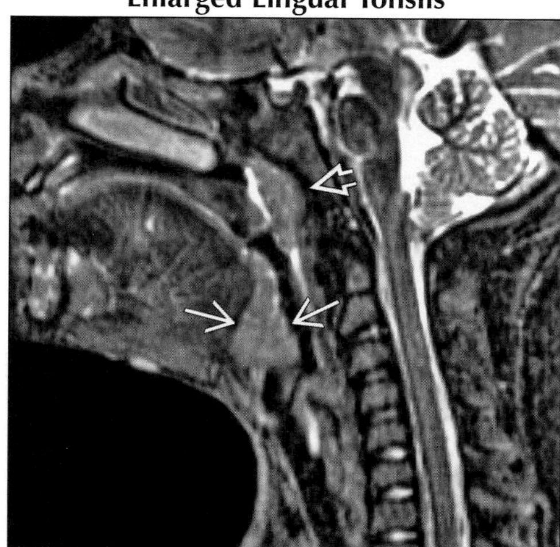

Enlarged Lingual Tonsils

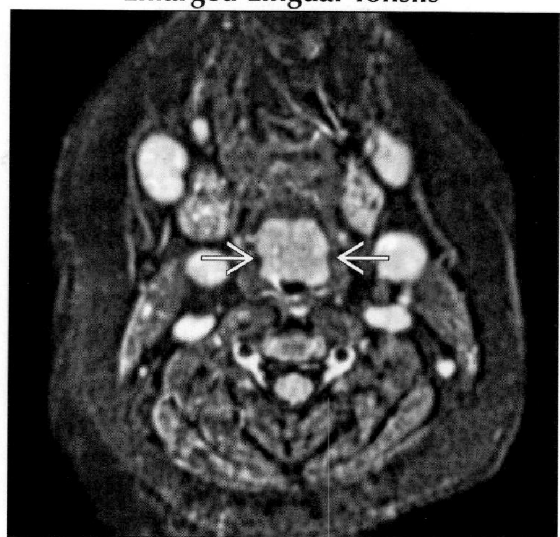

(Left) *Sagittal T2WI FSE MR shows a large mass ➔ located at the base of the tongue, consistent with marked enlargement of the lingual tonsils. The adenoid tonsils are also recurrent ➔.* ***(Right)*** *Axial T2WI FSE MR in the same patient shows markedly enlarged lingual tonsils ➔ filling the majority of the retroglossal airway.*

Enlarged Lingual Tonsils

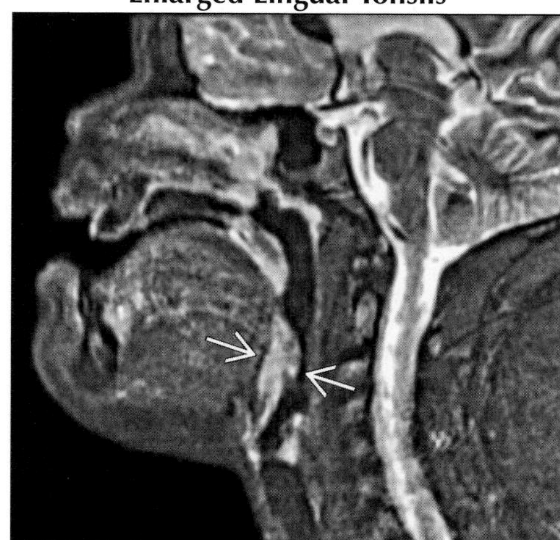

Enlarged Lingual Tonsils

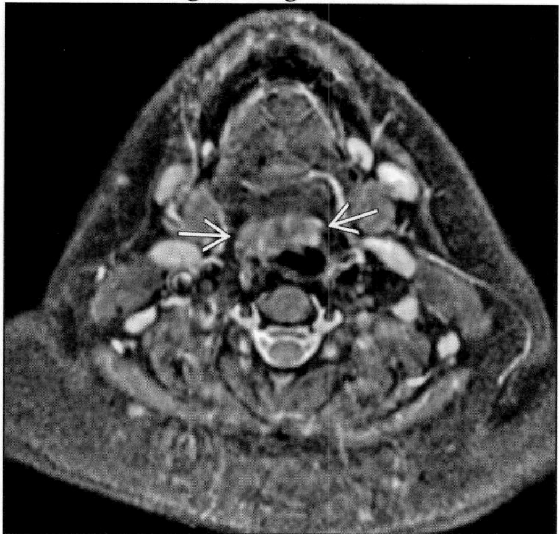

(Left) *Sagittal T2WI FSE MR shows enlarged lingual tonsils ➔ encroaching upon the retroglossal airway. Note encroachment upon retroglossal airway.* ***(Right)*** *Axial T2WI FSE MR in the same patient again shows enlarged lingual tonsils ➔ filling the majority of the retroglossal airway.*

Glossoptosis

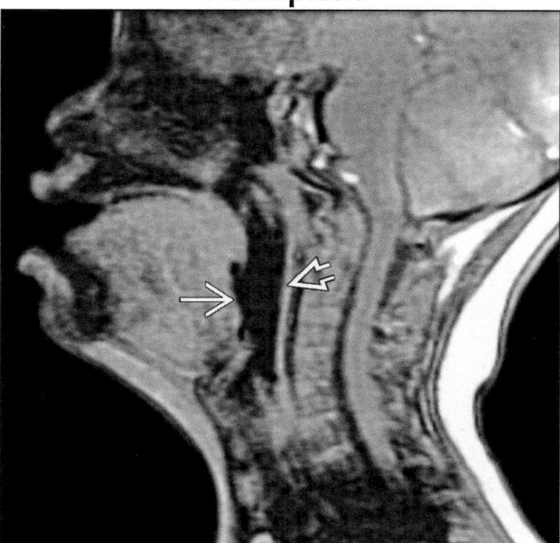

Glossoptosis

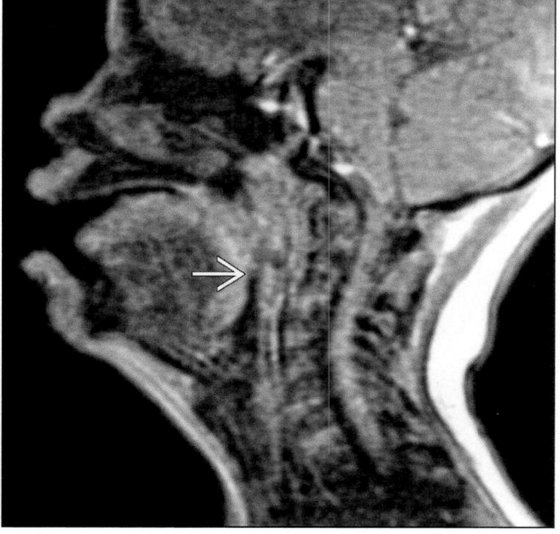

(Left) *Sagittal GRE MR at exhalation shows that the retroglossal airway ➔ is patent at this point, and the posterior aspect of the tongue ➔ is in normal position.* ***(Right)*** *Sagittal MR cine in the same patient at inspiration shows that the posterior wall of the tongue ➔ has moved posteriorly abutting the posterior pharyngeal wall and pushing soft palate posteriorly, obstructing both the retroglossal airway and posterior nasopharynx.*

OBSTRUCTIVE SLEEP APNEA

*(**Left**) Sagittal PDWI MR shows a posteriorly positioned tongue ➔ abutting the posterior pharyngeal wall, obstructing the retroglossal airway, consistent with glossoptosis. (**Right**) Axial GRE MR with cine image during exhalation in the same patient shows a small caliber retroglossal airway ➔ with the posterior aspect of the tongue positioned posteriorly.*

Glossoptosis

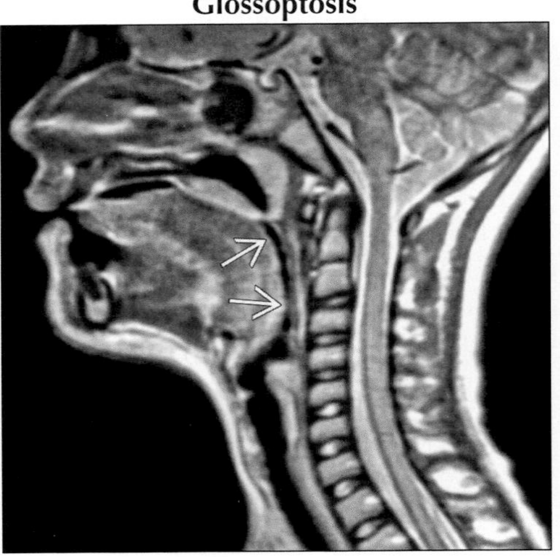

Glossoptosis

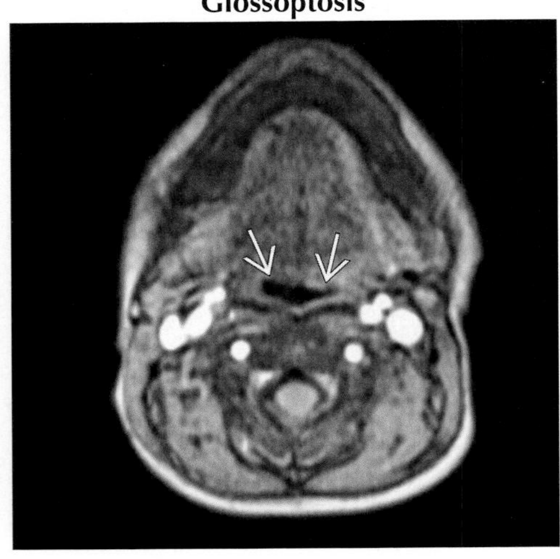

*(**Left**) Axial GRE MR with cine image during inspiration in the same patient shows an even smaller caliber retroglossal airway ➔ with the posterior aspect of the tongue further posteriorly positioned, consistent with glossoptosis. (**Right**) Sagittal GRE MR depicted in cine image at inspiration shows the retroglossal airway ➔ to be patent.*

Glossoptosis

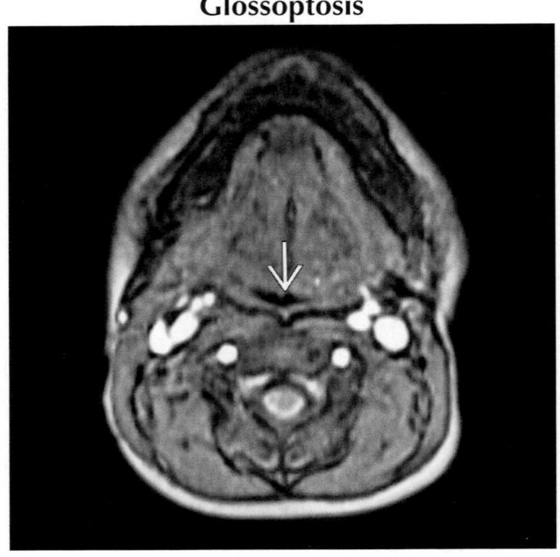

Hypopharyngeal Collapse

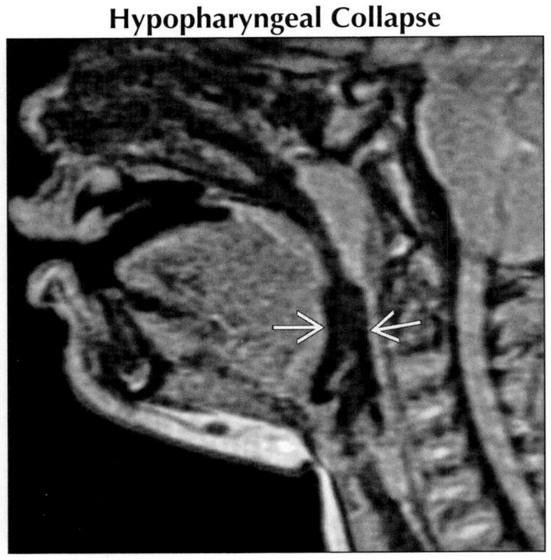

*(**Left**) Sagittal GRE MR depicted in cine image at exhalation in the same patient shows a collapsed retroglossal airway ➔. (**Right**) Axial GRE MR depicted in cine image at inspiration shows the retroglossal airway ➔ to be patent.*

Hypopharyngeal Collapse

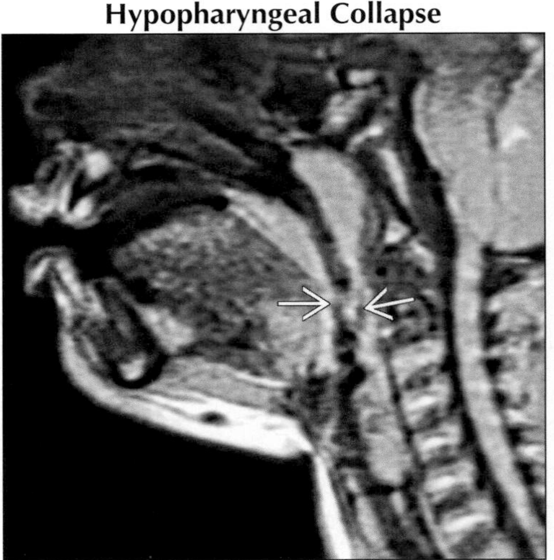

Hypopharyngeal Collapse

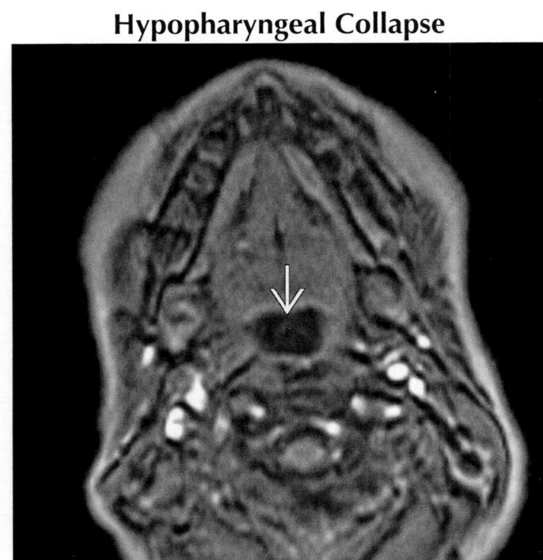

SECTION 2
Chest

OBSTRUCTIVE SLEEP APNEA

DIFFERENTIAL DIAGNOSIS

Common

- Enlarged Palatine Tonsils
- Enlarged Adenoid Tonsils
- Recurrent and Enlarged Adenoid Tonsils
- Enlarged Lingual Tonsils
- Glossoptosis
- Hypopharyngeal Collapse

Less Common

- Enlarged Soft Palate
- Macroglossia

Rare but Important

- Tongue-based Masses
- Thyroglossal Duct Cyst
- Artificial Airway (Mimic)

ESSENTIAL INFORMATION

Key Differential Diagnosis Issues

- MR sleep studies: Combination of T1WI (static) and T2WI (static and dynamic cine)
    - Depict both anatomic and dynamic motion abnormalities in children with obstructive sleep apnea (OSA)
    - Most often performed in children who have persistent OSA despite previous surgery
        - e.g., previous palatine tonsillectomy and adenoidectomy
    - When interpreting, it is important to identify both anatomic causes (enlarged tonsils) &/or collapse patterns (glossoptosis or hypopharyngeal collapse)
- 2 key anatomic areas for most causes of OSA
    - Posterior nasopharynx
        - Airway bordered by soft palate anteriorly, nasal turbinates anteriorly and superiorly, adenoids posteriorly
        - Inferior border defined by inferior tip of uvula
    - Retroglossal airway
        - a.k.a. hypopharynx
        - Aerated space bordered by posterior aspect of tongue anteriorly, posterior pharyngeal wall posteriorly, and inferior aspect of soft palate anteriorly
        - Inferior border is inferior extent (or base) of tongue

Helpful Clues for Common Diagnoses

- **Enlarged Palatine Tonsils**
    - Diagnosis made on physical inspection, not usually imaging diagnosis
        - Most patients referred for MR sleep studies already have had palatine tonsils removed
        - No published data on upper limits of normal measurement at imaging
    - Round, well-defined, high T2 signal masses within palatine tonsillar fossa
        - If appear prominent and "bob" centrally with respiration and obstruct airway → enlarged
    - Unlike adenoid tonsils, palatine tonsils do not recur after palatine tonsillectomy
- **Enlarged Adenoid Tonsils**
    - Natural history
        - Adenoid tonsils are absent at birth
        - Reach maximum size by 2-10 years
        - Shrink during 2nd decade of life
    - Upper limit of normal size is 12 mm
- **Recurrent and Enlarged Adenoid Tonsils**
    - Adenoids not encapsulated tonsil, so small amounts of lateral tonsillar tissue always left after surgery
        - Recurrence of adenoid 1 of more common causes of recurrent OSA
        - Postoperative appearance: Central wedge triangular defect in central portion of tonsil
    - > 12 mm in size and associated with intermittent collapse of posterior nasopharynx on cine images
        - Can be associated with secondary hypopharyngeal collapse secondary to negative pressure generated at obstruction of posterior nasopharynx
- **Enlarged Lingual Tonsils**
    - Previously thought to be rare cause of OSA, increasingly recognized as more common
    - Surgically treatable; important to identify
    - Not always easily appreciated on physical examination
    - In most normal children, lingual tonsils range from nonperceptible to several mm
    - In patients with previous palatine tonsillectomy and adenoidectomy, lingual tonsils can grow large
        - High propensity in patients with Down syndrome, obesity

- Appear as large, bilateral, high T2 signal masses at base of tongue
  - Can grow into 1 large dumbbell-shaped mass
  - Can grow superiorly into palatine fossa
  - Potentially confused with palatine tonsils if history of palatine tonsillectomy not known

- **Glossoptosis**
  - Defined as posterior motion of tongue during sleep
  - Tongue is posteriorly positioned, and posterior wall of tongue abuts posterior pharyngeal wall, obstructing retroglossal airway
    - Tongue may also displace soft palate posteriorly and obstruct nasopharynx
  - Occurs in children with macroglossia (large tongue), micrognathia (small mandible), or decreased muscular tone
    - e.g., Down syndrome, Pierre-Robin sequence, cerebral palsy
  - Axial cine images show posterior motion of tongue but no change in left-to-right transverse diameter of retroglossal airway
  - Important to differentiate glossoptosis from hypopharyngeal collapse as there are more and better surgical options for glossoptosis
- **Hypopharyngeal Collapse**
  - Primarily related to decreased muscular tone
  - Secondary to negative pressure, secondary to more superior obstruction (e.g., enlarged adenoids)
  - Axial cine images show dynamic and cylindrical narrowing of hypopharynx
    - All walls (left, right, anterior, posterior) collapse to center of retroglossal airway

Helpful Clues for Less Common Diagnoses

- **Enlarged Soft Palate**
  - Thickened and long soft palate possible cause of OSA
  - No established quantitative imaging criteria for when soft palate too long or thick
  - If soft palate draped over tongue and associated with collapse of airway on cine images → enlarged
  - Edema from snoring can occur
    - Appears as increased T2 signal in soft palate centrally
    - Soft palate normally same signal intensity of tongue musculature, dark on T2

Helpful Clues for Rare Diagnoses

- **Artificial Airway (Mimic)**
  - Obscures and distorts anatomic structures being evaluated
    - May simulate pathology
  - Try to avoid artificial airway when acquiring MR sleep studies

Enlarged Palatine Tonsils

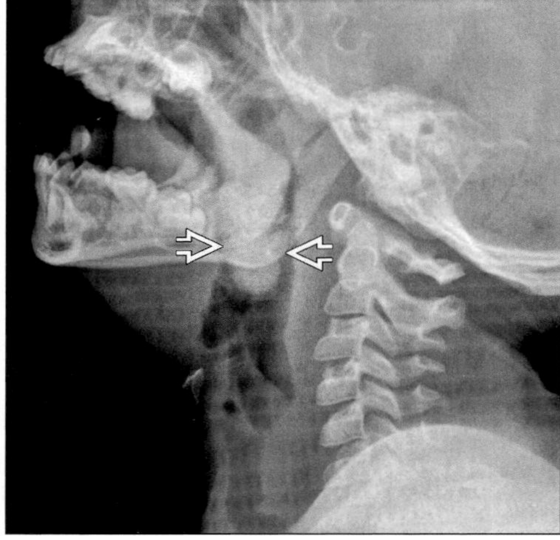

Sagittal radiograph shows enlarged palatine tonsils ➡, which appear as prominent soft tissue just inferior to the region of the soft palate.

Enlarged Palatine Tonsils

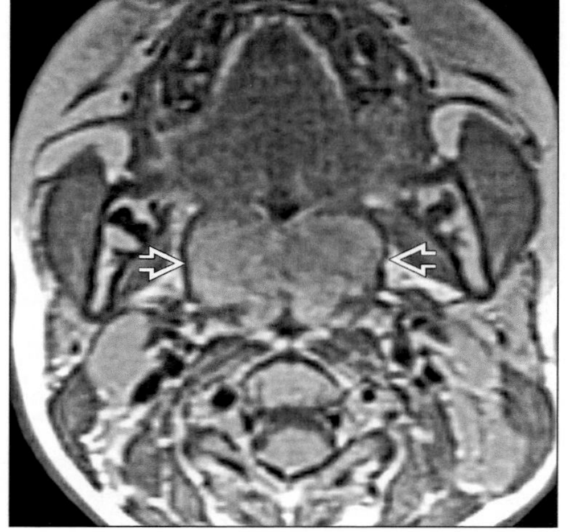

Axial PD FSE MR shows palatine tonsils as 2 round masses ➡ that meet at the midline, a phenomenon known as "kissing tonsils."

OBSTRUCTIVE SLEEP APNEA

*(**Left**) Sagittal T2WI FSE MR shows several high signal masses, which are enlarged adenoid and palatine tonsils. (**Right**) Sagittal GRE MR shows enlargement of the palatine and adenoid tonsils.*

Enlarged Palatine Tonsils

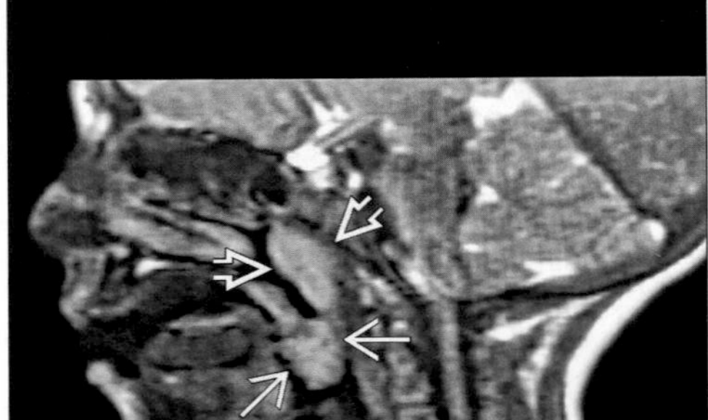

Enlarged Palatine Tonsils

*(**Left**) Sagittal T2WI FSE MR shows markedly enlarged adenoid tonsils encroaching upon the posterior nasopharynx. (**Right**) Axial T2WI FSE MR shows enlarged adenoid tonsils in a patient without a previous adenoidectomy. Note the smooth anterior surface of the adenoid tonsils.*

Enlarged Adenoid Tonsils

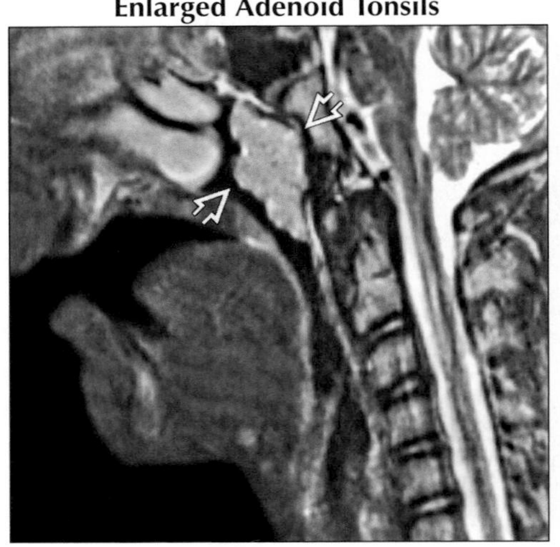

Enlarged Adenoid Tonsils

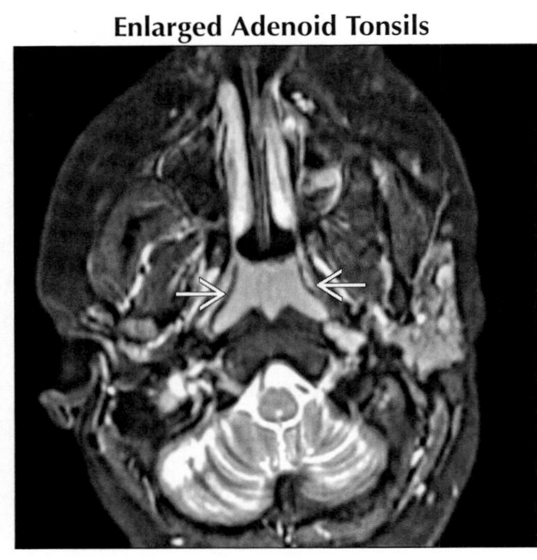

*(**Left**) Axial T2WI FSE MR shows recurrent and enlarged adenoid tonsils. Note the V-shaped wedge defect in the anterior margin of the adenoids, typical of the postresection appearance. (**Right**) Sagittal STIR MR shows a large mass located at the base of the tongue, consistent with marked enlargement of the lingual tonsils.*

Recurrent and Enlarged Adenoid Tonsils

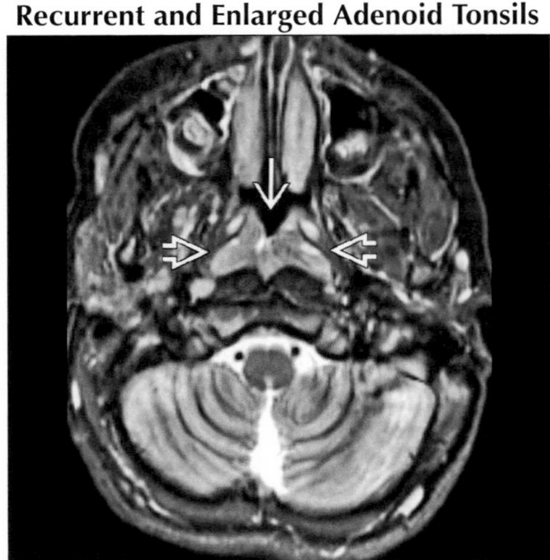

Enlarged Lingual Tonsils

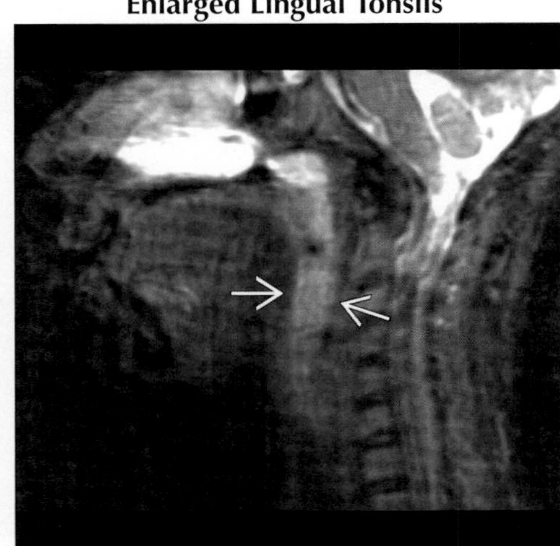

Hypopharyngeal Collapse

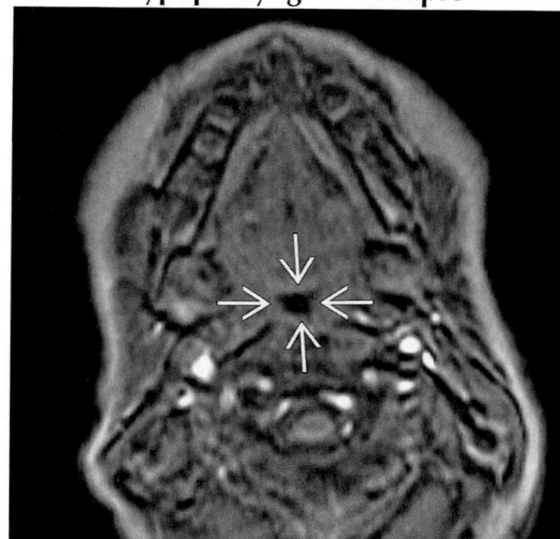

Enlarged Soft Palate

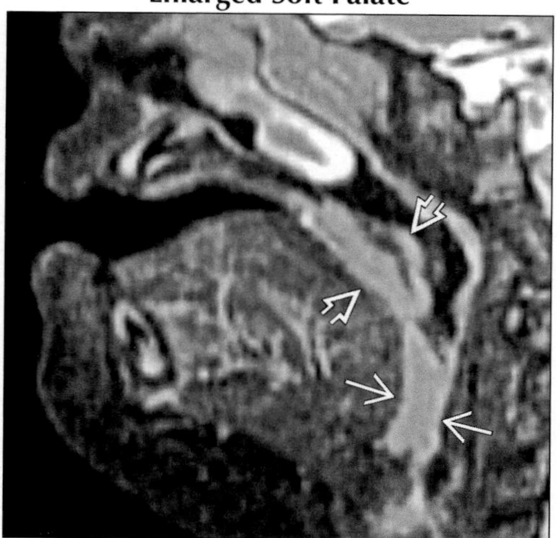

(Left) *Axial GRE MR in cine image at expiration in the same patient shows the collapsed retroglossal airway ➡. Note that all (left, right, anterior, posterior) walls of the airway collapse toward the center. This is different from the patent collapse seen in glossoptosis.* ***(Right)*** *Sagittal GRE MR shows an enlarged and high signal soft palate ➡, much brighter than the tongue musculature. The soft palate is normally similar in signal to the tongue. Also note the enlarged lingual tonsils ➡.*

Enlarged Soft Palate

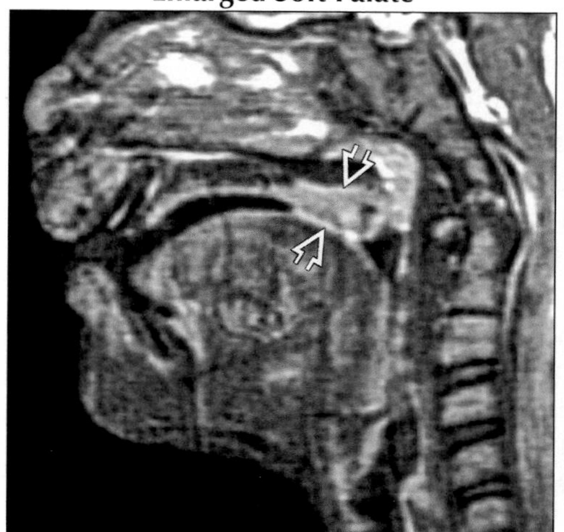

Artificial Airway (Mimic)

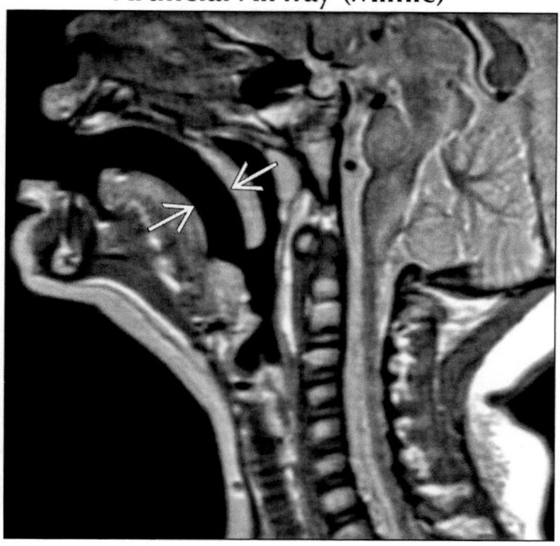

(Left) *Sagittal T2WI FS MR shows a high signal and thickened soft palate ➡. Note how bright the soft palate is compared to the tongue musculature.* ***(Right)*** *Sagittal PDWI MR shows the oral airway ➡ as a low signal tube causing distortion of the tongue. The region of interest is distorted and uninterpretable because of the presence of the oral airway. Artificial airways should be avoided in MR sleep studies.*

Artificial Airway (Mimic)

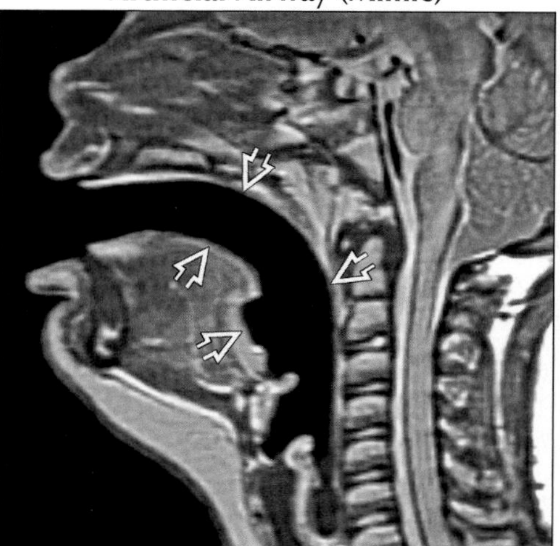

Artificial Airway (Mimic)

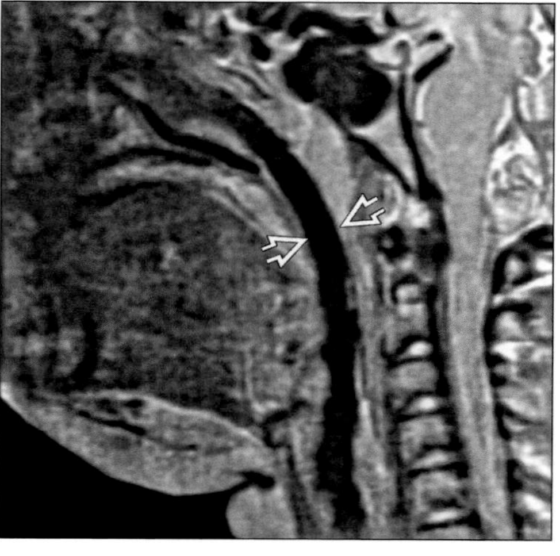

(Left) *Sagittal T2WI MR shows a laryngeal mask airway (LMA) in place ➡. The LMA pulls forward and distorts the tongue. This type of artificial airway obscures the anatomic structures being evaluated and should be avoided.* ***(Right)*** *Sagittal T2WI MR shows a nasopharyngeal trumpet (NT) in place. Note how little the NT ➡ distorts the regional anatomy compared to other artificial airways. If an artificial airway is absolutely necessary, a NT is recommended.*

INSPIRATORY STRIDOR

DIFFERENTIAL DIAGNOSIS

Common
- Croup
- Foreign Body, Esophagus
- Exudative Tracheitis
- Subglottic Hemangioma

Less Common
- Innominate Artery Compression Syndrome
- Congenital Tracheal Stenosis
- Iatrogenic Tracheal Stenosis

Rare but Important
- Epiglottitis, Child
- Right Arch with Aberrant Left SCA
- Foreign Body, Trachea

ESSENTIAL INFORMATION

Key Differential Diagnosis Issues
- Stridor: Variably pitched respiratory sound caused by tissue vibration through area of respiratory tract of decreased caliber

Helpful Clues for Common Diagnoses
- **Croup**
  - Key facts
    - Viral etiology; barky cough
    - Most common at age 6 months-3 years; peak 1 year
  - Imaging
    - AP radiograph: Symmetric subglottic tracheal narrowing produces lack of normal "shouldering" of subglottic trachea; results in "steeple" sign
    - Lateral radiograph: Hypopharyngeal distension and ill-defined narrow subglottic airway
    - Radiographs obtained to exclude other causes of stridor: Exudative tracheitis, epiglottitis, aspirated foreign body (FB), or subglottic hemangioma
- **Foreign Body, Esophagus**
  - Key facts
    - Coins are most common radiopaque FB in esophagus
    - If not passed, causes edema anterior to esophagus and around trachea; results in inspiratory stridor
    - Most common site: Upper thoracic esophagus followed by level of arch/carina and distal esophagus
    - Button batteries show 2-layered margin; require emergent removal to prevent caustic esophageal burn injury
  - Imaging
    - If radiodense, see FB posterior to trachea
    - ± thickening of soft tissue between esophagus and trachea
    - ± anterior displacement of trachea
    - ± tracheal narrowing at level of FB
- **Exudative Tracheitis**
  - Key facts
    - Purulent infection → intratracheal exudates may slough & occlude airway
    - Usually older than patients with croup
  - Imaging
    - Symmetric (or asymmetric) subglottic narrowing
    - ± linear, soft tissue densities (membranes) within trachea ± tracheal wall irregularities (plaques)
- **Subglottic Hemangioma**
  - Key facts
    - Inspiratory stridor, airway obstruction, hoarseness or abnormal cry; usually younger than 6 months
    - Associated with cutaneous hemangiomas in up to 50% of patients
    - 7% of patients with PHACE syndrome have subglottic hemangioma
  - Imaging
    - Asymmetric subglottic tracheal narrowing on radiographs
    - Enhancing soft tissue mass on CT or MR

Helpful Clues for Less Common Diagnoses
- **Innominate Artery Compression Syndrome**
  - Key facts
    - Infantile trachea lacks rigidity
    - Symptoms: Stridor, apnea, dyspnea; usually resolve as child grows
    - Increased incidence with esophageal atresia; dilated esophageal pouch deviates trachea forward, innominate artery compresses anterior trachea
  - Imaging
    - Anterior tracheal narrowing at crossing innominate artery; below thoracic inlet
- **Congenital Tracheal Stenosis**
  - Key facts

- Secondary to complete cartilaginous rings ± associated anomalies such as vascular ring
  - Imaging
    - Small caliber round (rather than horse shoe-shaped) trachea on cross sectional imaging
    - Inverted T-shaped carina on conventional radiograph or coronal reformatted CT images
    - Focal or diffuse stenosis possible
- **Iatrogenic Tracheal Stenosis**
  - Key facts: History of prior endotracheal tube (ET) intubation, tracheostomy, or other injury
  - Imaging: Subglottic tracheal narrowing at level of prior ET tube or tracheostomy tube
    - Smooth focal narrowing (ET tube) or irregular longer narrowing (tracheostomy secondary to granulation tissue ± structural damage to tracheal rings)

Helpful Clues for Rare Diagnoses

- **Epiglottitis, Child**
  - Key facts
    - Life threatening infectious inflammation and swelling of epiglottis and supraglottic structures
    - Abrupt onset of stridor, dysphagia, high fever, sore throat, dysphonia, hoarseness, and drooling
    - Symptoms of airway obstruction markedly increase when recumbent; do lateral radiograph in upright position
    - Incidence markedly decreased since *H. influenzae* vaccination became universal
  - Imaging
    - Enlargement of epiglottis & thickening of aryepiglottic folds on lateral X-ray
- **Right Arch with Aberrant Left SCA**
  - Key facts: 0.1% of general population but usually asymptomatic
    - Rarely associated with tightly constricting left ligamentum arteriosum; presents with congenital stridor
    - Posterior esophageal indentation by aberrant SCA may cause dysphagia or feeding difficulties in infants
  - Imaging
    - Posterior esophageal indentation by aberrant SCA on esophagram
    - Aberrant SCA coursing posterior to esophagus on CT or MR
- **Foreign Body, Trachea**
  - Key facts
    - Bronchial FB much more common than tracheal FB
    - Most airway FB not radiopaque; majority peanuts and carrots
    - Incident usually not witnessed
  - Imaging
    - If radiodense, identify FB in airway
    - When nonradiopaque FB aspiration, look for secondary signs: Hyperinflation, airtrapping, regional oligemia, atelectasis, pneumomediastinum, pneumothorax

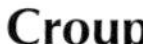

Croup

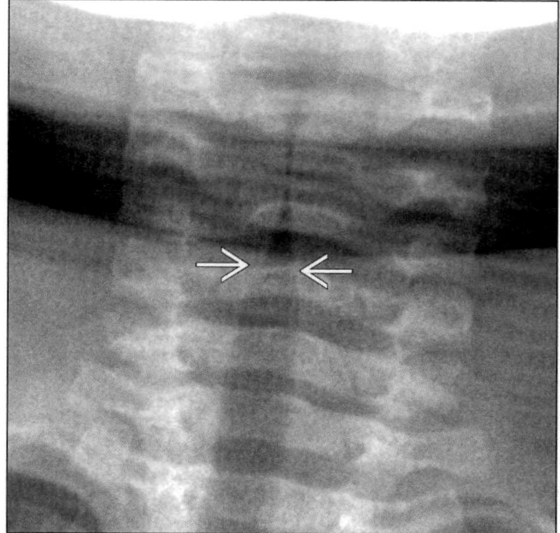

Anteroposterior radiograph shows loss of the normal shouldering of the subglottic airway, producing a "steeple sign" ➡.

Croup

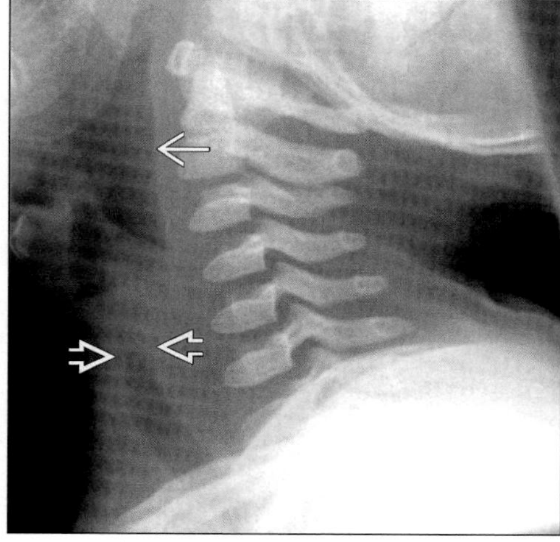

Lateral radiograph shows mild hypopharyngeal distention ➡ and a narrow subglottic airway ➡.

INSPIRATORY STRIDOR

(Left) *Lateral radiograph shows a radiopaque coin in the esophagus, a dilated proximal esophagus, and circumferential tracheal narrowing.* **(Right)** *Lateral radiograph shows mild irregularity of the subglottic trachea with an intraluminal linear density related to a plaque in an older child with exudative tracheitis.*

Foreign Body, Esophagus

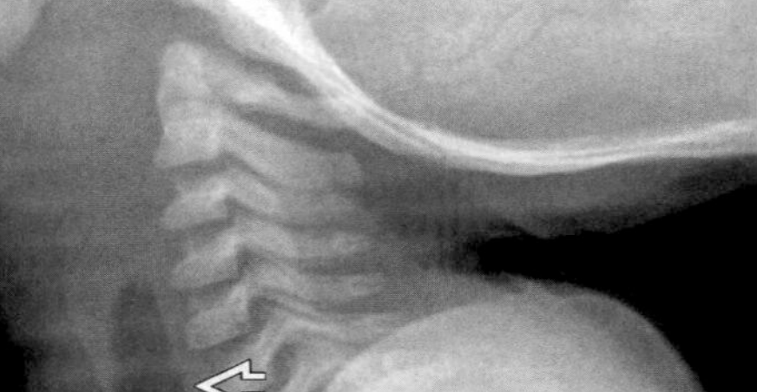

Exudative Tracheitis

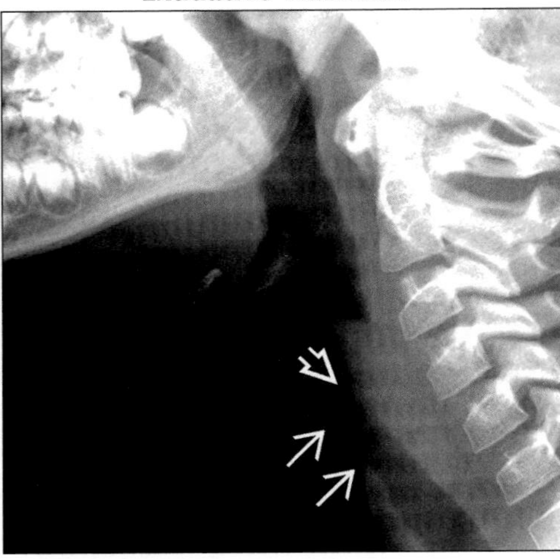

(Left) *Axial CECT demonstrates a small, intensely enhancing, subglottic mass. A submucosal airway hemangioma was visible on endoscopy.* **(Right)** *Sagittal CECT shows the posterior, enhancing mass resulting in focal tracheal narrowing. Not surprisingly, the infant presented with stridor.*

Subglottic Hemangioma

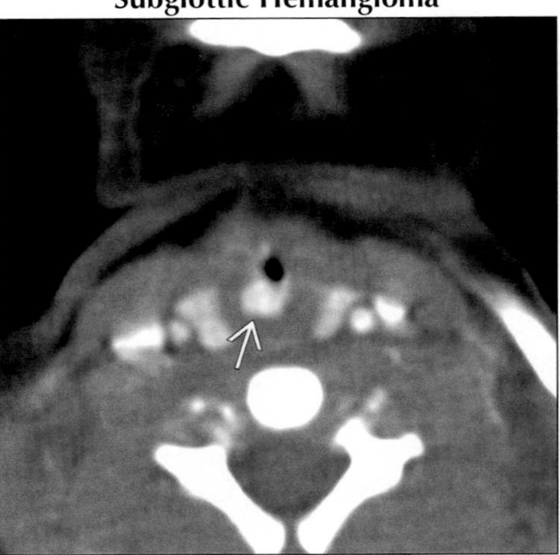

Subglottic Hemangioma

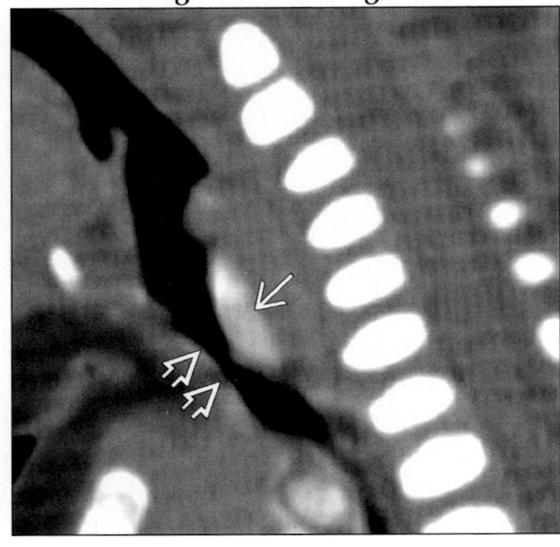

(Left) *Axial CECT reveals narrowing of the trachea at the level of the crossing innominate artery. A pH probe is also seen in the upper thoracic esophagus.* **(Right)** *Lateral esophagram shows anterior tracheal compression at the level of crossing innominate artery and a small esophageal stricture in a patient with prior esophageal atresia repair.*

Innominate Artery Compression Syndrome

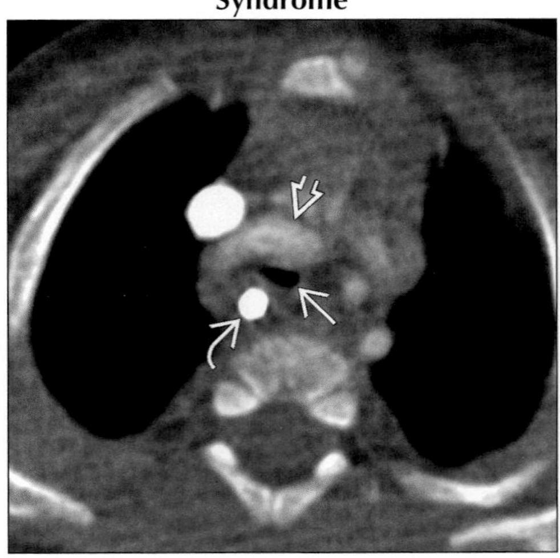

Innominate Artery Compression Syndrome

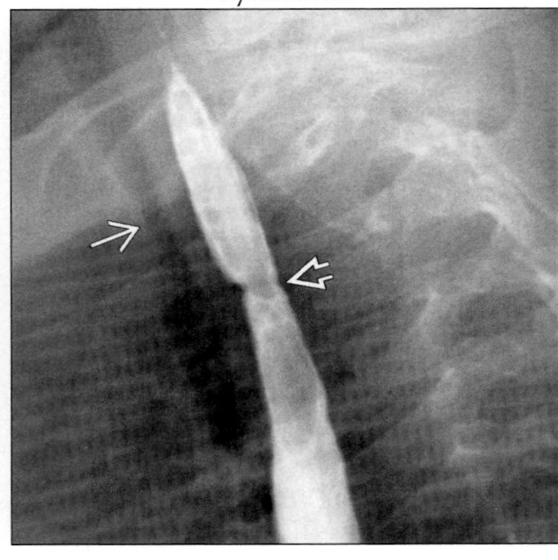

Congenital Tracheal Stenosis

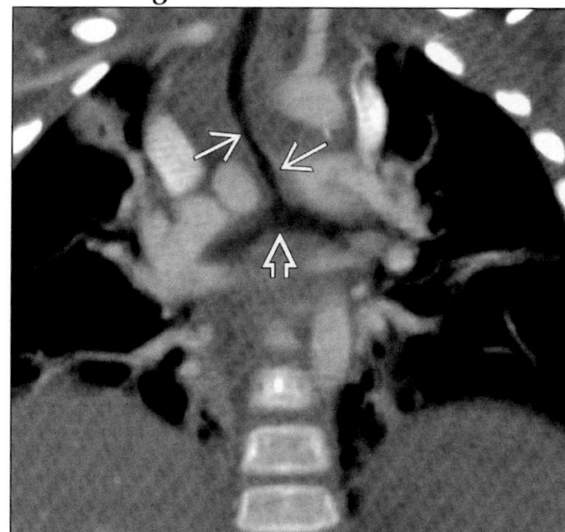

Congenital Tracheal Stenosis

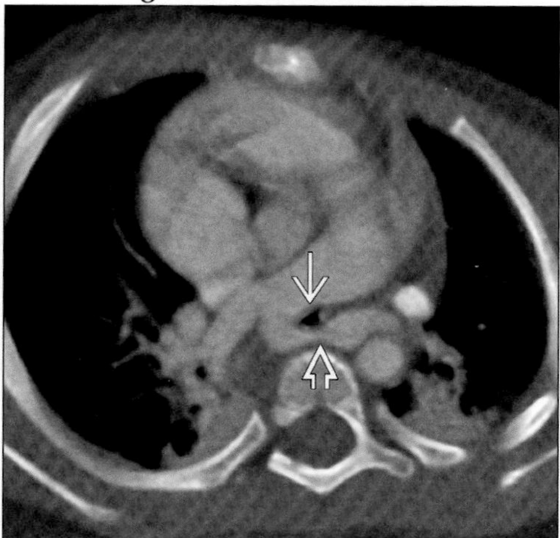

*(**Left**) Coronal CECT shows distal intrathoracic tracheal narrowing ➡ with a nearly 180° angle between mainstem bronchi, resulting in an inverted "T" appearance of the carina ➡. (**Right**) Axial CECT reveals a congenitally stenotic trachea ➡ in association with the aberrant left pulmonary artery ➡ arising from the right pulmonary artery and coursing posterior to the trachea.*

Iatrogenic Tracheal Stenosis

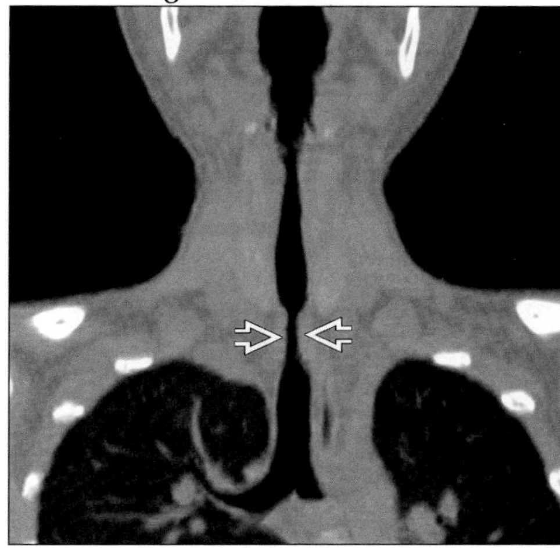

Epiglottitis, Child

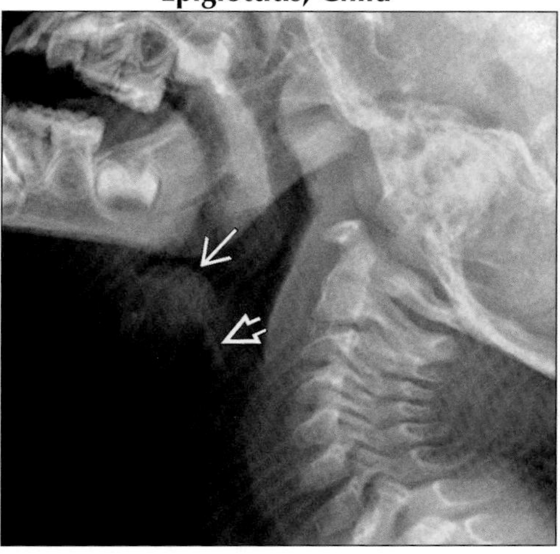

*(**Left**) Coronal bone CT demonstrates an abrupt shelf causing tracheal narrowing at the level of the thoracic inlet ➡. This child had a prior history of prolonged endotracheal intubation. (**Right**) Anteroposterior radiograph shows a markedly swollen epiglottis ➡ and thickened aryepiglottic folds ➡ diagnostic of epiglottitis.*

Right Arch with Aberrant Left SCA

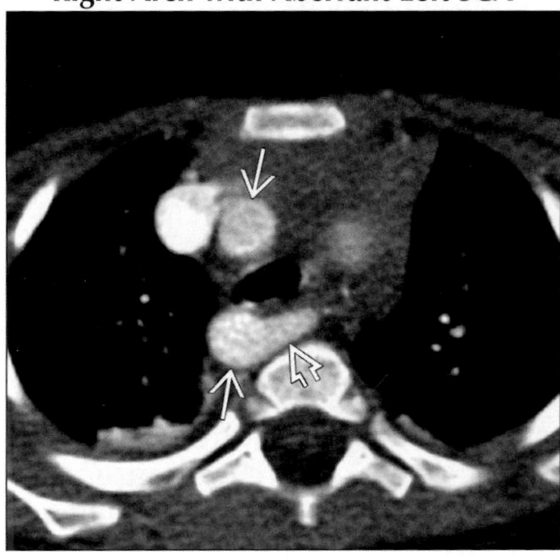

Foreign Body, Trachea

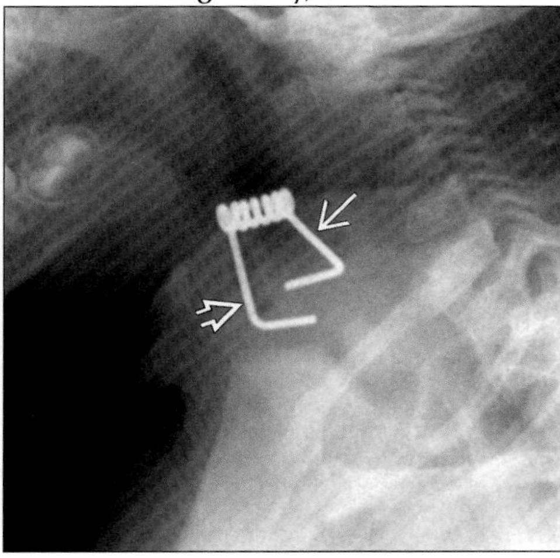

*(**Left**) Axial CECT shows the congenital right arch ➡ associated with an aberrant left subclavian artery ➡ coursing posterior to the trachea. (**Right**) Lateral radiograph reveals a radiopaque spring from a wooden clothes pin in the hypopharynx ➡ and larynx ➡.*

MEDIASTINAL WIDENING

DIFFERENTIAL DIAGNOSIS

Common
- Normal Thymus
- Lymphoma
- Reactive Lymphadenopathy

Less Common
- Bronchogenic Cyst
- Trauma
- Enlargement of Ascending Aorta

Rare but Important
- Germ Cell Tumor
- Neurofibromatosis Type 1
- Thyroid Carcinoma

ESSENTIAL INFORMATION

Key Differential Diagnosis Issues
- Normal pediatric mediastinum is wider than in adulthood due to thymus
- Trauma is uncommon cause of mediastinal widening in children

Helpful Clues for Common Diagnoses
- **Normal Thymus**
  - Most common mediastinal "mass" in neonates and infants
  - Most prominent in infancy
    - Has quadrilateral shape
  - Thymus increases in weight until adolescence when it begins to involute
    - Gradually becomes triangular-shaped in childhood and teenage years
  - Visible by radiograph until ~ 5 years of age
  - Appearance may change with respiration
  - Thymus can vary in size depending on intercurrent illness and stress
    - May ↓ in size during illness/stress and ↑ in size with recovery
  - Often asymmetric across midline
    - Usually more prominent on right side
    - Mimic upper lobe consolidation
  - Homogeneous appearance on CT and MR
    - Enhances homogeneously
  - Multiple linear echoes and discrete echogenic foci on ultrasound
- **Lymphoma**
  - 3rd most common malignancy in children after leukemia and brain tumors
  - Incidence increases with age
    - 25% of cancers in children 15-19 yo
  - Most common mediastinal mass in teens
  - Hodgkin lymphoma (HL) more common than non-Hodgkin lymphoma (NHL)
    - HL involves continuous nodal groups
    - NHL is more commonly extranodal
  - NHL is more common than HL in children < 10 years of age
  - Mediastinal disease is common in HL and NHL
    - Occurs in 2/3 with HL
  - Mediastinal mass can cause tracheal compression
- **Reactive Lymphadenopathy**
  - Most common organism depends on geographic location
  - Common causes: Tuberculosis (TB), histoplasmosis, coccidioidomycosis, and blastomycosis
    - TB and histoplasmosis may have lymph nodes with low-attenuation centers on contrast-enhanced CT in acute phase
    - Lymph node calcification in old disease
  - Enlarged lymph nodes can compress superior vena cava (SVC)
    - May cause SVC syndrome or fibrosing mediastinitis

Helpful Clues for Less Common Diagnoses
- **Bronchogenic Cyst**
  - May have bronchial or esophageal origin
  - Most common location: Paratracheal or subcarinal
  - May lead to bronchial compression
    - May cause atelectasis or hyperinflation
  - Round or oval with smooth contour
  - Homogeneous appearance
    - Typically fluid attenuation on CT
    - Can have higher density with ↑ protein content, hemorrhage, or infection
    - Wall of cyst is thin and does not enhance unless complicated by infection
  - Variable low T1 and homogeneously increased T2 signal on MR
    - Characteristically thin and nonenhancing wall unless infected
- **Trauma**
  - Most common cause of death in children
  - Mediastinal hematoma is cause of mediastinal widening in trauma
  - Traumatic aortic injuries are uncommon
    - Iatrogenic trauma is most common cause of aortic injury in children

- Aortic injury most common in teens
- Associated traumatic injuries are common

- **Enlargement of Ascending Aorta**
  - Aortic valve stenosis
    - Results in poststenotic dilatation
    - Can be valvular, subaortic, or supravalvular
    - Valvular aortic stenosis is most common
    - Can be seen in Turner syndrome and is associated with bicuspid aortic valve and coarctation of aorta
    - Supravalvar aortic stenosis is seen in Williams syndrome
  - Dilated aorta often caused by aneurysm
    - Causes of aortic aneurysm: Connective tissue disorders, vasculitis, trauma, or infection
  - Connective tissue disorders: Marfan syndrome, Ehlers-Danlos, Loeys-Dietz
    - Marfan and Ehlers-Danlos are disorders of collagen synthesis
    - Dilatation of sinus of Valsalva and ascending aorta
    - Other systemic manifestations
  - Vasculitis: Takayasu arteritis
    - Large vessel vasculitis
    - Affects aorta, its main branches, and pulmonary arteries
  - Mycotic aneurysm
    - Uncommon in children
    - Can occur in infants secondary to umbilical arterial line

Helpful Clues for Rare Diagnoses

- **Germ Cell Tumor**
  - Originate from germ cells that fail to complete migration from urogenital ridge
  - Mediastinum is 4th most common site for teratoma (ovary, sacrococcygeal, testis)
  - Often contain tissues that derive from germinal cell layers
  - Can be cystic
- **Neurofibromatosis Type 1**
  - Autosomal dominant disorder
  - Classical clinical findings of café au lait spots, axillary freckling, and dermal and plexiform neurofibromas
  - Plexiform neurofibromas can occur anywhere
  - Plexiform neurofibromas have targetoid appearance on MR
    - Loss of targetoid appearance should raise concern for degeneration into malignant peripheral nerve sheath tumor
- **Thyroid Carcinoma**
  - Uncommon in children
  - Most common pediatric endocrine tumor
  - Thyroid nodules seen in up to 1.5%
    - Nodules > 1 cm should be biopsied
  - Radiation exposure is risk factor

Normal Thymus

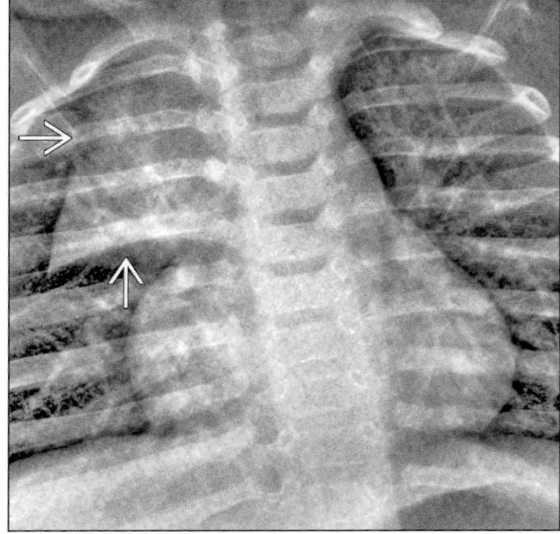

PA radiograph of the chest shows a sail-like appearance of the normal thymus ➡. The lateral border of the thymus typically has an undulating contour along the anterior lateral chest wall.

Normal Thymus

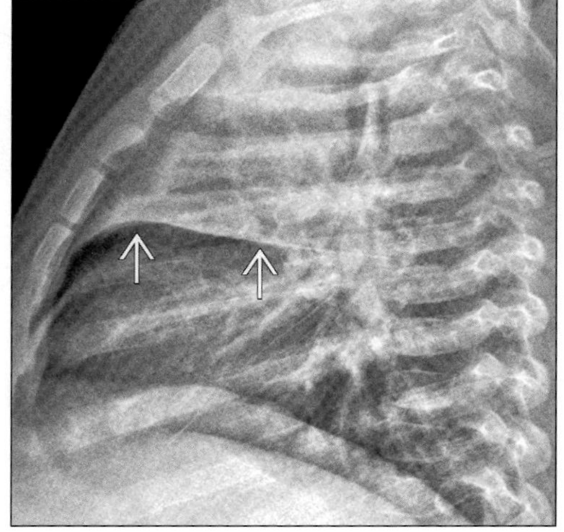

Lateral radiograph of the chest in the same patient shows the thymus in the anterior mediastinum filling in the retrosternal clear space ➡. This is a typical finding in young children.

MEDIASTINAL WIDENING

*(**Left**) Longitudinal ultrasound shows the normal thymus ➔ just below the anterior chest wall. On ultrasound, the thymus has multiple linear echoes and discrete echogenic foci. Ultrasound is useful to distinguish a normal thymus from a mediastinal mass. (**Right**) Axial CECT shows the normal thymus ➔ draped over the superior aspect of the heart. On CT, the thymus has a homogeneous soft tissue density with homogeneous enhancement.*

Normal Thymus

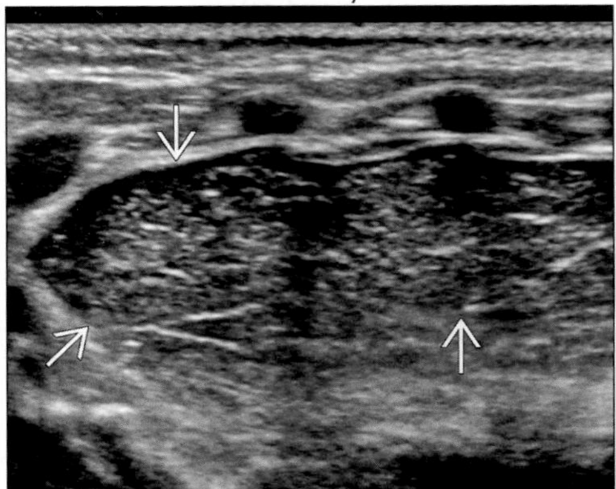

Normal Thymus

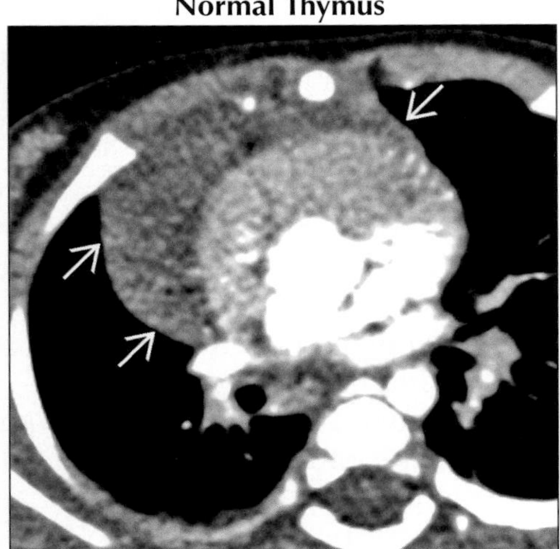

*(**Left**) PA radiograph of the chest shows abnormal widening of the mediastinum ➔ with bulging contours. Lymphoma is 3rd most common malignancy in children & the most common cause of mediastinal masses in teenagers. (**Right**) Axial CECT shows bulky mediastinal adenopathy ➔. Mediastinal disease can be present with both Hodgkin & non-Hodgkin lymphoma. The mediastinal mass can compress the trachea and lead to respiratory distress.*

Lymphoma

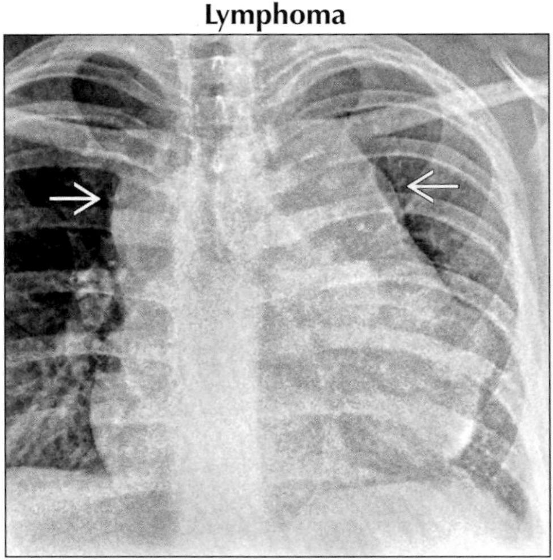

Lymphoma

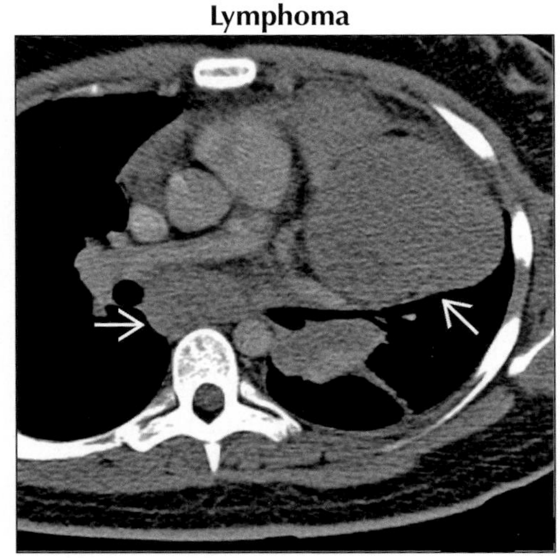

*(**Left**) Coronal PET/CT in the same patient shows extensive uptake of F18-FDG in the mediastinum ➔, left supraclavicular nodes ➔, and the spleen ➔. (**Right**) PA radiograph of the chest in a different pediatric patient shows left-sided mediastinal widening ➔. Lymphoma is more common in adolescents and young adults. Its incidence increases with age and accounts for 15% of all cancers in children 15-19 years old.*

Lymphoma

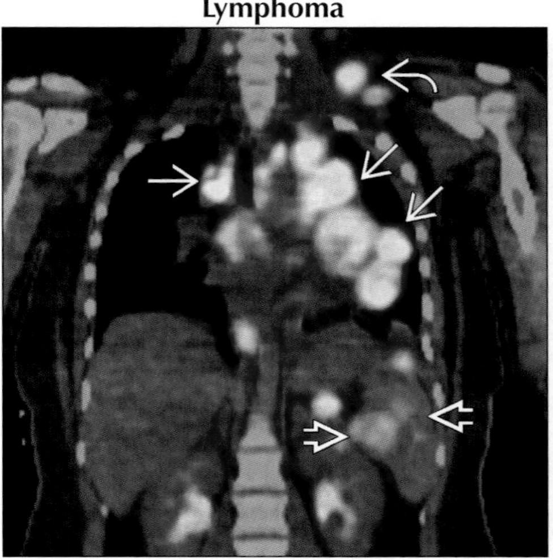

Lymphoma

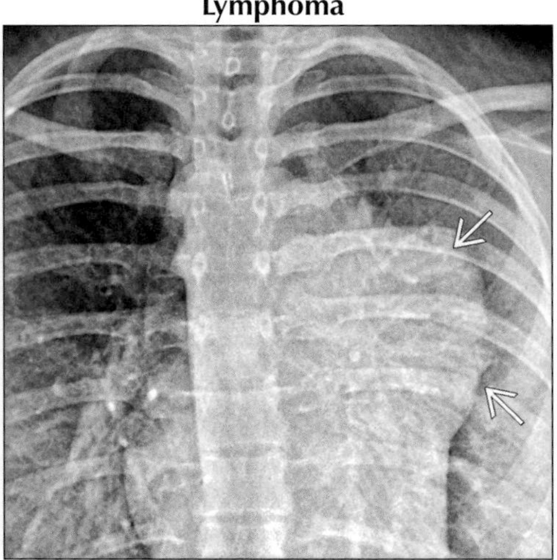

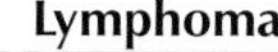

Lymphoma

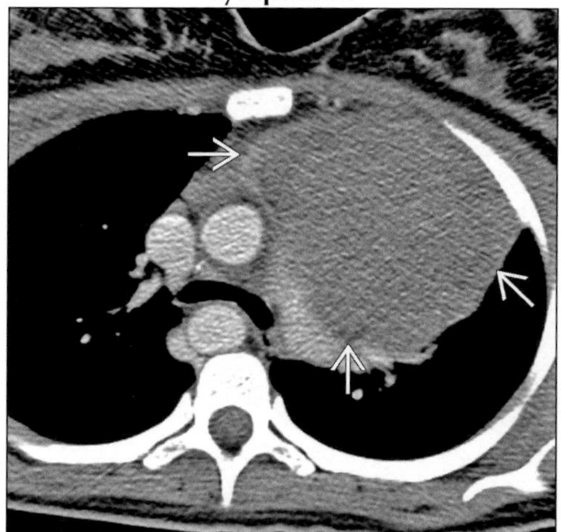

Lymphoma

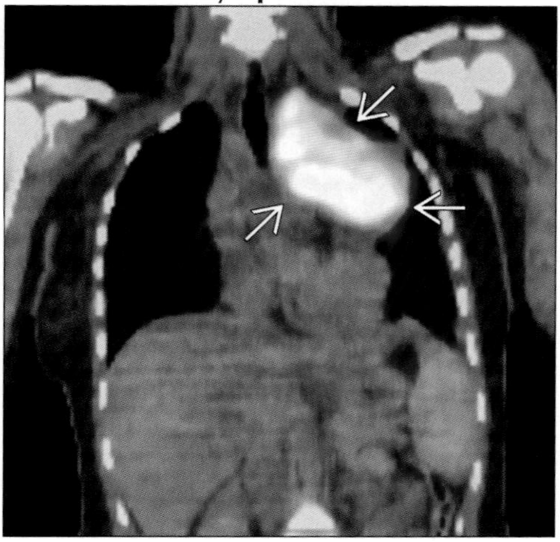

(Left) *Axial CECT in the same patient shows a large nodal mass in the anterior mediastinum →. The mass has a relatively homogeneous appearance, typical of lymphoma.* ***(Right)*** *Coronal PET/CT in the same patient shows intense F18-FDG uptake in the nodal mass within the left mediastinum →. PET/CT is a useful modality to evaluate lymphoma. In children, Hodgkin lymphoma is more common than non-Hodgkin lymphoma.*

Reactive Lymphadenopathy

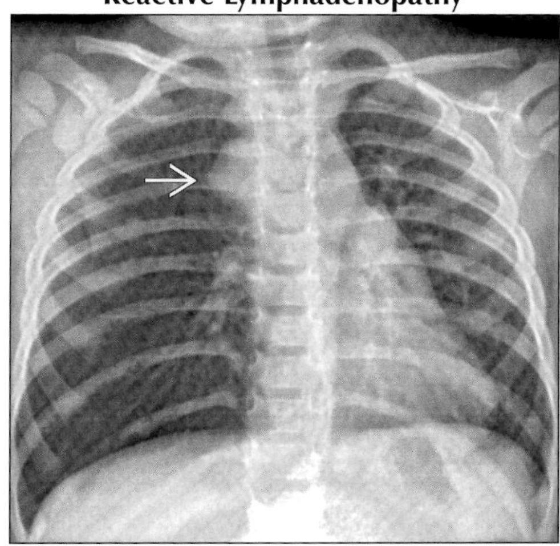

Reactive Lymphadenopathy

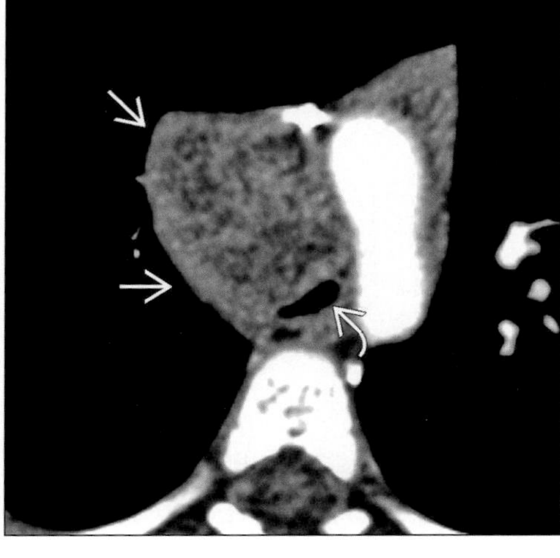

(Left) *PA radiograph shows a right paratracheal mass →. The mass is compressing the trachea displacing it to the left. The right lung is hyperinflated and more lucent than the left.* ***(Right)*** *Axial CECT in the same patient shows an enlarged right paratracheal lymph node → compressing the trachea ↷. A partially calcified pulmonary nodule was present in the right lower lobe (not shown). This reactive lymphadenopathy was caused by histoplasmosis.*

Bronchogenic Cyst

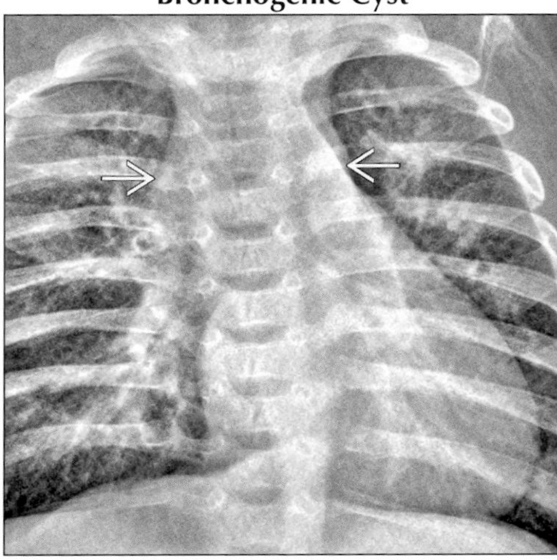

Bronchogenic Cyst

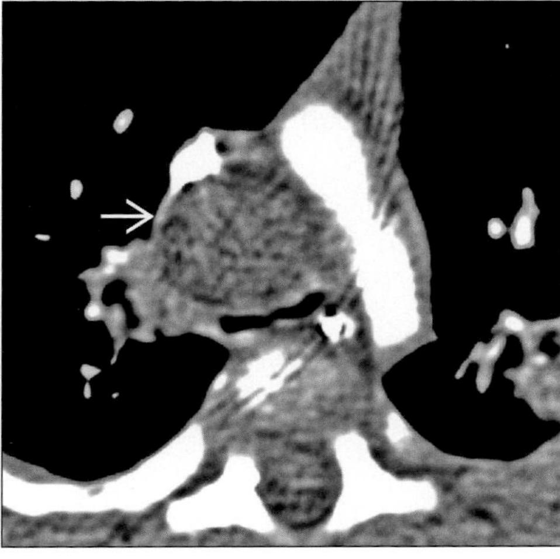

(Left) *PA radiograph of the chest shows widening of the upper mediastinum →. Bronchogenic cysts are usually located in a paratracheal or subcarinal location.* ***(Right)*** *Axial CECT shows a circular low-density mass in the pretracheal region →. The mass has a thin enhancing wall but otherwise has fluid density characteristic of a bronchogenic cyst. Bronchogenic cysts can cause compression of the airway leading to either atelectasis or hyperinflation.*

MEDIASTINAL WIDENING

(***Left***) *AP radiograph of the chest shows a widened mediastinum ➔ and a large right pneumothorax ↪. Traumatic aortic injuries are uncommon in children but become more frequent as they enter the late teen years.* (***Right***) *Axial CECT shows a mediastinal hematoma ➔ and hemothorax ↪. In older children and adults, the thymus normally has a concave border; mediastinal hematomas may cause the thymic border to become convex.*

Trauma

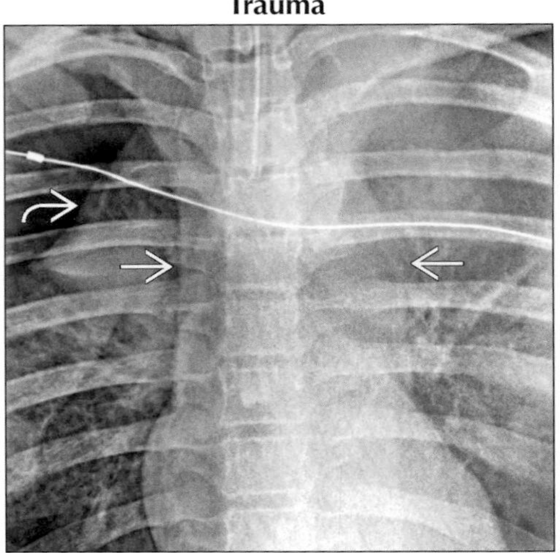

Trauma

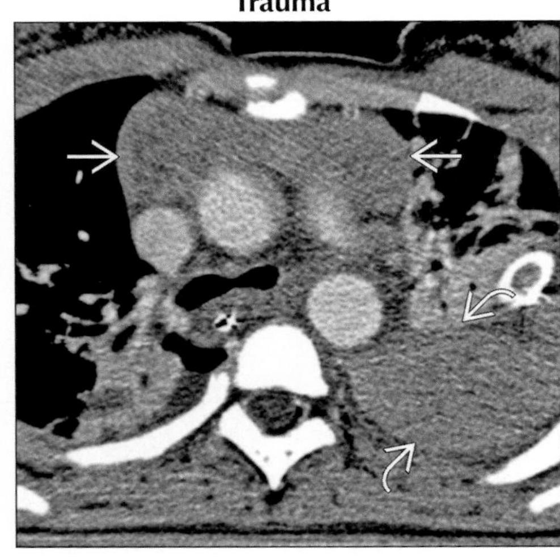

(***Left***) *AP scout image from a CT shows widening of the mediastinum ➔. Enlargement of the ascending aorta can have multiple causes.* (***Right***) *Axial CECT in a patient with Marfan syndrome shows marked dilation of the aortic root ➔. In children, common causes of an aortic aneurysm include connective tissue disorders, vasculitis, trauma, or infection. Marfan disease is a disorder of collagen synthesis.*

Enlargement of Ascending Aorta

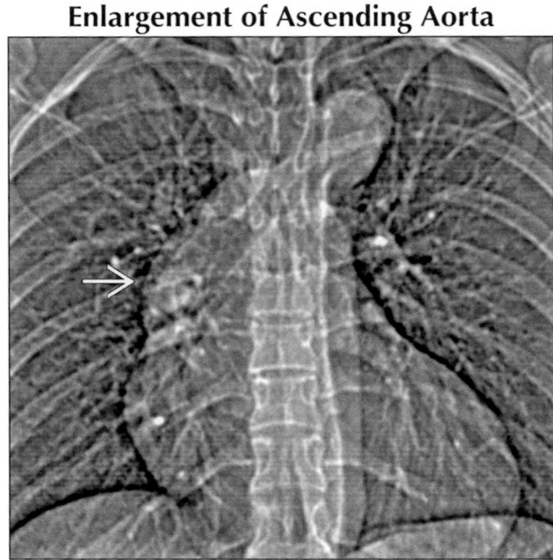

Enlargement of Ascending Aorta

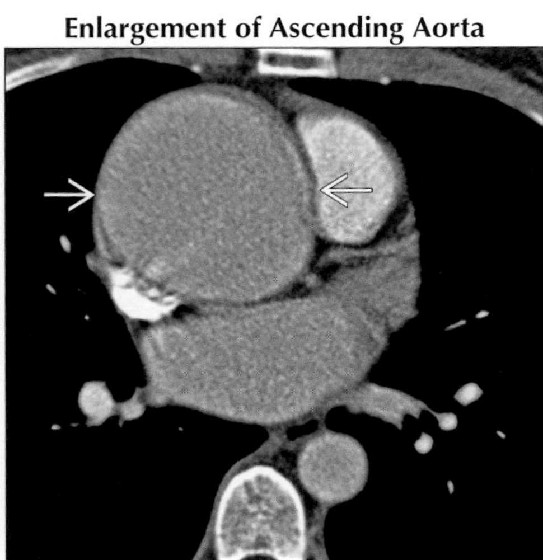

(***Left***) *Axial T1WI MR shows abnormal dilation of the ascending aorta. The wall of the aorta ➔ and right pulmonary artery ↪ are thickened. Takayasu arteritis is a large vessel vasculitis that affects the aorta, its branches, and the pulmonary arteries.* (***Right***) *Axial T1WI C+ FS MR shows enhancement and thickening of the wall of the descending aorta ➔. Takayasu arteritis is a chronic vasculitis of unknown etiology.*

Enlargement of Ascending Aorta

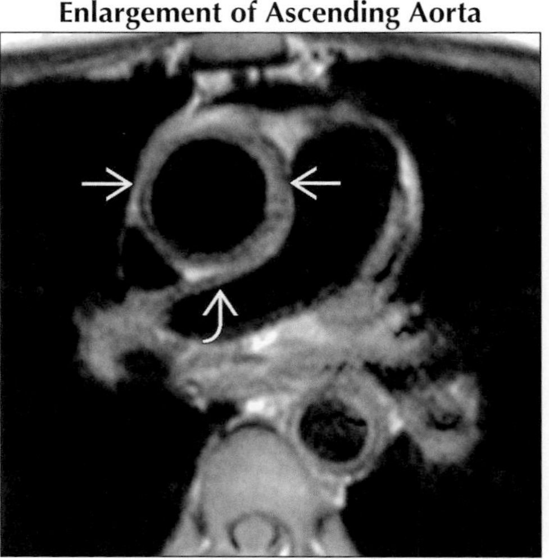

Enlargement of Ascending Aorta

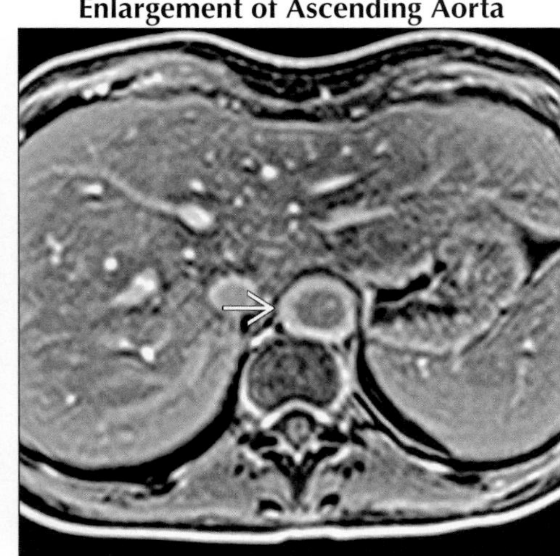

Germ Cell Tumor

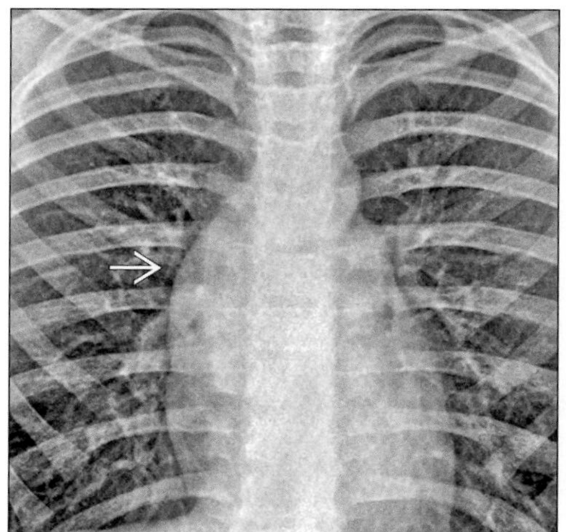

Germ Cell Tumor

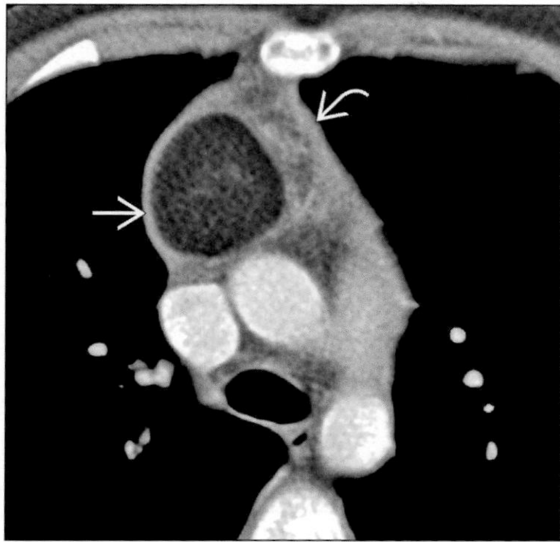

(Left) *PA radiograph of the chest shows an abnormal contour of the right heart border ➔. Germ cell tumors originate from germ cells that fail to complete migration from the urogenital ridge.* ***(Right)*** *Axial CECT shows a mass of the anterior mediastinum ➔. The mass has a mix of fat and soft tissue density ➔. The mediastinum is the 4th most common location for germ cell tumors after the ovaries, sacrococcygeal region, and testis.*

Neurofibromatosis Type 1

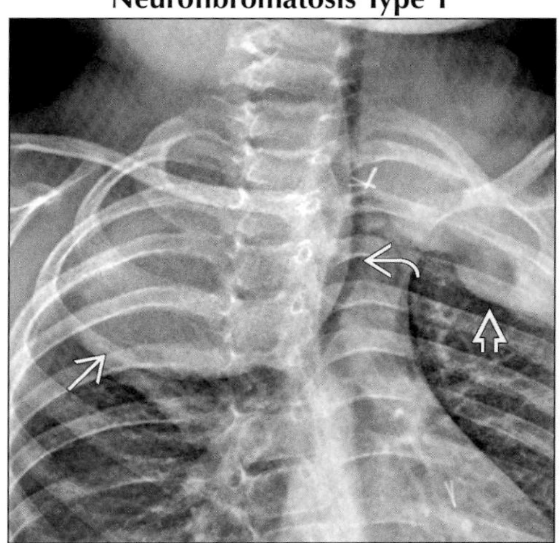

Neurofibromatosis Type 1

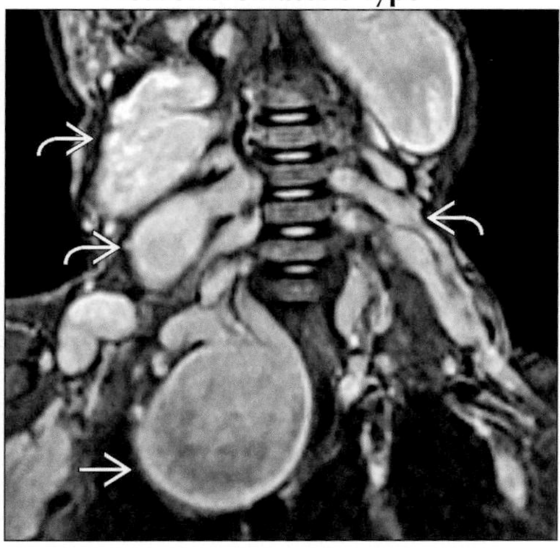

(Left) *PA radiograph of the chest shows a large mass in the upper chest/mediastinum ➔. The mass is displacing the trachea to the left ➔. A lobulated mass is also present in the left apex ➔. Neurofibromatosis type 1 is an autosomal dominant disorder.* ***(Right)*** *Coronal T2WI MR shows a large plexiform neurofibroma in the upper mediastinum ➔. There are extensive neurofibromas along every cervical nerve ➔.*

Thyroid Carcinoma

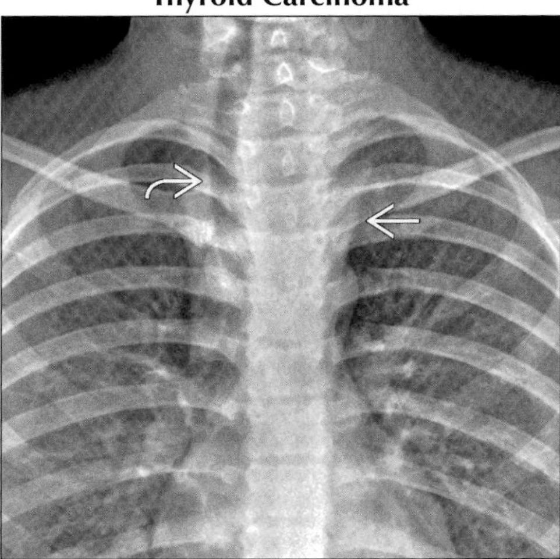

Thyroid Carcinoma

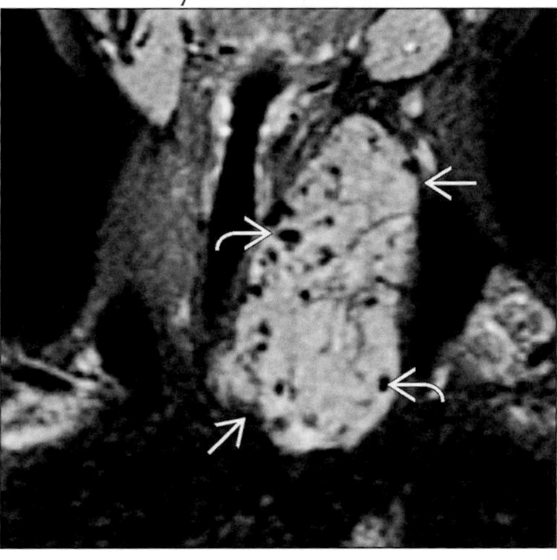

(Left) *PA radiograph of the chest shows a mass in the upper mediastinum ➔ displacing the trachea to the right ➔. Thyroid carcinoma is uncommon in children, although it is the most common pediatric endocrine tumor.* ***(Right)*** *Coronal T2WI MR shows a large hyperintense mass in the left neck ➔ with extent to the upper mediastinum. The mass has multiple flow voids ➔. Radiation exposure is a risk factor for development of thyroid carcinoma in children.*

ANTERIOR MEDIASTINAL MASS

DIFFERENTIAL DIAGNOSIS

Common
- Normal Thymus
- Rebound Thymic Hyperplasia
- Lymphoma

Less Common
- Germ Cell Tumor
- Lymphatic Malformation
- Thymic Cyst

Rare but Important
- Langerhans Cell Histiocytosis
- Morgagni Hernia

ESSENTIAL INFORMATION

Helpful Clues for Common Diagnoses
- **Normal Thymus**
  - Most common anterior mediastinal "mass" in neonates and infants
  - Has quadrilateral shape in infancy
  - Gradually becomes triangular-shaped in later childhood and teenage years
  - Thymus increases in weight until adolescence when it begins to involute
  - Most prominent in infancy
  - Visible on frontal radiograph until ~ 5 years of age
  - Appearance may change with phase of respiration
  - Look for "spinnaker sail" sign, "notch" sign, and "wave" sign
  - May be asymmetric across midline
  - Can extend inferiorly to drape over heart, superiorly into neck, or posteriorly to involute between great vessels and trachea
  - Homogeneous appearance on CT and MR, enhancing homogeneously following contrast administration
  - Typical sonographic appearance of multiple linear echoes and discrete echogenic foci
- **Rebound Thymic Hyperplasia**
  - Thymus can vary in size depending on intercurrent illness and stress
    - May decrease in size during illness/stress and with subsequent increase in size with recovery
    - Stressors include burns, surgery, and chemotherapy
  - Maintains normal attenuation and signal on CT and MR respectively
  - Maintains normal configuration on cross sectional imaging
  - Also maintains normal gross architecture and histologic appearance
- **Lymphoma**
  - Most common anterior mediastinal mass in teenagers
  - Distorts shape of thymus, which assumes lobulated or biconvex contour
  - Mass usually crosses midline
  - May be homogeneous or heterogeneous soft tissue mass on CT and MR
  - Positron emission tomography (PET) imaging best identifies involved nodes and extent of involvement elsewhere
  - May become more heterogeneous while it is being treated or if it rapidly enlarges and outgrows blood supply
  - May be associated with involvement of lymph nodes in hila and in other mediastinal compartments
  - Pleural and pericardial involvement, especially effusions, not uncommon; lung involvement is unusual
  - May displace trachea and vessels
  - Superior vena caval invasion and occlusion may cause SVC syndrome

Helpful Clues for Less Common Diagnoses
- **Germ Cell Tumor**
  - Pediatric patients (~ 66%) usually present with symptoms
  - 2nd most common extragonadal site after sacrococcygeal region
  - Occurs within or near thymus
  - Majority are mature teratomas (60%); seminoma is next most common
    - Less common are teratocarcinoma, endodermal sinus tumor, choriocarcinoma, and embryonal cell carcinoma
  - Tumors have lobulated or smooth contour on radiography; constituent elements may be identified, especially calcification
  - Intrinsic elements are better identified on CT

- CT appearances may be homogeneously cystic or soft tissue in appearance, contain well-demarcated fat, fluid, soft tissue, or calcific elements, or may have heterogeneous soft tissue appearance
- Calcifications are usually coarse
- May be well demarcated or inseparable from vascular structures
- Tumors are more commonly unilateral but may extend across midline

- **Lymphatic Malformation**
  - Formerly called cystic hygroma or lymphangioma
  - Usually detected on prenatal imaging or in neonatal period
  - Most often represents mediastinal extension from neck lesion but can be solely mediastinal
  - May be associated with more generalized lymphatic problem
  - Thin-walled fluid-filled structure, which may be focal but may also be multifocal or infiltrative and involve mediastinal compartments
- **Thymic Cyst**
  - May extend superiorly into neck between carotid artery and jugular vein
  - Usually thin walled and fluid filled
  - Rarely may have partial wall calcification
  - Can be congenital or postinflammatory

Helpful Clues for Rare Diagnoses

- **Langerhans Cell Histiocytosis**
  - Thymic involvement occurs commonly in multisystem disease
  - Most commonly presents as diffuse enlargement but can have focal lesion, usually cystic area on CT
  - Contour may be smooth or lobulated
  - Involved thymus is heterogeneous in appearance on CT and MR
  - Irregular calcifications and cystic lesions may be present
  - Calcifications are usually subtle in comparison to those seen in germ cell tumors and are usually only visible on CT
  - Enlarged, involved gland can displace trachea and great vessels, unlike normal thymus
  - Appearance of thymus reverts to normal with therapy
- **Morgagni Hernia**
  - Anteromedial parasternal defect of diaphragm, adjacent to xiphoid process
  - 90% occur on right side; right cardiophrenic angle on radiography
  - More commonly asymptomatic than Bochdalek type of congenital diaphragmatic hernia
  - Contents of hernia are variable but most commonly contain omentum with liver and bowel less common; contents determine radiographic appearance
  - Nature of contents is more easily assessed on CT and MR
  - Occasionally diagnosed on barium study

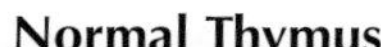

Normal Thymus

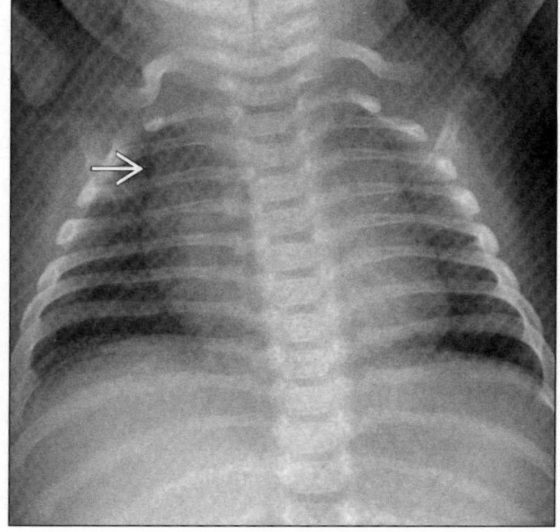

AP radiograph shows a quadrilateral shape to the thymus ➔ in a 5-week-old infant. The thymus can have a variety of appearances in infants and can be difficult to separate from the heart.

Normal Thymus

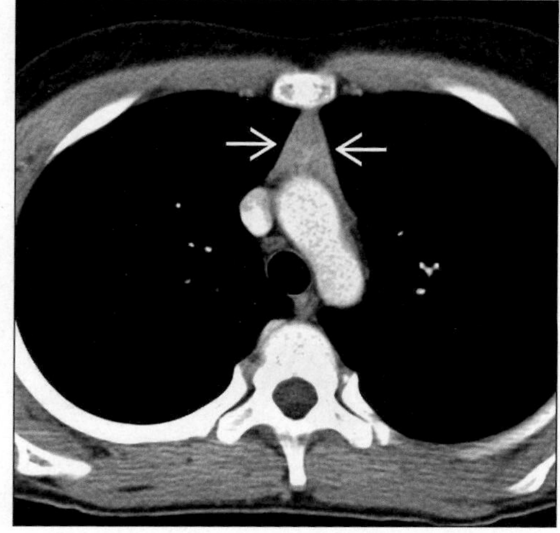

Axial CECT shows the normal appearance of the thymus in a teenager. The gland has a homogeneous attenuation and is triangular in shape with either straight or slightly concave borders ➔.

ANTERIOR MEDIASTINAL MASS

*(**Left**) Anteroposterior radiograph shows 2 signs of a normal thymus. The right lobe projects away from the heart and has a sharp inferior border → and a curved lateral border ↷, the "spinnaker sail" sign. Note the undulations of the lateral margin of the thymus ("wave" sign). (**Right**) AP radiograph shows the thymus ➦ extending to the left side of the mediastinum. Although a bilobed structure, the right lobe is more often prominent than the left.*

Normal Thymus

Normal Thymus

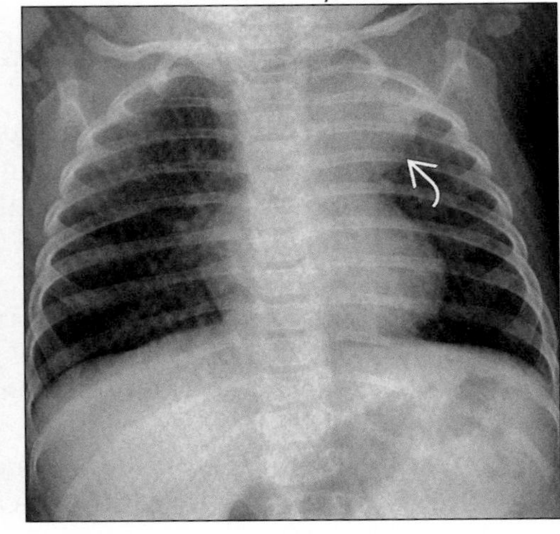

*(**Left**) Anteroposterior radiograph shows a large cardiomediastinal silhouette →. On a lateral view, this was seen to be confined to the anterior mediastinum. The thymus is variable in size and shape, which depends on multiple variables, including the age and health of the patient. It can extend into the neck or other compartments of the mediastinum. (**Right**) Coronal CECT shows the typical homogeneous attenuation of the thymus draping over the heart ➡.*

Normal Thymus

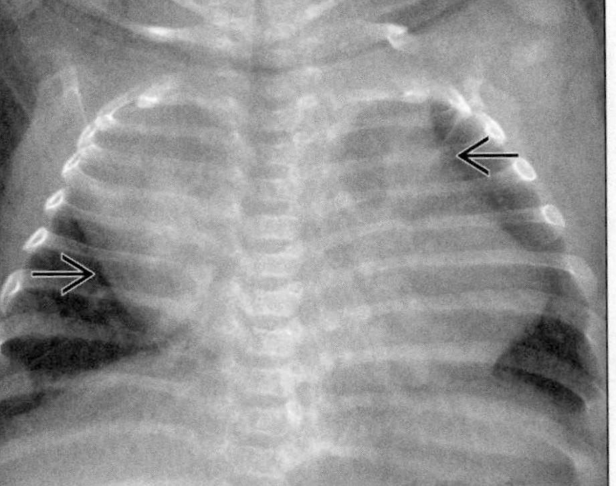

Normal Thymus

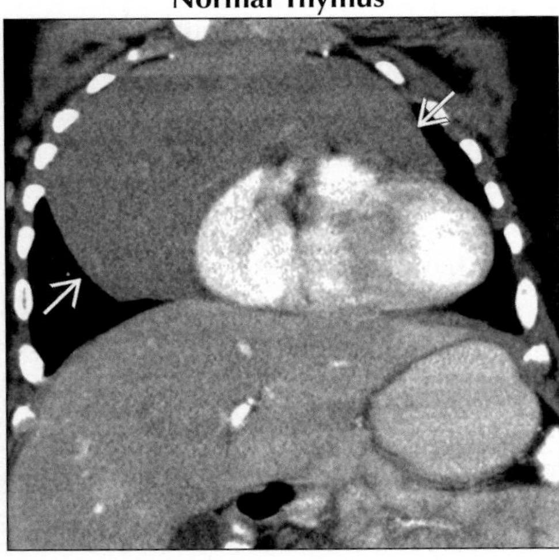

*(**Left**) Axial CECT shows the normal homogeneous attenuation of the thymus on CT. The thymus may extend superiorly into the neck or posteriorly ➦ between the SVC ➡ and trachea →. The thymus is soft and normally does not compress structures. (**Right**) Transverse ultrasound shows the normal sonographic appearance of the thymus with linear ➦ and speckled echoes ➡. The relatively large thymus of infants can often be imaged easily on ultrasound.*

Normal Thymus

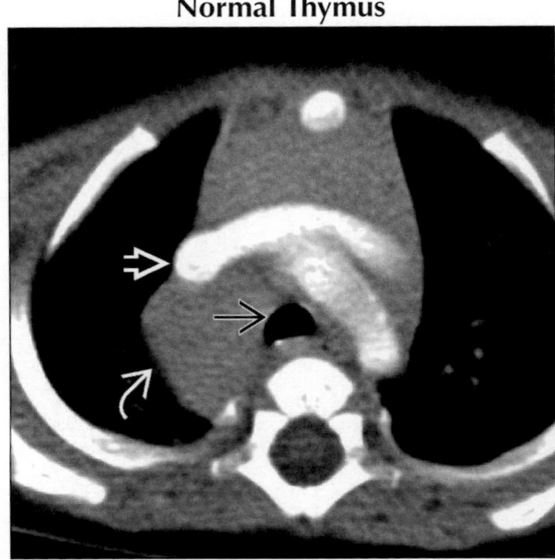

Normal Thymus

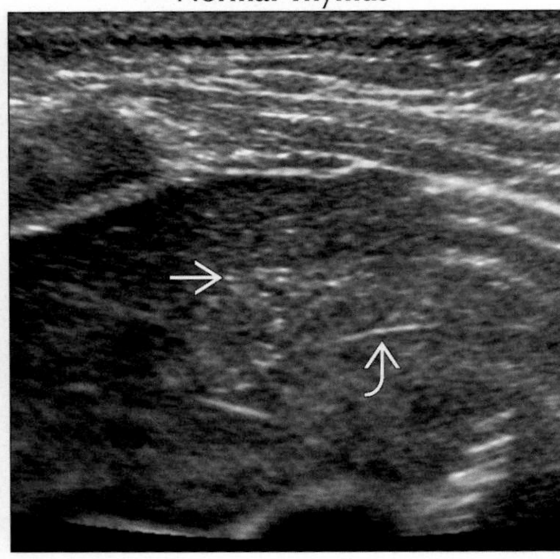

Rebound Thymic Hyperplasia

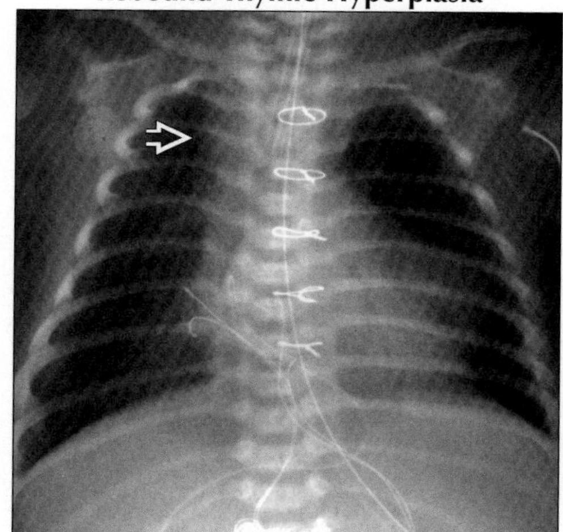

Rebound Thymic Hyperplasia

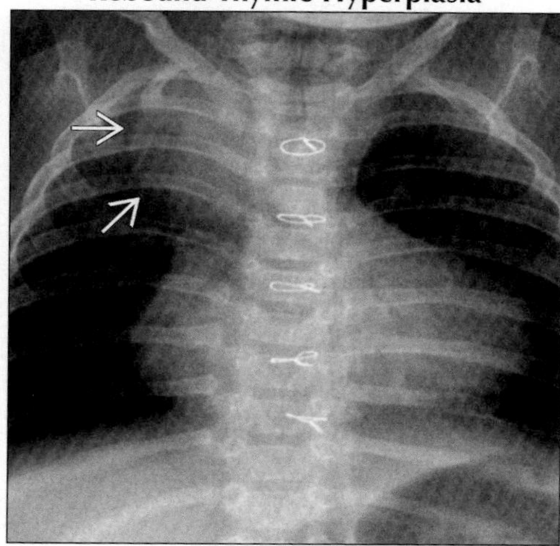

(Left) *Anteroposterior radiograph shows a mild convexity to the right side of the mediastinum ➔ in this patient 11 days following cardiac surgery. The thymus may decrease in size with stress, most often seen with chemotherapy, extensive burns, and following surgery.* ***(Right)*** *Anteroposterior radiograph shows a rebound increase in the size of the thymus ➔ 5 months following surgery in the same patient. This was confirmed as a normal thymus on ultrasound.*

Lymphoma

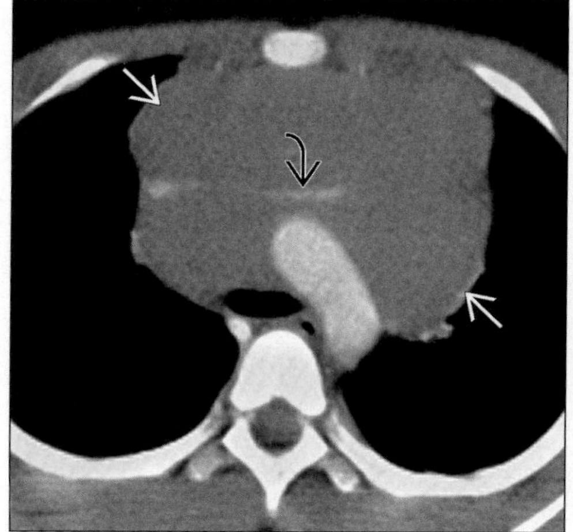

Lymphoma

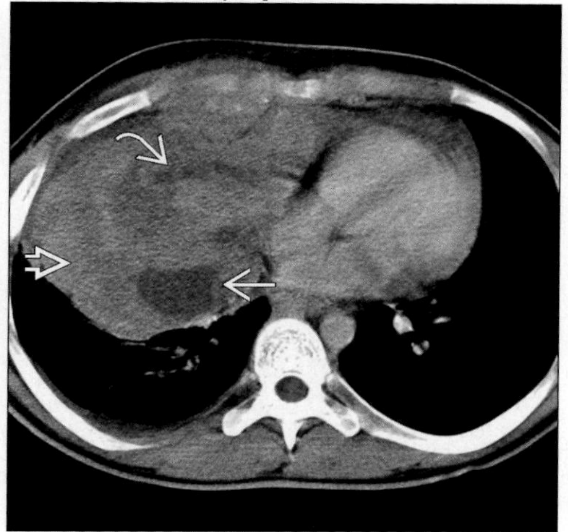

(Left) *Axial CECT shows a well-circumscribed homogeneous mass ➔ of soft tissue attenuation predominantly in the anterior mediastinum. This mass compresses the left brachiocephalic ➔ vein but does not occlude it.* ***(Right)*** *Axial CECT shows a heterogeneous mass in the anterior mediastinum. Areas of intermediate soft tissue attenuation material ➔ are interspersed with lower attenuation areas ➔. Some are cyst-like ➔, suggesting necrosis.*

Lymphoma

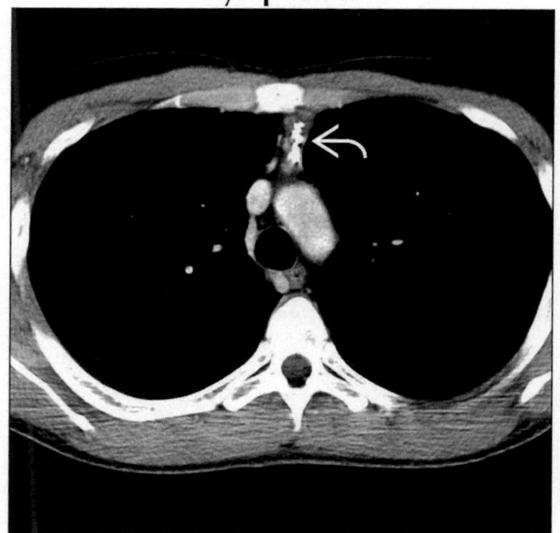

Lymphoma

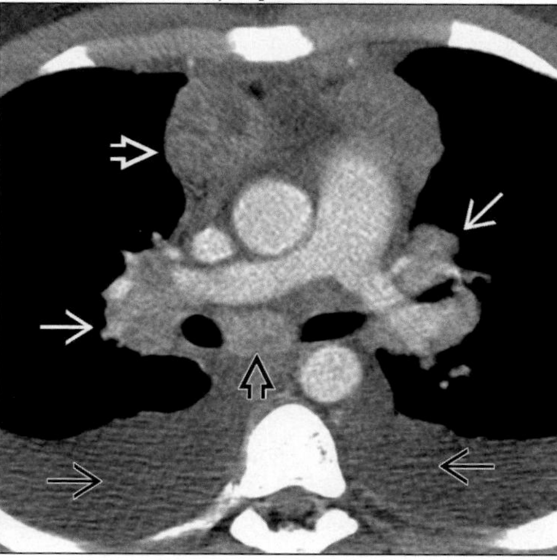

(Left) *Axial CECT shows coarse foci of calcification in the anterior mediastinum ➔ in a patient who had been treated successfully for lymphoma. Calcification may be seen in previously involved lymph nodes following therapy.* ***(Right)*** *Axial CECT shows multicompartment involvement with disease in the anterior mediastinum ➔, the middle mediastinum ➔, and the hila ➔, as well as bilateral pleural effusions ➔, findings that are consistent with lymphoma.*

ANTERIOR MEDIASTINAL MASS

(Left) *Axial NECT shows an area of fat attenuation ➔ in the anterior mediastinum. This is a good example of the superiority of CT over conventional radiography as this fatty lesion was not identified on a preceding radiograph.* **(Right)** *Axial CECT shows a partially fluid ➔, partially fatty ➔ mass. A mass in the anterior mediastinum containing multiple elements (soft tissue, fat, calcification, and fluid) is typical of a mature teratoma.*

Germ Cell Tumor

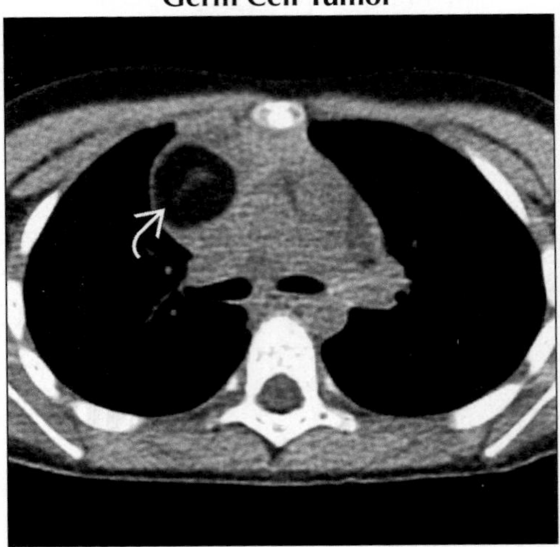

Germ Cell Tumor

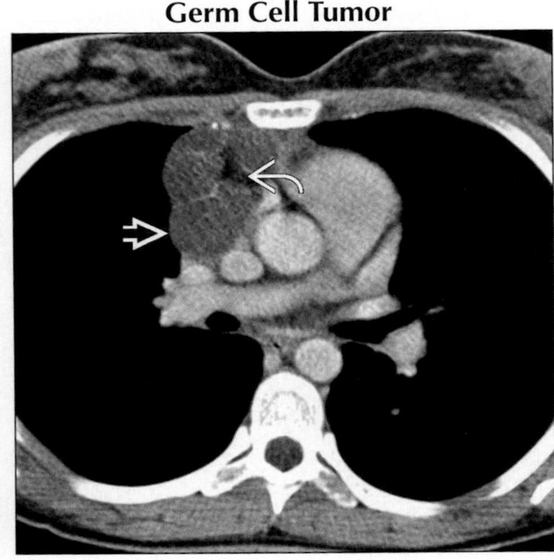

(Left) *Axial T2WI FS MR shows a lobulated mass of increased signal predominantly in the anterior mediastinum ➔ with a low signal septation →. These lesions are large and cause severe respiratory distress in the neonatal period due to pressure on the trachea.* **(Right)** *Coronal T1WI C+ FS MR shows the mass ➔ also involving the neck. Enhancement of multiple septations ➔ is typical. The pointed inferior ends of the thymus lobes are seen ➔.*

Lymphatic Malformation

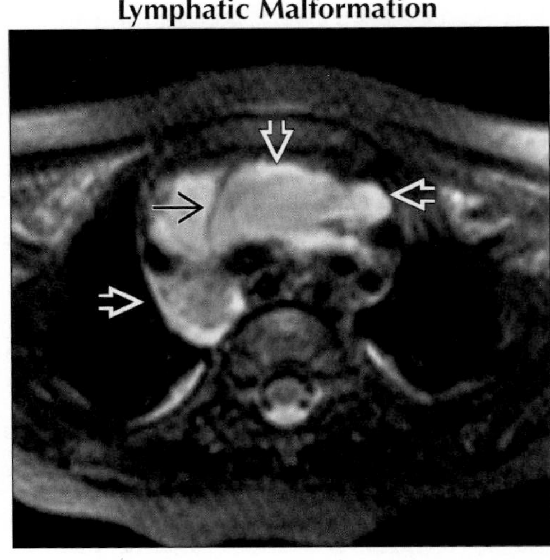

Lymphatic Malformation

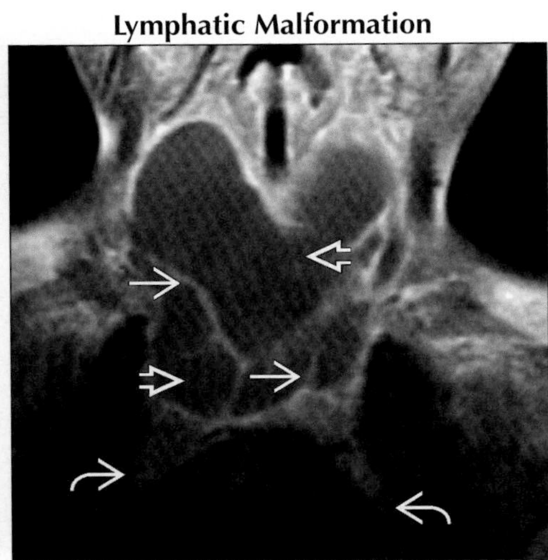

(Left) *Anteroposterior radiograph shows a narrowed trachea, which is deviated to the right ➔ in this neonate who presented with respiratory distress.* **(Right)** *Axial CECT shows a cystic mass ➔ extending into the anterior mediastinum in the expected location of the thymus. This cyst has an enhancing rim ➔, and the trachea is deviated to the right ➔. Thymic cysts, which grow into the neck, typically extend between the jugular vein and the carotid artery.*

Thymic Cyst

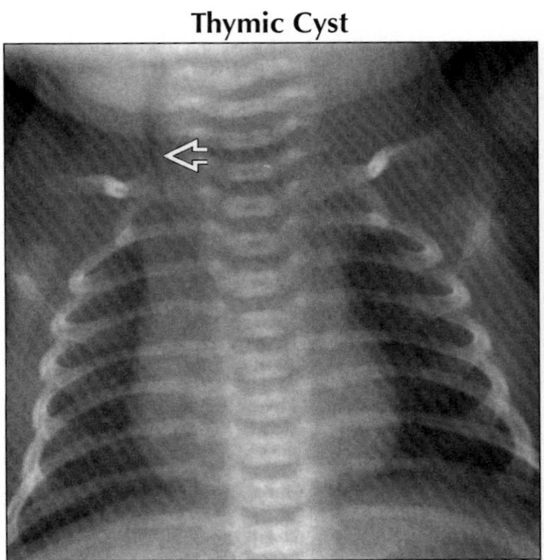

Thymic Cyst

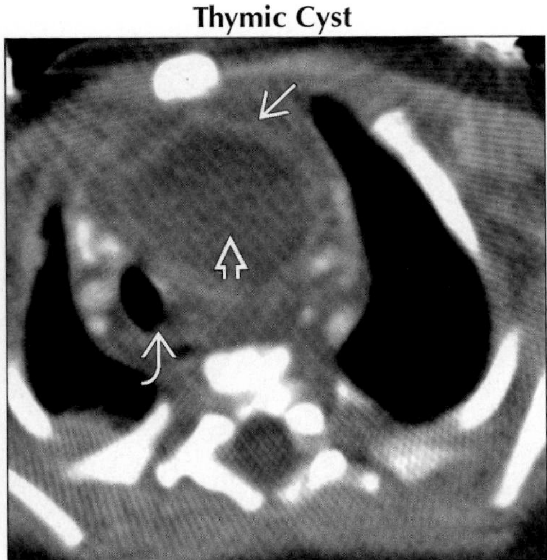

Langerhans Cell Histiocytosis

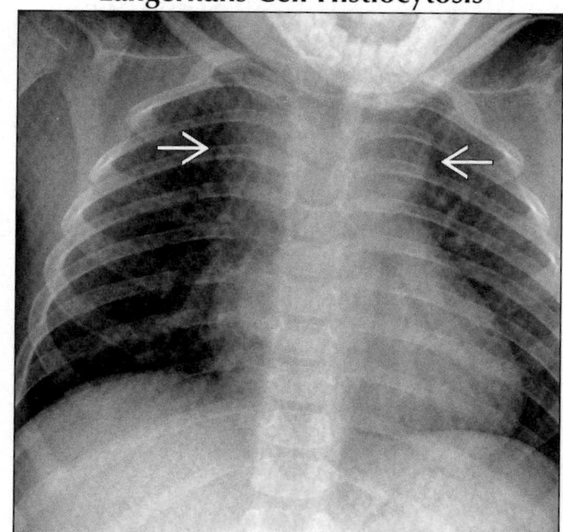

Langerhans Cell Histiocytosis

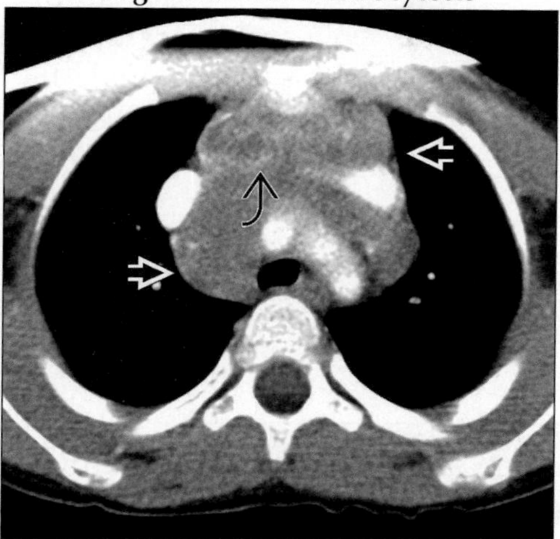

(Left) *Anteroposterior radiograph shows a convex appearance to both sides of the mediastinum ➔ in a young child. The mediastinum should have straighter margins. The patient also had osseous lesions, consistent with Langerhans cell histiocytosis.* ***(Right)*** *Axial CECT in the same patient shows a mass ➔ in the anterior mediastinum, which extends into the middle mediastinum. The mass demonstrates some lacy calcification anteriorly ➔.*

Langerhans Cell Histiocytosis

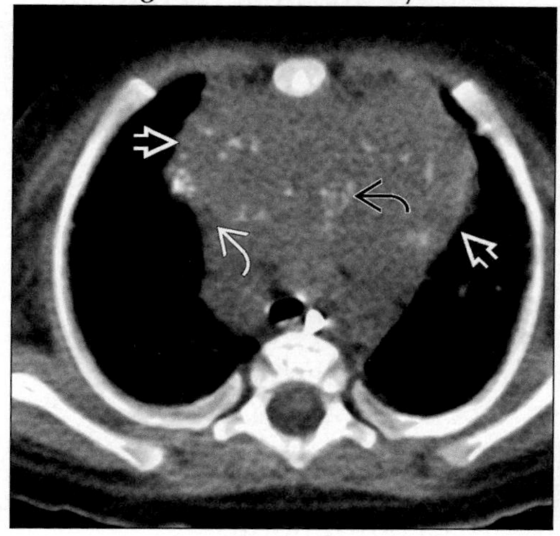

Langerhans Cell Histiocytosis

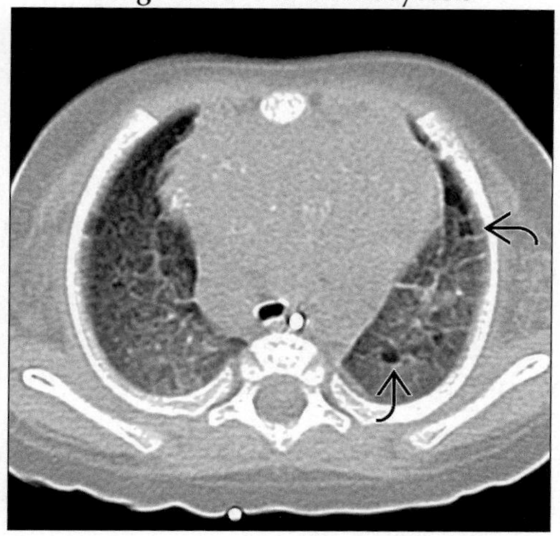

(Left) *Axial NECT shows a bulky mass ➔ in the anterior mediastinum. The mass caused lobulated diffuse enlargement of the thymus and is heterogeneous with foci of lace-like calcification ➔ and low-attenuation cystic areas ➔. The thymus is frequently involved in LCH when there are multiple organs involved.* ***(Right)*** *Axial NECT shows involvement of the lung parenchyma with small cysts ➔. Rupture of a peripheral cyst can lead to a pneumothorax.*

Morgagni Hernia

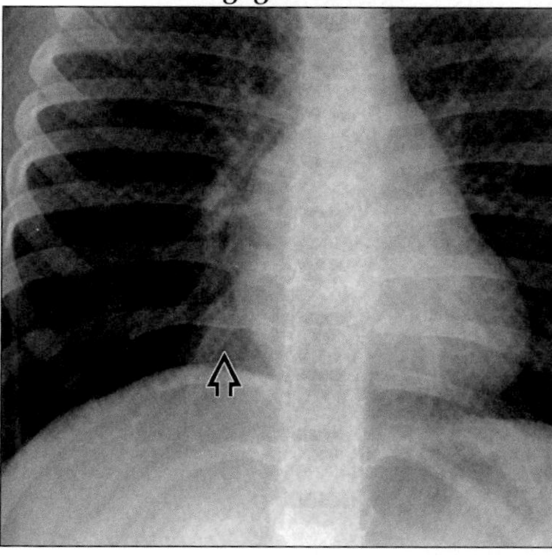

Morgagni Hernia

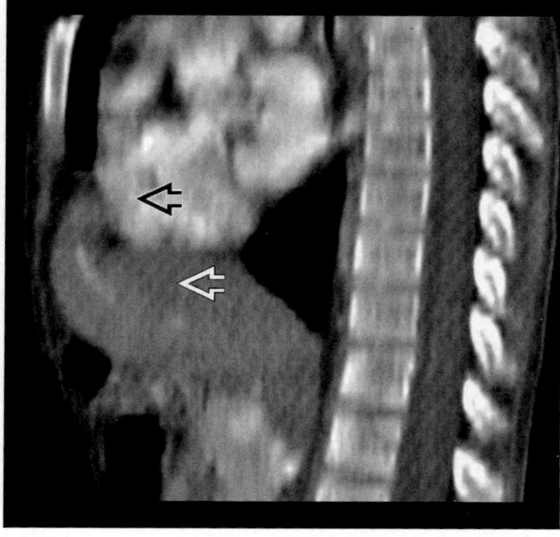

(Left) *Anteroposterior radiograph shows an opacity in the right cardiophrenic angle ➔, a typical location for a Morgagni hernia. A lateral radiograph (not shown) confirmed an anterior location.* ***(Right)*** *Sagittal CECT shows liver parenchyma ➔ extending superiorly anterior to the heart ➔. The content of the hernia is variable. Because of the location to the right of midline, herniation of the liver is common. Herniation of the bowel and omentum may also occur.*

MIDDLE MEDIASTINAL MASS

DIFFERENTIAL DIAGNOSIS

Common
- Lymphoma
- Bronchogenic Cyst

Less Common
- Lymphadenopathy
- Vascular Anomalies

Rare but Important
- Postoperative Complications
- Pericardial Lesions
- Malignant Tumors

ESSENTIAL INFORMATION

Helpful Clues for Common Diagnoses
- **Lymphoma**
  - Usually occurs with confluent multicompartment disease that involves anterior mediastinum
  - Most commonly involves paratracheal > hilar > subcarinal groups
  - Homogeneous or heterogeneous soft tissue attenuation and signal intensity on CT and MR
  - May compress or invade superior vena cava (SVC), esophagus, tracheobronchial tree, and pericardium
  - SVC more often compressed without associated obstruction, but invasion may lead to SVC syndrome
  - Bronchial involvement may lead to lobar collapse
  - Pericardial involvement can result in pericardial effusion
- **Bronchogenic Cyst**
  - May have bronchial or esophageal origin
  - Most commonly paratracheal or subcarinal
  - Collapse or hyperlucency may occur as result of bronchial compression
  - Usually round or oval with smooth contour
  - Homogeneous density on radiograph and attenuation on CT
    - Classically fluid attenuation but may be of higher attenuation due to high protein content
    - Wall of cyst is thin and does not enhance unless complicated by infection
  - Variable low T1 and homogeneously increased T2 signal on MR
    - Characteristically thin and nonenhancing wall unless infected

Helpful Clues for Less Common Diagnoses
- **Lymphadenopathy**
  - Usually related to infection in pediatric population
  - Most common inciting organism depends on geographic location
  - Consider primary tuberculosis (TB), histoplasmosis, coccidioidomycosis, and blastomycosis
    - TB and histoplasmosis may have lymph nodes with low-attenuation centers on contrast-enhanced CT in acute phase
    - Calcification of lymph nodes indicates more remote disease
- **Vascular Anomalies**
  - Most commonly due to congenital anomalies of aorta and its branches
    - Findings are more apparent on positive contrast studies of esophagus
    - Anomalous vessels are most easily seen on CT and MR
  - Convexity to right of trachea on radiograph may be due to right aortic arch or double aortic arch
  - Posterior impression/anterior bowing of trachea on lateral radiograph may be due to
    - Diverticulum of Kommerell related to aberrant subclavian artery
    - Passage of aorta across midline posterior to trachea and esophagus
  - Dilatation of ascending aorta
    - Seen in congenital aortic valvar or supravalvar stenosis (Turner syndrome and Williams syndrome)
    - Also may be seen in connective tissue disorders (Ehlers-Danlos and Marfan syndrome)
    - Convexity along right mediastinal border on chest radiograph
    - Dilatation of ascending aorta best seen on CT and MR
  - Pulmonary arterial lesions are less common
    - Anomalous origin of left pulmonary artery from right pulmonary artery (pulmonary arterial sling)
    - Left pulmonary artery passes between trachea and esophagus

- Passage of LPA between trachea and esophagus is best appreciated on CT and MR but also well seen on positive contrast studies of esophagus
  - Pulmonic valve stenosis may lead to poststenotic dilatation of main pulmonary arterial segment
    - Convexity in aortopulmonary window on radiography
    - Seen as dilatation of MPA on CT and MR
  - May also involve azygous vein and anomalous pulmonary venous drainage
    - Azygous vein enlargement leads to convexity above right main bronchus
    - Most commonly related to azygous continuation of IVC
    - May also be secondary to obstruction of SVC
    - Supracardiac type of anomalous pulmonary venous return leads to "snowman" appearance of mediastinum on radiograph

Helpful Clues for Rare Diagnoses

- **Postoperative Complications**
  - Some fluid always present in operative bed following cardiac surgery
    - Usually resolves in early days following surgery with gradual decrease in size of mediastinum
  - Concern if radiograph demonstrates increased widening of mediastinum
    - May be hematoma, seroma, or infection
  - Hematoma may be associated with pseudoaneurysm at surgical site
    - Contrast protrusion from vessel lumen on CT with signal changes of denatured blood and flow void on MR
- **Pericardial Lesions**
  - Pericardial effusion is seen as enlargement of cardiac silhouette with "water bottle" configuration on radiography
    - Lungs usually clear
    - "Fat pad" sign on lateral chest radiograph is rarely seen due to relative lack of fat in mediastinum in pediatric population
    - May be secondary to infection (most commonly viruses), following surgery or trauma, or related to neoplasia (lymphoma)
  - Pericardial cyst consists of various-sized loculations of fluid
    - Rounded convexity, most commonly in right cardiophrenic angle on radiography
    - Loculated fluid attenuation and signal on CT and MR respectively
  - Pericardial tumors are uncommon
- **Malignant Tumors**
  - Both primary and secondary malignant tumors are very rare, excluding lymphoma
  - Consider carcinoid, melanoma, rhabdomyosarcoma, malignant germ cell tumors, squamous cell carcinoma in patients with respiratory papillomatosis

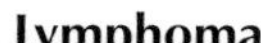

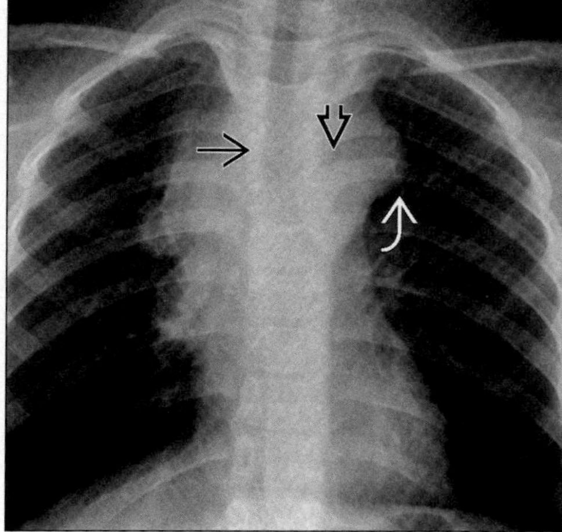

Posteroanterior radiograph shows a lobulated middle mediastinal mass with loss of the normal thin right paratracheal stripe and nonvisualization of the outline of the aortic arch.

Lymphoma

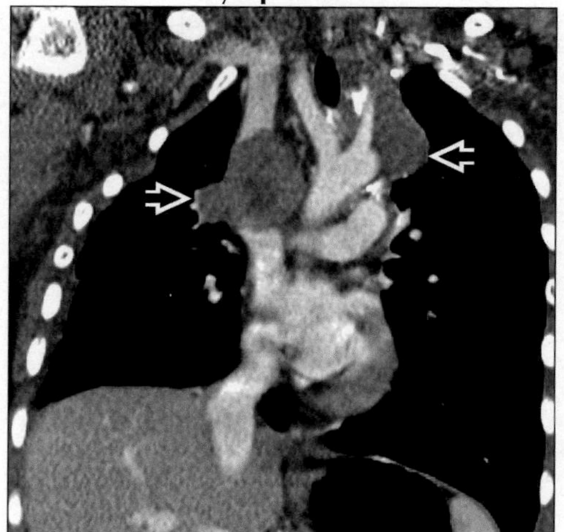

Coronal CECT shows the lobulated contour of the middle mediastinum due to involvement with lymphoma. Hodgkin and non-Hodgkin lymphoma cannot be differentiated by imaging.

MIDDLE MEDIASTINAL MASS

Lymphoma

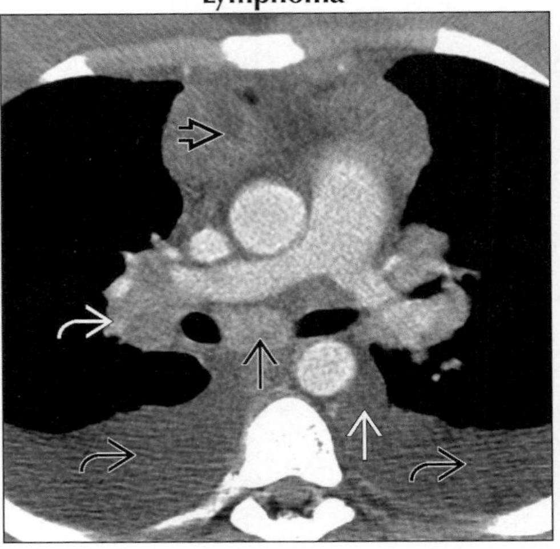

Lymphoma

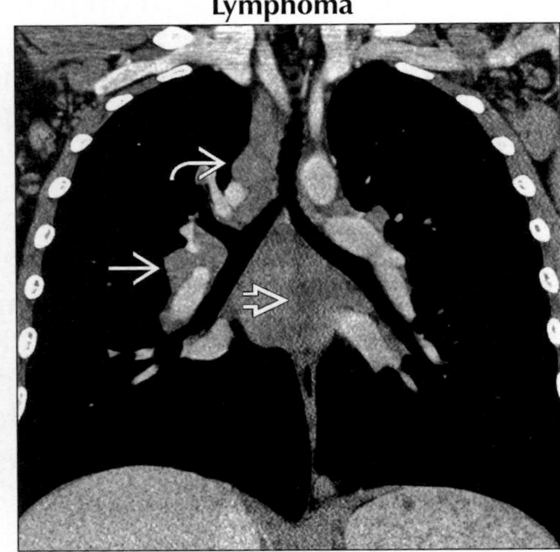

*(**Left**) Axial CECT shows a somewhat heterogeneous mass in the anterior, middle, and posterior mediastinum and in the right hilum. There are also bilateral pleural effusions. Lymphoma most commonly involves the anterior mediastinum but can involve the other mediastinal compartments. Pleural effusions are common. (**Right**) Coronal CECT shows the tumor involving the subcarinal, right paratracheal, and right hilar regions.*

Lymphoma

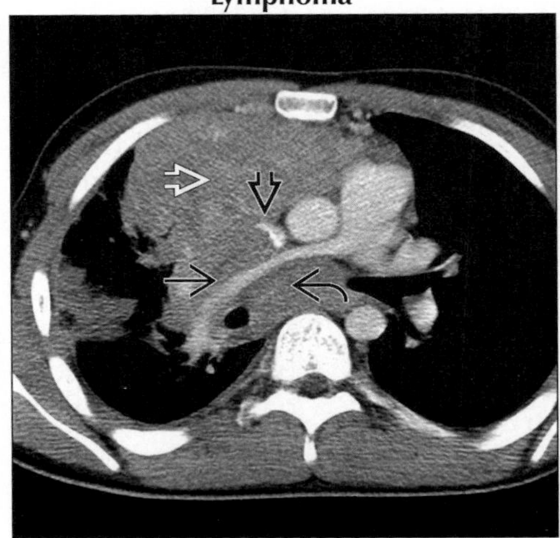

Lymphoma

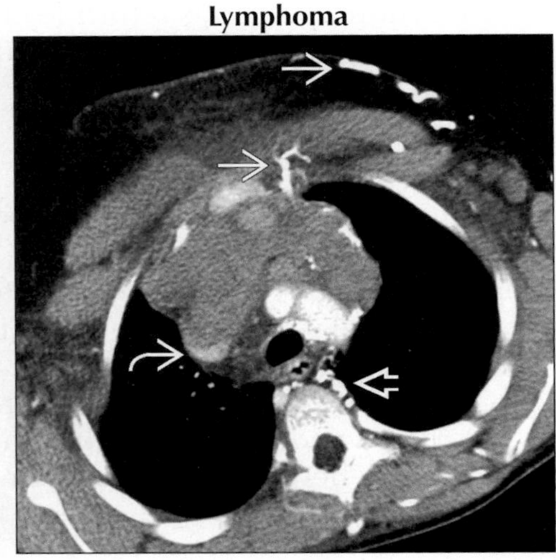

*(**Left**) Axial CECT shows a mass involving the anterior and middle mediastinum. The right pulmonary artery is stretched, and the SVC is compressed. Neither vessel was occluded. (**Right**) Axial CECT shows a nodal mass invading the superior vena cava. Note the numerous large collateral veins in the chest wall and in the paravertebral region. Lymphoma is the most common cause of SVC obstruction in pediatric patients.*

Lymphoma

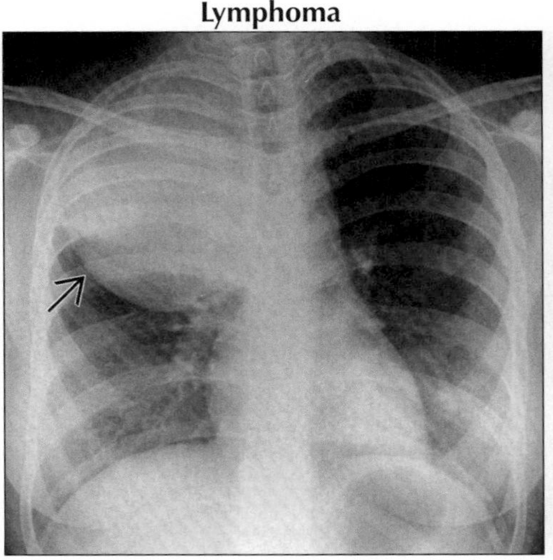

Lymphoma

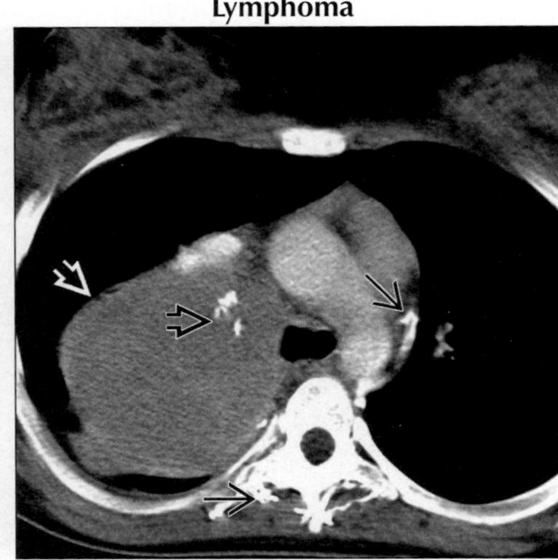

*(**Left**) Anteroposterior radiograph shows a large, well-circumscribed mass in the superior right hemithorax with loss of the paravertebral stripe. (**Right**) Axial CECT shows a soft tissue mass arising from the right paratracheal lymph nodes with collateral veins. There are calcifications within this mass related to prior infection. Calcifications in lymphoma are usually related to therapy or involvement of previously calcified nodes.*

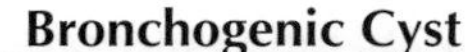

Bronchogenic Cyst | **Bronchogenic Cyst**

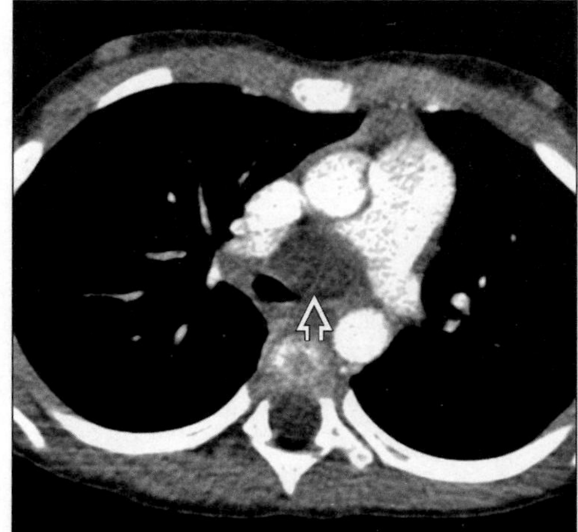

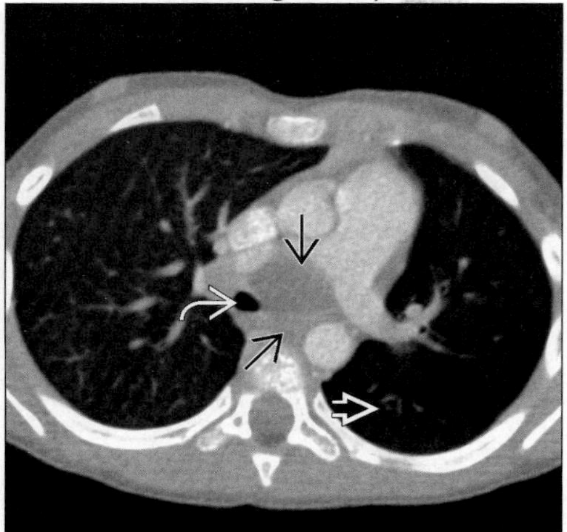

(Left) *Axial CECT shows a fluid attenuation mass in the subcarinal region. A bronchogenic cyst should be suspected when a thin-walled, fluid attenuation mass is seen in the middle mediastinum. The attenuation can be higher due to proteinaceous content.* ***(Right)*** *Axial CECT shows decreased attenuation of the left lung. The right main bronchus is visible, but the left is occluded due to compression from the cyst.*

Bronchogenic Cyst | **Bronchogenic Cyst**

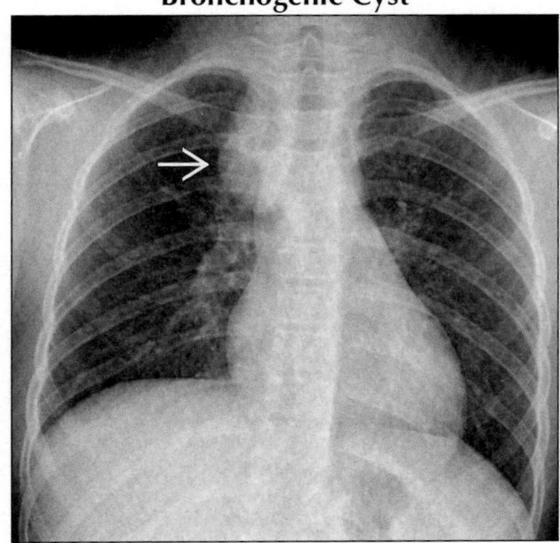

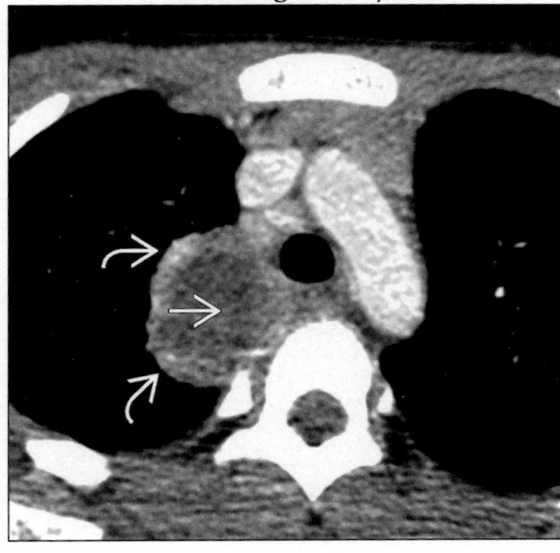

(Left) *Anteroposterior radiograph shows a well-circumscribed convexity in the right paratracheal region in a patient with a cough and fever.* ***(Right)*** *Axial CECT shows a low-attenuation mass in the right paratracheal region with a thick wall. At surgery, a bronchogenic duplication cyst was resected. A thickened wall indicates infection. The cyst may rarely contain air if there is a connection to a bronchus. Calcification has been described.*

Lymphadenopathy | **Lymphadenopathy**

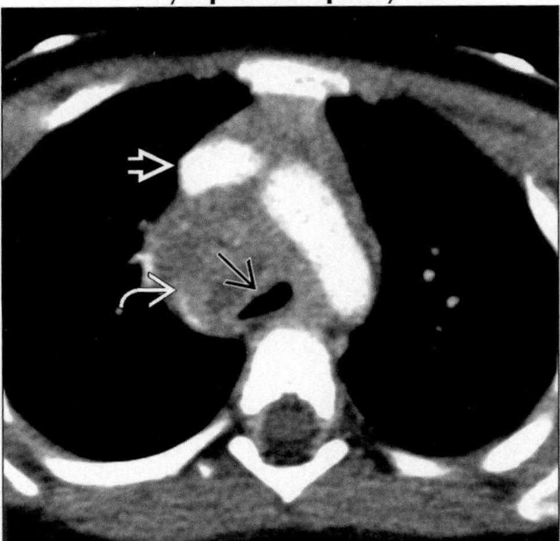

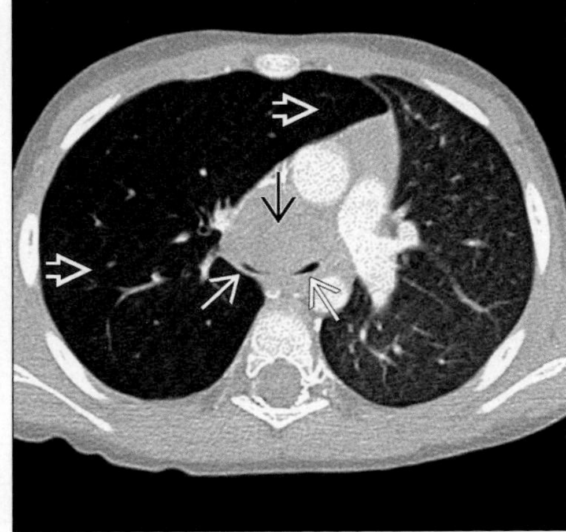

(Left) *Axial CECT shows a heterogeneous mass in the pretracheal region, which compresses the trachea and displaces the SVC anteriorly.* ***(Right)*** *Axial CECT shows the mass more inferiorly, causing compression of the right and left main bronchi. The narrowing of the right main bronchus is causing air-trapping in the right lung, which is low in attenuation and hyperinflated. These lymph nodes were enlarged due to a Histoplasma infection.*

MIDDLE MEDIASTINAL MASS

(**Left**) *Axial CECT shows low-attenuation nodes ➡ in the right paratracheal region. Note the enhancing rim. Worldwide, TB is the most common infectious cause for this appearance.* (**Right**) *Axial CECT shows coarse calcification of subcarinal lymph nodes ⇨. These are commonly seen in cases of remote infection with the fungus Histoplasma capsulatum, the organism that causes histoplasmosis. Calcification of lung parenchymal nodules is often seen in such cases.*

Lymphadenopathy

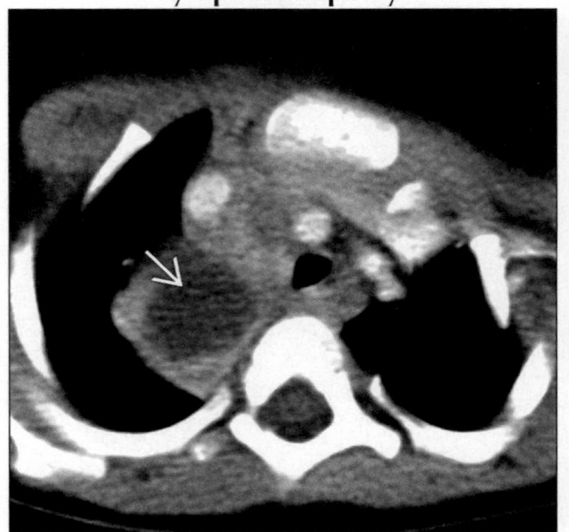

Lymphadenopathy

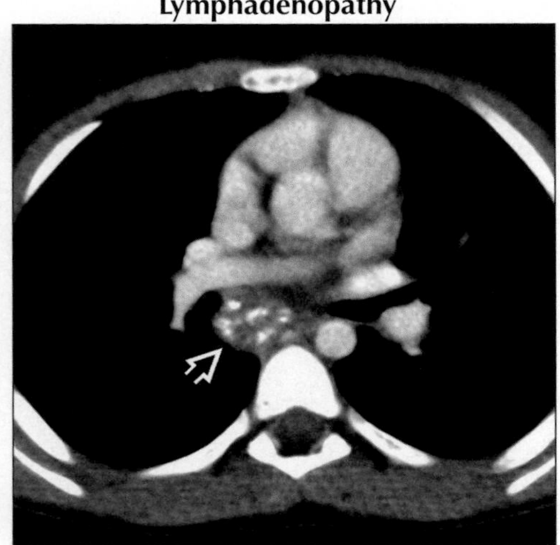

(**Left**) *Posteroanterior radiograph shows convexity along the right side of the mediastinum ➡ due to poststenotic dilatation in this patient with valvar aortic stenosis.* (**Right**) *Axial MRA shows dilatation of the ascending aorta ⇨ in a patient with Turner syndrome. The aorta was over 5 cm in diameter; compare to the size of the MPA ➡. Connective tissue disorders are another cause of dilatation of the ascending aorta in pediatric patients.*

Vascular Anomalies

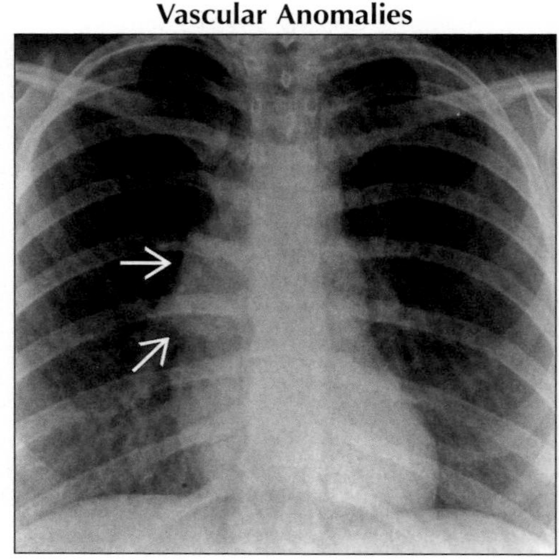

Vascular Anomalies

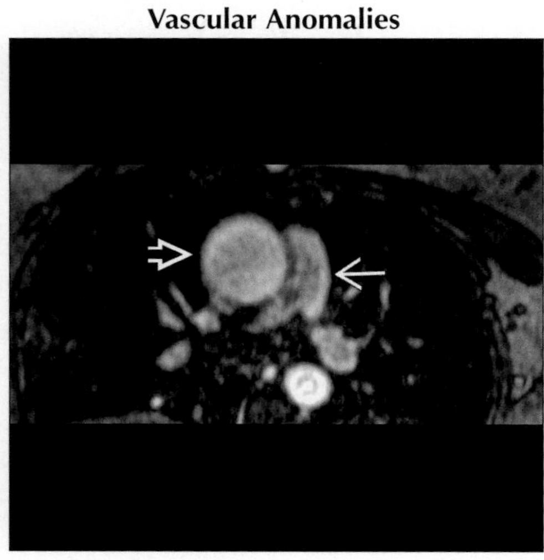

(**Left**) *Anteroposterior radiograph shows a biconvex enlargement of the mediastinum ⇨. In supracardiac types of total anomalous pulmonary venous return, this is called a "snowman" configuration.* (**Right**) *Anteroposterior radiograph shows an abnormal convexity ⇨ above the right main bronchus with thickening of the right paratracheal stripe. This patient had obstruction of the inferior vena cava, resulting in an enlarged azygous vein.*

Vascular Anomalies

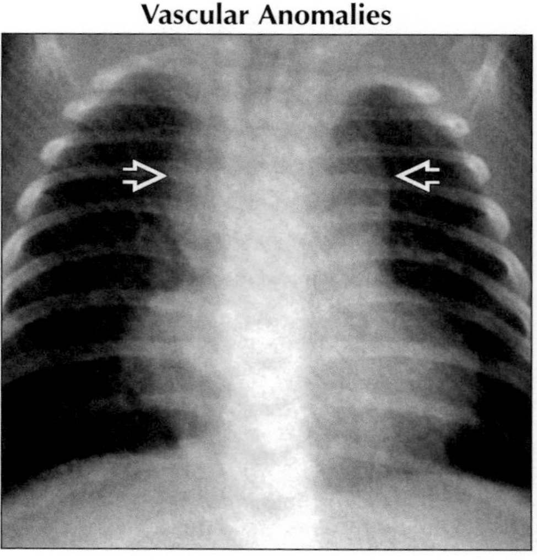

Vascular Anomalies

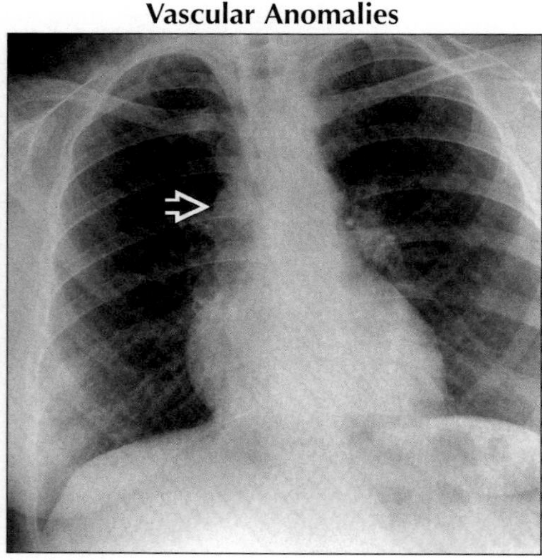

Postoperative Complications

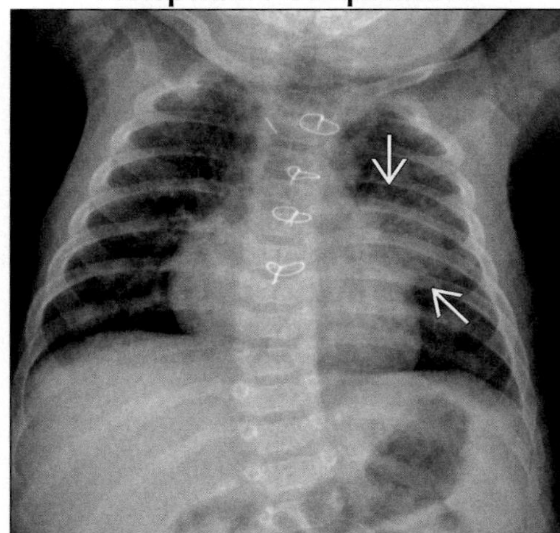

Postoperative Complications

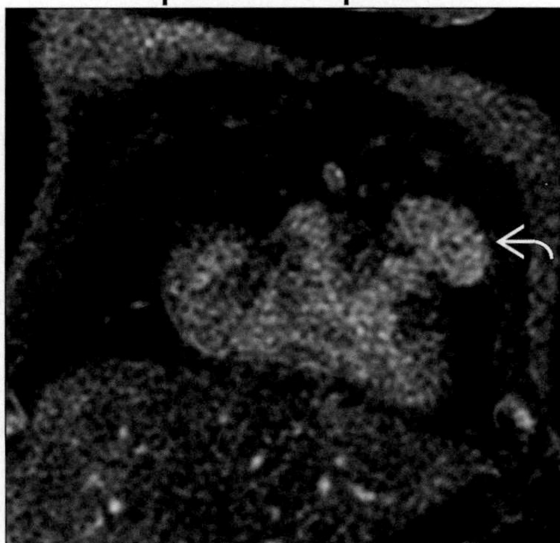

(Left) *Anteroposterior radiograph shows a rounded opacity ➡ adjacent to the left heart border. Perioperative radiographs had not demonstrated a mass.* ***(Right)*** *Coronal MRA shows filling of this lesion with blood ➡. This patient had a corrective procedure for hypoplastic left heart syndrome, and this represented a contained leak. Pseudoaneurysms should always be considered as a cause of a new mass in patients with prior vascular surgery.*

Pericardial Lesions

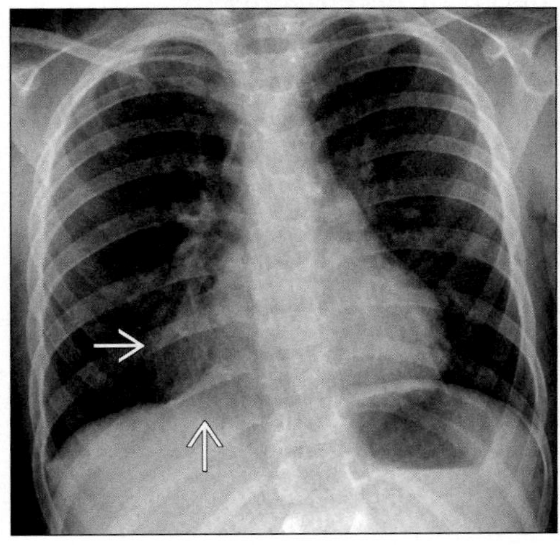

Pericardial Lesions

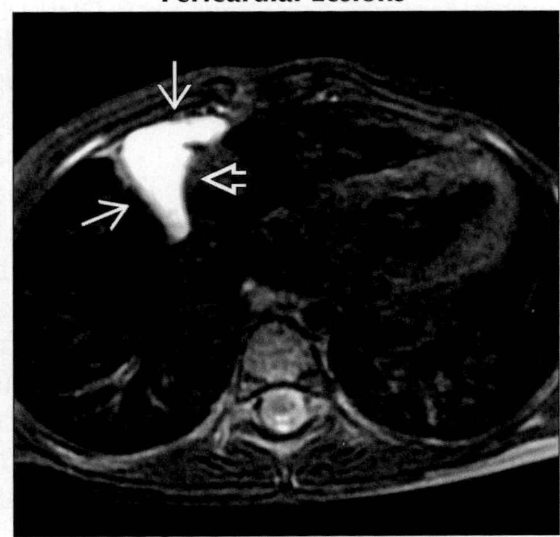

(Left) *Posteroanterior radiograph shows a mass in the right cardiophrenic angle ➡ obscuring the right heart border and the right hemidiaphragm.* ***(Right)*** *Axial T2WI MR shows a mass of homogeneously increased signal ➡ abutting the right heart border ➡. This lesion followed fluid signal on other sequences and did not enhance, consistent with a pericardial cyst. Pericardial tumors are another uncommon consideration for a mass in this region.*

Malignant Tumors

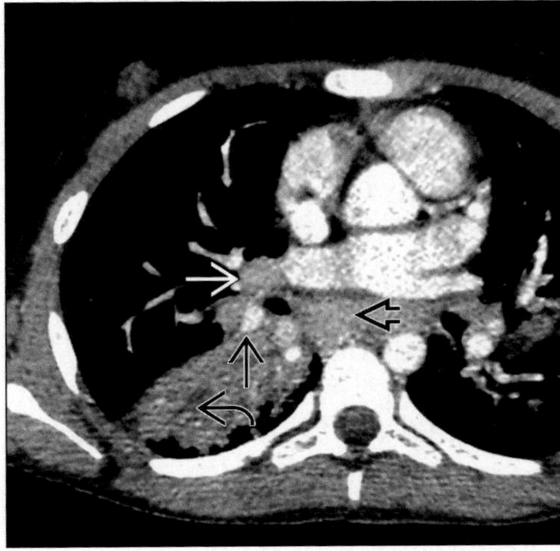

Malignant Tumors

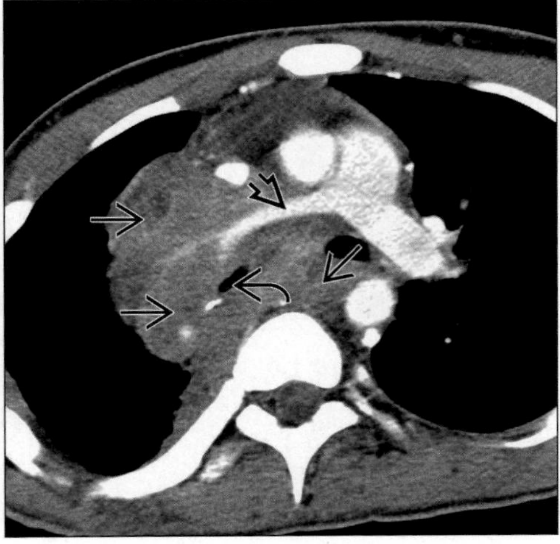

(Left) *Axial CECT shows an enhancing mass ➡ in the right lower lobe bronchus with associated hilar ➡ and mediastinal ➡ lymphadenopathy. Collapse of the left lower lobe ➡ is also present.* ***(Right)*** *Axial CECT shows extensive mediastinal lymphadenopathy ➡ in a patient with malignant melanoma. The right main pulmonary artery ➡ is narrowed as is the right main bronchus ➡. At another level, the tumor extended into a neural foramen.*

POSTERIOR MEDIASTINAL MASS

DIFFERENTIAL DIAGNOSIS

Common
- Neural Crest Tumors
- Lymphoma

Less Common
- Nerve Sheath Tumors
- Foregut Duplication Cyst

Rare but Important
- Neurenteric Cyst
- Meningocele
- Paraspinal Abscess
- Tumor
- Esophageal Varices
- Extramedullary Hematopoiesis

ESSENTIAL INFORMATION

Key Differential Diagnosis Issues
- Posterior mediastinal mass in young children should be considered neuroblastoma until proven otherwise

Helpful Clues for Common Diagnoses
- **Neural Crest Tumors**
  - Includes neuroblastoma, ganglioneuroma, and ganglioneuroblastoma, which demonstrate spectrum of cellular maturity and malignancy
    - Most neuroblastoma are immature, undifferentiated, and aggressive; occurs in younger population (median age < 2 years)
    - Ganglioneuroma most mature and least aggressive; occurs in older population (median age ~ 7 years)
    - Ganglioneuroblastoma intermediate between neuroblastoma and ganglioneuroma
  - Radiograph: Demonstrates elongated oval appearance with tapered borders in paraspinal location
  - Homogeneously solid or may contain foci of calcification, which may be fine or chunky in appearance
  - Separation or erosion of ribs and enlargement of neural foramina may be present
  - CT better demonstrates calcification (40%)
  - MR better demonstrates intraspinal extension
  - Nuclear medicine imaging with methyl-iodobenzylguanidine (MIBG) labeled with I-131 or I-123 and bone scintigraphy is mainstay of diagnosis and for monitoring response to therapy
  - PET/CT use is evolving and promising
- **Lymphoma**
  - Mediastinum is least common site of lymphoma
  - Nearly always associated with sites in other mediastinal compartments

Helpful Clues for Less Common Diagnoses
- **Nerve Sheath Tumors**
  - Includes neurilemoma (schwannoma), neurofibroma (plexiform and nonplexiform types), and malignant schwannoma
  - Sharply defined round, smooth, or lobulated paraspinal masses
  - Homogeneous or heterogeneous attenuation on CT with mild heterogeneous enhancement
  - Low to intermediate signal intensity on T1 with bright signal on T2 and mild enhancement following contrast administration
  - Neurofibromata may have "target" appearance on T2 and inversion recovery sequences
    - Higher signal peripherally and intermediate signal centrally
  - Neurofibromata are most commonly seen in neurofibromatosis type 1, where they are most commonly multiple
    - May be visible along intercostal nerves and in skin and subcutaneous tissues
    - Can distort ribs giving them ribbon-like appearance
  - Plexiform neurofibromas are more infiltrative and may extend into middle mediastinum
- **Foregut Duplication Cyst**
  - Rounded fluid-filled mass with thin wall associated with esophagus
  - Low attenuation on CT
    - No enhancement following contrast administration
  - In general, ↓ signal on T1 and ↑ signal on T2
    - May have higher signal on T1 due to high protein content of fluid

- In correct position, indistinguishable from bronchogenic cyst by imaging

Helpful Clues for Rare Diagnoses

- **Neurenteric Cyst**
  - Contains both neural and gastrointestinal elements
  - Associated with vertebral anomalies
- **Meningocele**
  - Herniation of leptomeninges through intervertebral foramen
  - May be anterior or lateral in addition to (more common) dorsal
  - Majority associated with neurofibromatosis, vertebral and rib anomalies
  - Associated with spinal anomalies; may lead to kyphosis or scoliosis
  - Fluid attenuation on CT
  - Low signal on T1 with high signal on T2 and no enhancement with contrast
- **Paraspinal Abscess**
  - Discitis more common in preschool children and vertebral osteomyelitis in older children
  - *Staphylococcus aureus* most common pyogenic organism; tuberculosis most common worldwide
  - Discitis and osteomyelitis
    - Disc space narrowing with indistinct end plates
    - Paravertebral soft tissue mass
  - Tuberculosis
    - Disc space narrowing often later than in pyogenic osteomyelitis
    - Gibbus deformity
- **Tumor**
  - Uncommon, except for lymphoma and neural tumors
  - Primary (e.g., rhabdomyosarcoma) and secondary tumors (e.g., malignant melanoma) that can occur at nearly any site in body should be considered
- **Esophageal Varices**
  - Most commonly secondary to portal hypertension
  - Paraspinal lobulated soft tissue mass
  - Flow voids on MR with enhancement on MRA
- **Extramedullary Hematopoiesis**
  - 1 or more lobulated soft tissue masses in lower thoracic paraspinal region
  - Homogeneous soft tissue attenuation on CT
  - Homogeneous signal on MR with mild to moderate enhancement
  - May have expanded ribs and vertebral bodies

Neural Crest Tumors

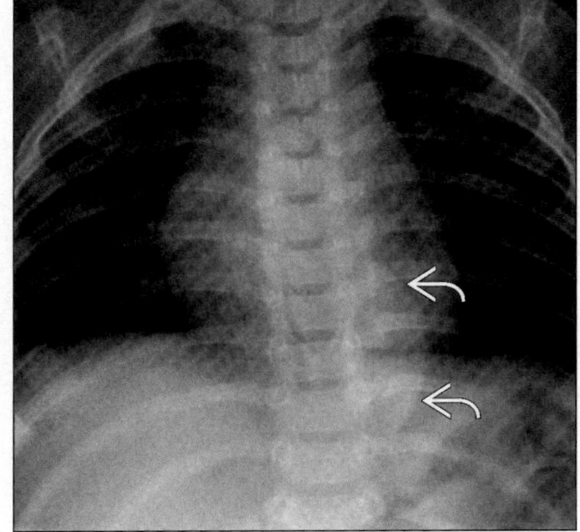

Anteroposterior radiograph shows a smoothly marginated oblong mass ➔ in the left paraspinal location. There is no rib destruction or expansion. Calcifications are not identified.

Neural Crest Tumors

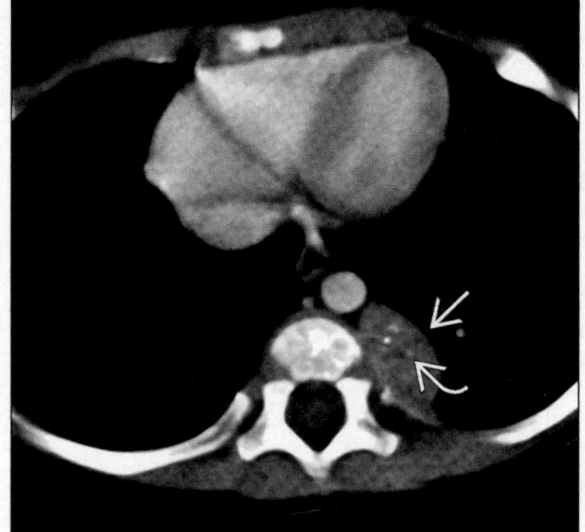

Axial CECT shows a well-circumscribed soft tissue mass ➔ in the posterior mediastinum. There are fine calcifications ➔ within the mass, consistent with a neuroblastoma.

POSTERIOR MEDIASTINAL MASS

Neural Crest Tumors

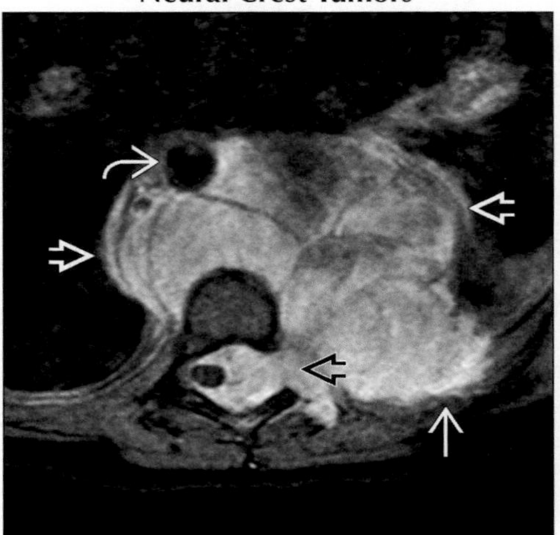

Neural Crest Tumors

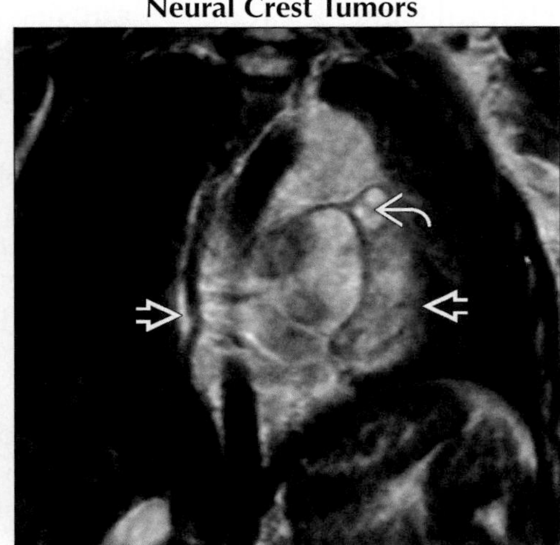

(Left) *Axial T1WI C+ MR shows the mass → crossing midline and elevating the aorta → and invading 1 of the neural foramina → on the left. There is also evidence of invasion of the posterior thoracic wall on the left →.* ***(Right)*** *Coronal T2WI FSE MR in the same child shows a large mass →, predominantly within the posterior mediastinum, deviating the aorta to the right. Cystic areas of degeneration → are seen in this ganglioneuroblastoma.*

Neural Crest Tumors

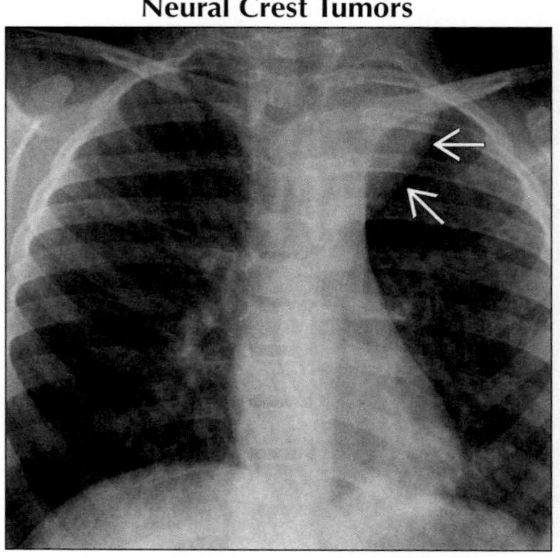

Neural Crest Tumors

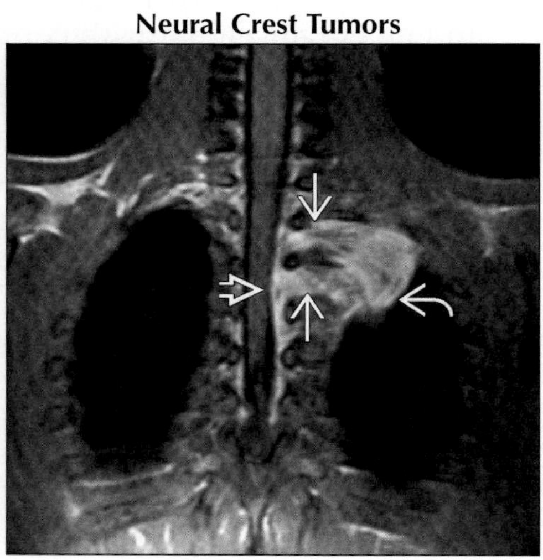

(Left) *Anteroposterior radiograph shows a smoothly marginated mass → in the superior left hemithorax.* ***(Right)*** *Coronal T1WI C+ FS MR shows an enhancing posterior mediastinal mass →. Note the neural foramina → with compression on the thecal sac →. MR is helpful in depicting neural foramina extension. Ganglioneuromas are benign tumors that may represent the end process of maturation of malignant neuroblastomas.*

Lymphoma

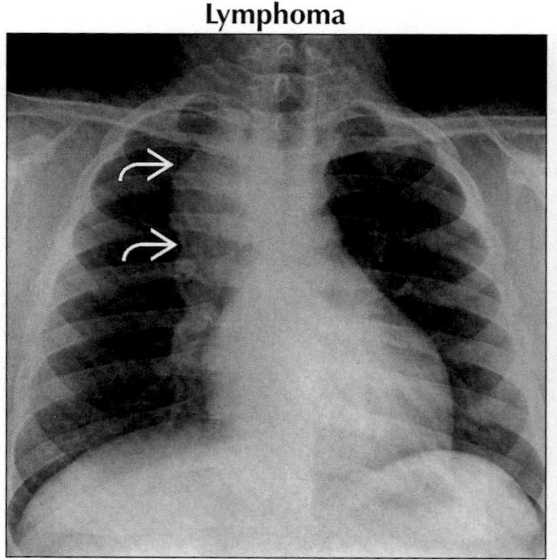

Lymphoma

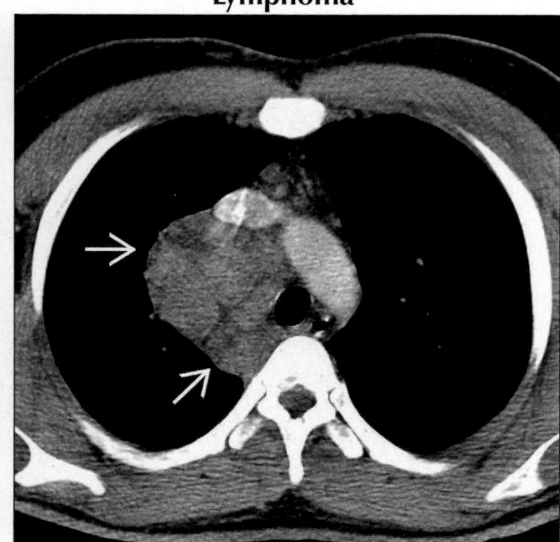

(Left) *Posteroanterior radiograph shows a lobulated mass → in the right side of the mediastinum.* ***(Right)*** *Axial CECT shows a multinodular mass → in the middle and posterior mediastinum. Lymphoma rarely is isolated to the posterior mediastinum and is the least common site of disease in the mediastinum. Lymphoma is uncommon in young children, the age group when neural crest tumors are usually detected.*

Nerve Sheath Tumors

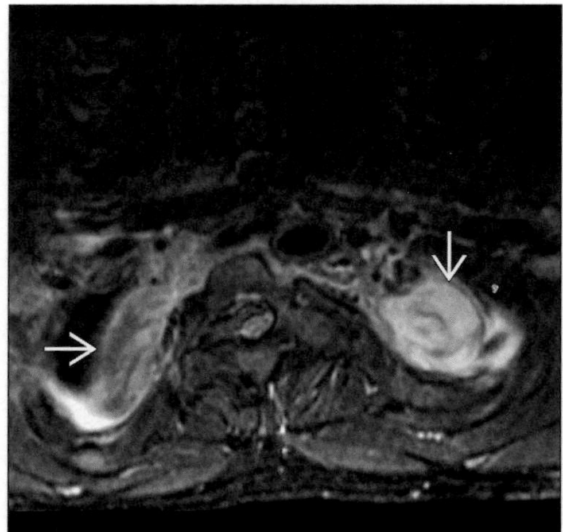

Nerve Sheath Tumors

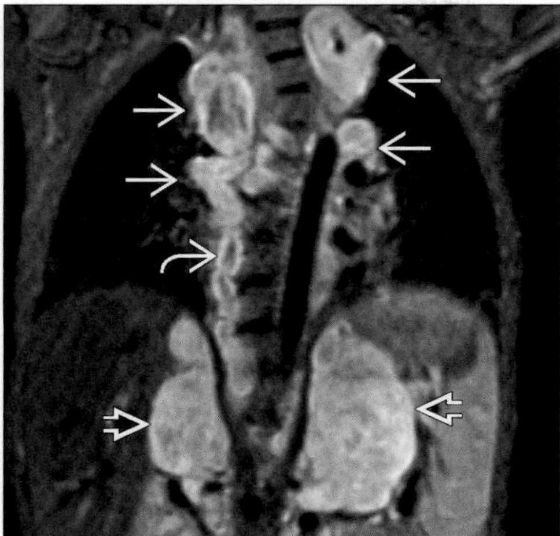

(Left) *Axial STIR MR shows bilateral heterogeneously increased signal masses ➡. The orientation of the spine suggests scoliosis, a common association with neurofibromatosis.* ***(Right)*** *Coronal STIR MR shows multiple masses in the posterior mediastinum ➡. Some of these ↪ have the typical "target" appearance with high signal on the periphery and relatively decreased signal centrally. Masses are also present in the retroperitoneum ⇨.*

Nerve Sheath Tumors

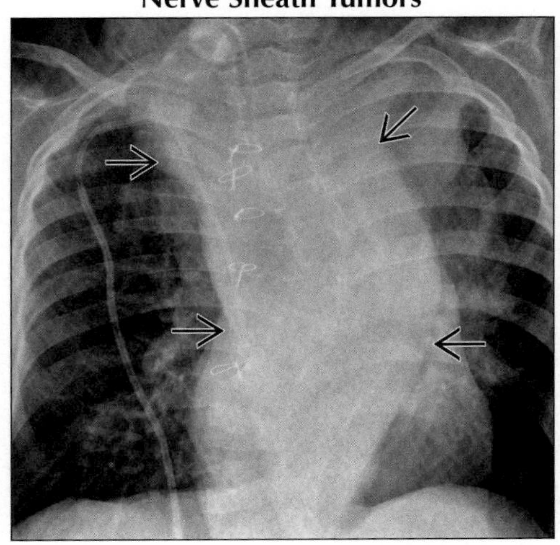

Nerve Sheath Tumors

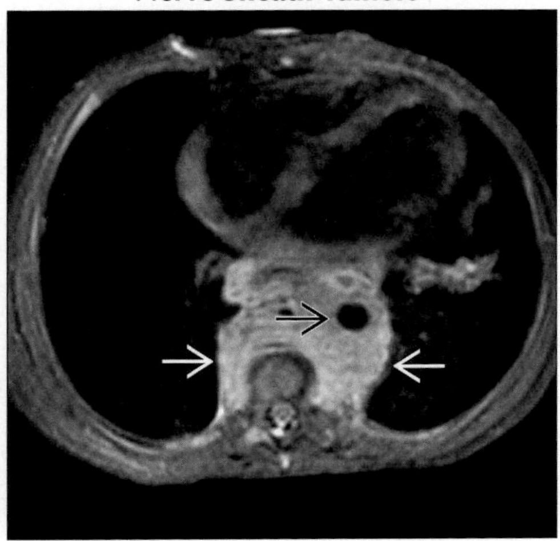

(Left) *Anteroposterior radiograph shows diffuse widening of the posterior mediastinum ➡. A significant scoliosis is present. The patient required a tracheostomy tube due to compromise of the airway by the neurofibromata.* ***(Right)*** *Axial STIR MR shows a high signal soft tissue mass ➡ that is surrounding the spine anteriorly and laterally. This plexiform neurofibroma is infiltrating the mediastinum and elevating the aorta ➡ away from the spine.*

Foregut Duplication Cyst

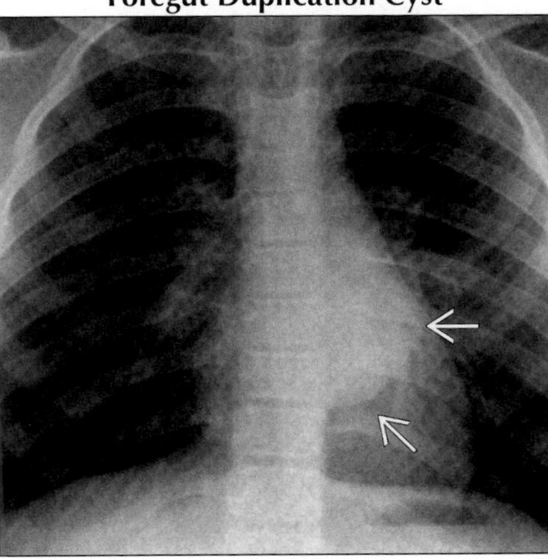

Foregut Duplication Cyst

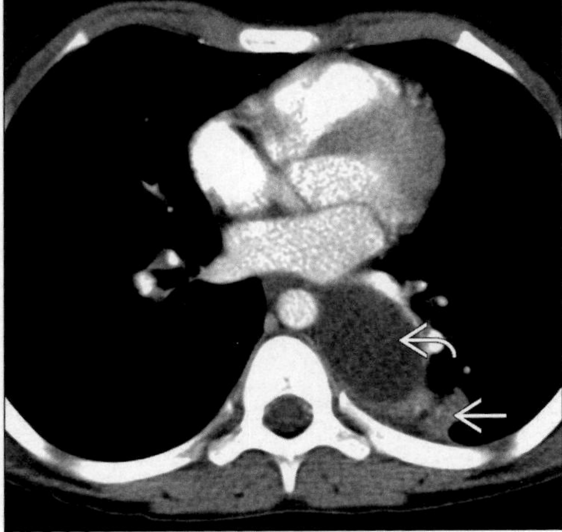

(Left) *Anteroposterior radiograph shows a left posterior mediastinal mass ➡. The patient had been diagnosed with recurrent "pneumonia" in the same location.* ***(Right)*** *Axial CECT shows a mass that has homogeneous fluid attenuation ↪. The mass has an imperceptibly thin wall. Some volume loss in the nearby lung is seen posteriorly ➡. At pathology, an esophageal duplication cyst was diagnosed.*

POSTERIOR MEDIASTINAL MASS

Neurenteric Cyst

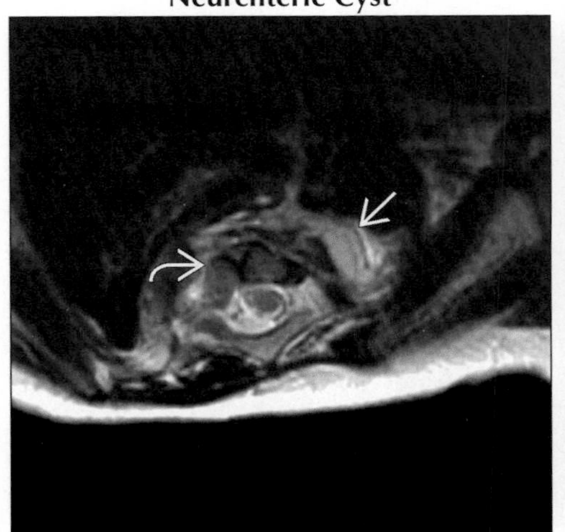

Neurenteric Cyst

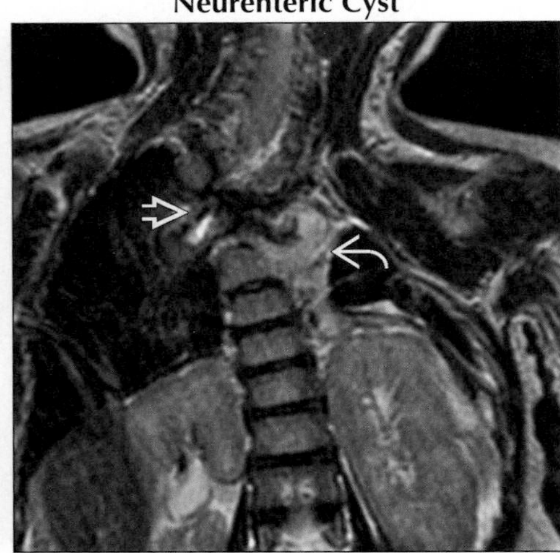

(Left) *Axial T2WI FSE MR shows a high signal mass ➡ in the left paravertebral location. Note the segmentation anomaly of the nearby vertebra ➡.* ***(Right)*** *Coronal T2WI FSE MR shows the high signal mass ➡ in the posterior mediastinum on the left. There is associated short-segment scoliosis ➡, consistent with vertebral segmentation anomalies. Neurenteric cysts contain neural and gastrointestinal elements and are connected to the meninges by a stalk.*

Meningocele

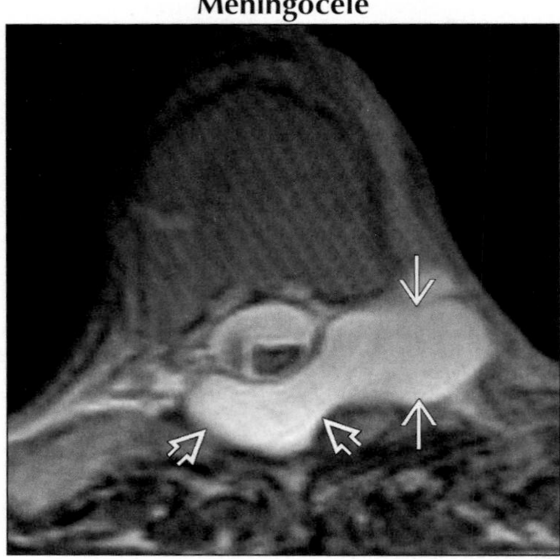

Meningocele

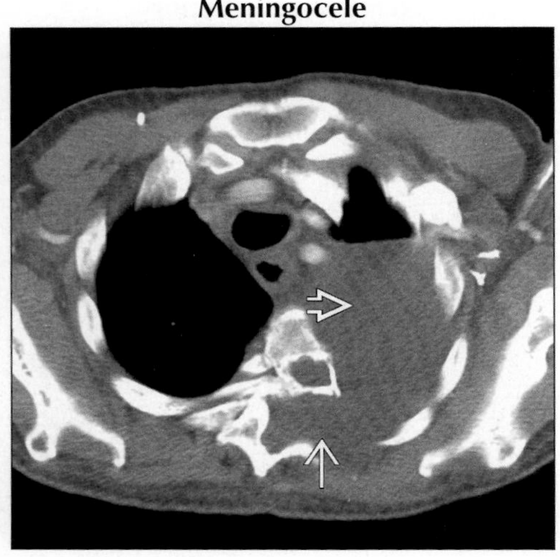

(Left) *Axial T2WI MR shows a meningocele extension through an expanded neural foramen ➡. There is also a meningocele component that extends dorsally within the spinal canal ➡, compressing and anteriorly displacing the thecal sac and spinal cord.* ***(Right)*** *Axial CECT shows a large fluid density mass ➡, which is contiguous with expansion of the foramen of the thoracic spine ➡ in a patient with neurofibromatosis type 1 with a large thoracic meningocele.*

Paraspinal Abscess

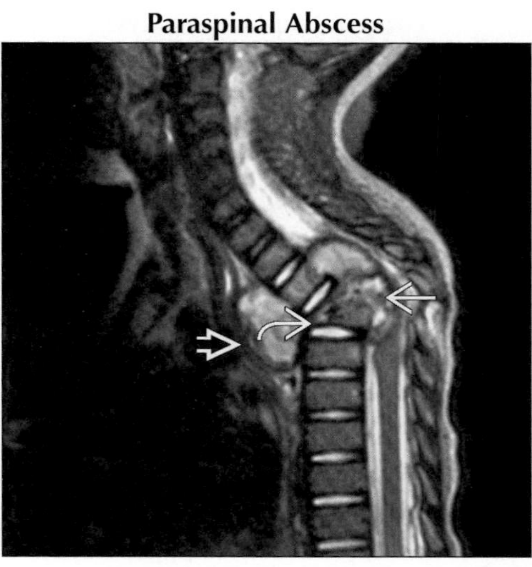

Paraspinal Abscess

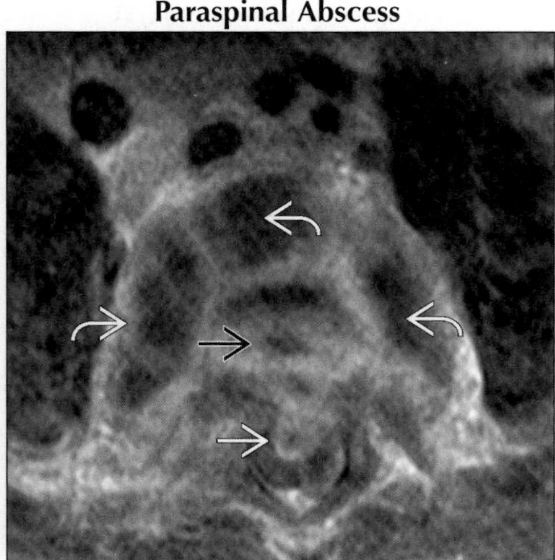

(Left) *Sagittal T2WI MR shows thoracic spinal TB with kyphotic deformity and large epidural ➡ and paraspinal ➡ abscesses. An intervertebral disc is absent with near complete destruction of 2 adjacent vertebral bodies ➡.* ***(Right)*** *Axial T1WI C+ MR shows large paravertebral abscesses ➡ and a spinal canal component ➡. There is also abnormal enhancement of the vertebral body ➡. TB is the most common cause or infectious spondylitis worldwide.*

POSTERIOR MEDIASTINAL MASS

Tumor

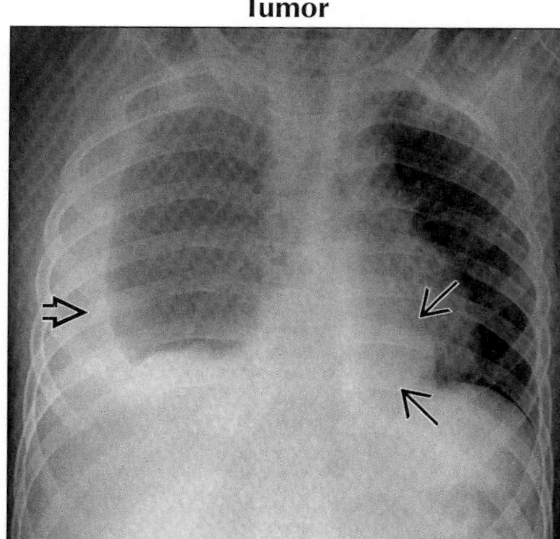

Tumor

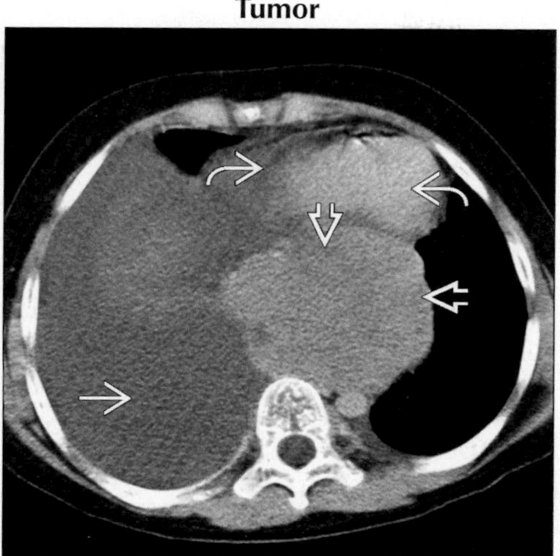

(Left) *Anteroposterior radiograph shows a soft tissue mass predominantly to the left of midline. A large right-sided pleural effusion is present. The heart is displaced slightly into the left hemithorax.* ***(Right)*** *Axial CECT shows a large homogeneous soft tissue mass, which is displacing the heart anteriorly. There is an associated large right pleural effusion. Pathology demonstrated a rhabdomyosarcoma.*

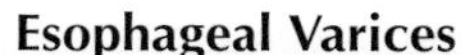

Esophageal Varices

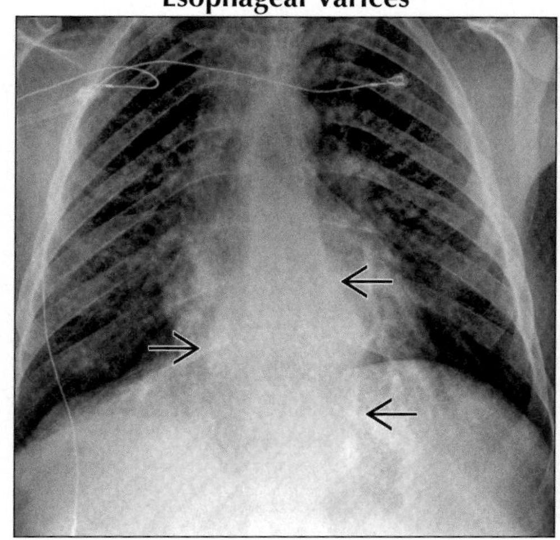

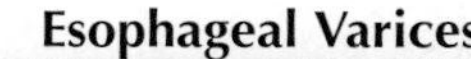

Esophageal Varices

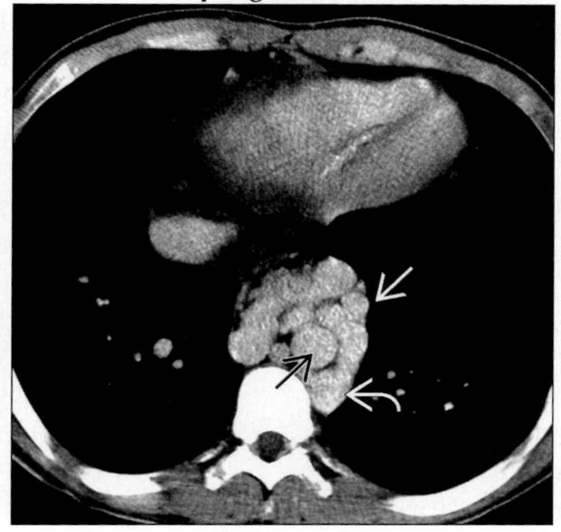

(Left) *Posteroanterior radiograph shows a soft tissue mass extending symmetrically across the midline.* ***(Right)*** *Axial CECT shows a mass that contains rounded and tubular lesions surrounding the aorta. These lesions are enhancing to the same degree as the aorta, consistent with vascular structures. The patient had portal hypertension secondary to sclerosing cholangitis.*

Extramedullary Hematopoiesis

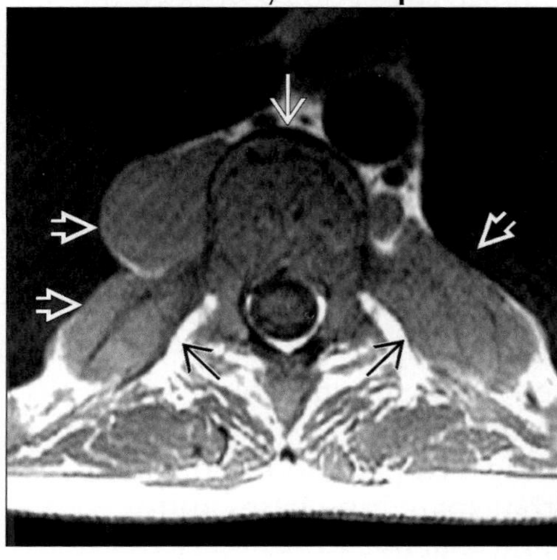

Extramedullary Hematopoiesis

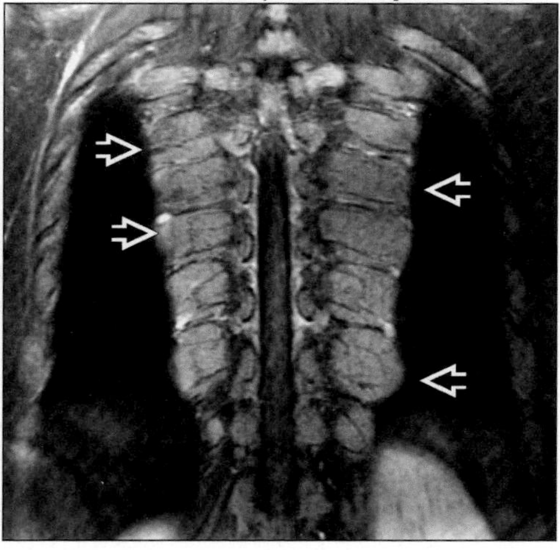

(Left) *Axial T1WI MR shows bilateral isointense paraspinal masses. Vertebral and bilateral rib marrow expansion is evident.* ***(Right)*** *Coronal T1WI C+ FS MR shows diffuse, mild to moderate enhancement of the bilateral paraspinal masses after intravenous gadolinium. These are typical MR appearances of extramedullary hematopoiesis. The masses are recruited tissue that produce red blood cells.*

RETICULONODULAR OPACITIES

DIFFERENTIAL DIAGNOSIS

Common

- Surfactant Deficient Disease
- Bronchiolitis
- Mycoplasma
- Pulmonary Edema

Less Common

- Langerhans Cell Histiocytosis
- Aspergillus
- Tuberculosis
- Pneumocystis jiroveci

Rare but Important

- Pulmonary Alveolar Proteinosis
- Systemic Lupus Erythematosus
- Niemann-Pick Disease
- Pulmonary Venoocclusive Disease

ESSENTIAL INFORMATION

Key Differential Diagnosis Issues

- Characterized by interstitial thickening and multiple small nodules
- Nonspecific pattern of disease

Helpful Clues for Common Diagnoses

- **Surfactant Deficient Disease**
  - a.k.a. respiratory distress syndrome, hyaline membrane disease
  - Most common cause of morbidity in premature infants
  - Most common in premature infants
    - Lack of mature type 2 pneumocytes
    - Most common in infants born at < 28 weeks fetal gestation
    - More common in males and infants of diabetic mothers
  - Radiograph: Decreased lung volume and diffuse reticulonodular opacities
    - Findings worst at 12-24 hours of life
  - Complications: Pneumothorax, pneumomediastinum, pulmonary interstitial emphysema
  - Treatment: Surfactant via endotracheal tube
  - Severe disease → bronchopulmonary dysplasia
- **Bronchiolitis**
  - Respiratory syncytial virus (RSV) is most common cause
  - Most common cause of hospitalization in infants
    - Usually self-limiting illness
  - Radiograph: Hyperinflation, atelectasis, and peribronchial cuffing
  - Risks for severe disease: Prematurity, age < 12 weeks, chronic lung disease, congenital heart disease, immunocompromised
- **Mycoplasma**
  - Common cause of community-acquired pneumonia
    - Most common cause of pneumonia in children > 5 years old
  - More severe presentation in children < 5 years old
  - Radiograph: Lobar consolidation, air bronchograms, or reticulonodular opacities
    - Reticulonodular opacities in 52%; more common in lower lobes
- **Pulmonary Edema**
  - 2 main causes: Cardiogenic and noncardiogenic
  - Cardiogenic pulmonary edema occurs when pulmonary capillary pressure is high
    - Overwhelms lymphatic system's ability to resorb fluid
    - Associated with congenital heart disease
    - Usually occurs in 1st 6 months of life
  - Noncardiogenic causes can be neurogenic, negative pressure, or miscellaneous
  - Neurogenic: Associated with head trauma
    - Onset within hours of injury
  - Negative pressure: Associated with upper airway obstruction
    - Rapid onset and resolves when obstruction is relieved
  - Other causes of noncardiogenic edema: Fluid overload, acute glomerulonephritis, inhalational injury, and allergic reaction

Helpful Clues for Less Common Diagnoses

- **Langerhans Cell Histiocytosis**
  - Unknown etiology
  - Strong association with cigarette smoking
  - Typically affects young adults between ages 20-40
    - Can affect any age
  - Can present with spontaneous pneumothorax
  - Early findings: Upper and middle lobe nodules that spare lung bases and costophrenic sulcus

- Late findings: Reticulonodular opacity and cystic changes
- **Aspergillus**
  - *Aspergillus fumigatus*: Fungus found in soil, water, and decaying organic material
  - Disease can be caused by allergic reaction or invasive disease
  - Often colonizes in patients with underlying airway disease
  - Aspergillomas grow in pulmonary cavities as with tuberculosis or cystic fibrosis
  - Invasive disease is associated with chronic granulomatous disease
- **Tuberculosis**
  - Caused by *Mycobacterium tuberculosis*
  - Pulmonary infection is most common manifestation
  - Infection in children is usually due to close contact with infected adult
  - Children are less resistant to organism and disseminated disease is more common
  - Hallmark of primary tuberculosis is large hilar or mediastinal adenopathy
- **Pneumocystis jiroveci**
  - a.k.a. *Pneumocystis carinii, Pneumocystis* pneumonia (PCP)
  - Increased incidence with AIDS and other immunocompromised states
  - Radiograph: Parahilar granular opacities, extensive consolidation, ground-glass opacity

Helpful Clues for Rare Diagnoses

- **Pulmonary Alveolar Proteinosis**
  - Characterized by intraalveolar accumulation of surfactant-like material
  - 3 types: Idiopathic, secondary, and congenital
  - Congenital type manifests in neonates; accounts for 2% of cases
  - Radiograph: Bilateral central and symmetric opacities with sparing of costophrenic angles and apices
    - Opacities can range from ground-glass to reticulonodular to consolidation
  - CT: "Crazy-paving" are thick septal lines superimposed on ground-glass opacity
  - Treatment: Whole-lung lavage, lung transplant
- **Systemic Lupus Erythematosus**
  - Systemic disease
  - Most common thoracic manifestation is pleuritis
  - Can cause interstitial lung disease
- **Niemann-Pick Disease**
  - Autosomal recessive disorder
  - Characterized by accumulation of sphingomyelin due to deficiency of sphingomyelinase
  - Radiograph: Diffuse reticulonodular pattern
- **Pulmonary Venoocclusive Disease**
  - Rare cause of pulmonary arterial hypertension
  - Characterized by occlusion of pulmonary venules by fibrous tissue
  - Findings: Nodular ground-glass opacity, septal lines, lymph node enlargement

Surfactant Deficient Disease

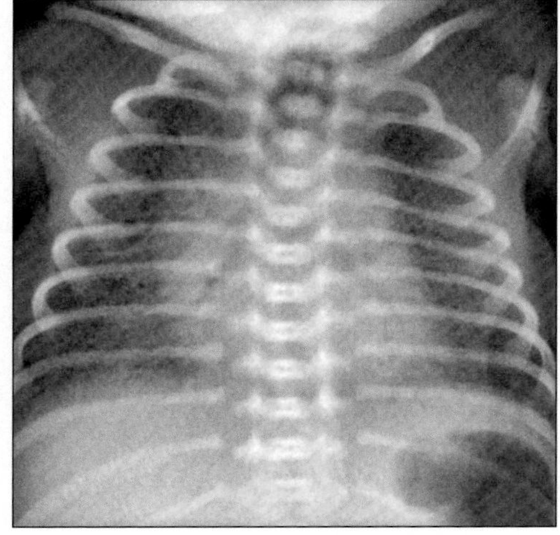

AP radiograph of the chest shows diffuse granular opacities of both lungs. Surfactant deficiency is the most common cause of morbidity in preterm infants.

Surfactant Deficient Disease

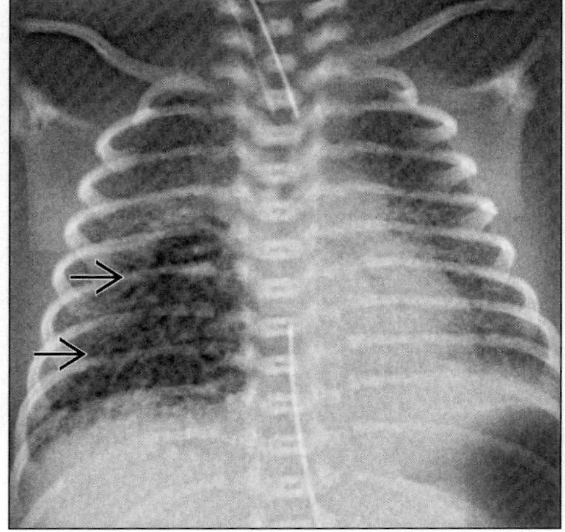

AP radiograph of the chest in the same patient 2 days later shows new branching lucencies in the right lower lobe ⇒. Pulmonary interstitial emphysema is a complication of surfactant deficiency.

RETICULONODULAR OPACITIES

(**Left**) *AP radiograph of the chest shows diffuse granular opacities in both lungs. Surfactant deficiency is most common in infants born at less than 28 weeks fetal gestation.* (**Right**) *AP radiograph of the chest in a different patient shows diffuse granular opacities of the right lung. Surfactant deficiency is caused by a lack of mature type 2 pneumocytes. It is treated with exogenous surfactant given by an endotracheal tube.*

Surfactant Deficient Disease

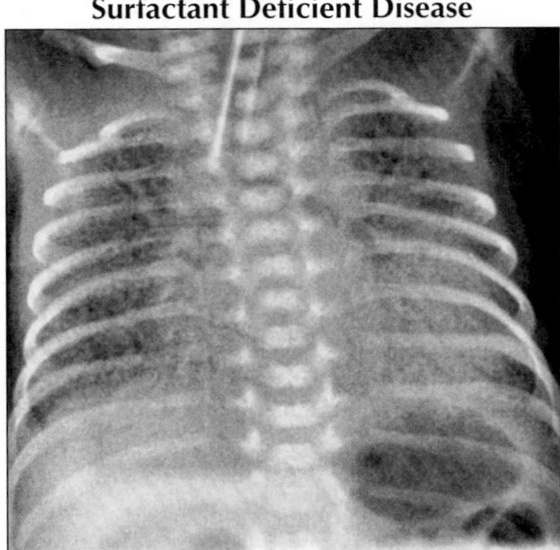

Surfactant Deficient Disease

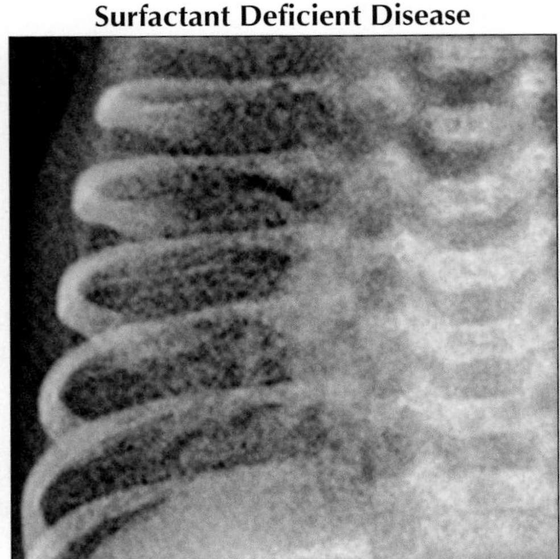

(**Left**) *AP radiograph of the chest shows hyperinflated lungs and streaky perihilar opacities ➔. Bronchiolitis is most commonly caused by respiratory syncytial virus (RSV). It is the most common cause of hospitalization in infants.* (**Right**) *Lateral radiograph of the chest shows hyperinflated lungs with flattening of the diaphragms ➔. Acute bronchiolitis is usually a self-limiting illness treated with supportive care.*

Bronchiolitis

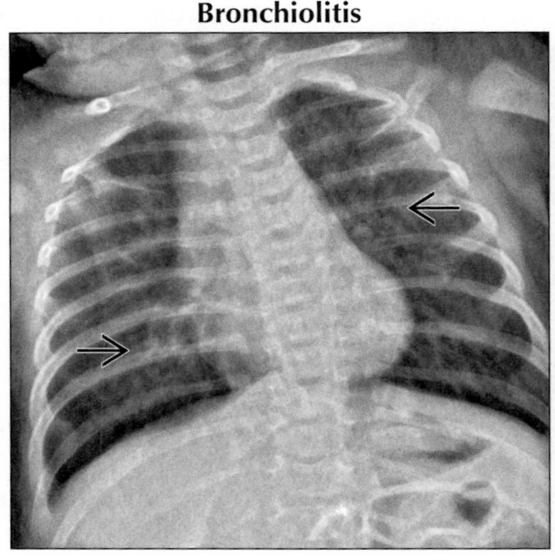

Bronchiolitis

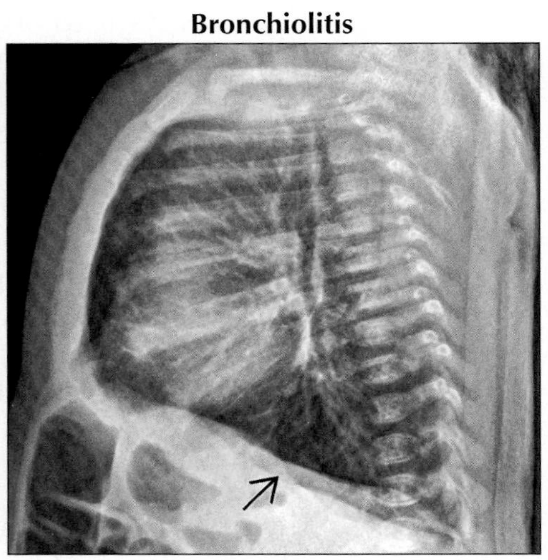

(**Left**) *AP radiograph of the chest shows a reticulonodular opacity in the right lower lobe ➔. Mycoplasma is the most common cause of pneumonia in children older than 5 years of age.* (**Right**) *AP radiograph of the chest in a different patient shows a reticulonodular opacity in the left lower lobe ➔. Reticulonodular opacities are seen in nearly half of the patients with Mycoplasma pneumonia.*

Mycoplasma

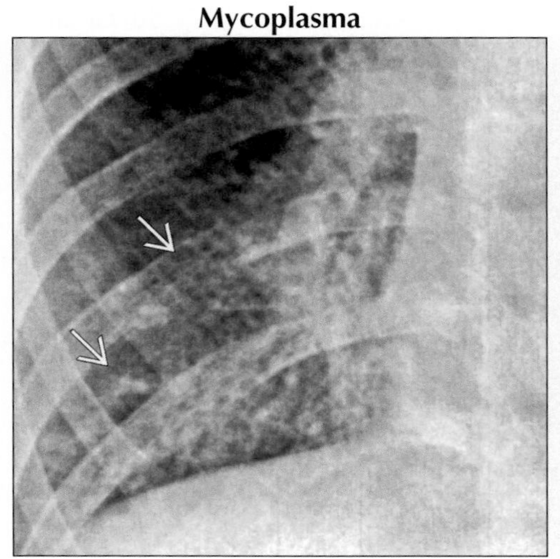

Mycoplasma

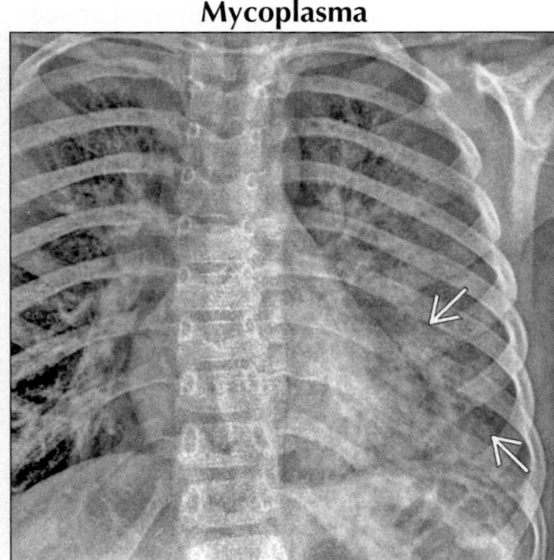

Pulmonary Edema

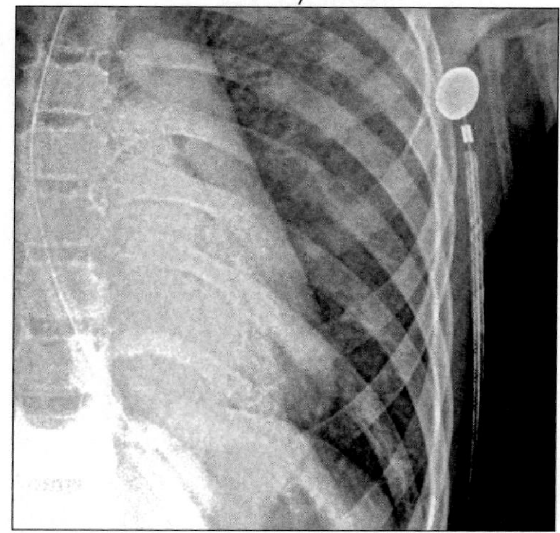

Pulmonary Edema

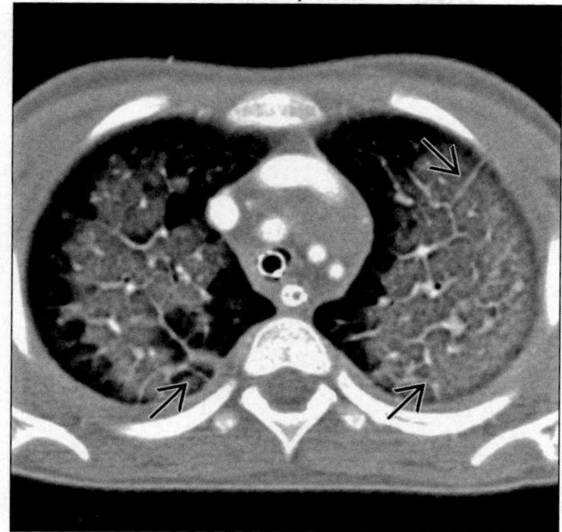

(Left) *AP radiograph of the chest shows fine nodules in the left lower lobe. The pulmonary vessels are indistinct with hazy opacities in the upper lung. There are 2 general categories of pulmonary edema: Cardiogenic and noncardiogenic.* ***(Right)*** *Axial CECT shows bilateral ground-glass opacity and thickening of the interlobular septa →. In children, cardiogenic pulmonary edema is associated with congenital heart disease (not shown in this case).*

Langerhans Cell Histiocytosis

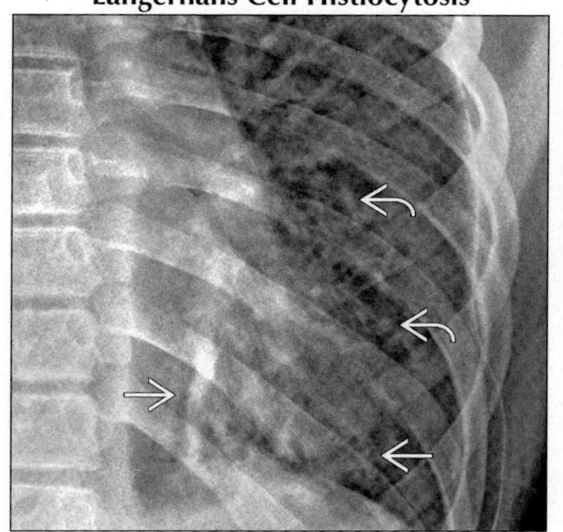

Langerhans Cell Histiocytosis

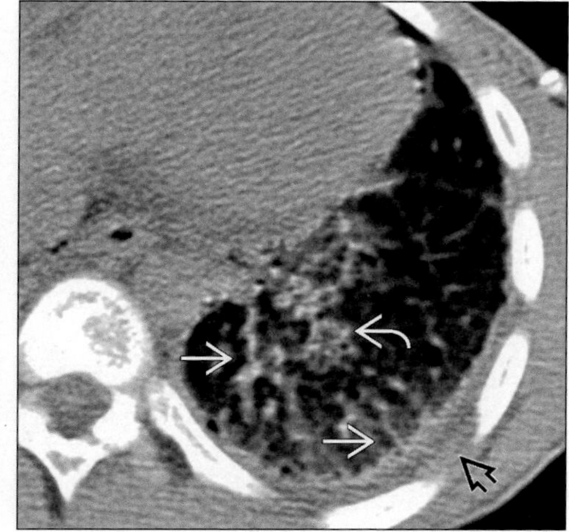

(Left) *AP radiograph of the chest shows thickened interstitial markings ➔ and multiple small nodules ↪. Langerhans cell histiocytosis can occur in children of any age. Patients can present with spontaneous pneumothorax.* ***(Right)*** *Axial NECT in the same patient shows interstitial thickening ➔ and multiple nodules ↪. A small pleural effusion is also present ⇨. In adults, Langerhans cell histiocytosis is associated with smoking.*

Aspergillus

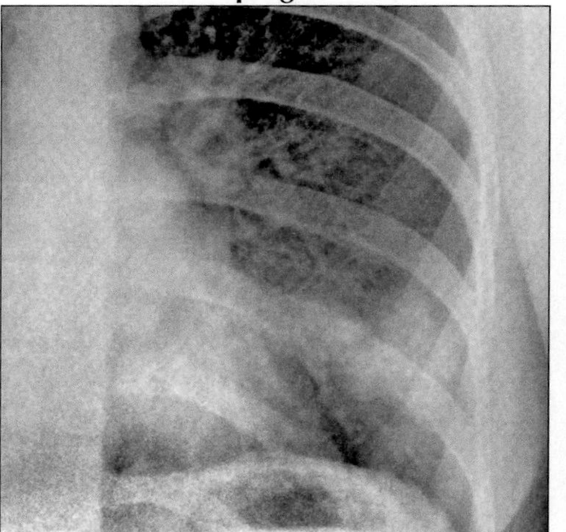

Aspergillus

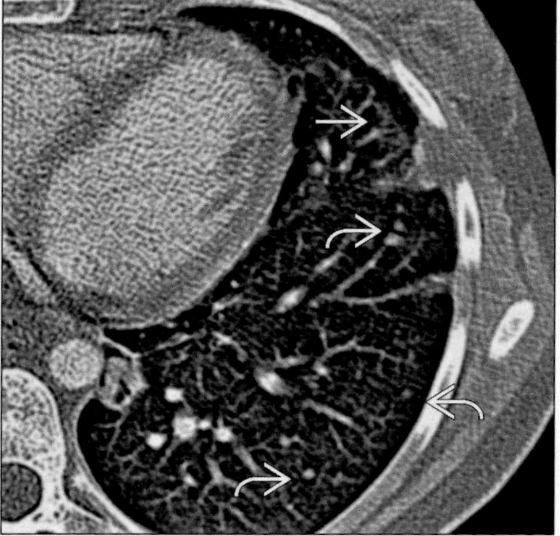

(Left) *AP radiograph of the chest shows a faint reticulonodular opacity at the left lung base. Aspergillus infection often occurs in patients who are immunocompromised or who have preexisting lung disease, such as cystic fibrosis or tuberculosis.* ***(Right)*** *Axial CECT shows a subtle reticulonodular opacity in the lingula ➔. Other small nodules are present in the left lower lobe ↪.*

RETICULONODULAR OPACITIES

Aspergillus

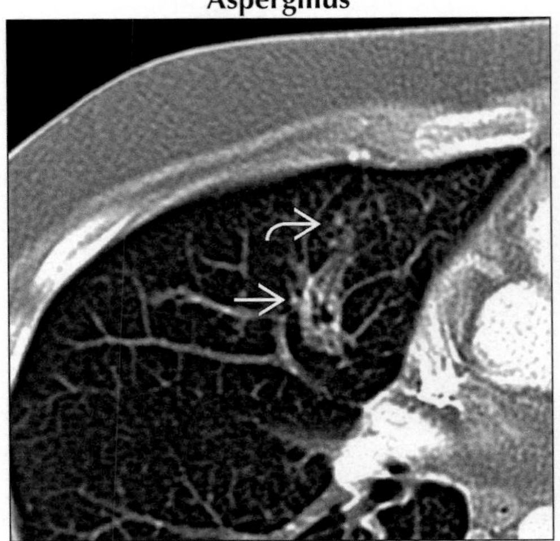

Tuberculosis

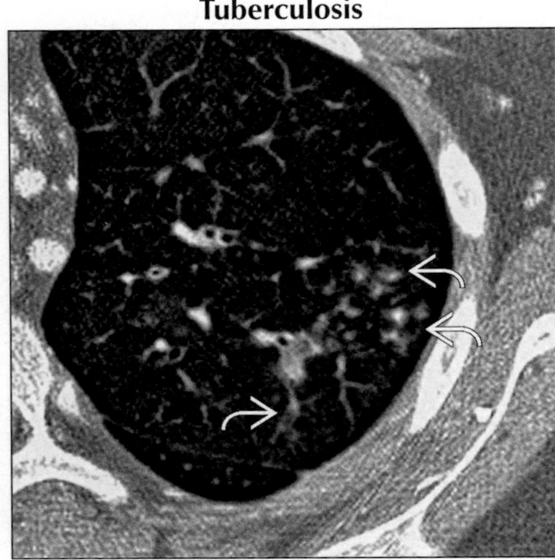

*(**Left**) Axial CECT shows a cavitary lesion in the right middle lobe → with small nodules at its periphery ↷. Invasive Aspergillus infection is a cause of cavitary lesion. (**Right**) Axial CECT shows a reticulonodular opacity in the left upper lobe ↷. Aspergillus infection is caused by a fungus found in soil, water, and decaying organic material.*

Tuberculosis

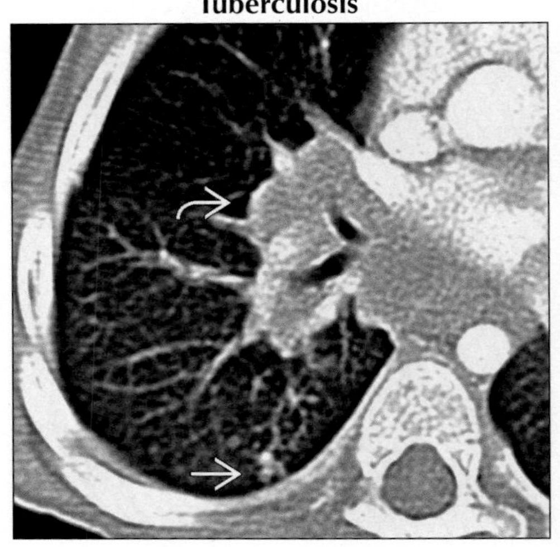

Pneumocystis jiroveci

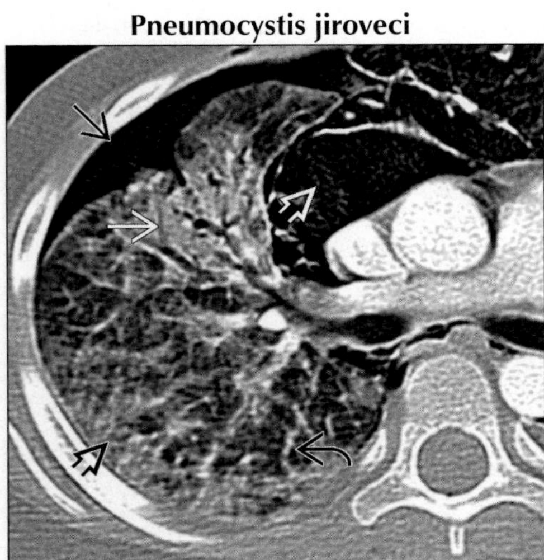

*(**Left**) Axial CECT shows multiple small nodules in the right lower lobe → and hilar adenopathy ↷. The most common manifestation of tuberculosis is pulmonary disease. Children are usually infected by close contact with an adult. (**Right**) Axial CECT shows extensive pneumothorax → and pneumomediastinum →. In addition, there are areas of consolidation with air bronchograms →, ground-glass opacity ⇨, and septal thickening ↷.*

Pulmonary Alveolar Proteinosis

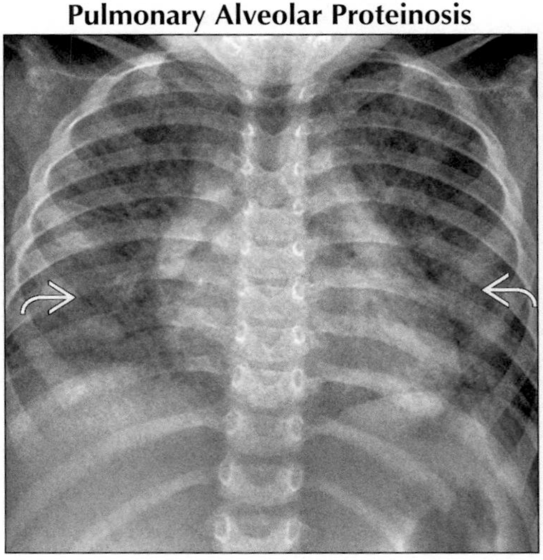

Pulmonary Alveolar Proteinosis

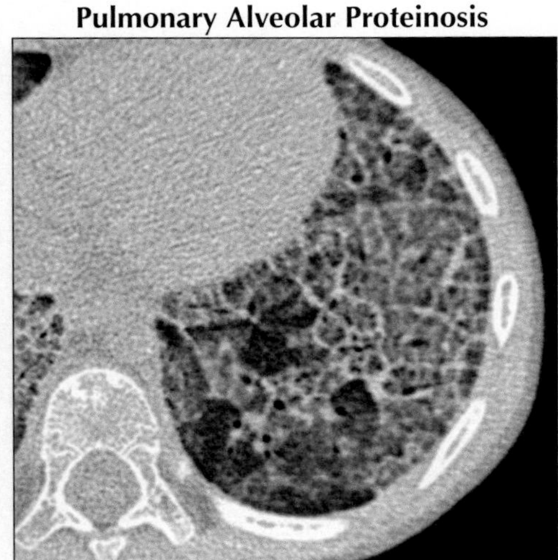

*(**Left**) AP radiograph of the chest shows bilateral ground-glass opacities of both lungs ↷. Pulmonary alveolar proteinosis is characterized by the intraalveolar accumulation of surfactant-like material. (**Right**) Axial NECT in the same patient shows the "crazy-paving" appearance of the left lower lobe with diffuse ground-glass opacity and thickened interlobular septa. Pulmonary alveolar proteinosis is treated with whole-lung lavage or transplant.*

RETICULONODULAR OPACITIES

Systemic Lupus Erythematosus

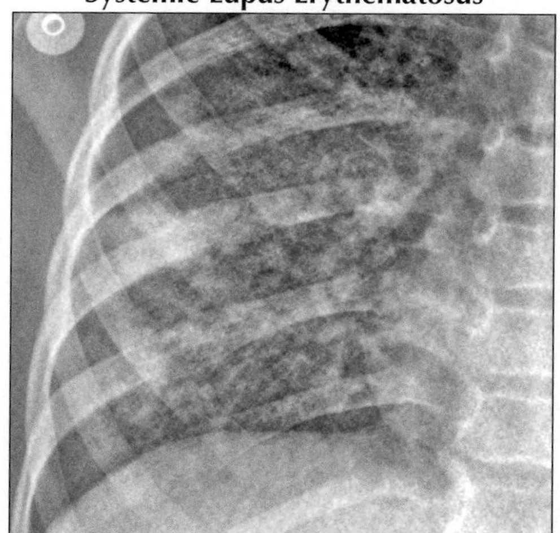

Systemic Lupus Erythematosus

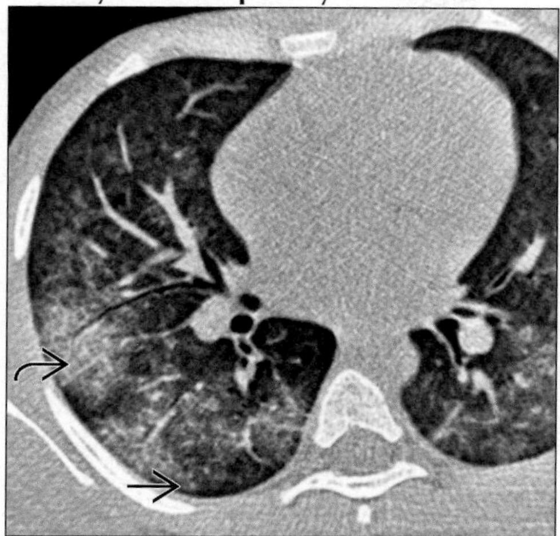

(Left) *AP radiograph of the chest shows a reticulonodular opacity in the right lung base. Systemic lupus erythematosus is an autoimmune disorder that can cause interstitial lung disease.* ***(Right)*** *Axial NECT in the same patient shows reticular nodular opacity in the right lower lobe. There are areas of ground-glass opacity, septal thickening ⤳, and small pulmonary nodules →. The most common thoracic manifestation of lupus is pleuritis.*

Niemann-Pick Disease

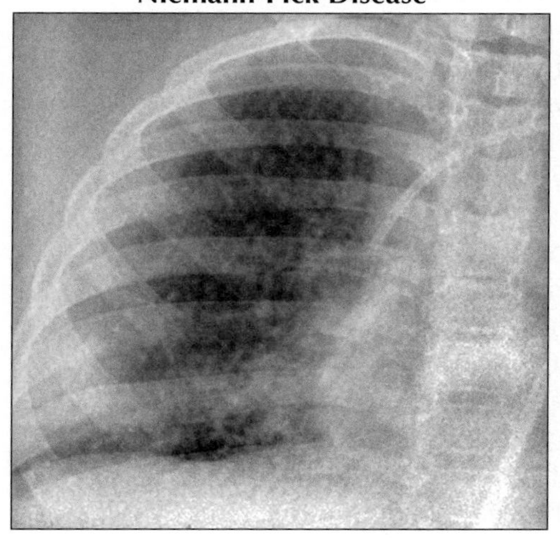

Niemann-Pick Disease

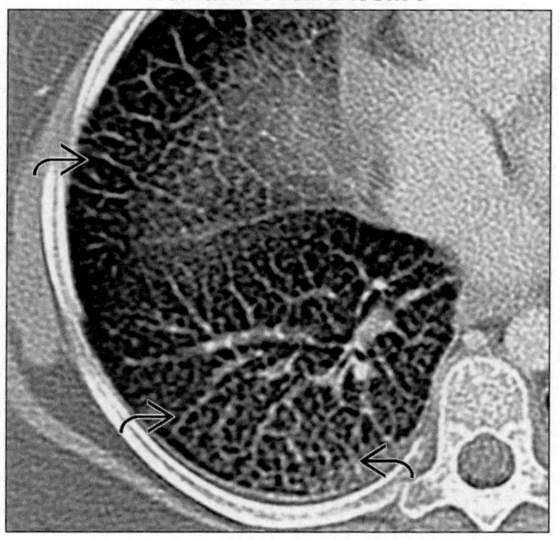

(Left) *AP radiograph of the chest shows prominent septal lines in the right lung base. Radiographs in patients with Niemann-Pick disease typically display a diffuse reticulonodular pattern.* ***(Right)*** *Axial CECT shows thickened interlobular septal lines ⤳ and multiple tiny nodules. Niemann-Pick disease is an autosomal recessive disorder that is characterized by accumulation of sphingomyelin.*

Pulmonary Venoocclusive Disease

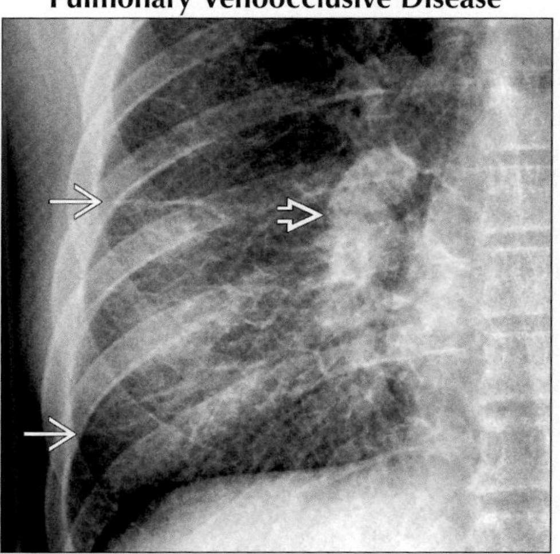

Pulmonary Venoocclusive Disease

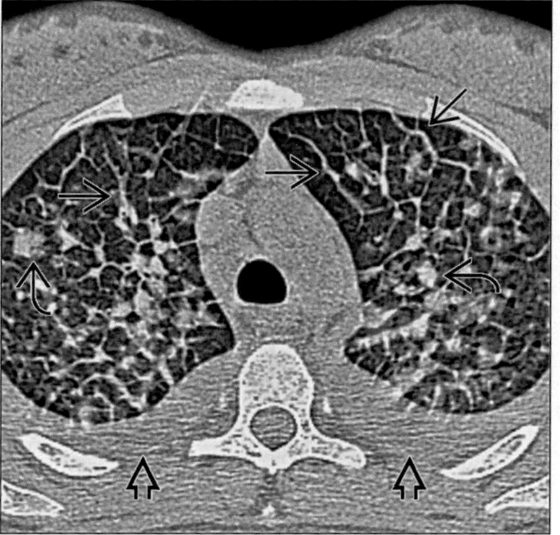

(Left) *AP radiograph of the chest shows septal lines ➡ throughout the right lung base. The right pulmonary artery is enlarged ➡.* ***(Right)*** *Axial NECT in the same patient shows diffuse interlobular septal thickening →, multiple pulmonary nodules ⤳, and small bilateral pleural effusions ⇨. Pulmonary venoocclusive disease is a rare cause of pulmonary artery hypertension and is characterized by occlusion of pulmonary venules by fibrous tissue.*

NEONATAL IRREGULAR LUNG OPACITIES

DIFFERENTIAL DIAGNOSIS

Common
- Transient Tachypnea of the Newborn
- Surfactant Deficient Disease
- Increased Pulmonary Vascularity
- Left-to-Right Cardiac Shunts

Less Common
- Pulmonary Interstitial Emphysema
- Meconium Aspiration Syndrome
- Neonatal Pneumonia
- Congenital Pulmonary Airway Abnormality
- Congenital Diaphragmatic Hernia

Rare but Important
- Total Anomalous Pulmonary Venous Return (TAPVR)
- Pulmonary Interstitial Glycogenosis
- Congenital Pulmonary Lymphangiectasia

ESSENTIAL INFORMATION

Helpful Clues for Common Diagnoses
- **Transient Tachypnea of the Newborn**
  - More common in patients born by cesarian section, by precipitous delivery, and to mothers with gestational diabetes
  - Resolves within 72 hours
  - Small amount of pleural fluid and linear opacities on radiography
- **Surfactant Deficient Disease**
  - Secondary to immaturity of lungs in premature infant
  - Initial diffuse bilateral hazy granular opacities are replaced by irregular opacities following treatment
  - Foci of collapsed terminal airspaces are intermixed with overinflated secondary pulmonary lobules
- **Increased Pulmonary Vascularity**
  - Pulmonary arterial blood flow or pulmonary venous congestion
  - May be cyanotic or acyanotic condition
- **Left-to-Right Cardiac Shunts**
  - May be intracardiac or extracardiac
  - Result in pulmonary overcirculation

Helpful Clues for Less Common Diagnoses
- **Pulmonary Interstitial Emphysema**
  - Result of air leak in patient on positive pressure ventilation
  - Most common in patients with surfactant deficiency and resultant "stiff lungs"
    - Pressure needed to ventilate lungs forces air into interstitium
  - Circular and linear lucencies, some of which are branching
  - Lucencies may be diffuse and bilateral, unilateral, or even lobar or segmental
  - May be associated with other manifestations of air leak, such as pneumomediastinum and pneumothorax
- **Meconium Aspiration Syndrome**
  - Usually in term infant
  - Complication of fetal stress with resultant defecation and aspiration of meconium
  - Relatively normal radiograph may worsen rapidly due to chemical pneumonitis
  - Lungs generally hyperinflated with areas of irregular opacification related to pneumonitis and atelectasis as well as regions of air-trapping
- **Neonatal Pneumonia**
  - Infection occurs shortly before, during, or shortly following birth
  - Classically caused by Group B *Streptococcus;* however, *Staphylococcus epidermidis* is now more common
    - *Escherichia coli* is becoming most common in very low birth weight infants (< 1,500 gm)
  - Varied appearance on radiography
    - Normal lung volumes with ill-defined foci of consolidation are most classic, but opacification may also be diffuse
- **Congenital Pulmonary Airway Abnormality**
  - Previously divided into congenital cystic adenomatoid malformation (CCAM) and pulmonary sequestration
    - Now seen as spectrum with both types often coexisting
  - May be visible on fetal imaging
  - 3 types of CCAM
    - Type 1 (most common): 1 or more cysts > 2 cm in diameter;
    - Type 2: Multiple small relatively numerous cysts < 2 cm in diameter
    - Type 3: Microscopic cysts that look solid on imaging
  - Sequestration may be intralobar (ILS) or extralobar (ELS) in type

- Both types have arterial supply from aorta
- Intralobar type is most common (75%); venous drainage to pulmonary veins and same pleural covering as parent lobe
- Extralobar type: Venous drainage to systemic vein and separate pleural covering
- Both are solid on initial imaging in postnatal period
- ILS shows gradual aeration over a few days, depending on amount of cystic disease present
- When ELS is aerated, typically has communication with foregut
- CTA best identifies type and extent of involvement
- MRA will equally identify arterial supply and venous drainage

- **Congenital Diaphragmatic Hernia**
  - Defect in diaphragm
    - Left side more common than right
  - Appearance depends on size of diaphragmatic defect and contents of hernia
    - Solid in appearance if liver or other solid organ is herniated
  - Herniated bowel may not be gas filled early and may appear homogeneous
    - Filling of bowel loops with gas leads to heterogeneous appearance
  - Associated with pulmonary hypoplasia from compression of lung
    - Also effects contralateral lung if there is significant deviation of mediastinum into contralateral hemithorax

Helpful Clues for Rare Diagnoses

- **Total Anomalous Pulmonary Venous Return (TAPVR)**
  - Pulmonary venous return may be obstructed, especially in infracardiac type
    - Common draining vein courses through diaphragm and anastomoses with portal vein, returning to heart via hepatic circulation
  - Obstruction is less common in other (supracardiac and cardiac) types of anomalous venous return
  - Obstruction results in pulmonary edema and pulmonary venous hypertension
  - Heart size is typically small due to lack of venous return
- **Pulmonary Interstitial Glycogenosis**
  - Usually term infants who present with tachypnea and hypoxemia
  - Well-inflated lungs with reticular interstitial opacities
  - Good prognosis
- **Congenital Pulmonary Lymphangiectasia**
  - Well-inflated lungs with interstitial reticular opacities
  - Interlobular septal thickening on CT
  - Persistent effusions, which can be chylous, are often present

Transient Tachypnea of the Newborn

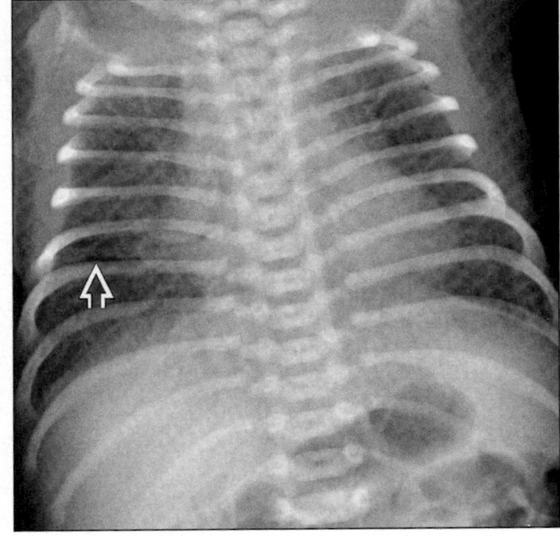

Anteroposterior radiograph shows mild hyperinflation with streaky opacities, especially in the perihilar regions. There is also a small amount of fluid in the horizontal fissure ➡.

Transient Tachypnea of the Newborn

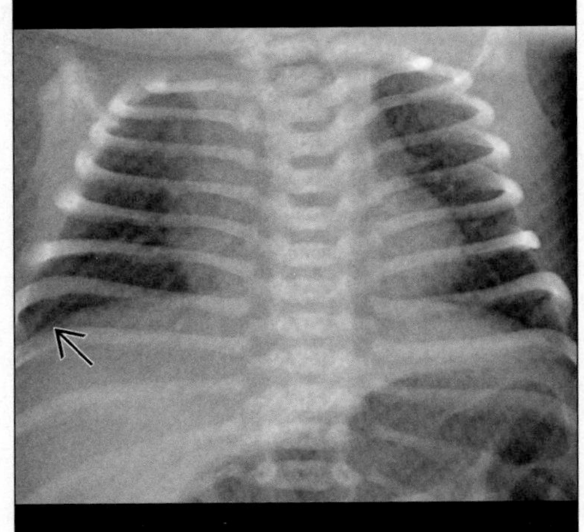

Anteroposterior radiograph shows mild hazy opacities bilaterally. In addition, there is a small amount of fluid in the right oblique fissure ➡. The appearance of transient tachypnea of the newborn are symmetrical.

NEONATAL IRREGULAR LUNG OPACITIES

Surfactant Deficient Disease

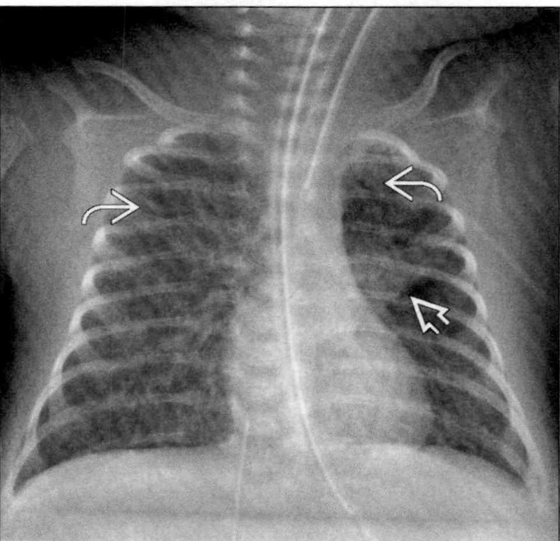

Surfactant Deficient Disease

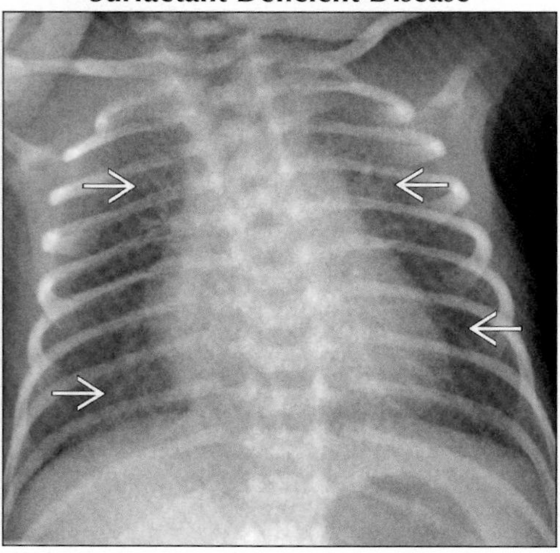

*(**Left**) AP radiograph shows coarse irregular opacities → throughout both lungs with a focal area of atelectasis → in the left perihilar region. The patient is intubated, likely contributing to the relative hyperinflation of the lungs, in this patient with RDS. (**Right**) AP radiograph shows linear opacities → throughout both lungs. Immediate postnatal radiographs in patients with RDS change from bilateral granular opacities to more irregular opacities following therapy.*

Left-to-Right Cardiac Shunts

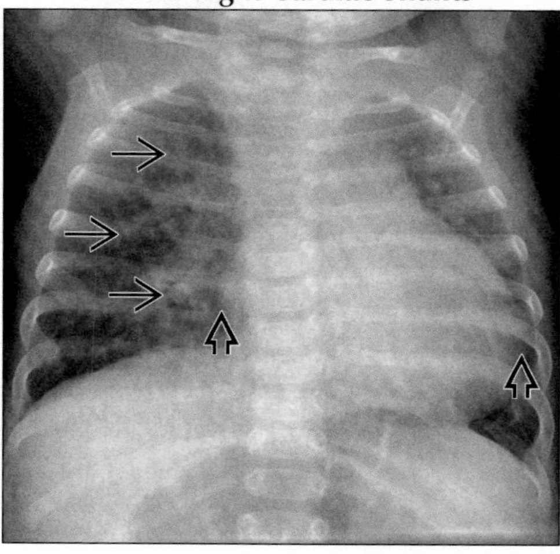

Left-to-Right Cardiac Shunts

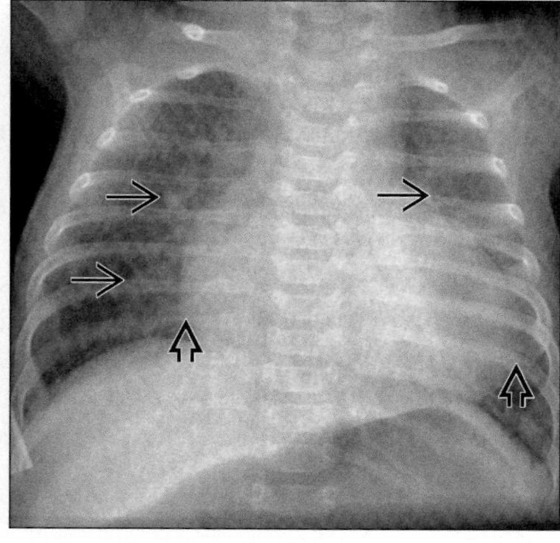

*(**Left**) Anteroposterior radiograph shows irregular opacities in the perihilar regions → consistent with enlarged vessels. The heart size is also prominent → in this newborn with a ventricular septal defect. (**Right**) Anteroposterior radiograph shows enlarged vessels → in the perihilar regions bilaterally. The heart is also enlarged →. This patient had an extracardiac shunt from a vein of Galen malformation. These shunts can lead to cardiac failure.*

Pulmonary Interstitial Emphysema

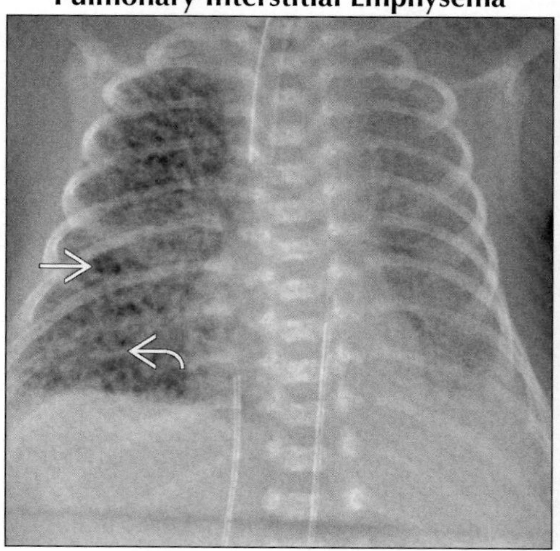

Pulmonary Interstitial Emphysema

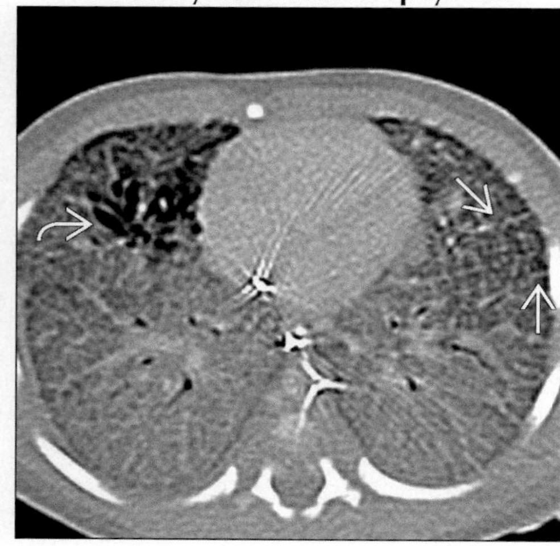

*(**Left**) AP radiograph in this patient with RDS shows coarse linear opacities → intermixed with lucencies →, almost exclusively in the right lung. (**Right**) Axial CECT shows collections of air in the interstitium of the middle lobe →. In neonates, pulmonary interstitial emphysema is nearly always seen in patients with RDS but can be seen with any condition that requires ventilatory support. This patient has TAPVR. Note the thickened interlobular septa →.*

NEONATAL IRREGULAR LUNG OPACITIES

Pulmonary Interstitial Emphysema

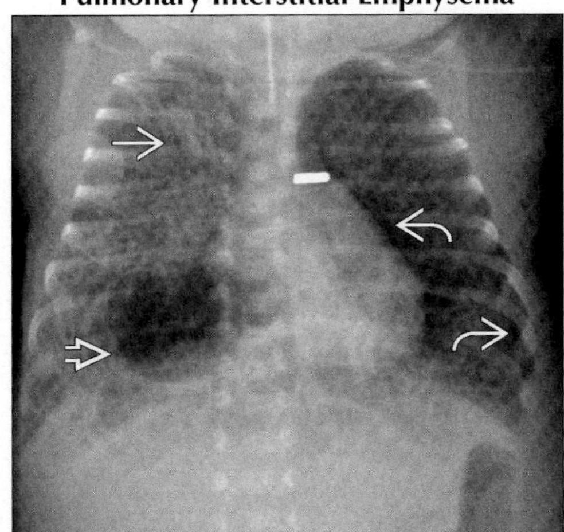

Pulmonary Interstitial Emphysema

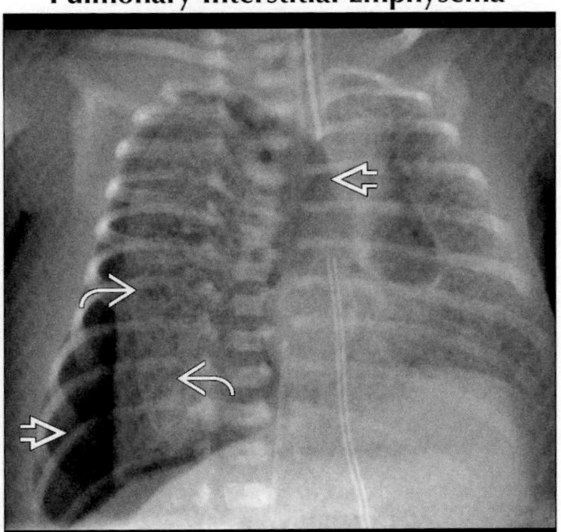

*(**Left**) Anteroposterior radiograph shows complications of PIE. The interstitial air is visible ➡, and there is now a pneumatocele in the right lung base ➡ and a left pneumothorax ➡. (**Right**) Anteroposterior radiograph shows a right tension pneumothorax ➡, identified by deviation of the mediastinum to the left and flattening of the right hemidiaphragm. PIE is seen in the right lung ➡. Tension pneumothoraces can develop rapidly.*

Meconium Aspiration Syndrome

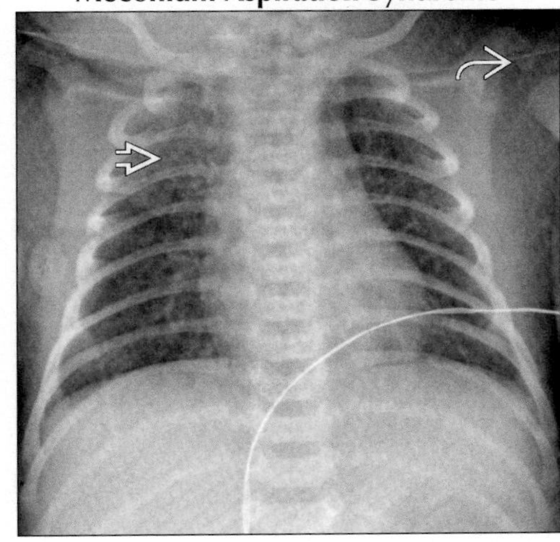

Meconium Aspiration Syndrome

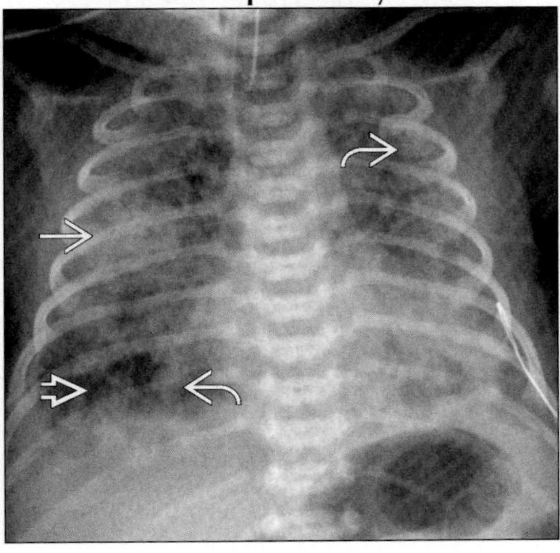

*(**Left**) AP radiograph shows coarse linear opacities bilaterally with volume loss in the right upper lobe ➡. The lungs are otherwise well inflated. The visible ossification center in the humeral heads ➡ indicates that the patient is a term infant. (**Right**) AP radiograph shows more advanced changes of meconium aspiration with focal opacities ➡, with more irregular coarse linear opacities ➡, and some more lucent areas ➡ related to air-trapping.*

Neonatal Pneumonia

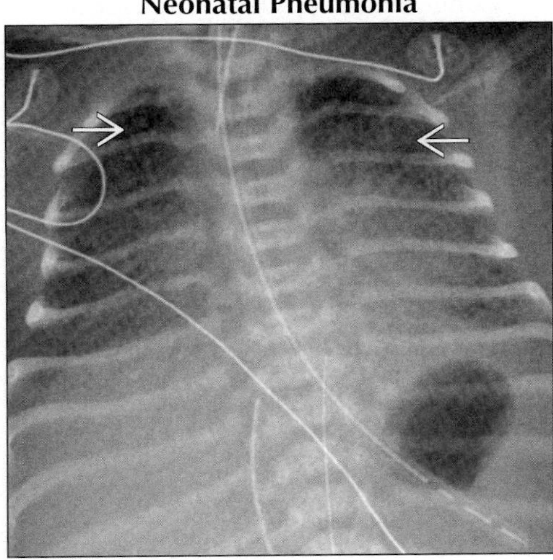

Neonatal Pneumonia

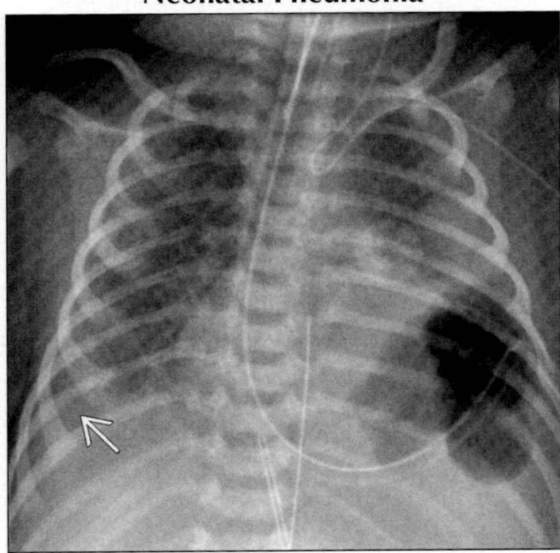

*(**Left**) AP radiograph shows low lung volumes with granular opacities bilaterally ➡, identical to surfactant deficiency. Other clinical data is needed to differentiate between the 2. (**Right**) AP radiograph shows a more heterogeneous appearance bilaterally with an area of consolidation in the right lower lobe ➡. Neonatal pneumonia can have a homogeneous/heterogeneous appearance. Effusions may also be present.*

NEONATAL IRREGULAR LUNG OPACITIES

Congenital Pulmonary Airway Abnormality

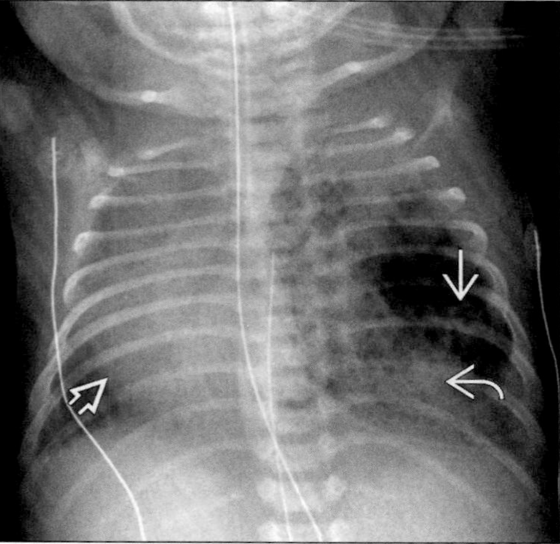

Congenital Pulmonary Airway Abnormality

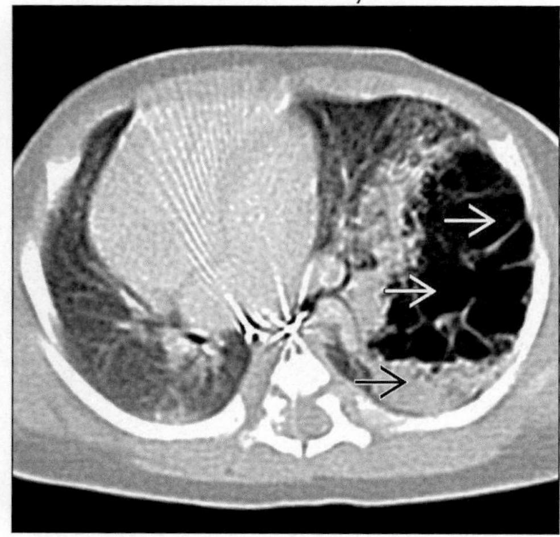

(Left) *AP radiograph shows a lucent lesion in the left lung with some irregular linear ➔ and more confluent ➔ foci of opacification. This lesion has mass effect deviating the heart ➔ to the right side.* ***(Right)*** *Axial CECT shows multiple thin-walled cysts in the left lung ➔ consistent with a type 2 CCAM. These cysts are fluid-filled at birth and become air-filled in the 1st few days of life. Some retained fluid ➔ is seen in the dependent cysts.*

Congenital Pulmonary Airway Abnormality

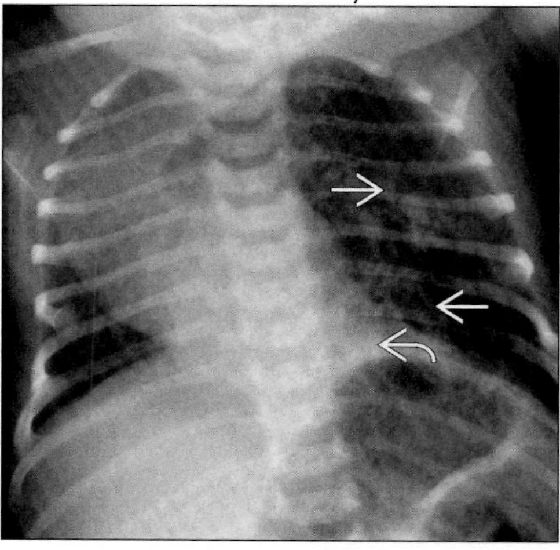

Congenital Pulmonary Airway Abnormality

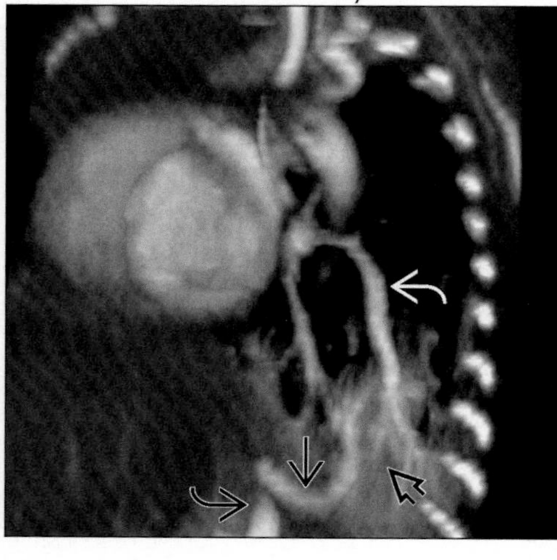

(Left) *AP radiograph shows irregular coarse opacities ➔ with more confluent opacification in the left lung base ➔. Mass effect is present with deviation of the heart to the left.* ***(Right)*** *Sagittal reformat CTA shows a large vessel ➔ arising from a similarly sized aorta ➔, supplying a mass ➔ in the left lower lobe. Venous drainage is through a large vein ➔ draining to the left atrium, consistent with intrapulmonary sequestration.*

Congenital Diaphragmatic Hernia

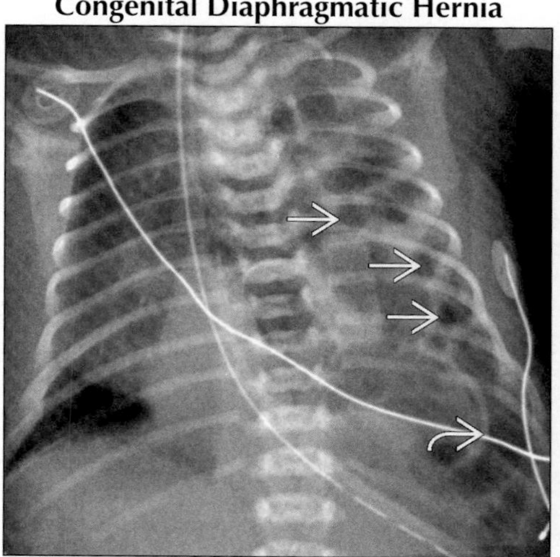

Congenital Diaphragmatic Hernia

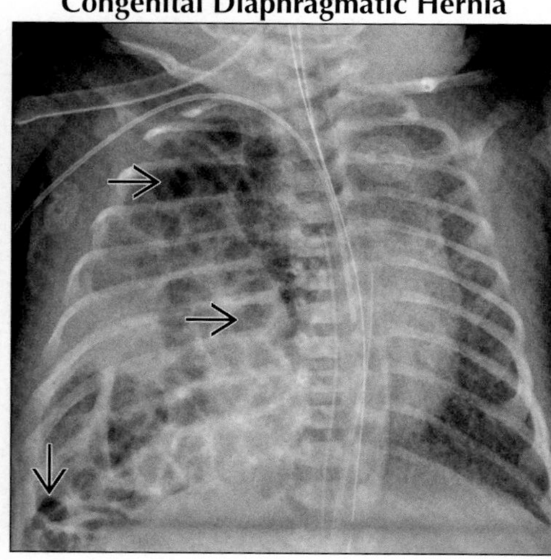

(Left) *AP radiograph shows multiple rounded lucencies ➔ in the left hemithorax. Some are elongated and tubular ➔, helping to identify the lucencies as gas-filled small bowel loops. Mass effect causes deviation of the mediastinum to the right.* ***(Right)*** *AP radiograph shows multiple similarly sized, rounded lucencies ➔ in the right hemithorax deviating the mediastinum to the left. Congenital diaphragmatic hernias are more common on the left side.*

Total Anomalous Pulmonary Venous Return (TAPVR)

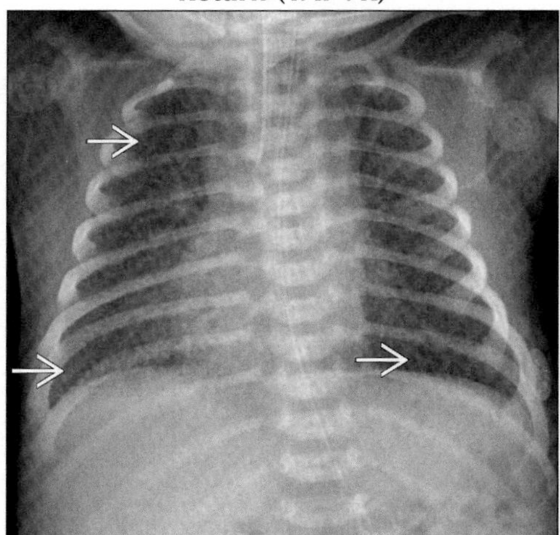

Total Anomalous Pulmonary Venous Return (TAPVR)

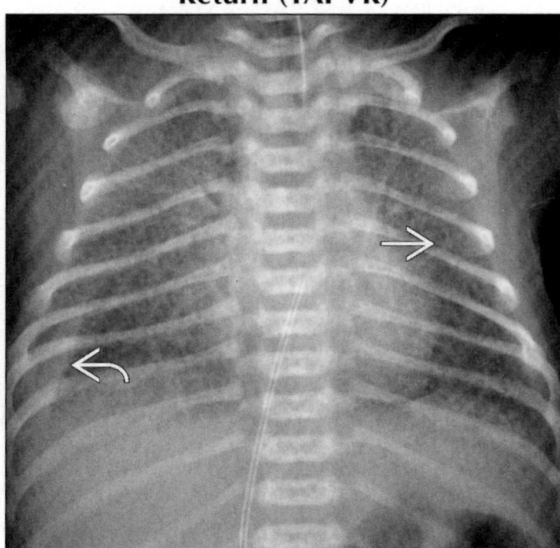

*(**Left**) AP radiograph shows symmetrical fine reticulonodular ➡ opacities. Note the relatively wide superior mediastinum in this patient with obstructed supracardiac TAPVR. (**Right**) Anteroposterior radiograph shows symmetrical fine reticulonodular opacities ➡. There is also a right-sided effusion ↪. The heart size is normal, and the superior mediastinum is not widened. These findings are in keeping with obstructed infradiaphragmatic TAPVR.*

Pulmonary Interstitial Glycogenosis

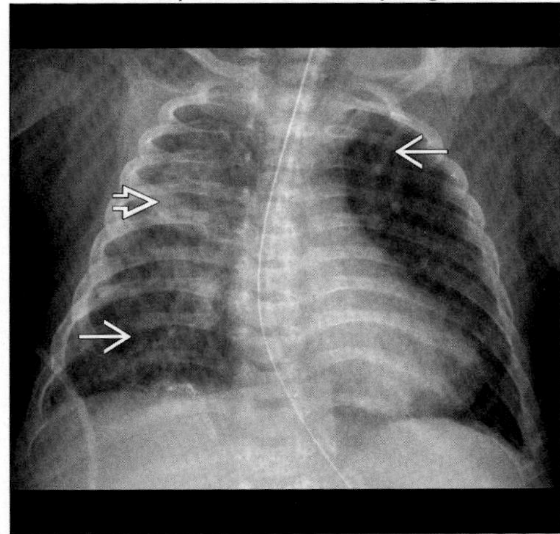

Pulmonary Interstitial Glycogenosis

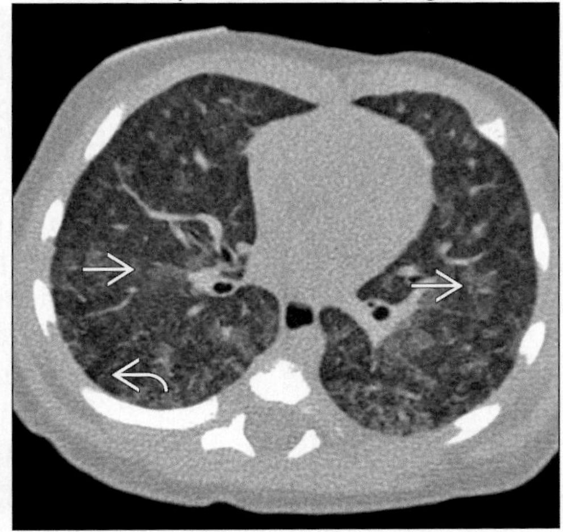

*(**Left**) Anteroposterior radiograph shows well-inflated lungs with irregular opacities in both. Some opacities are linear ➡ and some are more confluent ⇨. Initial fine reticular opacities change to more coarse reticular and linear opacities over the 1st few weeks of life. (**Right**) Axial HRCT shows scattered areas of ground-glass opacification ➡ in the lungs with a few linear opacities ↪. Over time, the linear opacities become more prominent.*

Congenital Pulmonary Lymphangiectasia

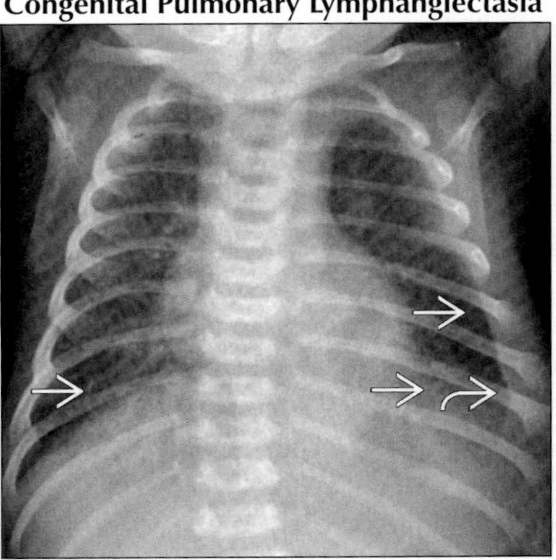

Congenital Pulmonary Lymphangiectasia

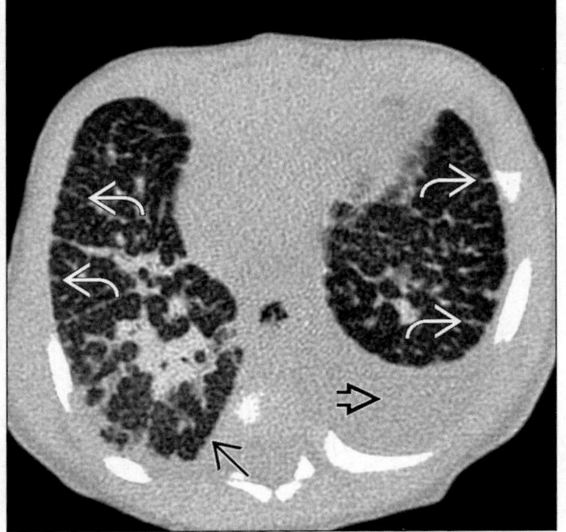

*(**Left**) Anteroposterior radiograph shows well-inflated lungs with fine reticular opacities ➡ bilaterally. A small left pleural effusion is present ↪. (**Right**) Axial HRCT shows fine interlobular septal thickening ↪ bilaterally and a moderate-sized left pleural effusion ⇨ and a small right effusion ➡. Patients may present with recurrent chylothorax, chylopericardium, or chylous ascites. The extent of involvement and the symptom severity varies.*

CONSOLIDATION

DIFFERENTIAL DIAGNOSIS

Common
- Infectious Pneumonia
- Aspiration Pneumonia
- Pulmonary Edema
- Atelectasis

Less Common
- Pulmonary Contusion
- Pulmonary Hemorrhage
- Pulmonary Infarct
- Lymphoma

Rare but Important
- Radiation Pneumonitis
- Hydrocarbon Aspiration
- Hypersensitivity Pneumonitis
- Pulmonary Alveolar Proteinosis
- Bronchiolitis Obliterans with Organizing Pneumonia
- Lymphoid Hyperplasia
- Near-Drowning
- Pulmonary Inflammatory Pseudotumor

ESSENTIAL INFORMATION

Key Differential Diagnosis Issues
- Blood, pus, protein, water, cells
- History extremely helpful

Helpful Clues for Common Diagnoses
- **Infectious Pneumonia**
  - Lung consolidation ± air bronchograms
  - Not associated with volume loss
  - ± associated parapneumonic effusion
  - Round pneumonia
    - Young children
    - Poorly developed collateral airway pathways
- **Aspiration Pneumonia**
  - Typically oral or gastric contents
  - Chemical pneumonitis, which can be superinfected
  - When upright, right lower lobe most frequent
  - When supine, posterior segments of upper lobes and superior segments of lower lobes most frequent
- **Pulmonary Edema**
  - Transudative fluid collecting in lung tissue
  - May result from
    - Increased hydrostatic gradient
    - Low oncotic pressure
    - Increased capillary permeability
  - Interstitial edema may progress to alveolar edema and consolidation
  - Pleural effusions
  - Cardiogenic vs. noncardiogenic (e.g., neurogenic, renal or hepatic disorders, toxins)
- **Atelectasis**
  - Airspace collapse resulting in increased lung density
  - Volume loss
    - Elevation of diaphragm
    - Cardiomediastinal shift
    - Shift of fissures
    - Crowding of vessels
  - Can be lobar, segmental, subsegmental, or plate-like
  - Frequently seen in inpatient settings, viral respiratory infections, and asthmatic patients

Helpful Clues for Less Common Diagnoses
- **Pulmonary Contusion**
  - Edema and hemorrhage collecting in area of lung trauma
  - Typically evolve on radiography over 24-48 hours
  - Typically resolve in 3-5 days
  - Look for other signs of trauma
    - Pneumothorax, mediastinal injury, fractures, pleural fluid
- **Pulmonary Hemorrhage**
  - Can be indistinguishable from other sources of consolidation on radiograph
  - May resolve fairly rapidly
  - Common causes in children include
    - Infection
    - Cystic fibrosis
    - Immunologic disorders (e.g., Goodpasture syndrome)
    - Wegener granulomatosis
    - Trauma
- **Pulmonary Infarct**
  - Usually result of pulmonary embolus
  - Peripheral, wedge-shaped consolidation
  - Hampton hump: Pleural-based, peripheral, wedge-shaped consolidation secondary to pulmonary embolus
- **Lymphoma**
  - Can present as chronic lung consolidation
  - Non-Hodgkin most frequent

- Consider AIDS-related primary pulmonary lymphoma
- Lymphadenopathy

Helpful Clues for Rare Diagnoses

- **Radiation Pneumonitis**
  - Typically requires at least 4500 rads
  - Acute
    - 1-8 weeks after radiation
    - Patchy consolidation confined to radiation portal
  - Chronic
    - 9-12 months after radiation and beyond
    - Consolidation and fibrosis/scarring
    - Bronchiectasis
- **Hydrocarbon Aspiration**
  - Gasoline, kerosene, lighter fluid
  - Severe chemical pneumonitis
  - Patchy consolidation develops over several hours
  - Edema
- **Hypersensitivity Pneumonitis**
  - a.k.a. extrinsic allergic alveolitis
  - Type 3 immune response to environmental antigen
    - Moldy hay, dust, pigeon droppings
  - Reticulonodular opacities typically seen on x-ray
  - Consolidation may occur during acute/subacute phase
  - HRCT may demonstrate ground-glass opacities, centrilobular nodules, and consolidation
- **Pulmonary Alveolar Proteinosis**
  - Accumulation of PAS-positive phospholipids in alveoli
  - Perihilar consolidation
  - "Crazy-paving" on CT
    - Ground-glass opacities and septal thickening
  - Diagnosis via bronchoalveolar lavage
- **Bronchiolitis Obliterans with Organizing Pneumonia**
  - a.k.a. cryptogenic organizing pneumonia
  - Granulation tissue in bronchioles and alveolar inflammation
  - Patchy alveolar consolidation, ground-glass opacification, centrilobular nodules
  - Diagnosis via tissue biopsy
- **Lymphoid Hyperplasia**
  - Nonneoplastic nodular proliferation
  - Nonspecific nodular areas of consolidation
  - Adenopathy
- **Near-Drowning**
  - Drowning 2nd most common cause of accidental death in children
  - Hypoxemia secondary to aspiration or laryngospasm
  - Pulmonary edema pattern on x-ray that may have delayed appearance
  - Edema typically resolves fairly rapidly
- **Pulmonary Inflammatory Pseudotumor**
  - a.k.a. plasma cell granuloma
  - Most common benign lung neoplasm in children
  - May involve mediastinum and pleura
  - Occasional calcifications

Infectious Pneumonia

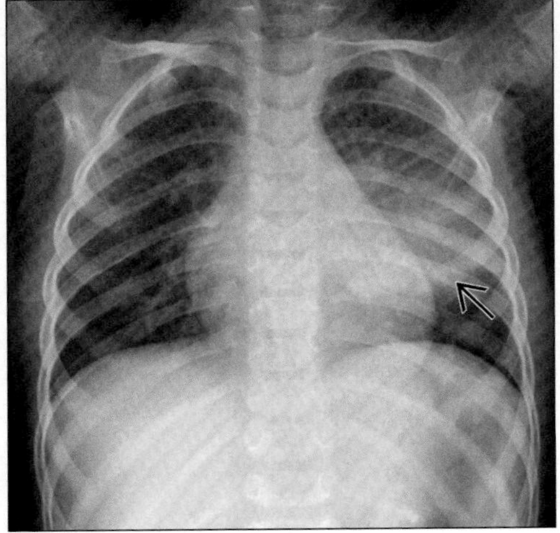

Frontal radiograph shows focal consolidation ➔ within the superior segment of the left lower lobe without associated volume loss, consistent with pneumonia in this toddler with a cough and fever.

Infectious Pneumonia

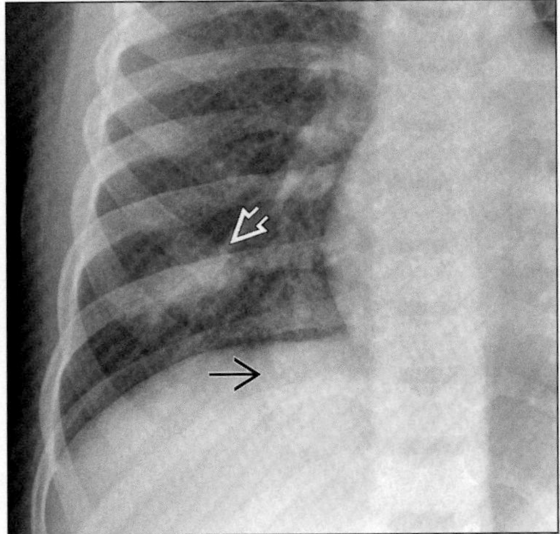

Frontal radiograph shows 2 areas of consolidation in the right lower lobe ➔. The more lateral density ➔ is consistent with a round pneumonia in this 6 year old with a cough and fever.

CONSOLIDATION

(Left) Frontal radiograph shows focal dense consolidation in left upper lobe without volume loss. After no response to antibiotics for presumed community-acquired bacterial pneumonia, a sputum culture in this 10-year-old child confirmed blastomycosis ➔. (Right) Frontal radiograph shows bibasilar, left greater than right, consolidation → that developed in the immediate postoperative period. This 3 year old aspirated following extubation.

Infectious Pneumonia

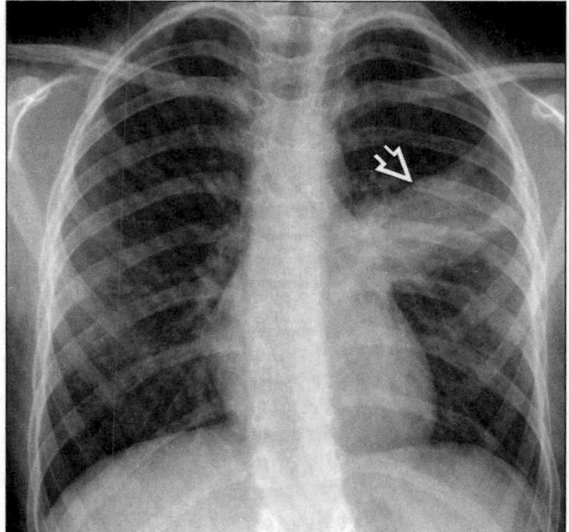

Aspiration Pneumonia

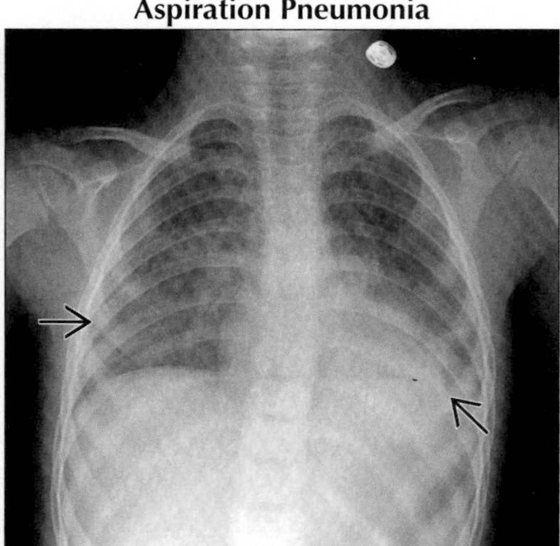

(Left) Frontal radiograph shows bilateral fluffy perihilar and basilar consolidation, consistent with pulmonary edema. In this child, the cause was noncardiogenic (neurogenic), secondary to a massive intracranial AVM hemorrhage. (Right) Lateral radiograph shows plate-like increased density → within the right middle lobe, abutting the major fissure. A chest x-ray taken the following day showed complete resolution of atelectasis in this 3 year old with asthma.

Pulmonary Edema

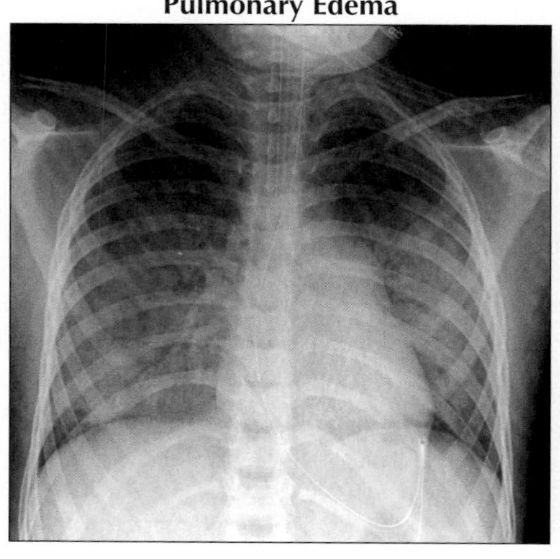

Atelectasis

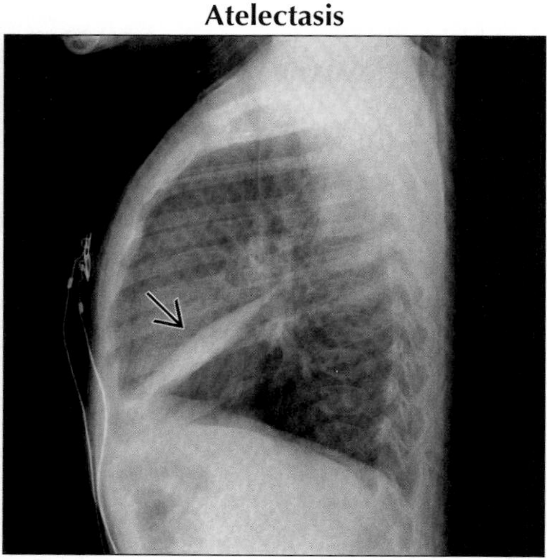

(Left) Frontal radiograph of a patient in a motor vehicle crash shows diffuse consolidation within the right lung, consistent with pulmonary contusion. Note the small anterior pneumothorax ➔, rib fractures ➔, and chest wall emphysema ➔. (Right) Axial NECT in the same patient several days later demonstrates decreased but residual consolidation in the right lower lobe →. There is early pneumatocele formation ➔ in some of the areas of contusion.

Pulmonary Contusion

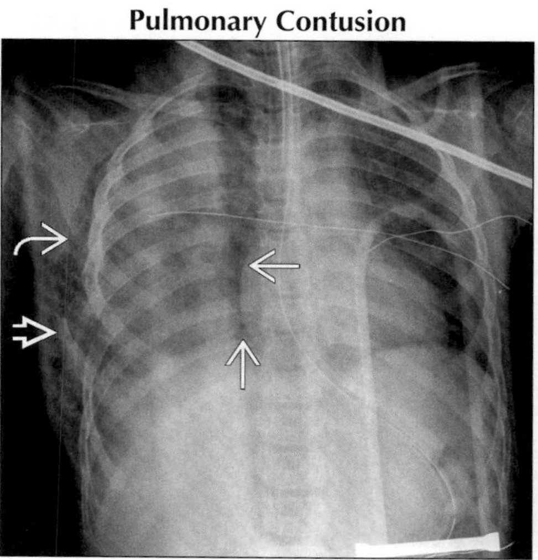

Pulmonary Contusion

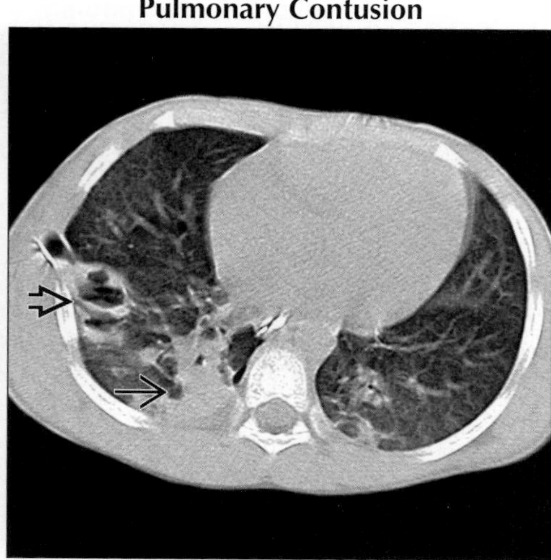

CONSOLIDATION

Pulmonary Hemorrhage

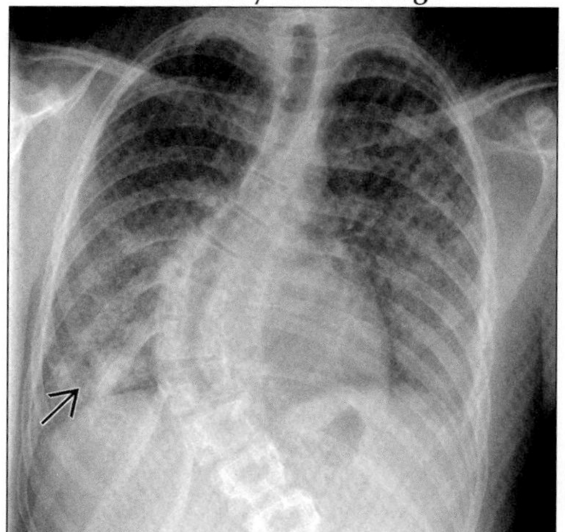

Pulmonary Hemorrhage

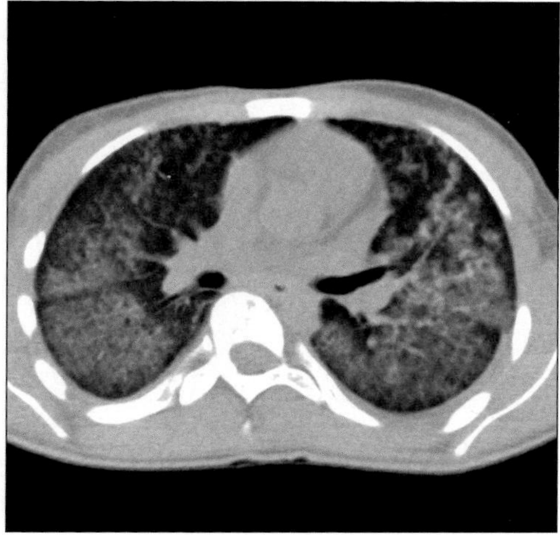

(Left) *Frontal radiograph shows diffuse multifocal areas of lung consolidation, particularly in the right lower lobe ➔. The consolidation is fluffy and alveolar in appearance.* ***(Right)*** *Axial NECT in the same patient better demonstrates the diffuse multifocal areas of alveolar consolidation. While nonspecific, the appearance is suspicious for hemorrhage, which was eventually confirmed by a bronchoscopy in this 15-year-old patient with Wegener granulomatosis.*

Pulmonary Infarct

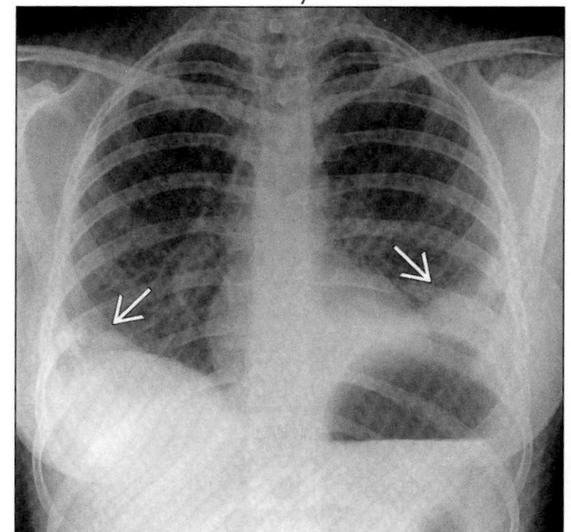

Pulmonary Infarct

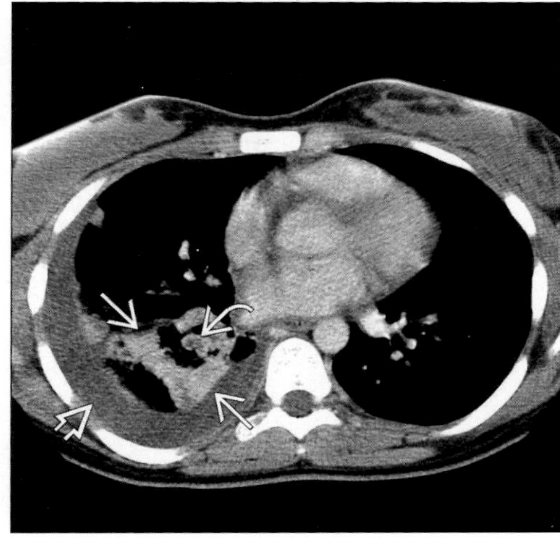

(Left) *Frontal radiograph shows peripheral, pleural-based areas of consolidation ➔ in both lower lobes. Though nonspecific, these findings are consistent with Hampton humps, which are associated with pulmonary emboli.* ***(Right)*** *Axial CECT in the same patient shows a peripheral wedge-shaped area of consolidation ➔ in the right lower lobe. There is an associated pleural effusion ➔. Note the emboli ➔ in the corresponding pulmonary arteries.*

Lymphoma

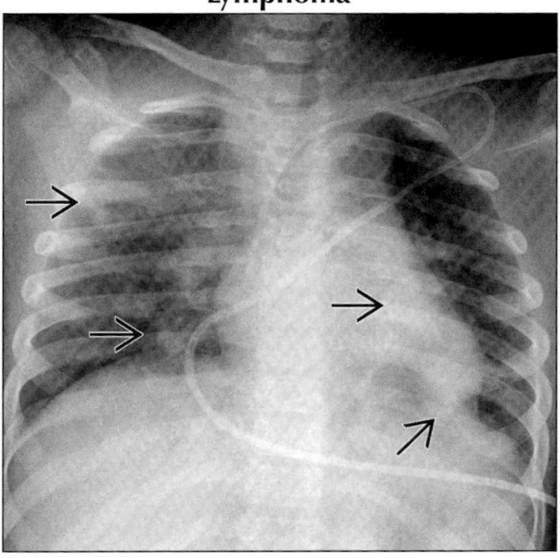

Lymphoma

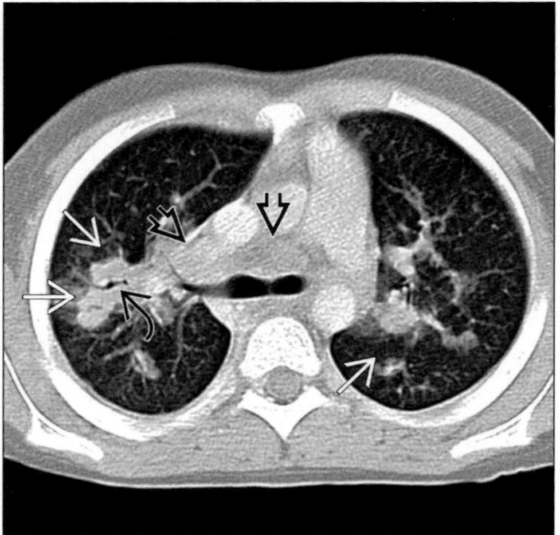

(Left) *Frontal radiograph shows multifocal areas of ill-defined lung consolidation ➔.* ***(Right)*** *Axial CECT in the same patient demonstrates multifocal areas of nonspecific lung consolidation ➔ with a few air bronchograms ➔. There is also hilar and mediastinal lymphadenopathy ➔. This adenopathy is better appreciated on mediastinal windows (not shown). This 9 year old had biopsy-proven pulmonary lymphoma.*

CONSOLIDATION

(Left) Coronal CECT shows well-demarcated consolidation in the right upper lung with volume loss, bronchiectasis ➔, and chest wall deformity in this 19 year old status post radiation therapy for an upper right chest wall Ewing sarcoma. *(Right)* Frontal radiograph shows dense consolidation in the lower lobes ➔, right greater than left, along with pulmonary vascular congestion. This 1 year old aspirated lighter fluid several hours prior to imaging.

Radiation Pneumonitis

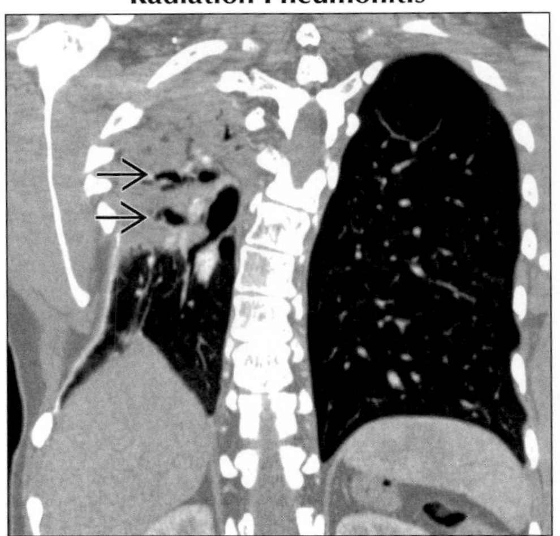

Hydrocarbon Aspiration

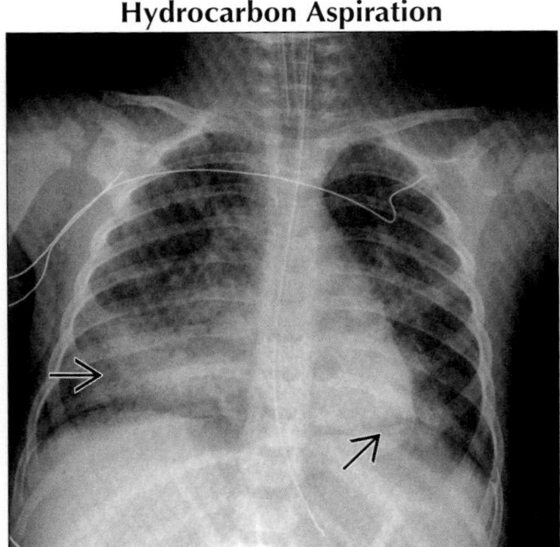

(Left) Frontal radiograph shows reticulonodular interstitial prominence and hazy mild bibasilar airspace consolidation ➔. *(Right)* Axial HRCT in the same patient shows bilateral lower lobe septal thickening, ground-glass opacities, scattered centrilobular nodules, and a small area of consolidation ➔. Other areas of consolidation, though present, are not shown. Bronchoalveolar lavage analysis confirmed hypersensitivity pneumonitis in this 8-year-old patient.

Hypersensitivity Pneumonitis

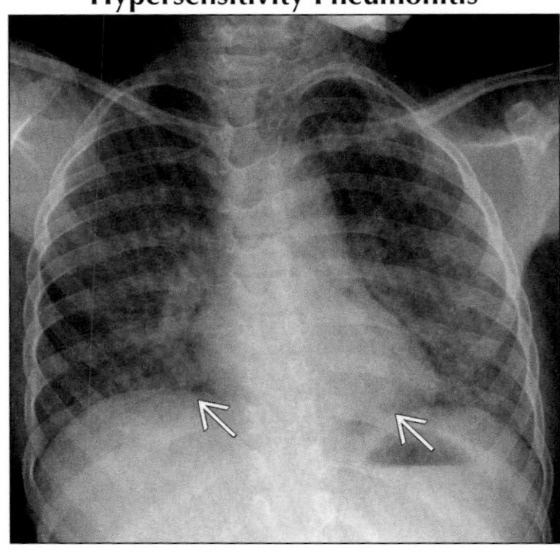

Hypersensitivity Pneumonitis

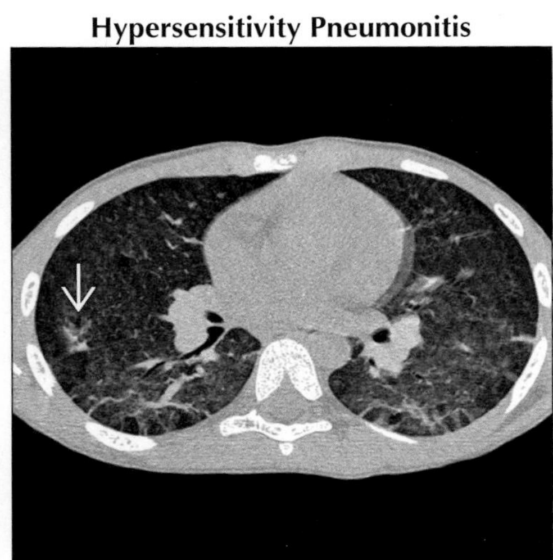

(Left) Frontal radiograph shows bilateral, symmetric, perihilar and basilar, predominantly fluffy airspace consolidation. The size of the heart is normal, and there are no pleural effusions. *(Right)* Axial HRCT in the same patient shows relatively symmetric, perihilar, ground-glass opacities combined with septal thickening in a "crazy-paving" pattern ➔. Bronchoalveolar lavage in this 19-year-old female confirmed pulmonary alveolar proteinosis.

Pulmonary Alveolar Proteinosis

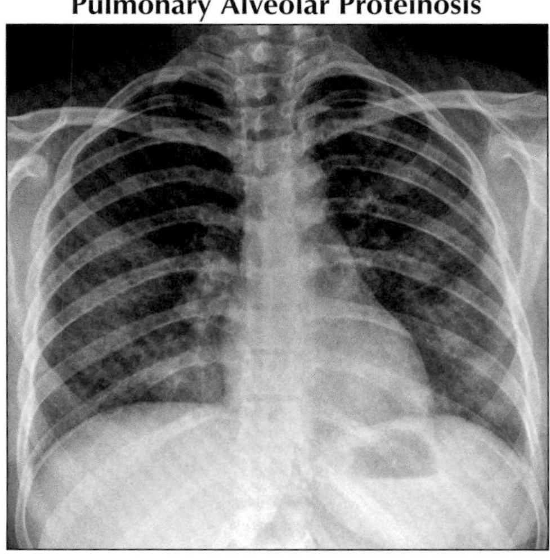

Pulmonary Alveolar Proteinosis

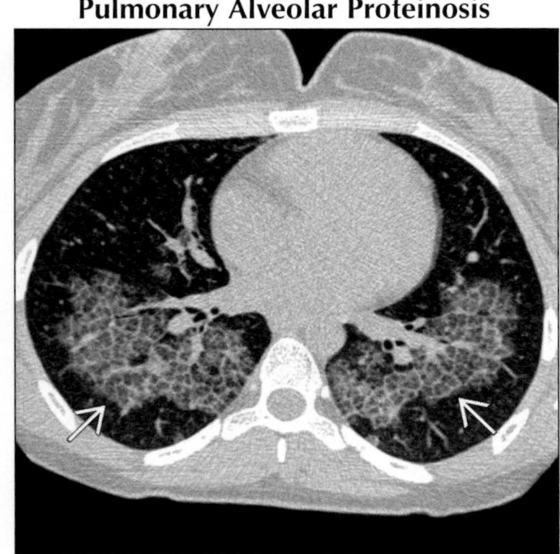

Bronchiolitis Obliterans with Organizing Pneumonia

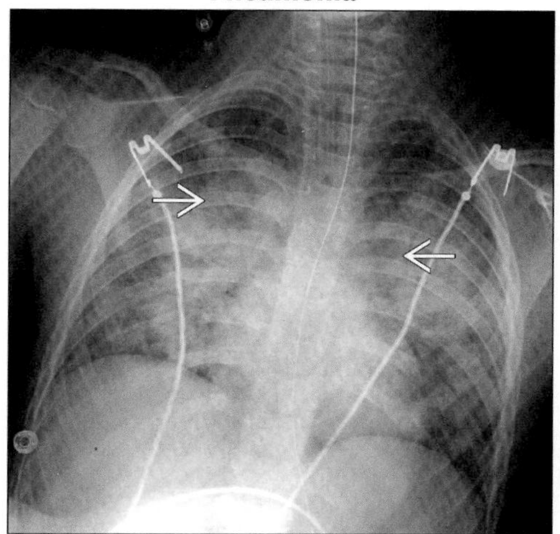

Bronchiolitis Obliterans with Organizing Pneumonia

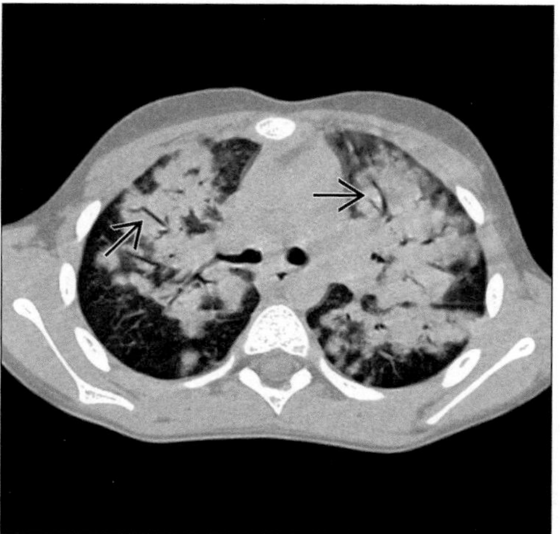

*(**Left**) Frontal radiograph shows bilateral, relatively symmetric consolidation within both lungs in this intubated patient. There are scattered air bronchograms ➡. (**Right**) Axial NECT in the same patient shows multifocal, relatively symmetric consolidation within both lungs with scattered air bronchograms ➡. Biopsy specimen showed findings consistent with bronchiolitis obliterans with organizing pneumonia in this 7 year old.*

Lymphoid Hyperplasia

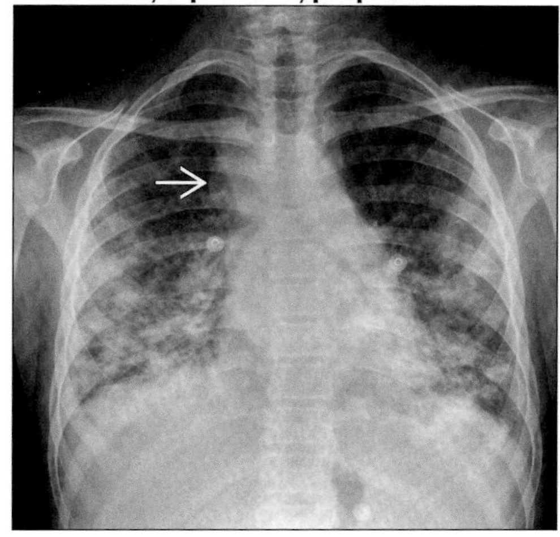

Lymphoid Hyperplasia

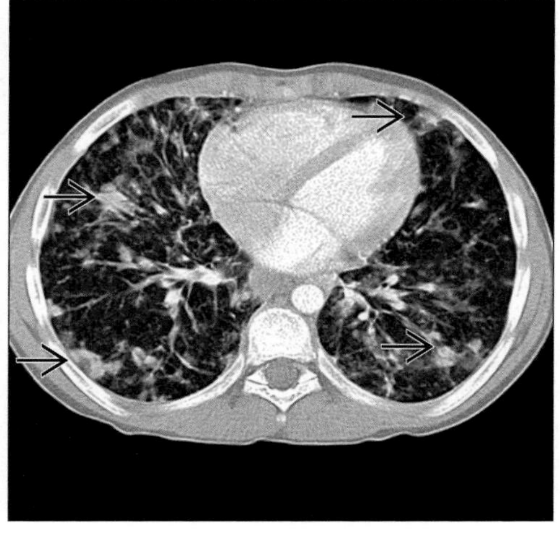

*(**Left**) Frontal radiograph shows relatively symmetric bibasilar areas of nodular consolidation. There is also mediastinal widening ➡, consistent with adenopathy. (**Right**) Axial CECT in the same patient shows multifocal areas of nodular consolidation bilaterally ➡. Mediastinal adenopathy was present (not shown). The imaging findings are nonspecific. Surgical pathology demonstrated benign nodular lymphoid hyperplasia in this 12-year-old child.*

Near-Drowning

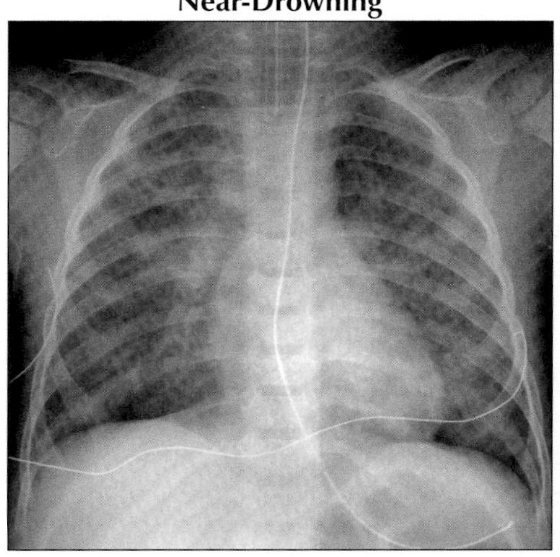

Pulmonary Inflammatory Pseudotumor

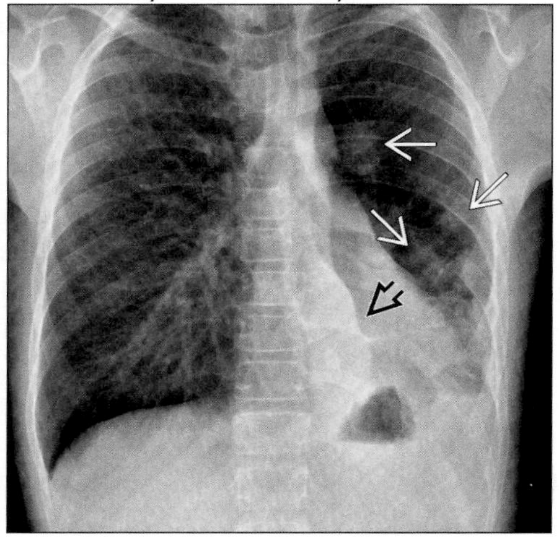

*(**Left**) Frontal radiograph shows nonspecific, bilateral, fluffy airspace opacification in this 2-year-old intubated patient. There is no cardiomegaly, and there are no pleural effusions. This chest x-ray was taken 1 day after a near-drowning event. (**Right**) Frontal radiograph shows a pleural-based mass ➡, as well as multiple areas of pulmonary consolidation ➡ on the left in this adolescent with a biopsy-proven pulmonary inflammatory pseudotumor.*

BUBBLY LUNGS

DIFFERENTIAL DIAGNOSIS

Common
- Pulmonary Interstitial Emphysema
- Cystic Adenomatoid Malformation
- Congenital Diaphragmatic Hernia
- Bronchopulmonary Dysplasia
- Pulmonary Cystic Fibrosis

Less Common
- Pneumatoceles
- Childhood Interstitial Lung Disease

Rare but Important
- Emphysema
- Tuberous Sclerosis Complex

ESSENTIAL INFORMATION

Key Differential Diagnosis Issues
- History is helpful in determining source of bubbly lung appearance
- CT may be necessary to narrow differential diagnosis

Helpful Clues for Common Diagnoses
- **Pulmonary Interstitial Emphysema**
  - Premature neonates
  - Background lung disease
    - Barotrauma from mechanical ventilation
    - Alveolar rupture with air leak into pulmonary interstitium
  - Reticular and cystic appearance
    - Can rapidly develop from 1 NICU chest x-ray to next
  - Can progress to pneumomediastinum and pneumothorax
  - Bilateral, unilateral, lobar, or segmental
  - May resolve quickly with change in ventilator settings
- **Cystic Adenomatoid Malformation**
  - a.k.a. congenital pulmonary airway malformation (CPAM)
  - Type 1
    - Single or multiple 2-10 cm cysts
    - Can present as bubbly lungs
    - May contain air-fluid levels
    - Good prognosis
  - Type 2
    - Multiple small (0.5-2 cm) cysts
    - Can present as bubbly lungs
  - Type 3
    - Innumerable microscopic cysts
    - Appears solid
    - Poorer prognosis
  - Evidence of associated mass effect
    - Mediastinal shift
    - Compression of adjacent normal lung
  - Can coexist with other pulmonary malformations
    - Sequestration
    - Bronchogenic cyst
  - Can become complicated by recurrent infections
  - Small malignancy risk
    - Pleuropulmonary blastoma
    - Rhabdomyosarcoma
- **Congenital Diaphragmatic Hernia**
  - Bochdalek hernia (90%)
    - Posterior
  - Morgagni hernia (10%)
    - Anterior
  - Left (75%), right (25%)
  - Bubbly chest appearance when gas-filled stomach/bowel involved
  - Associated mass effect
  - Associated pulmonary hypoplasia
  - Enteric tube may enter mass if stomach is herniated
- **Bronchopulmonary Dysplasia**
  - a.k.a. chronic lung disease of prematurity
  - Premature neonates with surfactant deficiency
  - Mechanical ventilation
  - High oxygen concentrations
  - Bubbly lung appearance begins to appear approximately 10 days after birth
    - Cystic changes
    - Streaky densities
    - Atelectasis
    - Air-trapping
  - Will not resolve on subsequent imaging exams
  - Wilson-Mikity syndrome
    - Similar radiographic appearance to bronchopulmonary dysplasia
    - No history of mechanical ventilation
- **Pulmonary Cystic Fibrosis**
  - Chronic hereditary lung disease
  - Defects in gene for cystic fibrosis transmembrane conductance regulator
    - Encodes protein of cell membrane chloride channel
  - Leads to exocrine gland dysfunction

- Lungs
- Liver
- Pancreas
- GI tract
- Radiographic findings include
  - Bronchiectasis
  - Bronchial wall thickening
  - Mucus plugging
  - Hyperinflation
  - Prominent hila
- Cystic bronchiectasis can give bubbly lung appearance

Helpful Clues for Less Common Diagnoses

- **Pneumatoceles**
  - Thin-walled cysts/cavities
  - May be secondary to trauma or infection/inflammation
  - Can resolve spontaneously
  - May become superinfected
  - When multiple, can appear as bubbly lungs
- **Childhood Interstitial Lung Disease**
  - Uncommon group of disorders
  - Can be idiopathic or secondary to known disorder (e.g., infection, drugs, exposure)
    - Possible association with systemic disease (e.g., connective tissue disease, vasculitis)
  - Neuroendocrine cell hyperplasia in infancy and pulmonary interstitial glycogenesis are unique to children
  - Radiographic findings
    - Include normal chest x-ray, ground-glass and reticulonodular opacities, hyperinflation
  - HRCT findings
    - Include septal thickening, air-trapping, nodules, ground-glass opacities, and honeycombing

Helpful Clues for Rare Diagnoses

- **Emphysema**
  - Alveolar destruction, which leads to obstructive pulmonary disease
  - Rare in children
  - Can be seen with α-1-antitrypsin disease and Marfan syndrome
  - Can also be idiopathic
  - Panacinar/panlobular
    - Due to alveolar destruction
    - More common in younger patients
  - Centroacinar/centrilobular
    - Due to terminal bronchiole destruction
    - Seen in adults/smokers
  - Hyperinflated lungs with true parenchymal destruction
  - Can mimic bubbly lung appearance
- **Tuberous Sclerosis Complex**
  - Lymphangioleiomyomatosis
    - Abnormal smooth muscle proliferation
    - Results in small airway and lymphatic obstruction
  - Small parenchymal cysts/bubbly lungs
  - Chylous pleural effusions
  - Cyst rupture can lead to pneumothorax

Pulmonary Interstitial Emphysema

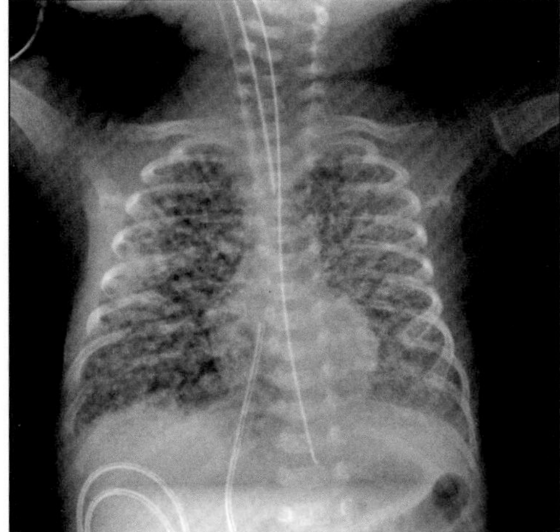

Frontal radiograph shows a diffuse bubbly lung appearance. The mixed reticular and cystic appearance is consistent with pulmonary interstitial emphysema in this mechanically ventilated neonate.

Pulmonary Interstitial Emphysema

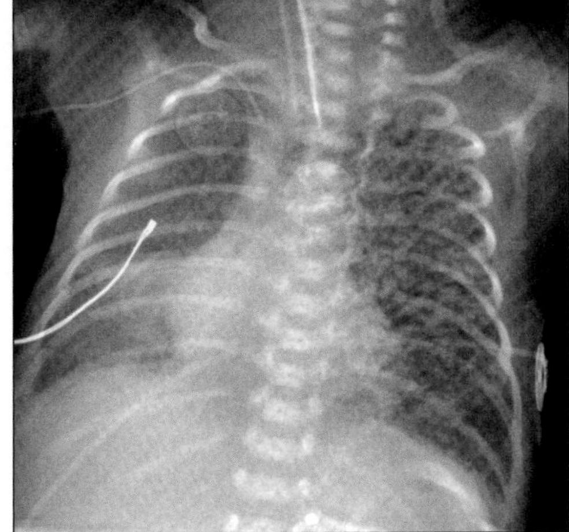

Frontal radiograph shows a unilateral left lung bubbly appearance in this mechanically ventilated premature neonate. Pulmonary interstitial emphysema can be asymmetric in its lung involvement.

BUBBLY LUNGS

*(**Left**) Frontal radiograph shows a focal bubbly lung appearance in the right base → in this mechanically ventilated premature neonate. The coarse reticular and cystic appearance is consistent with segmental pulmonary interstitial emphysema. The lungs are otherwise opacified due to surfactant deficiency and atelectasis. (**Right**) Frontal radiograph shows a bubbly appearance of the left lung with a rightward mediastinal shift → in this neonate with a type 1 CCAM.*

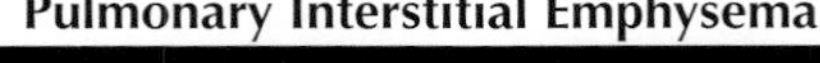

Pulmonary Interstitial Emphysema

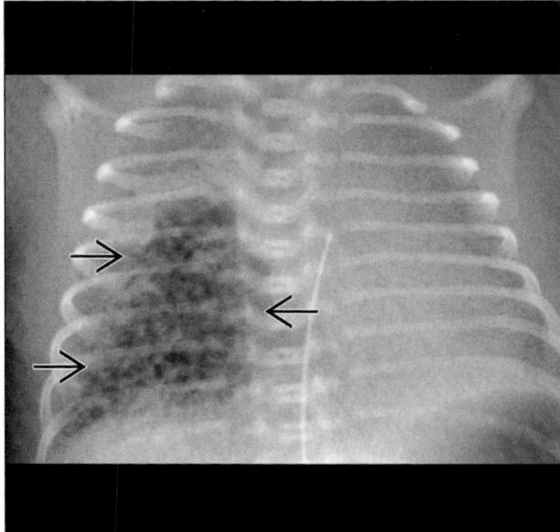

Cystic Adenomatoid Malformation

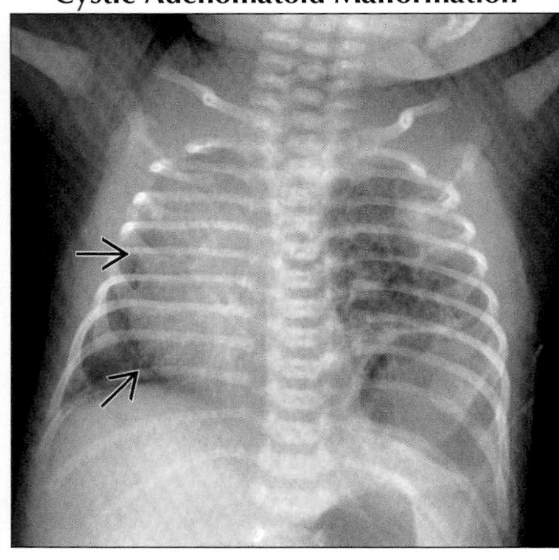

*(**Left**) Frontal radiograph shows a bubbly appearance to the left hemithorax due to herniated gas-filled bowel loops in this neonate on ECMO ➭. There is associated mass effect and pulmonary hypoplasia. (**Right**) Axial NECT shows hyperexpanded lungs with diffuse cystic changes. This 10 year old was a former premature neonate who developed severe chronic lung disease secondary to surfactant deficiency and mechanical ventilation with high oxygen concentrations.*

Congenital Diaphragmatic Hernia

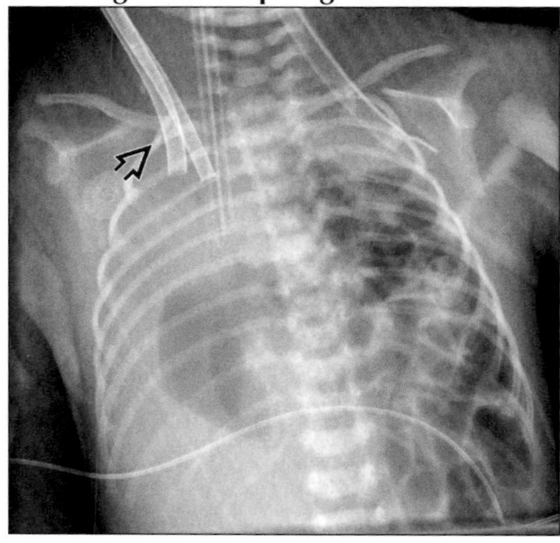

Bronchopulmonary Dysplasia

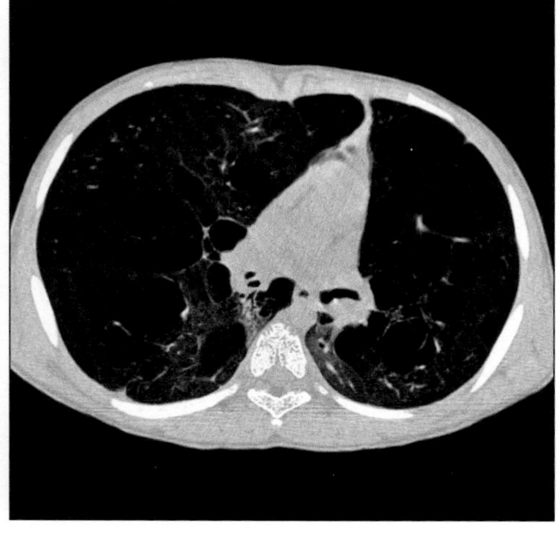

*(**Left**) Frontal radiograph in this 11-year-old patient with cystic fibrosis shows an upper lobe with a predominant bubbly lung appearance secondary to cystic bronchiectasis ➦ and bronchial wall thickening with overall hyperinflated lungs. Note the G-tube in the left upper quadrant →. (**Right**) Axial HRCT shows hyperexpanded lungs with diffuse bronchiectasis, bronchial wall thickening, and mucus plugging ➔ in this 14-year-old child with cystic fibrosis.*

Pulmonary Cystic Fibrosis

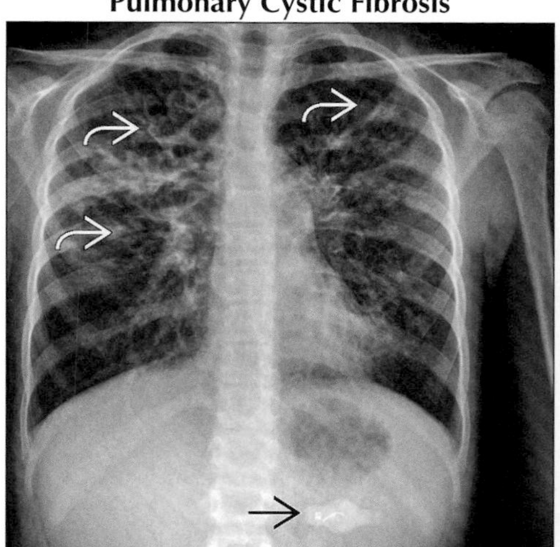

Pulmonary Cystic Fibrosis

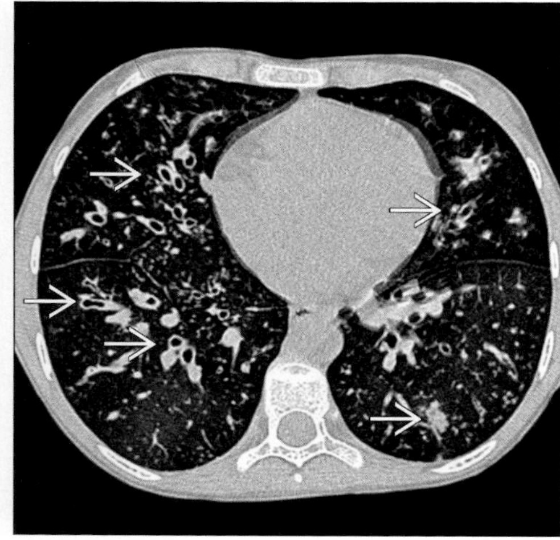

BUBBLY LUNGS

Pneumatoceles

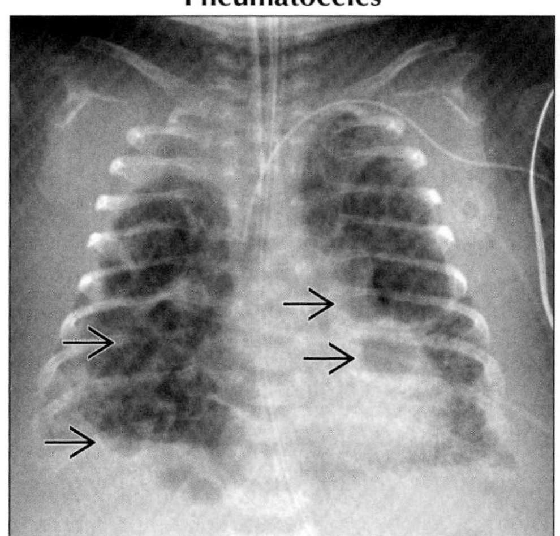

Pneumatoceles

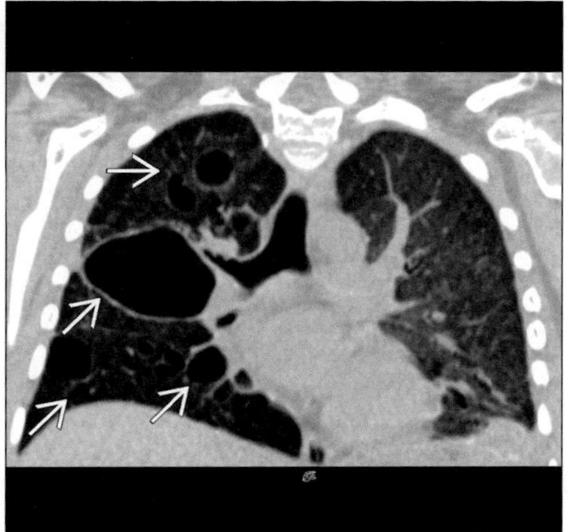

*(**Left**) Frontal radiograph shows bubbly lungs with multiple large cystic lucencies bilaterally ➔. The lucencies represent pneumatoceles in this 2 week old with pneumonia and sepsis. (**Right**) Coronal NECT shows multiple, large, thin-walled cystic spaces scattered throughout the right lung ➔. The cysts are consistent with pneumatoceles in this 12 year old with a remote history of a severe Staph pneumonia with cavitary necrosis in the right lung.*

Childhood Interstitial Lung Disease

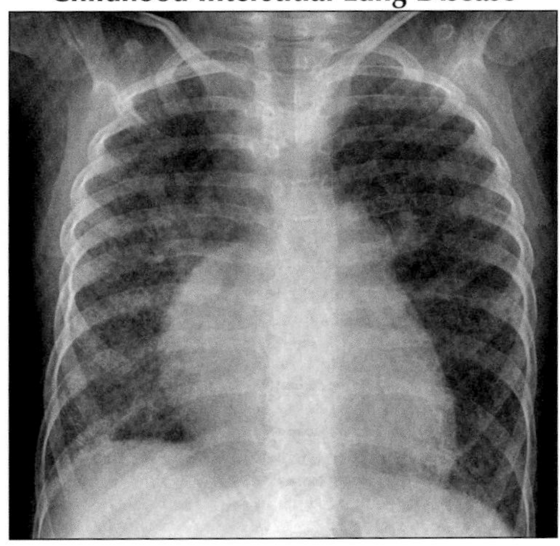

Childhood Interstitial Lung Disease

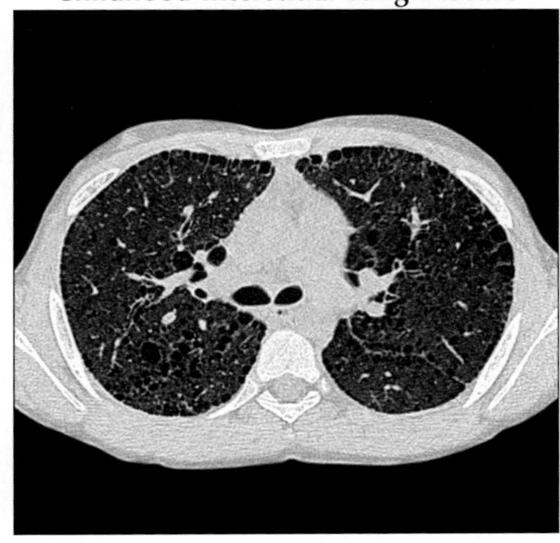

*(**Left**) Frontal radiograph shows hyperexpansion and diffuse reticular interstitial opacification, giving a fine bubbly appearance. A surgical pathology of a biopsy specimen in this child showed pulmonary fibrosis secondary to surfactant protein C deficiency. (**Right**) Axial HRCT shows a bubbly appearance of the lungs with innumerable tiny cystic spaces. Surgical pathology of a biopsy specimen in this 15 year old showed lymphocytic interstitial pneumonitis.*

Emphysema

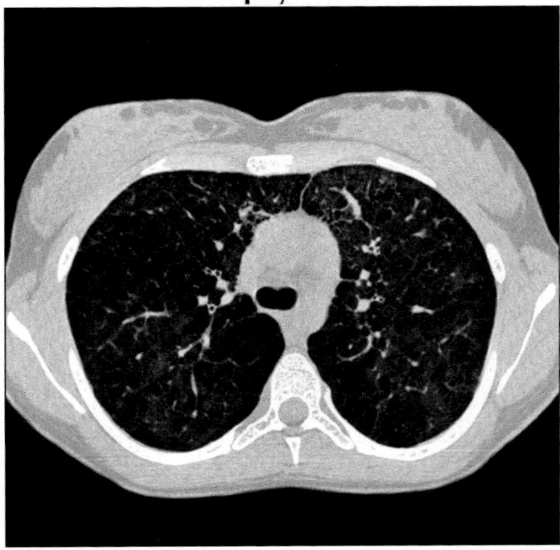

Tuberous Sclerosis Complex

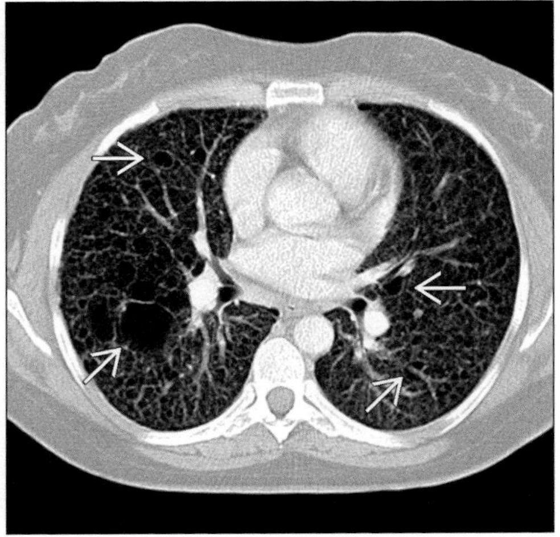

*(**Left**) Axial NECT shows diffuse emphysema giving a bubbly lung appearance. Note that this is true parenchymal destruction rather than lung cysts. The cause for this 16-year-old patient's emphysema could not be determined. (**Right**) Axial CECT shows innumerable parenchymal cysts of varying sizes ➔, creating a bubbly lung appearance. In this female adolescent with tuberous sclerosis, the appearance is consistent with lymphangioleiomyomatosis.*

UNILATERAL HYPERLUCENT LUNG

DIFFERENTIAL DIAGNOSIS

Common
- Endobronchial Obstruction/Foreign Body
- Asthma
- Pneumothorax

Less Common
- Swyer-James Syndrome
- Extrinsic Airway Compression by Mass Lesion
- Vascular Ring/Sling
- Scimitar Syndrome
- Bulla

Rare but Important
- Pulmonary Agenesis/Aplasia
- Poland Syndrome
- Pulmonary Embolus

ESSENTIAL INFORMATION

Key Differential Diagnosis Issues
- Appearance can result from variety of sources
  - Technical factors (rotation)
  - Chest wall abnormalities
  - Lung parenchymal abnormalities
  - Airway issues
  - Vascular abnormalities
- Appearance of unilateral hyperlucent lung may be result of compensatory hyperinflation due to contralateral lung abnormality
- Decubitus views can be helpful
- Chest CT may be necessary in confusing cases

Helpful Clues for Common Diagnoses
- **Endobronchial Obstruction/Foreign Body**
  - Food is most common aspirated foreign body
    - Peanuts most common food aspirated
  - Frequency of right vs. left bronchial tree involvement equal in young children
  - In adults, right > left
  - Air-trapping occurs distal to obstruction more commonly than atelectasis in children
  - Lateral decubitus radiographs helpful
    - Persistent air-trapping in obstructed lung
  - Fluoroscopy or expiratory images can also be utilized
- **Asthma**
  - Most common chronic childhood disease
  - Airway inflammation results in intermittent airflow obstruction
  - Chest radiograph typically obtained to rule out other etiologies or complications
    - May be normal
    - May show bilateral hyperinflated, hyperlucent lungs
  - When lungs are asymmetrically involved, unilateral hyperlucent lung appearance may result
    - Must consider aspirated foreign body in these situations
- **Pneumothorax**
  - Wide spectrum of etiologies in pediatric population
  - Can mimic appearance of unilateral hyperlucent lung
  - Radiolucent space lacking pulmonary markings
  - White pleural line visible

Helpful Clues for Less Common Diagnoses
- **Swyer-James Syndrome**
  - Postinfectious obliterative bronchiolitis
    - Viral
    - Bacterial
    - Mycoplasma
  - Arrest of progressive normal lung growth secondary to vascular compromise
  - Small hyperlucent lung
  - Attenuated pulmonary vascularity
  - Air-trapping during expiration on high-resolution chest CT
- **Extrinsic Airway Compression by Mass Lesion**
  - Any mass lesion in mediastinum or hila may compress tracheobronchial tree
    - Lymphadenopathy
    - Foregut duplication cysts
    - Neoplasm
  - Causative mass may not be apparent on plain radiograph
  - Chest CT may be necessary
    - 3D reformations can be helpful in identifying area of narrowing of tracheobronchial tree
- **Vascular Ring/Sling**
  - Common forms that cause tracheobronchial compression
    - Double aortic arch

- Right aortic arch with aberrant left subclavian
- Pulmonary artery sling
  - Results in air-trapping and hyperlucency
  - CT or MR angiography diagnostic
- **Scimitar Syndrome**
  - a.k.a. hypogenetic lung syndrome, pulmonary venolobar syndrome
  - Involved lung is hypoplastic
  - Systemic arterial supply
  - Venous return, typically to IVC
    - Resembles scimitar (Turkish sword)
  - Compensatory hyperinflation of contralateral lung
    - Appears hyperlucent
- **Bulla**
  - Thin-walled pulmonary parenchymal air-filled space
  - Commonly seen with emphysema
    - α-1-antitrypsin in children/adolescents
    - Idiopathic
  - Can be seen with connective tissue disorders, such as Marfan syndrome
  - Can rupture and lead to pneumothorax

Helpful Clues for Rare Diagnoses

- **Pulmonary Agenesis/Aplasia**
  - Agenesis
    - Absence of lung, bronchi, and vessels
  - Aplasia
    - Absence of lung and vessels
    - Rudimentary blind-ending bronchus present
  - Other associated congenital anomalies frequent
  - Compensatory hyperexpansion of contralateral lung
  - CT utilized to delineate anatomy and associated anomalies
- **Poland Syndrome**
  - Absent/underdeveloped unilateral chest wall
    - Absent/atrophic pectoralis musculature
  - Unilateral hyperlucent lung appearance
  - Other associated anomalies
    - Ipsilateral syndactyly
    - Sprengel deformity
    - Rhizomelia
    - Absent nipple/breast
    - Dextrocardia
  - M > F
  - Right > left
- **Pulmonary Embolus**
  - Uncommon in pediatric population
  - Chest radiograph typically normal
  - Rarely demonstrates hyperlucent lung on plain radiograph
    - Secondary to decreased vascular flow on involved side

Endobronchial Obstruction/Foreign Body

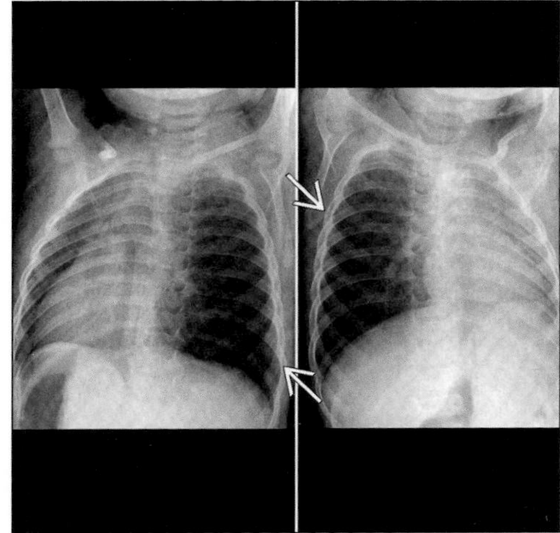

Bilateral decubitus radiographs show persistent hyperlucency of the right lung ➔ on both views. Subsequent bronchoscopy in this 2 year old revealed a peanut lodged in the right mainstem bronchus.

Endobronchial Obstruction/Foreign Body

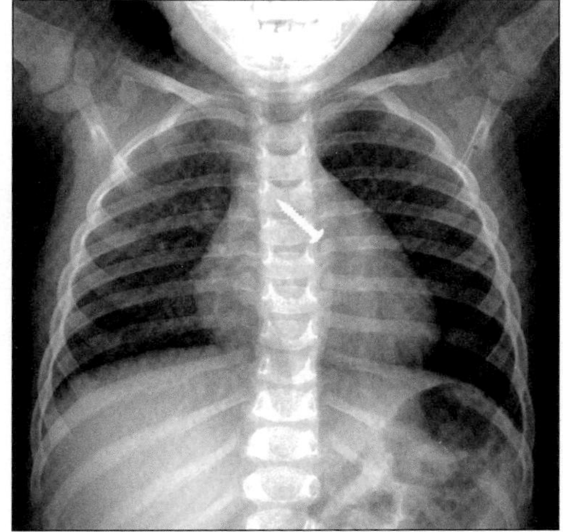

Frontal radiograph shows a metallic screw projected over the proximal left mainstem bronchus in this 2 year old. Note subtle diffuse relative lucency of the left lung compared to the right, consistent with mild air-trapping.

UNILATERAL HYPERLUCENT LUNG

(Left) Frontal radiograph shows diffuse relative hyperlucency and hyperexpansion of the right lung compared with the left in this 8 year old with known asthma. The appearance resolved after nebulizer treatment. **(Right)** Frontal radiograph in this 13 year old shows a large, right, spontaneous pneumothorax resulting in a hyperlucent right hemithorax. There is mild depression of the right hemidiaphragm ➢, indicating a tension component.

Asthma

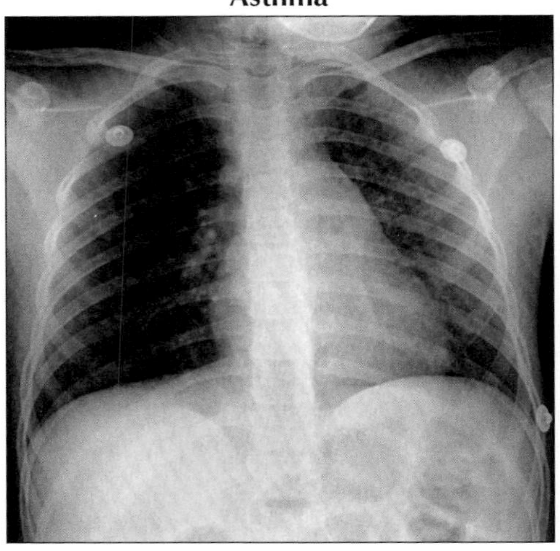

Pneumothorax

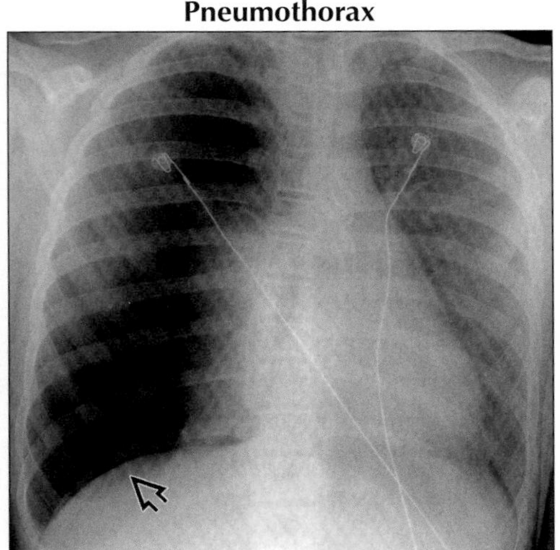

(Left) Frontal radiograph in this 14 year old with multiple prior respiratory infections shows a small, relatively hyperlucent right lung. There is attenuation of the right pulmonary vasculature and compensatory hyperinflation on the left. **(Right)** Frontal radiograph shows hyperlucency and hyperexpansion of the right lung. There is an abnormal soft tissue density bulge ➢ at the upper right mediastinal border in this 3 year old with dyspnea and a cough.

Swyer-James Syndrome

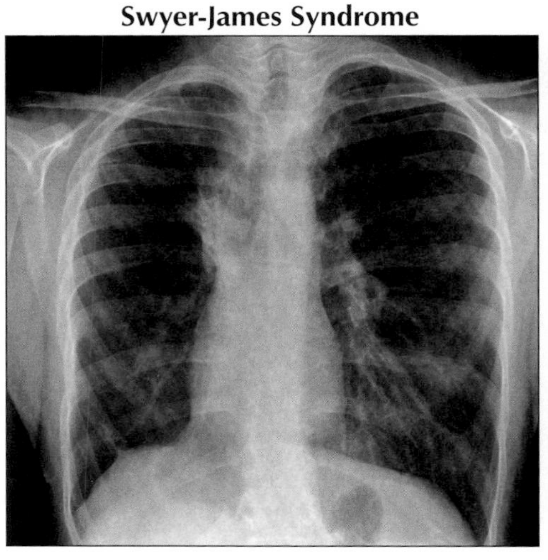

Extrinsic Airway Compression by Mass Lesion

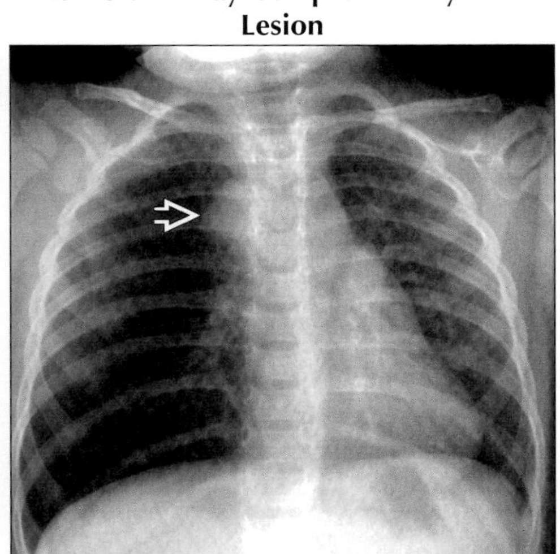

(Left) Coronal CECT in the same patient demonstrates the hyperlucent, hyperinflated right lung and the mediastinal mass ➢, which compresses the right mainstem bronchus. Surgical pathology demonstrated fibrosing mediastinitis. **(Right)** Frontal radiograph shows a hyperlucent and hyperexpanded left lung with a rightward mediastinal shift in this 2 year old. No cause is apparent.

Extrinsic Airway Compression by Mass Lesion

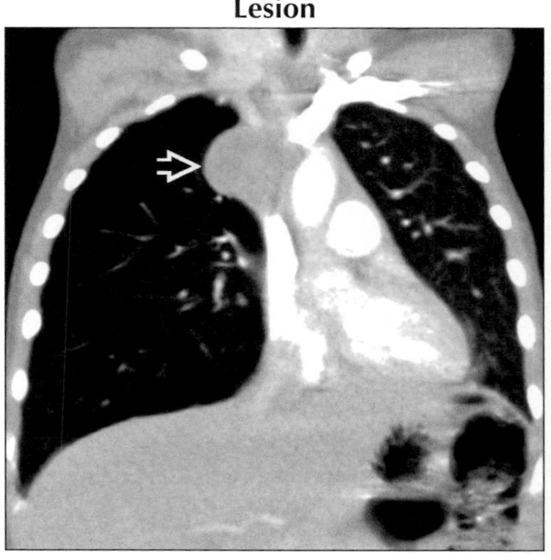

Vascular Ring/Sling

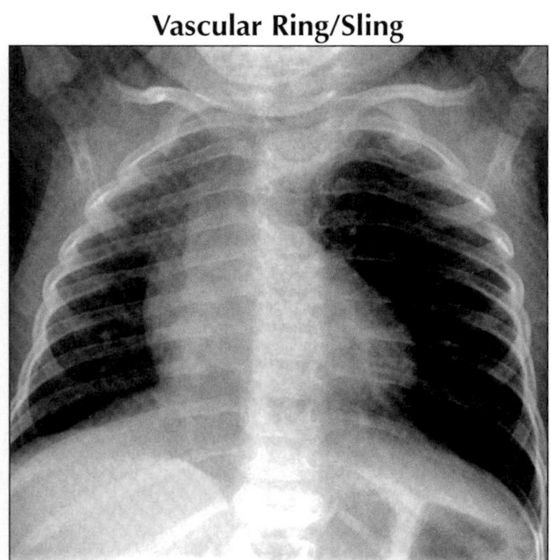

Vascular Ring/Sling

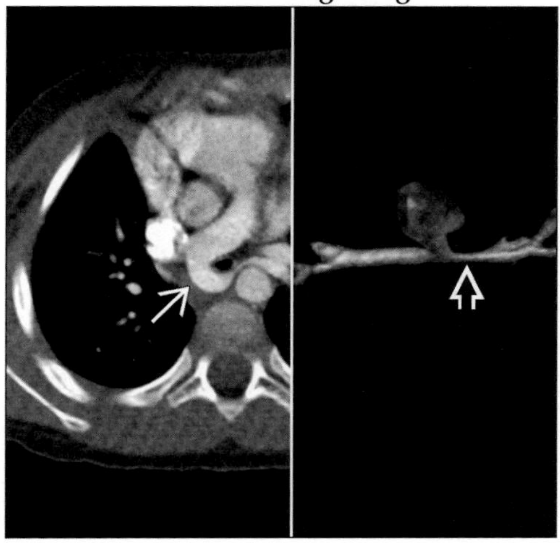

Scimitar Syndrome

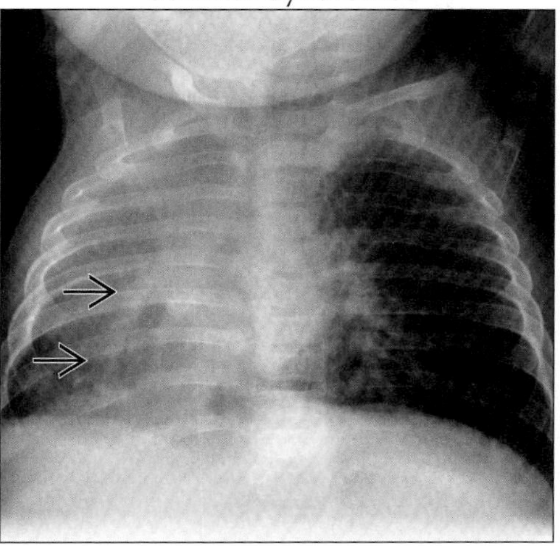

(Left) Axial CECT in the same child shows an aberrant left pulmonary artery originating from right pulmonary artery & coursing posterior to the trachea (pulmonary sling) ➡. 3D airway reformation shows narrowing of proximal left mainstem bronchus ➡, resulting in left lung hyperlucency. (Right) Frontal radiograph shows a hypoplastic right lung & hyperlucent, hyperexpanded left lung. Note anomalous draining vein ➡. Scimitar syndrome confirmed by CT angiography.

Bulla

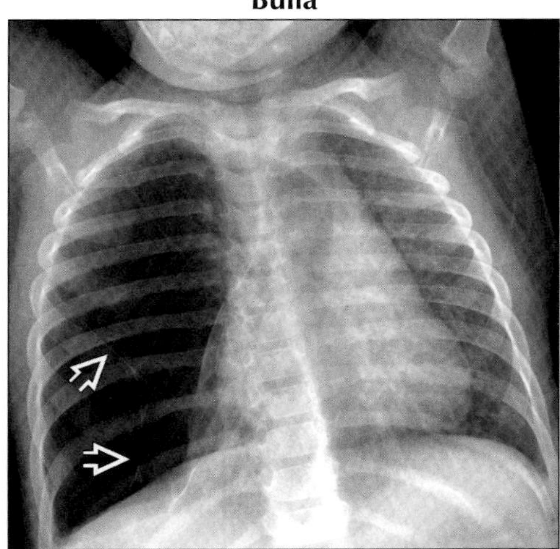

Pulmonary Agenesis/Aplasia

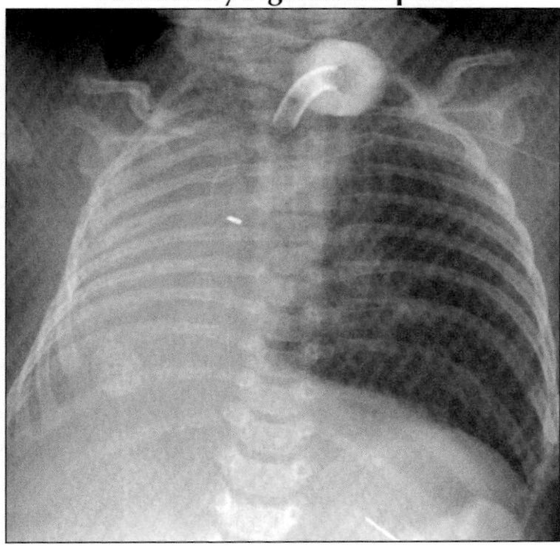

(Left) Frontal radiograph shows a hyperlucent right hemithorax. A right pneumothorax is present. In addition, the presence of multiple thin septations ➡ indicates the presence of a large bulla in this 3 year old. (Right) Frontal radiograph shows a hyperlucent and hyperexpanded left lung. No normal right lung parenchyma is identified. There is a rightward mediastinal shift. CECT (not shown) in this infant confirmed right pulmonary aplasia.

Poland Syndrome

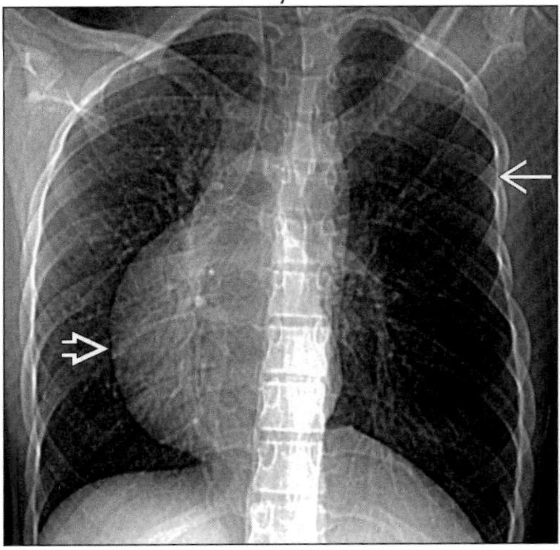

Poland Syndrome

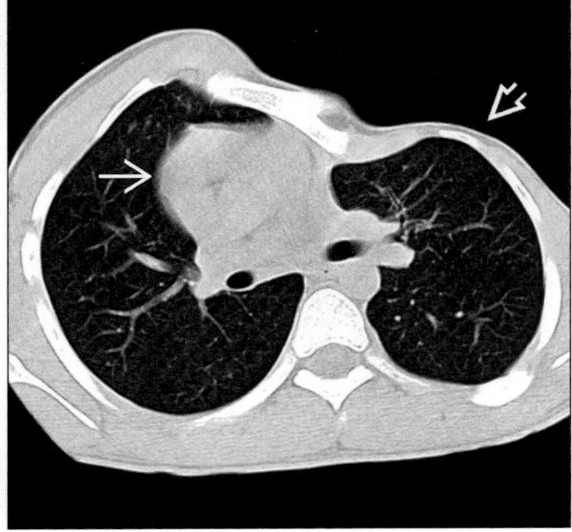

(Left) CT scout image in this adolescent male with Poland syndrome demonstrates relative hyperlucency of the left hemithorax compared to the right. There is dextrocardia ➡. Note the subtle deformity of the left chest wall ➡. (Right) Axial NECT in the same patient demonstrates absence of the left pectoralis musculature and chest wall deformity ➡, which resulted in the hyperlucent left lung appearance. Note the dextrocardia ➡.

BILATERAL HYPERLUCENT LUNG

DIFFERENTIAL DIAGNOSIS

Common
- Technical Factors
- Asthma
- Cyanotic Heart Disease

Less Common
- Foreign Body

Rare but Important
- Obliterative Bronchiolitis
- Emphysema

ESSENTIAL INFORMATION

Key Differential Diagnosis Issues
- Difficult diagnosis to make if appearance is symmetric
- If issue is not technical, look for clues of hyperaeration
  - e.g., small cardiomediastinal silhouette and depressed diaphragms
- Consider inspiratory/expiratory images

Helpful Clues for Common Diagnoses
- **Technical Factors**
  - Overexposed chest x-ray attenuates pulmonary markings, resulting in hyperlucent appearance of lungs
  - Good inspiratory effort can result in bilateral, hyperinflated, hyperlucent lungs
- **Asthma**
  - Airway inflammation results in intermittent airflow obstruction
  - During acute exacerbation, chest x-ray typically shows hyperinflated, bilateral, hyperlucent lungs
- **Cyanotic Heart Disease**
  - Decreased pulmonary vascularity can result in hyperlucent lung appearance
    - Patients with tetralogy of Fallot, pulmonary atresia, tricuspid atresia, Ebstein anomaly
  - Hyperinflated lungs due to cyanosis

Helpful Clues for Less Common Diagnoses
- **Foreign Body**
  - Tracheal foreign body may cause bilateral air-trapping and hyperlucent lungs
  - Esophageal foreign body can cause edema with resulting tracheal compression and hyperlucent lungs

Helpful Clues for Rare Diagnoses
- **Obliterative Bronchiolitis**
  - Bronchial inflammation resulting in airway obstruction
  - Due to toxic fumes, postinfectious and drug-related causes, connective tissue disorders, lung transplantation, bone marrow transplantation
  - Hyperlucent lungs with mosaic perfusion and ground-glass opacities on high-resolution chest CT
- **Emphysema**
  - Rare in children
  - Can be seen with Marfan syndrome, cutis laxa, and α-1-antitrypsin deficiency
  - Typically panacinar/panlobular

Technical Factors

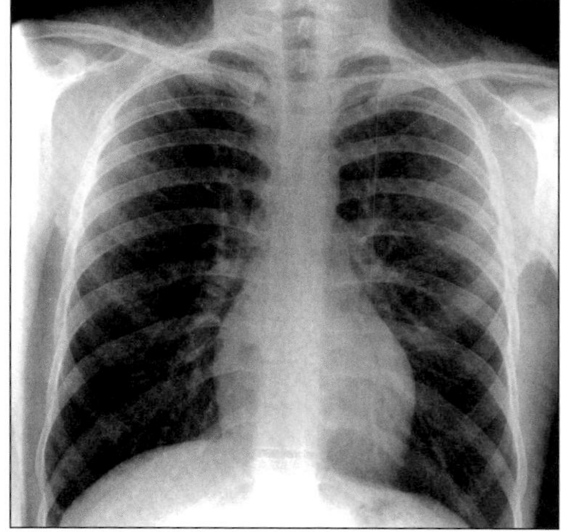

Frontal radiograph shows bilateral hyperlucent and hyperexpanded lungs. There were no respiratory symptoms. Older children are often exuberant in their inspiratory effort, as in this case.

Asthma

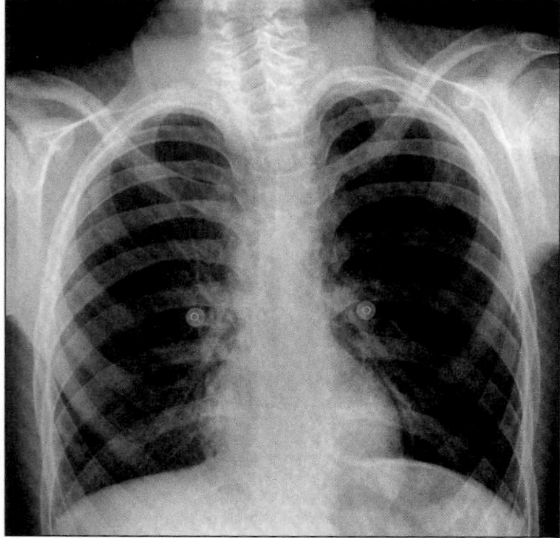

Frontal radiograph shows bilateral hyperlucent and hyperexpanded lungs in this child with acute onset wheezing and cough, no fever, and a known history of chronic asthma.

BILATERAL HYPERLUCENT LUNG

Cyanotic Heart Disease

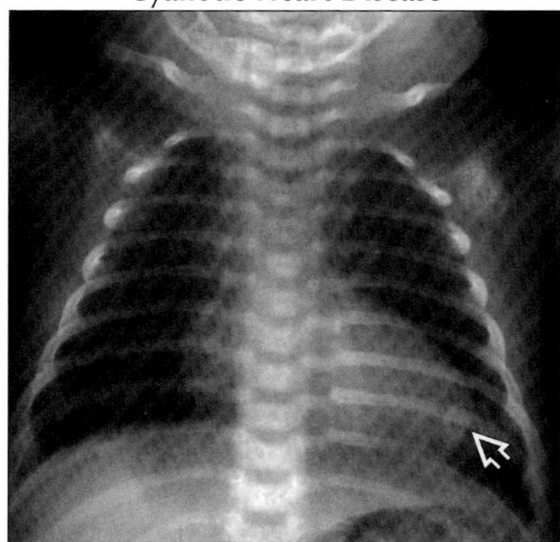

Foreign Body

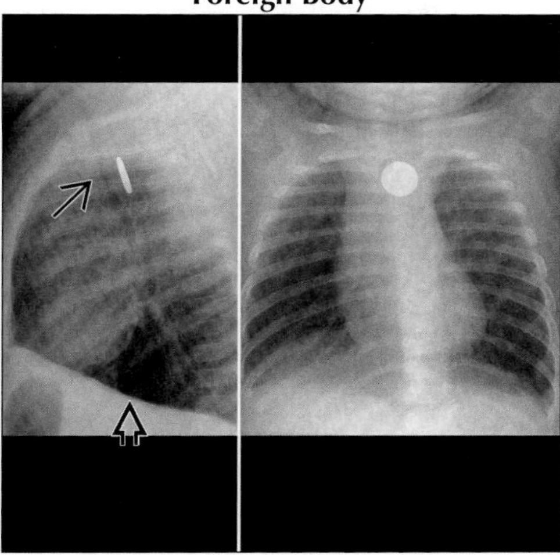

(Left) *Frontal radiograph shows bilateral hyperlucent lungs with decreased pulmonary vascularity. Notice the uplifted cardiac apex and boot-shaped heart in this neonate with tetralogy of Fallot.* ***(Right)*** *Lateral and frontal radiographs show a swallowed coin stuck in the proximal esophagus. The associated edema causes tracheal narrowing with resultant hyperlucency and hyperexpansion of the lungs in this 1 year old. Note the flattened diaphragms.*

Obliterative Bronchiolitis

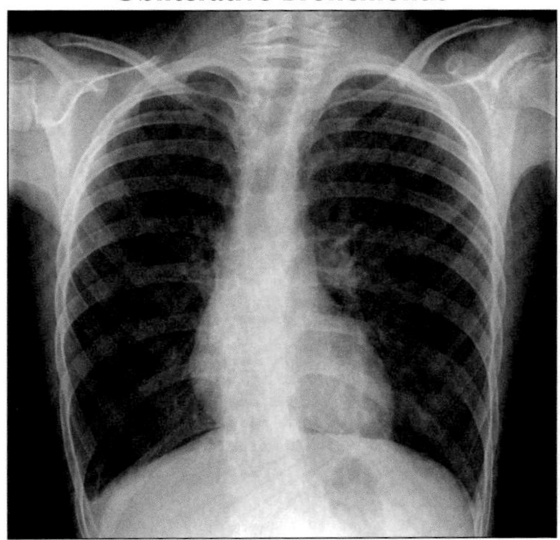

Obliterative Bronchiolitis

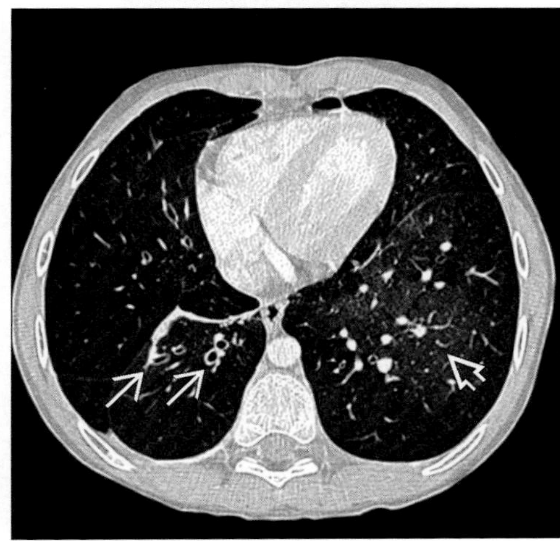

(Left) *Frontal radiograph shows hyperlucent and hyperinflated lungs. The pulmonary interstitial markings are diffusely decreased. This 12 year old had a history of multiple prior lung infections.* ***(Right)*** *Axial CECT in the same patient shows hyperexpanded, hyperlucent lungs with attenuated pulmonary vascularity. Note the scattered bronchiectasis and a representative focus of ground-glass attenuation in the left lower lobe.*

Emphysema

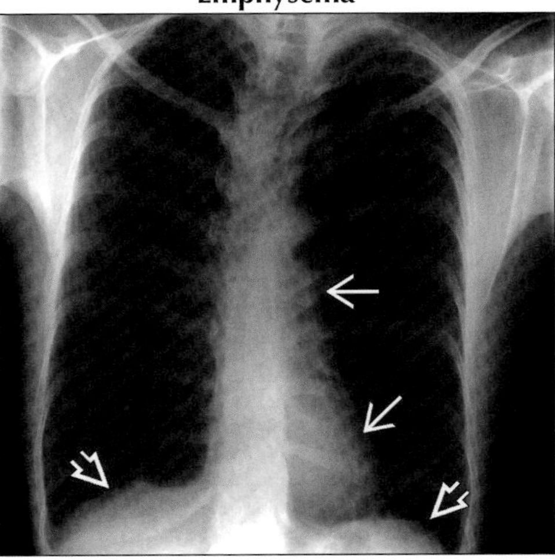

Emphysema

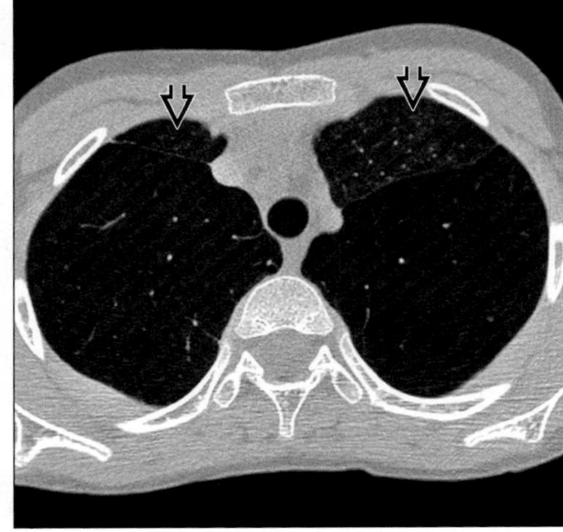

(Left) *Frontal radiograph shows hyperlucent and hyperexpanded lungs with a small cardiomediastinal silhouette and depressed diaphragms. This teenager had a history of Marfan syndrome with pulmonary emphysema.* ***(Right)*** *Axial HRCT shows bilateral hyperlucent and hyperexpanded lungs with diffuse emphysematous change. Note the relatively normal lung parenchyma anteriorly. The source of this teenager's emphysema was not determined.*

LUNG CAVITY

DIFFERENTIAL DIAGNOSIS

Common
- Pneumonia with Cavitary Necrosis
- Pulmonary Abscess
- Aspergillus Infection
- Tuberculosis
- Pneumatocele
- Cystic Adenomatoid Malformation

Less Common
- Septic Emboli

Rare but Important
- Metastatic Disease
- Wegener Granulomatosis
- Tracheobronchial Papillomatosis

ESSENTIAL INFORMATION

Key Differential Diagnosis Issues
- Cavitary lesions in children most frequently either infectious or congenital in nature
- History very helpful
- CT frequently necessary to narrow differential

Helpful Clues for Common Diagnoses
- **Pneumonia with Cavitary Necrosis**
  - *Strep* and *Staph* most common
  - Severely ill children
  - Complication of lobar pneumonia
  - Variable number of thin-walled cavities amidst area of consolidation
  - Plain radiography may underestimate degree of necrosis
  - Look for other signs of complicated pneumonia
    - Pleural effusion/empyema
    - Pulmonary abscess
  - Typically resolves completely with nonsurgical treatment
- **Pulmonary Abscess**
  - Frequently anaerobic infection from aspirated oral contents
  - Can also be seen with *Staph*, *Strep*, fungi, mycobacteria, and parasites
  - Irregularly shaped cavity with internal air-fluid level
    - Size of air-fluid level similar on frontal and lateral radiographs
  - Thick shaggy rind
  - Look for other signs of infection
    - Pleural effusion
    - Empyema
    - Lung consolidation
    - Cavitary necrosis
  - Typically resolves with IV antibiotics
    - Typically does not require surgical drainage
- **Aspergillus Infection**
  - Can cause 4 main pulmonary syndromes
    - Allergic bronchopulmonary aspergillosis
    - Chronic necrotizing pulmonary aspergillosis: Can present with lung cavity
    - Aspergilloma: Can present with lung cavity
    - Invasive aspergillosis
  - Chronic necrotizing pulmonary aspergillosis
    - Typically found in immunocompromised patients
    - Cavitary pulmonary consolidation
  - Aspergilloma
    - Fungal ball (mycetoma), which develops in preexisting lung cavity (e.g.,TB, cystic fibrosis, bullae, etc.)
    - Fungal ball within cavity may move with change in patient position
    - Air crescent sign
- **Tuberculosis**
  - Pulmonary infection with *Mycobacterium tuberculosis*
  - Primary infection
    - Adenopathy
    - Consolidation, which may cavitate
  - Post-primary infection
    - Consolidation typically involving apical posterior segments of upper lobes and superior segments of lower lobes
    - Cavitation common
    - Tuberculoma may form
  - Miliary infection
    - Innumerable punctate nodules
    - May cavitate
- **Pneumatocele**
  - Thin-walled cyst/cavity
  - Sequela of prior parenchymal insult
    - Trauma
    - Infection
  - Frequently resolve spontaneously
  - May become superinfected
- **Cystic Adenomatoid Malformation**

- Cystic types may become superinfected and appear as lung cavity
- Air-fluid level

Helpful Clues for Less Common Diagnoses

- **Septic Emboli**
  - Can reach lungs from variety of sources
    - Infected central lines
    - Peripheral septic thrombophlebitis
    - Infected heart valves
  - Immunocompromised patients at increased risk
  - Multiple nodules ± cavitation
  - Typically peripherally located
  - May see feeding vessel
  - Look for associated consolidation or pleural effusions
  - Lemierre syndrome
    - Oropharyngeal infection
    - Septic thrombophlebitis of jugular vein
    - Septic pulmonary emboli

Helpful Clues for Rare Diagnoses

- **Metastatic Disease**
  - Only ~ 4% of all lung metastases cavitate
  - Can be thin- or thick-walled depending on type of primary malignancy
  - Most common cavitating lung metastases from "adult" neoplasms
    - Squamous cell (lung, head and neck, esophagus, cervical)
    - Adenocarcinoma (colon, rectum)
  - Very rare in children
    - Can be seen with metastatic sarcomas (fibrosarcoma, osteosarcoma)
    - Has been reported with Wilms
  - History of primary neoplasm helpful
  - May be difficult to differentiate from infectious cavitary lesions
- **Wegener Granulomatosis**
  - Necrotizing granulomatous vasculitis
  - Primarily involves respiratory tract and kidneys
  - 40-70% of patients have lung nodules
  - 50% of nodules show cavitation
    - Thick or thin walled
    - 5 mm to 10 cm in size
    - Tend to be multiple
  - Look for associated chest findings
    - Pulmonary hemorrhage
    - Interstitial lung disease
    - Airway strictures
- **Tracheobronchial Papillomatosis**
  - Squamous papillomas of respiratory tract
  - 2/3 diagnosed prior to age 5
  - Infection with human papilloma virus, usually at birth
  - Thin-walled lung cavities
  - Airway papillomas
  - Increased risk of development of squamous cell carcinoma

Pneumonia with Cavitary Necrosis

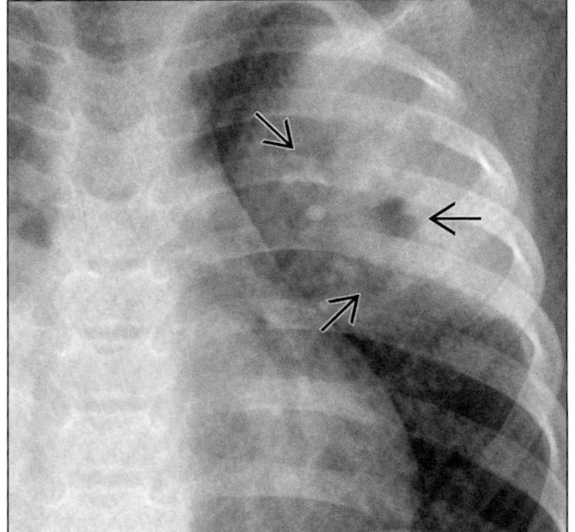

Frontal radiograph shows a focal area of consolidation in the left upper lobe in this 3-year-old patient with a fever and respiratory tract infection symptoms. Note the internal lucent foci →.

Pneumonia with Cavitary Necrosis

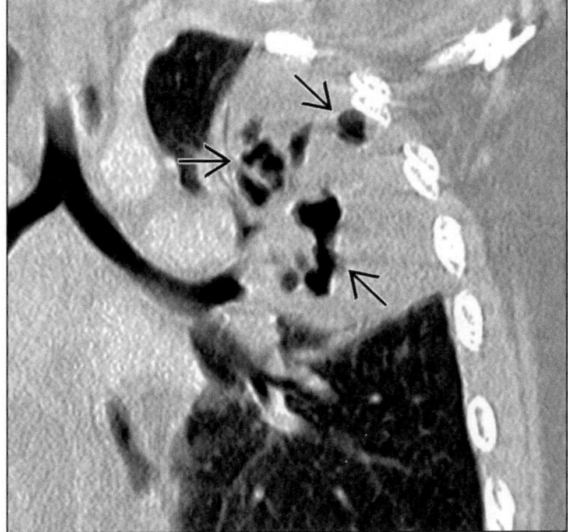

Coronal CECT in the same patient better illustrates the numerous irregularly shaped, thin-walled cavities → that represent regions of necrosis, complicating a lobar pneumonia.

LUNG CAVITY

(**Left**) Lateral and frontal plain radiographs in this 4 year old who presented with a fever and cough demonstrate a focal cavitary mass ➯ with a thick, shaggy rind and an internal air-fluid level ➡ in the left upper lobe. Note that the size of the air-fluid level within the cavity is similar on both projections. (**Right**) Axial CECT in the same patient re-demonstrates the left upper lobe cavitary mass with a thick shaggy rind ➡.

Pulmonary Abscess

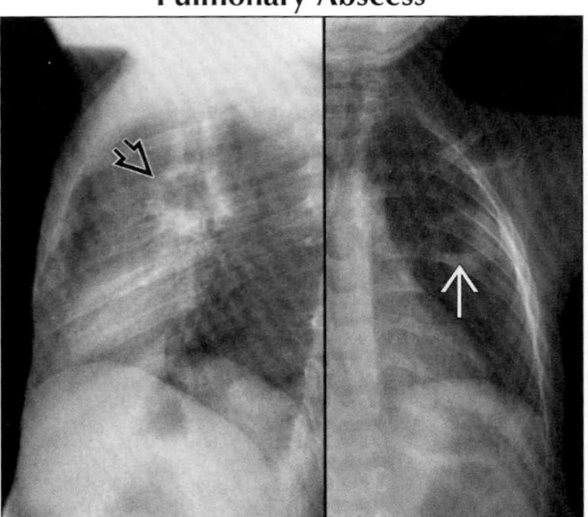

Pulmonary Abscess

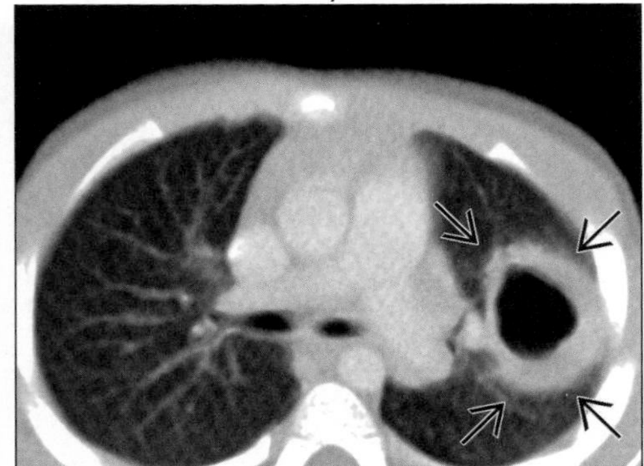

(**Left**) Frontal radiograph shows a large cavitary mass ➯ in the right upper lobe with internal soft tissue density ➡. Note that the soft tissue density lies within the dependent portion of the cavitary lesion. (**Right**) Axial CECT of the same patient shows the right upper lobe Aspergillus mycetoma in this 19-year-old leukemic patient status post bone marrow transplant. Note the presence of an air crescent sign ➯.

Aspergillus Infection

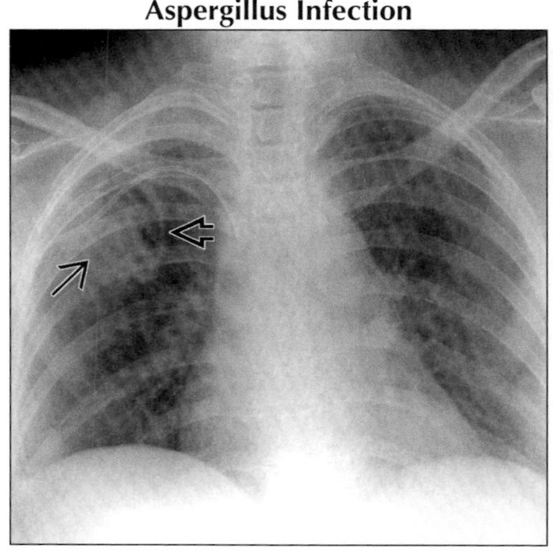

Aspergillus Infection

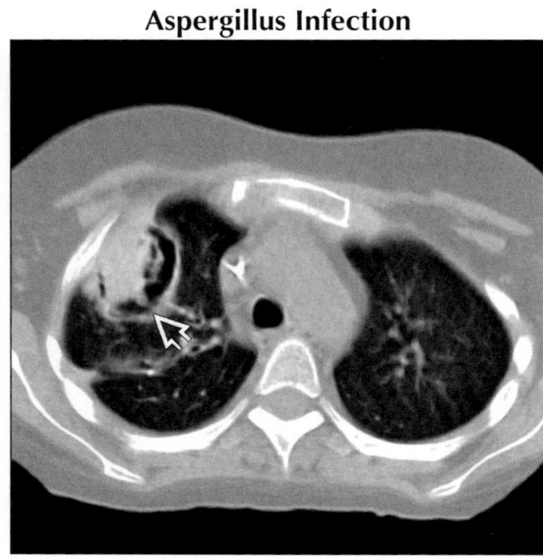

(**Left**) Axial CECT shows a small cavitary nodule ➡ within the right upper lobe. Note the large left pleural effusion ➡ and consolidated/atelectatic ➯ left lung. This 16-year-old adoptee from Cambodia was diagnosed with tuberculosis. (**Right**) Axial NECT shows a well-defined, thin-walled parenchymal cavity ➯ in the right upper lobe in this 7-year-old child with a remote history of right upper lobe pneumonia. There is also surrounding parenchymal scarring.

Tuberculosis

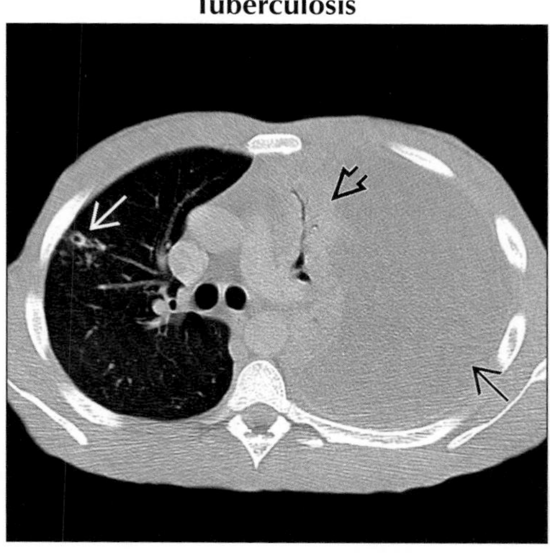

Pneumatocele

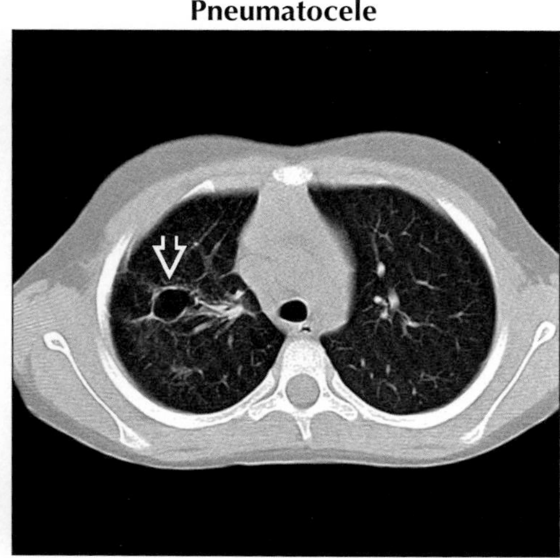

Cystic Adenomatoid Malformation

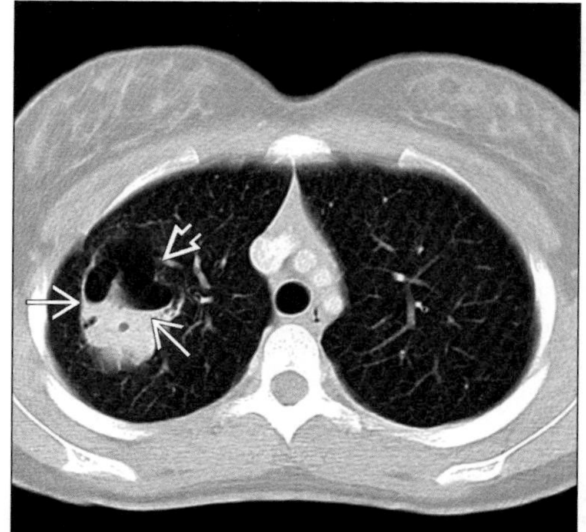

Septic Emboli

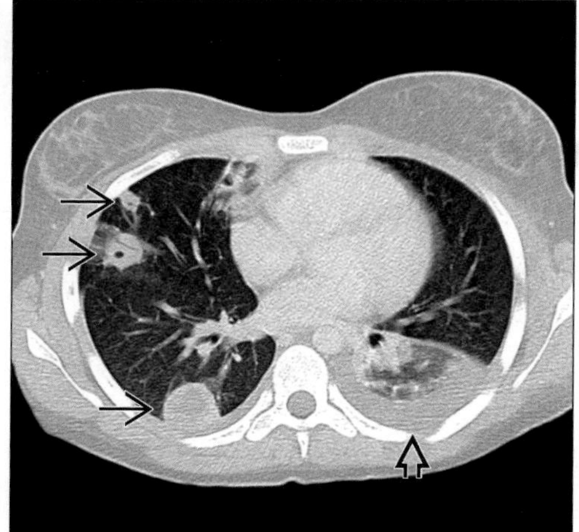

(Left) Axial CECT shows a large cavitary lesion ➡ in the right upper lobe. There are internal air-fluid levels ➡. Surgical pathology confirmed an infected cystic adenomatoid malformation in this 12 year old. (Right) Axial CECT shows multiple, peripheral, pulmonary nodules ➡ in the right lung, some of which are cavitary. There is also a left pleural effusion ➡. This 16-year-old female developed Lemierre syndrome following an oropharyngeal infection.

Wegener Granulomatosis

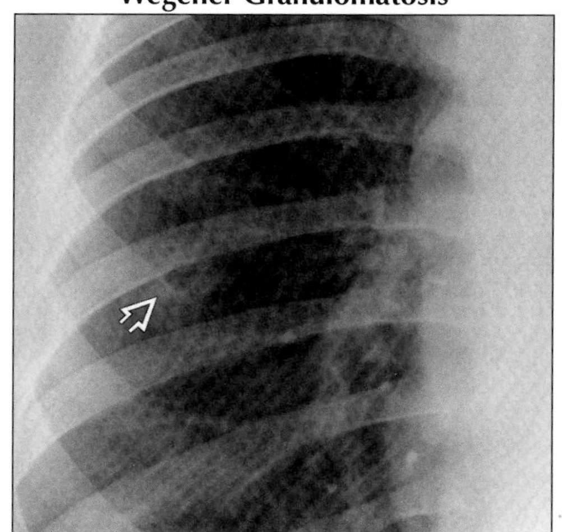

Wegener Granulomatosis

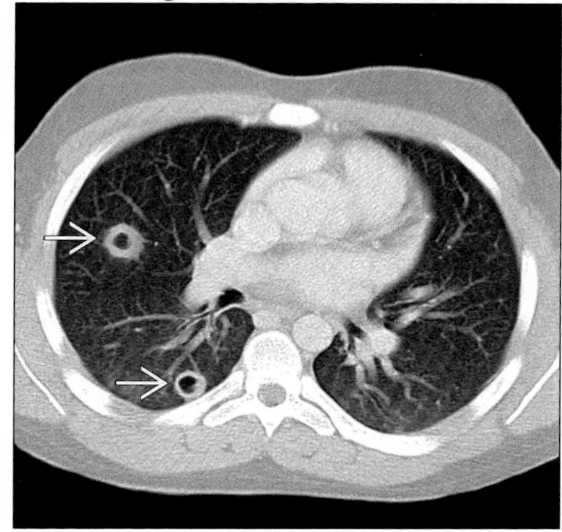

(Left) Frontal radiograph shows a small, thick-walled cavitary nodule ➡ within the right mid-lung. Other scattered similar-appearing nodules were also present. (Right) Axial CECT in the same patient shows 2 discrete cavitary nodules in the right lung ➡. The more anterior nodule has a thick wall, while the more posterior nodule has a thin wall. This 15 year old was diagnosed with Wegener granulomatosis.

Metastatic Disease

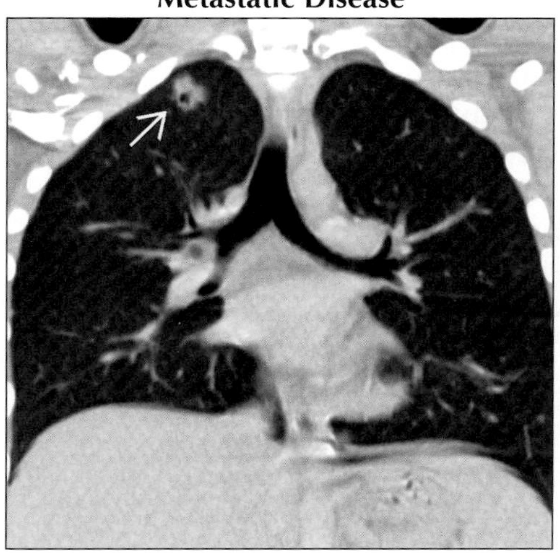

Tracheobronchial Papillomatosis

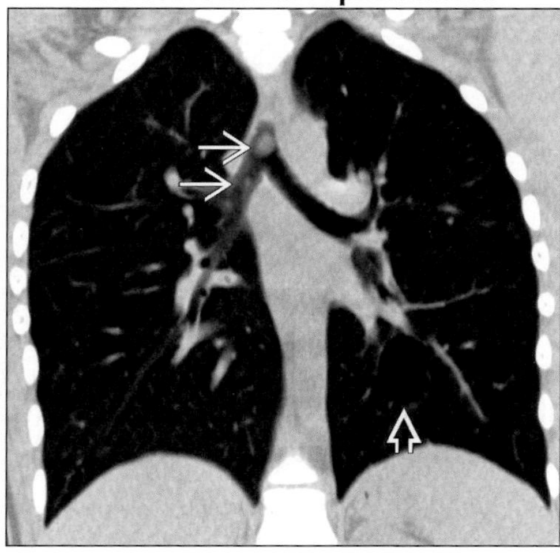

(Left) Coronal CECT shows a cavitary nodule in the right upper lobe ➡. The lesion shows a partial thin wall and a partial thick wall. Other similar lesions were present (not shown) in this 16 year old with biopsy-proven metastatic soft tissue sarcoma. (Right) Coronal NECT shows a thin-walled cavity in the left base ➡. Note the papillomas within the trachea and right mainstem bronchus ➡ in this 13 year old with tracheobronchial papillomatosis.

LUCENT LUNG MASS

DIFFERENTIAL DIAGNOSIS

Common
- Cystic Adenomatoid Malformation
- Congenital Lobar Emphysema
- Congenital Diaphragmatic Hernia
- Pneumatocele
- Pulmonary Abscess

Less Common
- Lung Contusion and Laceration
- Loculated Pneumothorax
- Bulla
- Bronchial Atresia

Rare but Important
- Traumatic Diaphragmatic Hernia
- Pleuropulmonary Blastoma

ESSENTIAL INFORMATION

Key Differential Diagnosis Issues
- Lucent lung masses in children most frequently either congenital or infectious in nature
- History very helpful
- CT frequently necessary to narrow differential

Helpful Clues for Common Diagnoses
- **Cystic Adenomatoid Malformation**
  - a.k.a. congenital pulmonary airway malformation (CPAM)
  - Diagnosis can be made prenatally with ultrasound and fetal MR
  - Type 1
    - Single or multiple 2-10 cm cysts
    - May contain air-fluid levels
    - Good prognosis
  - Type 2
    - Multiple small cysts (0.5-2 cm)
    - Variable prognosis
  - Type 3
    - Innumerable microscopic cysts
    - Appears solid
    - Poorer prognosis
  - Evidence of associated mass effect
    - Mediastinal shift
    - Compression of adjacent normal lung
  - Can coexist with other pulmonary malformations, such as sequestration
  - Infection risk
  - Small malignancy risk
    - Bronchioalveolar carcinoma
    - Pleuropulmonary blastoma
    - Rhabdomyosarcoma
- **Congenital Lobar Emphysema**
  - Overdistension of lobe of lung
    - Left upper > right middle > right upper lobe
  - Multifocal in only ~ 5%
  - During 1st few days of life, affected lobe may be opacified by lung fluid
  - Hyperlucent, hyperexpanded lobe thereafter
    - Evidence of associated mass effect
  - ~ 15% have associated congenital heart disease
- **Congenital Diaphragmatic Hernia**
  - Bochdalek (90%)
    - Posterior
  - Morgagni (10%)
    - Anterior
  - Left (75%), right (25%)
  - Multicystic mass in chest when stomach/bowel involved
  - Associated mass effect
  - Associated pulmonary hypoplasia
  - Enteric tube may enter mass
  - Diagnosis can be made prenatally with ultrasound and fetal MR
- **Pneumatocele**
  - Thin-walled cyst
  - Can be secondary to infection or trauma
  - Frequently resolves spontaneously
- **Pulmonary Abscess**
  - Frequently anaerobic infection from aspirated oral contents
  - Can also be seen with *Staph*, *Strep*, fungi, mycobacteria, and parasites
  - Irregularly shaped lucent mass with internal air-fluid level
    - Size of air-fluid level similar on frontal and lateral projections
  - Thick, shaggy rind
  - Look for other signs of infection
    - Pleural effusion/empyema
    - Lung consolidation
  - Typically resolve with IV antibiotics and do not require drainage

Helpful Clues for Less Common Diagnoses
- **Lung Contusion and Laceration**
  - Penetrating or blunt trauma with large shearing forces can result in laceration

- Commonly associated with pneumothorax
- Lucent lung cavity filled with air &/or fluid
- Complications
  - Bronchopleural fistula
  - Pulmonary abscess
  - Pneumatocele
  - Air embolism

- **Loculated Pneumothorax**
  - May mimic lucent lung mass
  - Typically found within fissure or in subpulmonic location
  - CT will confirm pleural rather than parenchymal source
- **Bulla**
  - Thin-walled pulmonary parenchymal air-filled space
  - Commonly seen with emphysema
    - α-1-antitrypsin in children/adolescents
    - Idiopathic
  - Can be seen with connective tissue disorders such as Marfan syndrome
  - Superinfection
    - Look for air-fluid level
  - Can rupture and cause pneumothorax
- **Bronchial Atresia**
  - Noncommunication of segmental bronchus with central airway
  - Likely a result of in utero vascular insult
  - Can coexist with other pulmonary malformations, such as sequestration
  - Left upper > left lower > right middle lobe
  - Hyperlucent and hyperexpanded lobe
  - Central tubular/branching density representing mucoid plugged bronchus
    - "Finger in glove" appearance

Helpful Clues for Rare Diagnoses

- **Traumatic Diaphragmatic Hernia**
  - Blunt or penetrating trauma
  - Left > right
  - High incidence of concomitant injuries
  - Plain radiographs may be insensitive
    - Distorted or elevated diaphragm
    - Abdominal contents in thorax
    - Enteric tube in thorax
  - CT higher sensitivity and specificity
    - Coronal and sagittal reformations very helpful
- **Pleuropulmonary Blastoma**
  - Rare childhood tumor
  - Can begin in lung parenchyma or pleura
  - Type 1 consists of cysts and can present as lucent lung mass
    - Better prognosis
  - Type 2 consists of mixed solid and cystic components
  - Type 3 is purely solid
    - Worst prognosis
  - Can arise from cystic adenomatoid malformation
  - Typically large mass with mediastinal shift and pleural effusion

Cystic Adenomatoid Malformation

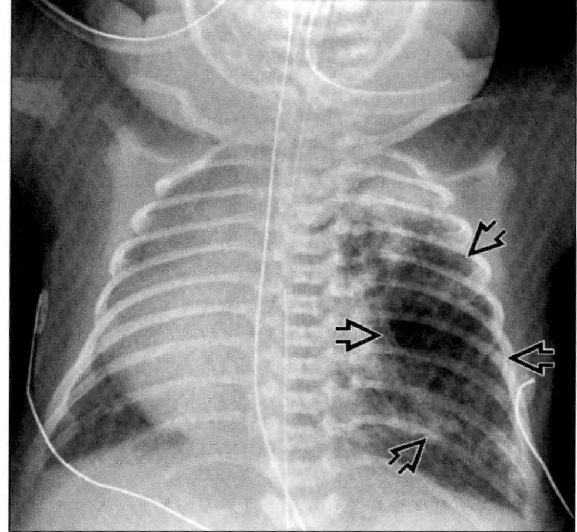

Frontal radiograph in a neonate shows a lucent mass in the left hemithorax ➪ with shift of the cardiomediastinum to the right. Surgical pathology demonstrated cystic adenomatoid malformation.

Cystic Adenomatoid Malformation

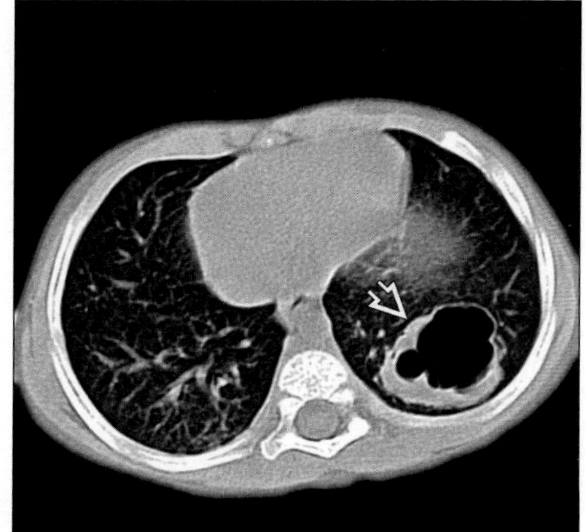

Axial NECT shows a well-circumscribed lucent mass ➪ in the left lower lobe with a thick rind and septations. Surgical pathology in this 2 year old showed cystic adenomatoid malformation.

LUCENT LUNG MASS

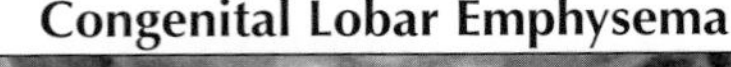

Congenital Lobar Emphysema

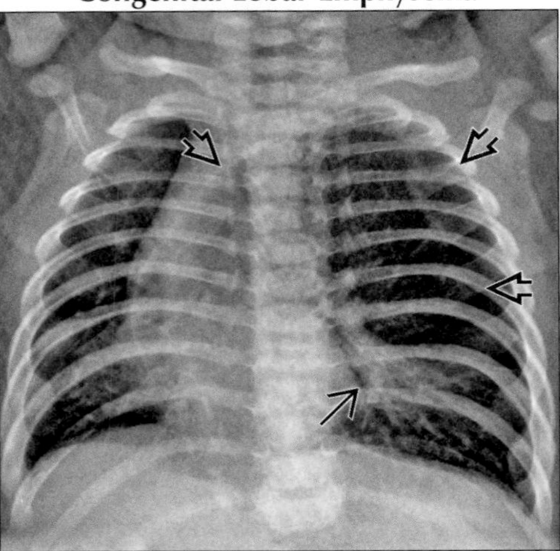

Congenital Lobar Emphysema

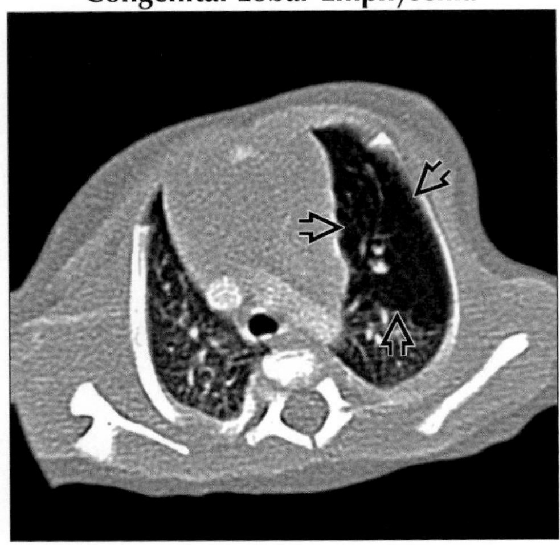

(Left) *Frontal radiograph shows hyperlucency and hyperexpansion of the left upper lobe ⇨ in this 4 month old with congenital lobar emphysema. Note the present but attenuated pulmonary vascularity. Also note the rightward mediastinal shift, the overall right lung volume loss, and the compressed left lower lobe →.* ***(Right)*** *Axial CECT shows hyperlucency and hyperexpansion of the left upper lobe ⇨ in another neonate with congenital lobar emphysema.*

Congenital Diaphragmatic Hernia

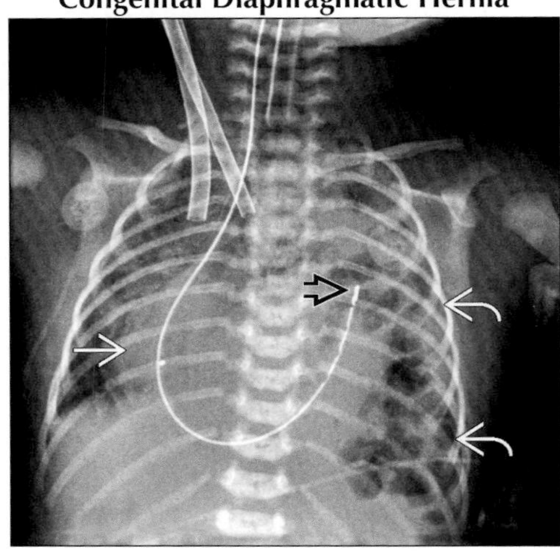

Congenital Diaphragmatic Hernia

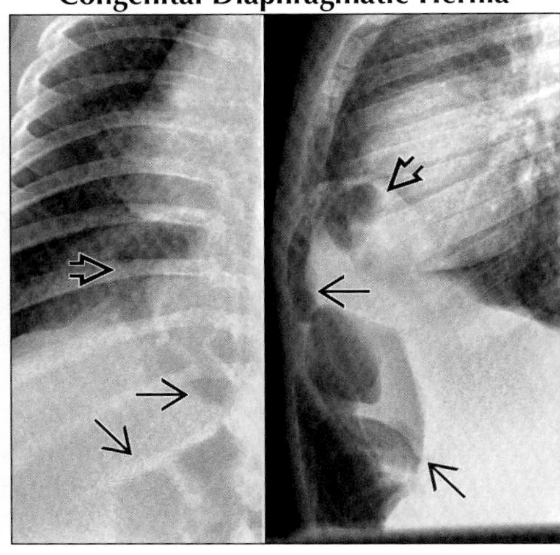

(Left) *Frontal radiograph shows a multicystic mass ➡ occupying the left hemithorax, consistent with congenital diaphragmatic hernia. Note rightward mediastinal shift ➡. An orogastric tube ⇨ enters the mass.* ***(Right)*** *Frontal and lateral radiographs in a 2-month-old infant show a multicystic mass crossing the diaphragm anteriorly ⇨. The mass is contiguous with bowel loops in the right upper quadrant → and is consistent with a Morgagni hernia.*

Pneumatocele

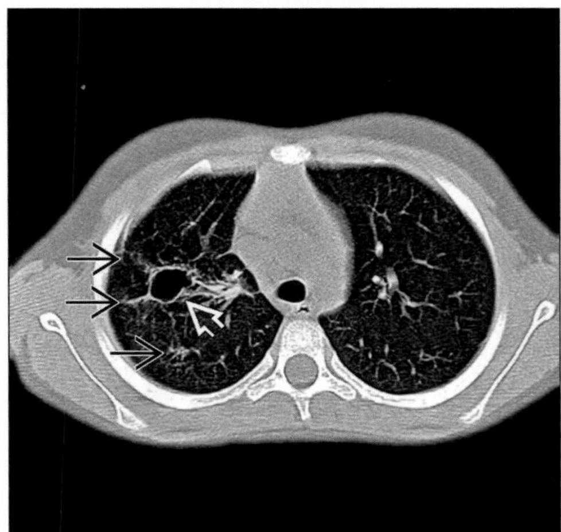

Pulmonary Abscess

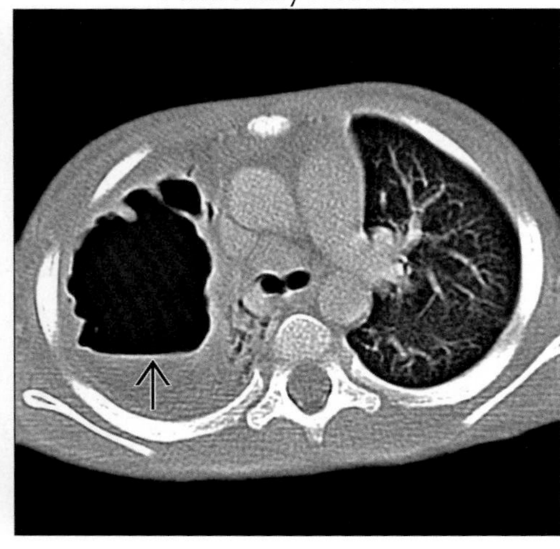

(Left) *Axial NECT shows a well-defined, thin-walled parenchymal cyst in the right upper lobe ➡ in this 7-year-old child with a history of prior right upper lobe pneumonia. Note the wispy areas of surrounding parenchymal scars →.* ***(Right)*** *Axial CECT shows a lucent mass with an air-fluid level → and irregular, thick walls. In this 2 year old with acute respiratory infection symptoms, the findings are consistent with a pulmonary abscess.*

LUCENT LUNG MASS

Lung Contusion and Laceration

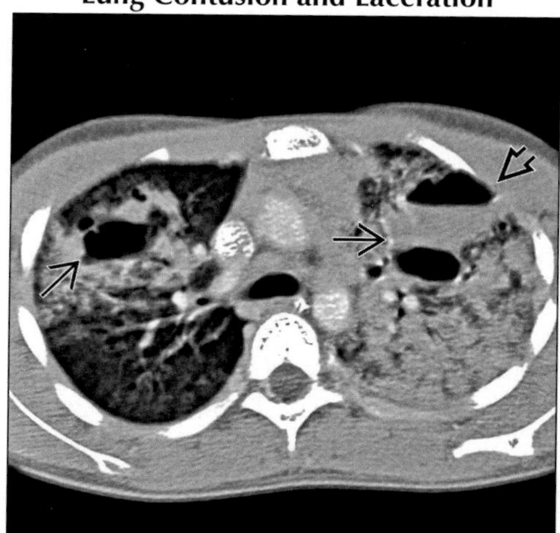

Loculated Pneumothorax

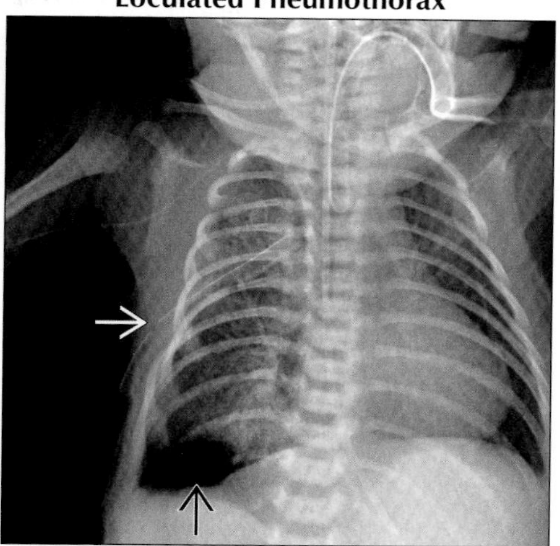

(Left) *Axial CECT shows several lucent masses ➔, including 1 with an air-fluid level ➔, surrounded by areas of contusion, consistent with pulmonary lacerations in this 14 year old who was in an ATV accident.* ***(Right)*** *Frontal radiograph shows a lucency within the right base ➔ that depresses the right hemidiaphragm, consistent with a loculated subpulmonic pneumothorax in this neonate. Note the chest tube side port outside of the pleural space ➔.*

Bulla

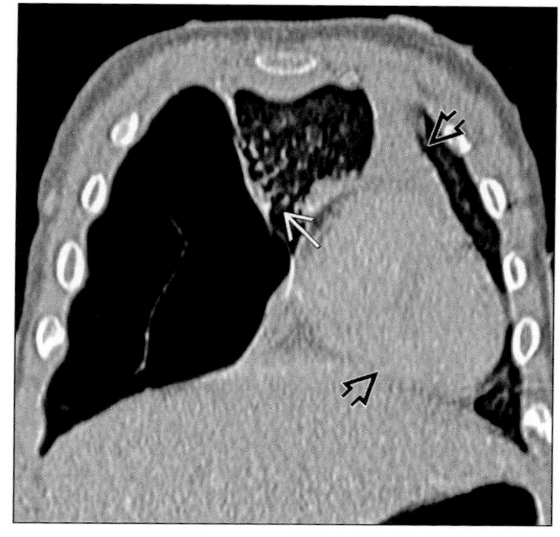

Bronchial Atresia

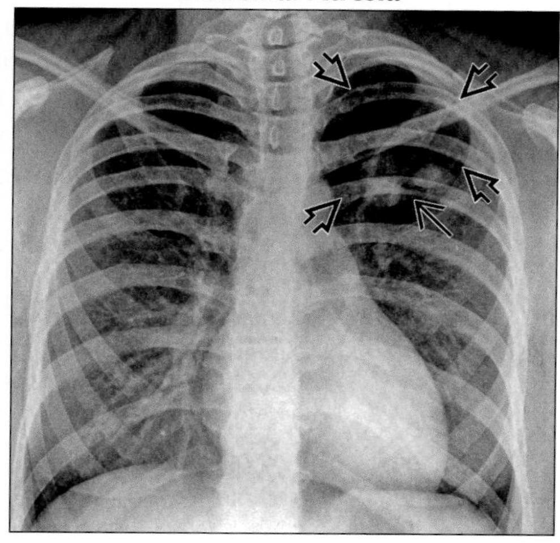

(Left) *Coronal CECT in a 3 year old shows large idiopathic bullae within the right lung causing mass effect on the right upper lobe ➔ and leftward mediastinal shift ➔.* ***(Right)*** *Frontal radiograph shows relative lucency in the left upper lobe ➔ with a central tubular/branching density ➔ representing impacted mucous within the noncommunicating bronchus ("finger in glove"). The findings are consistent with bronchial atresia in this 14 year old.*

Traumatic Diaphragmatic Hernia

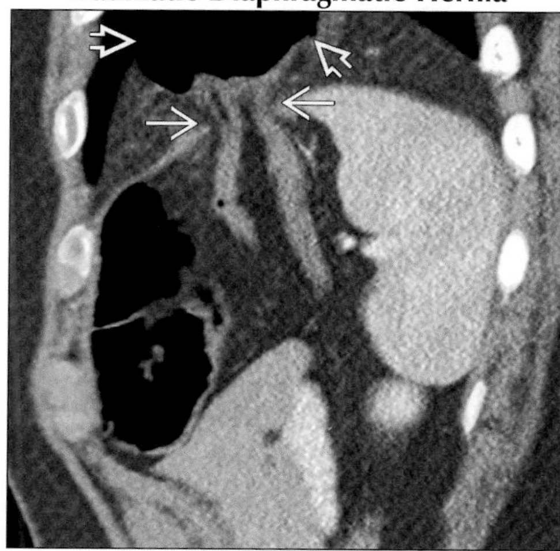

Pleuropulmonary Blastoma

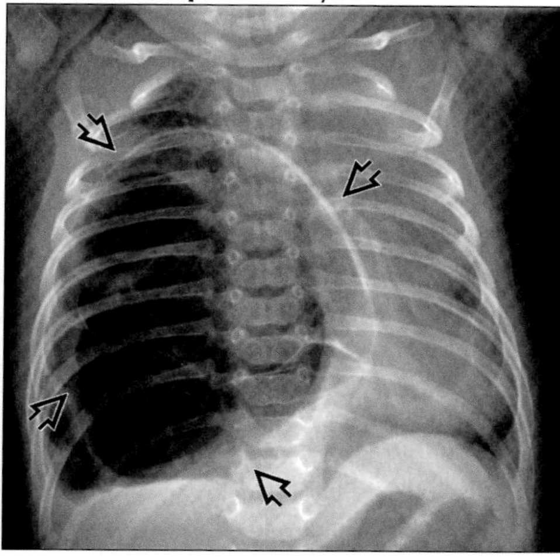

(Left) *Sagittal CECT shows a lucent mass ➔ within the left base surrounded by fat that communicates with the bowel in the intraabdominal cavity via a defect in the diaphragm ➔. This 14 year old suffered a stab wound to the left chest.* ***(Right)*** *Frontal radiograph shows a large lucent mass ➔ occupying the right hemithorax and causing a marked leftward mediastinal shift. Surgical pathology demonstrated a type 1 pleuropulmonary blastoma in this 1 month old.*

ROUNDED LUNG MASS

DIFFERENTIAL DIAGNOSIS

Common
- Round Pneumonia

Less Common
- Overlying Artifact
- Bronchogenic Cyst
- Congenital Cystic Adenomatoid Malformation (CCAM)
- Retrocaval Thymus
- Chest Wall Lesion
- Neuroblastoma
- Lung Abscess/Cavitary Necrosis
- Fungal Lesion
- Loculated Pleural Fluid (Pseudocyst)

Rare but Important
- Pleuropulmonary Blastoma

ESSENTIAL INFORMATION

Key Differential Diagnosis Issues
- Think round pneumonia
  - < 8 years of age (development of collateral circulation), solitary lesion, soft tissue density (without containing air-fluid levels)
  - Presence of fever and cough
  - Avoid unnecessary CT
- Look for underlying rib erosion or destruction
  - Consistent with neuroblastoma in young patients
  - Consider lesion arising from chest wall
- Look for sharp margins and unnatural geographic shapes (too round); think overlying artifact

Helpful Clues for Common Diagnoses
- **Round Pneumonia**
  - Most common cause of solitary round "lung mass" in child
    - In a study of 112 round lung densities in children suspected to have round pneumonia, 109 (97%) did prove to have round pneumonia
    - Other 3 had cavitary necrosis in pneumonia (2) and pleural pseudocyst (1) = no malignancies
  - When child has round density on chest radiograph and cough/fever, should be treated with antibiotics and repeat chest radiography obtained in several weeks
    - CT is not indicated to evaluate for other potential causes of mass in this clinical scenario
  - Mean age of round pneumonia is 5 years
    - Less common after 8 years of age
    - Thought to be related to poorly developed collateral circulation (channels of Lambert, pores of Kahn) that do not develop until ~ 8 years of age
    - Round lesions seen after 8 years of age should have increased suspicion of other underlying causes
  - Most common solitary lesions (98%), well-defined borders (70%)
  - Mean diameter = 3.8 cm
  - More common posteriorly (83%) and in lower lobes (65%)
  - Tend to resolve on follow-up imaging (95%) rather than progression to lobar pneumonia (4.6%)
  - May present with abdominal pain, rather than chest symptoms

Helpful Clues for Less Common Diagnoses
- **Overlying Artifact**
  - Should always be considered as potential cause of any round lung radiodensity
  - Often will be very round or other geometric shapes suggesting unnatural cause
  - Common causes include hair braids, buttons, shirt pocket contents, monitor leads, and other medical devices
- **Bronchogenic Cyst**
  - Much less common cause of round lung lesions than round pneumonia
  - Most bronchogenic cysts are hilar or mediastinal (around central airways); less common cause of round intralung parenchymal lesions
  - Typically are strictly fluid filled (no air-fluid levels) unless infection leads to wall breakdown
- **Congenital Cystic Adenomatoid Malformation (CCAM)**
  - Can appear as fluid only filled lesion early in life

- Later: More commonly air filled or air and fluid filled with air-fluid levels
- Uncommon to be unilocular "single" lesion
  - Much more commonly multicyst
- **Retrocaval Thymus**
  - Defined as present when portion of thymus extends between SVC and trachea into right paratracheal location
  - Most common aberrant location of thymus
  - Can have appearance as mass on chest radiograph or CT
  - Lesion should be contiguous with thymus, homogeneous and iso-signal (MR), or iso-attenuation (CT) with more anteriorly positioned normal thymus
- **Chest Wall Lesion**
  - Rib lesions can appear as round lung lesion on chest radiograph
  - Look for rib destruction or erosion to show chest wall origin of lesion
- **Neuroblastoma**
  - Most common cause of posterior mediastinal masses in young children
  - Most commonly will appear as obvious posterior mediastinal mass, particularly when occurring in inferior chest
  - Can appear as round lesion when large and in apex/superior chest; can be difficult at times to determine anatomic location
    - Look for associated rib erosion/destruction to identify lesion as posterior mediastinal mass
  - Often have calcifications
  - In young child (< 2 years of age), posterior mediastinal mass is neuroblastoma until proven otherwise
- **Lung Abscess/Cavitary Necrosis**
  - True lung abscesses are very uncommon in otherwise healthy children
  - Most commonly occur in children with underlying immunodeficiency or complex medical disorders
  - CT: Well-defined fluid collection with perceptible, enhancing wall
- **Fungal Lesion**
  - Uncommon in otherwise healthy children
  - Most commonly occur in children with underlying immunodeficiency or complex medical disorders
  - Typically multifocal, occur in cluster, poorly defined nodules
- **Loculated Pleural Fluid (Pseudocyst)**
  - Fluid can become loculated in pleural fissures and present as round-appearing mass
  - Fairly uncommon in children

Helpful Clues for Rare Diagnoses

- **Pleuropulmonary Blastoma**
  - Rare primary malignancy of childhood
  - Can appear as round mass but much more typically diagnosed late in disease and appears as large mass filling hemithorax, often with associated pleural disease

Round Pneumonia

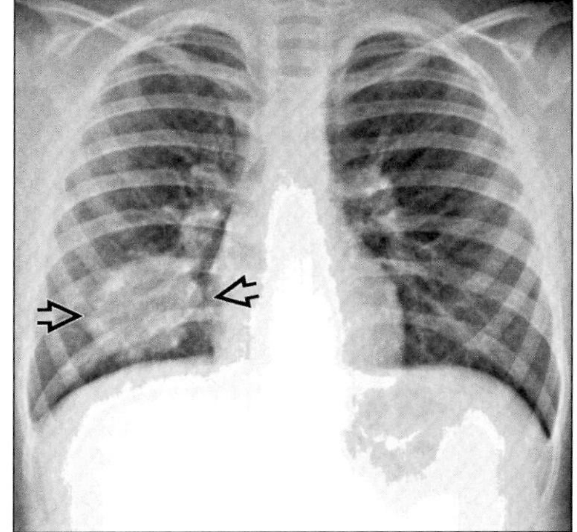

Frontal radiograph shows a very round mass-like lesion ➩ over the right lower lobe.

Overlying Artifact

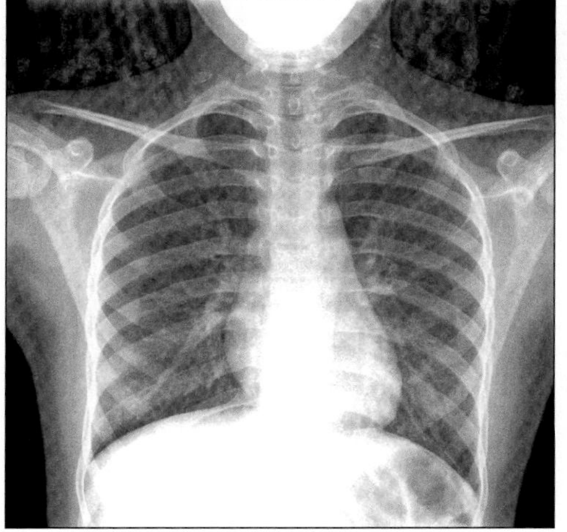

Frontal radiograph shows hair braids overlying the cervical region and lung apices. This case emphasizes the importance of considering an overlying artifact as a cause of any rounded radiodensity.

ROUNDED LUNG MASS

Round Pneumonia

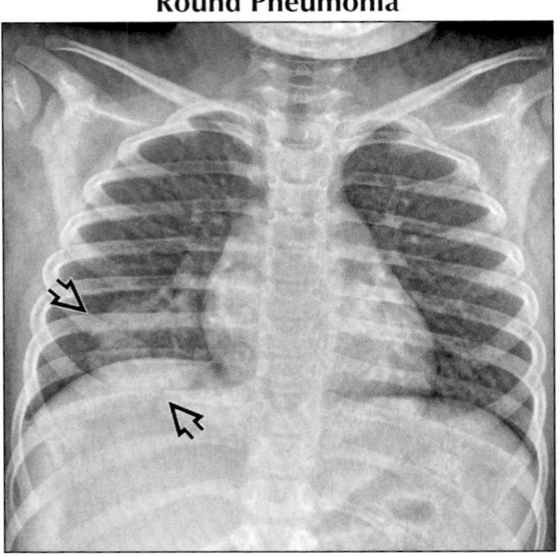

Round Pneumonia

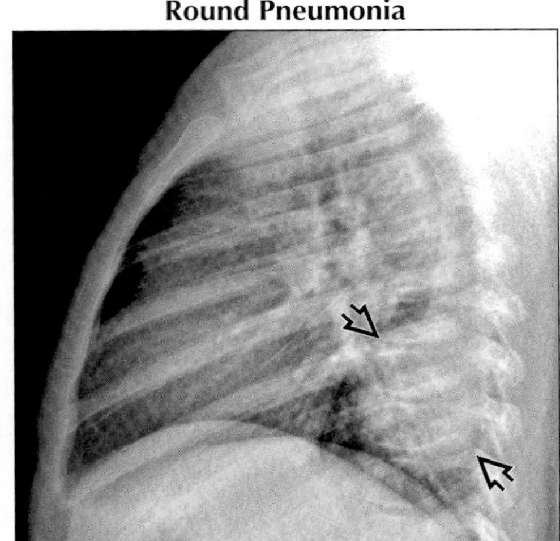

(Left) *Frontal radiograph shows round radiodensity ➩ in the right lower lobe in a young child with a fever. This patient responded to antibiotic therapy.* ***(Right)*** *Lateral radiograph in the same patient shows the round lung opacity ➩ to be posterior, located within the right lower lobe.*

Round Pneumonia

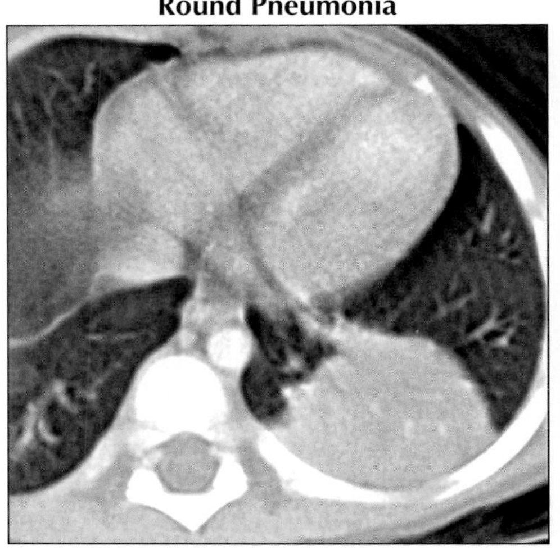

Round Pneumonia

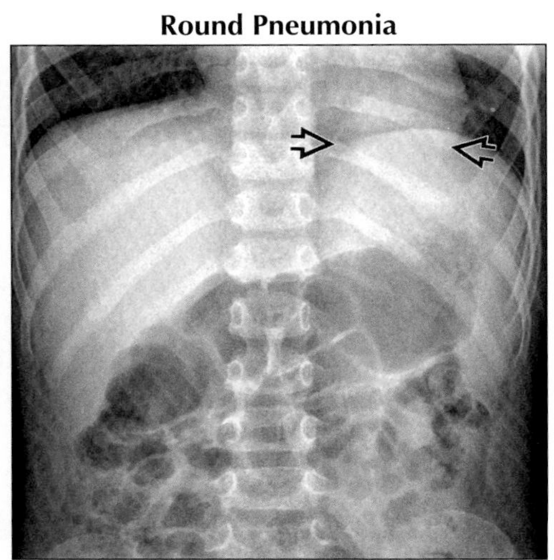

(Left) *Axial CECT performed in a young child for abdominal pain shows rounded left lower lobe consolidation consistent with round pneumonia. Round pneumonia can present with abdominal pain rather than chest symptoms.* ***(Right)*** *Frontal radiograph of the abdomen in the same patient shows left lower lobe lung opacification ➩ consistent with round pneumonia.*

Bronchogenic Cyst

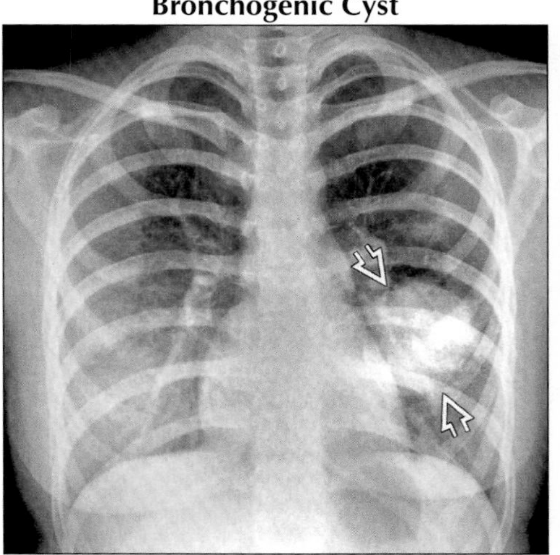

Bronchogenic Cyst

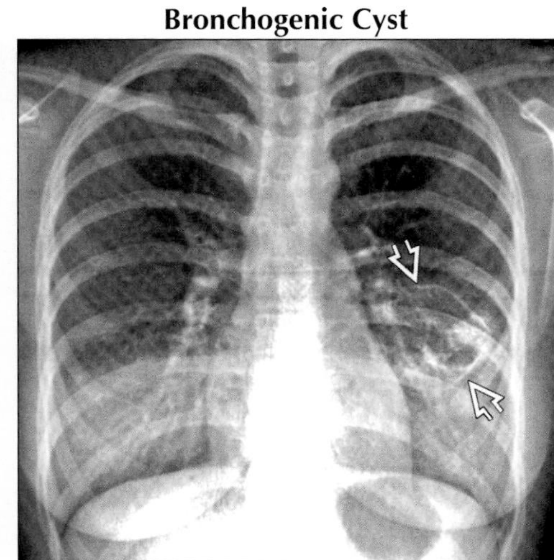

(Left) *Frontal radiograph in a patient with an infected congenital lesion shows soft tissue density in the left mid-lung ➡.* ***(Right)*** *Follow-up radiograph 3 weeks later in the same patient with an infected congenital lesion shows the thin-walled cyst ➡ present in area of previous opacification. This is most consistent with an underlying infected lesion, such as a bronchogenic cyst.*

Congenital Cystic Adenomatoid Malformation (CCAM)

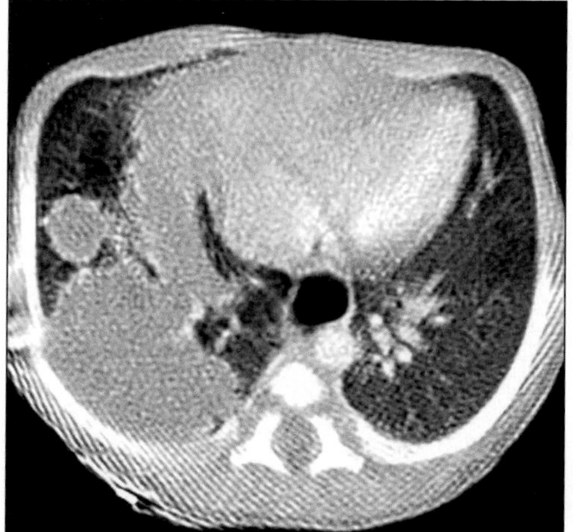

Congenital Cystic Adenomatoid Malformation (CCAM)

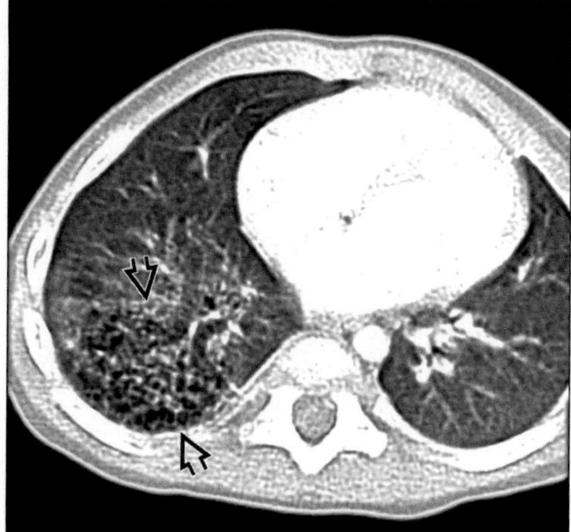

(Left) *Axial CECT in a newborn infant shows fluid-attenuation lesions in the right lower lobe. Note that the lesion is multifocal.* ***(Right)*** *Axial CECT in the same patient, now 2 months of age, shows fluid to have cleared. Now there is a multiple small cystic lesion ⇨ in the right lower lobe.*

Retrocaval Thymus

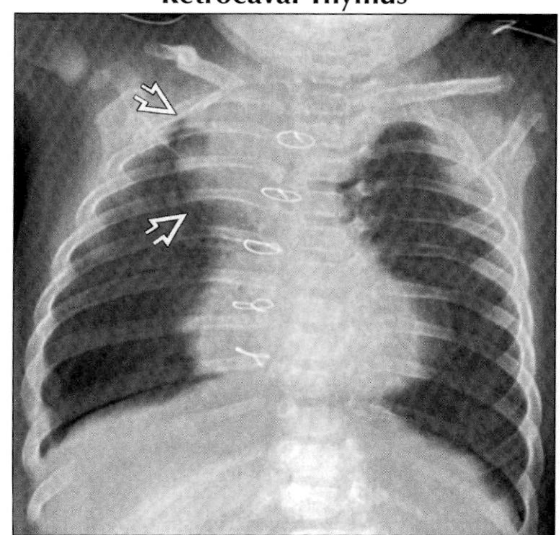

Retrocaval Thymus

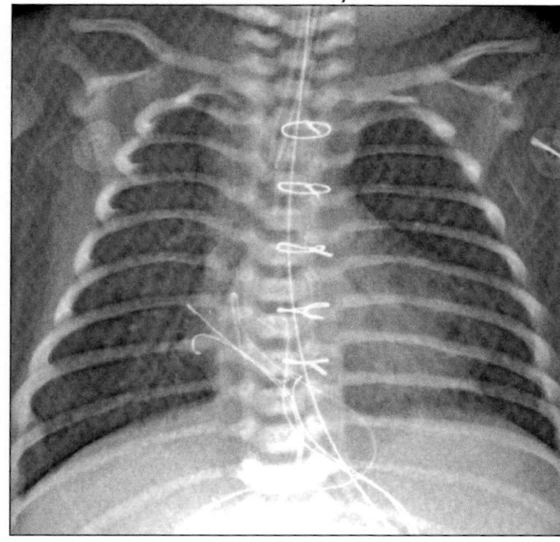

(Left) *Frontal radiograph in a child with a history of cardiac surgery shows a right superior mediastinal mass ⇨. Note the sternotomy wires.* ***(Right)*** *Frontal radiograph of baseline comparison in the same patient immediately after surgery shows that the right superior mediastinal mass is new.*

Retrocaval Thymus

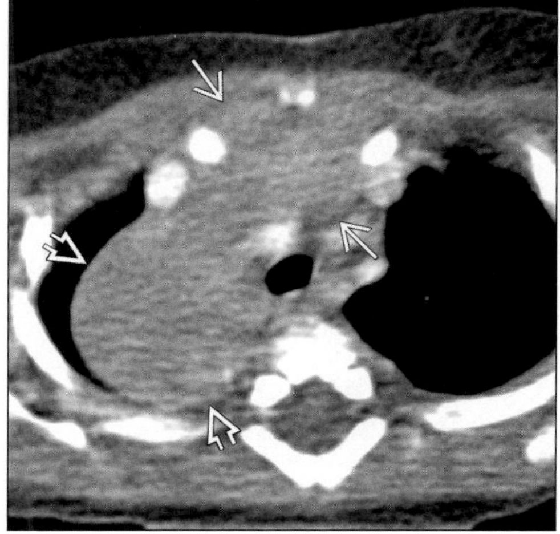

Fungal Lesion

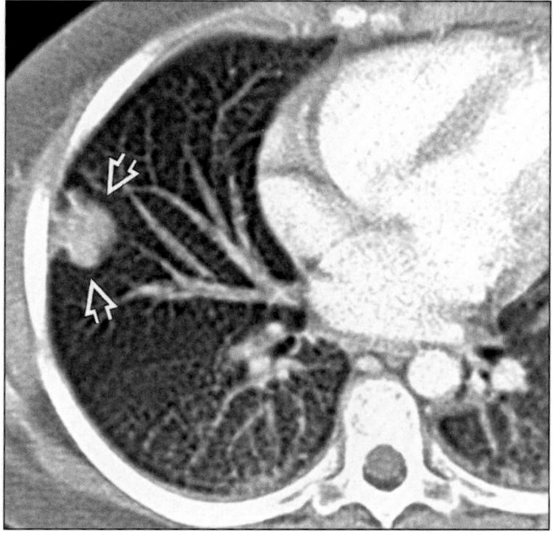

(Left) *Axial CECT in the same child shows a right paratracheal mass ⇨. The mass is contiguous and isodense with the thymus →. The thymus was small and immediately postoperatively related to stress and seen as small on the previous chest radiograph.* ***(Right)*** *Axial CECT in a child with underlying complex medical problems shows a multilobulated nodule ⇨ in the right upper lobe.*

ROUNDED LUNG MASS

(Left) Frontal radiograph shows an enchondroma of the rib as a rounded somewhat lobulated density ➔. Note there is erosion of the adjacent rib, which is a clue to the chest wall origins of this lesion. Note the metallic "BB" placed on the region of the palpable lesion during a physical examination. (Right) Sagittal NECT in the same patient shows enchondroma. Note the chondroid matrix and distortion of the adjacent rib.

Chest Wall Lesion

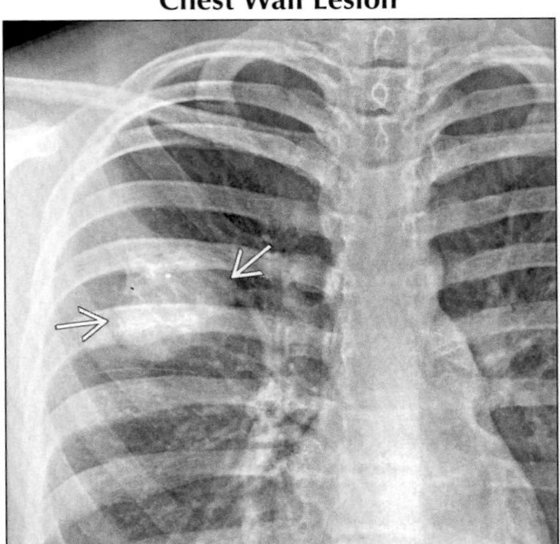

Chest Wall Lesion

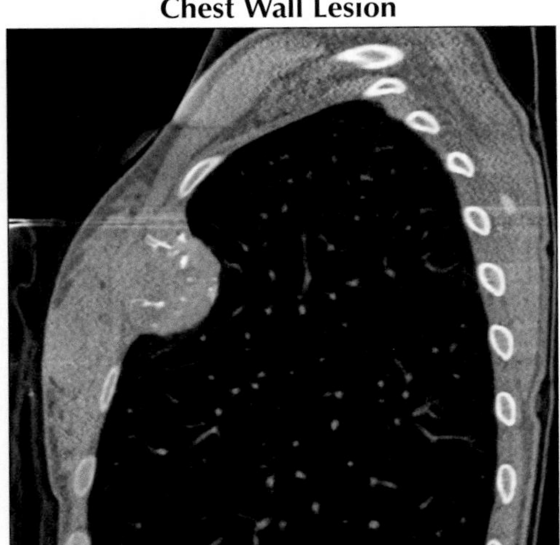

(Left) Frontal radiograph shows a large, round, soft tissue density mass overlying the apex of the right hemithorax. Note there is widening of the interspace between the right 3rd and 4th ribs, compared to the same interspace on the left. There is also erosion of the posterior right 3rd rib. (Right) Axial NECT in the same patient shows a large mass filling the apex of the right hemithorax. Note the mediastinal shift to the left and compression of the trachea ➔.

Neuroblastoma

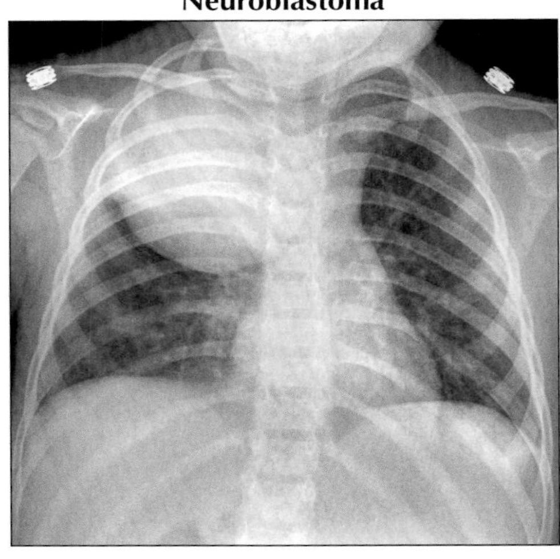

Neuroblastoma

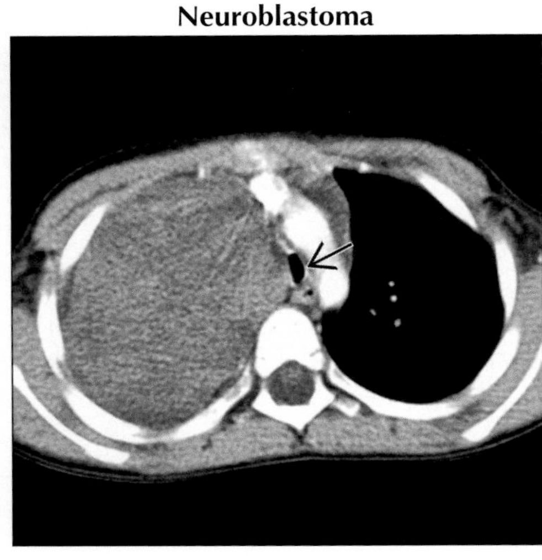

(Left) Frontal MIBG scintigraphy in the same patient shows increased uptake in the lesion ➲, consistent with neuroblastoma. Note the normal activity in the salivary glands, heart, and liver. (Right) Gross pathology in the same case shows the round encapsulated mass representing resected neuroblastoma.

Neuroblastoma

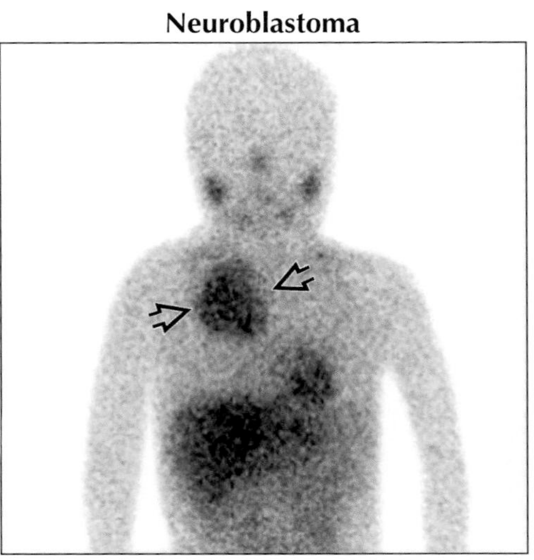

Neuroblastoma

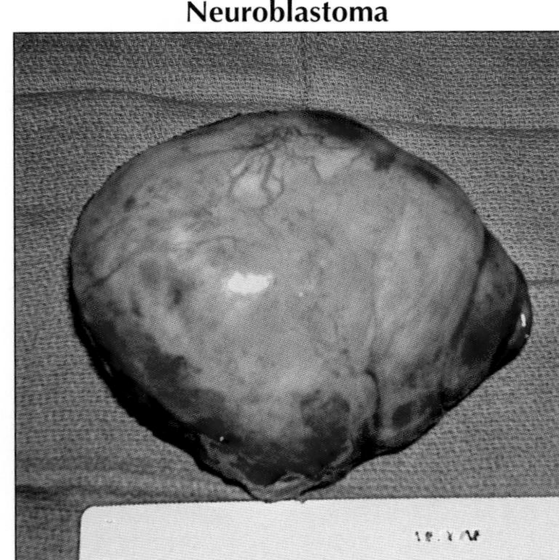

Lung Abscess/Cavitary Necrosis

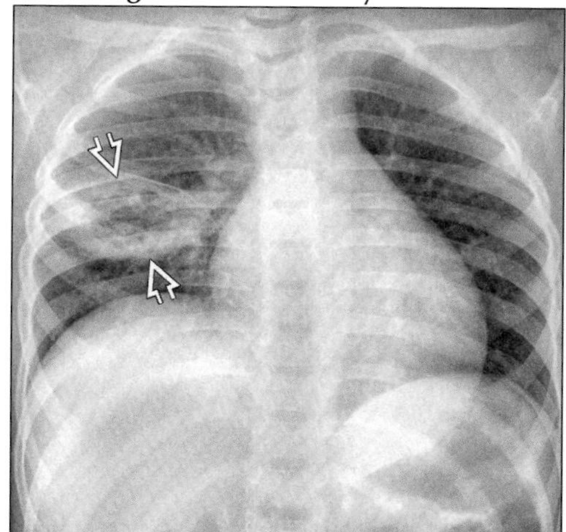

Lung Abscess/Cavitary Necrosis

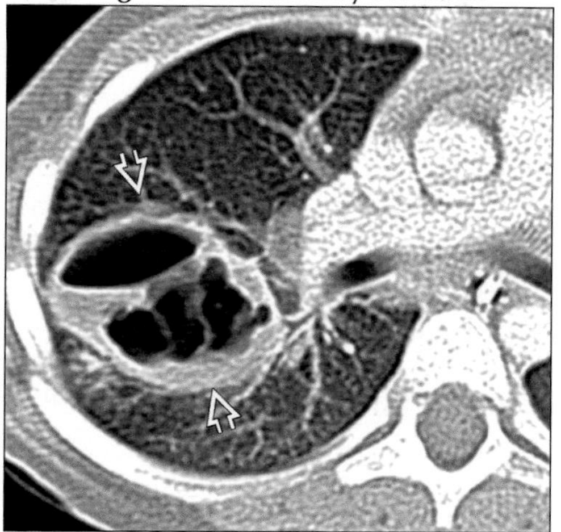

*(**Left**) Frontal radiograph of the chest in a patient with cavitary necrosis complicating pneumonia shows a cavitary-appearing lesion ➲ in the right mid-lung. (**Right**) Axial CECT in the same patient shows a multiseptated ➲ cavitary lesion in the right lung.*

Lung Abscess/Cavitary Necrosis

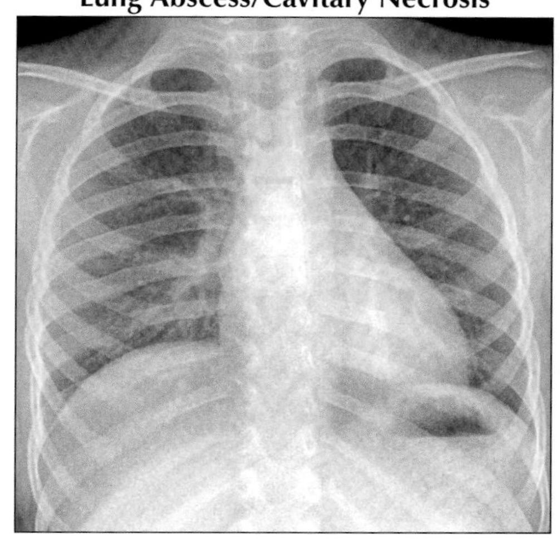

Lung Abscess/Cavitary Necrosis

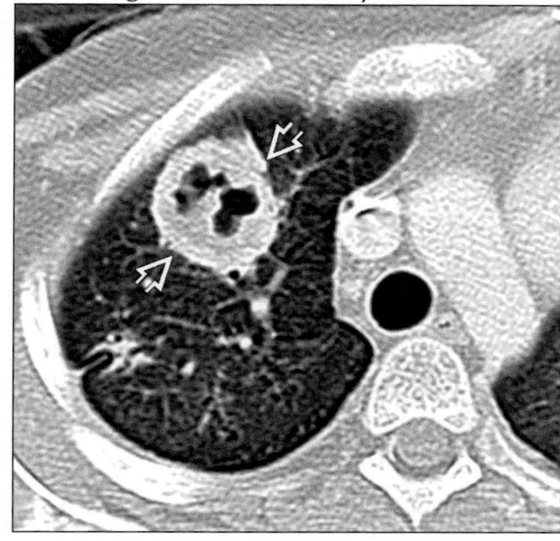

*(**Left**) Frontal radiograph follow-up in the same patient shows near resolution of the cavity, resolving cavitary necrosis. Most cases of cavitary necrosis will show near complete clearing on radiographs obtained after 40 days. Long-term follow-up imaging is not necessary unless clinical symptoms persist. (**Right**) Axial CECT in an immunocompromised child shows a thick-walled cavity ➲ containing air in the right upper lobe. Note the lack of surrounding consolidated lung.*

Pleuropulmonary Blastoma

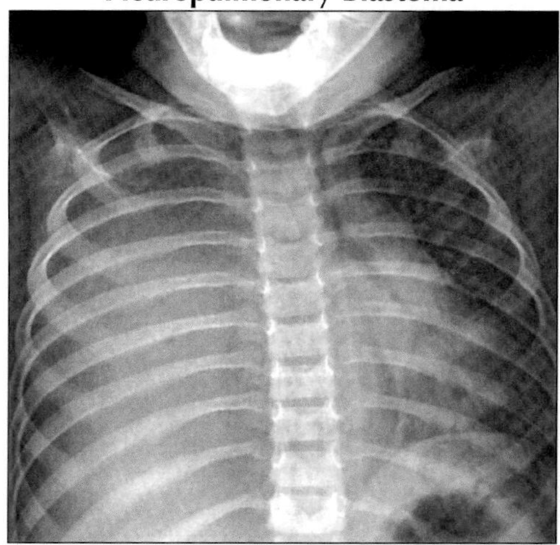

Pleuropulmonary Blastoma

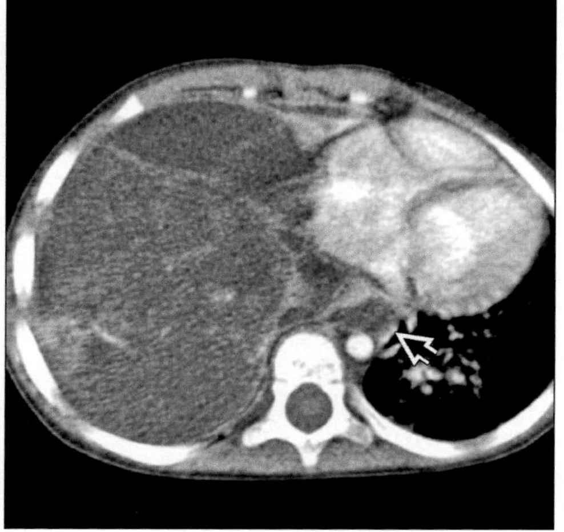

*(**Left**) Frontal radiograph shows opacification of the right hemithorax with a mediastinal shift to the left. The left lung is clear. (**Right**) Axial CECT in the same patient shows a large, heterogeneous, low-attenuation mass in the right hemithorax. The mass extends into the azygoesophageal recess ➲. Note displacement of the heart to the left.*

MULTIPLE PULMONARY NODULES

DIFFERENTIAL DIAGNOSIS

Common

- Fungal Infection
- Mycoplasma Infection

Less Common

- Tuberculosis (TB)
- Viral Infection
- Septic Emboli
- Metastatic Disease
- Lymphoproliferative Disease
- Post-Transplant Lymphoproliferative Disorder
- Langerhans Cell Histiocytosis, Pulmonary
- Wegener Granulomatosis
- Sarcoid

Rare but Important

- Hypersensitivity Pneumonitis
- Thoracic Lymphoma

ESSENTIAL INFORMATION

Key Differential Diagnosis Issues

- Location within pulmonary parenchyma
  - Centrilobular vs. random
  - Upper vs. lower lobe predominant
- Tendency to present as cavitary lesions
  - Septic emboli, *Aspergillus*, Wegener, papillomatosis
- Patient demographic/clinical considerations
  - High risk TB population?
  - Regional endemic fungal infections?
  - Immunocompromised patient?
- Many primary neoplasms metastasize to lungs; usually there is known primary when lung metastases are detected

Helpful Clues for Common Diagnoses

- **Fungal Infection**
  - Histoplasmosis
    - Common in midwestern USA
    - Variable appearance: Multiple nodules, alveolar, ill-defined peripheral opacities
    - Coarsely calcified mediastinal/hilar lymph nodes are common
    - Pulmonary nodules often calcify
  - *Candida*
    - Typically seen in patients with multiple underlying medical conditions
    - Variable parenchymal pattern: Nodules, segmental consolidation, ± cavitation
    - Look for other systemic disease: Spleen, liver, bloodstream, sinuses
  - *Aspergillus*
    - Allergic: Typically seen in asthma or cystic fibrosis patients; ill-defined consolidation or branching mucoid plugs
    - Saprophytic: Preexisting architectural abnormality (bronchiectasis, cavity); classic fungus ball
    - Mildly invasive: Chronically ill patients; focal infiltrate or fungus ball in cavity
    - Frankly invasive: Immunocompromised patients; variable appearance of peripheral consolidation, "halo" sign, cavitary lesions
  - Coccidiomycosis
    - Imaging appearance compared to TB
    - Highly variable appearance: Nodules, infiltrates, or thin-walled cavities
    - Pleural effusions, adenopathy possible
  - Blastomycosis
    - Rare in children
    - More severe infection/multiorgan involvement if immunocompromised
    - Variable pattern: Nodules, peripheral consolidation, interstitial opacities
- **Mycoplasma Infection**
  - Wide spectrum of radiologic and clinical presentations
    - May manifest as bronchopneumonia, atelectasis, or interstitial opacities
    - Typical in older school-aged children

Helpful Clues for Less Common Diagnoses

- **Tuberculosis (TB)**
  - Secondary tuberculosis may present as diffuse bilateral < 3 mm nodular opacities
    - May be associated with pleural effusions, lymphadenopathy
    - Consider concomitant solid visceral or CNS involvement
- **Viral Infection**
  - Cytomegalovirus
    - Typically seen after bone marrow transplant
    - Bilateral, diffusely distributed, small nodular opacities
  - Human papillomavirus
    - Endobronchial spread of laryngeal papillomatosis
    - Bilateral nodules of varying size, may cavitate

MULTIPLE PULMONARY NODULES

- **Septic Emboli**
  - Common organisms: *Staphylococcus aureus*, *Streptococcus*
  - Search for underlying source: Soft tissue infection, osteomyelitis, central line infection, endocarditis
  - Imaging
    - Multiple, basilar-predominant, nodular or ill-defined opacities
    - Eventual cavitation common
    - Source vessel may be identified
- **Metastatic Disease**
  - Wilms tumor
    - Lungs are most common site of mets
    - Pulmonary: Multiple pulmonary nodules, masses
    - Cardiovascular: Tumor extension into renal vein, IVC, right atrium
  - Ewing sarcoma
    - Lungs are most common site of metastatic disease; metastases may be seen at diagnosis or years later
  - Rhabdomyosarcoma
    - Common tumor in children arising from GU tract, orbits, chest wall
    - Lungs are most common site of metastatic disease
  - Osteosarcoma
    - Most common malignant bone tumor in children
    - Lungs are most common site of metastases: Nodules that may be ossified; spontaneous pneumothorax; hemothorax
- **Lymphoproliferative Disease, Post-Transplant Lymphoproliferative Disorder**
  - Variable appearance: Infiltrates or nodules
  - Hilar/mediastinal adenopathy may be seen
- **Langerhans Cell Histiocytosis, Pulmonary**
  - Parenchymal findings: Nodule that cavitates; thick- or thin-walled cysts
  - Other thoracic features: Pneumothorax, adenopathy, fibrosis
- **Wegener Granulomatosis**
  - Vasculitis, cavitating nodules (basilar predominant), ± ground-glass halo
  - Other respiratory/thoracic manifestations: Rhinorrhea, epistaxis, mucosal ulcerations, airway stenosis, pleural effusions, pulmonary hemorrhage
  - Other visceral manifestations: Glomerulonephritis, splenic lesions
- **Sarcoid**
  - Pulmonary: Small reticulonodular opacities
  - Thoracic: Hilar, paratracheal adenopathy

Helpful Clues for Rare Diagnoses

- **Hypersensitivity Pneumonitis**
  - Variable pattern of fine nodules, alveolar or interstitial opacities
- **Thoracic Lymphoma**
  - Pulmonary nodules more common in Hodgkin vs. non-Hodgkin
  - Typically seen with mediastinal/hilar adenopathy
  - Variable pattern of round nodules or ill-defined opacities

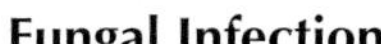

Fungal Infection

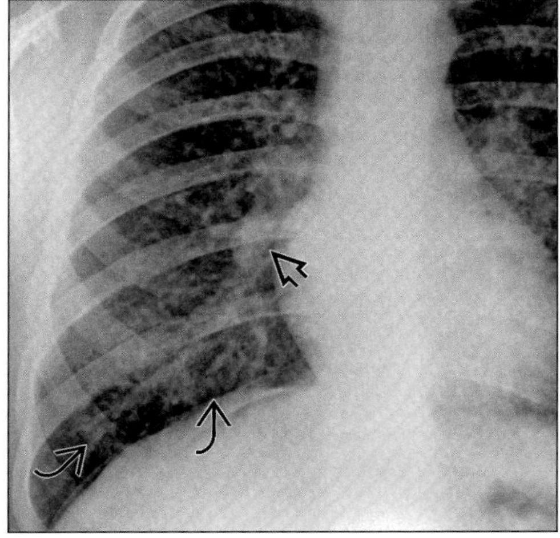

AP radiograph shows numerous, small, indistinct, nodular opacities [arrow] in this 15-year-old boy with biopsy-proven histoplasmosis. There is right hilar adenopathy [arrow].

Fungal Infection

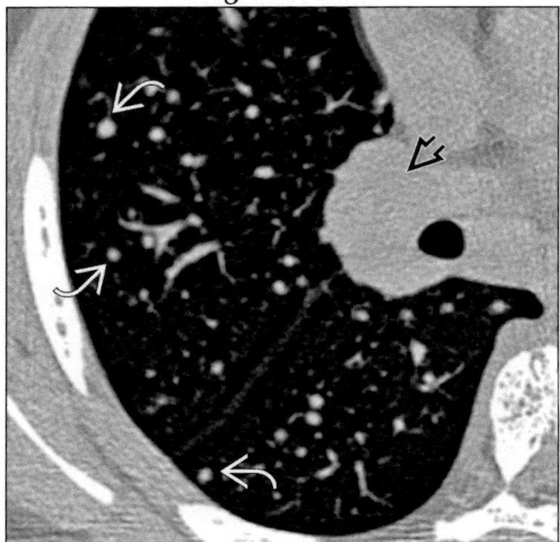

Axial CECT in the same patient shows the typical appearance of the small pulmonary nodules [arrow] at the lung base. Bulky right hilar adenopathy [arrow] is redemonstrated.

MULTIPLE PULMONARY NODULES

*(**Left**) Axial CECT shows the early presentation of histoplasmosis infection in this 10-year-old child. There are ill-defined nodular opacities at the lung bases. (**Right**) Axial NECT shows the appearance of the lung bases in the same child 2 years later. The remaining pulmonary nodules are now smaller and well defined in appearance. Note the stippled calcifications in the hilar and mediastinal lymph nodes.*

Fungal Infection

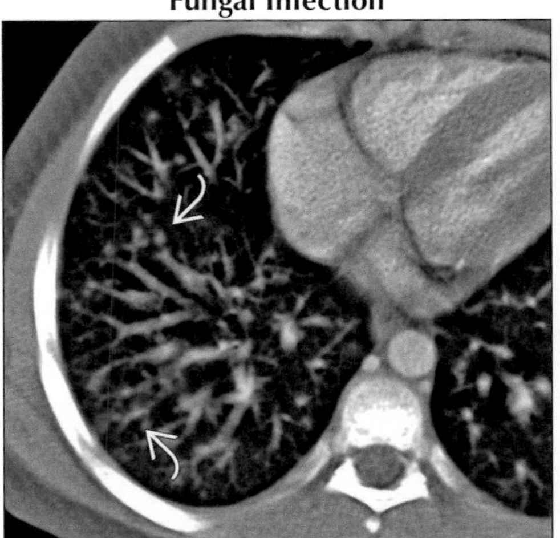

Fungal Infection

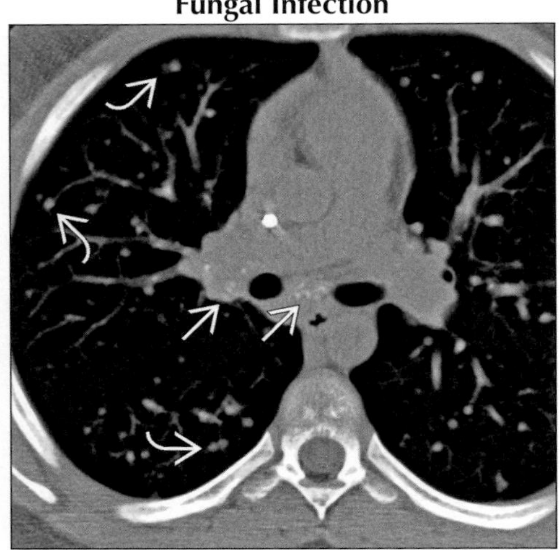

*(**Left**) Axial CECT shows 2 of many basilar predominant pulmonary nodular opacities in this 14-year-old girl with relapsed acute lymphocytic leukemia who presented with abdominal pain and fever. This was a biopsy-proven candidal infection. (**Right**) Axial CECT in the same patient demonstrates multiple, small, low-attenuation foci of candidal fungal infection in the liver and spleen.*

Fungal Infection

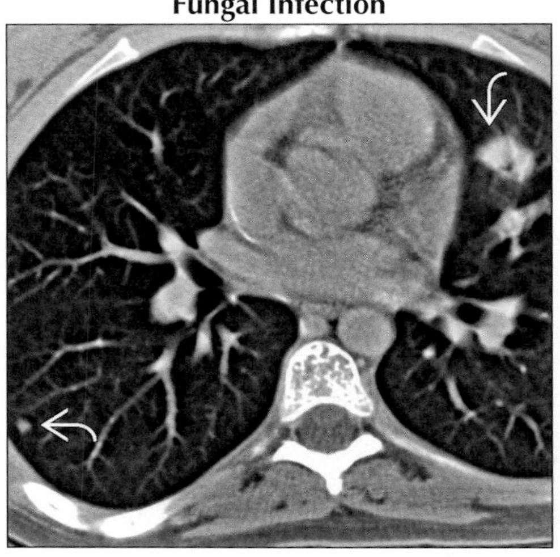

Fungal Infection

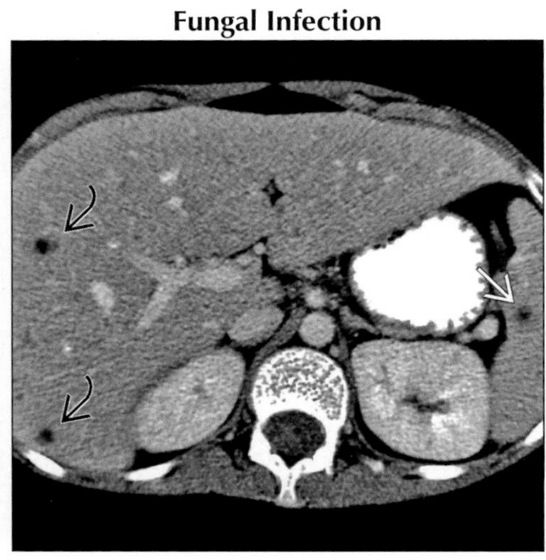

*(**Left**) Axial NECT shows 2 of the many nodular opacities in this immunosuppressed teenager with a fever and cough due to an Aspergillus infection. Central clearing within the nodules consistent with early cavitation is noted. (**Right**) Axial NECT shows the same right upper lobe lesion 2 months later, now larger in size with progression of cavitation and an organized fungal ball internally.*

Fungal Infection

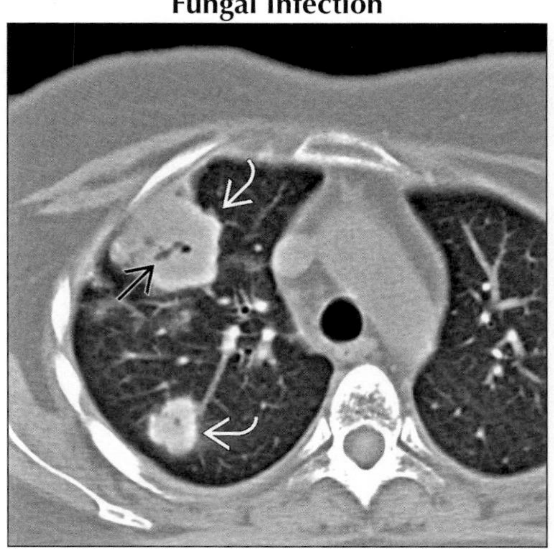

Fungal Infection

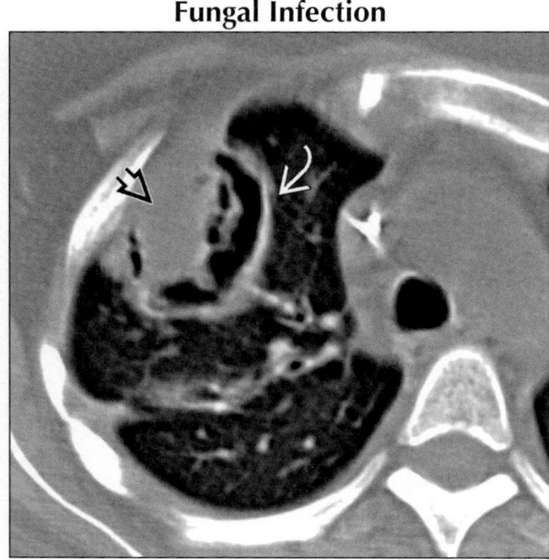

Viral Infection

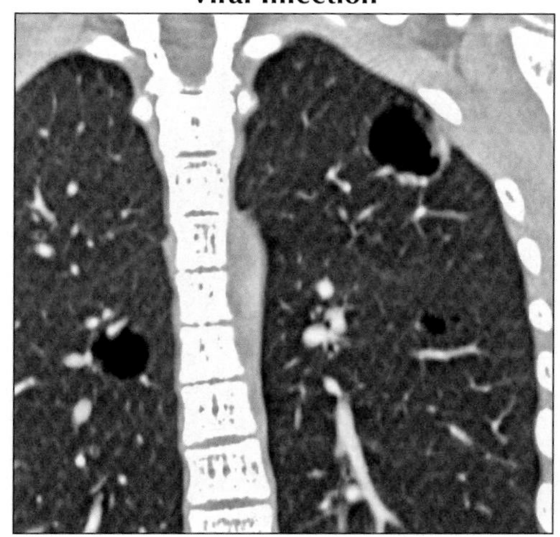

Viral Infection

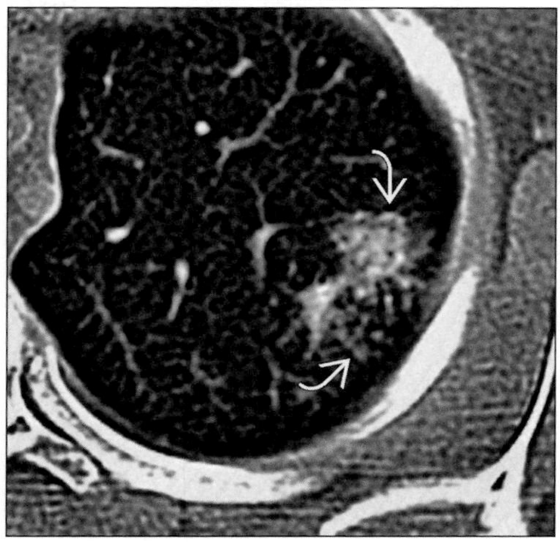

(Left) *Coronal NECT shows scattered lesions throughout both lungs in this 14-year-old female with recurrent laryngeal papillomatosis. These lesions start as nodules but may eventually cavitate and become thin-walled cystic lesions such as these. Rarely, malignant transformation may occur.* ***(Right)*** *Axial NECT shows small, peripheral, nodular opacities ➔ in this 9 year old with a Cytomegalovirus infection related to a prior bone marrow transplant.*

Septic Emboli

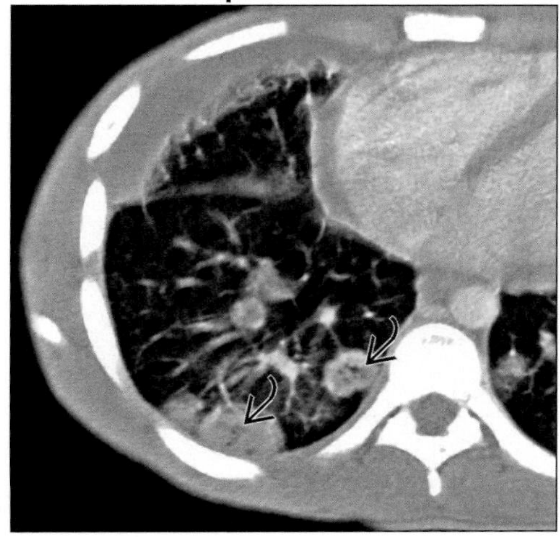

Septic Emboli

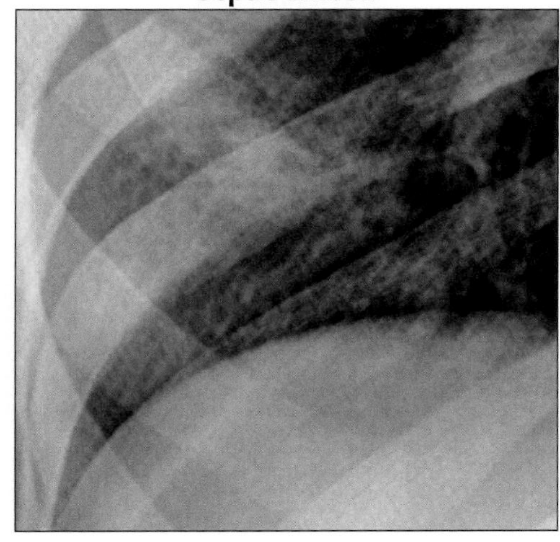

(Left) *Axial CECT shows nodules with early cavitation evidenced by central clearing ➔ in this 17-year-old boy with Lemierre syndrome, septic thrombophlebitis of the internal jugular veins. The patient presented with group C streptococcal pharyngeal infection.* ***(Right)*** *Frontal radiograph shows the lung nodules in the same patient. This image was obtained 1 day before the CT, demonstrating the limits of radiographs in nodule detection.*

Metastatic Disease

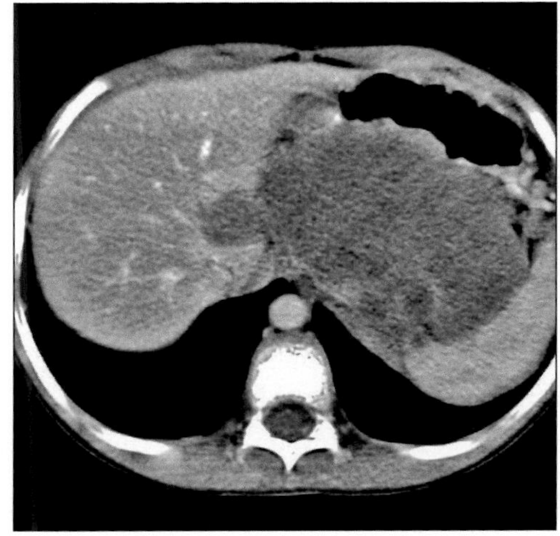

Metastatic Disease

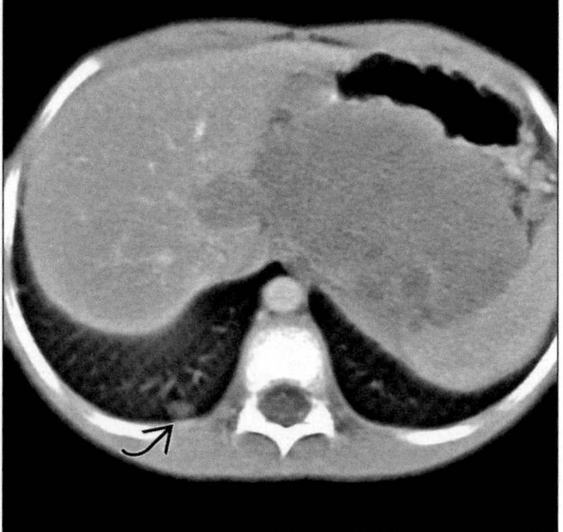

(Left) *Axial CECT shows a stage IV Wilms tumor arising from the left kidney in this 8-year-old girl. No left renal vein or IVC invasion was seen.* ***(Right)*** *Axial CECT at the same level in lung windows shows scattered metastatic nodules ➔ at the lung bases.*

MULTIPLE PULMONARY NODULES

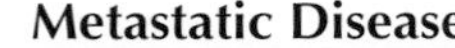

*(**Left**) Axial NECT shows micronodular metastatic disease at the lung bases in this 13-year-old girl with papillary thyroid cancer. (**Right**) Axial NECT shows calcified right infrahilar and noncalcified pleural-based metastases in this teenager with osteosarcoma of the right mandible.*

Metastatic Disease

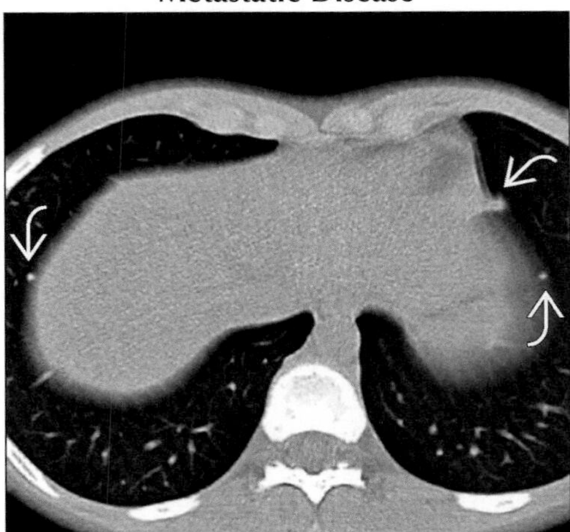

Metastatic Disease

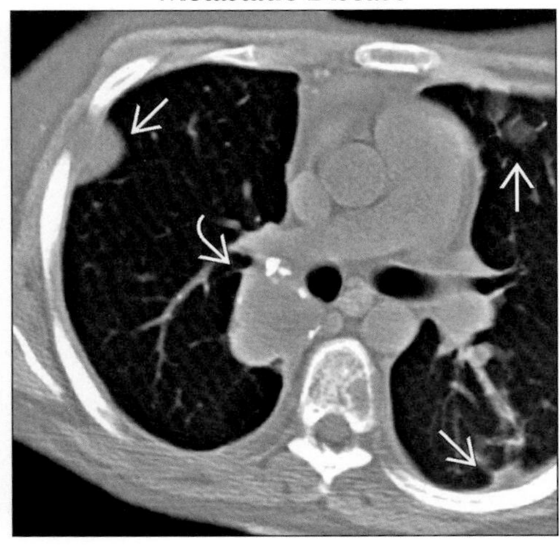

*(**Left**) Lateral noncontrast CT scout view shows a large soft tissue prominence arising in the parieto-occipital region in this 12-year-old boy with an incidental history of minor trauma 2 months previously. This was a pathologically proven rhabdomyosarcoma. (**Right**) Axial CECT shows numerous bilateral pulmonary nodules in the same patient, consistent with widely metastatic disease.*

Metastatic Disease

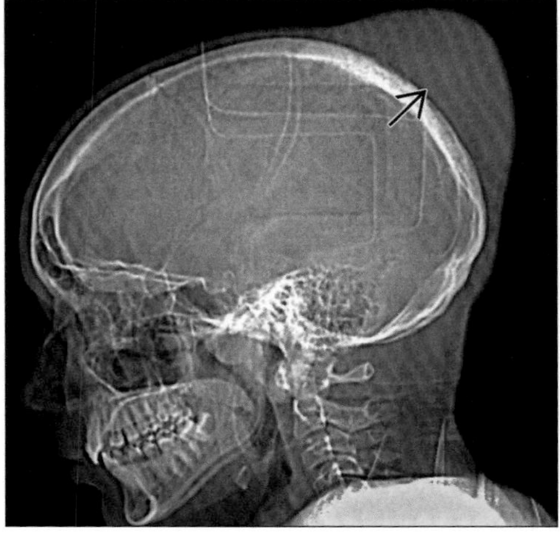

Metastatic Disease

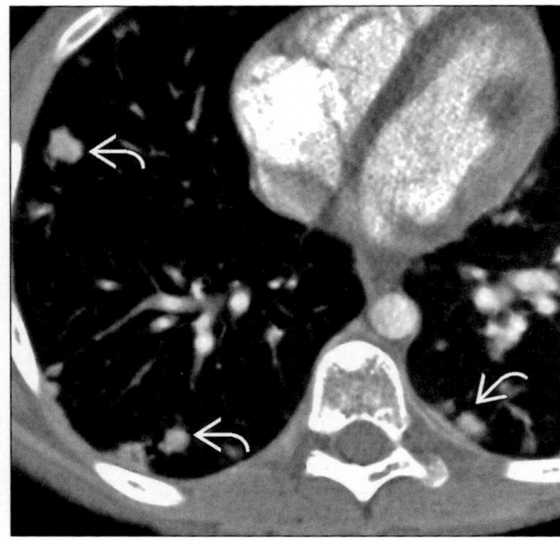

*(**Left**) Axial CECT shows multiple pulmonary nodules at the lung bases in this 17 year old with metastatic osteosarcoma. At the left anterior lung base is a pneumothorax, and the prominent lesion at the right anterior lung base has a faintly seen ossified rim, features that are highly characteristic of osteosarcoma. (**Right**) Frontal radiograph shows the appearance of the pulmonary nodules in the same patient.*

Metastatic Disease

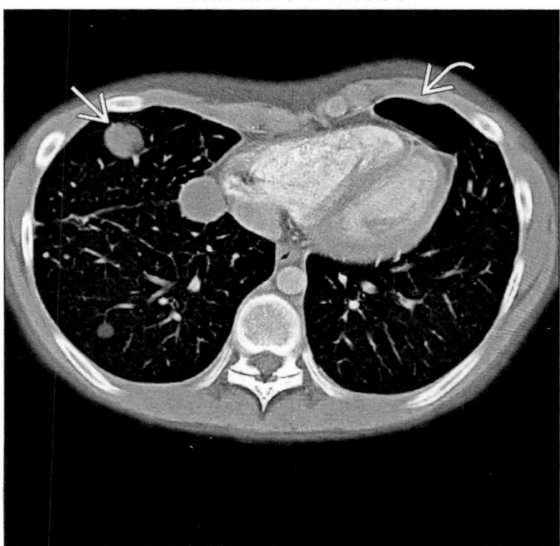

Metastatic Disease

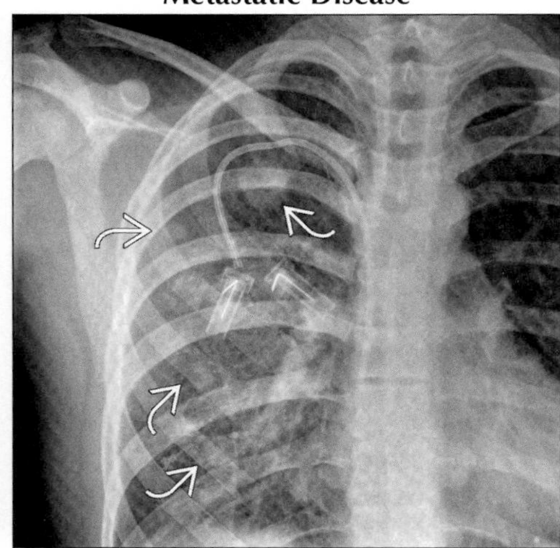

Lymphoproliferative Disease

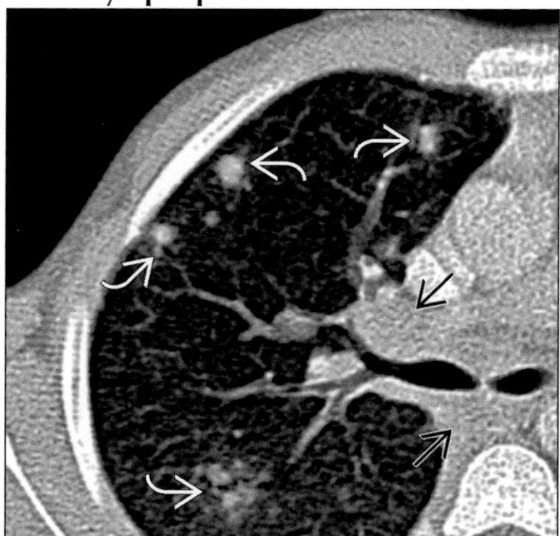

Lymphoproliferative Disease

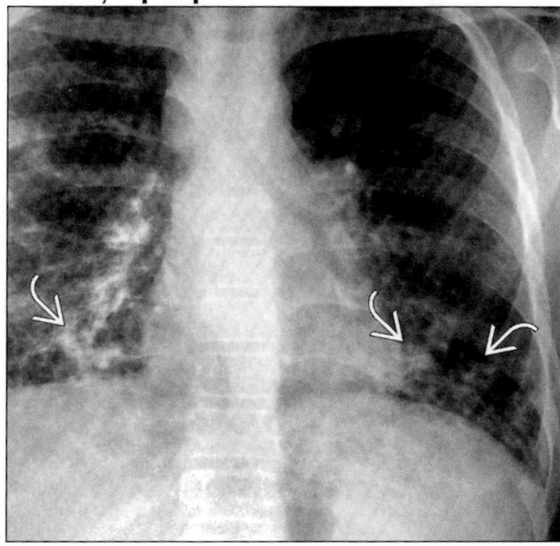

*(**Left**) Axial CECT shows multiple, randomly distributed, pulmonary nodules ➔ in this 10-year-old boy with lymphoproliferative disorder. Note the bulky mediastinal and hilar lymphadenopathy ➔. (**Right**) Frontal radiograph shows numerous, indistinct, pulmonary nodules ➔ at the bilateral lung bases in an 11-year-old boy with common variable immunodeficiency syndrome with lymphoproliferative features.*

Wegener Granulomatosis

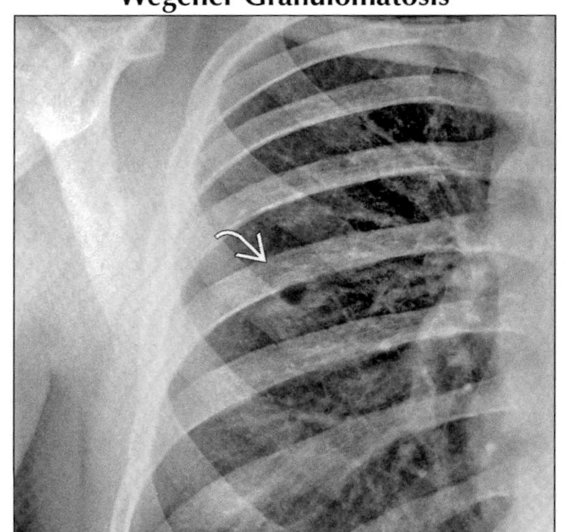

Wegener Granulomatosis

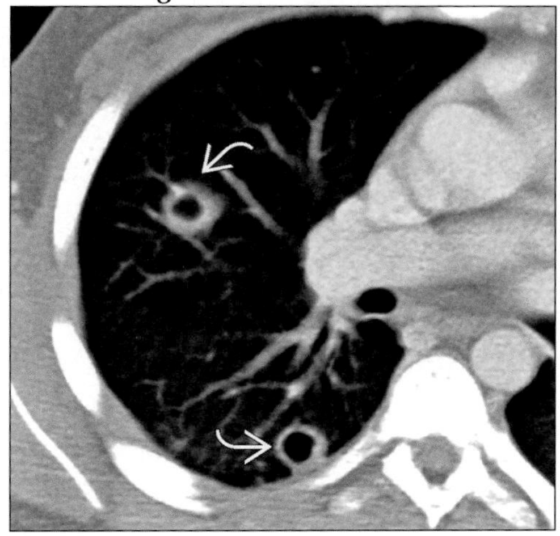

*(**Left**) Frontal radiograph shows a thick-walled cavitary pulmonary nodule ➔ in the right upper lobe in this 15-year-old boy who presented with dyspnea and suspected granulomatous disease of the nose. (**Right**) Axial CECT shows the cavitary right upper lobe lesions ➔ of the same patient in more detail. These lesions eventually resolved.*

Wegener Granulomatosis

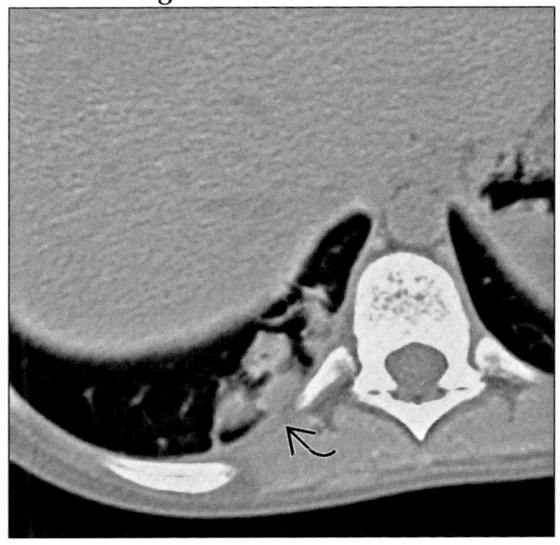

Wegener Granulomatosis

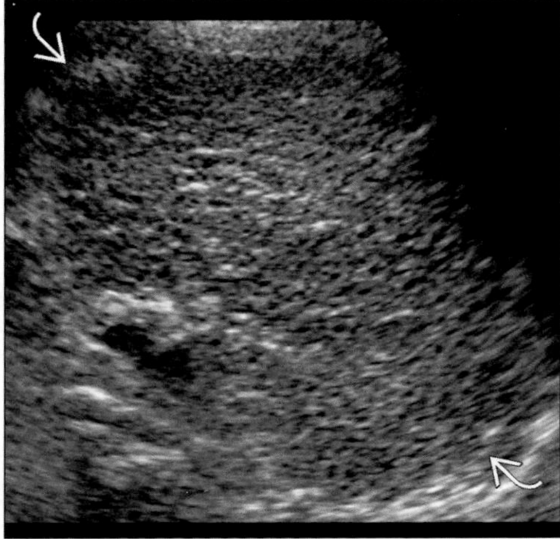

*(**Left**) Axial NECT shows a cluster of lobulated, nonspecific-appearing, basilar pulmonary nodules ➔ in this 13-year-old girl who presented with a fever and weight loss. (**Right**) Transverse ultrasound shows the diffusely coarsened and heterogeneous appearance of the splenic parenchyma in the same patient. The margins of the spleen ➔ are usually well defined, but in this case are very poorly defined. The spleen is infrequently involved in Wegener granulomatosis.*

NEONATAL CHEST MASS

DIFFERENTIAL DIAGNOSIS

Common
- Cystic Adenomatoid Malformation
- Pulmonary Sequestration
- Congenital Diaphragmatic Hernia
- Congenital Lobar Emphysema

Less Common
- Thoracic Neuroblastoma
- Foregut Duplication Cyst

Rare but Important
- Pleuropulmonary Blastoma
- Mesenchymal Hamartoma

ESSENTIAL INFORMATION

Key Differential Diagnosis Issues
- Neonatal lung masses are typically congenital lesions
  - Neonatal lung neoplasms extremely rare
  - Infectious lung masses in neonatal period uncommon
- Review of prenatal studies can aid in forming differential for neonatal lung mass
- Mediastinal and chest wall masses can mimic lung masses
- CT often necessary to narrow differential

Helpful Clues for Common Diagnoses
- **Cystic Adenomatoid Malformation**
  - a.k.a. congenital pulmonary airway malformation (CPAM)
  - Diagnosis can be made prenatally with ultrasound and fetal MR
  - Type 1
    - Single or multiple 2-10 cm cysts
    - May contain air-fluid levels
    - Good prognosis
  - Type 2
    - Multiple, small (0.5-2 cm) cysts
    - Variable prognosis
  - Type 3
    - Innumerable microscopic cysts
    - Appears solid on CT and ultrasound
    - Poorer prognosis
  - Evidence of associated mass effect
    - Mediastinal shift
    - Compression of adjacent normal lung
  - Can coexist with other pulmonary malformations
    - Sequestration
    - Bronchogenic cyst
  - Can become complicated by recurrent infections
  - Small malignancy risk
    - Pleuropulmonary blastoma
    - Rhabdomyosarcoma
- **Pulmonary Sequestration**
  - Extralobar variety in neonate
  - No normal connection to tracheobronchial tree
  - Enhancing mass near diaphragm
    - May be subdiaphragmatic in location
  - Mass invested by its own pleura
  - Look for systemic arterial feeder (typically originating from aorta near diaphragmatic hiatus)
    - Perform CT evaluation as CT angiography protocol
  - Typically systemic venous drainage to inferior vena cava
  - Associated anomalies
    - Other bronchopulmonary foregut malformations
    - Cardiac defects
  - Can be detected prenatally with ultrasound and fetal MR
- **Congenital Diaphragmatic Hernia**
  - Bochdalek (90%)
    - Posterior
  - Morgagni (10%)
    - Anterior
  - Left (75%), right (25%)
  - Multiloculated lucent mass in chest when stomach/bowel involved
  - Associated mass effect
  - Associated pulmonary hypoplasia
  - Enteric tube may enter mass
  - Can be detected prenatally with ultrasound and fetal MR
- **Congenital Lobar Emphysema**
  - Overdistension of lobe of lung
    - Left upper > right middle > right upper lobe
  - Multifocal in only ~ 5%
  - During 1st few days of life, affected lobe may be opacified by lung fluid
  - Hyperlucent, hyperexpanded lobe thereafter
    - Associated mass effect
  - ~ 15% have congenital heart disease

Helpful Clues for Less Common Diagnoses

- **Thoracic Neuroblastoma**
  - Most common malignant tumor in neonates
  - Adrenal location most common
    - ~ 20% are thoracic in location
    - 3rd most common location after adrenal and extraadrenal retroperitoneum
  - May be diagnosed prenatally with ultrasound or fetal MR
  - Thoracic/mediastinal location can mimic lung mass
  - Soft tissue density mass in posterior mediastinum
  - Calcifications common
  - Frequent involvement of neural foramina
    - MR well suited for evaluation
  - Associated osseous erosions and rib splaying
  - Favorable outcome profile vs. abdominal neuroblastoma
- **Foregut Duplication Cyst**
  - Bronchogenic cyst
  - Esophageal duplication cyst
  - Neurenteric cyst
  - Typically mediastinal in location but can mimic lung mass
    - ~ 15% located within lung
  - Typically homogeneous, fluid-attenuating mass
  - Well defined, rounded
  - Thin walled
  - Nonenhancing
  - May become superinfected

Helpful Clues for Rare Diagnoses

- **Pleuropulmonary Blastoma**
  - Rare childhood tumor
  - Can present in neonatal period
  - Can begin in lung parenchyma or pleura
  - Type 1 consists of cysts and can present as lucent lung mass
    - Better prognosis
  - Type 2 consists of mixed cystic and solid components
    - Variable prognosis
  - Type 3 is purely solid
    - Worst prognosis
  - Can arise from cystic adenomatoid malformation
  - Typically large mass at presentation
  - Mediastinal shift
  - Pleural effusion
- **Mesenchymal Hamartoma**
  - Rare benign lesion of infancy/childhood
  - May be present at birth
  - Can mimic lung mass
  - Arises from rib
  - Large expansile mass
  - Associated calcifications
  - Distortion of chest wall
  - Rib erosion/destruction
  - May contain hemorrhagic/cystic areas

Cystic Adenomatoid Malformation

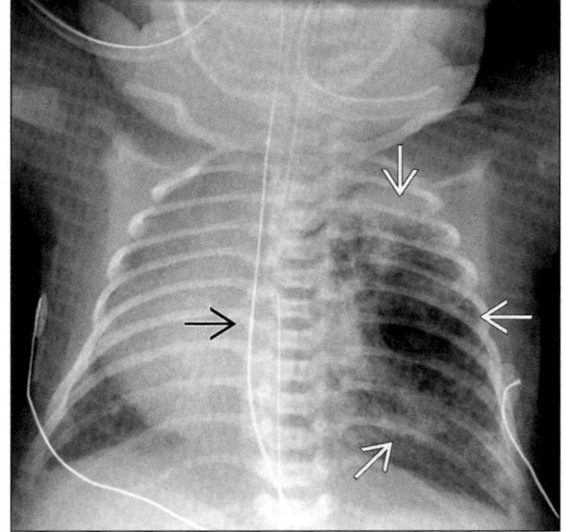

Frontal radiograph in a neonate shows a mass ➔ in the left hemithorax with mixed areas of lucency and soft tissue density. Note the rightward mediastinal shift, including the enteric tube ⇨.

Cystic Adenomatoid Malformation

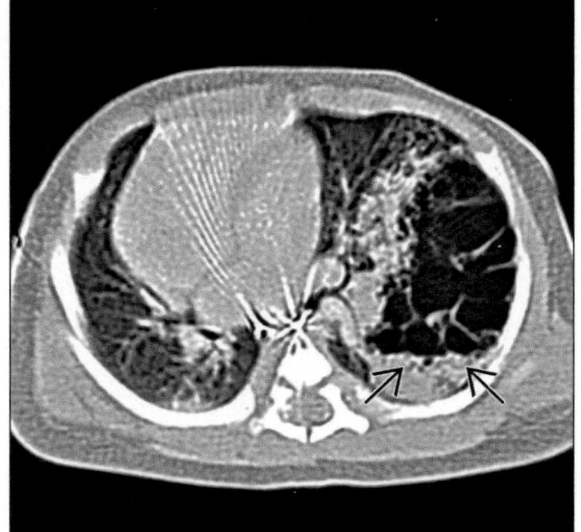

Axial CECT in the same patient shows a multiloculated cystic mass with internal air-fluid levels ⇨ in the left lung. Surgical pathology confirmed a type 1 cystic adenomatoid malformation.

NEONATAL CHEST MASS

(**Left**) Axial NECT in a 14 day old shows a soft tissue density mass ➲ in the left lower lobe. There is mild associated mass effect. Surgical pathology confirmed a type 3 cystic adenomatoid malformation. (**Right**) Axial CECT shows an enhancing mass in the left lung base ➡. There is a systemic arterial feeding vessel originating from the descending thoracic aorta ➡. The appearance is consistent with sequestration in this neonate.

Cystic Adenomatoid Malformation

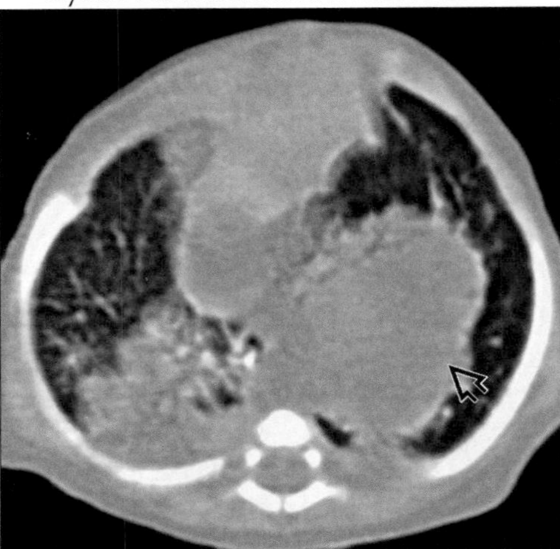

Pulmonary Sequestration

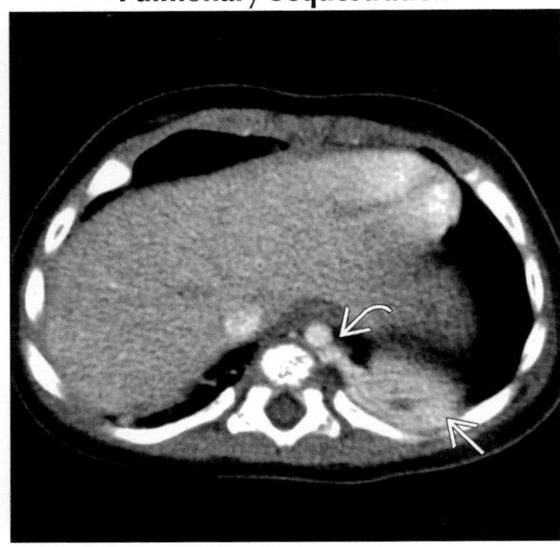

(**Left**) Axial CECT shows an enhancing mass in the left lung base ➡. There is a systemic arterial feeding vessel originating from the descending thoracic aorta ➡. The appearance is consistent with sequestration in this neonate. (**Right**) Frontal radiograph shows a heterogeneous, mixed lucent and soft tissue density mass encompassing the entire left hemithorax in this neonate. The mass causes a rightward mediastinal shift and pulmonary hypoplasia.

Pulmonary Sequestration

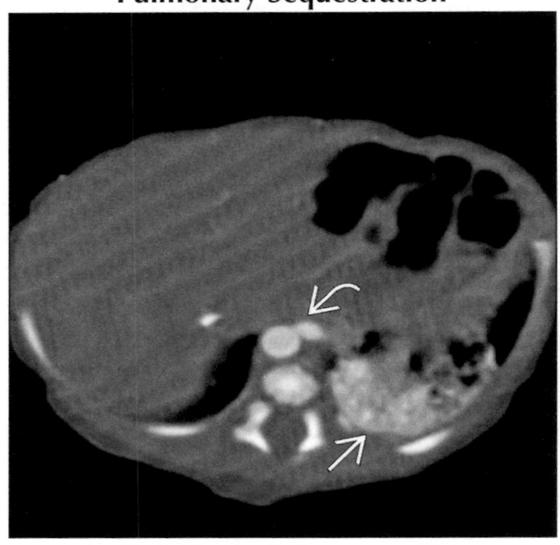

Congenital Diaphragmatic Hernia

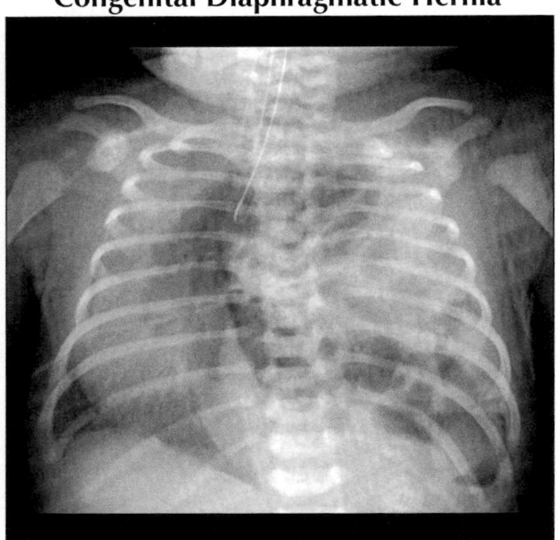

(**Left**) Frontal radiograph in a neonate shows a multiloculated lucent mass within the left hemithorax. The mass causes a rightward mediastinal shift ➡ and pulmonary hypoplasia. Note the ECMO catheters ➲, as well as the orogastric tube entering the herniated stomach ➡. (**Right**) Axial CECT in this neonate with classic congenital lobar emphysema shows well-demarcated hyperlucency and hyperexpansion confined to the left upper lobe ➲.

Congenital Diaphragmatic Hernia

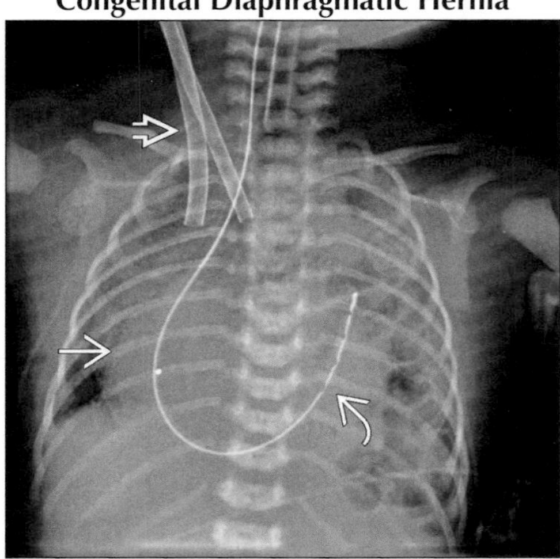

Congenital Lobar Emphysema

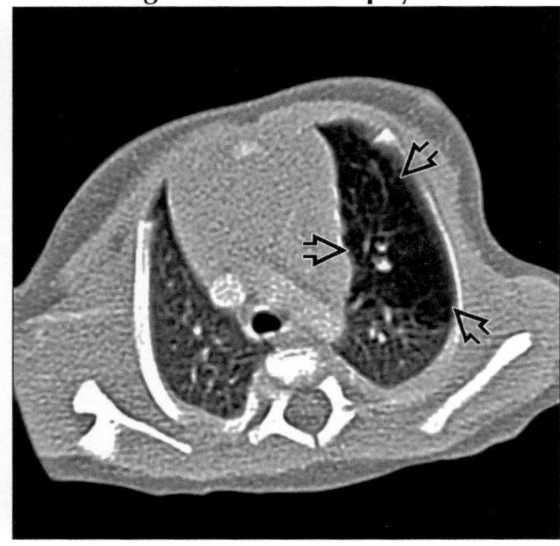

Thoracic Neuroblastoma

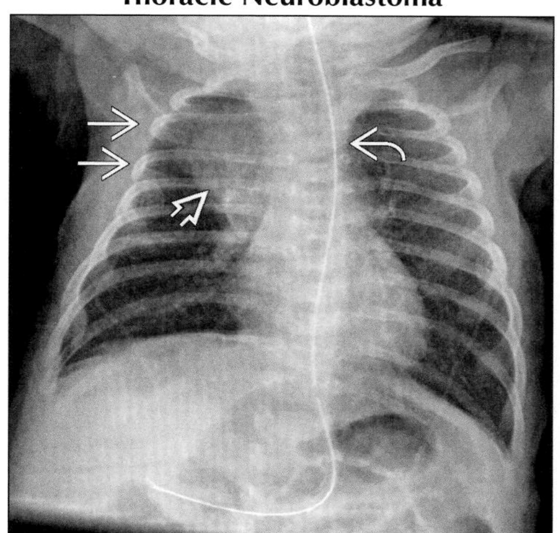

Thoracic Neuroblastoma

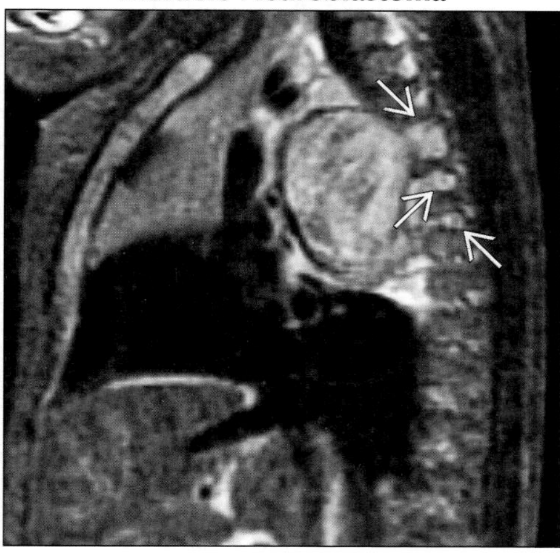

(Left) *Frontal radiograph shows a focal opacity → in the right upper thorax in this 4 week old. There is splaying between the posterior right 3rd and 4th ribs → compared with the left. Note also the subtle shift of the enteric tube to the left → at the level of the lesion, indicating associated mass effect.* ***(Right)*** *Sagittal T2WI MR in the same neonate demonstrates the thoracic neuroblastoma with multilevel neural foraminal encroachment →.*

Foregut Duplication Cyst

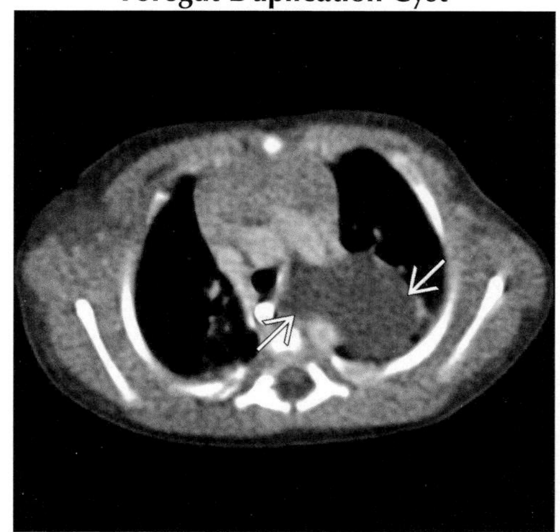

Pleuropulmonary Blastoma

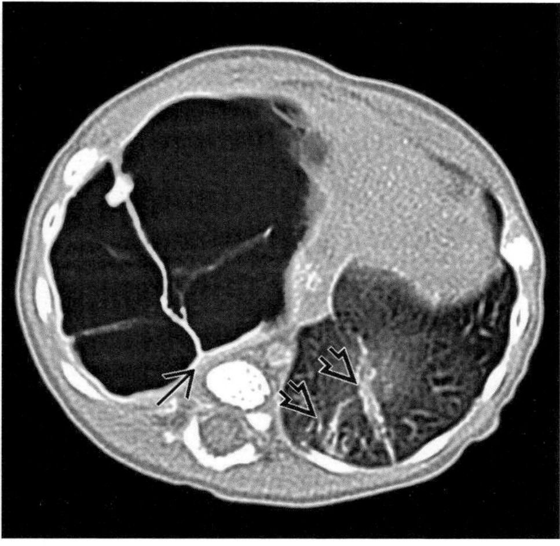

(Left) *Axial CECT shows a nonenhancing, homogeneous, fluid density mass → originating from the mediastinum and extending into the left hemithorax. Surgical pathology revealed a foregut duplication cyst.* ***(Right)*** *Axial CECT in this 1 month old shows a septated cystic mass with minimal associated pleural thickening → in the right lung. There is a rightward mediastinal shift and left lung atelectasis →. Surgical pathology showed a pleuropulmonary blastoma.*

Mesenchymal Hamartoma

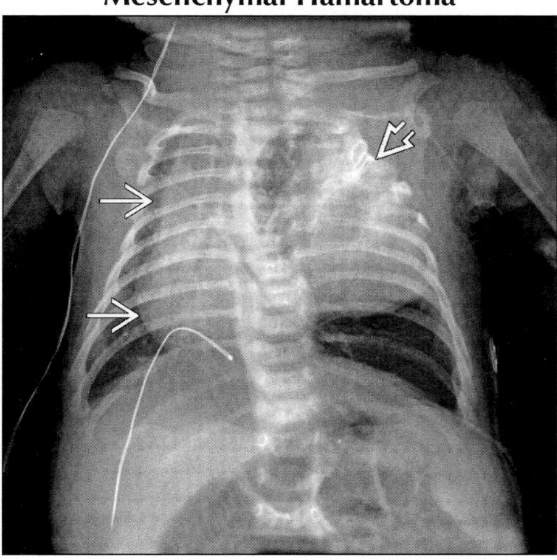

Mesenchymal Hamartoma

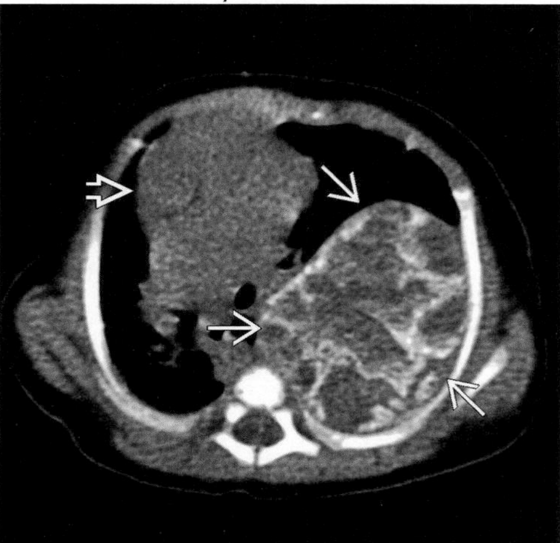

(Left) *Frontal radiograph shows a large left upper hemithorax mass. The mass distorts the chest wall → and causes a rightward mediastinal shift → in this 3-week-old neonate.* ***(Right)*** *Axial NECT in the same patient shows the large mass → based in the left chest with areas of calcification and associated cardiomediastinal shift to the right →. Surgical pathology revealed a mesenchymal hamartoma.*

CHEST WALL MASS

DIFFERENTIAL DIAGNOSIS

Common
- Normal Variants
- Infantile Hemangioma
- Abuse: Subacute Rib Fractures

Less Common
- Osteomyelitis
- Venous Malformation
- Lymphatic Malformation
- Arteriovenous Malformation
- Ewing Sarcoma
- Neuroblastoma
- Other Aggressive Lesions
  - Langerhans Cell Histiocytosis
  - Osteosarcoma
  - Aggressive Fibromatosis
- Benign Bone Tumors
  - Enchondroma

Rare but Important
- Mesenchymal Hamartoma of Chest Wall

ESSENTIAL INFORMATION

Helpful Clues for Common Diagnoses
- **Normal Variants**
  - Anatomic variations leading to palpable masses
    - Asymmetric costal cartilage, tilted sternum, asymmetric rib anterior convexity, paracartilaginous cartilage rests, etc.
    - Variations of minor pectus abnormalities may cause bony or cartilaginous protuberance
    - Asymmetries of anterior chest wall occur in up to 1/3 of children
    - Most likely diagnosis in children with asymptomatic palpable anterior chest wall lesions
    - Such variations are easily demonstrated by US, CT, or MR
  - Asynchronous ossification of sternal segments
    - 1st 4 sternal segments (manubrium = 1, xiphoid = 5) ossified at birth; 5th sternal segment (xiphoid) ossifies later in childhood in up to 32% of cases
    - Delayed ossification of 2nd (1.5% of population) and 4th (1.5% of population) sternal segments may occur
    - "Missing" sternal ossification centers should not be mistaken for destructive bony processes
- **Infantile Hemangioma**
  - Most common tumor of childhood
    - Occurs in 12% of all infants
  - Characteristic 2-state growth and regression
    - Small at birth, rapidly progresses in size over 1st several months of life, then begins to involute
  - Most require no therapy
    - Can cause Kasabach-Merritt syndrome (consumptive coagulopathy), compression of vital structures, and fissure/ulceration
  - Imaging shows discrete lobulated mass, often isolated to subcutaneous tissues
    - High vascularity with diffuse enhancement; prominent vessels within and around mass (draining veins)
- **Abuse: Subacute Rib Fractures**
  - Estimated 1,000,000 children seriously injured and 5,000 killed each year in USA related to child abuse
  - Most victims < 1 year of age
  - Subacute rib fractures form prominent periosteal reaction and present as palpable lump or mass seen at imaging
  - Posterior medial rib fractures are highly suspicious for child abuse
  - Identification of unsuspected rib fractures should initiate process of investigation, including skeletal radiographic survey

Helpful Clues for Less Common Diagnoses
- **Osteomyelitis**
  - Primarily disease of infants and young children
    - 1/3 of cases in children < 2 years, 1/2 of cases in children < 5 years
  - 1 of most common destructive lesions of chest wall in young children
- **Venous Malformation**
  - Present at birth and grow proportionate to child
  - MR: Collection of serpentine structures that demonstrate enhancement but no evidence of high velocity flow on gradient echo images
  - Often involve multiple tissue types without respect for fascial planes

- **Lymphatic Malformation**
  - Present at birth and grow proportionate to child
  - Typically appear as mass with multicystic components
  - Cystic areas do not enhance, unlike venous malformations
  - Often involve multiple tissue types without respect for fascial planes
- **Arteriovenous Malformation**
  - Much less common than hemangioma, venous malformation, or lymphatic malformation
  - "High flow" vascular malformation
  - At imaging, appear as "tangle" of vessels that show flow void on most MR sequences and high flow on gradient echo images
  - Minimal associated soft tissue mass but can have edema and fibro-fatty stroma surrounding tangle
- **Ewing Sarcoma**
  - 2nd most common primary malignancy of bone in children after osteosarcoma
  - Most common in teenage years
  - Unheard of prior to 5 years of age
  - Ribs not uncommon location (after femur, pelvis, tibia, and humerus)
  - Aggressive appearance on radiographs (bony destruction, aggressive periosteal reaction)
  - Often prominent associated soft tissue mass shown on MR
- **Neuroblastoma**
  - Posterior mediastinal mass invading posterior chest wall in infant is considered neuroblastoma
  - Look for rib erosion, rib splaying, calcification, and extension into spinal canal
- **Other Aggressive Lesions**
  - **Langerhans Cell Histiocytosis**
    - Often involves ribs (2nd most common location after skull involvement)
  - **Osteosarcoma**
    - Most common primary bone tumor of childhood, most common in teenagers; involves ribs less commonly than Ewing sarcoma
  - **Aggressive Fibromatosis**
    - Like fibrosarcoma but locally invasive without distant metastatic disease
- **Benign Bone Tumors**
  - Enchondroma common
  - Any benign bone lesion can also occur in ribs

Helpful Clues for Rare Diagnoses

- **Mesenchymal Hamartoma of Chest Wall**
  - Rare but very specific imaging appearance
  - Most commonly presents in infancy
  - Arises from ribs
  - Often involves multiple ribs
  - Majority have internal mineralization
  - Large expansile rib lesion with associated extrapleural soft tissue mass
    - Simulates aggressive appearance

Normal Variants

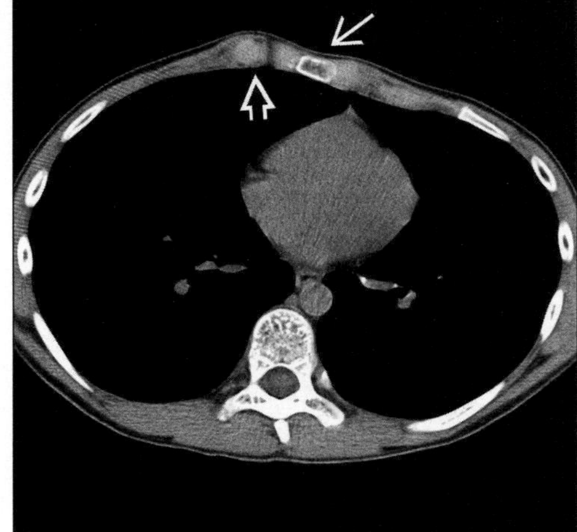

Axial NECT in a child with a palpable mass found on physical exam shows a tilted sternum ➡ and associated asymmetric costal cartilage ⇨ as the cause. There is no presence of a soft tissue mass.

Normal Variants

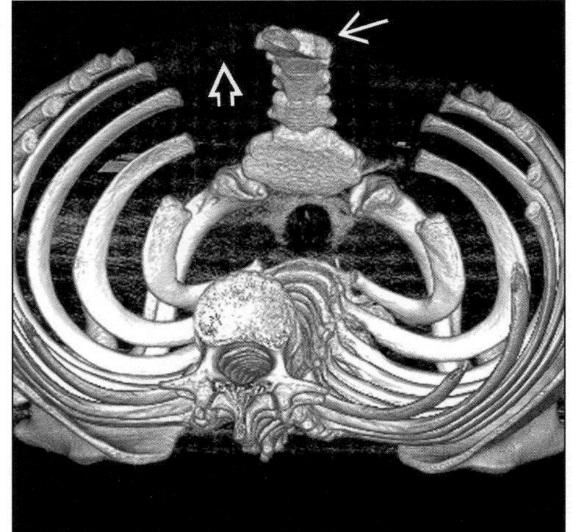

3D CT in the same child shows the tilted sternum ➡ to greater advantage, with the right more anterior than the left, and associated asymmetric costal cartilage ⇨ as the cause of the palpable mass.

CHEST WALL MASS

(**Left**) *Axial ultrasound in a child with a palpable mass on a physical examination shows anterior convex costal cartilage ➯ as the cause. There is no presence of a soft tissue mass.* (**Right**) *Lateral radiograph shows lack of ossification of the 2nd sternal segment ➯. This is a normal variant that occurs in 1.5% of children and should not be mistaken for a destructive bony process.*

Normal Variants

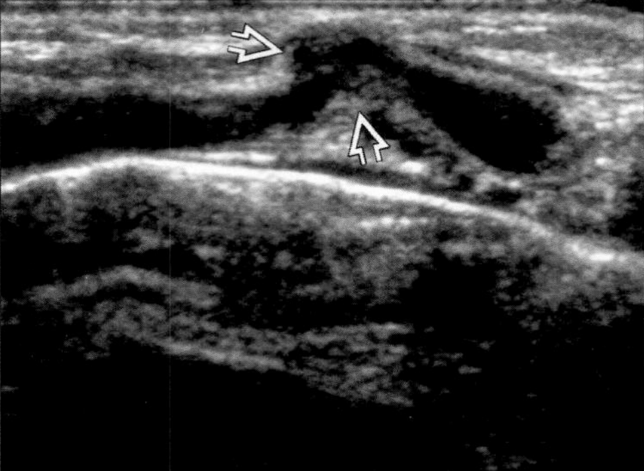

Normal Variants

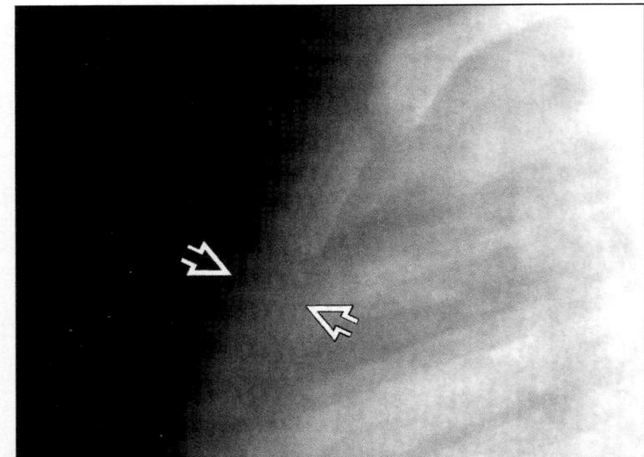

(**Left**) *Sagittal T2WI MR shows a lobulated soft tissue mass ➯ in the superior chest wall, extending into the mediastinum. Note the well-defined, lobulated borders and flow-void vessels within the mass.* (**Right**) *Axial CECT in an infant shows a subacute rib fracture ➯ with abundant callus formation. There are also acute rib fractures ➔ without callus formation. The presence of multiple rib fractures and rib fractures of varying ages is consistent with abuse.*

Infantile Hemangioma

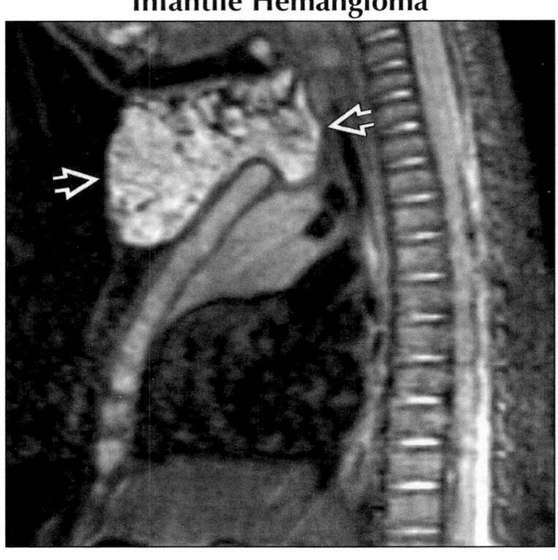

Abuse: Subacute Rib Fractures

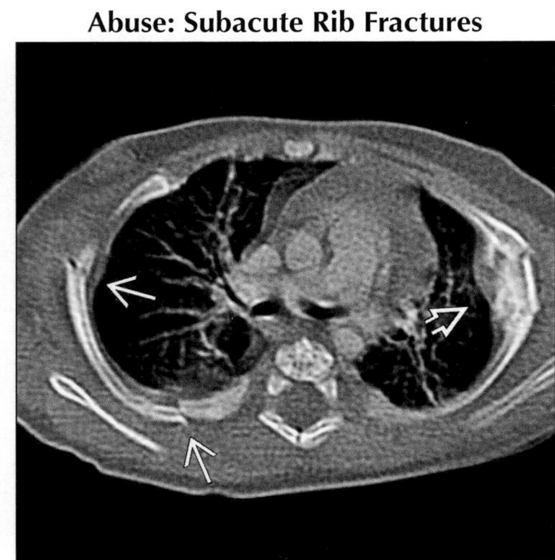

(**Left**) *Clinical photograph shows skin involvement by venous malformation. Note the soft tissue enlargement with associated multiple venous structures.* (**Right**) *Sagittal T2WI MR in the same patient shows multiple serpentine structures ➯ that are high in signal.*

Venous Malformation

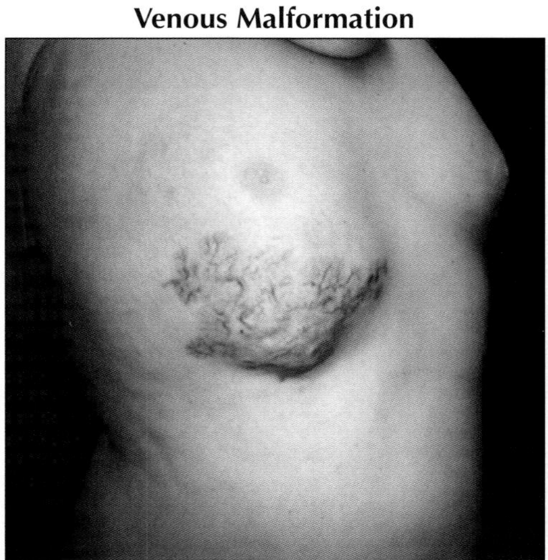

Venous Malformation

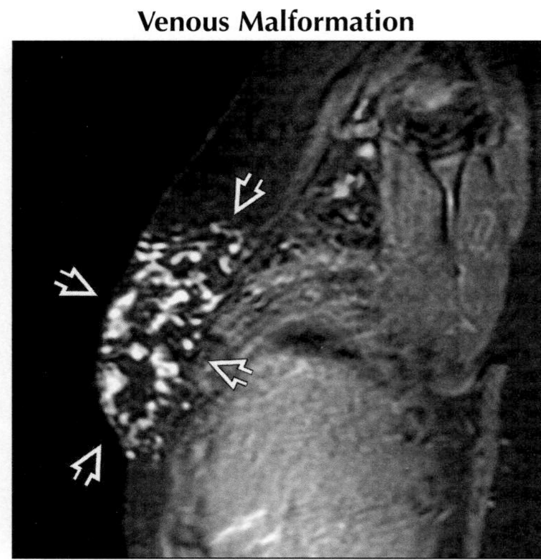

Venous Malformation

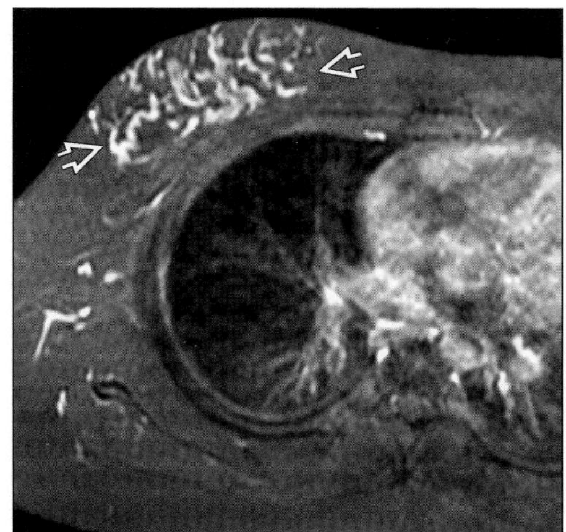

Venous Malformation

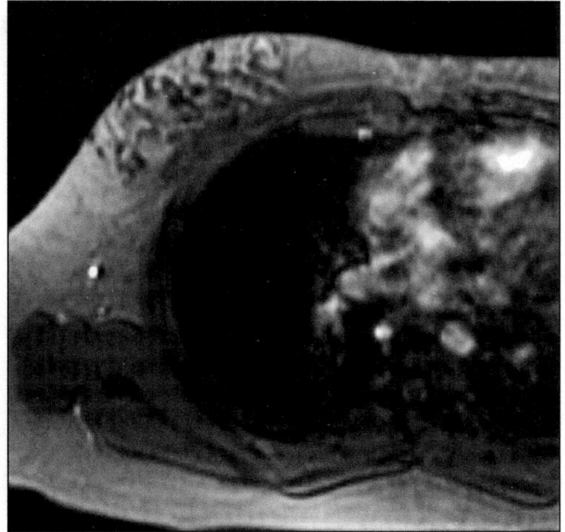

(Left) *Axial T1WI C+ FS MR in the same patient shows diffuse enhancement of the multiple serpentine structures ➩.* ***(Right)*** *Axial GRE MR in the same patient shows no high signal in multiple serpentine structures. Therefore, there is no evidence of high flow, and the findings are consistent with a venous malformation.*

Lymphatic Malformation

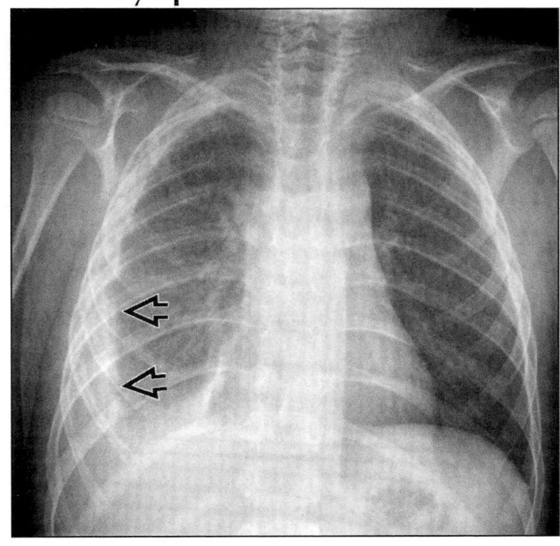

Lymphatic Malformation

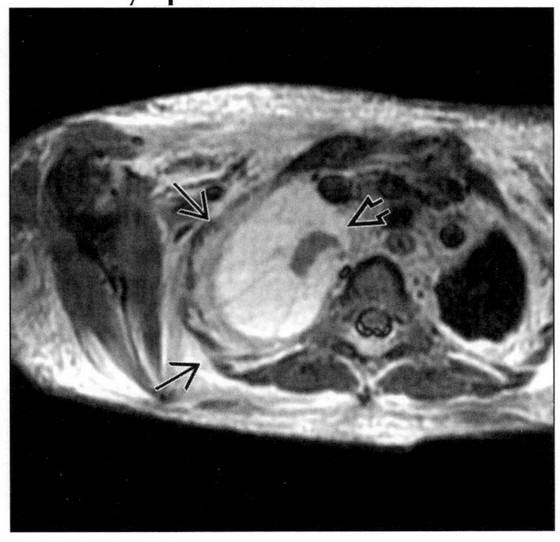

(Left) *Frontal radiograph shows right pleural effusion ➩, sclerosis of the ribs, and rotation and deformity of the right scapula.* ***(Right)*** *Axial T2WI MR in the same patient shows diffusely abnormal high T2 signal throughout the subcutaneous tissues and involving muscle groups. The right ribs are deformed →. There is a cystic collection involving the right pleural space ➩.*

Arteriovenous Malformation

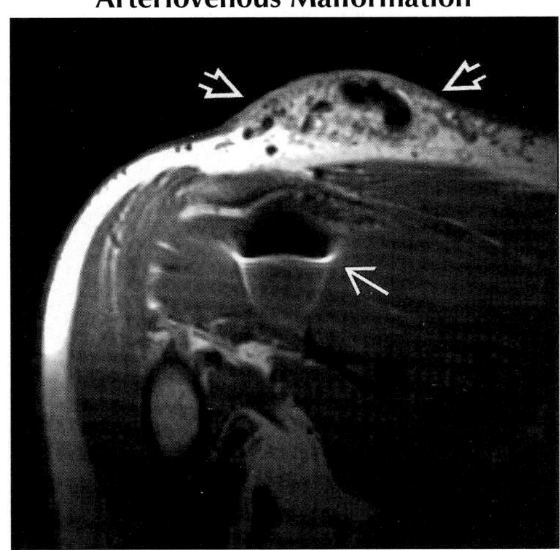

Arteriovenous Malformation

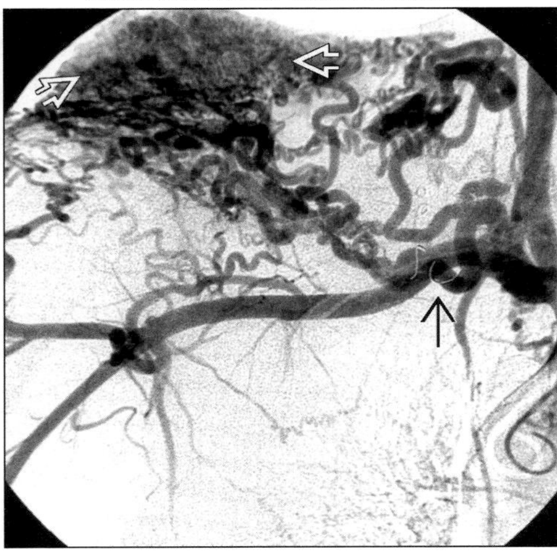

(Left) *Coronal T1WI MR shows a tangle of flow void vessels ➩ in the subcutaneous tissues of the right shoulder. Note the artifact from a previous embolization coil ➔.* ***(Right)*** *Anteroposterior angiography shows a large vascular tangle ➩ AVM within the right shoulder. Several coils → are seen from prior embolization procedures.*

CHEST WALL MASS

Ewing Sarcoma

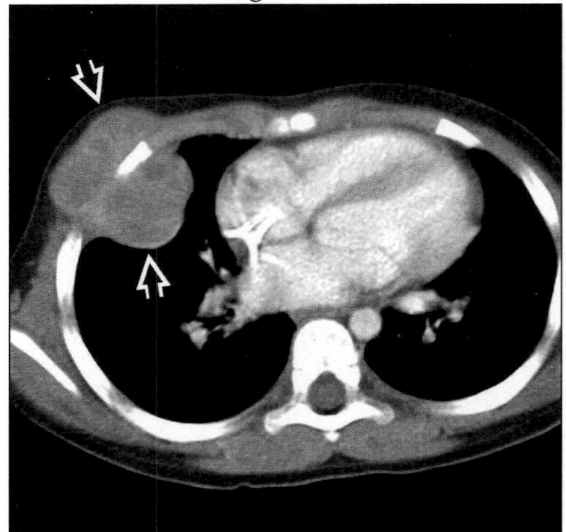

Ewing Sarcoma

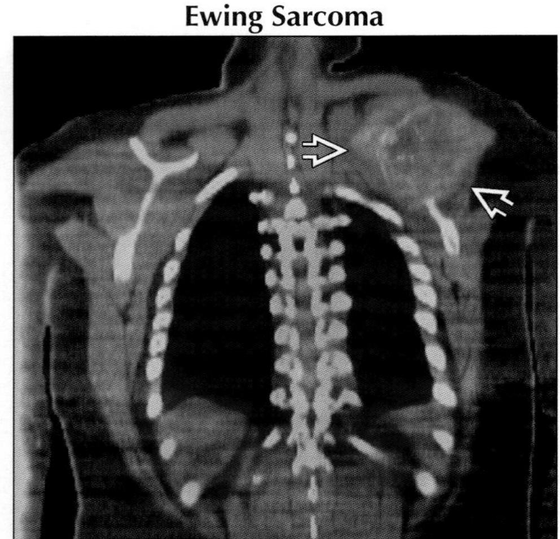

*(**Left**) Axial CECT shows an aggressive mass ⊳ emanating from the ribs with soft tissue components extending both internally and externally. The mass is heterogeneous. (**Right**) Coronal PET CT shows high metabolic activity (orange) ⊳ emanating from a destructive mass of the left scapula.*

Ewing Sarcoma

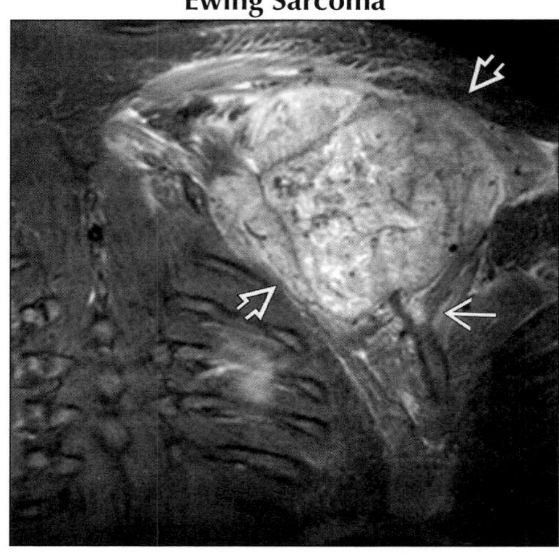

Ewing Sarcoma

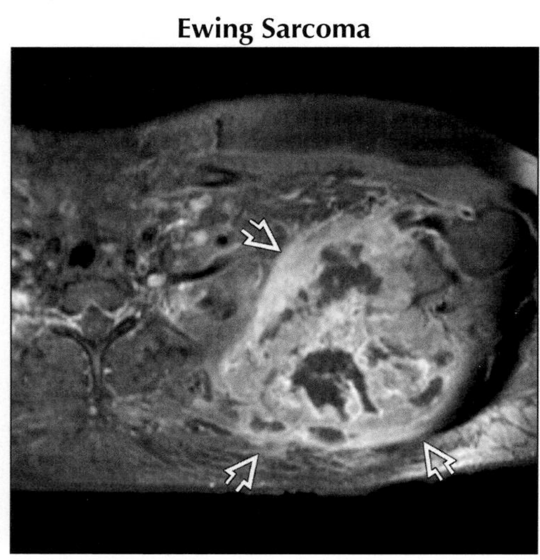

*(**Left**) Coronal T2WI MR in the same patient shows a large soft tissue mass ⊳ emanating from the left scapula. Note the destruction ➔ of the scapula along the margin of the soft tissue mass. (**Right**) Axial T1WI C+ FS MR in the same patient shows heterogeneous enhancement ⊳ of the soft tissue mass. Areas not enhancing are consistent with necrosis.*

Neuroblastoma

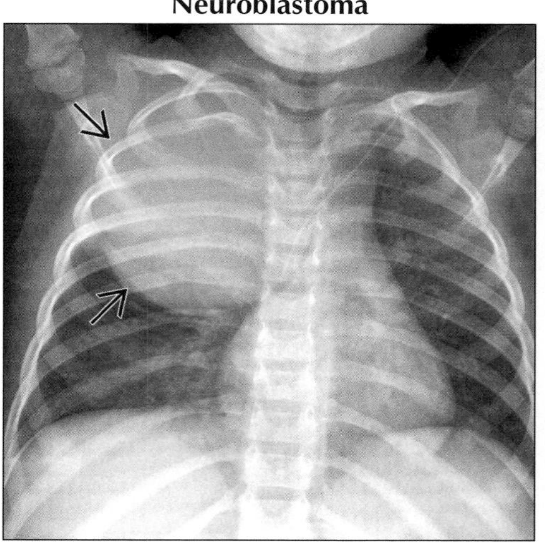

Neuroblastoma

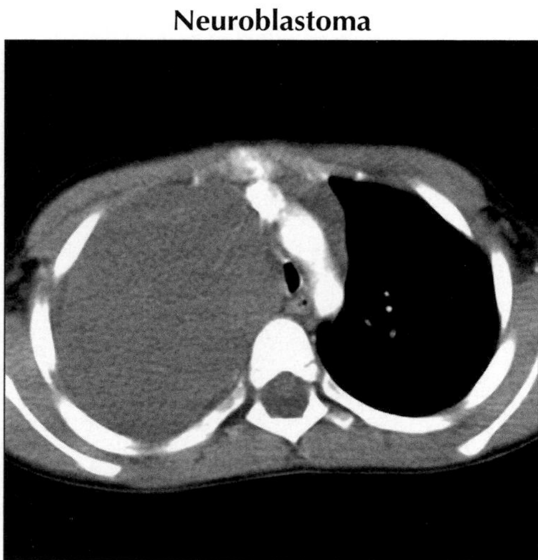

*(**Left**) Frontal radiograph shows a soft tissue mass ➔ with associated rib erosions and asymmetric widening of the intercostal spaces of the adjacent ribs. These findings are consistent with a posterior mediastinal mass invading the chest wall. In a child < 1 year old, these findings are consistent with neuroblastoma. (**Right**) Axial CECT in the same child shows a large mass in the superior right hemithorax with mediastinal shift to the left and compression of the trachea.*

CHEST WALL MASS

Aggressive Fibromatosis

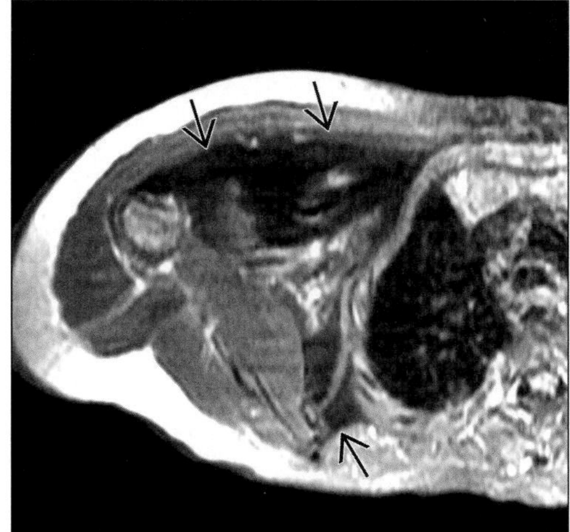

Enchondroma

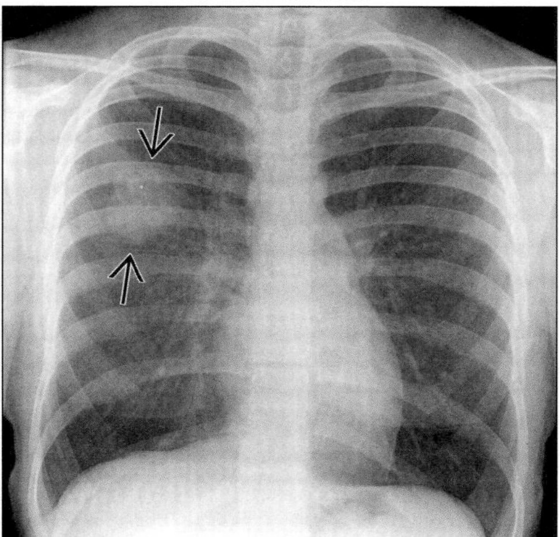

(Left) *Axial T1WI MR in a child with aggressive fibromatosis shows abnormal low signal diffusely involving a number of muscle groups →. The fibrotic nature of these lesions can cause a low signal appearance, but some cases also demonstrate high signal.* ***(Right)*** *Frontal radiograph of a child with enchondroma shows a rounded soft tissue mass → overlying the right upper hemithorax. There is some deformity of the adjacent associated rib.*

Enchondroma

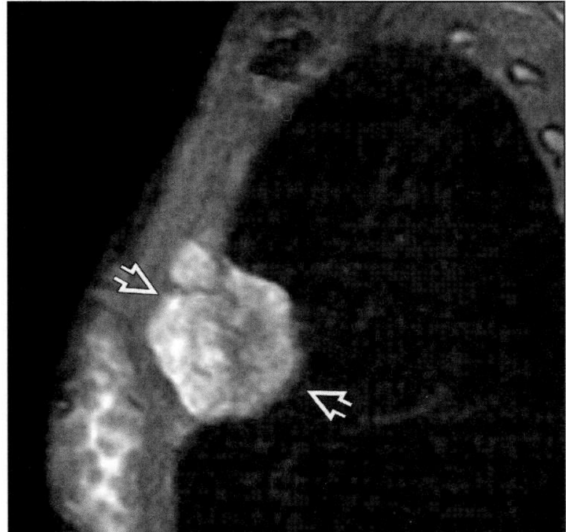

Enchondroma

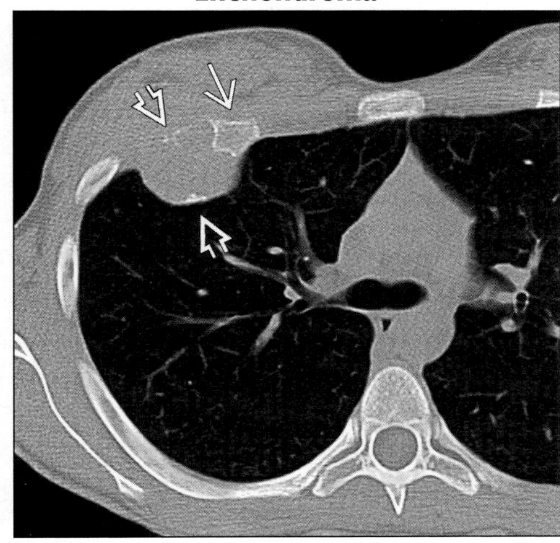

(Left) *Sagittal T2WI MR in the same child shows the lobulated mass ➡ with heterogeneous T2W signal. The mass protrudes from the chest wall.* ***(Right)*** *Axial NECT in the same child shows erosion of the adjacent rib ➡ and some chondroid matrix calcifications ➡.*

Mesenchymal Hamartoma of Chest Wall

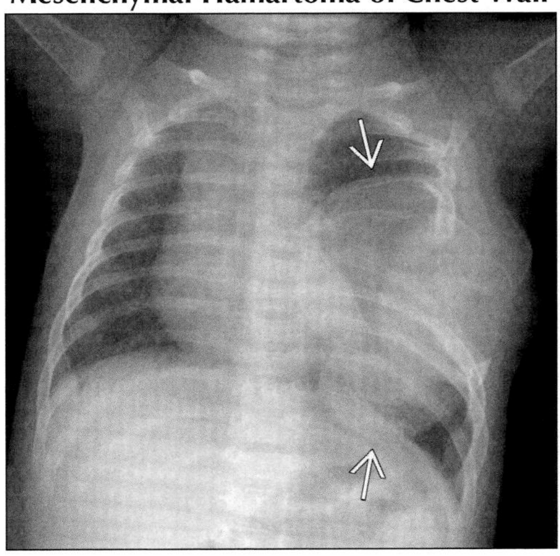

Mesenchymal Hamartoma of Chest Wall

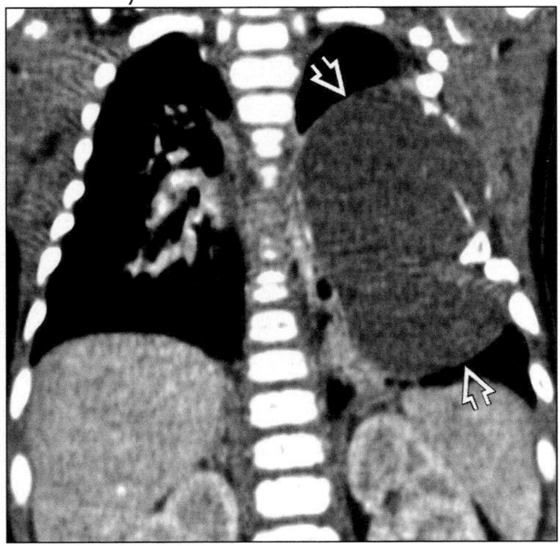

(Left) *Frontal radiograph in an infant shows a large soft tissue mass ➡. There is deformity and erosion of multiple associated ribs.* ***(Right)*** *Coronal CECT in the same infant shows the large mass ➡. Note the multiple deformed ribs laterally.*

RIB LESION

DIFFERENTIAL DIAGNOSIS

Common
- Normal Variant
- Healing Rib Fracture

Less Common
- Enchondroma
- Osteochondroma
- Metastasis
- Osteomyelitis
- Fibrous Dysplasia
- Langerhans Cell Histiocytosis
- Osteoblastoma

Rare but Important
- Ewing Sarcoma
- Aneurysmal Bone Cyst
- Lymphoma/Leukemia

ESSENTIAL INFORMATION

Key Differential Diagnosis Issues
- If palpable chest wall mass, image with chest radiograph 1st, ± rib radiographs
  - Asymmetric costochondral cartilage, congenital fused or bifid anterior rib
  - Many have characteristic diagnostic features and need no additional imaging

Helpful Clues for Common Diagnoses
- **Normal Variant**
  - Bifid or fused ribs
  - Relatively common, up to 3% of population (supernumerary > agenesis/aplasia > errors of segmentation)
  - May present with firm or hard anterior chest wall mass
  - Chest radiograph is diagnostic
- **Healing Rib Fracture**
  - Should be differentiated from pathologic fracture
  - If multiple posterior rib fractures, nonaccidental trauma should be excluded

Helpful Clues for Less Common Diagnoses
- **Enchondroma**
  - Age: 15-40 years old
  - Lytic, well-defined with chondroid matrix, endosteal scalloping, marginal sclerosis, no periosteal reaction or soft tissue mass
  - Most commonly small tubular bones of hands and feet
  - Ollier disease
    - Nonhereditary
    - More common in boys
    - Multiple enchondromas
    - Mostly unilateral, predilection for appendicular skeleton
    - Sarcomatous transformation (5%)
  - Maffucci syndrome
    - Nonhereditary
    - Multiple enchondroma and soft tissue venous malformation
    - Unilateral involvement of hands and feet
    - Malignant transformation (15-25%)
- **Osteochondroma**
  - Age: 10-25 years old
  - Most commonly around knee (35%)
  - Metaphysis of long bones (70%)
  - Pedunculated or sessile; grows away from joint
  - Multiple hereditary exostoses
  - Cartilage cap thickness is variable during childhood
  - Malignant degeneration
    - 1% in solitary
    - 3-5% in multiple hereditary exostoses
    - Should consider if rapid growth, indistinct lesion margin, osseous destruction, &/or soft tissue mass
- **Metastasis**
  - Most commonly neuroblastoma
  - Lymphoma/leukemia
    - More commonly metastatic than primary involvement
  - Usually known malignancy
- **Osteomyelitis**
  - Over 50% occur in preschool age children
  - *Staphylococcus aureus* most common pathogen for osteomyelitis in children (followed by *Streptococcal pneumonia*, *Streptococcal pyogenes*)
    - Most common pathogen in neonates
  - If more aggressive infection present, also consider actinomycosis (especially after dental procedures)
    - Aspiration of saliva
    - Pulmonary infiltrate/mass may spread to pleura, pericardium, chest wall
  - MRSA &/or ORSA becoming common cause of osteomyelitis
  - Chronic recurrent multifocal osteomyelitis (CRMO)

- Unknown pathogen; not bacterial infection
- Metaphyseal lesion but can occur anywhere
- Pustulous dermatosis (psoriasis, acne, palmar or plantar pustulosis)
- Pustulous dermatosis occurs in children/adolescents (25%) and adults (50%) with CRMO

- **Fibrous Dysplasia**
  - Monostotic or polyostotic
  - Expansile, endosteal scalloping, lucent to ground-glass appearance
  - Sarcomatous degeneration in up to 0.5%
  - McCune-Albright: Female, precocious puberty, café au lait spots, and unilateral fibrous dysplasia
- **Langerhans Cell Histiocytosis**
  - Flat bones (70%)
  - Monostotic (50-75%)
  - Well-defined or ill-defined margin, lytic ± sclerotic margin
  - Beveled edges in skull
- **Osteoblastoma**
  - Benign osseous lesion with osteoid production
  - Age: 10-20 years old
  - > 1.5 cm (range 1-10 cm)
  - Most commonly located in posterior elements of spine
  - Expansile, lytic, cortex usually preserved ± internal calcification
  - May present with painful scoliosis

Helpful Clues for Rare Diagnoses

- **Ewing Sarcoma**
  - Age: 10-25 years old
    - 90% before age 20 years
    - Caucasians (96%)
  - Soft tissue or bone
  - Slight male predominance
  - Diaphysis of long bones (70%)
  - Ill-defined, lytic, permeative, moth-eaten, large, soft tissue mass; aggressive periosteal reaction ("onion skin," "sunburst")
  - Fever, leukocytosis, elevated ESR, soft tissue mass, localized pain
  - Other sarcomas
    - Ewing family of tumors, synovial cell sarcoma, chondrosarcoma, osteosarcoma, malignant peripheral nerve sheath tumor, primitive neuroectodermal tumor
    - Chest wall tumor ± rib involvement
- **Aneurysmal Bone Cyst**
  - Expansile
  - Septated with fluid-fluid levels (CT or MR) ± periosteal reaction
  - Can present with pain and swelling
  - Often associated with other benign tumors
- **Lymphoma/Leukemia**
  - Usually disseminated disease

Normal Variant

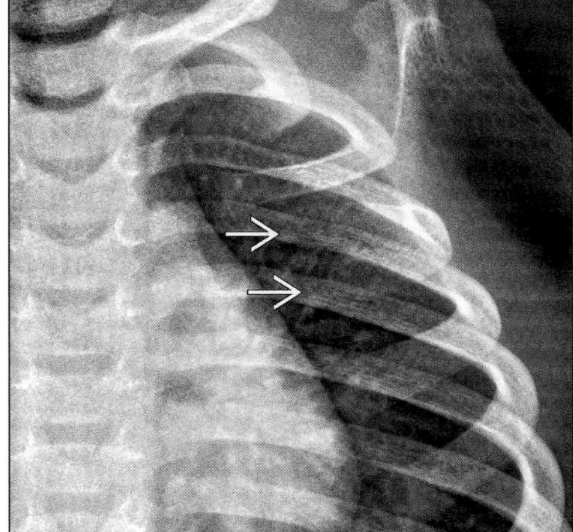

Anteroposterior radiograph shows an ill-defined, fork-shaped left anterior 3rd rib ➡. Rib anomalies are present in approximately 3% of the population.

Normal Variant

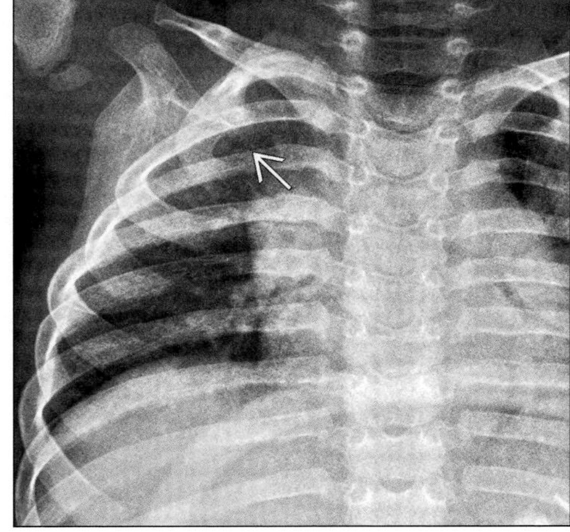

Anteroposterior radiograph shows congenital fusion ➡ of the anterior right 1st and 2nd ribs. In this young child, such fusion could present as a hard palpable supraclavicular mass.

RIB LESION

(**Left**) Anteroposterior radiograph shows an expanded, bifid, anterior, left-sided rib ➡ in a 1-year-old girl who presented with a fever and dyspnea. (**Right**) Anteroposterior radiograph in this 1 month old shows multiple bilateral posterior rib fractures ➡. This female infant had posterior rib and metaphyseal corner fractures (not shown), which are highly specific signs of child abuse. CT can add increased sensitivity in detecting rib fractures.

Normal Variant

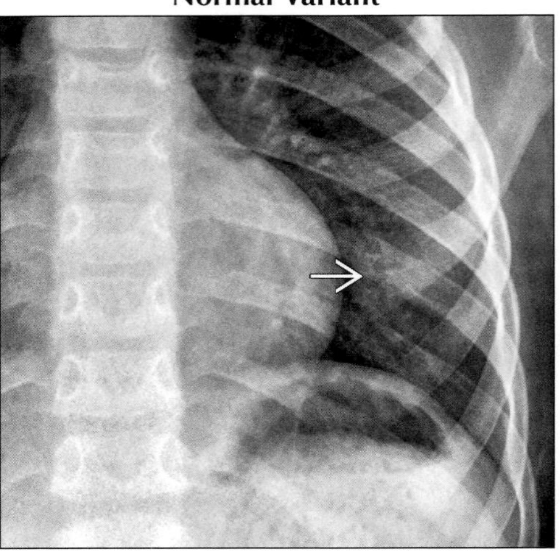

Healing Rib Fracture

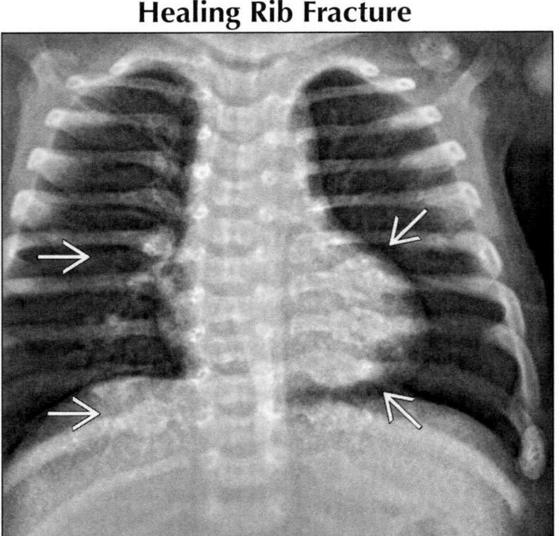

(**Left**) Anteroposterior radiograph shows a rounded mass inseparable from an anterior rib. Small metallic BB was placed over the palpable anterior chest wall mass. The palpable mass was noticed a few days prior. (**Right**) Axial NECT shows an irregular, expanded, cupped anterior rib ➡ at the costochondral junction. Notice the small calcification within the soft tissue mass ↪. This mass was resected and pathologically proven to be enchondroma.

Enchondroma

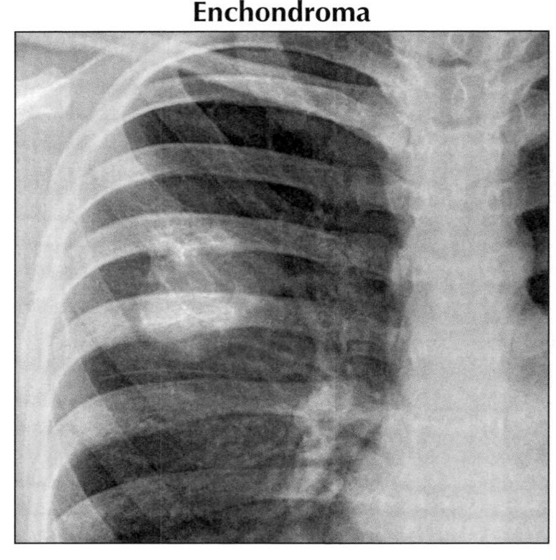

Enchondroma

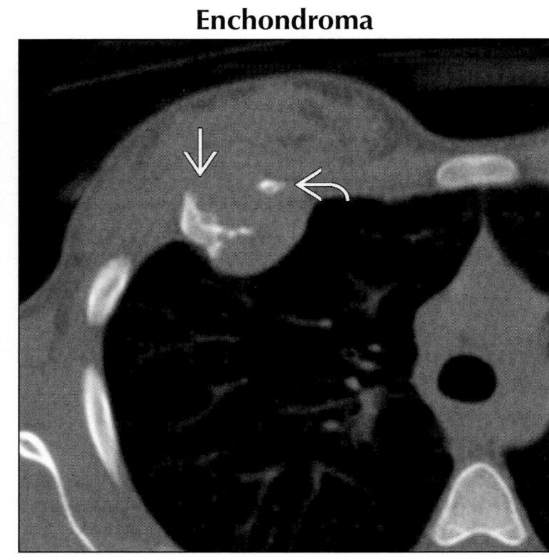

(**Left**) Coronal CECT shows posterior rib head exostosis ➡ in a 15 year old with a history of total body radiation for a neuroblastoma as a 1 year old. The prevalence of radiation-induced osteochondromas is approximately 12% compared to less than 1% for those that occur spontaneously. (**Right**) Coronal T2WI FS MR in the same patient shows a subtle, thin, hyperintense cartilaginous cap ➡ of an osteochondroma.

Osteochondroma

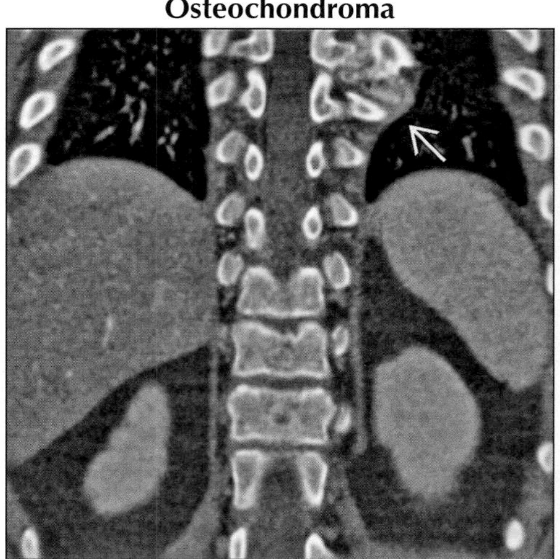

Osteochondroma

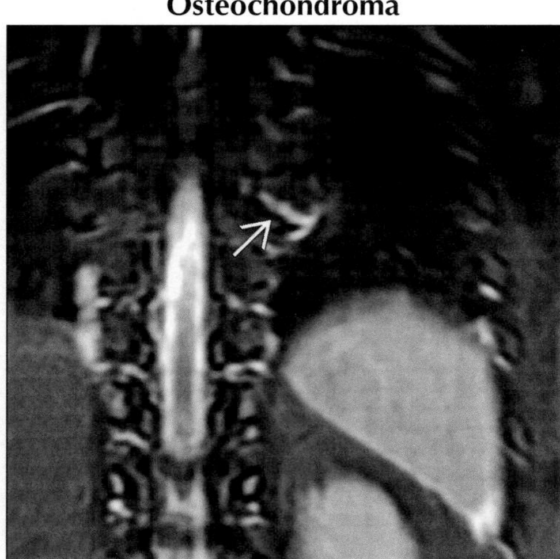

Metastasis

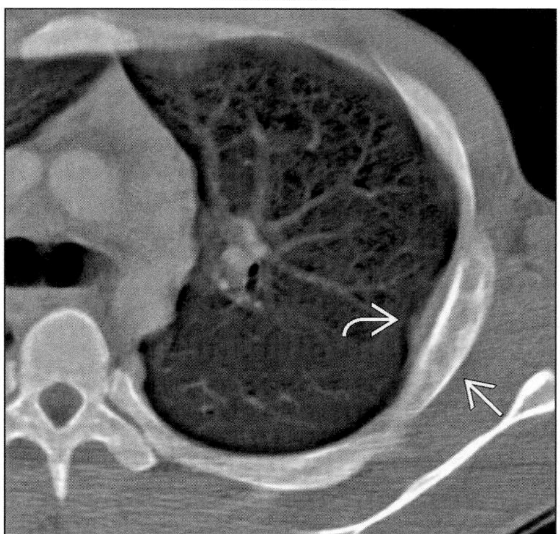

Metastasis

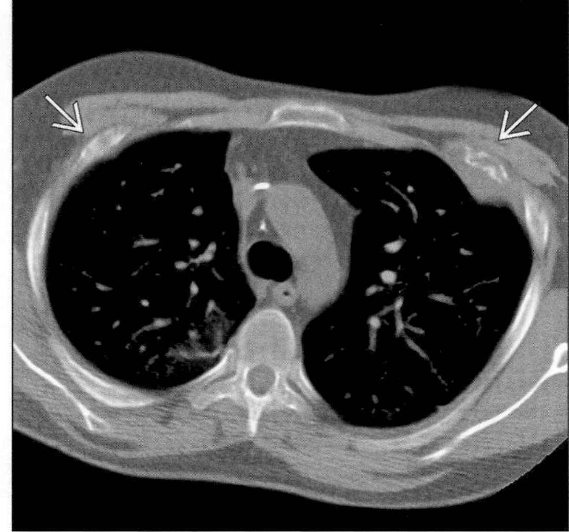

(Left) *Axial CECT in this 16-year-old boy shows an expanded, posterior, lateral 4th left rib ➡. Notice the endosteal scalloping and adjacent pleural reaction ↗. On other CECT images, innumerable bone metastases and diffuse lymphadenopathy were seen in this teenager later diagnosed with Hodgkin lymphoma.* ***(Right)*** *Axial CECT shows destruction of bilateral anterior ribs ➡ from metastatic disease in this patient with mandibular osteosarcoma.*

Osteomyelitis

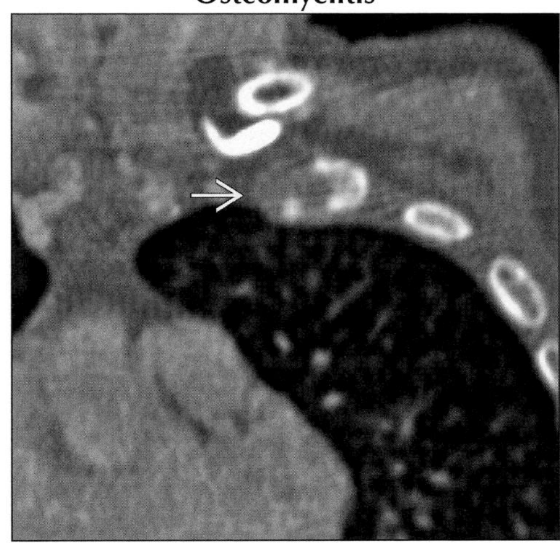

Osteomyelitis

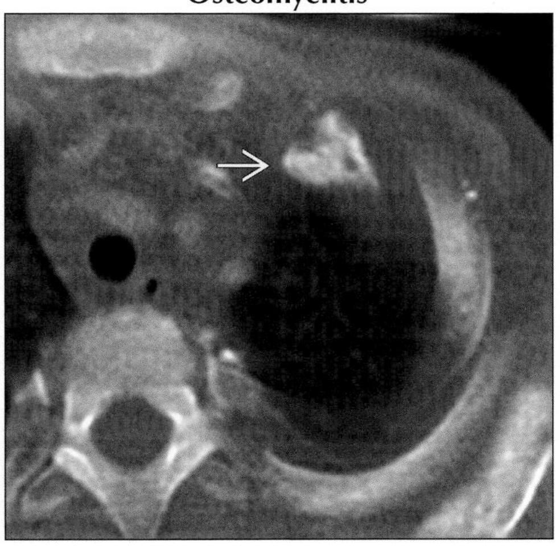

(Left) *Coronal CECT in an 8-year-old child with Gaucher disease shows cupping, fraying, and fragmentation ➡ of the anterior left 1st rib. This patient also had similar findings in the left 2nd rib (not shown).* ***(Right)*** *Axial CECT in the same patient 4 months later shows increased sclerosis ➡ and healing of the anterior rib osteomyelitis. Staphylococcus aureus is the most common cause of osteomyelitis in children.*

Osteomyelitis

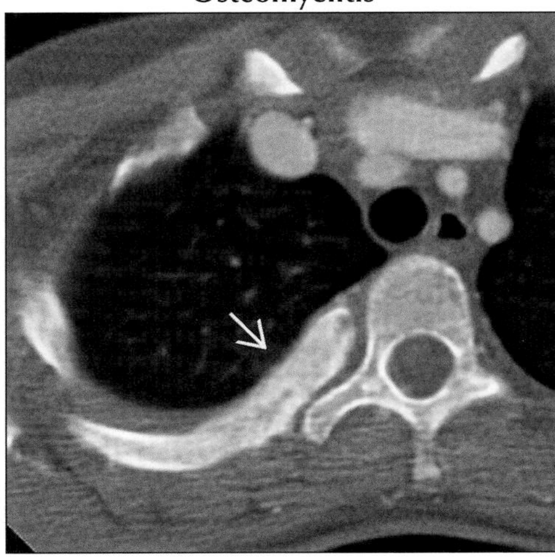

Osteomyelitis

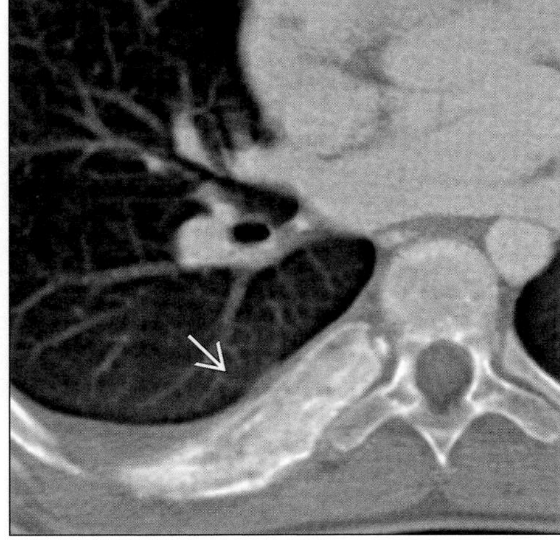

(Left) *Axial CECT in this 11 year old presenting with posterior lateral rib pain shows expansion and sclerosis ➡ of the right posterior 3rd rib.* ***(Right)*** *Axial CECT in the same child shows similar expansion and mild destruction ➡ of the right 7th posterior rib. No pathogen was cultured in this patient with chronic recurrent multifocal osteomyelitis.*

RIB LESION

Osteomyelitis

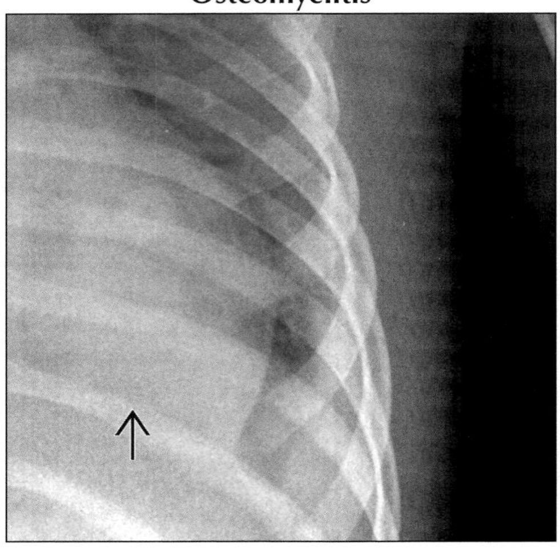

Osteomyelitis

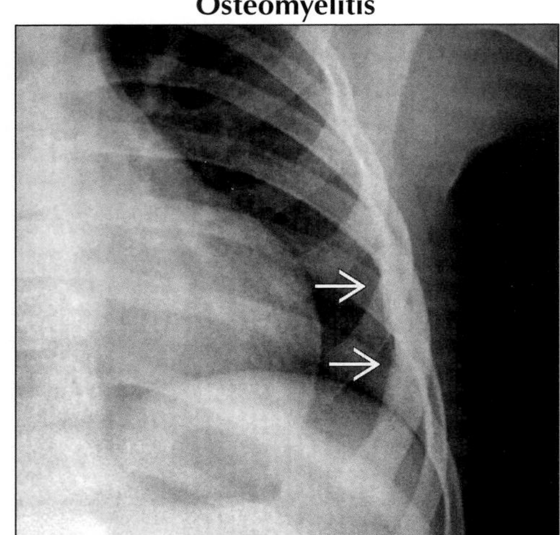

(Left) *Anteroposterior radiograph in this 5-year-old child with a history of pneumonia and pericarditis shows no focal rib abnormality. Notice the loss of definition of the left hemidiaphragm ⇨, lower lobe pneumonia, and left-sided effusion.* ***(Right)*** *Anteroposterior radiograph 6 months later shows diffuse sclerosis and expansion of a left lateral rib ➡. This patient was diagnosed with MRSA osteomyelitis.*

Fibrous Dysplasia

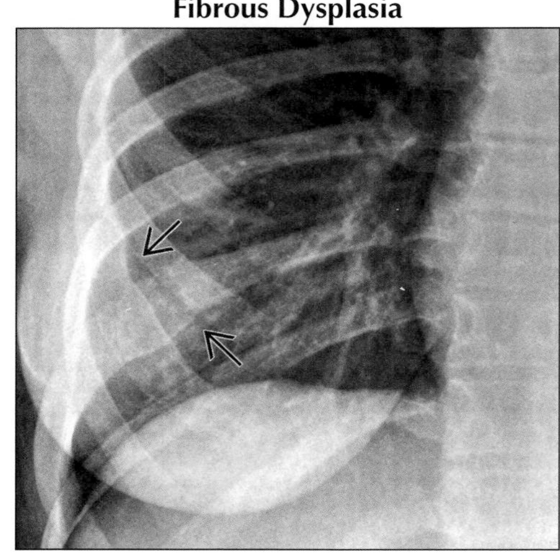

Fibrous Dysplasia

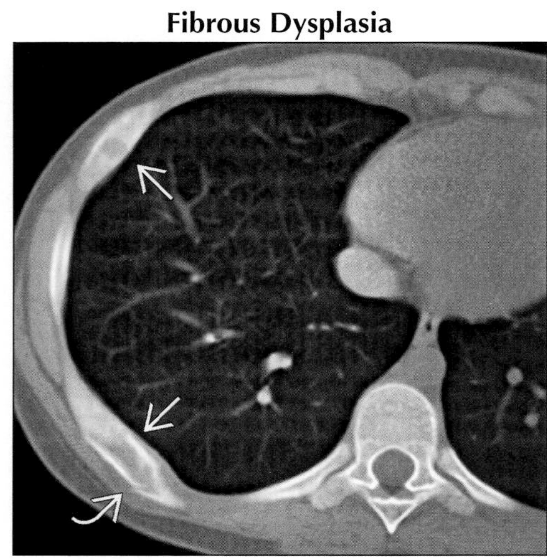

(Left) *Anteroposterior radiograph in this 15-year-old teenager with chest wall pain and swelling shows expansile lesions of 2 overlapping ribs ⇨.* ***(Right)*** *Axial CECT in the same patient shows focal expansion of 2 right-sided ribs ➡. The more posterior rib lesion demonstrates a pathologic fracture ➡. This teenager also had right-sided scapular, femoral, and tibial fibrous dysplasia lesions.*

Langerhans Cell Histiocytosis

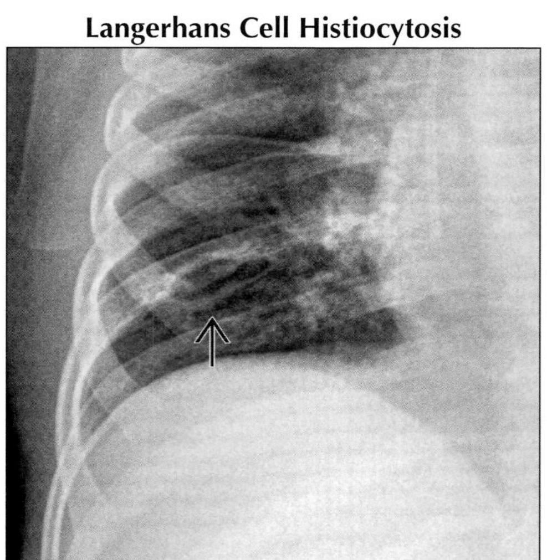

Langerhans Cell Histiocytosis

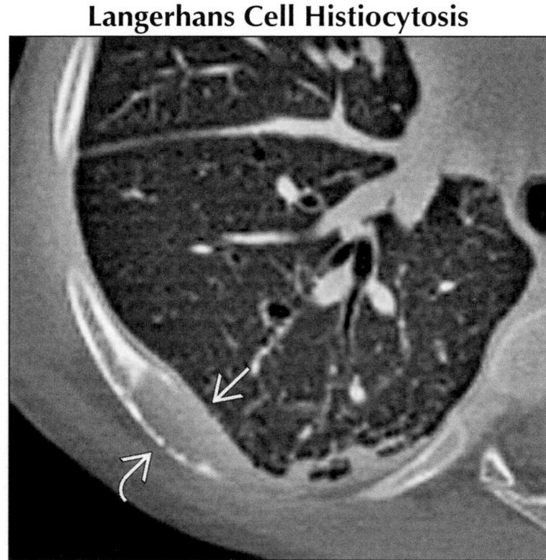

(Left) *Anteroposterior radiograph in this 2-year-old boy shows inferior expansion ⇨ of the right posterior 7th rib.* ***(Right)*** *Axial NECT shows a lucent expansile posterior 7th rib lesion. Notice its permeation through the posterior cortex ➡ and absent inner cortical margin ➡. There were multiple lesions throughout the skeleton detected on bone scintigraphy and skeletal survey (not shown).*

RIB LESION

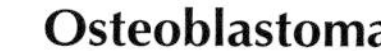

Osteoblastoma

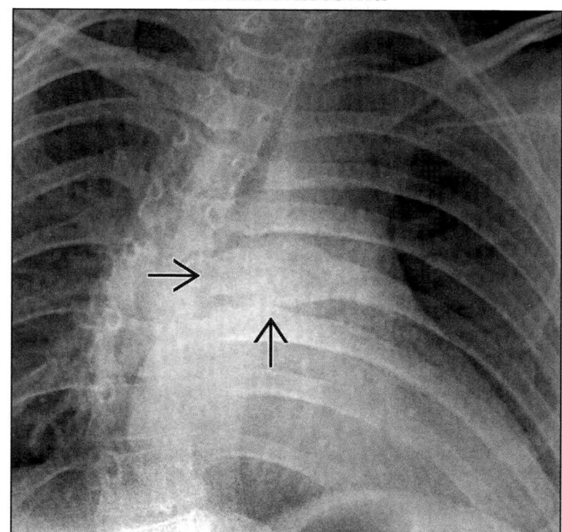

Osteoblastoma

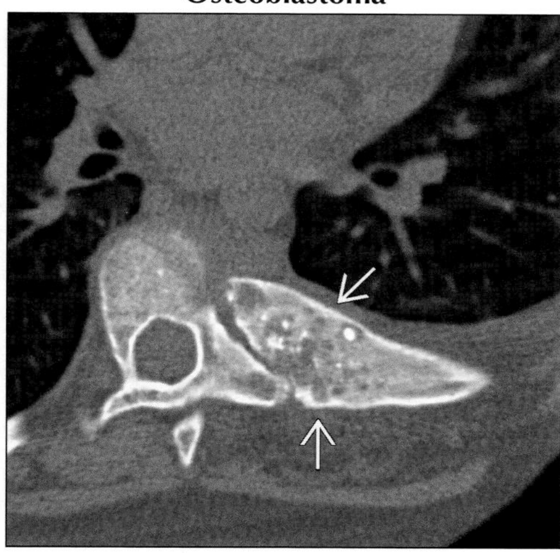

(Left) *Anteroposterior radiograph in a 10 year old with scoliosis and left upper back pain shows a focal bulbous expansile lesion → of the left 7th posterior rib. Notice the dextroscoliotic curvature.* ***(Right)*** *Axial NECT in the same patient shows expansion → of the posterior rib. Notice the mixed lucency and bone matrix contained within this osteoblastoma. Osteoblastomas of the spine can present with painful scoliosis.*

Ewing Sarcoma

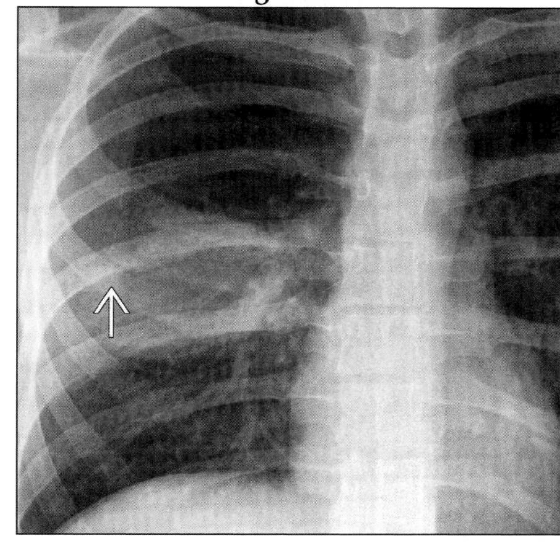

Ewing Sarcoma

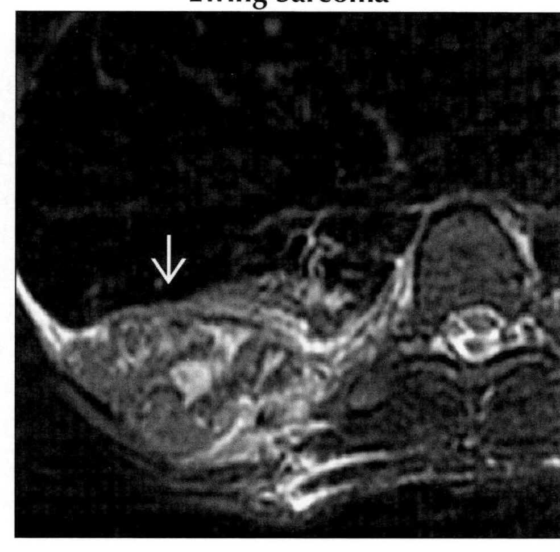

(Left) *Anteroposterior radiograph in this 15-year-old male shows splaying of the right 7th and 8th posterior ribs (widened posterior interspace). Subtle scalloping → of the posterior inferior 7th rib is shown.* ***(Right)*** *Axial T2WI FS MR shows a large, heterogeneous chest wall mass → with subpleural extension. Patients with Ewing sarcoma often present with a disproportionately larger soft tissue mass compared to the severity of bone destruction.*

Aneurysmal Bone Cyst

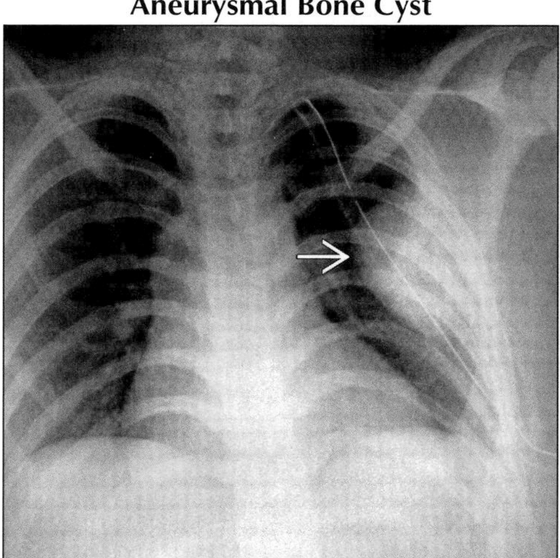

Aneurysmal Bone Cyst

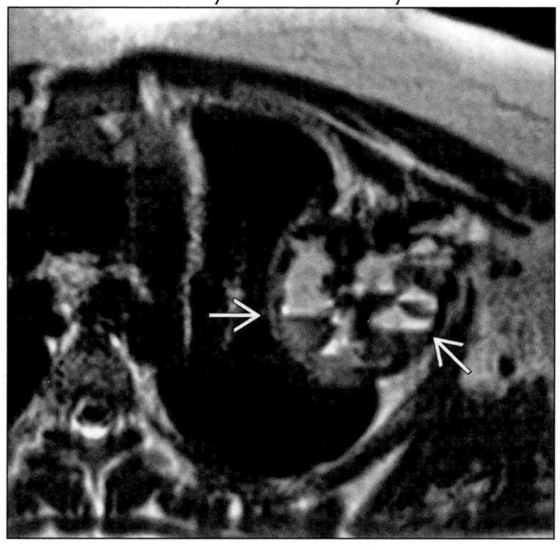

(Left) *Anteroposterior radiograph in a 13 year old shows a large left chest wall mass →.* ***(Right)*** *Axial T2WI FS MR shows numerous fluid-fluid levels → within this expansile anterior rib mass. The multiple fluid-fluid levels without a soft tissue mass are characteristic of ABC. ABCs may be associated with other preexisting osseous lesions (i.e., fibrous dysplasia, chondroblastoma, giant cell tumor).*

PNEUMOMEDIASTINUM

DIFFERENTIAL DIAGNOSIS

Common
- Asthma
- Straining against Closed Glottis
- Aspiration
- Blunt Chest Trauma
- Iatrogenic
- Surfactant Deficiency Disease
- Pulmonary Interstitial Emphysema

Less Common
- Infection
- Extension of Pneumoperitoneum or Pneumoretroperitoneum

Rare but Important
- Esophageal Tear

ESSENTIAL INFORMATION

Key Differential Diagnosis Issues
- Potential sources for pneumomediastinum
  - Trachea and bronchi
  - Lung
  - Esophagus
  - Pleural space
  - Head/neck
  - Peritoneal space
  - Retroperitoneal space
- Helpful radiographic signs in pneumomediastinum
  - Thymic sail sign: Elevation of thymus by large amount of pneumomediastinum
  - Continuous diaphragm: Air trapped posterior to pericardium
  - Ring around artery sign: Air surrounding pulmonary artery branch
  - Air in inferior pulmonary ligament: Retrocardiac extension of pneumomediastinum
  - Double wall sign: Intramural gas along proximal airways
  - Associated pneumothorax, pneumopericardium, or subcutaneous emphysema
- Pneumomediastinum is frequently asymptomatic and self-limited
- History is extremely helpful in determining possible source of pneumomediastinum
  - Is there trauma history?
  - Is there history of recent instrumentation?
  - Is the patient asthmatic?

Helpful Clues for Common Diagnoses
- **Asthma**
  - Airway narrowing and mucous plugging leads to air-trapping and alveolar rupture
  - History of asthma exacerbation helpful in making diagnosis
  - Hyperinflated lungs
- **Straining against Closed Glottis**
  - History helpful
    - Vomiting
    - Giving birth to child
    - Weight-lifting
  - No specific imaging features
- **Aspiration**
  - Results from air-trapping and alveolar rupture
  - Meconium aspiration
    - History of meconium-stained amniotic fluid helpful
    - Coarse interstitial and patchy opacities
    - Hyperinflation
  - Foreign body aspiration
    - Peanuts most common in children
    - Frequency of right vs. left bronchial tree involvement is equal in young children
    - Right > left bronchial tree involvement in older children and adults
    - Unilateral hyperinflation
    - Atelectasis
    - Decubitus views can be helpful if radiolucent foreign body is suspected
- **Blunt Chest Trauma**
  - History helpful
    - Motor vehicle crash
    - Fall
    - Sports injury
  - Alveolar rupture &/or tracheobronchial injury
  - Other signs of trauma
    - Fractures
    - Pulmonary contusions
    - Mediastinal injuries
    - Pleural effusions
- **Iatrogenic**
  - Mechanical ventilation
  - Instrumentation can result in
    - Tracheobronchial injury
    - Esophageal injury
  - Postoperative patients
  - History helpful
- **Surfactant Deficiency Disease**

- Premature neonates
- Reticulogranular opacities
- Air leak from alveolar rupture can lead to pneumomediastinum

- **Pulmonary Interstitial Emphysema**
  - Premature infants
  - Barotrauma from mechanical ventilation
  - Reticular and cystic opacities
  - Alveolar rupture with air leak into pulmonary interstitium
  - Can progress to pneumomediastinum and pneumothorax

Helpful Clues for Less Common Diagnoses

- **Infection**
  - Mycoplasma pneumonia
    - Common cause of community-acquired pneumonia in children
    - Typically good prognosis
    - Typically reticulonodular opacities
    - Can be complicated by alveolar destruction and rupture leading to pneumomediastinum
  - *Pneumocystis* pneumonia
    - History helpful
    - AIDS-defining illness
    - Bilateral ground-glass and reticulonodular opacities
    - Can result in parenchymal lung cysts, which can rupture and lead to pneumomediastinum
- **Extension of Pneumoperitoneum or Pneumoretroperitoneum**
  - No direct constant communication between peritoneal space and mediastinum
  - Direct communication exists between retroperitoneal space and mediastinum
    - Esophageal hiatus
    - Aortic hiatus
  - Pneumomediastinum can result from extension of peritoneal or retroperitoneal gas
    - Perforation of hollow viscous
    - Laparoscopy

Helpful Clues for Rare Diagnoses

- **Esophageal Tear**
  - History is helpful
  - Iatrogenic is most common cause
  - Other causes
    - Vomiting/retching
    - Blunt trauma
    - Foreign bodies
    - Toxic ingestion
  - Lack of serosa increases vulnerability to tear
  - Reflux esophagitis increases risk
  - Naclerio "V" sign: Mediastinal air separates parietal pleura from left hemidiaphragm
  - Look for associated pleural effusion
  - Contrast esophagram helpful in diagnosis

Asthma

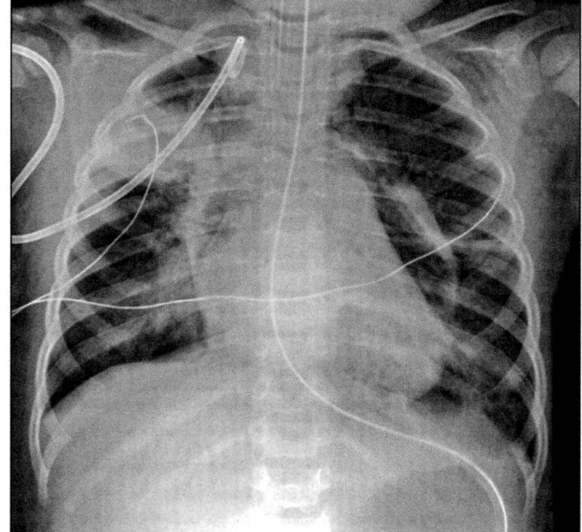

Frontal radiograph shows extensive pneumomediastinum resulting in a thymic sail sign in this 2 year old in the midst of an acute asthma exacerbation.

Straining against Closed Glottis

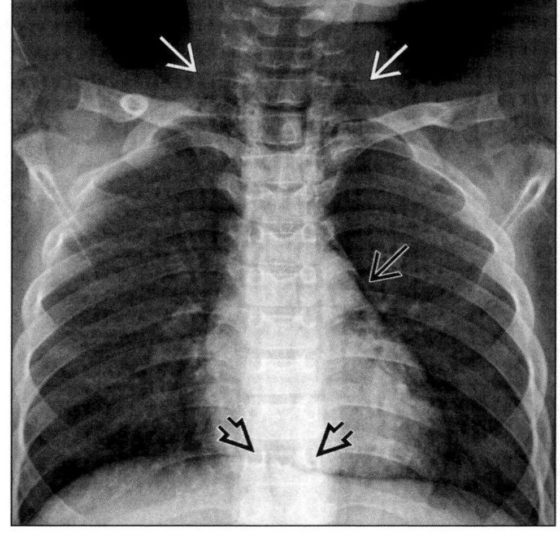

Frontal radiograph shows pneumomediastinum along the left mediastinal border ⇒, subcutaneous emphysema ➡ in the neck, and a continuous diaphragm sign ⇨ in this 9 year old with vomiting.

PNEUMOMEDIASTINUM

*(**Left**) Frontal radiograph shows extensive pneumomediastinum uplifting the thymus ➙. Note the diffuse coarse interstitial opacities in this neonate with meconium aspiration. (**Right**) Left lateral radiograph shows hyperinflation of the left lung, pneumomediastinum ➙, and subcutaneous emphysema ➙ in this 2 year old who aspirated a peanut into the left mainstem bronchus.*

Aspiration

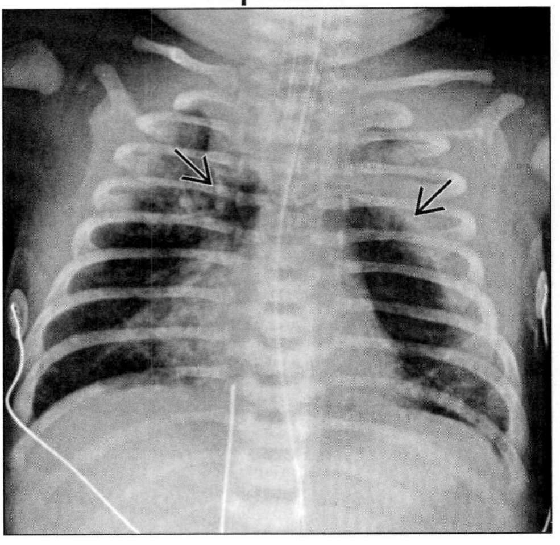

Aspiration

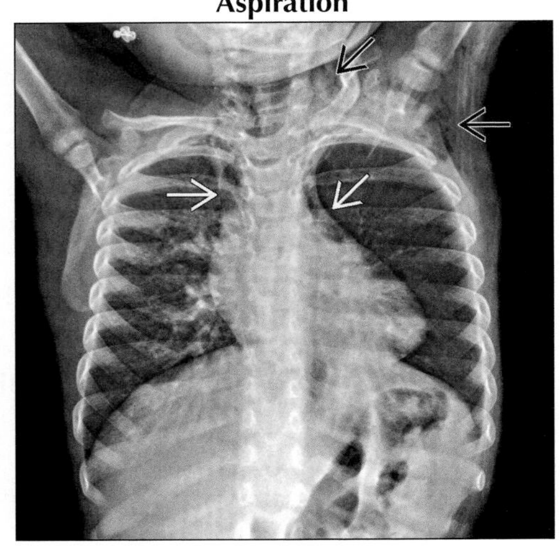

*(**Left**) Axial CECT shows pneumomediastinum in this 15-year-old patient who suffered blunt chest trauma from a tackle during football practice and presented with chest pain. (**Right**) Anteroposterior radiograph shows pneumomediastinum with a thymic sail sign ➙ and continuous diaphragm sign ➙, as well as subcutaneous emphysema ➙ in this 2 year old who fell 2 stories.*

Blunt Chest Trauma

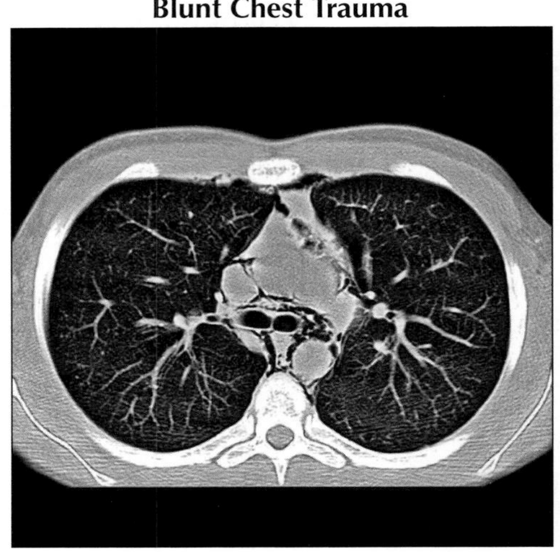

Blunt Chest Trauma

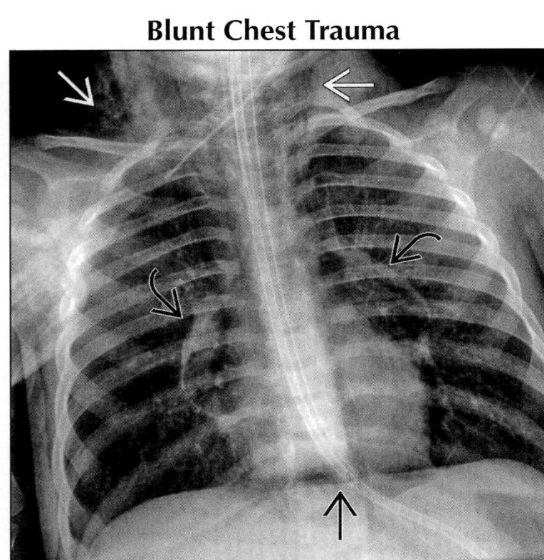

*(**Left**) Frontal radiograph shows pneumomediastinum with air extending along the inferior pulmonary ligament ➙ in this 6-month-old, postoperative patient with a tracheostomy. There is a small right pneumothorax ➙ as well. (**Right**) Axial NECT shows extensive pneumomediastinum and subcutaneous emphysema in this 15-year-old patient status post-traumatic right mainstem intubation and airway laceration. Note the irregular appearance of the carina ➙.*

Iatrogenic

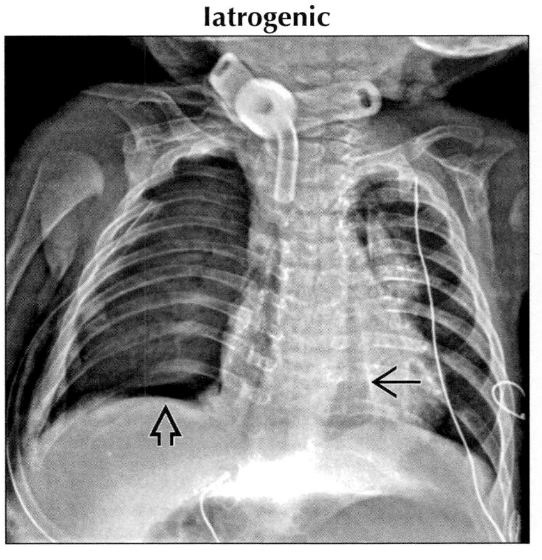

Iatrogenic

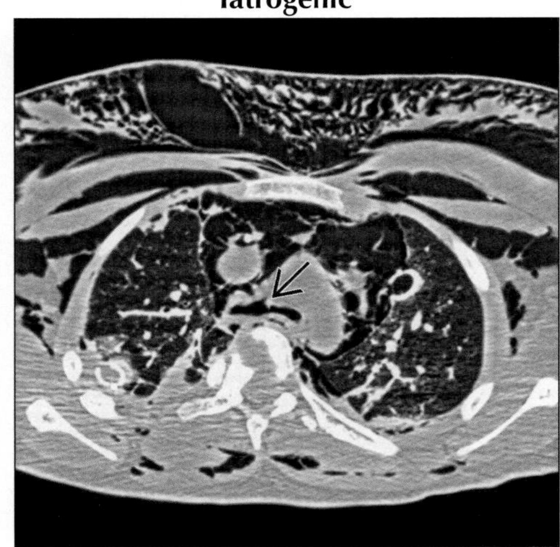

Surfactant Deficiency Disease

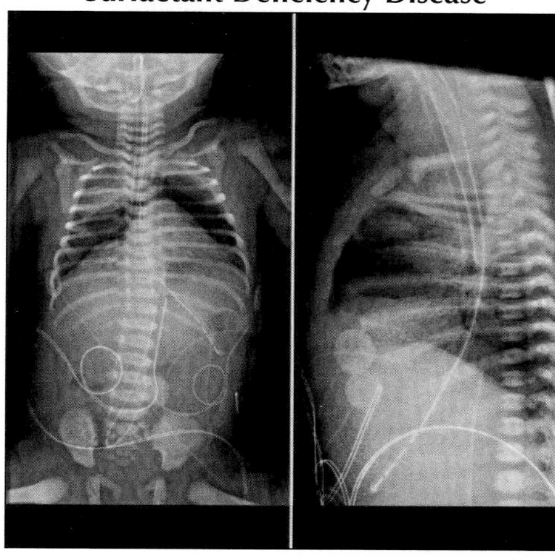

Pulmonary Interstitial Emphysema

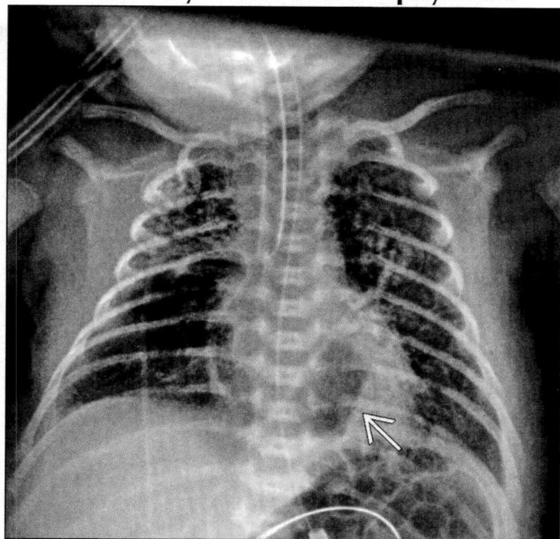

(Left) *Frontal and lateral radiographs demonstrate a large amount of pneumomediastinum, which causes a thymic sail sign in this premature neonate with surfactant deficiency disease.* ***(Right)*** *Anteroposterior radiograph shows reticular opacities and cystic areas in this intubated premature neonate, consistent with pulmonary interstitial emphysema. There is pneumomediastinum with air extending into the inferior pulmonary ligament ➡.*

Infection

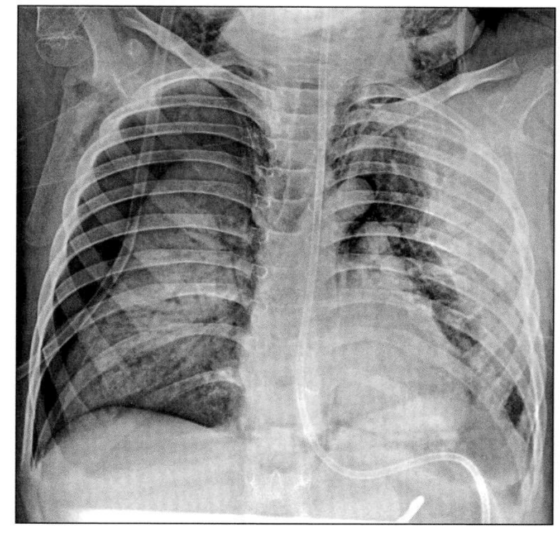

Infection

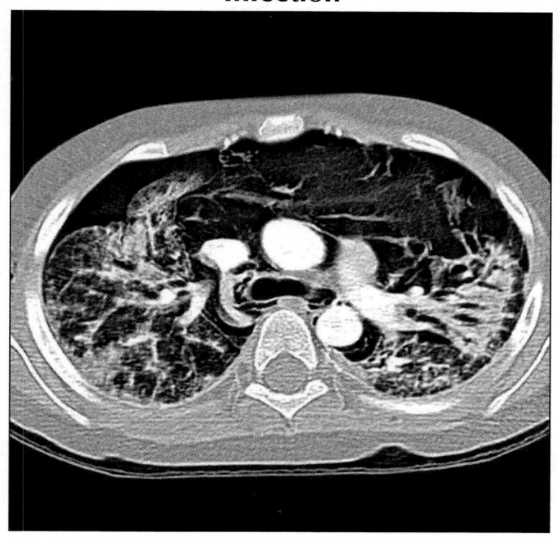

(Left) *Frontal radiograph shows extensive pneumomediastinum, subcutaneous emphysema, right-sided pneumothorax, and diffuse parenchymal lung opacification.* ***(Right)*** *Axial CECT of the same patient shows extensive pneumomediastinum and pneumothorax. There are diffusely scattered areas of airspace density, which indicate nonspecific underlying pulmonary parenchymal disease, in this 6 year old with Pneumocystis pneumonia.*

Extension of Pneumoperitoneum or Pneumoretroperitoneum

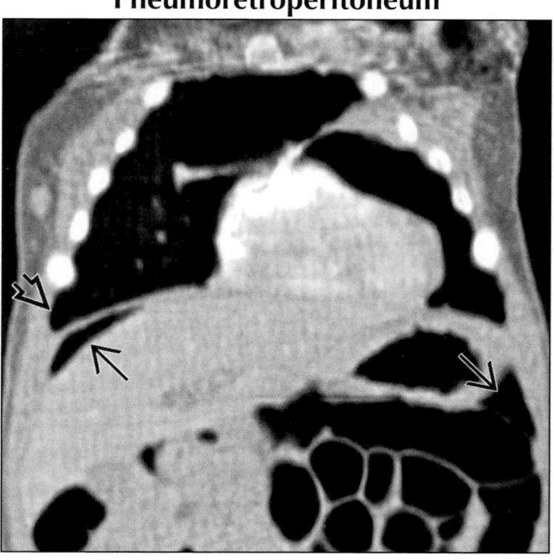

Esophageal Tear

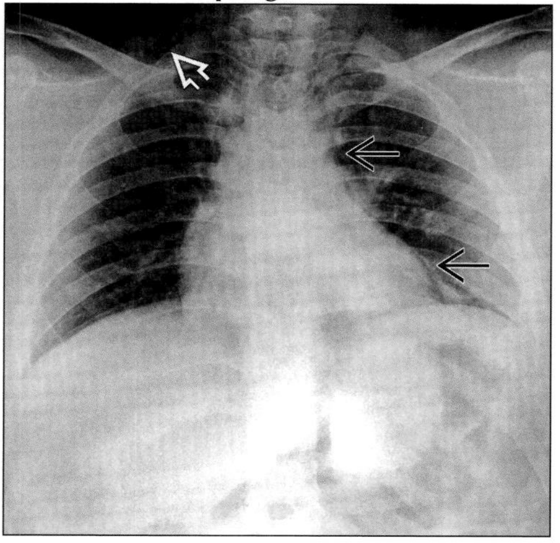

(Left) *Coronal CECT shows pneumomediastinum that presumably extended from the pneumoperitoneum → in this 8-week-old abused child with a pancreatic laceration and duodenal injury (not shown). There is a tiny right pneumothorax as well ⇨.* ***(Right)*** *Frontal radiograph shows pneumomediastinum along the left cardiomediastinal border →, as well as subcutaneous emphysema ➡, in this 13 year old with an esophageal tear following stricture dilatation.*

PNEUMOTHORAX

DIFFERENTIAL DIAGNOSIS

Common
- Pulmonary Hypoplasia
- Surfactant Deficiency Disease
- Meconium Aspiration Syndrome
- Pulmonary Interstitial Emphysema
- Asthma
- Cystic Fibrosis, Lung
- Iatrogenic
- Spontaneous
- Trauma
- Skin Fold (Mimic)

Less Common
- Langerhans Cell Histiocytosis
- Tuberous Sclerosis Complex
- Ruptured Bulla/Blebs

Rare but Important
- Metastatic Neoplasm
- Infection
- Marfan Syndrome
- Ehlers-Danlos Syndrome

ESSENTIAL INFORMATION

Key Differential Diagnosis Issues
- History is extremely helpful in determining possible source of pneumothorax
  - Is there history of trauma? asthma? recent instrumentation?
- Appearance of pneumothorax depends on position of patient and amount of pleural gas
  - In supine patient, air collects anteromedially
    - Sharp, well-delineated cardiac and mediastinal borders
  - In upright patient, air collects laterally and apically
    - Radiolucent space lacking pulmonary vascular markings
    - White pleural line visible
- Size of pneumothorax difficult to accurately estimate on chest x-ray
- Signs of tension pneumothorax
  - Depressed/inverted hemidiaphragm
  - Contralateral shift of mediastinum
  - Expansion of spaces between ribs
- Expiratory, decubitus, and cross-table lateral views may all aid in diagnosis in equivocal cases
- Skin folds and pneumomediastinum can mimic pneumothorax

Helpful Clues for Common Diagnoses
- **Pulmonary Hypoplasia**
  - Potter syndrome
    - Oligohydramnios related to fetal urinary system problems
    - Resultant pulmonary aplasia and typical abnormal facies
  - Pneumothorax may result from progressive air leaks &/or mechanical ventilation
- **Surfactant Deficiency Disease**
  - Premature neonates
  - Reticulogranular opacities
  - Air leak from alveolar rupture can lead to pneumothorax
- **Meconium Aspiration Syndrome**
  - History of meconium-stained amniotic fluid helpful
  - Coarse interstitial and patchy opacities
  - Hyperinflation
  - Pneumothorax may result from air-trapping and alveolar rupture
- **Pulmonary Interstitial Emphysema**
  - Premature neonates
  - Barotrauma from mechanical ventilation
  - Reticular and cystic opacities
  - Alveolar rupture results in pneumothorax
- **Asthma**
  - Airway narrowing and mucous plugging leads to air-trapping and alveolar rupture
  - History of asthma exacerbation helpful
  - Hyperinflated lungs
- **Cystic Fibrosis, Lung**
  - Chronic lung disease can lead to airway obstruction and alveolar rupture
  - Superimposed infection increases pneumothorax risk
  - Pneumothorax indicates poor prognosis
  - Bronchiectasis, bronchial wall thickening, mucus plugging, hyperinflation, prominent hila
- **Iatrogenic**
  - Mechanical ventilation
  - Instrumentation, such as central line placement or thoracentesis
  - Postoperative patients
  - History helpful
- **Spontaneous**
  - Diagnosis of exclusion
  - No distinguishing radiologic features

PNEUMOTHORAX

- **Trauma**
  - Pneumothorax may result from acute blunt or penetrating trauma
  - May also result from rupture of pneumatocele from old trauma
  - Motor vehicle crashes, falls, sports injuries
  - Other signs of trauma
    - Fractures
    - Pulmonary contusions
    - Mediastinal injuries
    - Pleural effusions
- **Skin Fold (Mimic)**
  - Frequently seen in neonates in NICU
  - Can be difficult to differentiate from pneumothorax
    - Linear interface with Mach line
    - No white pleural line
  - Consider decubitus or cross-table lateral views in equivocal cases

Helpful Clues for Less Common Diagnoses

- **Langerhans Cell Histiocytosis**
  - Small pulmonary nodules and parenchymal lung cysts
  - Apical reticulonodular pattern
  - Lung cysts may rupture and result in pneumothorax
- **Tuberous Sclerosis Complex**
  - Lymphangioleiomyomatosis
  - Small parenchymal cysts
  - Chylous pleural effusion
  - Pneumothorax in ~ 70%
- **Ruptured Bulla/Blebs**
  - Small pleural blebs and parenchymal bulla may spontaneously rupture and lead to pneumothorax
  - CT can be very helpful in these cases

Helpful Clues for Rare Diagnoses

- **Metastatic Neoplasm**
  - Pneumothorax may occur in presence of metastases, especially when present on pleural surface
  - Seen in children with osteosarcoma and Wilms tumor
- **Infection**
  - Any infection that causes alveolar destruction can lead to pneumothorax
  - Particularly seen with tuberculosis and *Pneumocystis* infection
- **Marfan Syndrome**
  - Autosomal dominant connective tissue disorder
  - At risk for spontaneous pneumothorax
  - Look for associated findings
    - Aortic aneurysms
    - Kyphoscoliosis
    - Arachnodactyly
- **Ehlers-Danlos Syndrome**
  - Connective tissue disorder
  - At risk for spontaneous pneumothorax

Pulmonary Hypoplasia

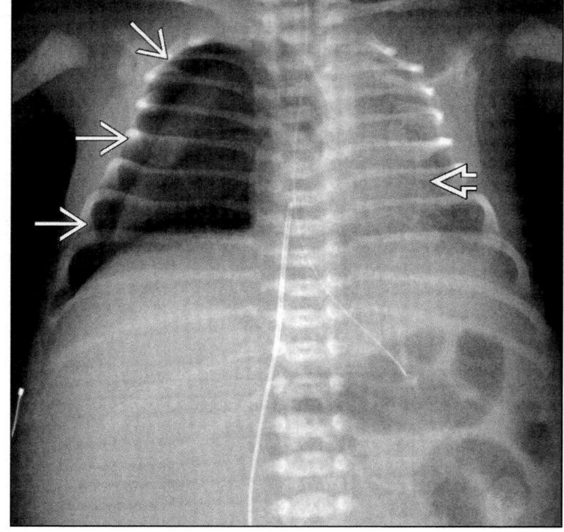

Frontal radiograph in this neonate with Potter syndrome shows a moderate right pneumothorax ➔. Note the shift of cardiomediastinal silhouette to the left ➔, evidence of a tension component.

Surfactant Deficiency Disease

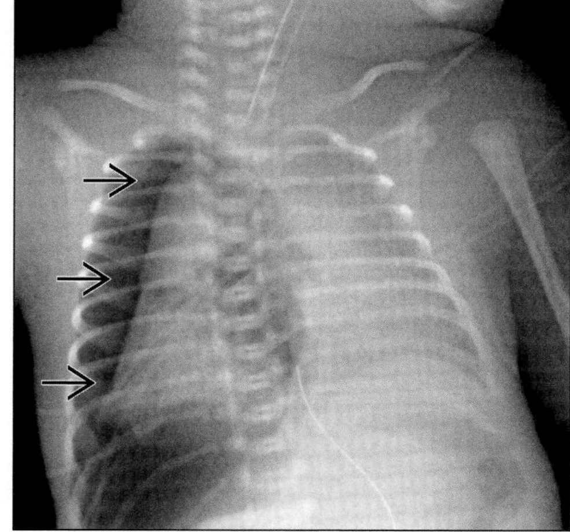

Frontal radiograph shows a large right-sided tension pneumothorax ➔ in this premature neonate with surfactant deficient disease. Note the granular opacities throughout the lungs.

PNEUMOTHORAX

(*Left*) *Frontal radiograph shows bilateral pneumothoraces in this neonate with meconium aspiration. Note the bilateral, coarse, interstitial lung opacities. The left pneumothorax is loculated* → *& the right pneumothorax is under tension with depression of the diaphragm* ⇨. (*Right*) *Frontal radiograph shows a left pneumothorax* → *in this premature neonate with pulmonary interstitial emphysema. Note diffuse, coarse, reticular opacities.*

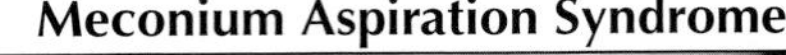

Meconium Aspiration Syndrome

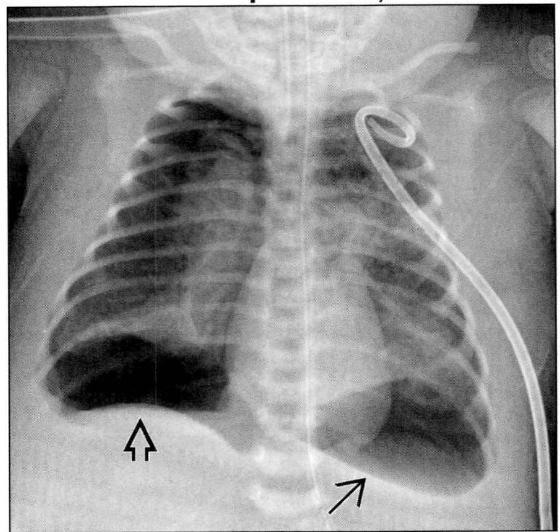

Pulmonary Interstitial Emphysema

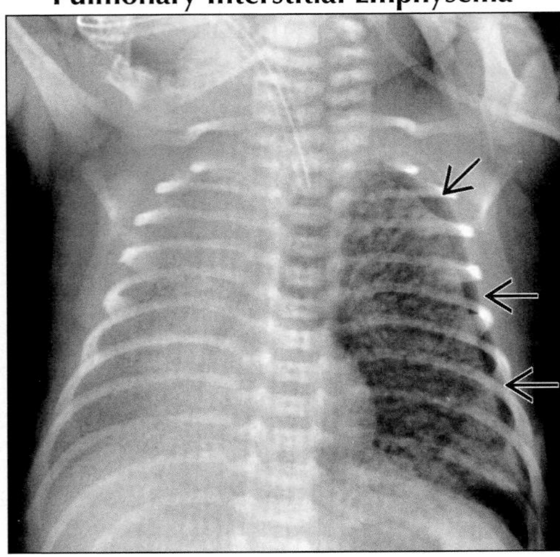

(*Left*) *Frontal radiograph shows a left apical pneumothorax in a 14 year old suffering an asthma attack. Note the white pleural line* ➡ *and lack of pulmonary markings superolateral to this line when the patient is upright.* (*Right*) *Frontal radiograph shows a small, left, apical pneumothorax in this adolescent with cystic fibrosis. Note the white pleural line* ➡, *background bronchiectasis/bronchial wall thickening* ➡, *and left hilar prominence* →.

Asthma

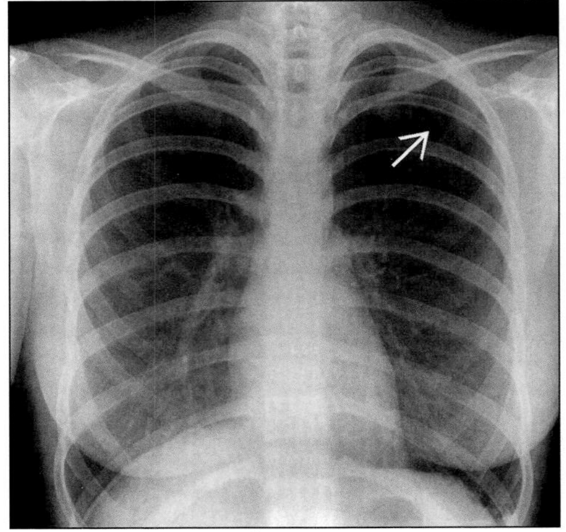

Cystic Fibrosis, Lung

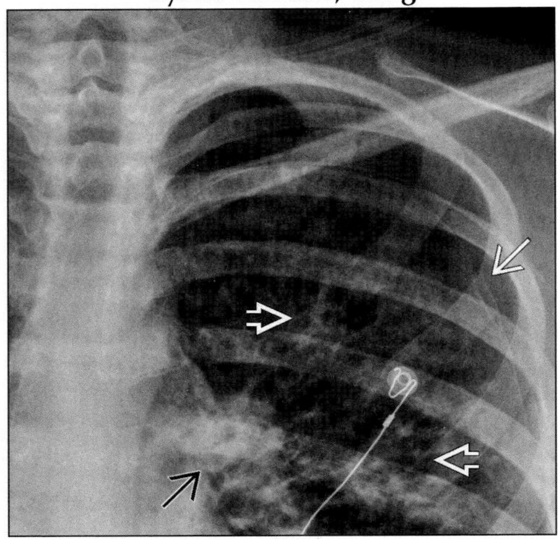

(*Left*) *Frontal radiograph shows a small anteromedial right pneumothorax in this infant status post bilateral thoracostomy tube placement for pleural fluid drainage. Note the sharp, well-demarcated right cardiac border* →. (*Right*) *Coronal MRA shows a small left pneumothorax* ➡ *in this 14-year-old patient being evaluated for central vascular access. Immediately preceding this study, multiple attempts at central line placement failed.*

Iatrogenic

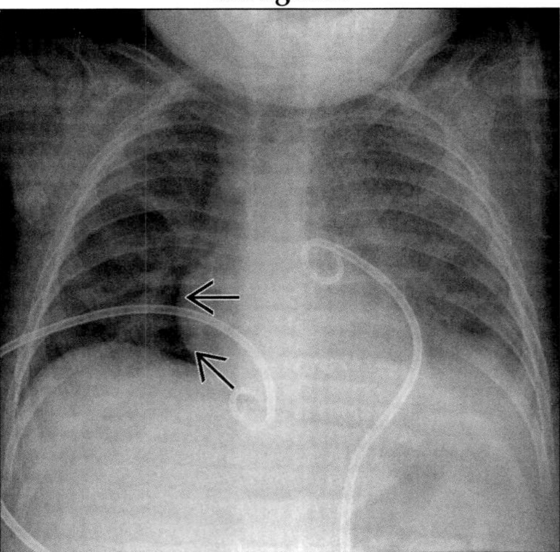

Iatrogenic

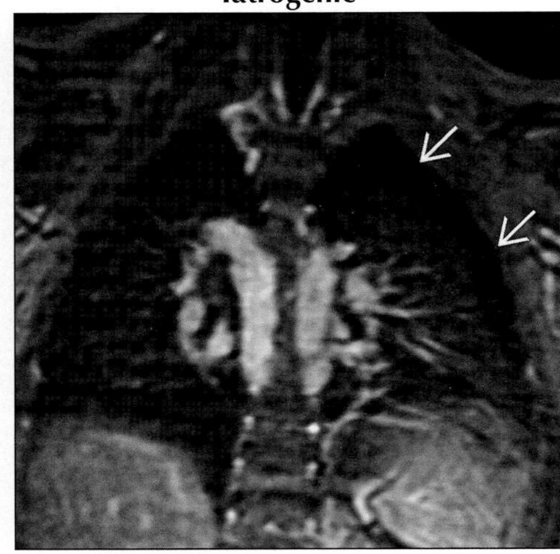

PNEUMOTHORAX

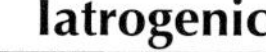
Iatrogenic

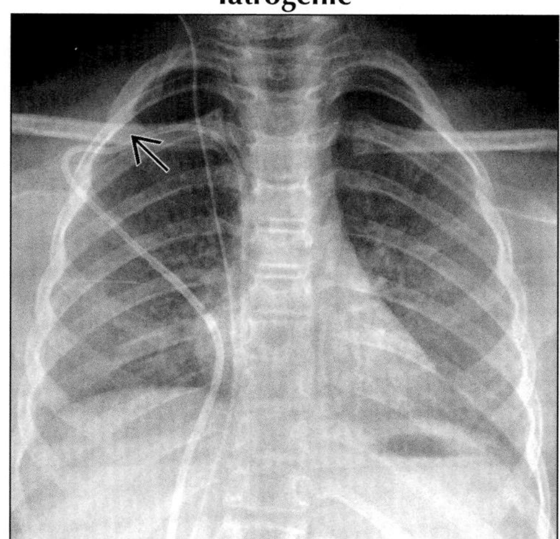

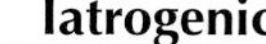
Iatrogenic

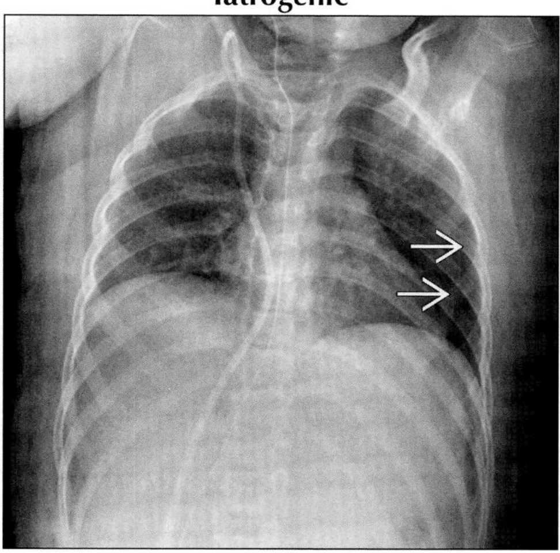

(Left) *Frontal radiograph shows a subtle small, right, apical pneumothorax ➡ in this 10-year-old patient following central line placement with right subclavian approach. A left pneumothorax was not suspected.* ***(Right)*** *Decubitus radiographs were performed on the same patient. The left decubitus radiograph (not shown) confirmed a right pneumothorax. This right decubitus radiograph shows a small left pneumothorax ➡. Decubitus views can be helpful in difficult cases.*

Spontaneous

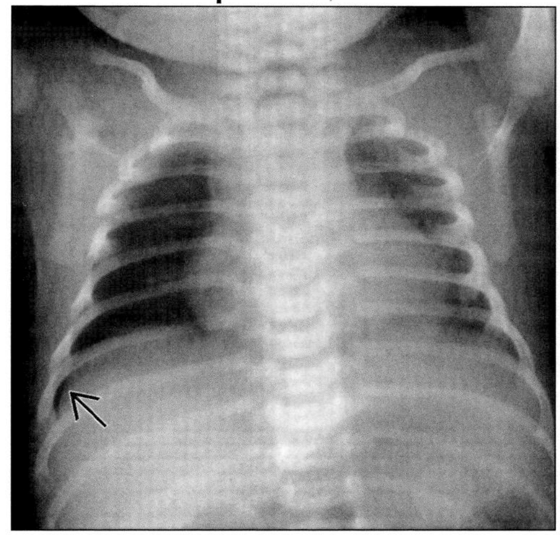

Spontaneous

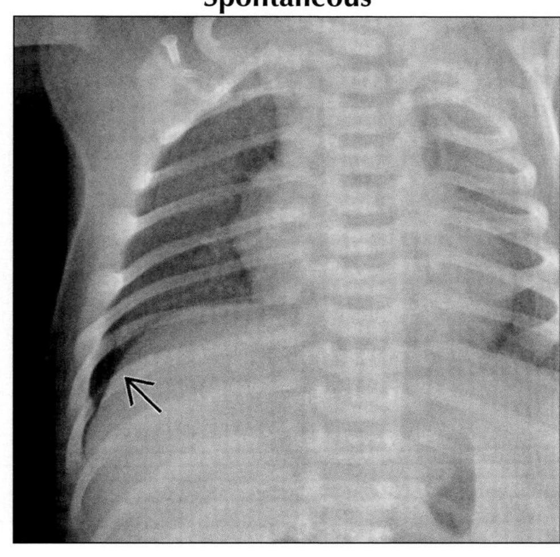

(Left) *Frontal radiograph shows a deep right costophrenic angle ➡. In a supine patient, pleural gas may collect anteriorly and basally. When this air collects laterally, it abnormally deepens the costophrenic angle.* ***(Right)*** *Left lateral decubitus radiograph in the same patient better demonstrates the deep right costophrenic angle ➡ secondary to an anterolateral pneumothorax. No cause was determined; a diagnosis of spontaneous pneumothorax was made.*

Trauma

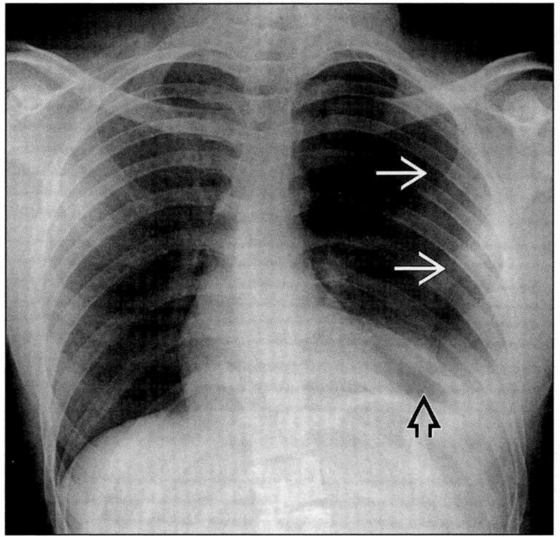

Trauma

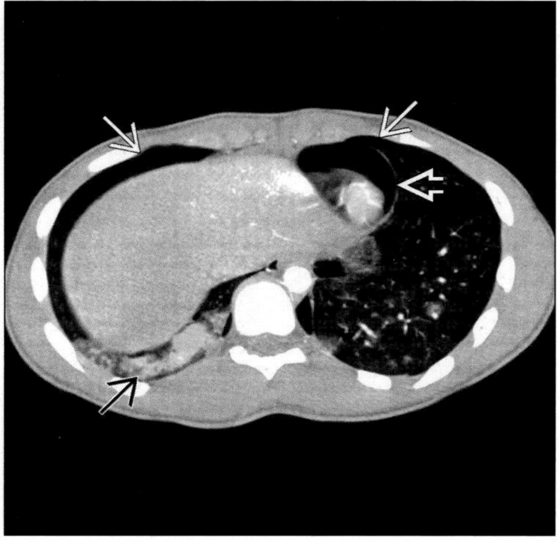

(Left) *Frontal radiograph shows a moderate-sized to large left pneumothorax in this 16 year old following a stab wound. Notice the white pleural line ➡ and lack of pulmonary markings beyond this line. The left basilar opacity ⇨ was a combination of atelectasis and pleural fluid.* ***(Right)*** *Axial CECT shows bilateral small pneumothoraces ➡, pneumomediastinum ⇨, and pulmonary contusions ➡ in this 17-year-old patient involved in a motor vehicle crash.*

PNEUMOTHORAX

(**Left**) Frontal radiograph shows a linear interface over the right hemithorax →. Note the presence of pulmonary markings lateral to this interface. Subsequent images confirmed that this was a skin fold, not a pneumothorax. (**Right**) Frontal radiograph shows a linear interface over the right hemithorax →. Note the presence of pulmonary markings lateral to this interface and the absence of a distinct white pleural line. A decubitus view confirmed a skin fold.

Skin Fold (Mimic)

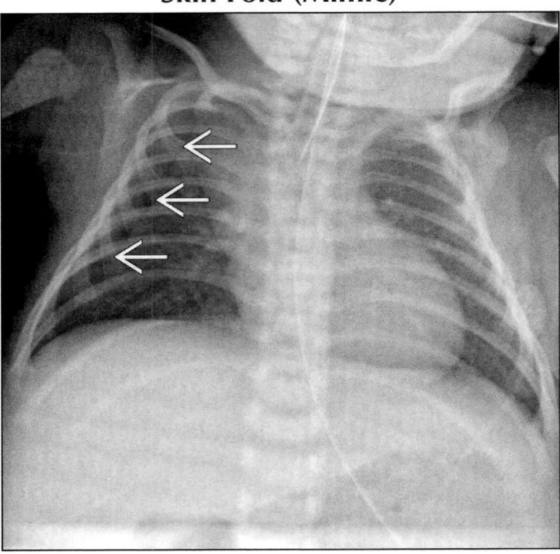

Skin Fold (Mimic)

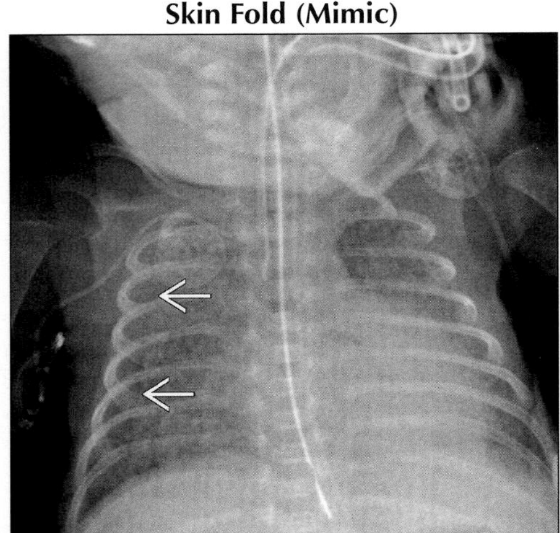

(**Left**) Coronal NECT shows diffuse reticulonodular parenchymal lung disease →, multiple calcified lymph nodes →, and a small right apical pneumothorax → in this 16-year-old patient with Langerhans cell histiocytosis. (**Right**) Axial NECT shows a small anterior left pneumothorax → in this adolescent patient with tuberous sclerosis. Note the innumerable small parenchymal lung cysts → bilaterally, consistent with lymphangioleiomyomatosis.

Langerhans Cell Histiocytosis

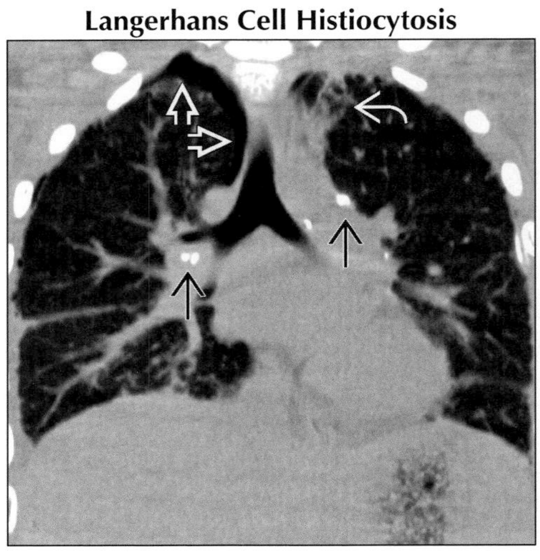

Tuberous Sclerosis Complex

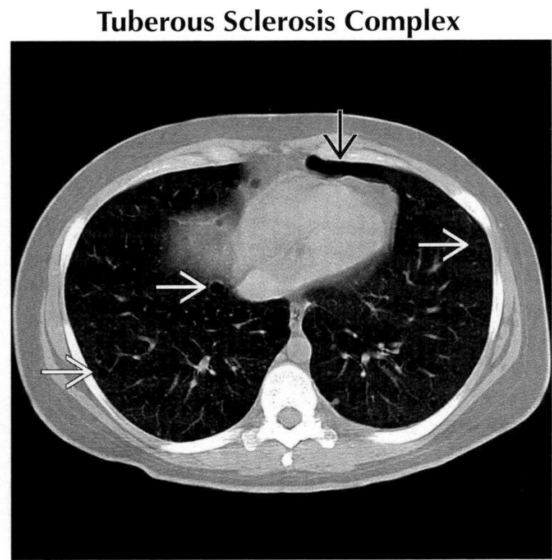

(**Left**) Axial NECT shows a small to moderate-sized left-sided pneumothorax →, the result of a spontaneous rupture of tiny pleural blebs → posteriorly in this 17-year-old patient. (**Right**) Coronal NECT shows a small right-sided apical pneumothorax → in this 16-year-old patient. Note the multiple tiny apical pleural blebs that likely underwent a spontaneous rupture →.

Ruptured Bulla/Blebs

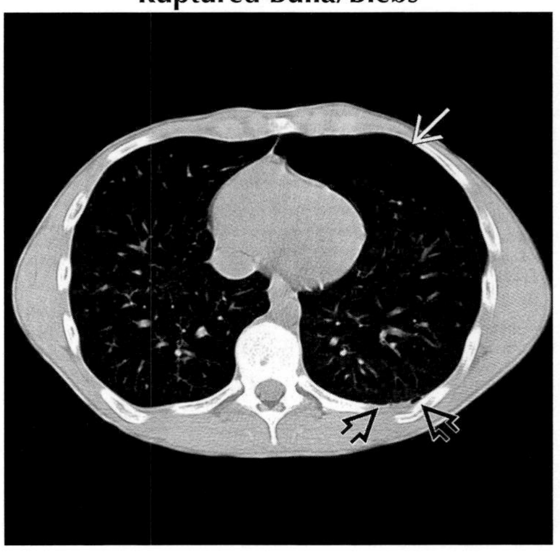

Ruptured Bulla/Blebs

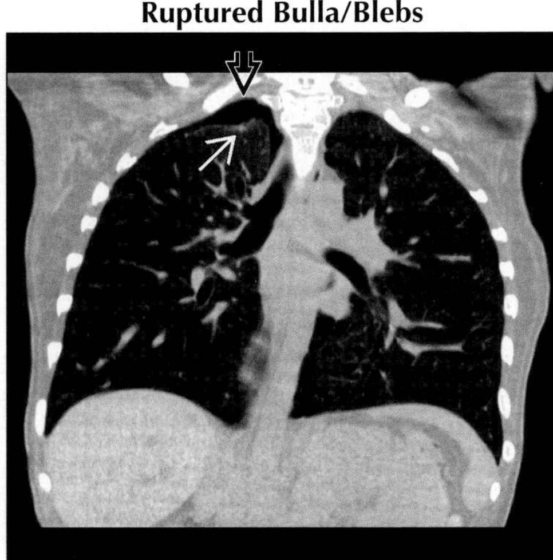

PNEUMOTHORAX

Ruptured Bulla/Blebs

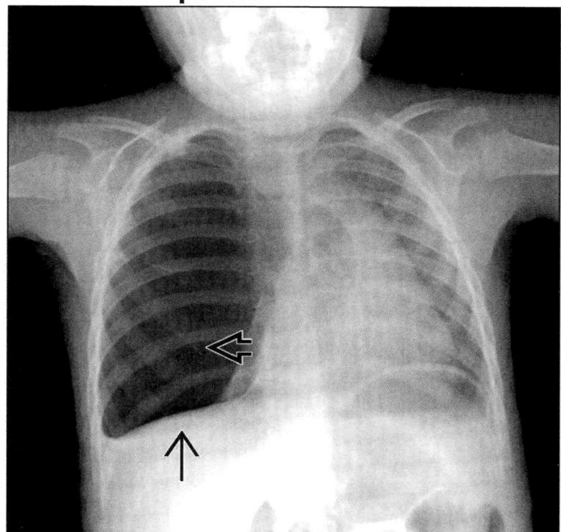

Metastatic Neoplasm

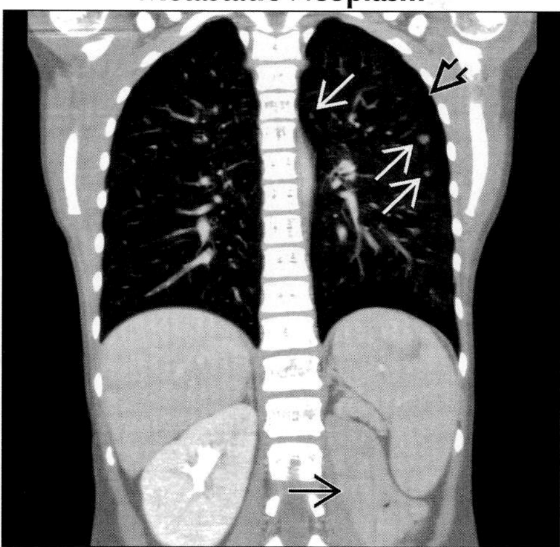

*(**Left**) Frontal radiograph shows a right tension pneumothorax with depression of the diaphragm → and contralateral mediastinal shift in this 3 year old. Note the presence of septations on the right →, indicating the presence of a bulla. (**Right**) Coronal CECT shows a small left pneumothorax → and 3 small pulmonary nodules in the left lung →. Note the absence of the left kidney → in this patient with metastatic Wilms tumor status post nephrectomy.*

Infection

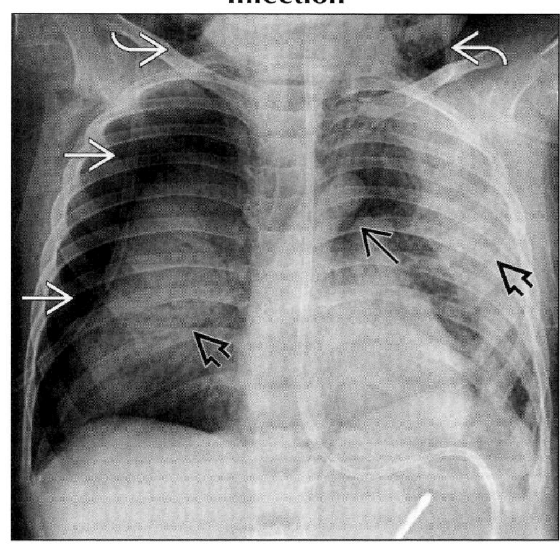

Infection

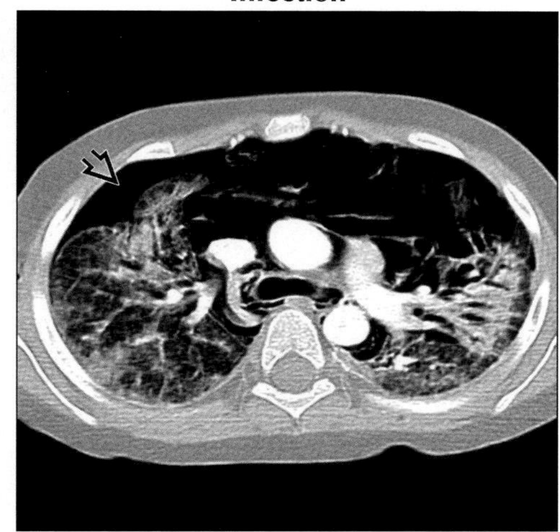

*(**Left**) Frontal radiograph shows pneumomediastinum →, subcutaneous emphysema →, and a right pneumothorax →. Note the dense consolidative lung disease → with air bronchograms in this 6 year old with Pneumocystis pneumonia. (**Right**) Axial CECT of the same patient shows extensive pneumomediastinum and a right pneumothorax →, associated with scattered areas of parenchymal consolidation and ground-glass opacities.*

Marfan Syndrome

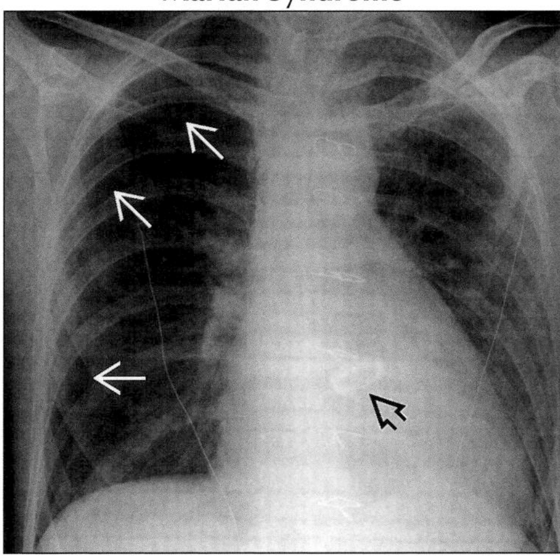

Ehlers-Danlos Syndrome

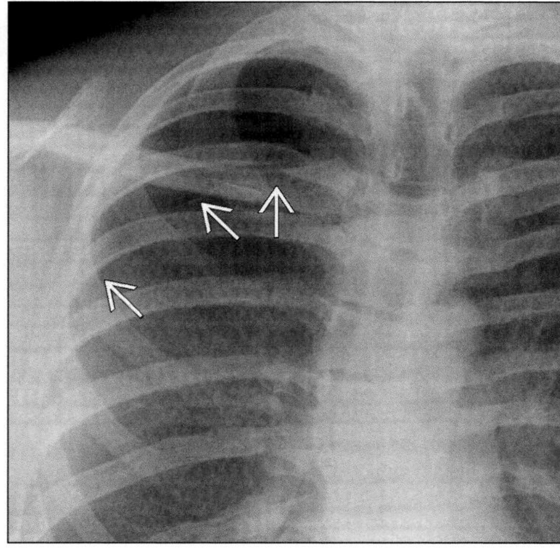

*(**Left**) Frontal radiograph shows a right-sided pneumothorax → in this 18-year-old patient with Marfan syndrome. Note the median sternotomy wires and prosthetic aortic valve →, clues to the presence of cardiac disease. (**Right**) Frontal radiograph shows a right apical pneumothorax in this 19-year-old patient with Ehlers-Danlos syndrome. Note the white pleural line → and lack of pulmonary markings superolateral to this line.*

SECTION 3
Gastrointestinal

ACUTE ABDOMEN IN INFANTS AND CHILDREN

DIFFERENTIAL DIAGNOSIS

Common
- Appendicitis
- Inguinal Hernia
- Midgut Volvulus
- Intussusception
- Adhesions
- Crohn Disease

Less Common
- Ovarian Torsion
- Pelvic Inflammatory Disease
- Ectopic Pregnancy
- Meckel Diverticulum
- Nonaccidental Trauma/Child Abuse
- Henoch-Schönlein Purpura
- Foreign Body Ingestion

Rare but Important
- Gastric Volvulus
- Wandering Spleen

ESSENTIAL INFORMATION

Key Differential Diagnosis Issues
- Gender
- Bilious emesis vs. nonbilious emesis
- Presence or absence of bowel obstruction
- If bowel obstruction, proximal or distal
- Skin: Rash or bruising

Helpful Clues for Common Diagnoses
- **Appendicitis**
  - Fever, leukocytosis, anorexia are expected but none are universal
  - Radiograph
    - Findings range from right lower quadrant air-fluid levels to frank small bowel obstruction
    - Useful for excluding free air
  - US
    - Noncompressible tubular structure > 7 mm in diameter
    - In children, may obviate CT and avoid radiation
    - Pitfall: Must see entire length of appendix to exclude tip appendicitis
  - CT
    - Hyperemic walls, inflammatory stranding in fat
- **Inguinal Hernia**
  - Radiograph may demonstrate loops of bowel in scrotal sac
  - US: Peristalsing bowel within scrotal sac
- **Midgut Volvulus**
  - With midgut malrotation
    - Typical presentation in neonate with bilious emesis but may present at any age
    - Usually a proximal obstruction
  - Without midgut malrotation
    - Lead points include adhesions, Meckel diverticulum, or other abdominal lesions
    - Proximal or distal obstruction
- **Intussusception**
  - Radiographs (notoriously unreliable) may suggest intussusception with rounded soft tissue density
  - US sensitive and specific for ileocolic intussusception
    - Bowel and mesenteric fat trapped within colon create "doughnut" sign if seen in transverse plane
- **Adhesions**
  - Presents as partial, complete, or intermittent bowel obstruction
  - Adhesions not seen but transition point from dilated to collapsed bowel may be identified on CT
- **Crohn Disease**
  - Marked bowel wall thickening, often with skip areas
  - Perirectal inflammation/abscess easily missed on imaging

Helpful Clues for Less Common Diagnoses
- **Ovarian Torsion**
  - US: Torsed ovary is generally large, heterogeneous, predominantly hypoechoic
    - Pitfall: Blood flow on US may confound diagnosis due to intermittent torsion or multiplicity of blood supply to ovaries
  - Obvious size/volume discrepancy between ovaries is virtually always present
    - In postmenarchal patient, torsed ovarian volume often > 20 mL
    - In premenarchal patient, ovarian volumes markedly discrepant, but torsed ovarian volume may be < 20 mL
  - Consider underlying ovarian mass or cyst
- **Pelvic Inflammatory Disease**
  - Early PID shows nonspecific inflammatory changes

- Tuboovarian abscess may be seen with US or CT
- **Ectopic Pregnancy**
  - Look for extrauterine gestational sac
  - If ruptured, appears as complex cystic/solid mass with echogenic peritoneal fluid
- **Meckel Diverticulum**
  - May present as bleeding, intussusception, or bowel obstruction
  - CT: Small bowel obstruction, inflammatory changes around bowel loops, hyperemic tubular structure
- **Nonaccidental Trauma/Child Abuse**
  - Abdomen CT obtained when laboratory values are abnormal (liver, pancreatic enzymes, CK-MB)
    - Abdomen CT: Duodenal hematoma, jejunal perforation, liver laceration, pancreatic laceration, pericardial effusion
    - Scrutinize images for fractures
  - Rectal prolapse is uncommon but known presentation
- **Henoch-Schönlein Purpura**
  - Small vessel vasculitis
  - Acute abdominal findings may precede rash, arthralgia, hematuria
  - CT findings may prompt clinical consideration
    - Marked bowel wall thickening predominantly in jejunum and ileum, with skip areas
    - Intussusception, ascites
    - Mesenteric lymphadenopathy and vascular engorgement
- **Foreign Body Ingestion**
  - May cause perforation, erosion, obstruction
  - Multiple magnets retain attraction to each other, cause pressure erosion, perforation

Helpful Clues for Rare Diagnoses

- **Gastric Volvulus**
  - Radiograph: Large spherical gastric bubble
  - Fluoroscopic upper gastrointestinal (UGI) study considered definitive
  - Mesenteroaxial gastric volvulus
    - Stomach folds and twists
    - Higher association with vascular compromise and obstruction in children
    - Pylorus near/above gastroesophageal junction
    - May be associated with congenital diaphragmatic or abdominal abnormalities
  - Organoaxial gastric volvulus
    - Stomach flips upside down
    - Lower likelihood of vascular compromise or acute obstruction in children
    - Greater curvature above lesser curvature; downward pointing pylorus
  - Mixed mesenteroaxial/organoaxial
- **Wandering Spleen**
  - Spleen absent from usual position in left upper quadrant due to lax or absent splenic ligaments
    - Risk of torsion of long vascular pedicle
    - Higher risk of injury in minor accidents when not protected by thoracic cage

Appendicitis

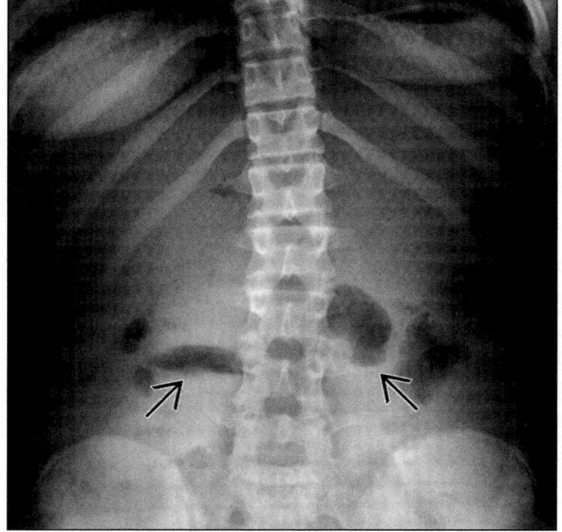

Frontal radiograph shows a nonspecific bowel gas pattern with air-fluid levels ⇒, hinting at trouble in the right lower quadrant. Note the patient is bending slightly, splinting from pain.

Appendicitis

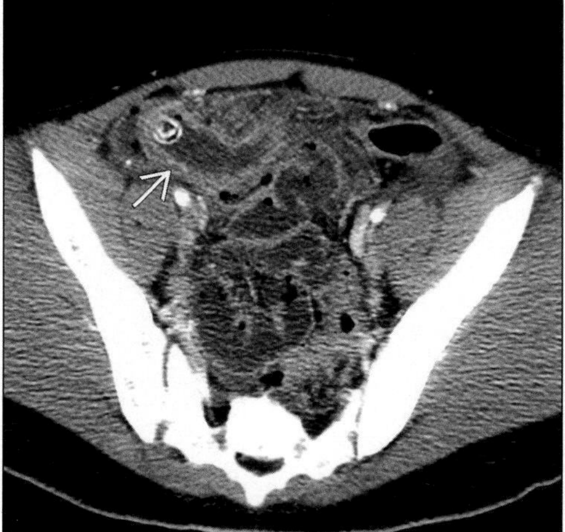

Axial CECT of the same patient shows a dilated hyperemic tubular structure ➡ and lamellated appendicolith in the right lower quadrant, consistent with acute appendicitis.

ACUTE ABDOMEN IN INFANTS AND CHILDREN

(**Left**) Longitudinal ultrasound shows an elongated dilated noncompressible tubular structure ➔ in the right lower quadrant. (**Right**) Axial CECT shows diffuse severe bowel wall thickening ➔, free fluid ➔, flattened IVC, and small caliber aorta ➔ in a 3 year old with perforated appendicitis who presented in septic shock with abdominal compartment syndrome. The patient survived after multiple abdominal washouts.

Appendicitis

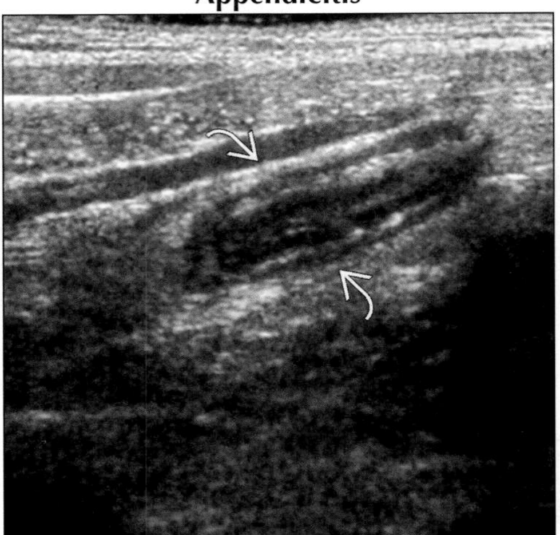

Appendicitis

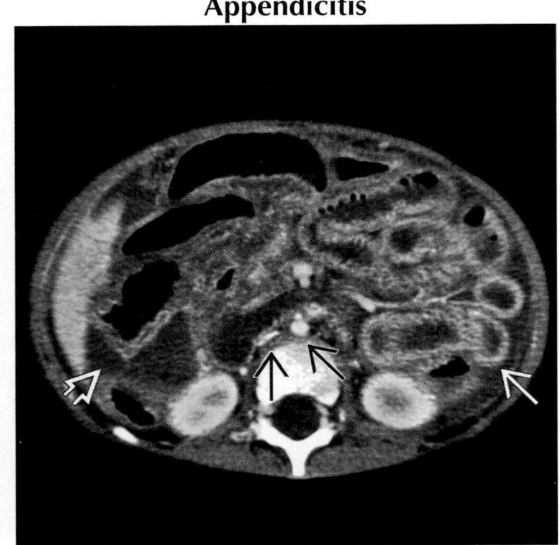

(**Left**) Frontal radiograph shows multiple moderately dilated loops of small bowel in the central mid-abdomen, suspicious for obstruction. There is a distinct paucity of distal bowel gas. Note the marked soft tissue fullness of the right hemiscrotum ➔. (**Right**) Transverse ultrasound of the same patient shows fluid-filled loops of peristalsing bowel ➔ in the scrotum, a normal right testis ➔, and reactive hydrocele ➔.

Inguinal Hernia

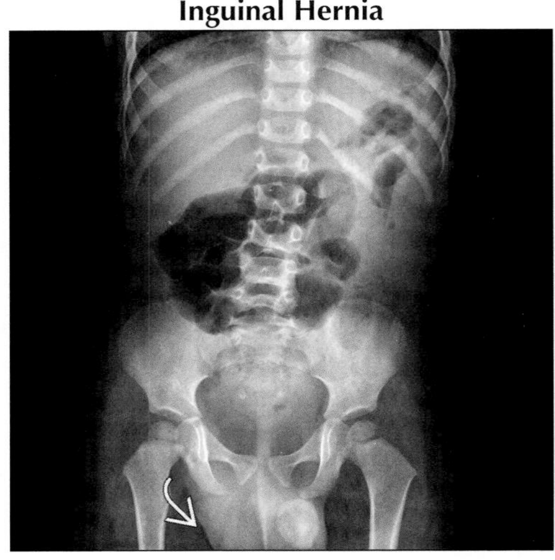

Inguinal Hernia

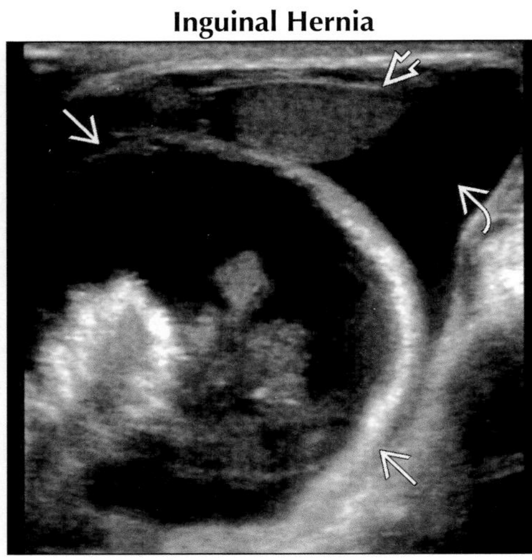

(**Left**) Frontal radiograph shows moderately dilated loops of proximal small bowel ➔ and modest distal air in this 5 day old with midgut malrotation and volvulus presenting with bilious emesis. (**Right**) Lateral fluoroscopic spot radiograph shows the typical corkscrew appearance of the duodenum in midgut malrotation with volvulus in another infant with bilious emesis. Note the more prominent caliber of air-filled distal small bowel compared with the previous image.

Midgut Volvulus

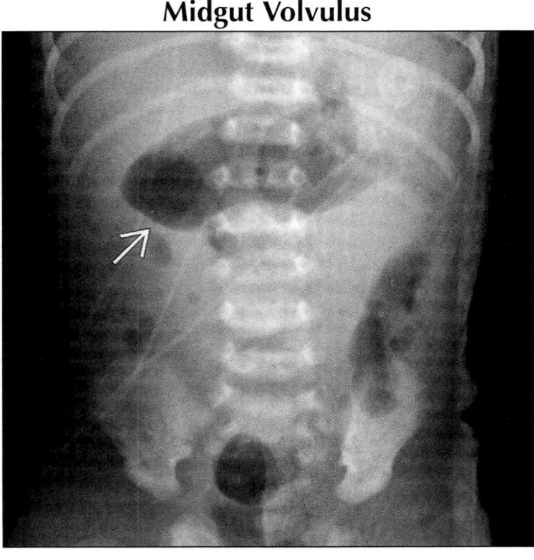

Midgut Volvulus

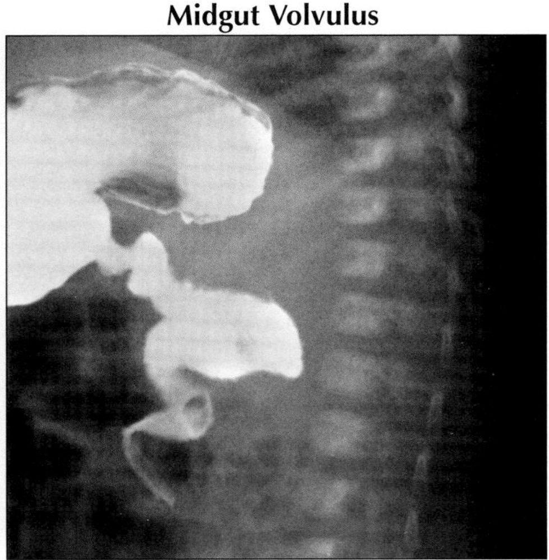

Intussusception

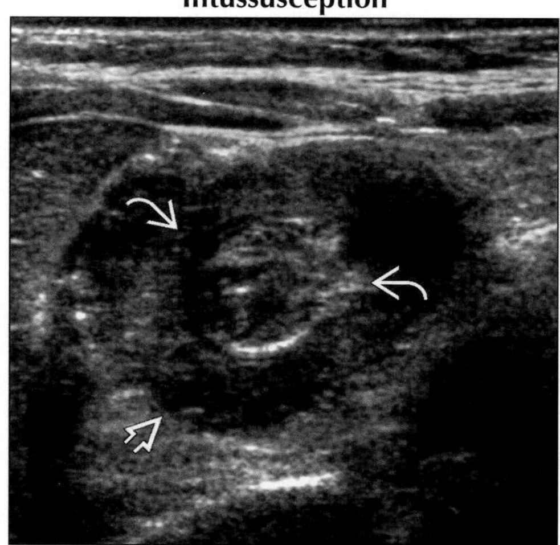

Crohn Disease

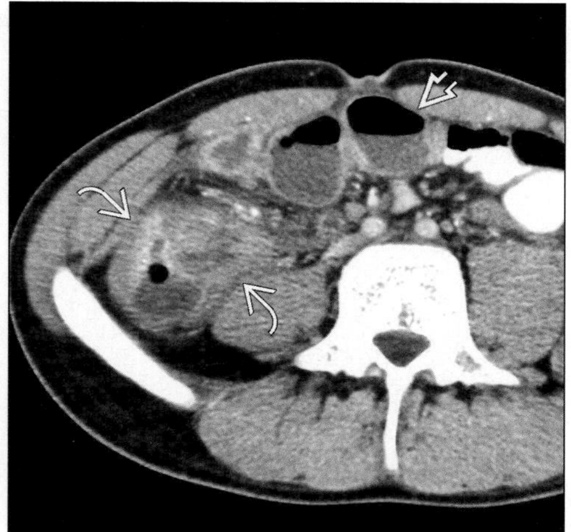

(Left) *Transverse ultrasound shows the target-like or "pseudokidney" appearance of a small bowel and mesentery ➢ trapped within the colon ➡, consistent with ileocolic intussusception.* ***(Right)*** *Axial CECT shows right lower quadrant bowel wall thickening and inflammatory change ➢ in this teenager with newly diagnosed but advanced Crohn disease. There is also partial small bowel obstruction ➡. This was originally thought to be appendicitis.*

Ovarian Torsion

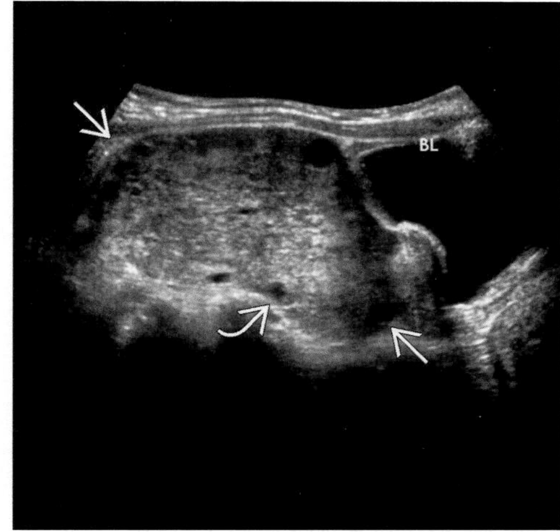

Ovarian Torsion

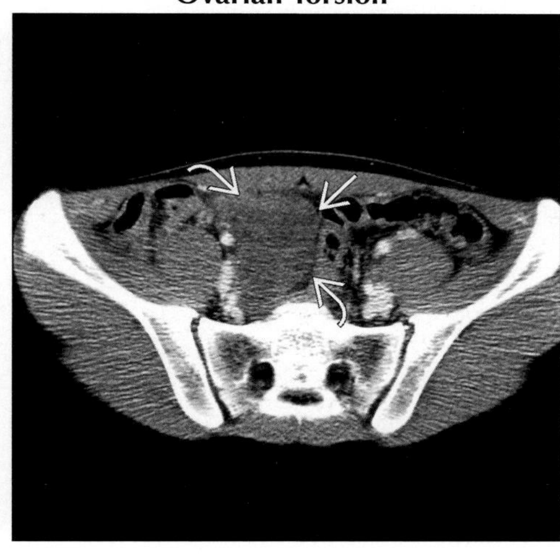

(Left) *Longitudinal ultrasound shows a massively enlarged right ovary ➡ with a few peripheral follicles ➢ in this 12 year old complaining of pain for 1 day. No flow was seen. A torsed infarcted right ovary and fallopian tube were removed.* ***(Right)*** *Axial CECT shows an oval, low- to intermediate-attenuation 4.5 cm x 7 cm pelvic mass ➢. This was a torsed right ovary, which also had a 9 cm cyst (not shown). Note the peripheral follicles ➡.*

Pelvic Inflammatory Disease

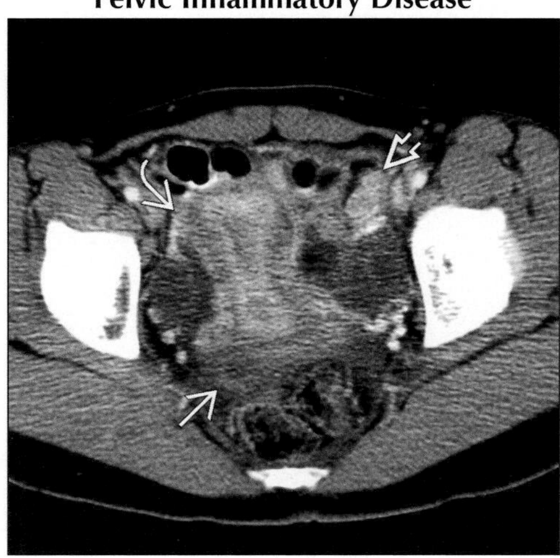

Pelvic Inflammatory Disease

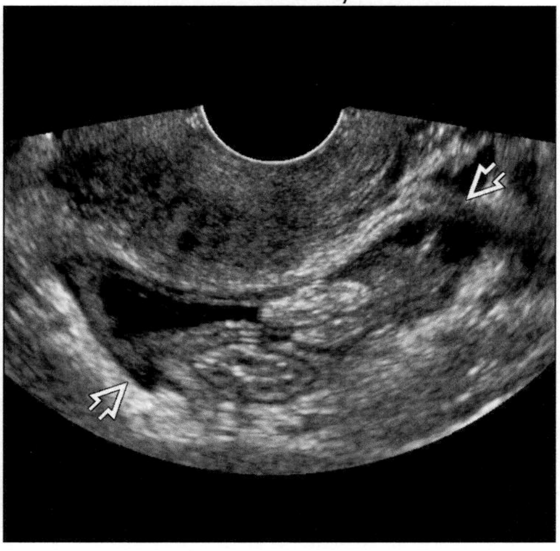

(Left) *Axial CECT shows an inflamed uterus ➢ surrounded by fluid and a hyperemic left fallopian tube ➡ in this teenager with cervical cultures positive for gonorrhea and chlamydia. The ovaries are both seen, as well as part of the tuboovarian abscess ➡.* ***(Right)*** *Transverse transvaginal ultrasound in the same patient shows the complex, mixed cystic and solid appearance of the thick-walled tuboovarian abscess ➡.*

ACUTE ABDOMEN IN INFANTS AND CHILDREN

(**Left**) *Longitudinal transvaginal ultrasound shows an extrauterine thick-walled ring structure ➡ with a small yolk sac. The large volume of heterogeneous pelvic fluid ➡ is consistent with rupture of this ectopic pregnancy.* (**Right**) *Axial CECT shows an inflamed blind-ending tube in the right lower quadrant ➡. A normal appendix (not shown) was identified. Small bowel obstruction ➡ is present.*

Ectopic Pregnancy

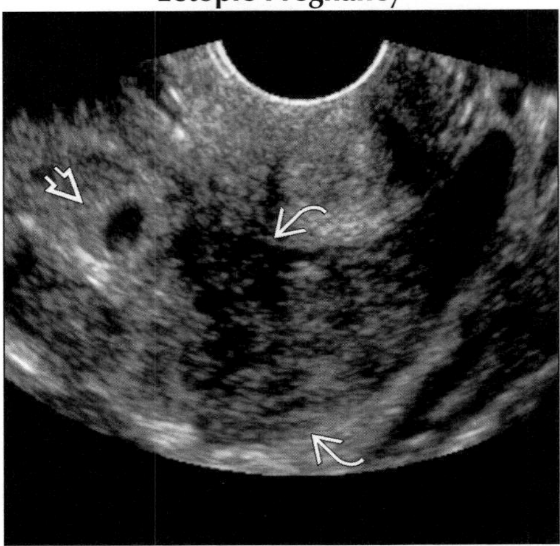

Meckel Diverticulum

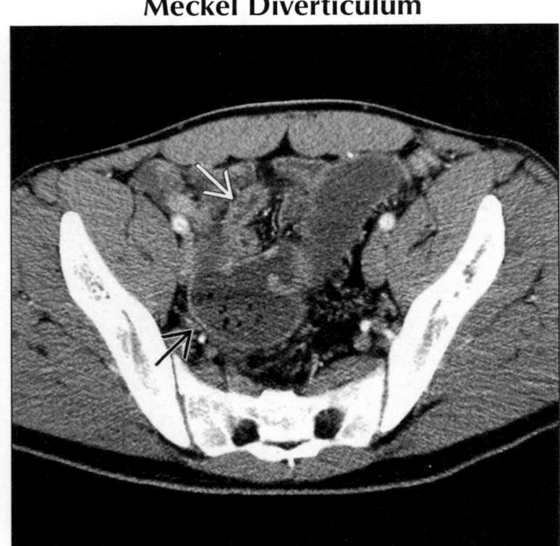

(**Left**) *Frontal radiograph shows a nonspecific, possibly partially obstructed bowel gas pattern in this 9 month old who presented with recurrent rectal prolapse. Note many (but not all) of the lateral and posterior rib fractures ➡.* (**Right**) *Axial CECT shows a branching, low attenuation structure ➡ in the hepatic parenchyma, consistent with a laceration in this 4-year-old child who presented with failure to thrive and elevated liver enzymes.*

Nonaccidental Trauma/Child Abuse

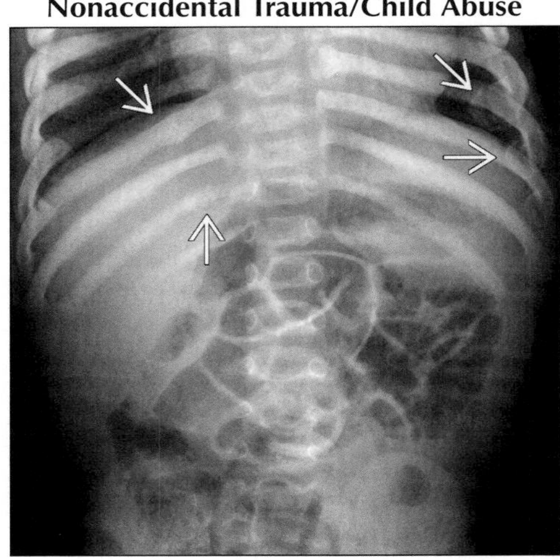

Nonaccidental Trauma/Child Abuse

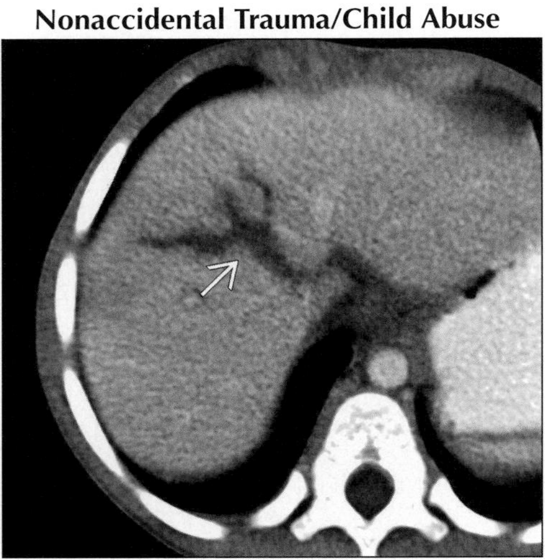

(**Left**) *Axial CECT shows a healing rib fracture ➡, hemoperitoneum ➡, pneumoperitoneum ➡, dense adrenal glands ➡, & a heterogeneously enhancing liver with laceration ➡ in this hemodynamically unstable 4 year old with multiple bruises. Duodenal & jejunal perforations were found at surgery.* (**Right**) *Axial CECT shows a globular low-attenuation area ➡, consistent with right adrenal hematoma in this 3 year old with multiple bruises & lacerations.*

Nonaccidental Trauma/Child Abuse

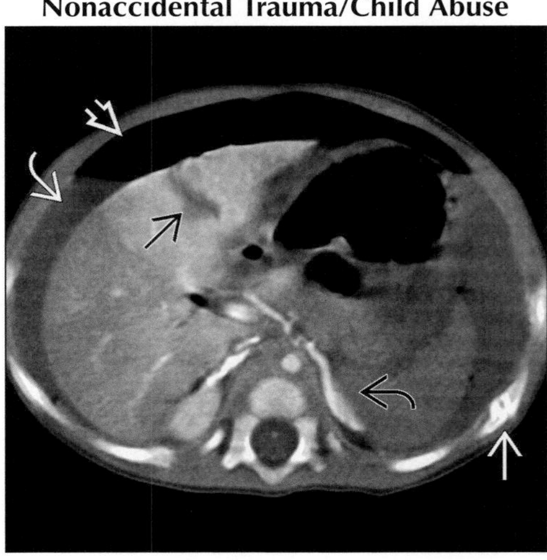

Nonaccidental Trauma/Child Abuse

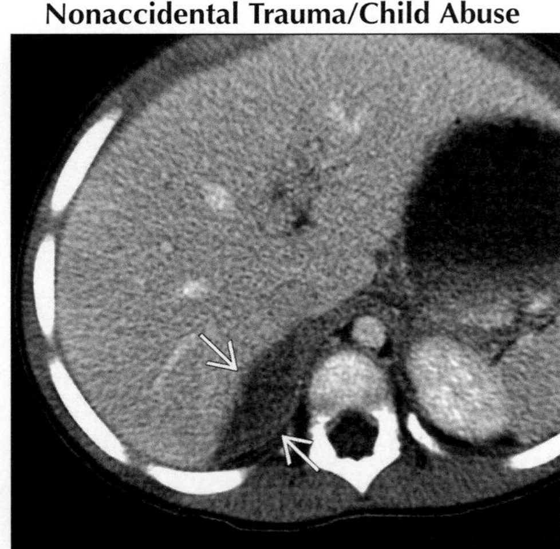

Henoch-Schönlein Purpura

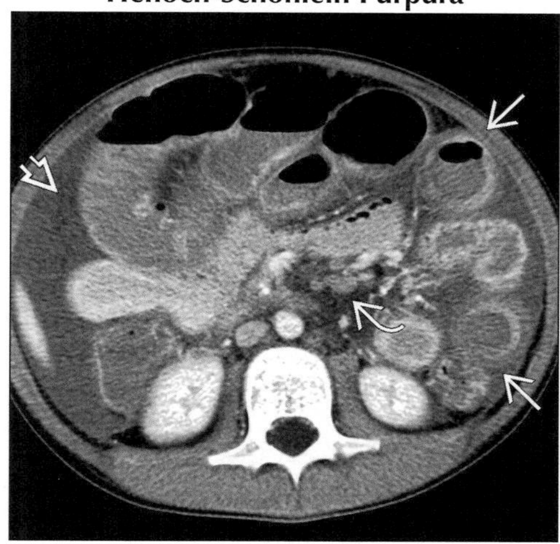

Foreign Body Ingestion

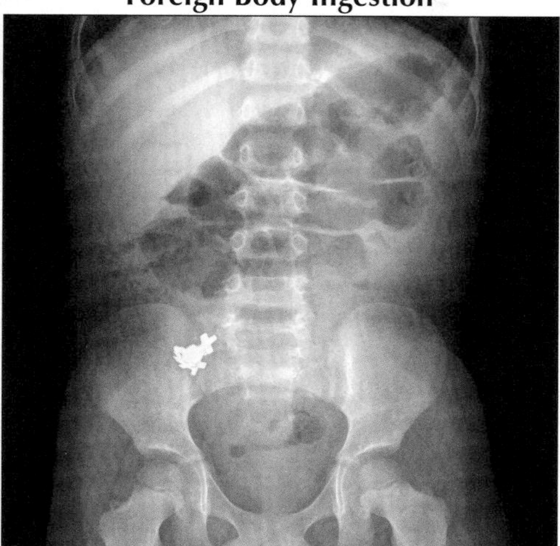

(Left) *Axial CECT shows dilated thick-walled hyperemic loops of small bowel ➔ throughout the abdomen, free intraperitoneal fluid ➔, and mesenteric adenopathy ➔. These abdominal findings preceded the classic skin lesions of Henoch-Schönlein purpura.* ***(Right)*** *Frontal radiograph shows clustered right lower quadrant magnets. Continued attraction of magnets in adjacent loops of the bowel caused pressure erosion and perforation.*

Gastric Volvulus

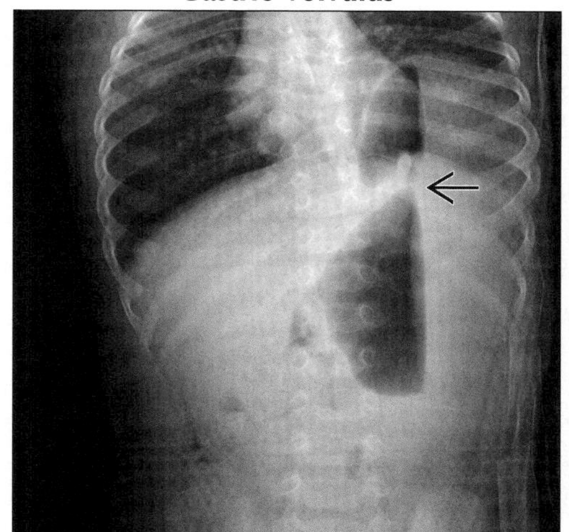

Gastric Volvulus

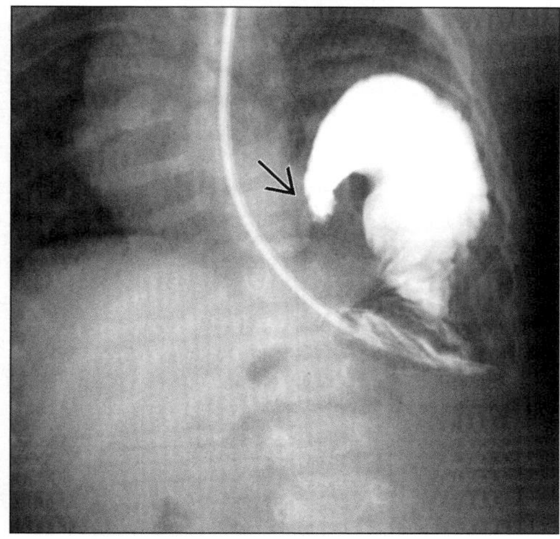

(Left) *Left lateral radiograph shows the mid-gastric body twist ➔ in this 6 month old with acute mesenteroaxial gastric volvulus who presented with abrupt onset nonbilious emesis.* ***(Right)*** *Frontal fluoroscopic spot radiograph in the same patient shows mesenteroaxial gastric volvulus with diaphragmatic defect, gastric outlet obstruction, and pylorus ➔ above the GE junction.*

Wandering Spleen

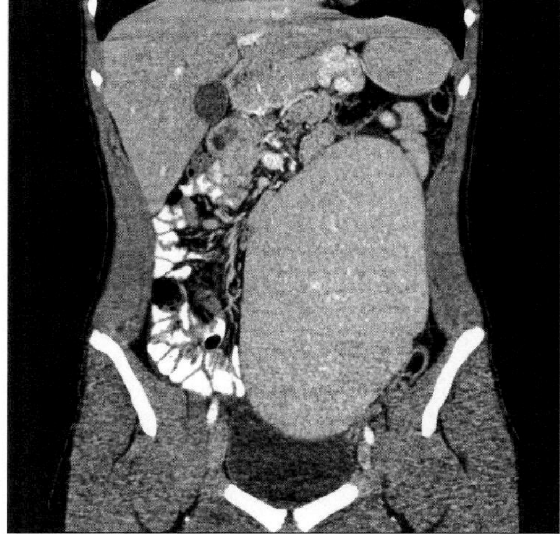

Wandering Spleen

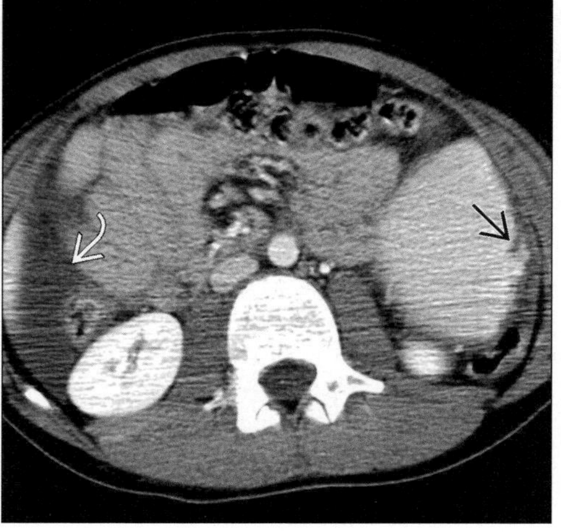

(Left) *Coronal CECT shows a massively enlarged spleen in the lower anterior abdomen in this teenaged girl. Subtle low-attenuation branching structures are seen within the parenchyma. The pathology report described extensive venous congestion, probably from intermittent torsion given the clinical presentation.* ***(Right)*** *Axial CECT shows a lacerated ➔ low-positioned unprotected spleen in this boy after a sledding accident. Note the hemoperitoneum ➔.*

RIGHT LOWER QUADRANT PAIN

DIFFERENTIAL DIAGNOSIS

Common

- Appendicitis
- Enteritis
  - *Yersinia enterocolitica*, *Escherichia coli* 0157:H7, *Salmonella enteritidis*, *Clostridium difficile*, *Shigella*, *Campylobacter*
- Crohn Disease
- Mesenteric Adenitis

Less Common

- Renal/Ureteral Calculus, Obstructing
- Pyelonephritis
- Pneumonia
- Epiploic Appendagitis (Appendicitis Epiploica)
- Pelvic Inflammatory Disease
- Ovarian Torsion
- Ectopic Pregnancy
- Meckel Diverticulum
- Typhlitis

Rare but Important

- Tuberculosis

ESSENTIAL INFORMATION

Key Differential Diagnosis Issues

- Surgical abdomen (toxic appearing) vs. nonsurgical abdomen
- Male vs. female
- Prior medical or surgical history

Helpful Clues for Common Diagnoses

- **Appendicitis**
  - Radiograph: Findings range from right lower quadrant air-fluid levels to small bowel obstruction
    - Helpful to quickly exclude free air; appendicolith in up to 10%
  - US: Noncompressible tubular structure
    - Useful modality in children, may obviate CT and avoid radiation
    - ≥ 7 mm diameter with surrounding inflammatory change
    - If 6-7 mm equivocal size, considered positive if noncompressible with increased blood flow
    - Pitfall: Inflammation may involve only tip; must see entire length of appendix
  - CT: Hyperemic walls, fat stranding, non-filling with contrast
    - Pitfall: Early ruptured appendix may still appear intact on imaging
- **Enteritis**
  - Thickened bowel walls, air-fluid levels, modest free fluid
  - Often involves longer segments of bowel
- **Crohn Disease**
  - Abdominal inflammatory changes more widespread
    - Marked circumferential bowel wall thickening
    - Common to see skip areas of bowel involvement
  - Perirectal inflammation easily missed by CT
  - Psoas abscess also not uncommonly seen
- **Mesenteric Adenitis**
  - Nonsurgical abdomen, clinically more benign
  - Minimal bowel changes, large cluster of mesenteric and RLQ lymph nodes

Helpful Clues for Less Common Diagnoses

- **Renal/Ureteral Calculus, Obstructing**
  - US may obviate CT and save patient radiation
    - Asymmetric hydronephrosis
    - Absence of ipsilateral ureteral jet at ureterovesicular junction
  - CT findings sensitive, specific; may identify multiple calculi & specific sizes
    - Asymmetric hydronephrosis
    - Delayed nephrogram: Affected kidney enhances later than normal side
    - Delayed images may provide more information about partial vs. complete obstruction
- **Pyelonephritis**
  - US may be utilized to exclude renal abscess
    - US color/power Doppler may demonstrate focal absence of flow but is neither sensitive nor specific
  - CT is sensitive and specific for acute pyelonephritis
    - Striated nephrogram of low-attenuation stripes or smudgy areas
    - Perinephric stranding often seen
    - Usually results from ascending infection; if pyelonephritis is bilateral, consider possibility of hematogenous source
- **Pneumonia**

- Lower OR upper lobe pneumonia may present as right upper OR lower quadrant pain
- Scrutinize abdominal radiographs at lung bases
- CT scout view may reveal lung base pneumonia

- **Epiploic Appendagitis (Appendicitis Epiploica)**
  - Hyperdense ring surrounding fatty nodule
  - No bowel obstruction
- **Pelvic Inflammatory Disease**
  - Even at younger ages: Consider abuse; recommend skeletal survey if indicated
  - US: Superior for earlier findings such as tubal inflammation
  - CT: Nonspecific pelvic inflammatory changes
  - Either CT or US may show tubo-ovarian abscess
- **Ovarian Torsion**
  - Obvious size/volume discrepancy between ovaries virtually always present
    - In postmenarchal patient, torsed ovarian volume often > 20 mL
    - In premenarchal patient, ovarian volumes markedly discrepant but torsed ovarian volume may be < 20 mL
  - US: Torsed ovary generally large, heterogeneous, predominantly hypoechoic
  - CT: Torsed ovary generally large, heterogeneous, predominantly low attenuation
  - Pitfall: Demonstration of blood flow by US may confound diagnosis due to intermittent torsion or multiplicity of blood supply to ovaries
- **Ectopic Pregnancy**
  - Extremely uncommon to rare in teenager
  - Hemorrhage and blood products in peritoneum often seen with rupture
  - US: May be thick-walled cystic structure or solid heterogeneous mass
- **Meckel Diverticulum**
  - Many nonspecific imaging presentations
    - Small bowel obstruction with normal appendix with no prior surgery
    - Intussusception (consider underlying lesion such as Meckel diverticulum, polyp, or adenopathy if intussusception occurs at atypical age or is irreducible)
    - Lower GI bleeding
- **Typhlitis**
  - Thickened bowel wall
  - Well seen on radiograph; CT to confirm and determine extent
  - Pitfall: Distended bowel with fluid stool and air bubbles against bowel wall can mimic pneumatosis, may require follow-up exam to confirm or exclude diagnosis

Helpful Clues for Rare Diagnoses

- **Tuberculosis**
  - Suspect based on patient information specifics, such as living in endemic areas or prior history

Appendicitis

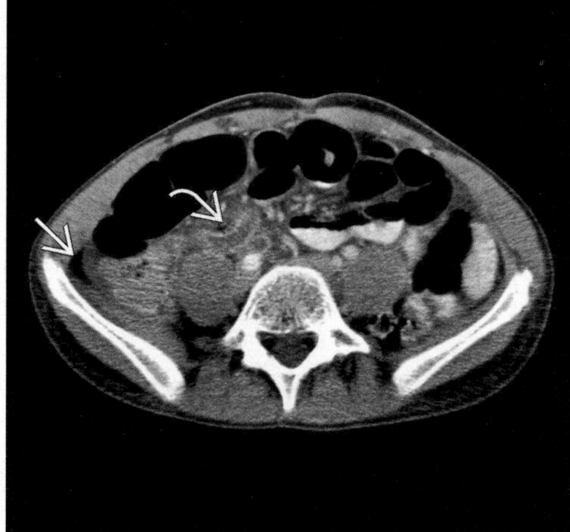

Axial CECT shows a dilated and hyperemic appendix ➔ measuring 11 mm in diameter. There is also a small amount of free intraperitoneal fluid ➔.

Appendicitis

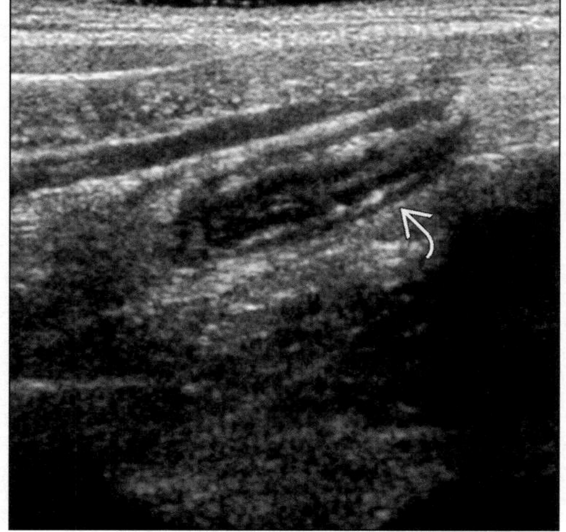

Longitudinal ultrasound shows a blind-ending tubular structure ➔ with surrounding inflammatory changes.

RIGHT LOWER QUADRANT PAIN

*(**Left**) Transverse US shows a dilated appendix (calipers), which was noncompressible and corresponded to the patient's site of pain. (**Right**) Longitudinal ultrasound shows the base of the appendix ➔ that still appeared totally normal, a pitfall in this diagnosis. Visualization of the tip of the appendix is important in excluding appendicitis. This 8-year-old girl had intraoperatively confirmed perforated tip appendicitis. Note the adjacent lymph node ⇨.*

Appendicitis

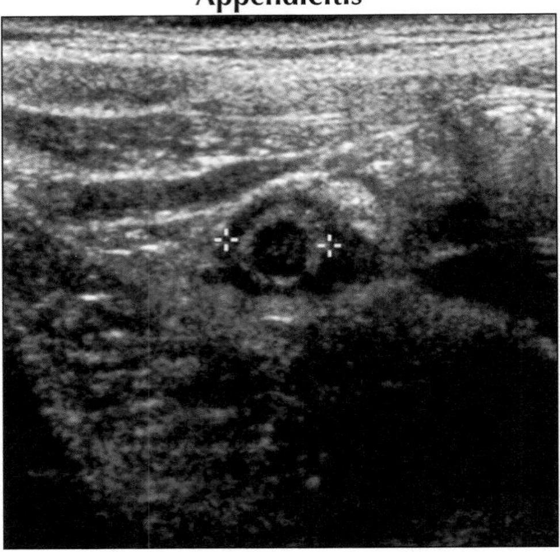

Appendicitis

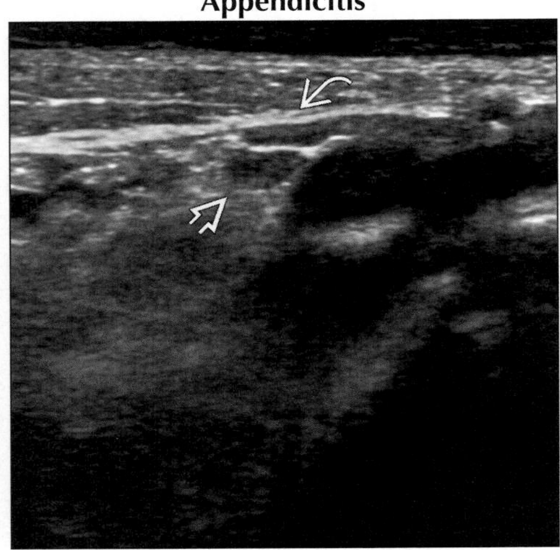

*(**Left**) Longitudinal ultrasound shows an asymmetrically enlarged, echogenic, right ovary ➔ in the same 8 year old with tip appendicitis. Blood flow to the ovary was normal. Intraoperatively, the adnexa were found to be inflamed. (**Right**) Axial CECT shows right lower quadrant bowel wall thickening ➔. Compare to the left lower quadrant ↪, which shows normal bowel wall thickness. This teenage girl's stool culture was positive for Salmonella.*

Appendicitis

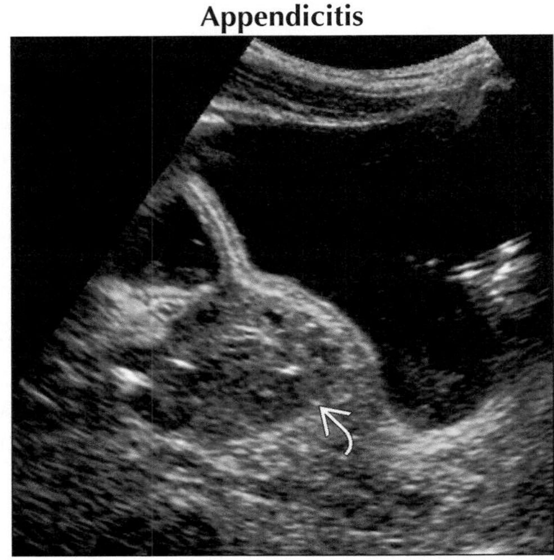

Enteritis

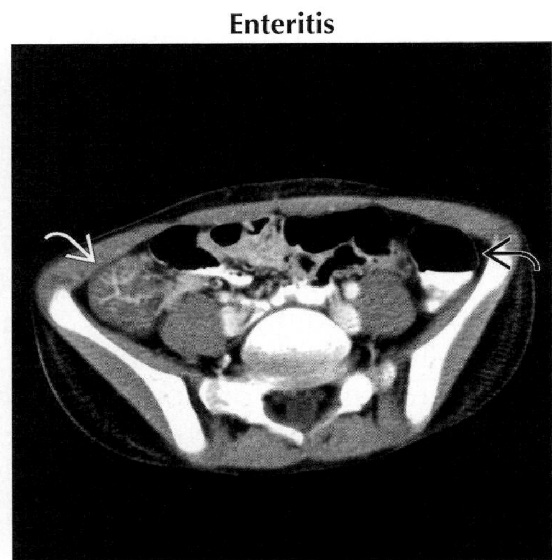

*(**Left**) Axial CECT shows marked bowel wall thickening and fluid and inflammatory change in the right lower quadrant in the region of the cecum ➔. This 17-year-old male patient was originally thought to have perforated appendicitis. (**Right**) Axial CECT shows an inferior image from the same 17 year old. Perirectal inflammatory changes have organized into an abscess ➔, a finding that should raise suspicion for Crohn disease, particularly in this location.*

Crohn Disease

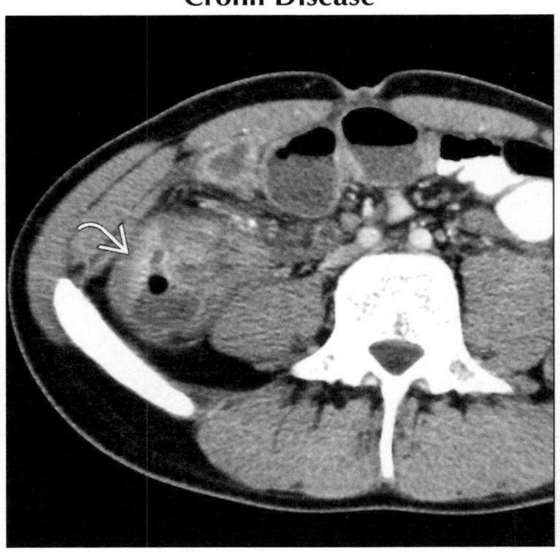

Crohn Disease

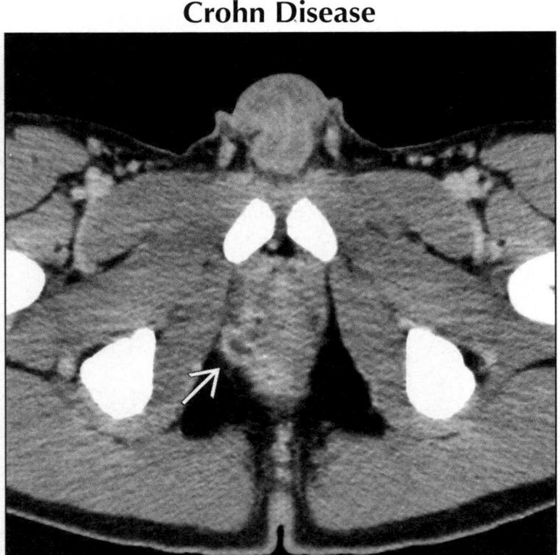

Crohn Disease

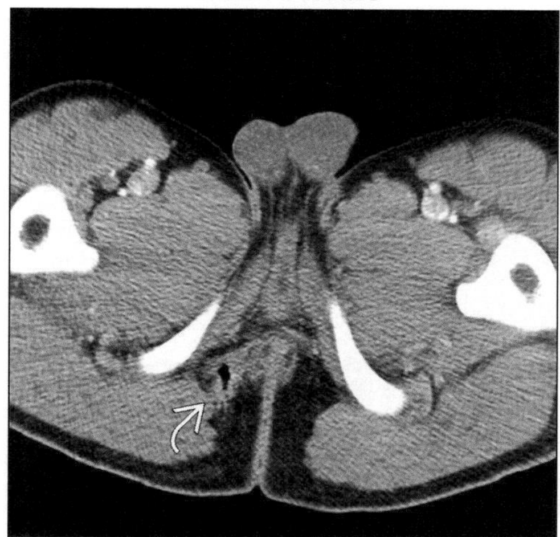

Crohn Disease

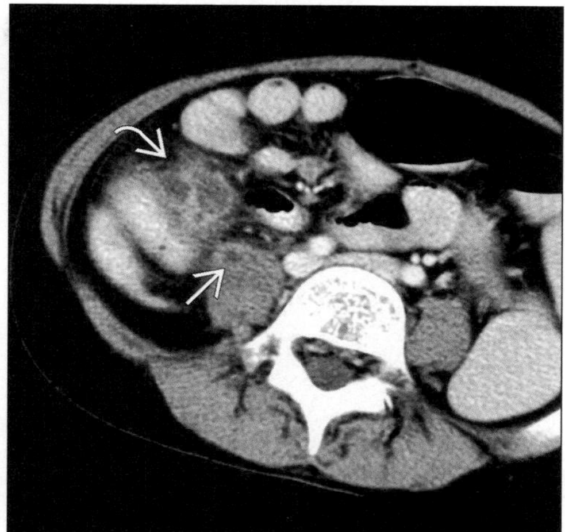

(Left) *Axial CECT 4 months later shows progression of the same perirectal abscess ➢. It fistulized extensively, from the perirectal region to the medial gluteal skin surface. If Crohn is suspected, consider extending imaging caudally to exclude abscess or fistula.* ***(Right)*** *Axial CECT shows a small right psoas intramuscular abscess ➔ adjacent to the right lower quadrant inflammatory change related to Crohn disease ➢ in this patient.*

Mesenteric Adenitis

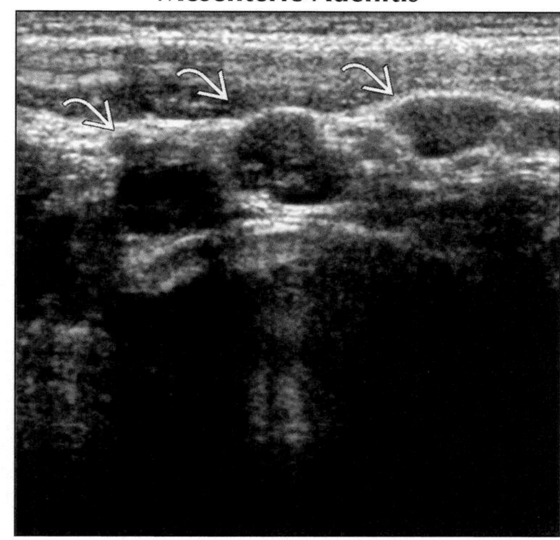

Renal/Ureteral Calculus, Obstructing

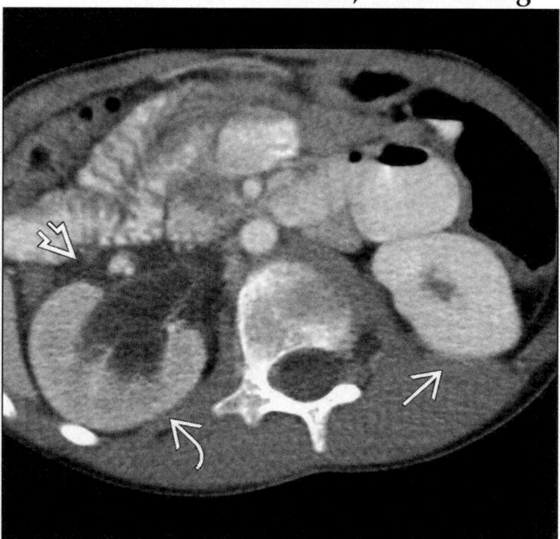

(Left) *Axial ultrasound shows a cluster of lymph nodes ➢ in the right lower quadrant. This qualifies as mesenteric adenitis, with more than 3 lymph nodes with ≥ 5 mm short axis diameter.* ***(Right)*** *Axial CECT shows an obstructed, enlarged right kidney with delayed parenchymal enhancement ➢ relative to the left kidney ➔. Notice collecting system dilation and perinephric fluid ⇨. A 1 cm mid-ureteral calculus (not shown) was identified on this study.*

Pyelonephritis

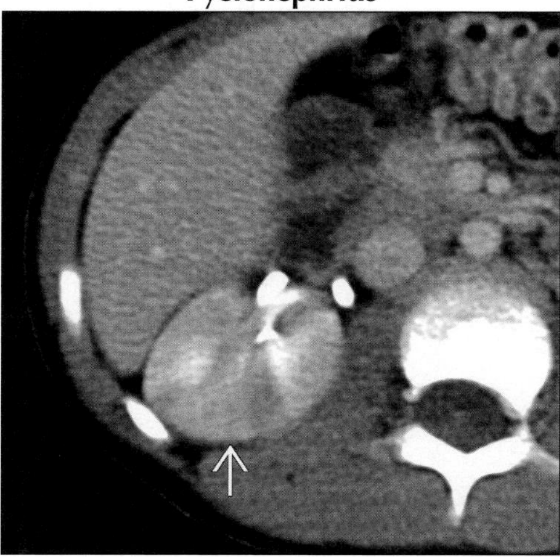

Pyelonephritis

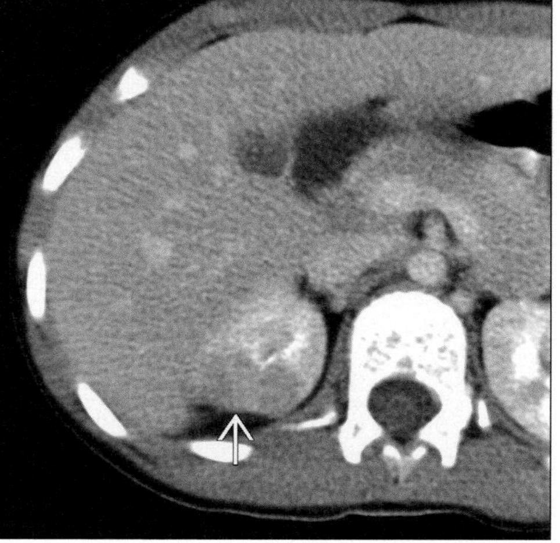

(Left) *Axial CECT shows an example of the striped appearance of the "striated nephrogram" ➔ commonly seen with acute pyelonephritis. No abscess or perinephric fluid was detected on this study.* ***(Right)*** *Axial CECT in the same patient shows an ill-defined peripheral mass-like region of diminished attenuation ➔ within the lower pole of the right kidney. No intrarenal abscess was found.*

RIGHT LOWER QUADRANT PAIN

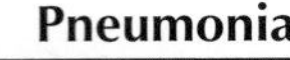

(**Left**) *Frontal radiograph shows an oval opacity at the medial right lung base. This was a right lower lobe pneumonia in a child who presented with abdominal pain.* (**Right**) *Axial CECT shows a torsed epiploic appendage that appears as a rounded, ring-shaped, fat-containing structure in the right lower quadrant, surrounded by mild hazy inflammatory stranding. A normal appendix (not shown) was also seen.*

Pneumonia

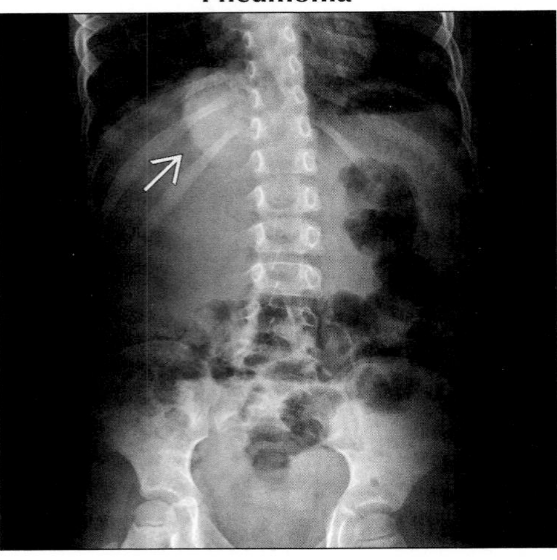

Epiploic Appendagitis (Appendicitis Epiploica)

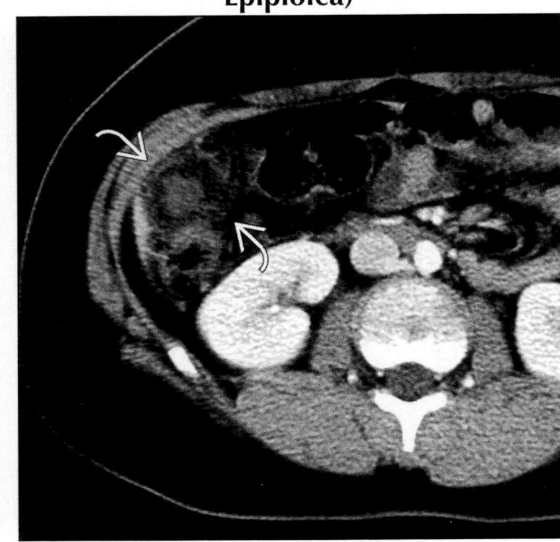

(**Left**) *Transverse ultrasound shows an extensive complex phlegmon composed of thick-walled cystic areas alternating with solid areas, consistent with a tuboovarian abscess. The cervical cultures were positive for gonorrhea and chlamydia in this 17 yo.* (**Right**) *Axial CECT shows an inflamed, edematous uterus surrounded by fluid. The left fallopian tube is thickened and hyperemic. A portion of the posterior cul-de-sac abscess is also seen.*

Pelvic Inflammatory Disease

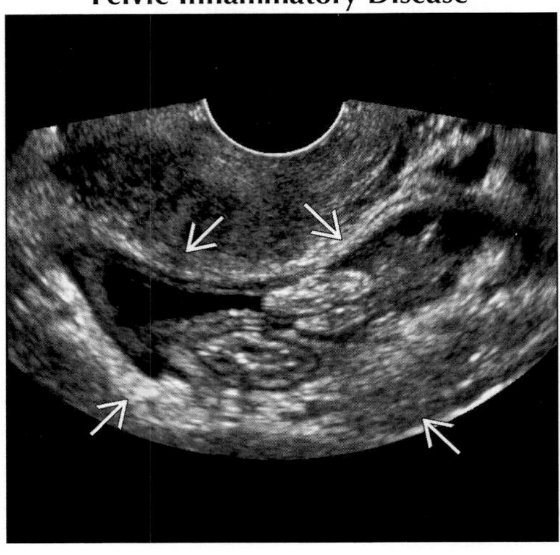

Pelvic Inflammatory Disease

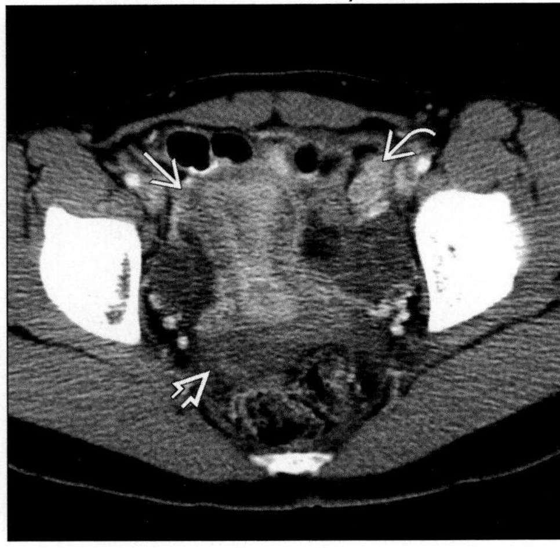

(**Left**) *Longitudinal ultrasound shows an enlarged right ovary with scattered peripheral follicles in this 12 year old complaining of pain for 1 day. No blood flow was seen on Doppler. A torsed, infarcted ovary and tube were removed at surgery.* (**Right**) *Transverse transvaginal ultrasound shows the thick-walled gestational sac as well as a large, heterogeneous, predominantly hypoechoic acute hematoma in the cul-de-sac.*

Ovarian Torsion

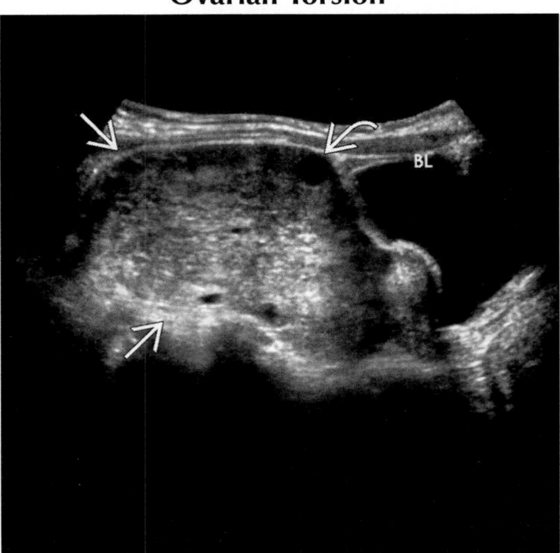

Ectopic Pregnancy

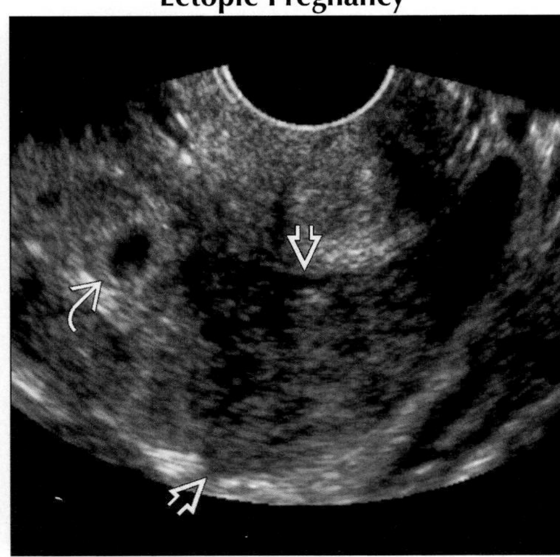

Meckel Diverticulum

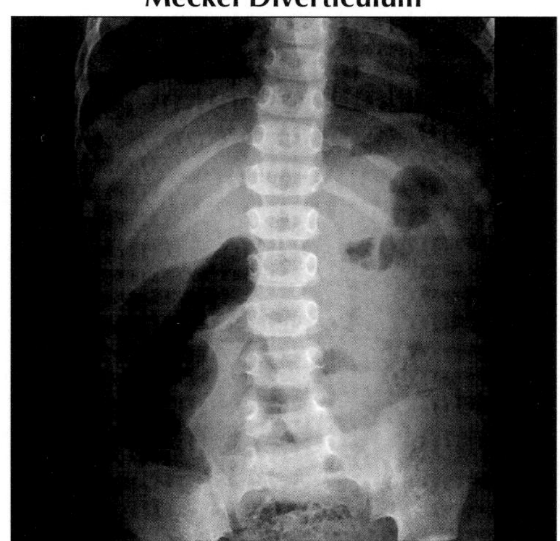

Meckel Diverticulum

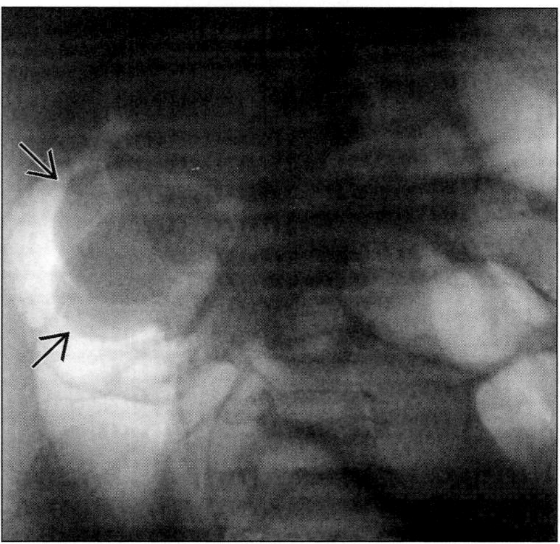

*(**Left**) Frontal radiograph shows a nonspecific bowel gas pattern. Though it is not frankly obstructive in appearance, there are abnormally distended loops of bowel in the right mid-abdomen. (**Right**) Frontal fluoroscopic spot radiograph shows a persistent, lobulated, soft tissue mass ⇒ preventing successful air reduction of an ileocolic intussusception. Intraoperatively, Meckel diverticulum was identified as the lead point.*

Meckel Diverticulum

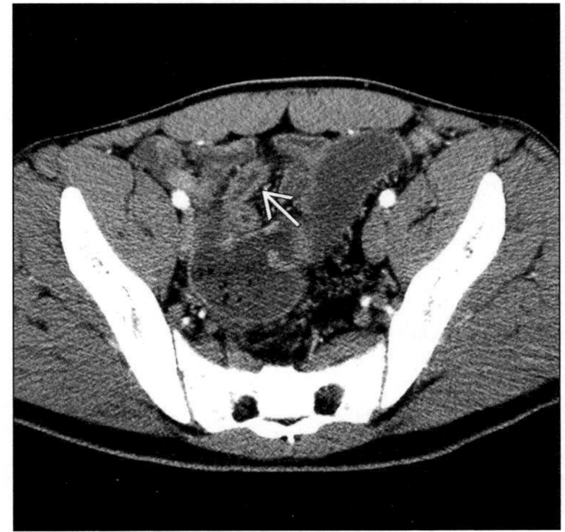

Meckel Diverticulum

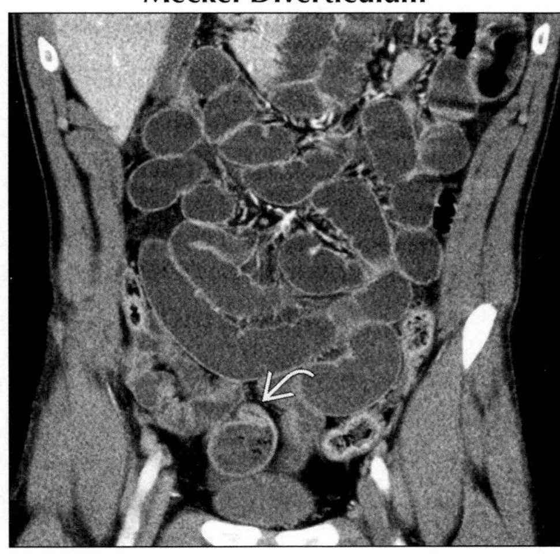

*(**Left**) Axial CECT shows a blind-ending tubular structure with thickened, hyperemic walls ➡ in the right lower quadrant. A normal appendix, not shown here, was also present. A Meckel diverticulum was identified at surgery. (**Right**) Coronal CECT shows the same Meckel diverticulum ↪. These are often difficult to identify prospectively. Coronal reformatted images are sometimes helpful.*

Typhlitis

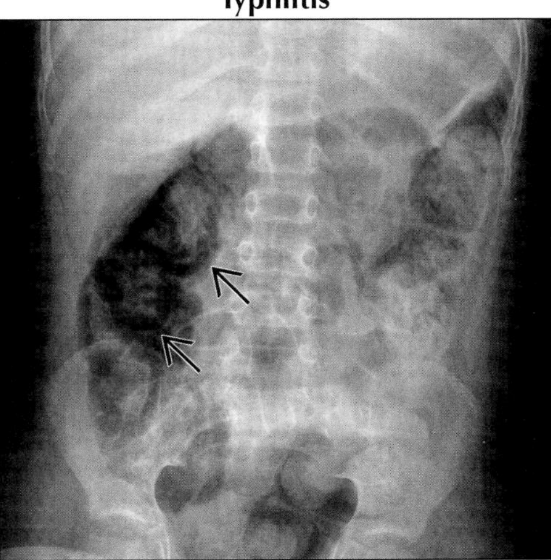

Typhlitis

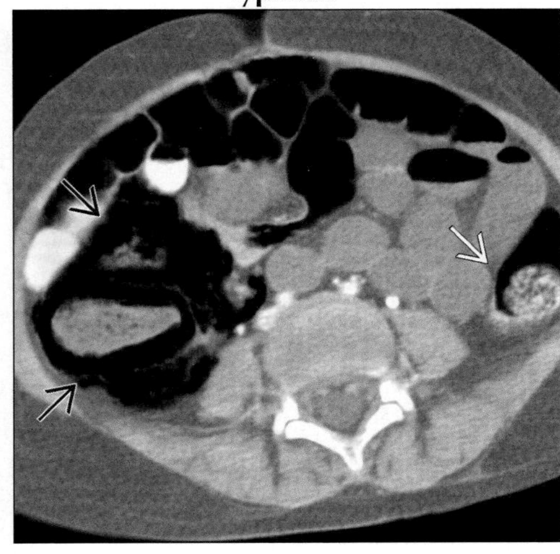

*(**Left**) Frontal radiograph shows extensive pneumatosis involving the ascending colon ⇒ in this 7-year-old child with relapsed ALL. (**Right**) Axial CECT shows air distributed circumferentially within the wall of the ascending colon ⇒, consistent with pneumatosis in this 7-year-old child with relapsed leukemia. Compare this with the normal appearance of the descending colon wall ➡. No bowel wall thickening, abscess, or ascites was detected in this child.*

EXTRINSIC DEFECTS ON ESOPHAGUS

DIFFERENTIAL DIAGNOSIS

Common
- Aortic Arch
- Left Mainstem Bronchus
- Left Atrium

Less Common
- Right Arch with Aberrant Left Subclavian Artery
- Left Aortic Arch with Aberrant Right Subclavian Artery
- Double Aortic Arch

Rare but Important
- Pulmonary Sling
- Bronchogenic Cyst
- Gastrointestinal Duplication Cysts

ESSENTIAL INFORMATION

Key Differential Diagnosis Issues
- Children may present with stridor due to impingement on trachea
- Chest radiograph
  - 1st step in evaluation of stridor
  - Evaluate position and contour of trachea
    - Is there a right or left aortic arch?
    - Is there symmetry in lung aeration?
- UGI
  - Delineates extrinsic impressions on esophagus contour
- CTA
  - Best for evaluation of vascular anatomy

Helpful Clues for Common Diagnoses
- **Aortic Arch**
  - Upper GI
    - Smooth crescentic impression upon proximal esophagus is best visualized on frontal projection
    - Extrinsic impression correlates to position of right/left aortic arch on plain film
- **Left Mainstem Bronchus**
  - Upper GI
    - Smooth tubular impression on mid-esophagus just below aortic arch
    - Frontal projection: Impression courses in oblique manner, mirroring course of left mainstem bronchus
    - Lateral projection: Smooth crescentic impression on anterior esophagus just below level of aortic arch
- **Left Atrium**
  - Upper GI
    - Large, smooth, crescentic impression on anterior aspect of lower esophagus
    - Best visualized on lateral view

Helpful Clues for Less Common Diagnoses
- **Right Arch with Aberrant Left Subclavian Artery**
  - Most common anomaly of aortic arch
  - Ligamentum arteriosum completes vascular ring
    - May compress trachea
  - Symptomatic (stridor) in 5% of cases
  - Conventional radiograph
    - Right aortic arch deviates trachea to left
    - Lateral view: Posterior impression caused by aberrant subclavian artery upon esophagus/trachea
  - Upper GI
    - Frontal view: Extrinsic defect upon proximal esophagus that courses from right inferior to left superior
    - Lateral view: Extrinsic defect upon posterior aspect of proximal esophagus
  - CT angiogram
    - Dilatation of origin of aberrant subclavian artery (diverticulum of Kommerell) in 60% of cases
    - Evaluate for compression upon trachea
- **Left Aortic Arch with Aberrant Right Subclavian Artery**
  - Mirrors anatomy of right arch with aberrant left subclavian artery
  - Aberrant subclavian artery courses from left inferior to right superior
  - Rarely symptomatic
- **Double Aortic Arch**
  - Plain film findings
    - Trachea may have straight midline position
  - Upper GI
    - Smooth bilateral indentations upon upper esophagus on frontal view
    - Right arch is most often larger and more cranial in orientation
    - Lateral view will show smooth indentation upon posterior proximal esophagus

- CT angiogram
  - Complete vascular ring that encircles trachea and esophagus
  - Right arch is dominant with descending left aorta in 75% of cases
  - Each arch gives off separate anterior carotid artery with posterior subclavian artery, "4 vessel" sign

Helpful Clues for Rare Diagnoses

- **Pulmonary Sling**
  - Plain film
    - Asymmetric hyperinflation of lungs (right > left)
    - Lateral chest radiograph: Round soft tissue density positioned between trachea and esophagus
  - Upper GI
    - Only vascular ring with smooth indentation upon anterior/mid-esophagus
  - CT angiogram
    - Left pulmonary artery arises from proximal right pulmonary artery
    - Left pulmonary artery crosses between trachea and esophagus
    - May be associated with complete tracheal rings
    - In tracheal rings, trachea will have round instead of oval configuration
- **Bronchogenic Cyst**
  - Plain film
    - Well-defined, soft tissue mass predominantly mediastinal (paratracheal, carinal, or hilar region)
    - Pulmonary involvement usually restricted to medial 1/3 of lung
    - May have mass effect on trachea, causing air-trapping
  - Upper GI
    - May find incidental small external impression on esophagus
  - CT
    - Attenuation varies with composition of cyst
  - MR
    - Typically hyperintense T2 signal
- **Gastrointestinal Duplication Cysts**
  - ~ 18% of duplication cysts are associated with esophagus
  - More common on right side than left side
  - Plain film
    - Well-defined soft tissue mass
  - Ultrasound shows classic appearance, including
    - Echogenic inner mucosal layer
    - Hypoechoic muscular layer
    - Echogenic outer serosal layer

Aortic Arch

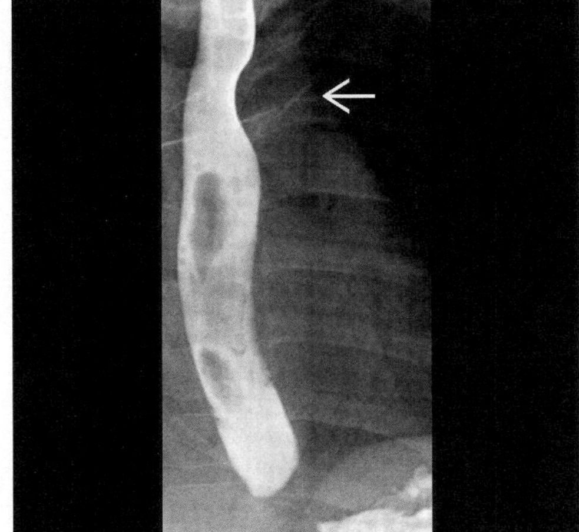

Frontal upper GI demonstrates a smooth extrinsic impression ➔ on the proximal left esophagus. This extrinsic impression correlated with the left arch on chest radiograph (not shown).

Left Mainstem Bronchus

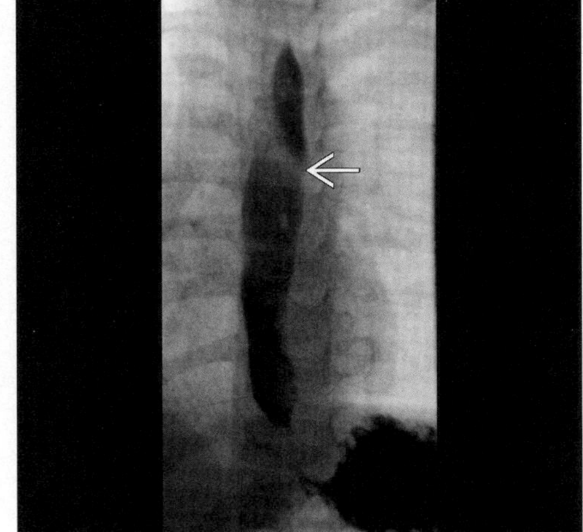

Frontal upper GI demonstrates an oblique tubular impression ➔ on the esophagus by the left mainstem bronchus. This impression is located below the aortic arch.

EXTRINSIC DEFECTS ON ESOPHAGUS

*(**Left**) Lateral upper GI demonstrates a smooth crescentic impression on the anterior esophagus ➡. This impression is below the level of the aortic arch and above the impression by the left atrium. (**Right**) Lateral upper GI demonstrates a smooth extrinsic impression on the anterior aspect of the distal esophagus ➡. This impression is caudal to the impression made by the left mainstem bronchus ↪.*

Left Mainstem Bronchus

Left Atrium

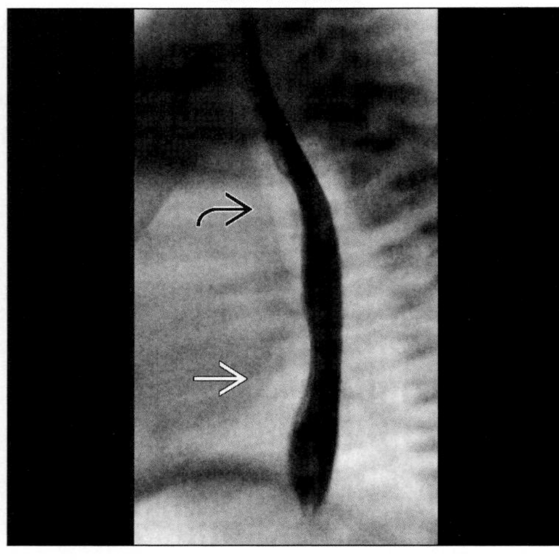

*(**Left**) Lateral upper GI demonstrates an aberrant left subclavian artery crossing posterior to the esophagus →. This is only symptomatic in a minority of children; 5% can be symptomatic. The ligamentum arteriosum completes the ring. (**Right**) Axial CECT demonstrates a right aortic arch ➡. The aberrant left subclavian artery courses posterior to the esophagus ↪.*

Right Arch with Aberrant Left Subclavian Artery

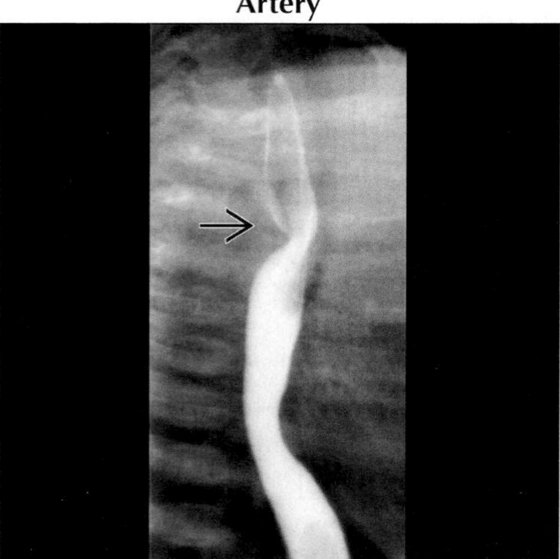

Right Arch with Aberrant Left Subclavian Artery

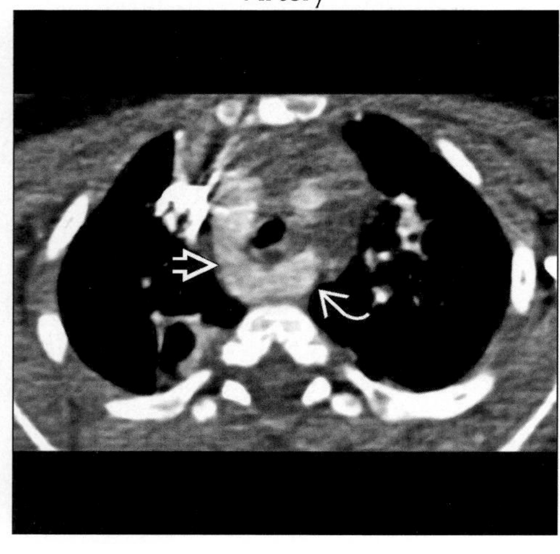

*(**Left**) Lateral radiograph demonstrates mass effect on the posterior aspect of the tracheal air column ↪. (**Right**) Axial CECT demonstrates a left arch ➡. The aberrant right subclavian artery ↪ courses posterior to the esophagus.*

Left Aortic Arch with Aberrant Right Subclavian Artery

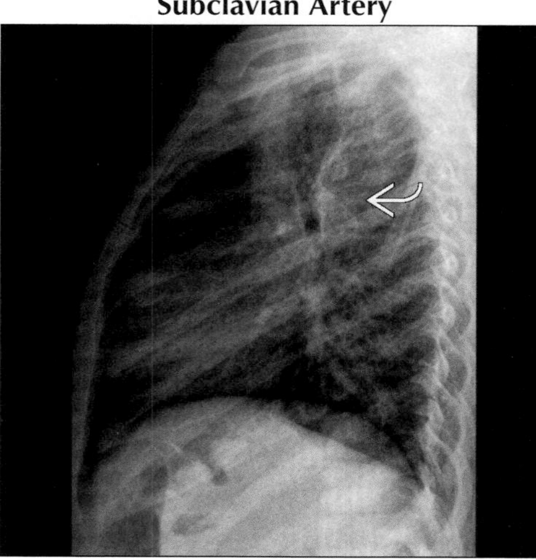

Left Aortic Arch with Aberrant Right Subclavian Artery

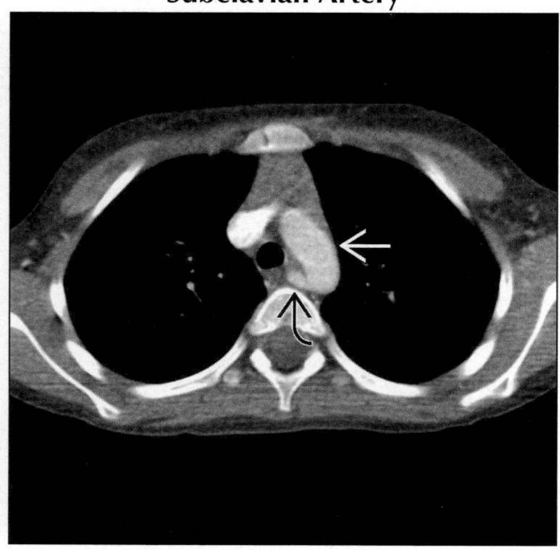

Double Aortic Arch

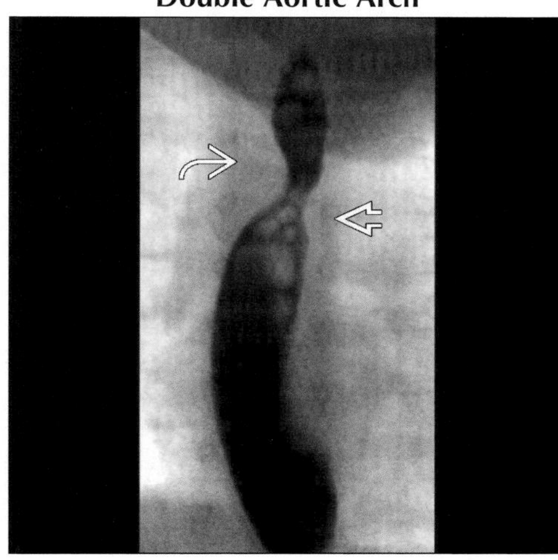

Double Aortic Arch

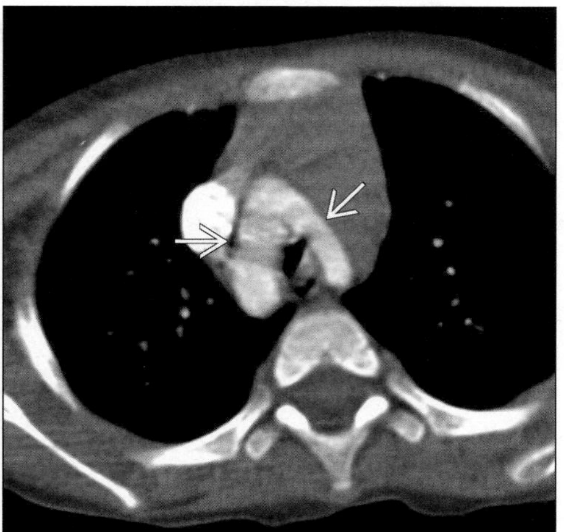

(Left) *Frontal upper GI demonstrates the extrinsic defect by the right arch to be dominant and higher in position ➔. The extrinsic defect by the left arch is smaller and more inferior in position ➔. These findings are typical for a double aortic arch.* ***(Right)*** *Axial CECT demonstrates 2 arches ➔ that completely encircle the trachea and esophagus.*

Pulmonary Sling

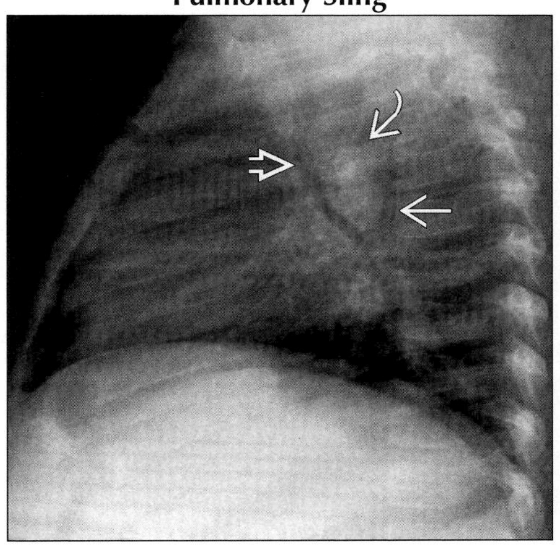

Pulmonary Sling

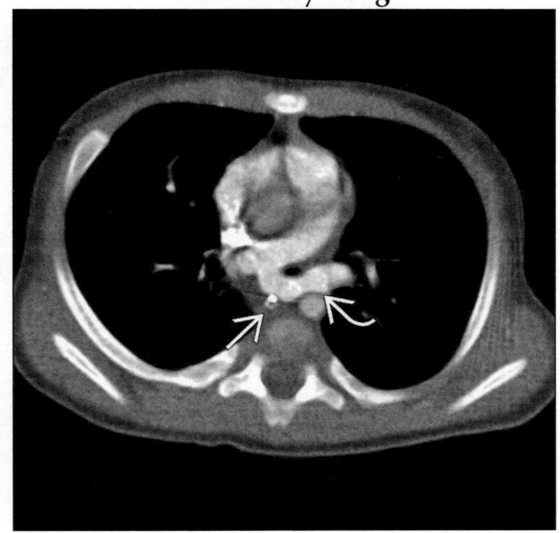

(Left) *Lateral radiograph demonstrates an aberrant left pulmonary artery ➔ coursing between the trachea ➔ and the esophagus ➔.* ***(Right)*** *Axial CECT demonstrates an aberrant left subclavian artery ➔ coursing anterior to the esophagus ➔ and posterior to the trachea.*

Bronchogenic Cyst

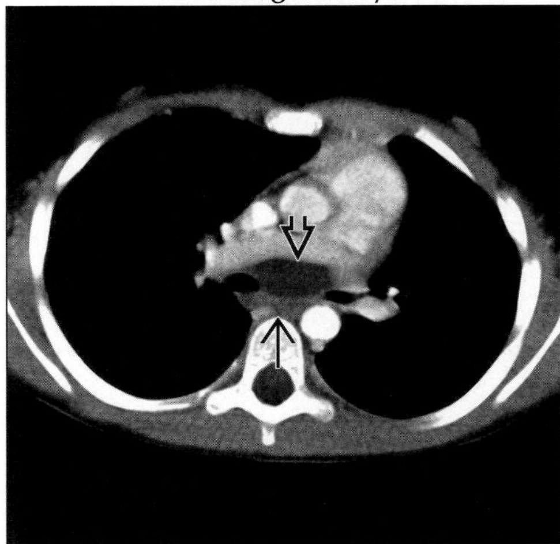

Gastrointestinal Duplication Cysts

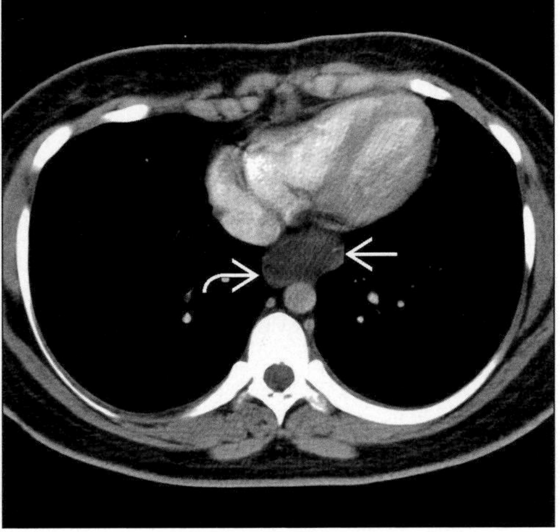

(Left) *Axial CECT demonstrates a subcarinal bronchogenic cyst ➔. The cyst is equal to fluid in density. Its subcarinal position causes mass effect on the anterior aspect of the esophagus ➔.* ***(Right)*** *Axial CECT demonstrates a paraesophageal duplication cyst ➔. The cyst causes mass effect on the left lower esophagus ➔.*

DILATED STOMACH

DIFFERENTIAL DIAGNOSIS

Common
- Aerophagia
- Hypertrophic Pyloric Stenosis
- Midgut Volvulus

Less Common
- Duodenal Hematoma
- Duodenal Atresia or Stenosis
- Bezoar
- Ileus

Rare but Important
- Gastric Volvulus
- Gastrointestinal Duplication Cysts

ESSENTIAL INFORMATION

Key Differential Diagnosis Issues
- Abdominal obstructions should be divided between proximal and distal etiologies
- Dilated stomach is considered a proximal obstruction
- Plain film findings include
  - Air-filled, distended stomach; minimal to no distal bowel gas
  - Patient may present with nonbilious emesis
- Age of patient may help to narrow differential diagnosis
- Trauma history also help to limit different etiologies

Helpful Clues for Common Diagnoses
- **Aerophagia**
  - Swallowed air usually associated with crying
  - Most common cause for distended stomach in pediatric patients
  - Nonobstructive bowel gas pattern, with air distal to distended stomach
- **Hypertrophic Pyloric Stenosis**
  - Presents with nonbilious projectile vomiting
  - Age range is 2-12 weeks
  - Conventional radiographic findings
    - Air-filled distended stomach, excessive gastric motility ("caterpillar" sign), minimal to no distal bowel gas
  - Ultrasound findings
    - Preferred modality for diagnosis
    - Single wall thickness > 3.0 mm, channel length > 16 mm
    - No passage of fluids from stomach into duodenal bulb on cine images
    - **Note**: Spasm of gastric antrum mimics pyloric stenosis but does not persist on delayed images
- **Midgut Volvulus**
  - Surgical emergency
    - Twisting of small bowel about superior mesenteric artery can result in obstruction and ischemia/infarction

Helpful Clues for Less Common Diagnoses
- **Duodenal Hematoma**
  - Most common cause is blunt trauma to abdomen (i.e., handle bar injury)
    - Other etiologies include child abuse, biopsy, bleeding disorder, and Henoch-Schönlein purpura
  - Most commonly located in 2nd or 3rd portion of duodenum
  - Plain film may show air-filled distended stomach with minimal or no distal bowel gas
  - CT findings
    - Duodenal hematoma may be eccentric or circumferential with narrowing of bowel lumen
    - May be distention of stomach and proximal duodenum with minimal distal bowel gas
    - Acute hematoma is high in attenuation and decreases with time
    - Signs of perforation include extraluminal air, extraluminal contrast, and retroperitoneal fluid
- **Duodenal Atresia or Stenosis**
  - Conventional radiographic findings
    - Dilated stomach and duodenal bulb, "double bubble" sign
    - Duodenal atresia has no distal bowel gas (→ low probability for midgut volvulus in differential)
    - Duodenal stenosis has some degree of air in distal bowel (midgut volvulus cannot be excluded from differential)
  - Fluoroscopic findings
    - Upper GI is not often performed for duodenal atresia; plain film diagnosis

- Duodenal stenosis requires upper GI to confirm diagnosis and exclude midgut volvulus from differential
- **Bezoar**
  - Mottled-appearing filling defect in distended stomach
  - Bezoar is compliant and conforms to contour of stomach
  - Food debris may have similar mottled appearance
  - Upper GI may help to further delineate size and extent of bezoar
- **Ileus**
  - Postoperative, drugs, metabolic, etc.

Helpful Clues for Rare Diagnoses

- **Gastric Volvulus**
  - Organoaxial volvulus
    - Most common type of gastric volvulus
    - Rotation of stomach along longitudinal axis extending from cardia to pylorus
    - Stomach is dilated with minimal to no distal bowel gas
    - Greater curvature of stomach is situated more cranially than lesser curvature
    - Organoaxial volvulus may occur with hernia of stomach into thorax
    - Poor gastric emptying on fluoroscopic exam
  - Mesenteroaxial volvulus
    - Rotation of stomach along craniocaudal axis
    - Gastroesophageal junction is lower and further right than normal
    - Stomach usually demonstrates massive dilatation
    - Minimal to no distal bowel gas
    - Reversal of gastric antrum and cardia
    - Antrum is situated higher and further left than normal
    - 2 air-fluid levels on plain film, higher one is antrum and lower one is cardia
    - Poor emptying of stomach on fluoroscopic exam
    - Antrum may show beaking on upper GI study due to twisting
- **Gastrointestinal Duplication Cysts**
  - Duplication cysts can occur anywhere along GI tract
    - Jejunum/ileum (53%), esophagus (18%), colon (13%), stomach (7%), and duodenum (6%)
  - Gastric duplication cysts are usually associated with greater curvature of stomach as well as posterior gastric wall
  - Duodenal duplication cysts are usually associated with 2nd/3rd portion of duodenum
  - Classic duplication cysts demonstrate bowel signature on ultrasound
    - Inner echogenic mucosal layer
    - Middle hypoechoic muscular layer
    - Outer echogenic serosal layer

Aerophagia

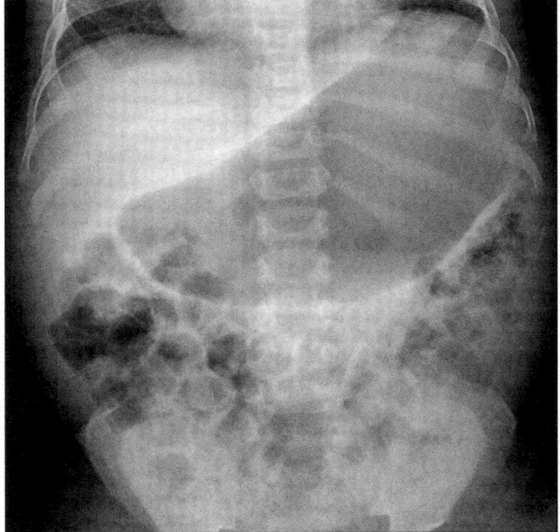

AP radiograph demonstrates an air-filled distended stomach. There is air distally in nondilated large and small bowel.

Hypertrophic Pyloric Stenosis

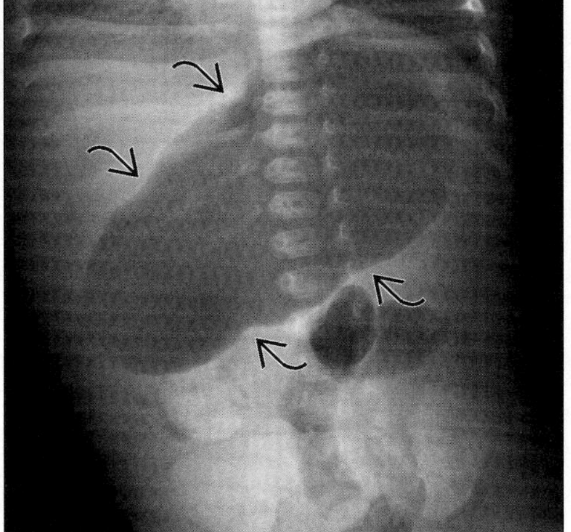

Frontal radiograph demonstrates a dilated stomach in a 4-week-old patient. There is also increased peristalsis against the thickened pylorus, creating a "caterpillar" stomach ➔.

DILATED STOMACH

(Left) and (Right) images:

Hypertrophic Pyloric Stenosis

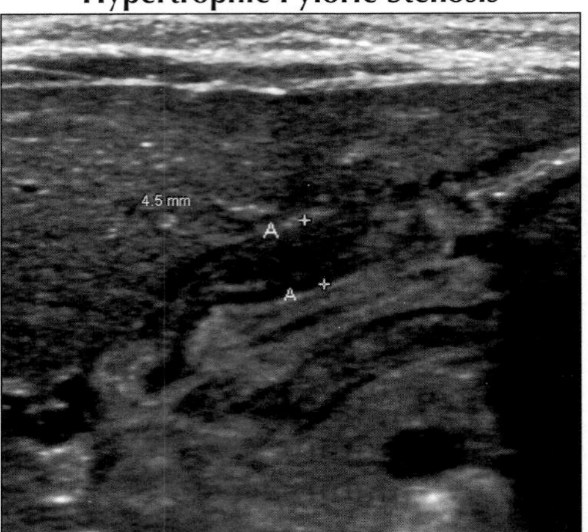

Hypertrophic Pyloric Stenosis

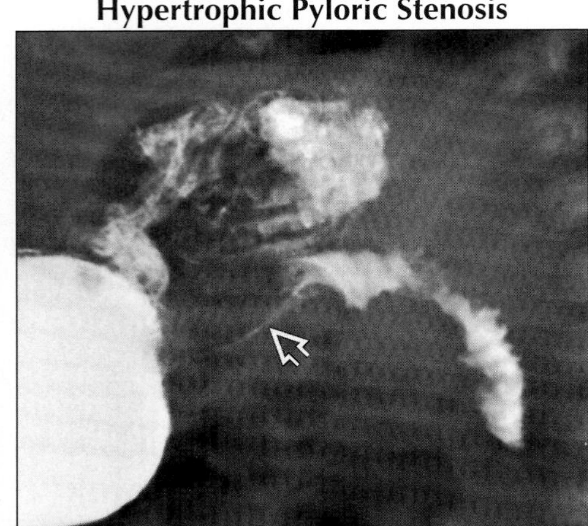

(Left) *Longitudinal oblique ultrasound demonstrates a thickened pyloric channel. The single wall thickness of the pyloric channel exceeds 3 mm. The pyloric channel is also elongated. Note the classic bowel signature, echogenic mucosa, and hypoechoic muscular layer.* ***(Right)*** *Oblique upper GI demonstrates a narrow and elongated pyloric channel . This is the classic "string" sign associated with hypertrophic pyloric stenosis.*

Midgut Volvulus

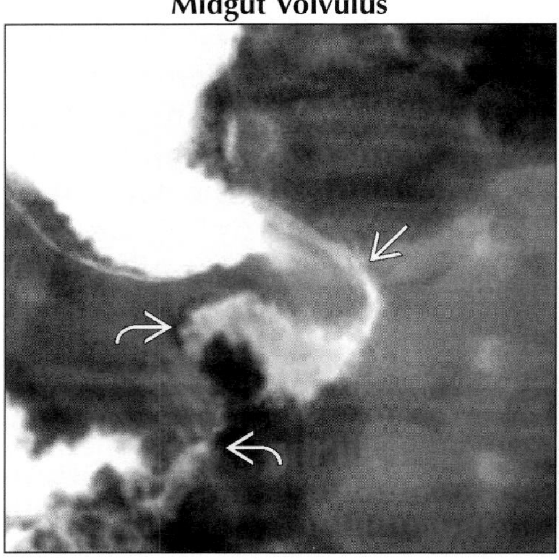

Duodenal Hematoma

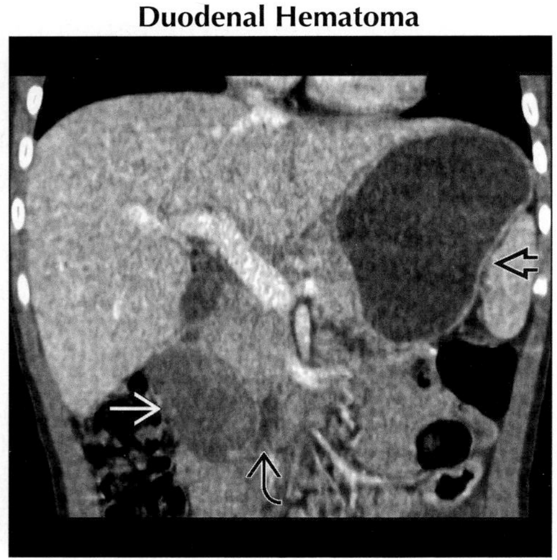

(Left) *Fluoroscopic spot radiograph shows an abnormally positioned duodenojejunal junction , with a corkscrew appearance of the proximal bowel .* ***(Right)*** *Coronal CECT demonstrates an eccentric duodenal hematoma with mass effect upon the lumen of the 2nd portion of the duodenum . The hematoma is subacute in nature, as shown by its mixed attenuation. Note the distended fluid-filled stomach .*

Duodenal Hematoma

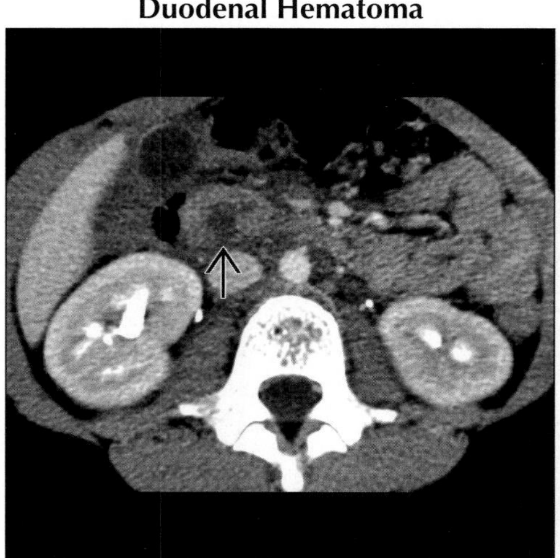

Duodenal Atresia or Stenosis

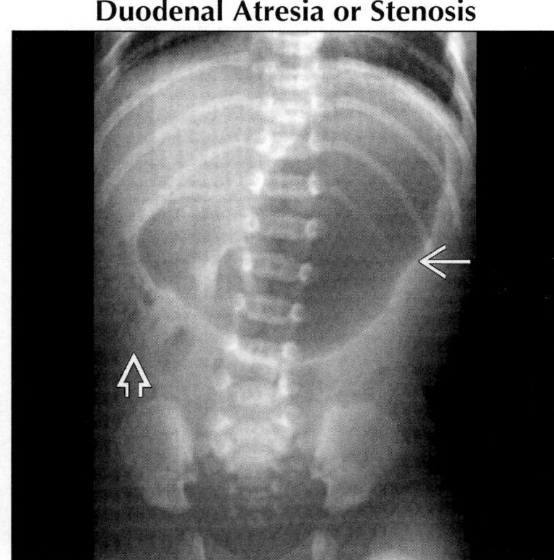

(Left) *Axial CECT demonstrates circumferential thickening of the 2nd portion of the duodenum after handle bar trauma to the abdomen. There is also a focal duodenal laceration .* ***(Right)*** *Coronal radiograph demonstrates a dilated stomach . There is minimal air in the proximal small bowel , which is suspicious for duodenal stenosis. An upper GI tract series was recommended.*

Duodenal Atresia or Stenosis

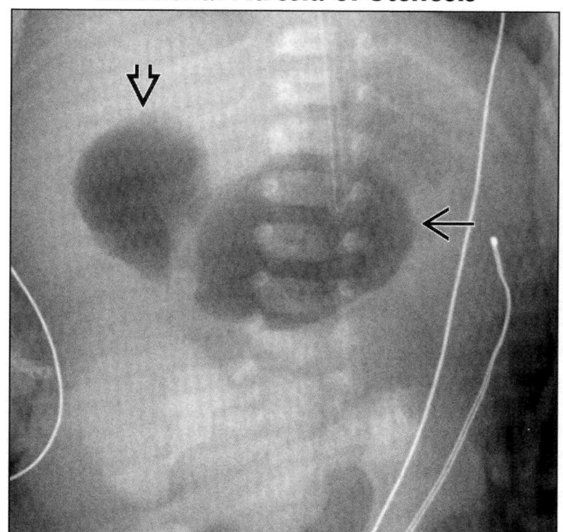

Bezoar

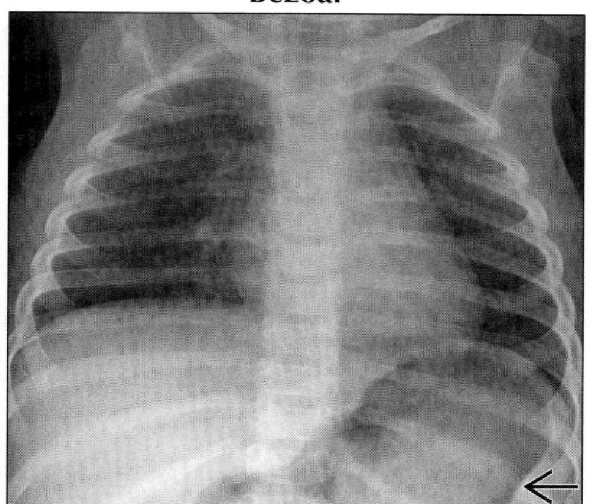

*(**Left**) Coronal radiograph demonstrates a distended stomach ⇨ and duodenal bulb ⇨. This represents the classic "double bubble" sign. There is no distal bowel gas, which is suspicious for duodenal atresia. Duodenal atresia is a plain film diagnosis, and an upper GI series is not usually performed. (**Right**) Frontal radiograph of the chest demonstrates an incidental mottled filling defect within the stomach, suspicious for a bezoar ⇨.*

Gastric Volvulus

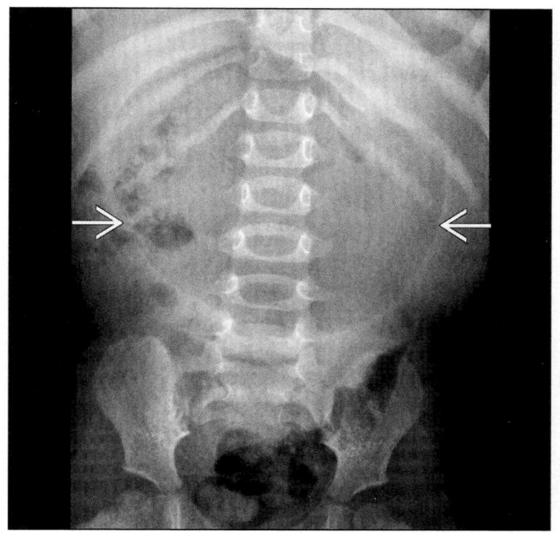

Gastric Volvulus

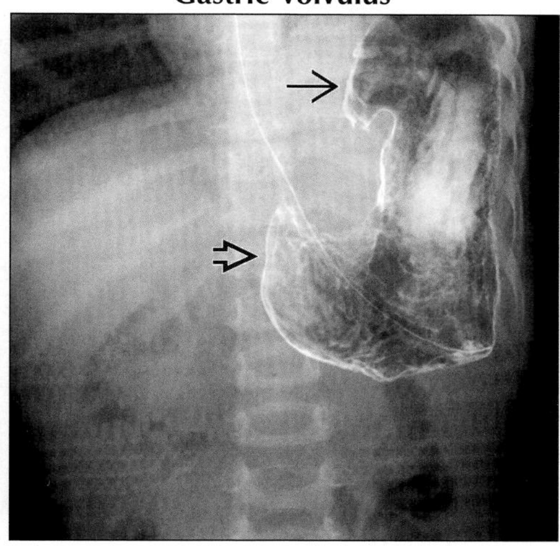

*(**Left**) Frontal radiograph shows a massively dilated stomach ⇨. This indicates minimal distal bowel gas. (**Right**) Frontal upper GI shows a mesenteroaxial gastric volvulus. The antrum of the stomach ⇨ is positioned more cranially and to the left than normal. The gastric antrum also demonstrates "beaking." The fundus of the stomach ⇨ is positioned more caudally and to the right than normal. No contrast progressed into the duodenum on upper GI series.*

Gastric Volvulus

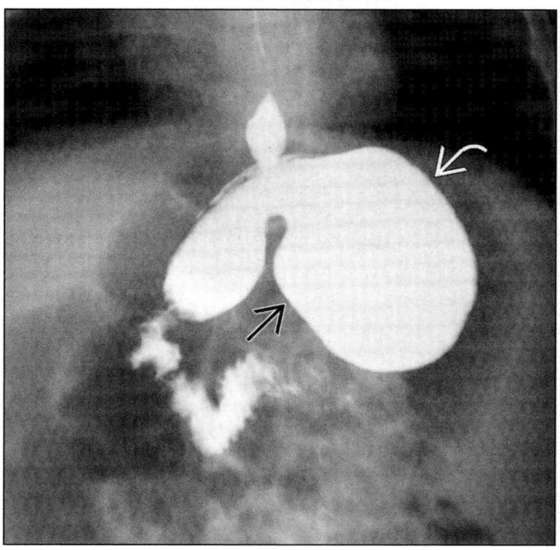

Gastrointestinal Duplication Cysts

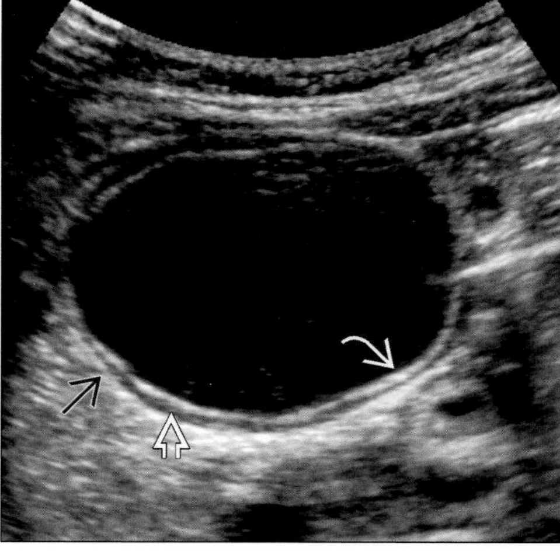

*(**Left**) AP fluoroscopy demonstrates organoaxial positioning of the stomach. The greater curvature ⇨ of the stomach is cranial relative to the lesser curvature ⇨. There is no obstruction on this UGI. (**Right**) Longitudinal ultrasound demonstrates the classic bowel signature: Inner echogenic mucosa ⇨, isoechoic muscular ⇨ layer, and outer echogenic serosa ⇨.*

DUODENAL OBSTRUCTION

DIFFERENTIAL DIAGNOSIS

Common
- Malrotation/Midgut Volvulus
- Duodenal Atresia
- Duodenal Stenosis/Web

Less Common
- Jejunal Atresia
- Superior Mesenteric Artery (SMA) Syndrome
- Duodenal Hematoma
- Gastrointestinal Duplication Cyst

Rare but Important
- Bezoar
- Lymphoma
- Annular Pancreas

ESSENTIAL INFORMATION

Key Differential Diagnosis Issues
- Differentiate between proximal (high) or distal (low) obstruction in neonates
  - High (proximal) obstruction
    - Malrotation/midgut volvulus
    - Duodenal atresia or stenosis
    - Duodenal web
    - Duodenal hematoma
    - Annular pancreas
    - Jejunal atresia (proximal portion)
    - Extrinsic compression from mass or cyst
  - Mid-level obstruction
    - Jejunal atresia
    - Extrinsic compression from mass or cyst
  - Low (distal) obstruction
    - Anorectal malformation/anal atresia
    - Hirschsprung disease
    - Meconium plug syndrome (small left colon syndrome)
    - Ileal atresia
    - Meconium ileus
    - Extrinsic compression from mass or cyst
- Duodenal obstruction falls into proximal (high) obstruction differential
- Conventional radiograph may show distention of stomach, duodenum, or a few proximal small bowel loops
- Midgut volvulus must be urgently excluded in patients presenting with bilious emesis
- UGI is initial radiographic exam for evaluation of proximal (high) obstruction

Helpful Clues for Common Diagnoses
- **Malrotation/Midgut Volvulus**
  - Malrotation: Abnormal fixation of duodenum to retroperitoneum; prone to twisting upon itself
  - Midgut volvulus: Twisting of malrotated bowel that may result in obstruction, ischemia, and bowel necrosis
    - Malrotation with midgut volvulus must be excluded in patients who present with bilious emesis
  - Radiographic findings range from normal abdominal x-ray to distended stomach and proximal duodenum
  - UGI is next step in work-up
    - Entire duodenal sweep must course through retroperitoneum on UGI lateral view
    - Duodenojejunal junction must be situated to left of spinal pedicle and at same level as duodenal bulb
  - **Note**: Volvulus may occur in normally rotated patients who have other bowel pathology, such as mass or cyst, adhesions, inspissated meconium, etc.
- **Duodenal Atresia/Stenosis/Web**
  - Accepted etiology is failure of canalization of lumen in utero rather than vascular insult (as with other atresias)
  - Distended, air-filled stomach and duodenum appear as "double bubble" sign
  - Distal bowel gas
    - Usually absent in duodenal atresia
    - Present in varying amounts in duodenal stenosis or web
  - Normal caliber colon on contrast enema (unless ileal atresia is present)
  - Associated with other anomalies
    - Down syndrome (25%)
    - Other GI anomalies, such as malrotation, pancreatic and biliary anomalies, Meckel diverticulum, other atresias, gastrointestinal duplications (25%)
    - Vertebral or rib anomalies (> 33%)
    - Congenital heart disease
    - Assess for VACTERL sequence anomalies

Helpful Clues for Less Common Diagnoses
- **Jejunal Atresia**
  - Few distended loops of bowel may appear as "triple bubble" sign

- Intrauterine vascular insult is commonly accepted cause
- Associated with other abnormalities
  - Malrotation/volvulus
  - Anterior abdominal wall defects
- Other, more distal atresias may be present; contrast enema should be performed
  - If colon caliber is normal, ileal atresia very unlikely
  - If there is microcolon, other distal (ileal) atresias are present

- **Superior Mesenteric Artery (SMA) Syndrome**
  - Often in older children with recent history of weight loss
  - 3rd portion of duodenum compressed by overlying superior mesenteric artery
  - Best diagnosed with upper GI
    - Proximal half of duodenum often mildly distended
    - Contrast material has difficulty passing beyond middle of 3rd portion of duodenum, sloshes back and forth
    - Contrast column halts at vertical linear extrinsic compression caused by SMA
    - Expect difficulty passing feeding tube beyond this point
- **Duodenal Hematoma**
  - Typically traumatic in nature
    - Handlebar injury, direct blow/punch
    - May result from endoscopy/biopsy
  - Variable appearance
    - Focal intramural bulge into lumen
    - Circumferential wall thickening narrowing lumen
- **Gastrointestinal Duplication Cyst**
  - Typically round or tubular, highly variable size, commonly present with obstruction
    - US: Contents may be anechoic, hypoechoic, or complex with debris; may demonstrate bowel wall layers
    - CT: Low-attenuation contents
  - Most do not communicate with true bowel lumen

Helpful Clues for Rare Diagnoses

- **Bezoar**
  - Foreign body bezoar
    - Appearance is commonly swirled or mottled; depends on what patient has eaten (hair, soil/sand, plant matter, household products)
- **Lymphoma**
  - Nonspecific soft tissue mass
    - CT: Homogeneous or mildly heterogeneous, low to intermediate attenuation
    - US: Homogeneous or mildly heterogeneous, hypoechoic
- **Annular Pancreas**
  - Usually seen in conjunction with other anomalies, such as duodenal web/stenosis

Malrotation/Midgut Volvulus

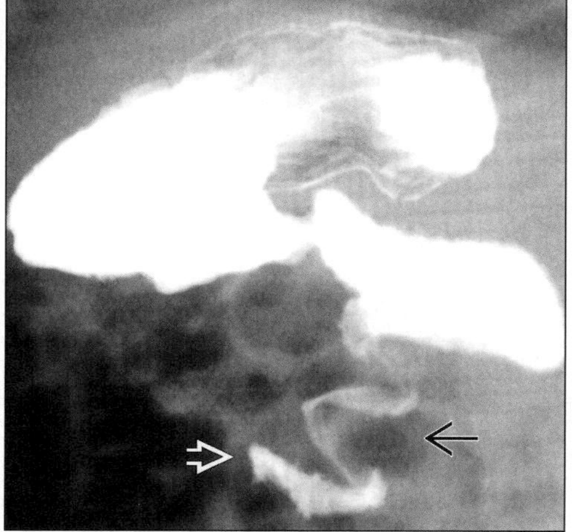

Lateral upper GI shows the "corkscrew" sign ➔ associated with midgut volvulus. There is abrupt termination of contrast material at the point of the volvulus ➔.

Malrotation/Midgut Volvulus

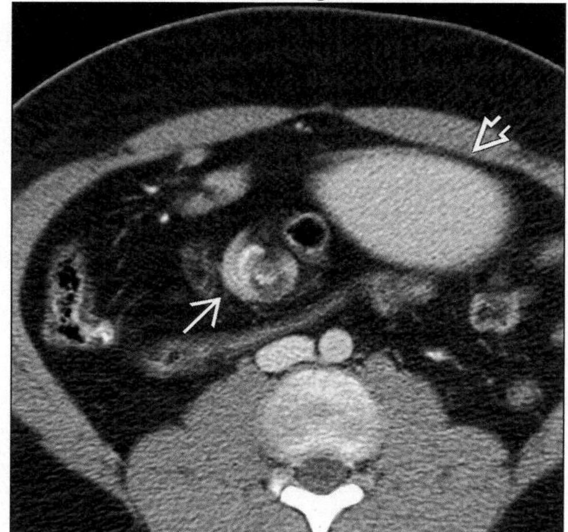

Axial CECT shows the swirled appearance of twisted mesenteric vessels ➔ in a teenager who presented with nonspecific abdominal pain. Note the dilated loop of contrast-filled obstructed bowel located proximally ➔.

DUODENAL OBSTRUCTION

*(**Left**) Axial CECT shows abnormally reversed positions of the mesenteric artery and vein. In this patient with midgut malrotation and volvulus, the mesenteric artery is on the right, and the mesenteric vein is on the left. (**Right**) Frontal radiograph shows a dilated stomach and duodenal bulb, together demonstrating the classic "double bubble" sign of duodenal atresia. Note that there is no distal bowel gas.*

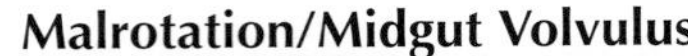

Malrotation/Midgut Volvulus

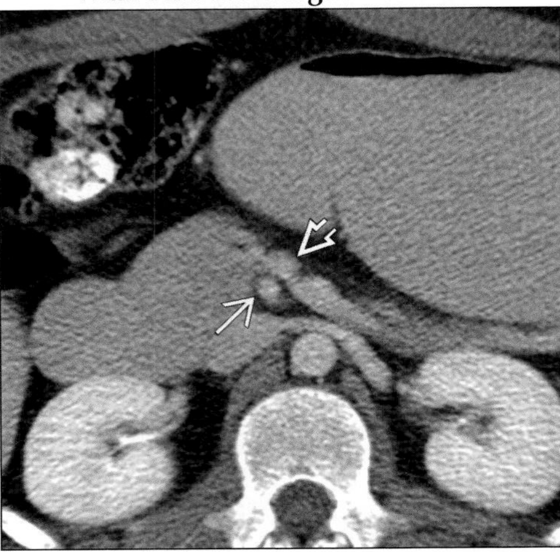

Duodenal Atresia

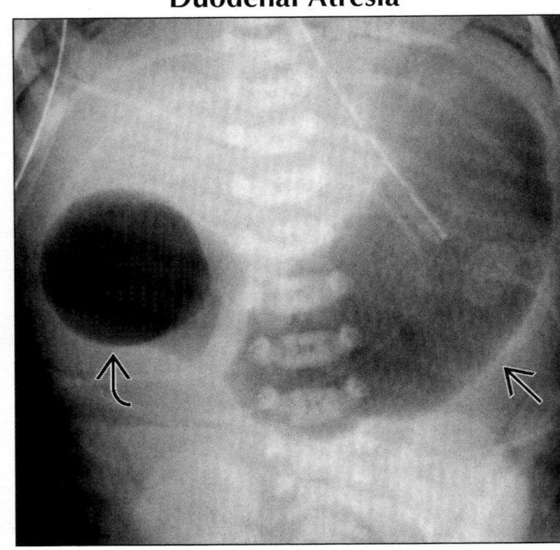

*(**Left**) Coronal T2WI MR shows a fetus with a dilated stomach and duodenum, consistent with duodenal atresia. There is subjectively increased amniotic fluid, common in a fetus with impaired swallowing. This child was known to have trisomy 21. (**Right**) Frontal radiograph shows the same infant at birth. Note the dilated stomach and duodenum, 11 pairs of ribs, and an enlarged heart due to congenital heart disease.*

Duodenal Atresia

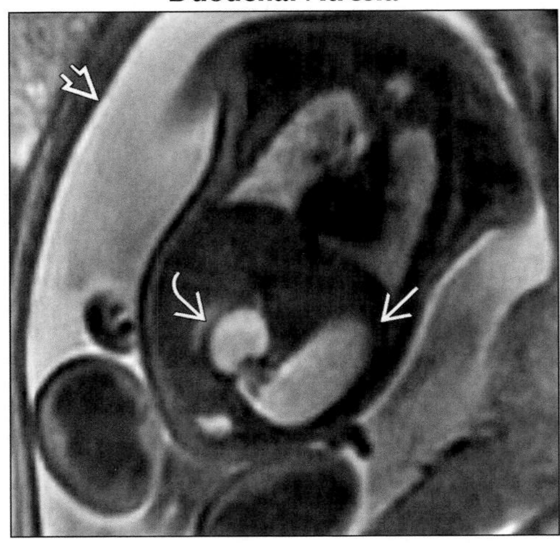

Duodenal Atresia

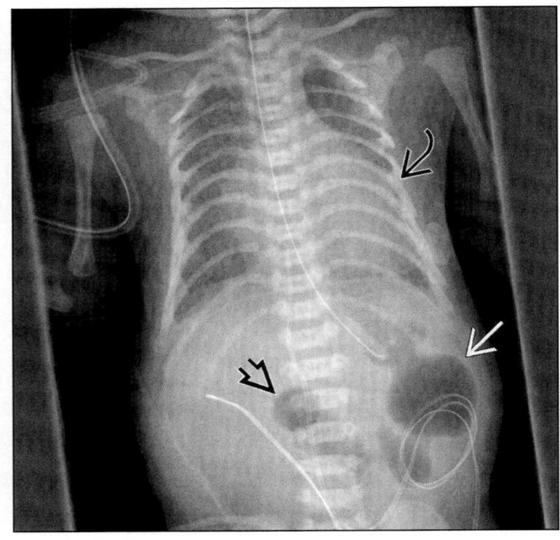

*(**Left**) Frontal fluoroscopic spot radiograph of an upper GI tract demonstrates that no contrast material passes beyond the duodenal bulb in this patient with duodenal atresia. (**Right**) Frontal radiograph shows a markedly dilated stomach and proximal duodenum in this 2-day-old infant without any other abnormalities.*

Duodenal Atresia

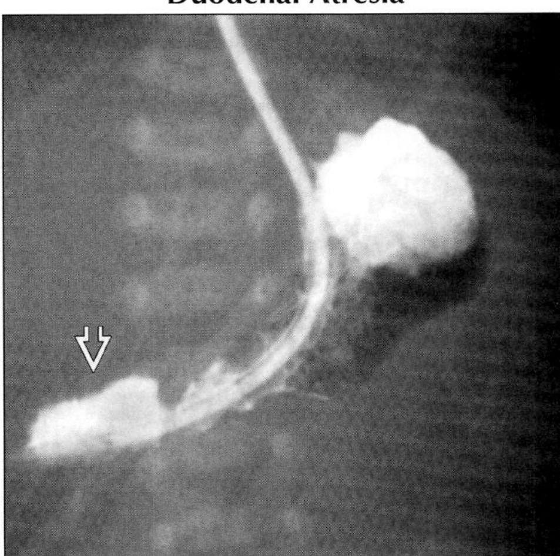

Duodenal Atresia

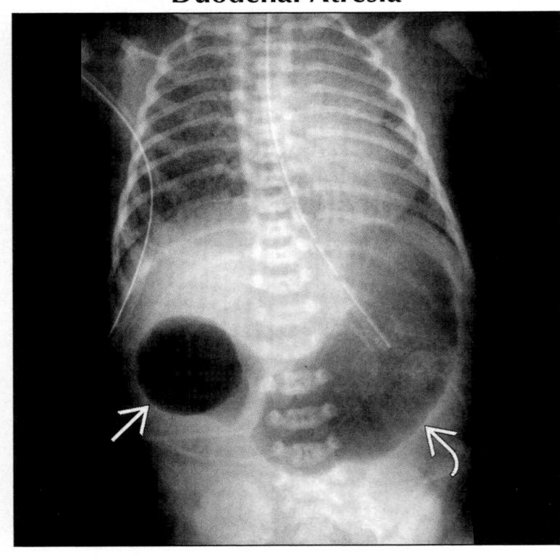

DUODENAL OBSTRUCTION

Duodenal Stenosis/Web

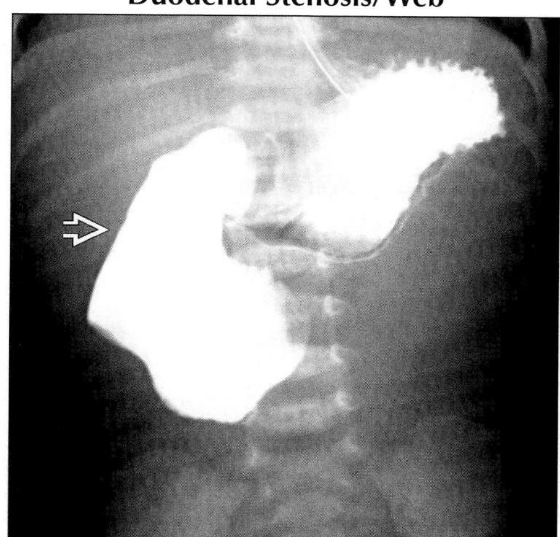

Duodenal Stenosis/Web

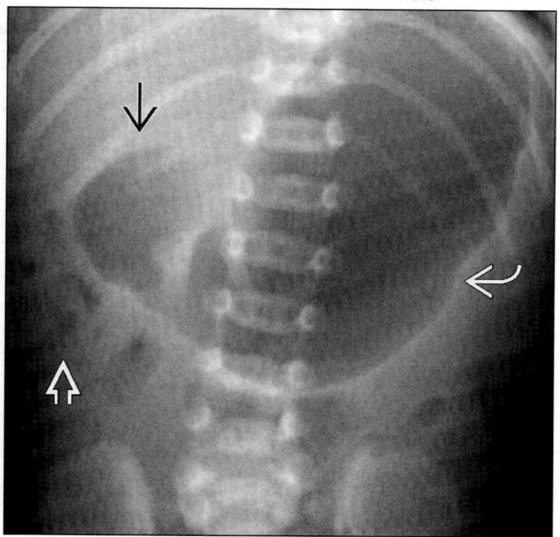

(Left) *Frontal upper GI shows the dilated proximal duodenum secondary to a surgically proven duodenal web in the 3rd portion of the duodenum.* ***(Right)*** *Frontal radiograph shows a very dilated stomach and proximal duodenum. Note that there is a small amount of distal bowel gas present.*

Duodenal Stenosis/Web

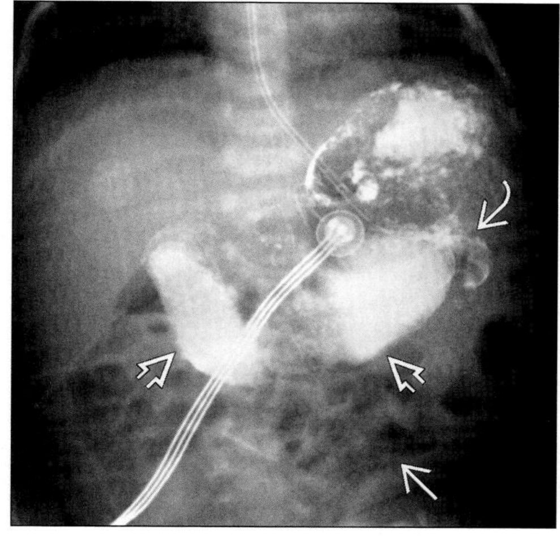

Jejunal Atresia

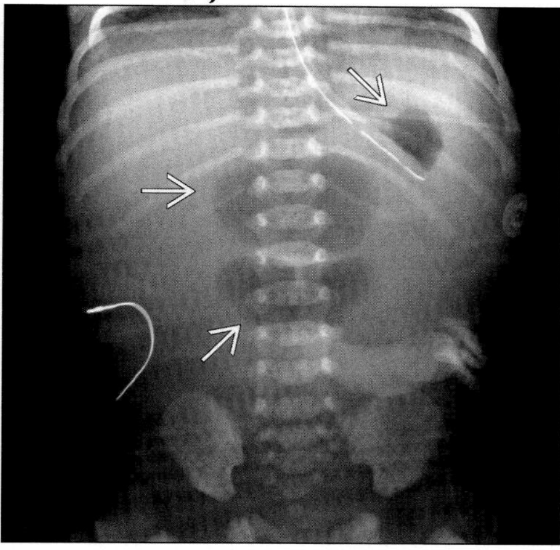

(Left) *AP fluoroscopic spot radiograph shows markedly dilated duodenum and abrupt beak-like tapering at the duodenal-jejunal junction. This 5-day-old child had a high-grade obstruction due to webs. Note the normal gas-filled loops of bowel distally.* ***(Right)*** *AP radiograph shows the "triple bubble" pattern in a newborn. Note the absence of distal bowel gas. In such a proximal level of obstruction, an upper GI is the appropriate initial work-up.*

Superior Mesenteric Artery (SMA) Syndrome

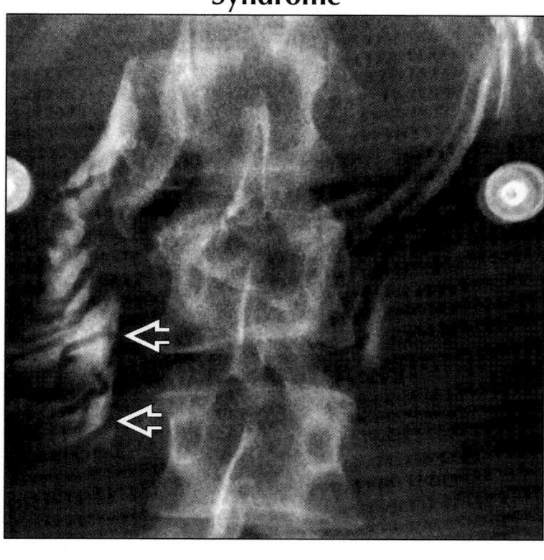

Superior Mesenteric Artery (SMA) Syndrome

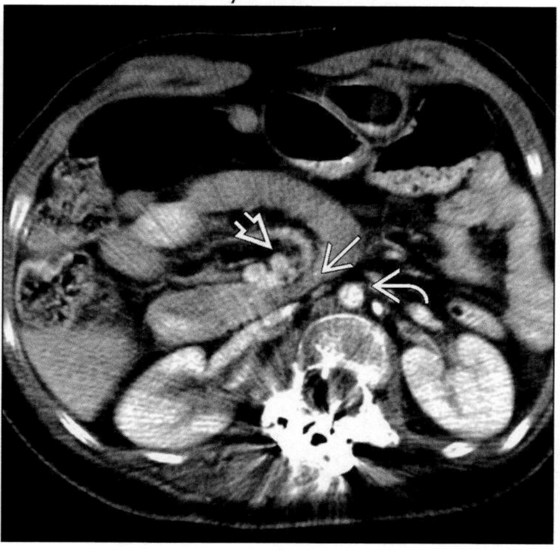

(Left) *AP fluoroscopic spot radiograph shows contrast material in the stomach and proximal duodenum terminating abruptly as the contrast encounters vertical extrinsic compression. This 18-year-old female presented with weight loss and vomiting with a history of posterior spinal fusion for scoliosis.* ***(Right)*** *Axial CECT shows bowel compression between the aorta and superior mesenteric artery. This condition is often caused or exacerbated by scoliosis, as seen here.*

DUODENAL OBSTRUCTION

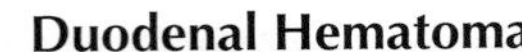

Duodenal Hematoma | **Duodenal Hematoma**

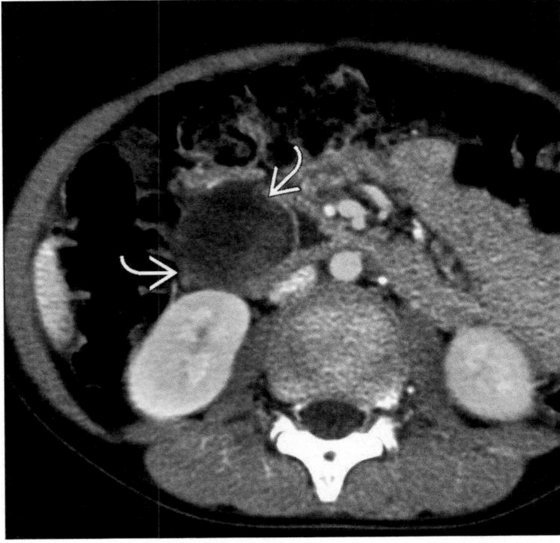

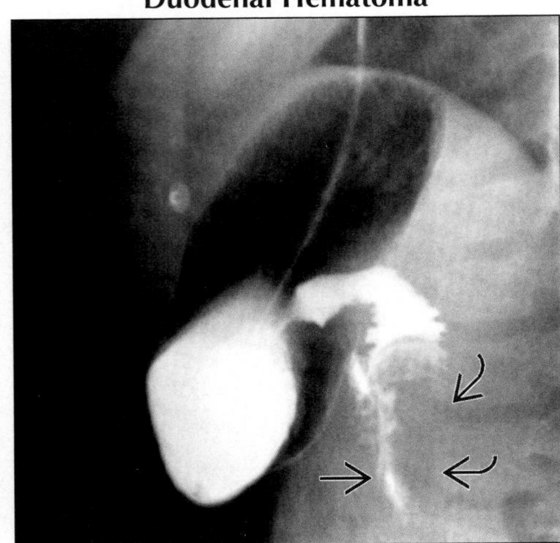

(Left) *Axial CECT shows a large, round, mixed-attenuation lesion → within the bowel wall and obstructing the 2nd portion of the duodenum. This 6-year-old boy sustained a handlebar injury but still managed to eat dinner afterwards.* ***(Right)*** *Lateral fluoroscopic spot radiograph of the same child shows a small stream of contrast material → sneaking past the obstructing hematoma, which causes the filling defect → in the duodenum.*

Duodenal Hematoma | **Duodenal Hematoma**

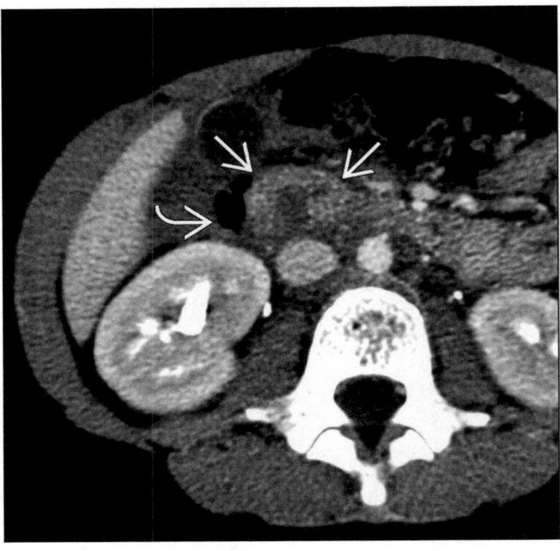

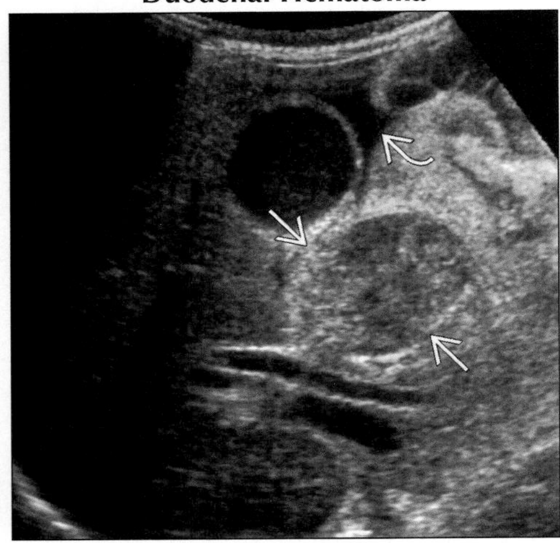

(Left) *Axial CECT shows hyperattenuating circumferential thickening of the duodenal wall → in this 8 year old who sustained a handlebar injury. Note the free retroperitoneal air from perforation →.* ***(Right)*** *Longitudinal oblique ultrasound shows a circumscribed, heterogeneous collection → in the RUQ in this 2 year old who recently underwent an endoscopy with duodenal biopsy. There is also a small amount of free fluid adjacent to the liver →.*

Gastrointestinal Duplication Cyst | **Gastrointestinal Duplication Cyst**

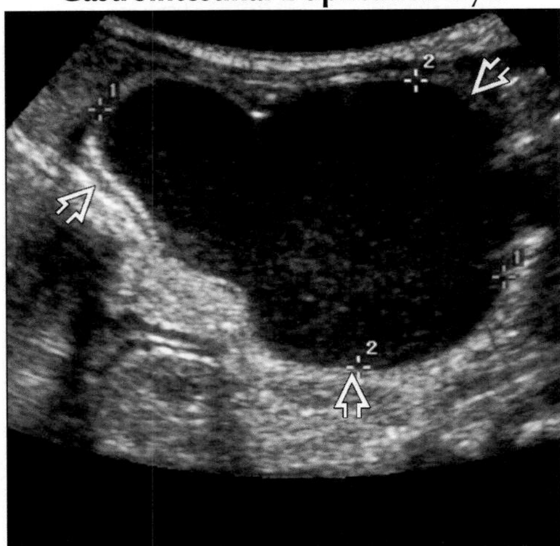

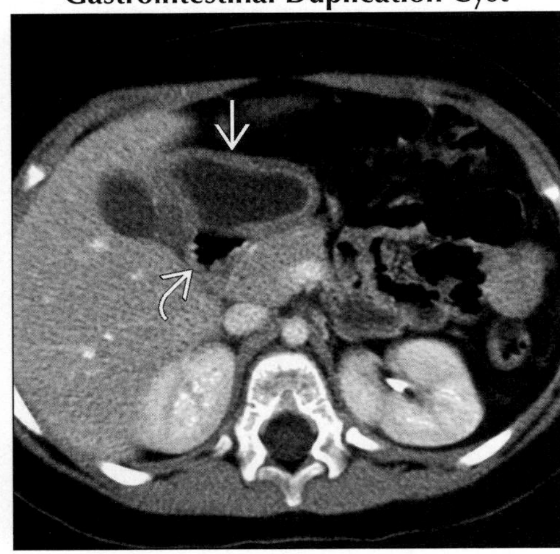

(Left) *Transverse ultrasound shows a lobular, circumscribed lesion bound by what resembles a bowel wall →. This was a duodenal duplication cyst in a newborn with a palpable mass. Note the internal debris.* ***(Right)*** *Axial CECT shows a thick-walled duplication cyst → associated with the 2nd portion of the duodenum →. Note that the contents are more hyperattenuating than simple fluid would be.*

Bezoar

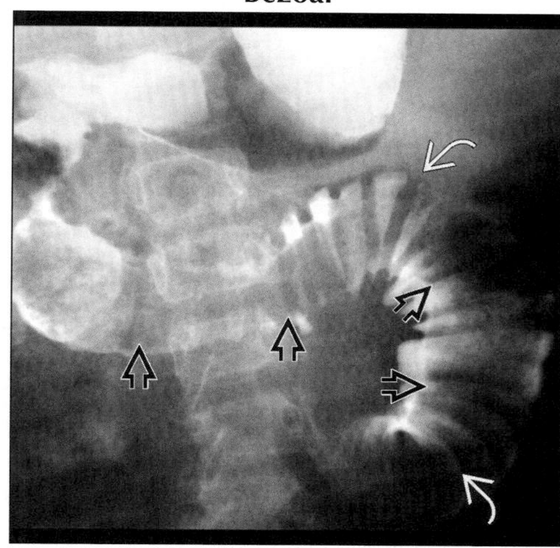

Bezoar

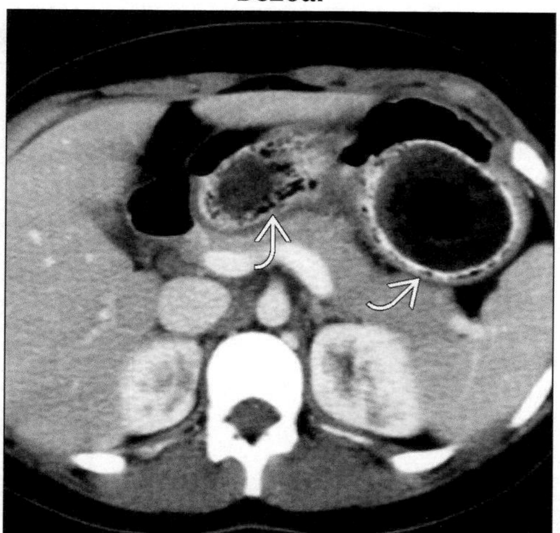

(Left) *Frontal upper GI shows a long filling defect extending through the duodenum and proximal jejunum ⇨, which are mildly dilated with thickened folds ➔.* ***(Right)*** *Axial CECT in this 17 year old with trichotillomania shows the typical, swirled, foamy appearance of hair with entrapped debris and air bubbles filling the stomach and duodenum ➔. The patient presented with complaints of abdominal fullness.*

Lymphoma

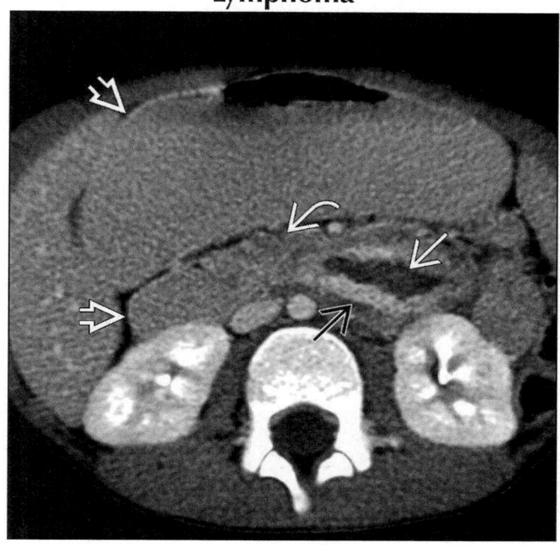

Lymphoma

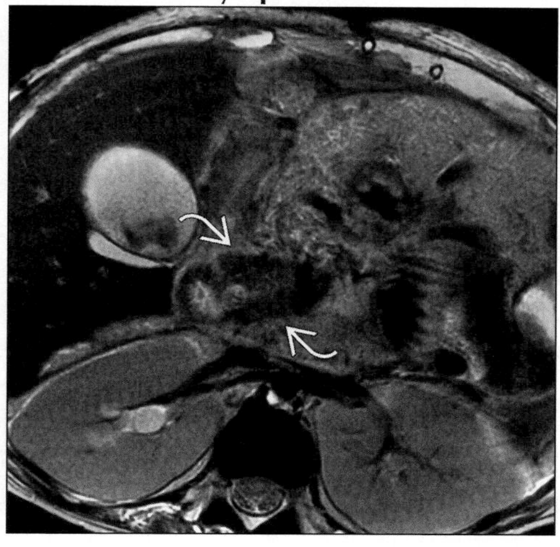

(Left) *Axial CECT shows an abnormally thickened duodenal wall →, prominent periduodenal soft tissue ➔, and abnormal material filling the duodenal lumen ➔ in this 4 year old with T-cell lymphoma. The stomach and proximal duodenum are noticeably distended ⇨.* ***(Right)*** *Axial T2WI MR in the same patient shows the poorly defined, intermediate signal soft tissue surrounding the 3rd portion of the duodenum ➔.*

Annular Pancreas

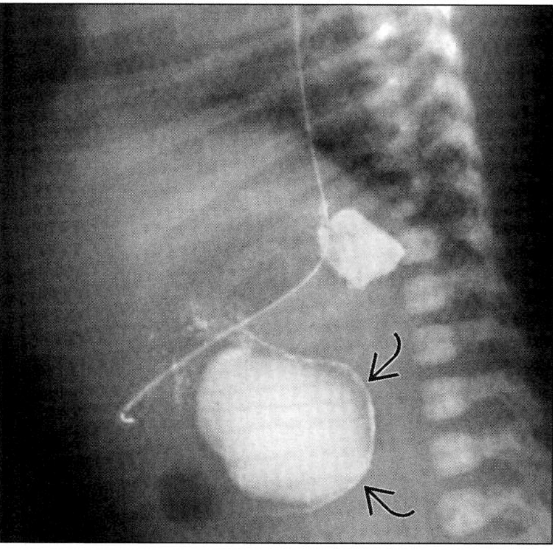

Annular Pancreas

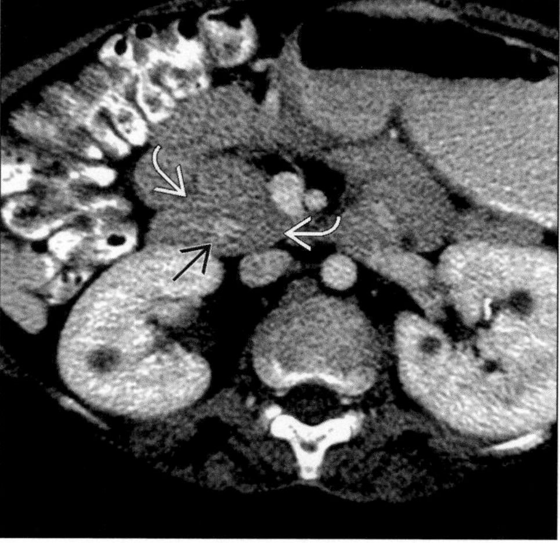

(Left) *Lateral fluoroscopic spot radiograph shows abrupt termination of the column of contrast material filling a dilated duodenum ➔ in this 4-day-old patient with trisomy 21, malrotation (without volvulus), and Ladd bands, in addition to an annular pancreas.* ***(Right)*** *Axial CECT shows a narrow caliber duodenum filled with oral contrast material → encircled by somewhat bulky-appearing pancreatic head parenchyma ➔ in a 12 year old with chronic abdominal pain.*

NEONATAL PROXIMAL BOWEL OBSTRUCTION

DIFFERENTIAL DIAGNOSIS

Common
- Esophageal Atresia (EA)
- Duodenal Atresia (DA) or Stenosis (DS)
- Duodenal Web (DW)
- Jejunal Atresia

Less Common
- Hiatal Hernia
- Midgut Volvulus (MV)
- Annular Pancreas
- Preduodenal Portal Vein

Rare but Important
- Gastric Atresia

ESSENTIAL INFORMATION

Key Differential Diagnosis Issues
- Many neonates diagnosed prenatally by US or MR
- Inability to pass nasogastric tube suggests EA
  - Neonate usually has difficulty swallowing secretions
  - Look for other radiologic findings of VATER or VACTERL
    - Vertebral anomalies, anorectal malformation, renal anomalies, radial ray anomalies, congenital heart defects
- Radiographs can be diagnostic for duodenal atresia
  - "Double bubble" (rounded duodenum)
  - Air-filled duodenum without complete distention → immediate upper GI to exclude MV (surgical emergency)
  - Look for signs of Down syndrome
    - 11 rib pairs
    - Cardiomegaly, shunt physiology
- Duodenal dilation with distal gas in face of bilious emesis is suspicious for midgut volvulus
  - Immediate upper GI required
- Radiographs show "triple bubble" of jejunal atresia
  - Contrast enema sometimes to assess for distal atresia (suggested by microcolon)
- Radiograph showing retrocardiac lucency suggests hiatal hernia
  - UGI can confirm
  - Frequently associated with gastric volvulus
- Annular pancreas almost always associated with DA
- Preduodenal portal vein rarely found in isolation
- Gastric atresia usually with other atresias, not isolated

Helpful Clues for Common Diagnoses
- **Esophageal Atresia (EA)**
  - Intermittent fluid distention of proximal esophagus on fetal imaging
    - High T2 signal in distended pouch on fetal MR
    - Anechoic fluid distention of pouch on fetal US
  - Air-filled esophageal pouch on newborn chest radiograph
    - Nasogastric tube tip upper esophagus
  - Sometimes associated tracheoesophageal fistula (TEF); preoperative esophagram
    - Lateral position esophagram to show fistula
    - Fistula usually just above carina; extends anterior and superior toward trachea
  - Sometimes associated with laryngotracheal cleft
  - Faulty division of foregut
  - 50-75% have associated anomalies
  - 5 types
    - Proximal EA with distal TEF (82%)
    - EA without TEF (10%)
    - Isolated TEF (H type) (4%)
    - EA with proximal and distal TEF (2%)
    - EA with proximal TEF (2%)
- **Duodenal Atresia (DA) or Stenosis (DS)**
  - Dilated, round proximal duodenum and stomach "double bubble" on fetal imaging
    - Anechoic, high T2 signal in round D1-2 segment on fetal US/MR
  - Air-filled "double bubble"; no distal gas on neonatal radiograph
    - If duodenum initially not rounded (partially distended), cannot exclude MV; immediate upper GI indicated
  - Most common upper bowel obstruction in neonate
  - Failure of vacuolization (recanalization) during embryogenesis
  - Up to 33% also have annular pancreas
  - Up to 33% also have Down syndrome
  - Up to 28% also have malrotation
- **Jejunal Atresia**
  - "Triple bubble" on neonatal radiographs

- Dilated air-filled stomach, duodenum, and proximal jejunum without distal gas
- No other imaging generally required
- Microcolon on water-soluble enema suggests additional distal atresia

- Dilated fluid-filled proximal bowel loops on fetal sonography or MR
- Absence or complete occlusion of intestinal lumen of segment of jejunum
- Likely due to in utero ischemic event

Helpful Clues for Less Common Diagnoses

- **Hiatal Hernia**
  - Neonatal radiography shows retrocardiac density overlying mid to right heart
  - Upper GI shows gastroesophageal junction and stomach above diaphragm
    - Sliding hiatal hernia does not usually cause bowel obstruction
  - Traction or torsion (volvulus) of stomach is common
  - Can be associated with congenital short esophagus
- **Midgut Volvulus (MV)**
  - Abnormal twisting of small bowel around superior mesenteric artery causing obstruction ± bowel ischemia/necrosis
  - Most frequent finding on abdominal radiography is normal bowel pattern
    - Multiple dilated bowel loops is later finding, likely due to ischemic ileus
    - Late findings: Pneumatosis, portal venous gas, gasless abdomen, free intraperitoneal air
  - UGI
    - Duodenal dilation to 2nd segment of duodenum
    - Cone-shaped appearance of D2 segment with decompressed D3 and distal bowel
    - Usually duodenojejunal junction (DJJ) low and not at, or to left of, left vertebral pedicle on AP image (malrotation)
    - Rare cases of MV with normal duodenal rotation
    - Corkscrew appearance of duodenum and proximal jejunum
    - If contrast obstructed at D2, cannot exclude MV; may indicate surgical exploration at surgeon's discretion
    - If enema performed, may show nonrotation with spiral course of colon involved in volvulus
- **Annular Pancreas**
  - Similar radiographic and UGI findings as DA, DW, MV
  - Band of pancreatic tissue surrounds D2
- **Preduodenal Portal Vein**
  - Radiographic and UGI findings similar to DA, DW, MV

Helpful Clues for Rare Diagnoses

- **Gastric Atresia**
  - No gas beyond stomach; UGI: Gastric outlet obstruction
  - Usually with multiple intestinal atresias
  - Enema: Usually microcolon due to distal atresias

Esophageal Atresia (EA)

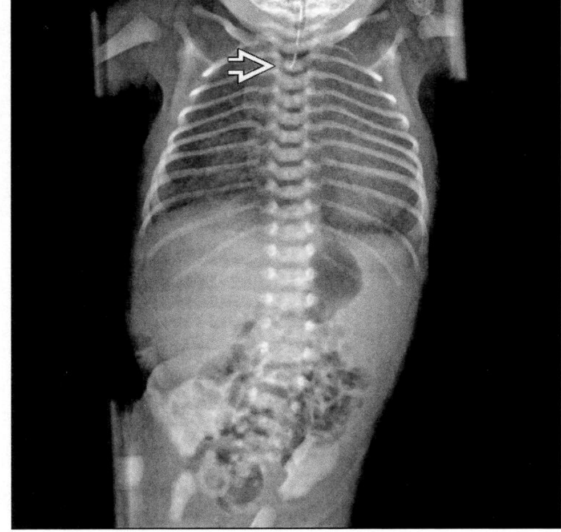

AP radiograph shows feeding tube tip overlying thoracic inlet ➡ due to EA. The abdominal gas indicates a TEF. Ribs are gracile. No vertebral anomalies. Question congenital heart disease.

Esophageal Atresia (EA)

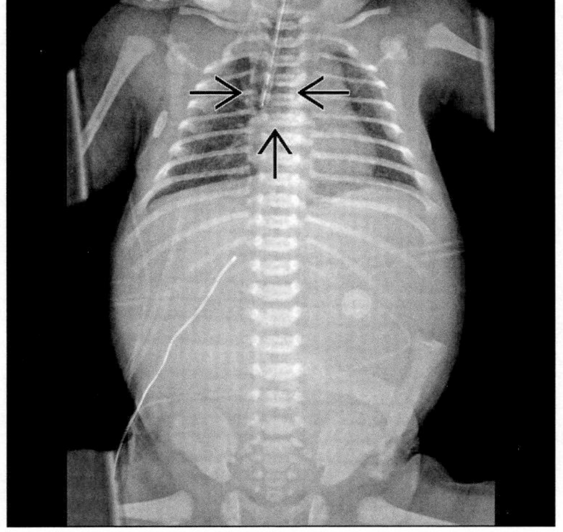

AP radiograph of the chest/abdomen in another patient shows EA pouch ➡ without fistula; there is no gas beyond atretic esophagus.

NEONATAL PROXIMAL BOWEL OBSTRUCTION

(Left) *Anteroposterior radiograph of a newborn shows a dilated, air-filled stomach and dilated, spherical proximal duodenum ➪ with no distal gas, consistent with DA. The presence of cardiomegaly, pulmonary edema, and 11 rib pairs suggests Down syndrome.* **(Right)** *Anteroposterior radiograph shows a "double bubble" sign of duodenal atresia: Dilated, air-filled stomach and round, obstructed proximal duodenum ➡.*

Duodenal Atresia (DA) or Stenosis (DS)

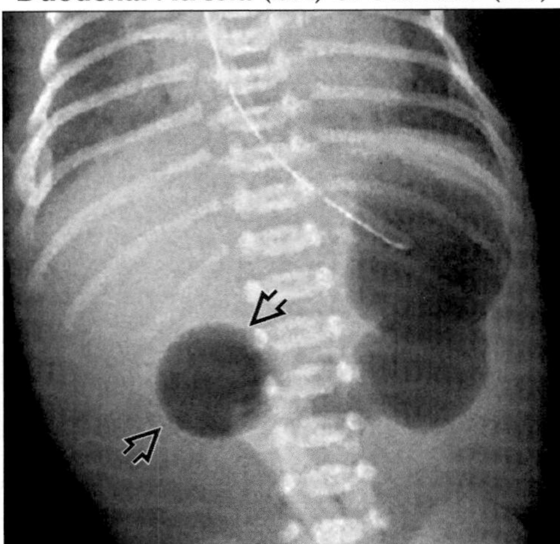

Duodenal Atresia (DA) or Stenosis (DS)

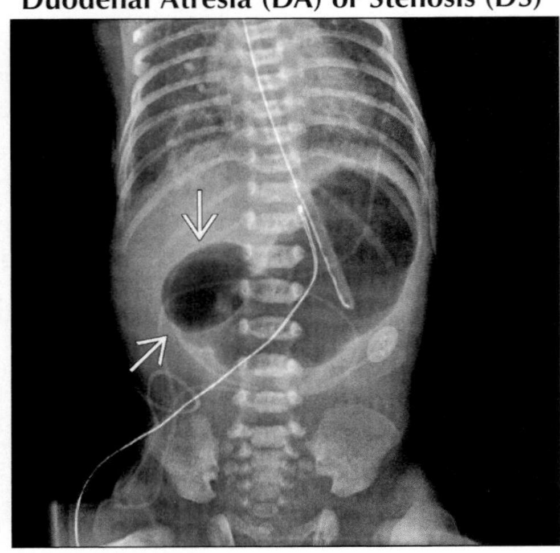

(Left) *Anteroposterior radiograph of the abdomen shows a dilated, nonspherical proximal duodenum ➪ due to prior suctioning of the stomach. Also consider antenatal midgut volvulus. UGI is recommended.* **(Right)** *Lateral upper GI shows partial obstruction with dilation of the 2nd segment of the duodenum ➪. The duodenum distal to stenosis is decompressed but still appears somewhat retroperitoneal in location.*

Duodenal Atresia (DA) or Stenosis (DS)

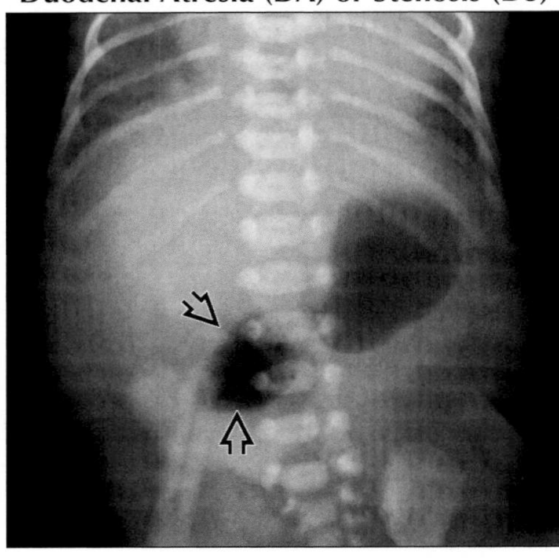

Duodenal Atresia (DA) or Stenosis (DS)

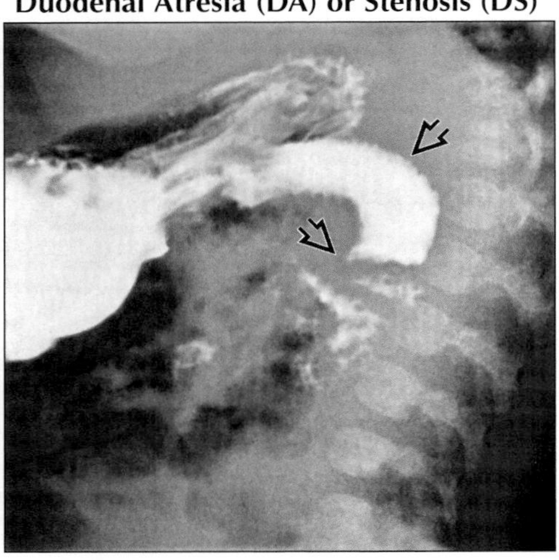

(Left) *Anteroposterior upper GI in the same patient shows positioning of the duodenojejunal junction in the midline ➪, consistent with malrotation. MV cannot be excluded preoperatively. At surgery, malrotation without volvulus was confirmed.* **(Right)** *Lateral upper GI left side down shows a dilated duodenum with a "teet" ➪ in the center of the obstructed duodenum. At surgery, a duodenal web with a very tiny orifice was found.*

Duodenal Atresia (DA) or Stenosis (DS)

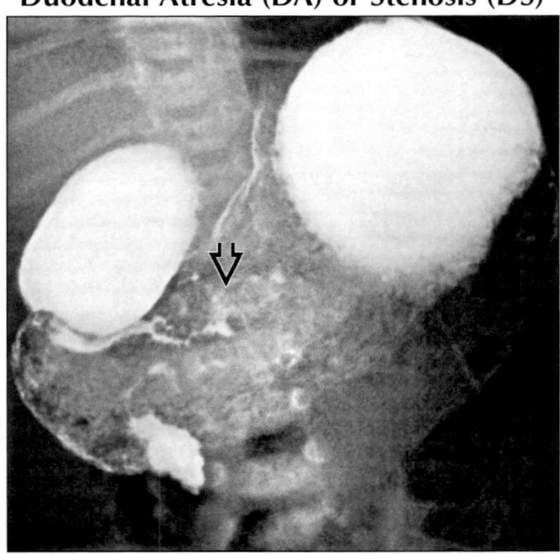

Duodenal Web (DW)

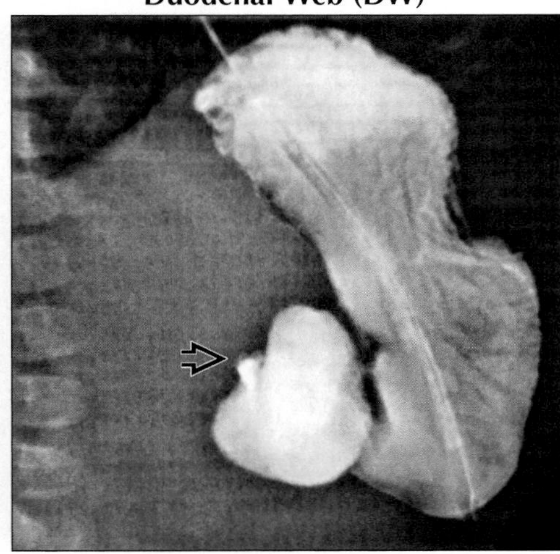

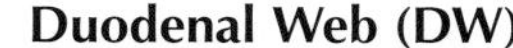

Duodenal Web (DW)

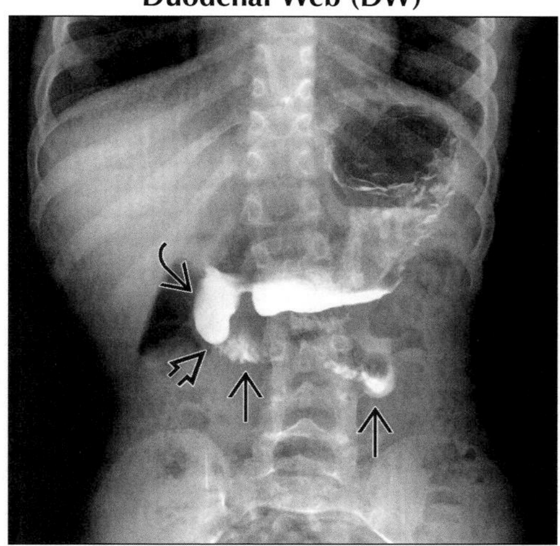

Hiatal Hernia

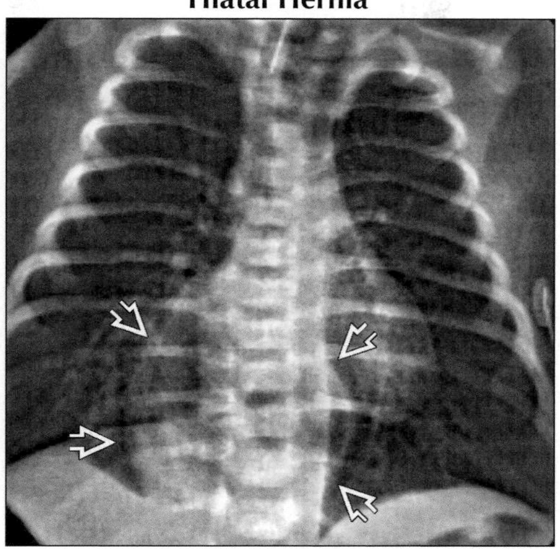

(Left) *Anteroposterior upper GI in this older child with a long history of vomiting shows dilation of the 2nd duodenal segment, a windsock or web appearance of the obstructed segment, with decompression of the distal duodenum and proximal jejunum.* ***(Right)*** *Anteroposterior radiograph of the chest at birth shows round lucent density in the midline retrocardiac region, suggestive of a hiatal hernia.*

Hiatal Hernia

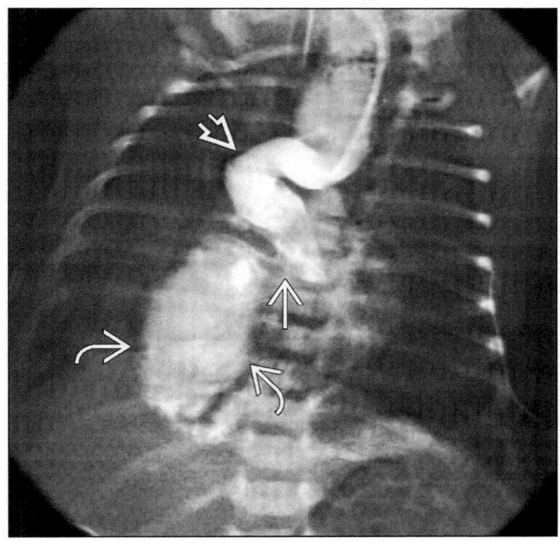

Midgut Volvulus (MV)

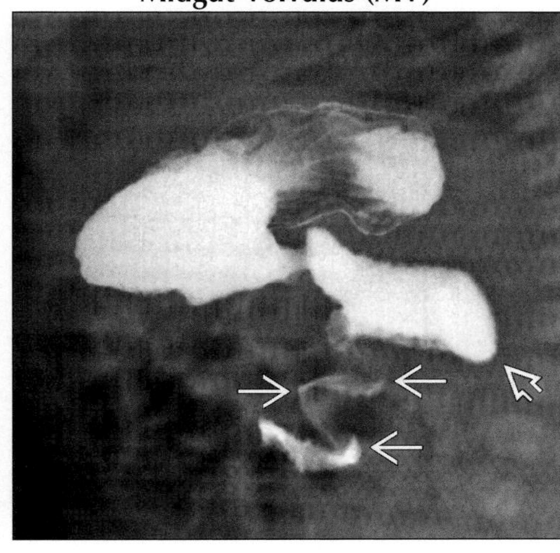

(Left) *Anteroposterior upper GI shows a dilated tortuous esophagus, gastroesophageal junction above the diaphragm, and most of the stomach located in the right chest. Most severe neonatal hiatal hernias are associated with volvulus of the stomach.* ***(Right)*** *Lateral upper GI shows duodenal dilation up to D2-3 segment and corkscrew appearance of distal intraperitoneal duodenum, consistent with midgut volvulus due to midgut malrotation.*

Midgut Volvulus (MV)

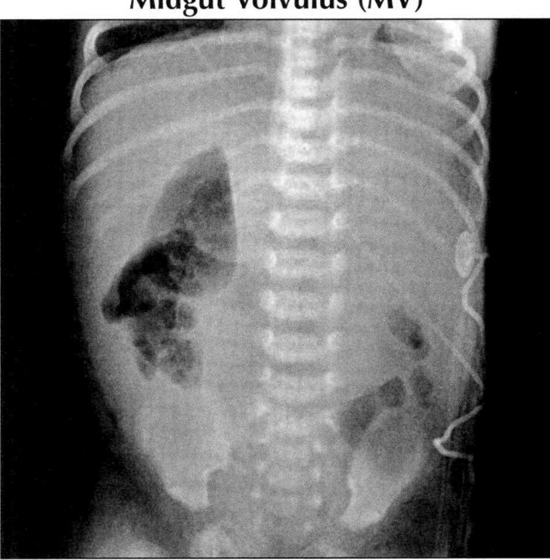

Midgut Volvulus (MV)

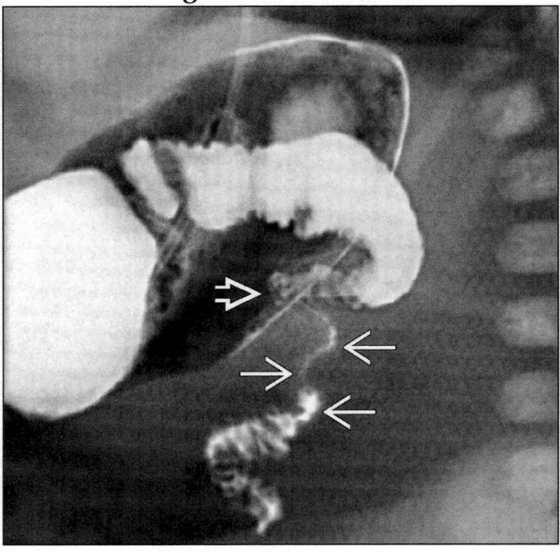

(Left) *Anteroposterior radiograph in left decubitus position in a newborn with bilious emesis shows air-fluid level in the dilated proximal duodenum with distal gas. This should prompt an immediate UGI to exclude MV.* ***(Right)*** *Lateral upper GI in the same patient shows a dilated duodenum with partial obstruction of 2nd portion duodenum and corkscrew appearance of the remainder of the duodenum, coursing intraperitoneal and caudad, consistent with midgut volvulus.*

NEONATAL PROXIMAL BOWEL OBSTRUCTION

Midgut Volvulus (MV)

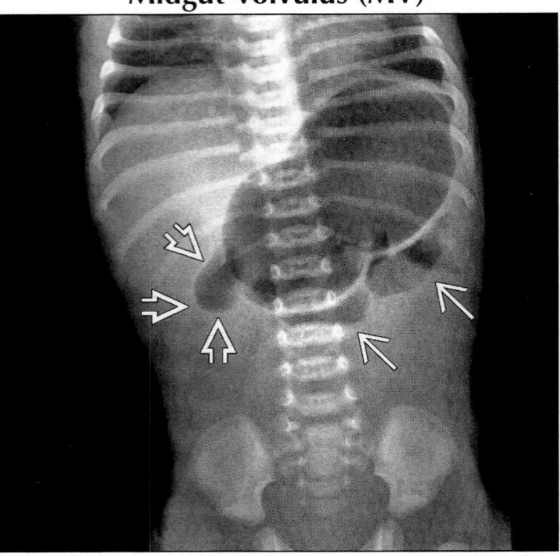

Midgut Volvulus (MV)

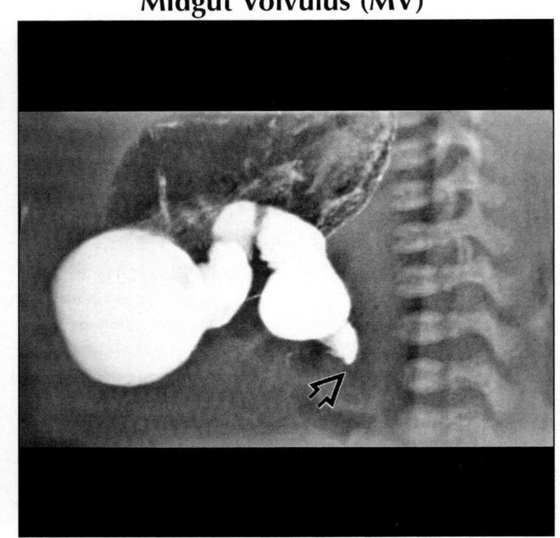

__(Left)__ Anteroposterior radiograph shows a dilated air-filled stomach and a less distended duodenum ➡ with a small amount of distal gas ➡, an abnormal pattern in an infant 1-2 days old who presented with bilious vomiting. The entire bowel should be filled with gas in the non-fed day-old neonate. __(Right)__ Lateral upper GI shows duodenal dilation to the D2 segment. The end of the contrast bolus is cone-shaped ⇨, suggesting volvulus until proven otherwise.

Midgut Volvulus (MV)

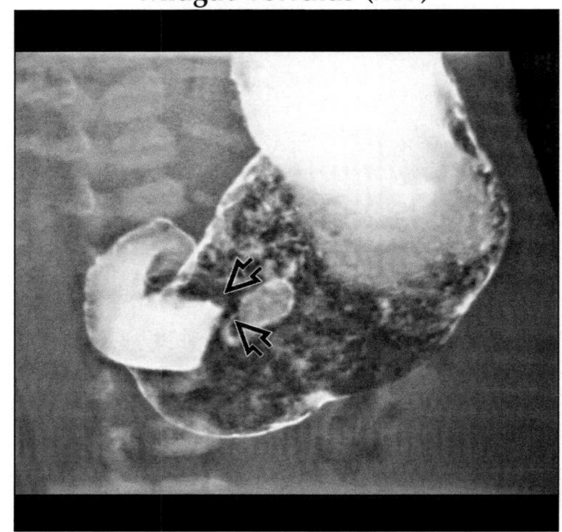

Midgut Volvulus (MV)

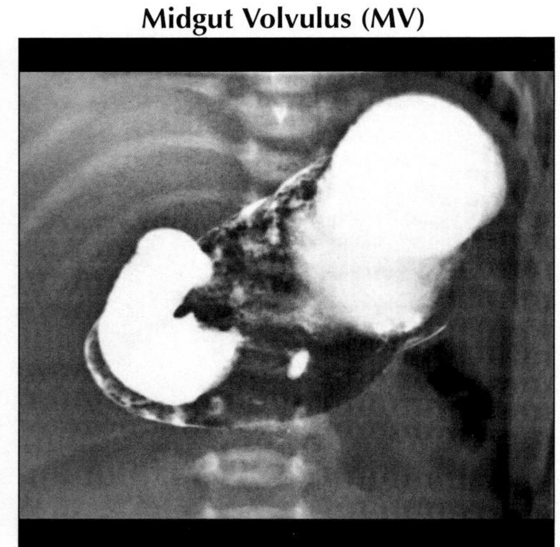

__(Left)__ Oblique upper GI left posterior side down shows a dilated duodenum, which ends in a point or arrowhead configuration ⇨ with a small amount of contrast passing through. Without better definition of the distal loops, the most important diagnostic consideration is midgut volvulus. __(Right)__ Anteroposterior upper GI shows duodenal obstruction proximal to the DJJ, indeterminate rotation, and findings suspicious for midgut volvulus, which was found at operation.

Midgut Volvulus (MV)

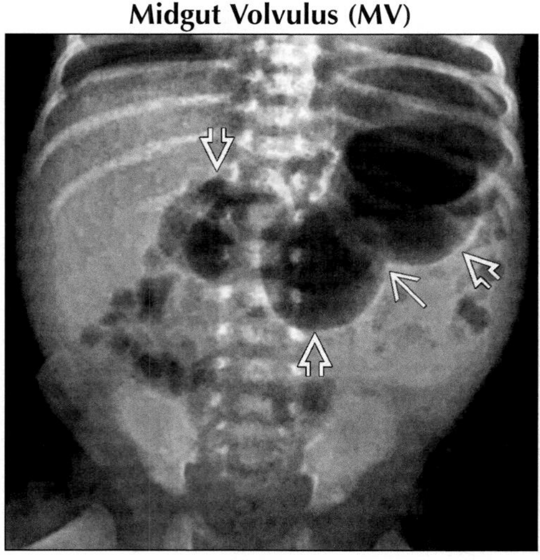

Midgut Volvulus (MV)

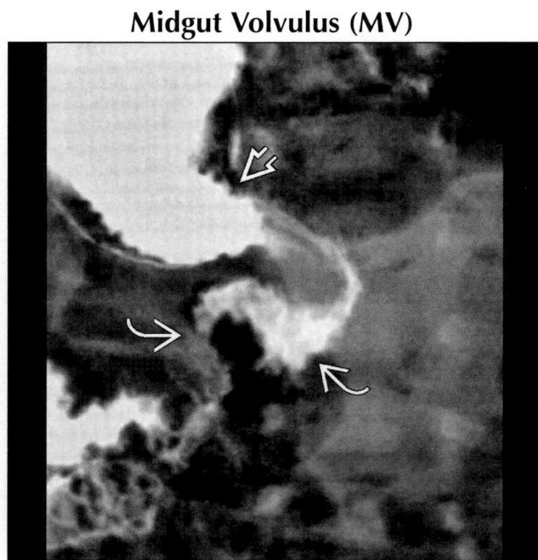

__(Left)__ Anteroposterior radiograph in another patient shows the stomach and duodenum distended with air ➡, out of proportion to remainder of the bowel, and a clinical history of bilious emesis. Prominent peristaltic contraction of the stomach ➡ may suggest upper bowel obstruction. __(Right)__ Anteroposterior upper GI shows proximal duodenal dilation ➡, abnormally located DJJ, and a corkscrew sign ➡ of midgut volvulus, confirmed at surgery. The bowel was viable.

Annular Pancreas

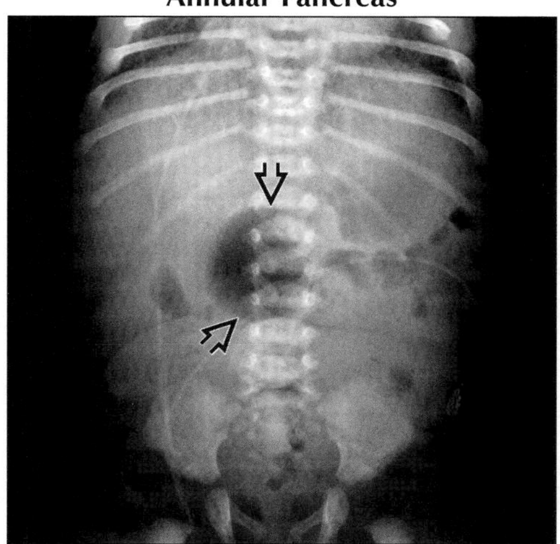

Annular Pancreas

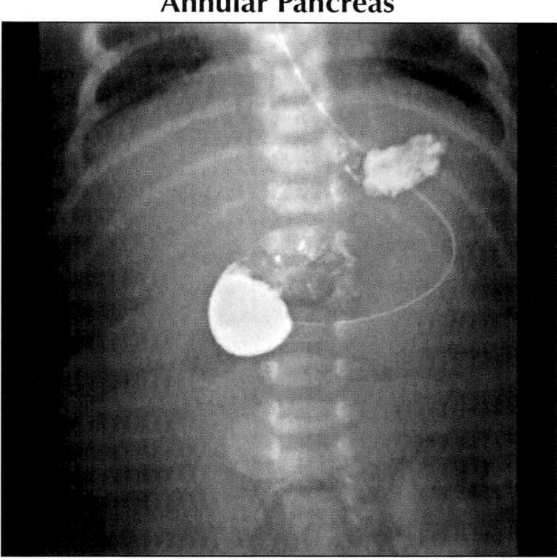

*(**Left**) Anteroposterior radiograph of this 1-day-old patient who presented with bilious vomiting shows a rounded air collection in the mid-abdomen in the expected location of the duodenum ⇨, with distal gas suggestive of partial duodenal obstruction. (**Right**) Anteroposterior upper GI follow-up radiograph shows a dilated duodenum with little, if any, contrast distally.*

Annular Pancreas

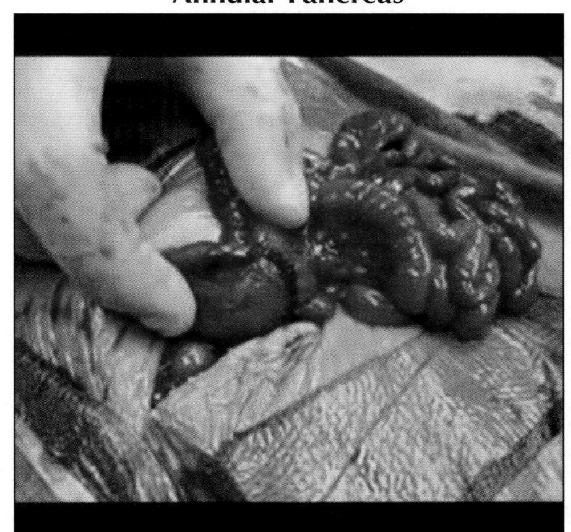

Preduodenal Portal Vein

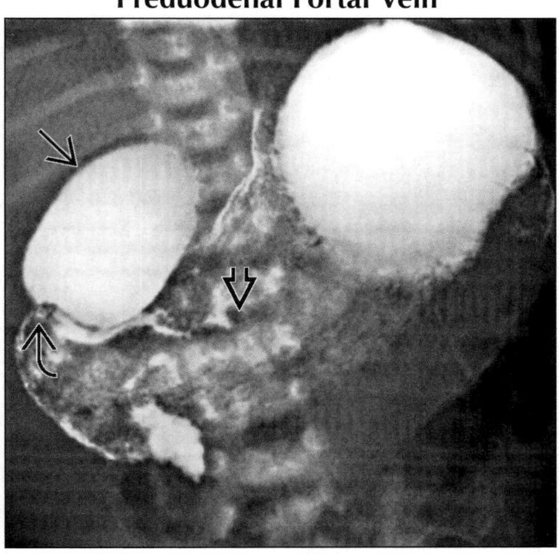

*(**Left**) Surgical photograph in the same patient shows the pancreas completely surrounding the duodenum, consistent with annular pancreas. (**Right**) Anteroposterior upper GI shows malrotation with DJJ in midline ⇨ and proximal duodenal dilation → to D2 ↗, which at surgery was found to be due to duodenal stenosis with Ladd bands and a preduodenal portal vein. The previous images demonstrate the difficulty of differentiating DS from MV preoperatively.*

Gastric Atresia

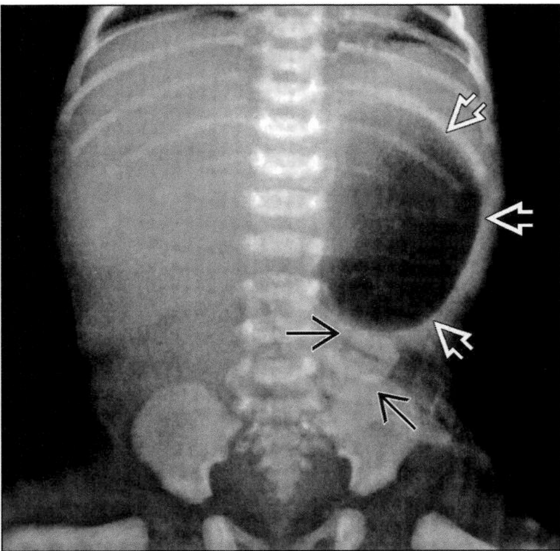

Gastric Atresia

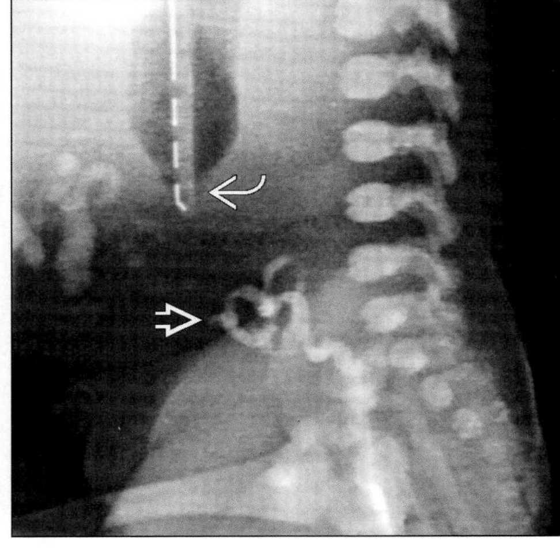

*(**Left**) Anteroposterior radiograph shows air-filled stomach ➡ without distal gas. The umbilical cord → is still attached. There is no other bowel gas seen. (**Right**) Lateral contrast enema shows a Replogle tube ➡ in the stomach, which was distended with additional air. An enema was performed with water-soluble contrast showing microcolon with abrupt termination of the sigmoid/descending colon ➡ suggestive of colonic atresia. Gas never emptied from the stomach.*

SMALL BOWEL OBSTRUCTION

DIFFERENTIAL DIAGNOSIS

Common

- Appendicitis
- Adhesions
- Ileocolic Intussusception
- Midgut Volvulus
- Inflammatory Bowel Disease (Crohn Disease)
- Incarcerated Inguinal Hernia

Less Common

- Hirschsprung Disease
- Meconium Plug Syndrome (Small Left Colon Syndrome)
- Meckel Diverticulum
- Jejunoileal Atresia
- Meconium Ileus
- Gastrointestinal Duplication Cysts

Rare but Important

- Distal Intestinal Obstructive Syndrome

ESSENTIAL INFORMATION

Key Differential Diagnosis Issues

- In **neonates**, differentiate between high (proximal) and low (distal) obstruction
  - Common causes of proximal obstruction
    - Malrotation/midgut volvulus
    - Duodenal atresia
    - Duodenal stenosis/web
    - Diagnostic work-up starts with upper GI
  - Common causes of mid-bowel obstruction
    - Jejunal atresia/web
    - Volvulus ± malrotation
    - Diagnostic work-up usually involves upper GI and contrast enema
  - Low (distal) obstruction
    - Hirschsprung disease
    - Meconium plug syndrome (small left colon syndrome)
    - Ileal atresia
    - Meconium ileus
    - Work-up starts with contrast enema
- Common differential considerations for obstruction in **older children**
  - Appendicitis
  - Adhesions
  - Intussusception
  - Incarcerated inguinal hernia
  - Inflammatory bowel disease
  - Meckel diverticulum

Helpful Clues for Common Diagnoses

- **Appendicitis**
  - Radiograph
    - Appendicitis should be considered with appendicolith on plain film
    - Classic small bowel obstruction is common presentation: Dilated loops, multiple air-fluid levels on upright or decubitus views
    - Early appendicitis may be subtle with distal bowel gas and stool, scattered air in small bowel
  - Ultrasound
    - Iliac artery/vein useful landmark for locating appendix, which often lies near/over vessels
    - Noncompressible blind-ending tube, ≥ 7 mm diameter, echogenic periappendiceal fat
    - If significant amount of free intraperitoneal fluid, suspect perforation
  - CT
    - Inflamed, hyperemic tubular structure; does not fill with oral contrast
    - Look for signs of longstanding/perforated appendicitis: Free fluid, free air, inflammatory phlegmon
- **Adhesions**
  - Almost never directly visualized; diagnosis made intraoperatively
  - Wide range of severity on any modality (radiograph, CT, US)
    - Nonspecific increased small bowel air with fluid levels, distal bowel gas if mild/partial/intermittent obstruction
    - Dilated small bowel loops, absent distal gas, air-fluid levels if high-grade or complete obstruction
- **Ileocolic Intussusception**
  - Majority of cases occur between age 3 months to 3 years
    - If well outside this age range or recurrent, consider pathologic lead point
  - Radiograph
    - Bowel gas pattern ranges from nonspecific to frank obstruction
    - Intussusceptum may be identifiable as right lower quadrant soft tissue density
  - Ultrasound is sensitive and specific tool to confirm or exclude intussusception

- Alternating hypo-/hyperechoic rings
- **Midgut Volvulus**
  - Must be excluded in patients with bilious emesis
  - Bowel gas pattern ranges from nonspecific/normal to ominously dilated loops of proximal bowel with paucity of distal bowel gas
- **Inflammatory Bowel Disease (Crohn Disease)**
  - Findings may manifest anywhere from mouth to anus
  - CT
    - Segmental, circumferentially thickened bowel wall with luminal narrowing
    - Fatty proliferation, engorged vessels, inflammatory stranding around bowel
    - Abscesses, especially perirectal
  - Fluoroscopic
    - "String" sign of narrowed lumen
    - Fistulae to skin or adjacent bowel loops
    - Thickened mucosal folds
    - Cobblestone pattern: Longitudinal and transverse ulcers
- **Incarcerated Inguinal Hernia**
  - Diagnosed with loops of bowel in scrotum
    - Detected clinically, easily confirmed by ultrasound

Helpful Clues for Less Common Diagnoses

- **Hirschsprung Disease**
  - Abnormal rectosigmoid ratio (R/S diameter < 1) on contrast enema may be clue
- **Meconium Plug Syndrome (Small Left Colon Syndrome)**
  - Contrast enema: Transition point between dilated proximal and narrow distal colon
- **Meckel Diverticulum**
  - Mimics appendicitis: Thickened, blind-ending tubular structure in abdomen/pelvis
  - Rule of 2s: 2% of population, within 2 feet of ileocecal valve, symptoms before age 2
  - Tc-99m pertechnetate scan demonstrates focus of activity in lower abdomen
- **Jejunoileal Atresia**
  - Ileal atresia contrast enema: Microcolon
  - Jejunal atresia contrast enema: Normal caliber colon
    - If microcolon on contrast enema, expect presence of other distal atresias
- **Meconium Ileus**
  - Radiograph: Distal bowel obstruction
  - Fluoroscopy: Microcolon, meconium pellets in terminal ileum
    - Meconium ileus not excluded until contrast refluxes into terminal ileum
- **Gastrointestinal Duplication Cysts**
  - Most common location is terminal ileum
  - Ultrasound: Round, hypoechoic structure with bowel wall signature

Helpful Clues for Rare Diagnoses

- **Distal Intestinal Obstructive Syndrome**
  - Meconium ileus equivalent
  - Must be suspected with small bowel obstruction in cystic fibrosis population

Appendicitis

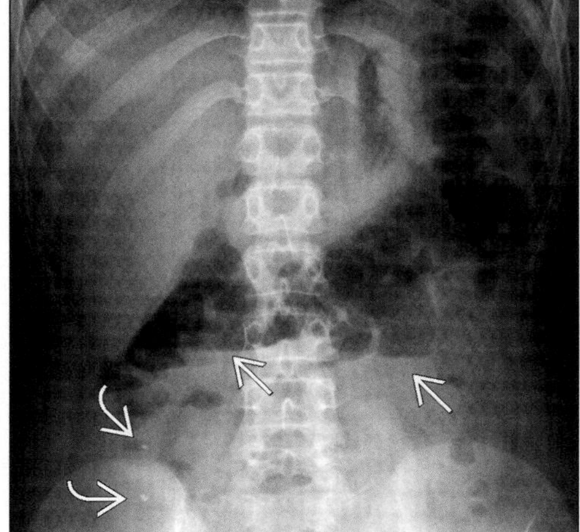

Frontal radiograph shows mildly dilated loops of small bowel with air-fluid levels ➡ on the the upright view. Note the appendicoliths ➡ in the right lower quadrant.

Appendicitis

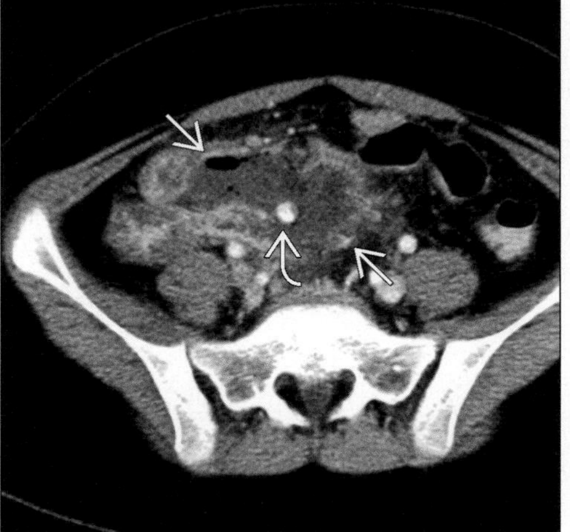

Axial CECT in the same patient shows the large abscess ➡ resulting from perforation. Note 1 of several appendicoliths ➡. The patient presented after 8 days of fever.

SMALL BOWEL OBSTRUCTION

Appendicitis

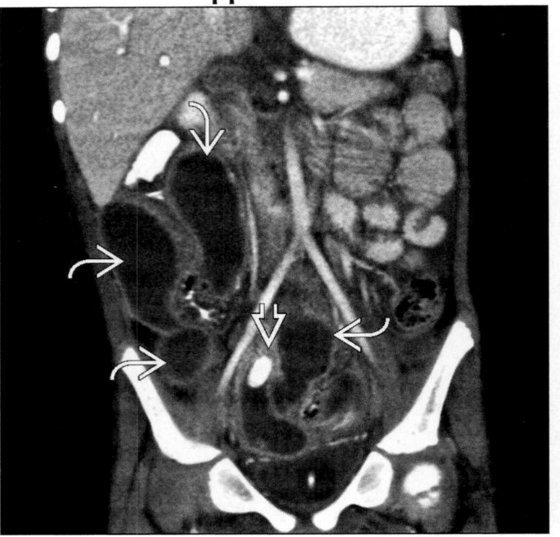

Appendicitis

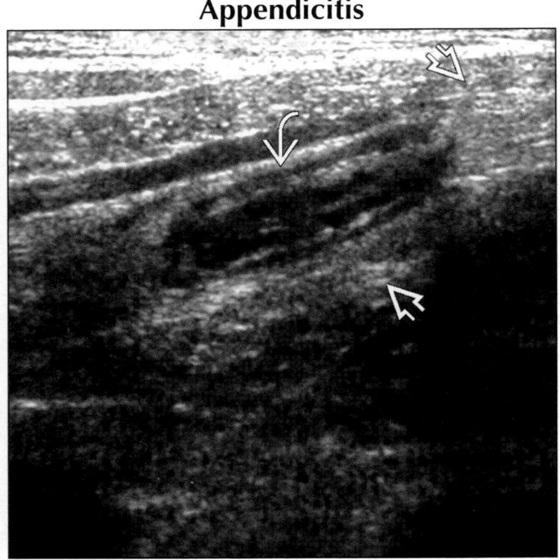

(Left) *Coronal CECT shows numerous, rim-enhancing, loculated fluid collections ➔ interspersed among the loops of bowel, consistent with intraperitoneal abscesses resulting from a ruptured appendicitis. Note the sizable appendicolith ➔.* ***(Right)*** *Longitudinal ultrasound shows a dilated, noncompressible, tubular structure ➔ in the RLQ, surgically confirmed to be an appendicitis. Note the surrounding echogenic and inflamed periappendiceal fat ➔.*

Ileocolic Intussusception

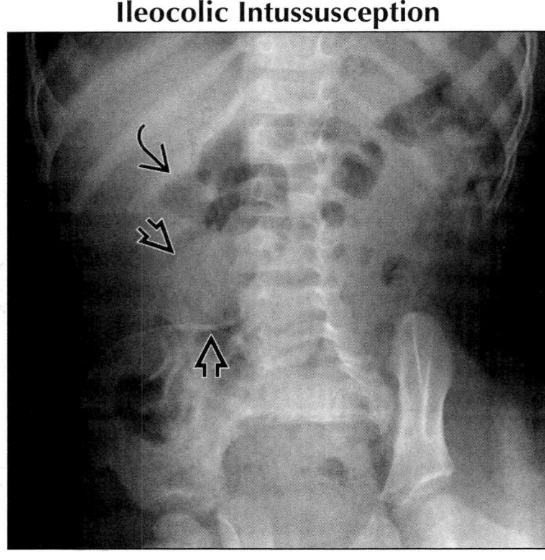

Ileocolic Intussusception

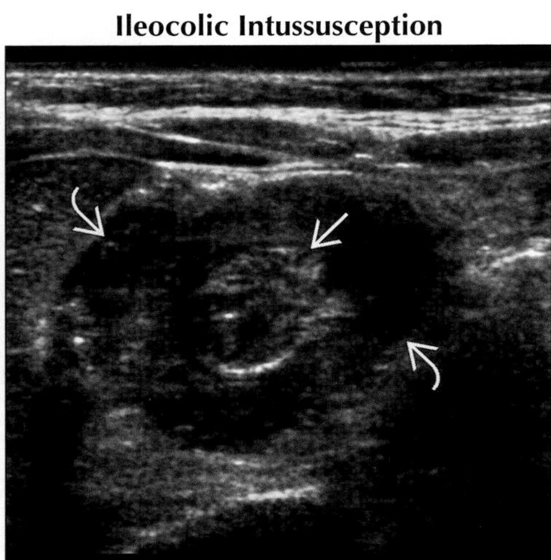

(Left) *Frontal radiograph shows a rounded soft tissue mass ➔ in the right mid-abdomen. Note that the bowel gas pattern is nonspecific, with air-filled loops of small bowel proximally ➔.* ***(Right)*** *Transverse ultrasound shows an outer hypoechoic rim of the bowel wall ➔ and trapped echogenic material internally ➔, representing mesenteric fat in this right mid-abdomen ileocolic intussusception.*

Ileocolic Intussusception

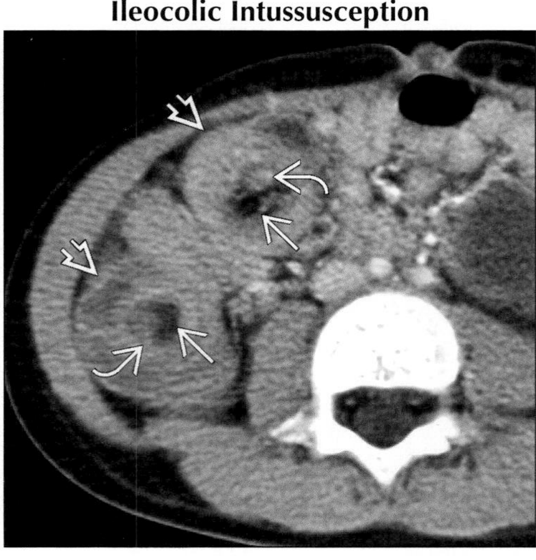

Ileocolic Intussusception

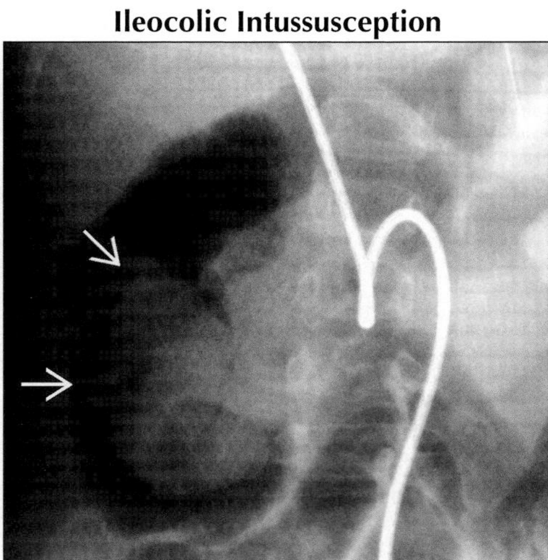

(Left) *Axial CECT shows low-attenuation mesenteric fat ➔ and small bowel ➔ trapped within a thick-appearing ascending colon ➔ in this 4-year-old boy who presented with severe abdominal pain and in frank septic shock. This is an atypical presentation, and it was not the expected diagnosis.* ***(Right)*** *Frontal air enema in the same patient shows reduction of the intussusception. The small bowel is pushed back by the air column ➔.*

Midgut Volvulus

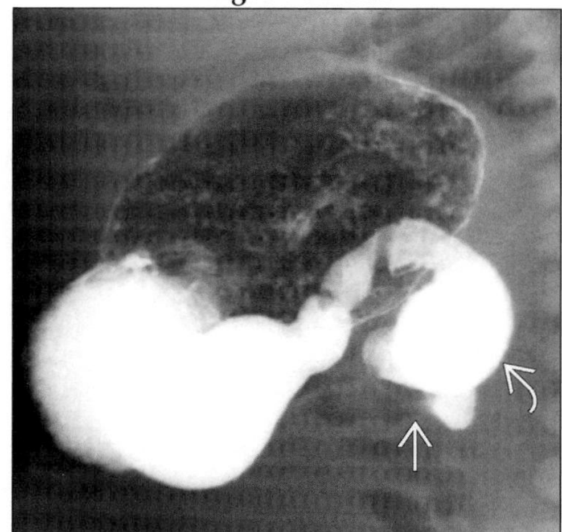

Midgut Volvulus

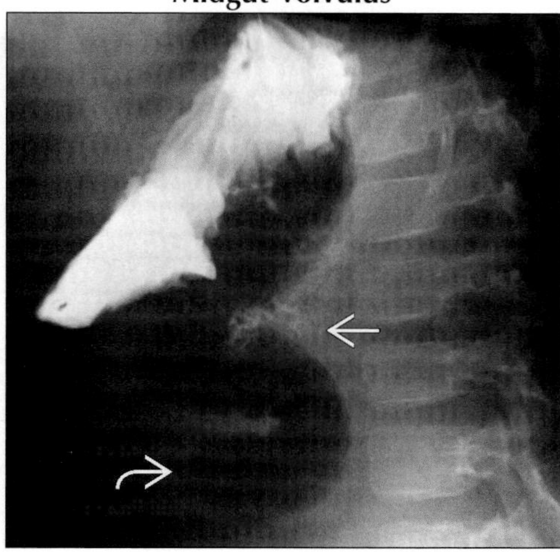

*(**Left**) Lateral fluoroscopic spot radiograph shows a distended duodenum ➨. The contrast column ends abruptly. Note the "beaking" at the point of volvulus ➨. (**Right**) Lateral fluoroscopic spot radiograph shows revolvulus in the same patient 8 years later. Faint contrast material is seen in the duodenum ➨. Air in the dilated proximal small bowel demonstrates the same abruptly twisted-off appearance ➨. One could argue that the contrast study was not needed.*

Midgut Volvulus

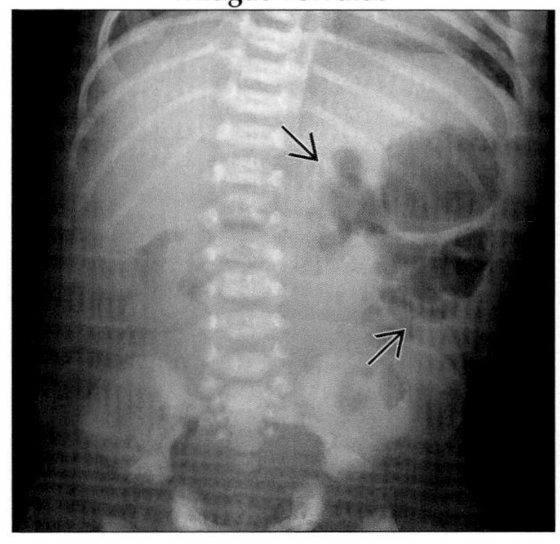

Midgut Volvulus

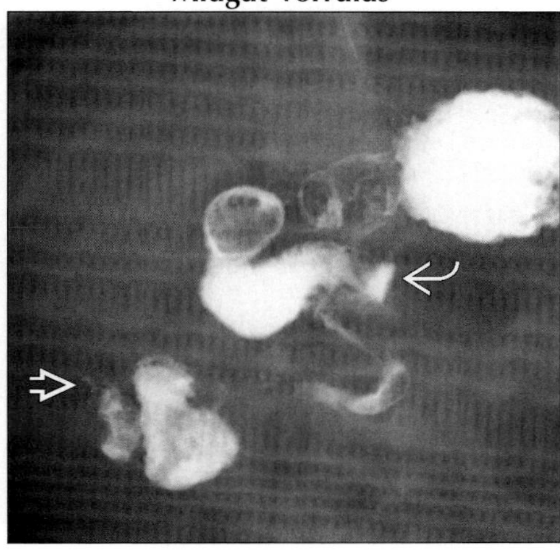

*(**Left**) Frontal radiograph shows a nonspecific appearance of air-filled bowel loops ➨ in a 4-day-old female with bilious emesis. Although not entirely normal, the bowel gas pattern does not necessarily indicate obstruction. (**Right**) Frontal upper GI in the same patient shows the duodenal-jejunal junction to be low in position ➨, below the level of the duodenal bulb. There is no antegrade flow of contrast material beyond this point in the mid-jejunum ➨.*

Inflammatory Bowel Disease (Crohn Disease)

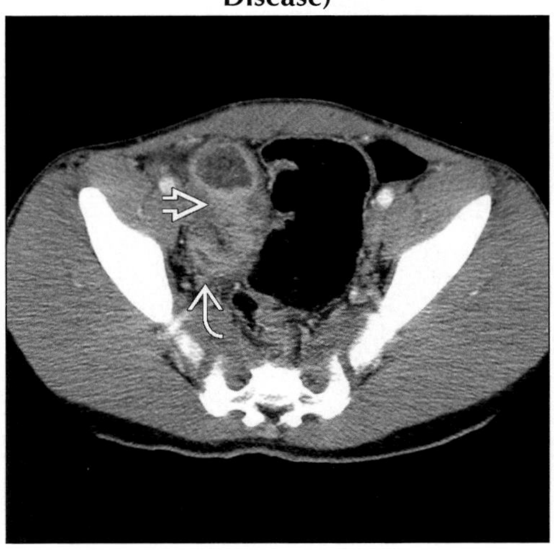

Inflammatory Bowel Disease (Crohn Disease)

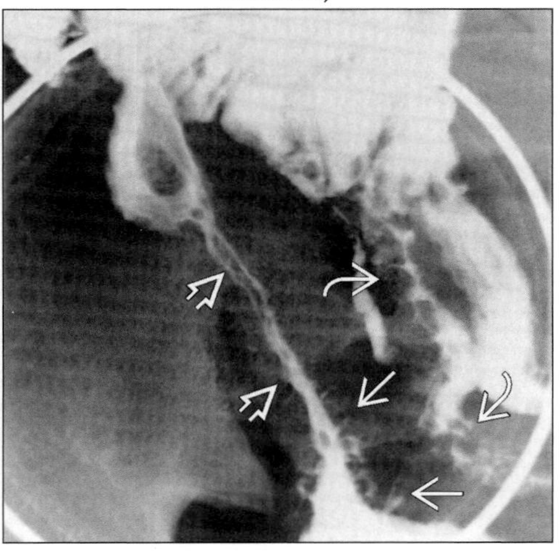

*(**Left**) Axial CECT shows the transition point ➨ in the distal ileum between the dilated proximal small bowel and inflamed terminal ileum. Note the abruptly narrowed lumen of the terminal ileum ➨. (**Right**) Frontal fluoroscopic spot radiograph shows a long segment of terminal ileum with a significantly narrowed lumen ➨ in a "string" sign. Close inspection also reveals a "cobblestone" pattern ➨ and wisps of contrast-filling transmural fissures ➨.*

SMALL BOWEL OBSTRUCTION

*(**Left**) Coronal CECT shows a fluid-filled bowel loop in the scrotum in a 2 month old who presented with extremis and then coded. Note the multiple loops of dilated bowel . (**Right**) Lateral contrast enema shows the rectum to be smaller in caliber than the sigmoid colon . This represents reversal of the rectosigmoid ratio. In normal patients, the rectosigmoid ratio should always be greater than 1, with the rectum larger than the sigmoid colon.*

Incarcerated Inguinal Hernia

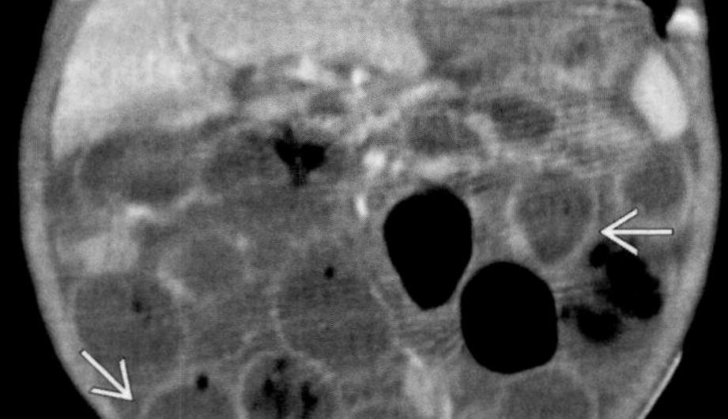

Hirschsprung Disease

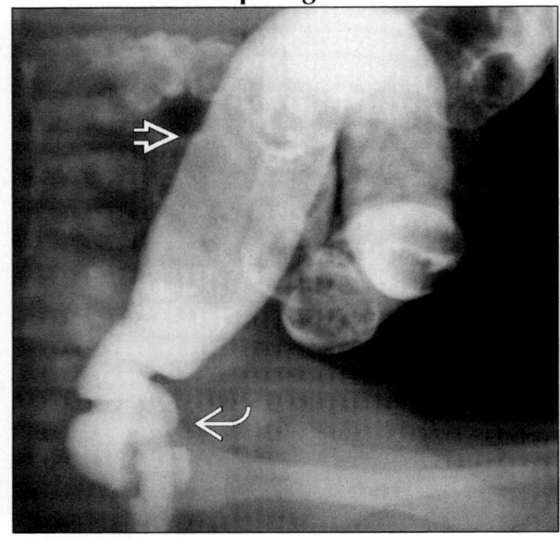

*(**Left**) Frontal contrast enema shows the transition zone between the normal caliber colon and the abnormally narrow colon in the region of the splenic flexure. Numerous lucent filling defects represent retained meconium. (**Right**) Coronal Meckel scan shows a focus of increased activity in the lower mid-abdomen . The activity is equivalent to that of gastric mucosa and increases with time. Note the physiologic bladder activity .*

Meconium Plug Syndrome (Small Left Colon Syndrome)

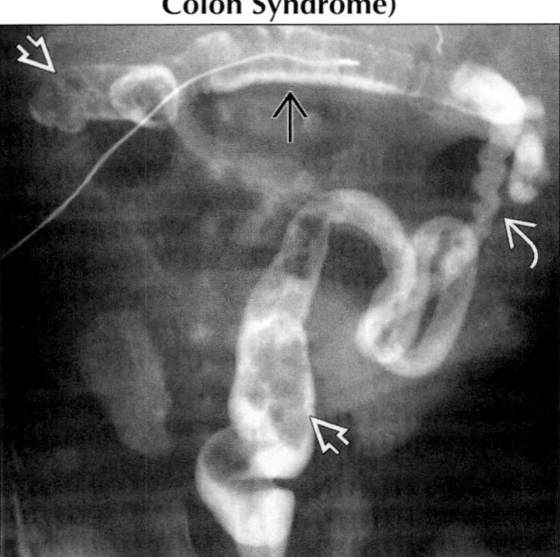

Meckel Diverticulum

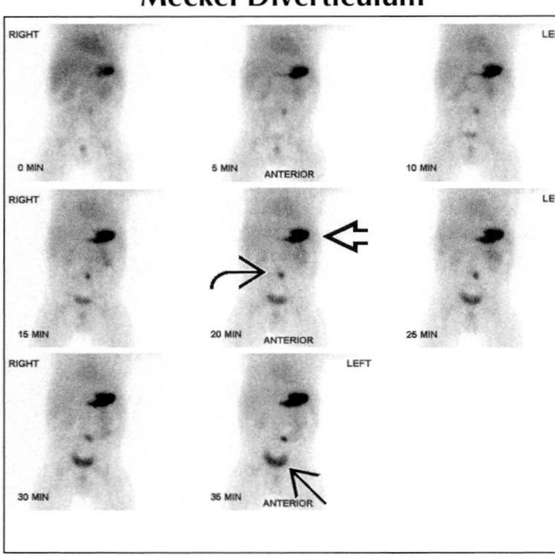

*(**Left**) Frontal radiograph shows several severely dilated bowel loops in a 2-day-old newborn with increasing abdominal distension after feedings. (**Right**) Frontal contrast enema in the same patient shows a classic appearance of a microcolon . The patient had proximal jejunal atresia with additional, more distal atresias discovered at surgery, which explains a microcolon in a patient with proximal jejunal atresia. Minimal meconium is seen .*

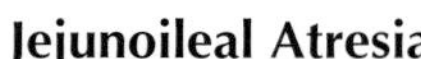

Jejunoileal Atresia

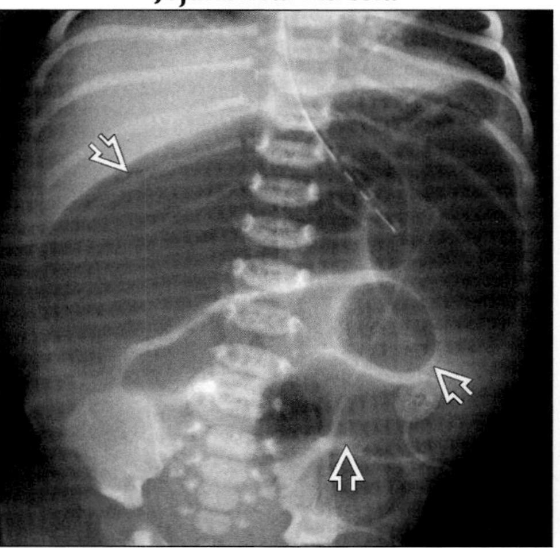

Jejunoileal Atresia

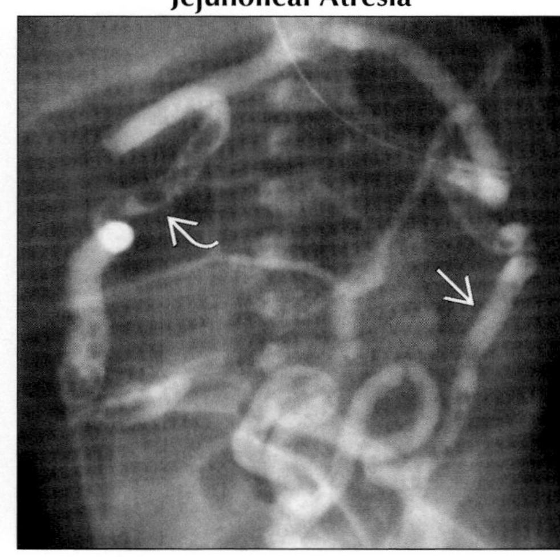

SMALL BOWEL OBSTRUCTION

Jejunoileal Atresia

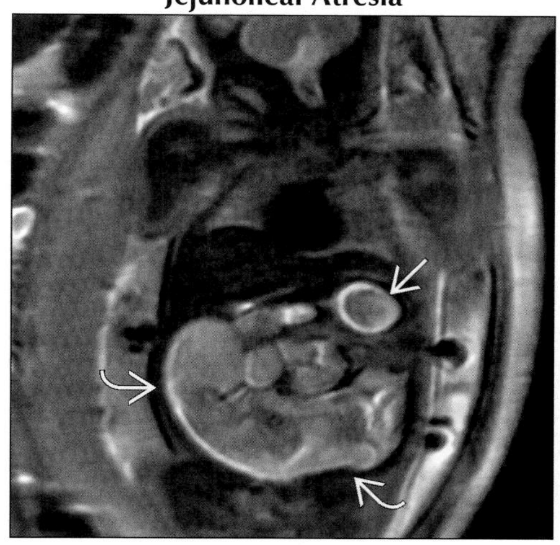

Jejunoileal Atresia

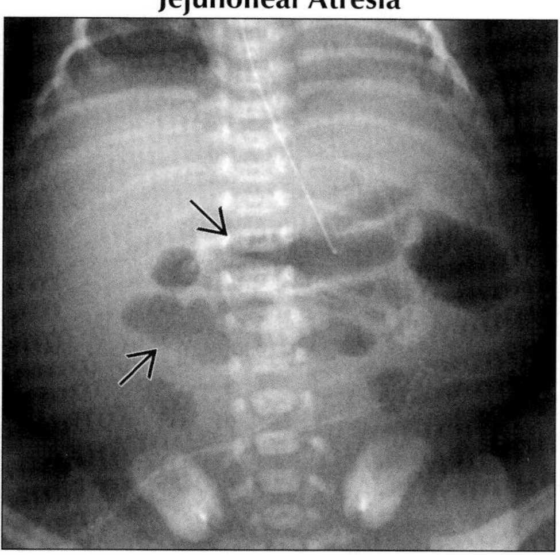

*(**Left**) Coronal T2WI MR shows a severely dilated loop of bowel → in the mid-abdomen in this fetus with mid-jejunal atresia. Note the stomach →. The level of atresia was distal, and no meconium was seen in the rectum on T1WI (not shown). (**Right**) AP radiograph shows several air-filled, mildly distended, mid-abdominal bowel loops → in a 1 day old with bilious emesis. Although only several loops of distended bowel are seen, the atresia was distal.*

Meconium Ileus

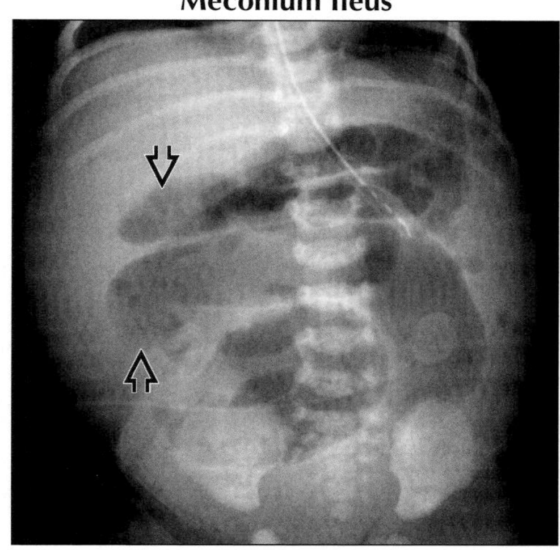

Meconium Ileus

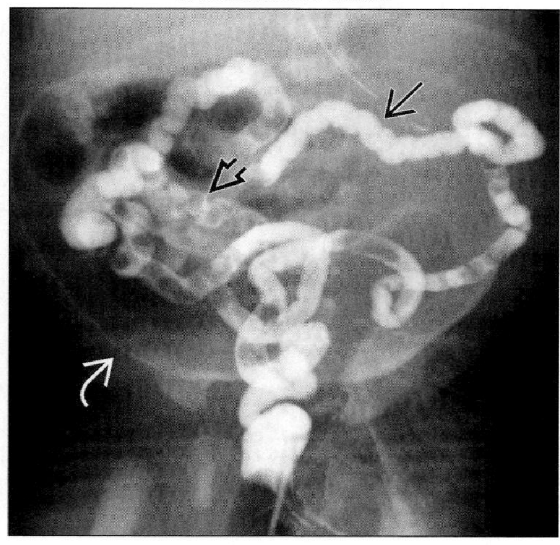

*(**Left**) Frontal radiograph with multiple dilated small bowel loops is consistent with a distal obstruction. Note the mottled bowel gas pattern in the right hemi-abdomen → reflecting inspissated meconium. (**Right**) Frontal contrast enema shows a microcolon →. Multiple filling defects seen in the distal ileum represent meconium →. This meconium ileus is complicated by bowel perforation; note the intraperitoneal contrast spillage →.*

Gastrointestinal Duplication Cysts

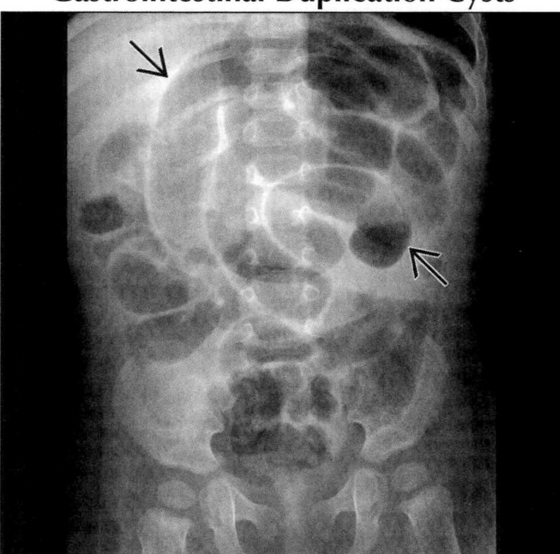

Gastrointestinal Duplication Cysts

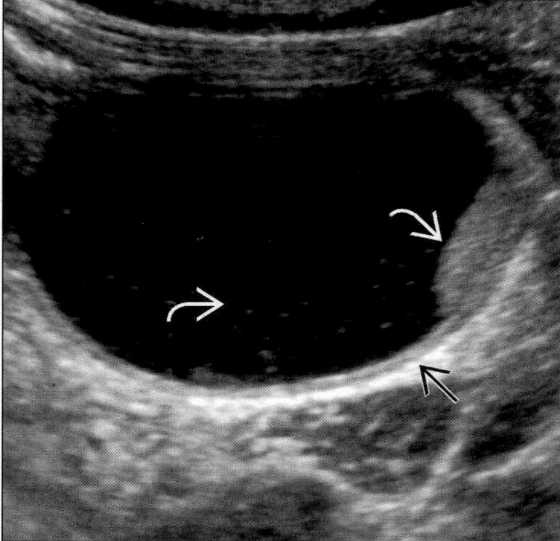

*(**Left**) Frontal radiograph shows multiple dilated bowel loops →, suggesting a distal obstructive process in this child who is clearly not a newborn based on skeletal maturation. (**Right**) Longitudinal ultrasound in a different patient shows an enteric duplication cyst palpated by the patient's clinician. Note the bowel wall layers →, as well as floating and layering echogenic debris →.*

NEONATAL DISTAL BOWEL OBSTRUCTION

DIFFERENTIAL DIAGNOSIS

Common
- Hirschsprung Disease (HD)
- Meconium Plug Syndrome (MPS)

Less Common
- Meconium Ileus (MI)
- Jejunoileal Atresia

Rare but Important
- Anorectal Malformation (ARM)
- Midgut Volvulus (MV)
- Omphalomesenteric Duct Remnant Obstruction
- Rectal Atresia
- Colonic Atresia

ESSENTIAL INFORMATION

Key Differential Diagnosis Issues
- Findings of contrast enema (CE) limit differential diagnosis: Colonic vs. small bowel process
- Antenatal or prenatal midgut volvulus late in natural history (ischemia); ileus can mimic distal bowel obstruction
- Hirschsprung disease more common in patients with Down syndrome
- Consider meconium ileus if family history of cystic fibrosis
- Meconium plug syndrome associated with maternal Mg++ therapy, maternal diabetes
- No rectal opening in male or single perineal opening in female patient with ARM
- Abdominal radiographs: Many dilated bowel loops
  - ± air-fluid levels
  - If dilated bowel loops but no air-fluid levels, suspect meconium ileus
- If CE and upper GI (UGI) normal in face of obstruction, consider omphalomesenteric duct remnant anomaly

Helpful Clues for Common Diagnoses
- **Hirschsprung Disease (HD)**
  - Often presents at birth with distal bowel obstruction
  - Contrast enema primary findings
    - Rectosigmoid ratio < 1
    - Transition most commonly sigmoid
    - Transition often missed if at anorectal verge; enema misinterpreted as normal
  - Other supporting CE findings
    - Distal colonic spasm
    - Colitis
    - Irregular contractions
    - Mucosal irregularity
    - Delayed evacuation
  - Total colonic Hirschsprung
    - Small colon without transition ± intraluminal terminal ileal calcification
  - Higher incidence in Down syndrome, especially total colonic disease
  - Radiologic transition not equivalent to histologic transition, especially in long-segment HD
- **Meconium Plug Syndrome (MPS)**
  - Nonpathologic diagnosis
  - Association with Mg++ therapy for preeclampsia and diabetic mother
  - Presents clinically similar to Hirschsprung disease
  - Enema findings
    - Rectosigmoid ratio > 1
    - Small left colon, abrupt transition to dilated bowel at splenic flexure, colonic meconium pellets
    - Evacuation of meconium during and after enema

Helpful Clues for Less Common Diagnoses
- **Meconium Ileus (MI)**
  - Possible radiographic findings
    - "Soap bubble" densities in right lower quadrant
    - Multiple dilated loops of air-filled bowel likely indicates simple MI
    - Air-fluid levels within bowel loops less likely due to thick meconium
    - Gasless abdomen indicates high risk of complicated MI
    - Peritoneal calcifications indicate meconium peritonitis (evidence of bowel perforation, complicated MI)
  - Contrast enema findings
    - Microcolon
    - Small terminal ileum (TI) filled with meconium pellets
    - Dilated ileum proximal to obstructing meconium
  - Possible ultrasound findings
    - Echogenic bowel loops
    - Meconium pseudocyst
    - Peritoneal calcifications

- Almost always associated with cystic fibrosis
- **Jejunoileal Atresia**
  - Possible radiographic findings
    - Multiple, dilated, air-filled bowel loops
    - Air-fluid levels within bowel loops
    - Gasless abdomen suggests bowel perforation
    - Peritoneal calcifications suggest meconium peritonitis due to bowel perforation
  - Contrast enema findings
    - Rectosigmoid ratio > 1
    - Microcolon
    - Normal caliber TI without meconium
    - Refluxed contrast in TI abruptly terminates in ileum or distal jejunum

Helpful Clues for Rare Diagnoses

- **Anorectal Malformation (ARM)**
  - Imperforate anus or anteriorly located stenotic rectal orifice on physical exam in male
  - Anterior stenotic rectal orifice or single perineal orifice on physical exam in female
  - Distal bowel obstruction
    - Colon generally more compliant; dilates more than small bowel
- **Midgut Volvulus (MV)**
  - Late presentation: Dilated bowel due to ischemic ileus
  - Radiographs show multiple dilated bowel loops
    - Sometimes pneumatosis or bowel wall thickening
  - Normal caliber colon on CE
  - UGI shows duodenal obstruction
    - Partial: Corkscrew with dilation of proximal duodenum
    - Complete: No contrast distal to obstruction
- **Omphalomesenteric Duct Remnant Obstruction**
  - Radiographs show dilated bowel loops of distal obstruction
  - Contrast enema: Usually normal caliber colon; reflux contrast into beak-shaped, obstructed terminal ileum
  - Normal duodenal rotation on UGI
  - Volvulus of omphalomesenteric duct remnant
- **Rectal Atresia**
  - Radiographs show dilated bowel loops of distal obstruction
  - Colonic loops usually dilate more than small bowel loops
  - Contrast enema: Abrupt obstruction of colon just above anorectal verge
  - Considered by some to be a type of anorectal malformation
- **Colonic Atresia**
  - Findings on radiographs similar to rectal atresia
  - Contrast enema: Obstruction of colon proximal to rectum
  - Etiology: Ischemic event in utero similar to small bowel atresias

Hirschsprung Disease (HD)

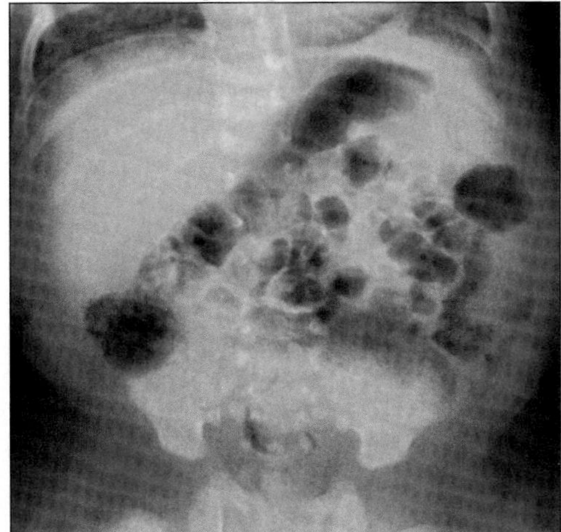

Anteroposterior fluoroscopic spot radiograph scout in an infant with infrequent stooling shows moderate to large stool load without other specific abnormality. The bones appear normal.

Hirschsprung Disease (HD)

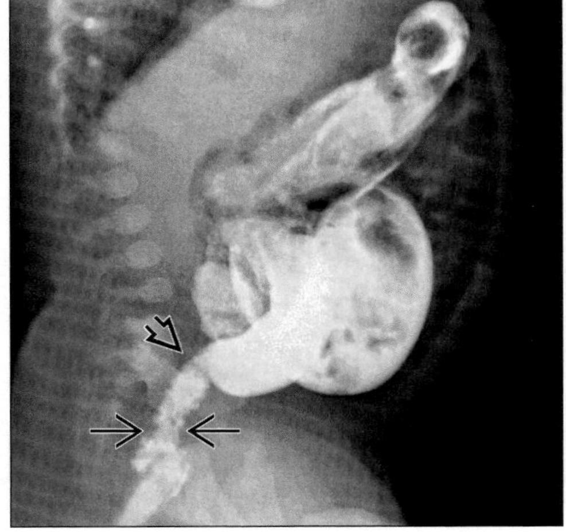

Lateral contrast enema in the same patient shows a narrow rectum with transition ⇨ to the dilated colon at the rectosigmoid junction consistent with Hirschsprung disease. Note the spasm → in the distal segment.

NEONATAL DISTAL BOWEL OBSTRUCTION

Hirschsprung Disease (HD)

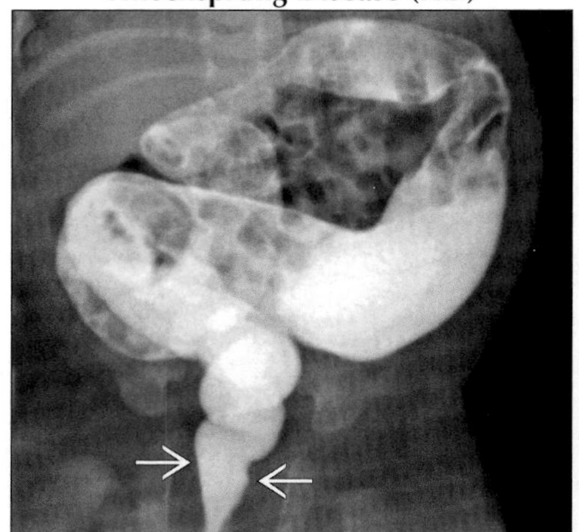

Hirschsprung Disease (HD)

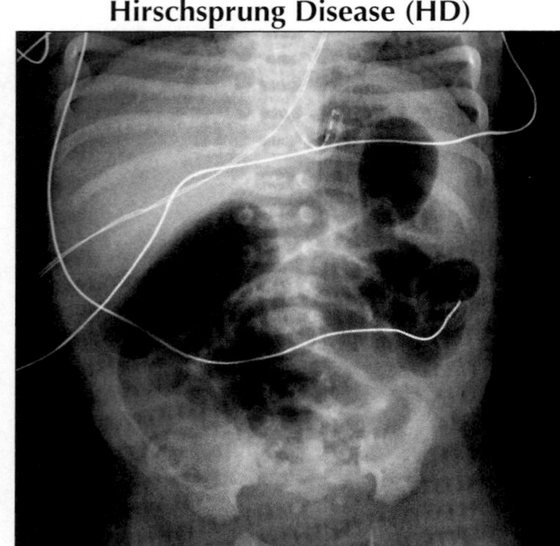

(Left) *AP contrast enema in the same patient shows the catheter has been removed. There is less spasm, but there is still a small rectum ➔ (RS ratio < 1). The initially distended lateral view of the colon to the splenic flexure is the key view for a well-performed enema.* ***(Right)*** *AP radiograph shows multiple dilated loops of bowel throughout abdomen, most consistent with a distal bowel obstruction. There are no calcifications, free air, pneumatosis, or soft tissue masses.*

Hirschsprung Disease (HD)

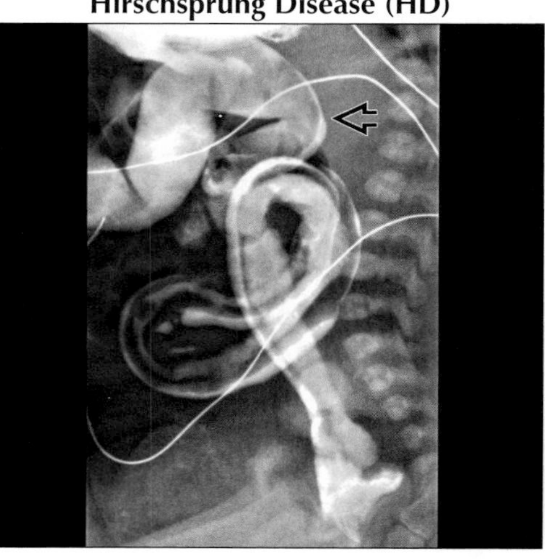

Hirschsprung Disease (HD)

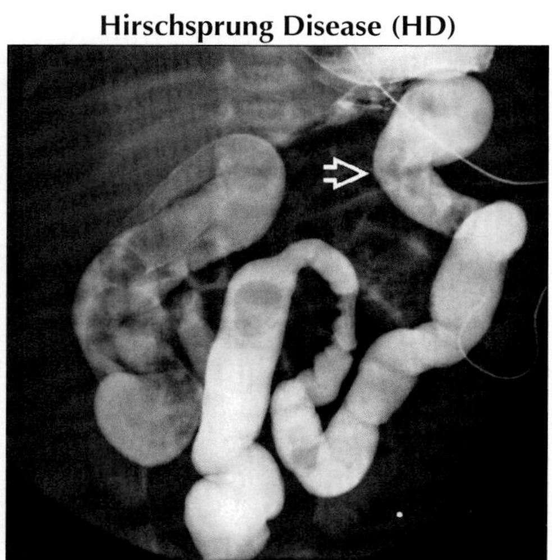

(Left) *Lateral contrast enema shows borderline RS ratio, meconium within the small left colon, and a transition zone at the splenic flexure ⇨, suggesting MPS. Symptoms did not improve, and biopsy was performed in this pathologically proven HD.* ***(Right)*** *AP contrast enema in the same child shows transition at splenic flexure ➔ and evacuation of meconium. However, rectal biopsy showed no ganglion cells, consistent with HD. MPS and HD can be indistinguishable on enema.*

Hirschsprung Disease (HD)

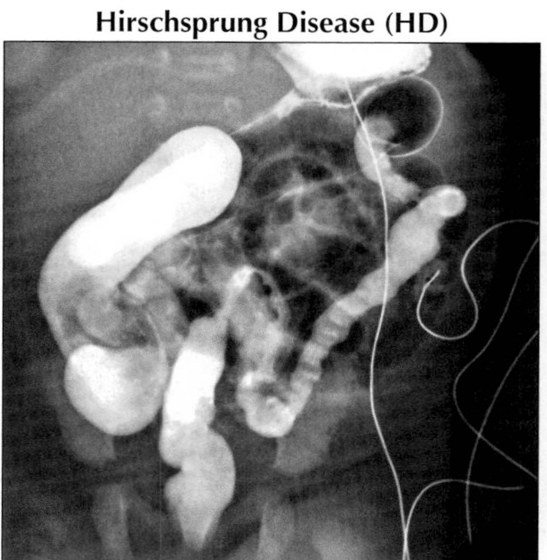

Meconium Plug Syndrome (MPS)

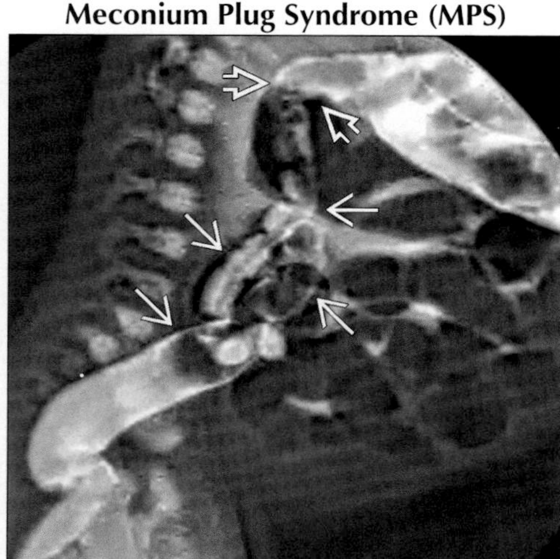

(Left) *AP contrast enema shows findings suggestive of MPS. At operation, total-colonic HD was found. In high-colonic HD, an enema transition is unreliable in estimating histologic transition.* ***(Right)*** *Lateral contrast enema shows a rectosigmoid ratio > 1, meconium plugs in the small left colon ➔, and a splenic flexure transition ➔ to the dilated transverse colon of MPS.*

NEONATAL DISTAL BOWEL OBSTRUCTION

Meconium Plug Syndrome (MPS)

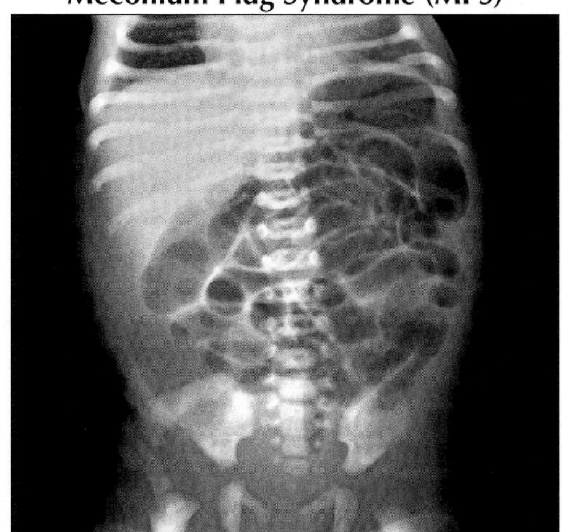

Meconium Plug Syndrome (MPS)

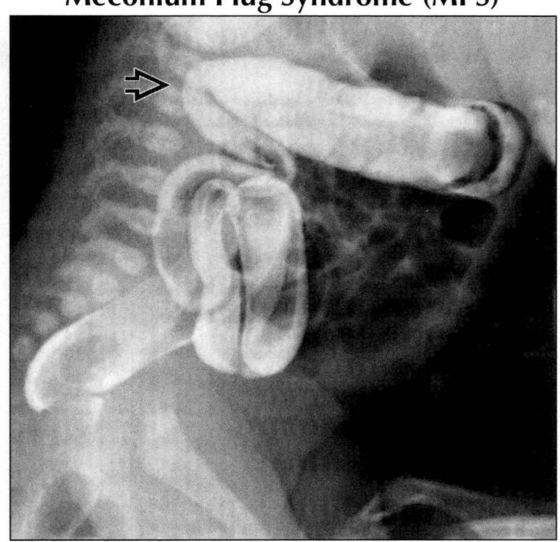

(Left) *AP radiograph in a 2-day-old infant shows multiple air-filled dilated loops of bowel, consistent with neonatal distal intestinal obstruction.* ***(Right)*** *Lateral contrast enema in the same patient shows a RS ratio > 1, a small left colon, a transition to dilated colon at the splenic flexure ➡, and multiple large tubular meconium plugs in the entire colon, consistent with meconium plug (a.k.a. small left colon) syndrome.*

Meconium Plug Syndrome (MPS)

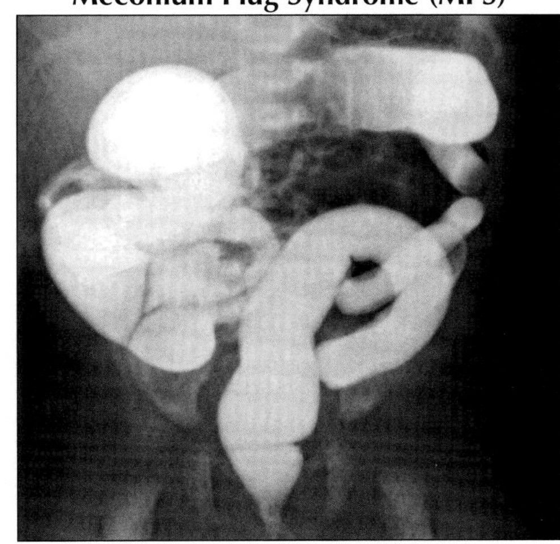

Meconium Ileus (MI)

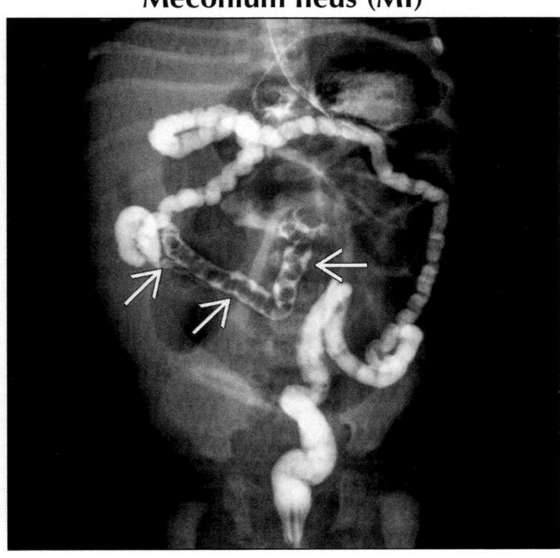

(Left) *AP contrast enema in the same infant shows that the meconium plugs seen on the earlier study have passed; the enema in most cases of MPS is curative. High Hirschsprung is also possible.* ***(Right)*** *Anteroposterior contrast enema shows a microcolon with meconium plugs lined up in the terminal ileum like "pearls on a string" ➡ and small bowel obstruction of the meconium ileus.*

Meconium Ileus (MI)

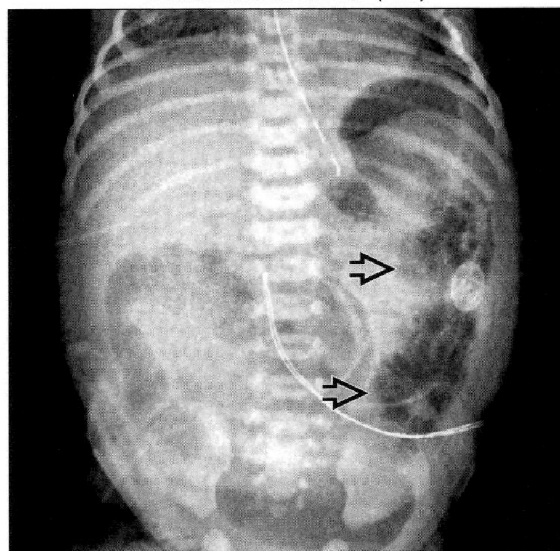

Meconium Ileus (MI)

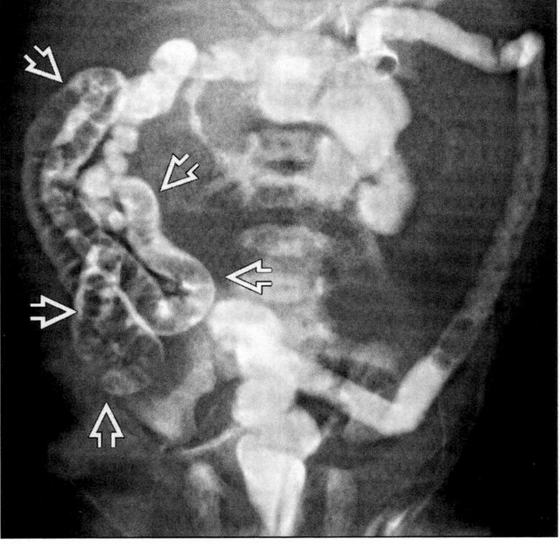

(Left) *AP fluoroscopic spot radiograph scout image in a neonate shows findings of distal obstruction and bubbly lucencies ➡ in the abdomen. When this pattern is seen, consider complications of obstruction or meconium ileus (MI).* ***(Right)*** *AP contrast enema shows a microcolon devoid of significant meconium and a terminal ileum filled with pellets of meconium ➡, diagnostic of MI and almost always of underlying cystic fibrosis.*

NEONATAL DISTAL BOWEL OBSTRUCTION

*(**Left**) AP fluoroscopic spot radiograph in a 2-day-old infant shows multiple loops of bowel, suggestive of distal obstruction, with soft tissue density ➡ in the right lower abdomen. (**Right**) AP contrast enema shows a microcolon with reflux into terminal ileum (TI), abrupt termination of the contrast head ➡, and dilated proximal air-filled bowel, consistent with ileal atresia. Note that there is no meconium in TI ⇨, differentiating this from MI.*

Jejunoileal Atresia

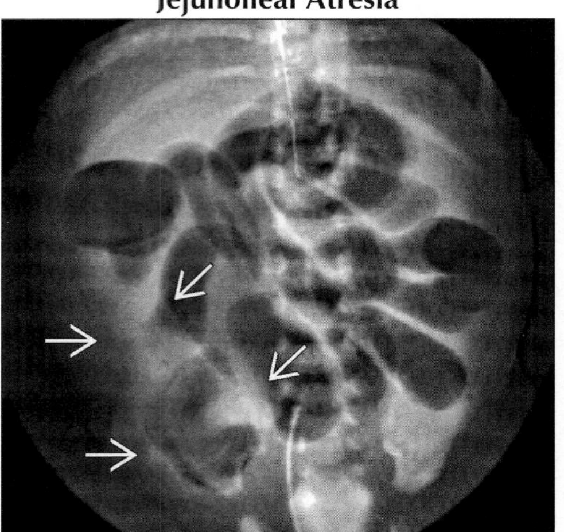

Jejunoileal Atresia

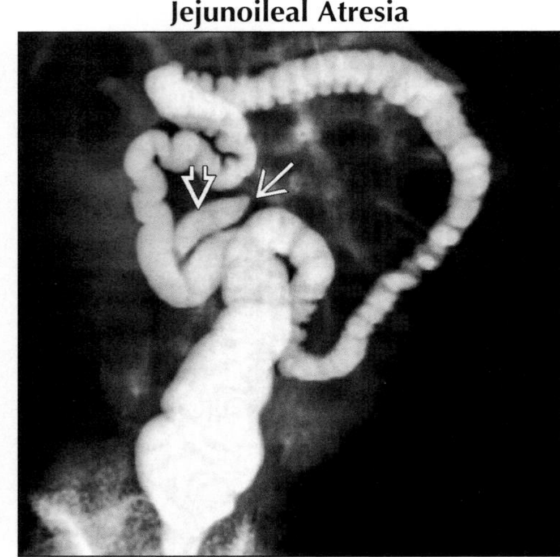

*(**Left**) AP radiograph on this 1-day-old male neonate shows multiple dilated loops, consistent with distal obstruction all the way to the rectum ➡ in this patient who has no anal opening on the perineum, clinically consistent with ARM. (**Right**) Lateral x-table prone radiograph shows a dilated rectum ➡ very close to the expected location of the anal sphincter ⇨, a low ARM. This image positioning is used when the level of ARM is clinically occult.*

Anorectal Malformation (ARM)

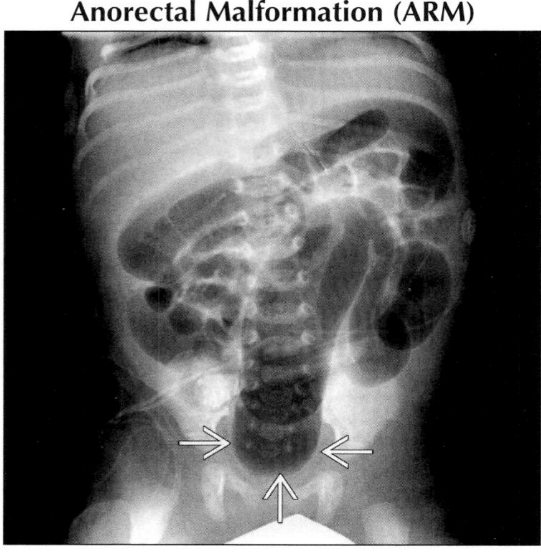

Anorectal Malformation (ARM)

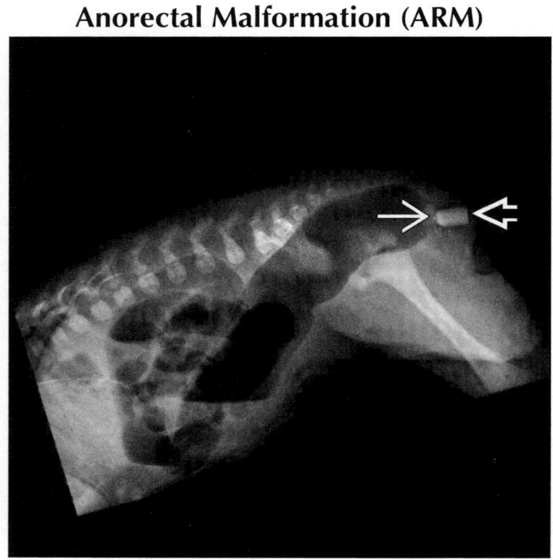

*(**Left**) AP radiograph in a 1-day-old neonate with bilious emesis shows multiple distended bowel loops in the mid and right abdomen and a nasogastric suction tube. A contrast enema is recommended to exclude distal bowel obstruction. (**Right**) AP contrast enema in the same patient shows an essentially normal colon caliber without explanation for bilious emesis; therefore, an upper GI was recommended to exclude MV, which could mimic distal obstruction.*

Midgut Volvulus (MV)

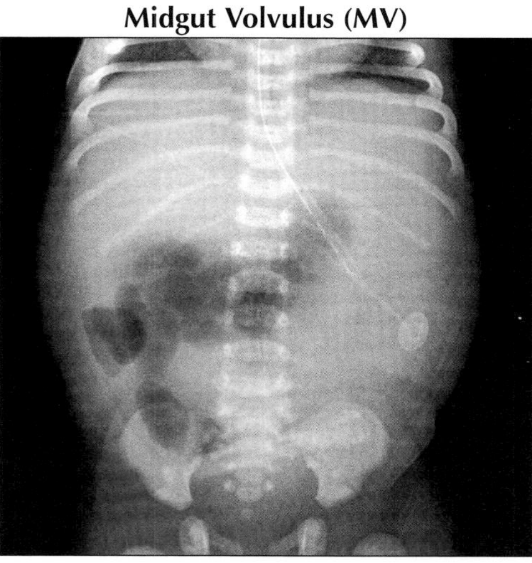

Midgut Volvulus (MV)

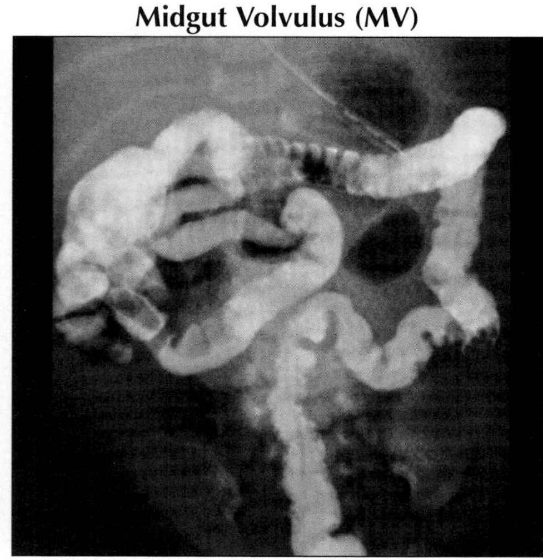

Midgut Volvulus (MV)

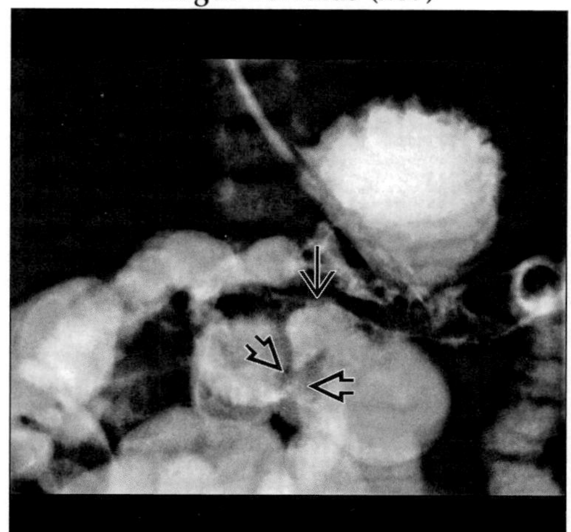

Omphalomesenteric Duct Remnant Obstruction

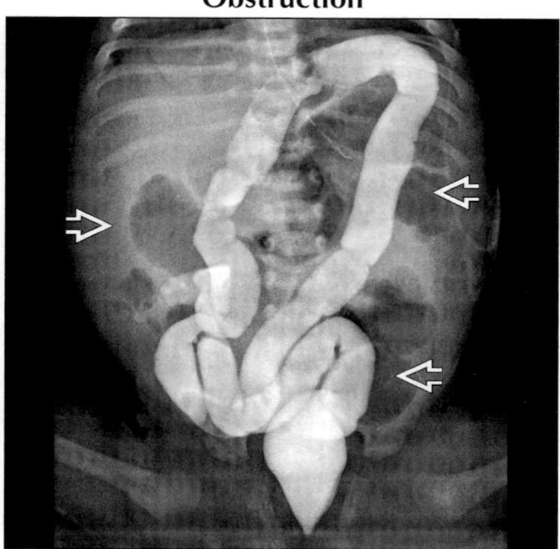

*(**Left**) AP upper GI in the same child shows a low duodenojejunal ➔ and "beaked" appearance of D3 to D4 segment ➢, suggesting a twist. Given the findings of possible malrotation, the patient was taken for surgical exploration, which yielded a midgut volvulus. (**Right**) AP contrast enema in another patient shows a normal rectosigmoid and a normal to smallish colon on a background of small bowel obstruction ➢.*

Omphalomesenteric Duct Remnant Obstruction

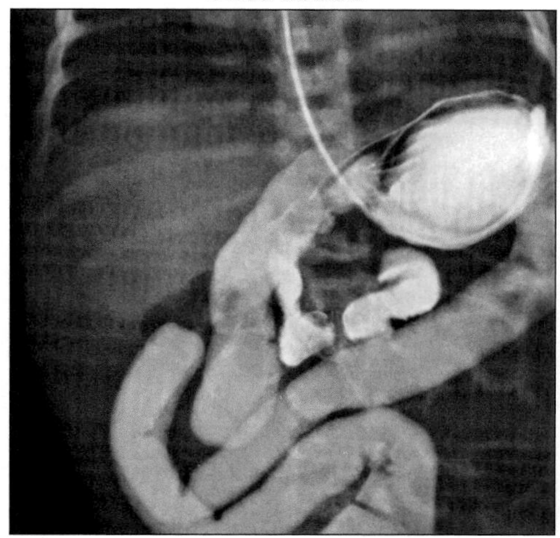

Rectal Atresia

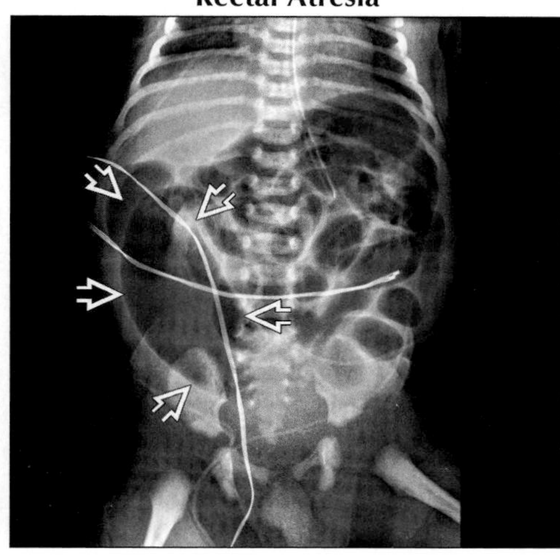

*(**Left**) AP upper GI in the same child shows normal rotation; the duodenum was retroperitoneal on lateral view (not shown). With a smallish colon and normal upper GI, one should consider omphalomesenteric duct remnant obstruction, which was found at surgery. (**Right**) AP radiograph shows dilated bowel loops with an asymmetrically dilated loop ➢, out of proportion to the surrounding bowel, possibly representing the colon.*

Rectal Atresia

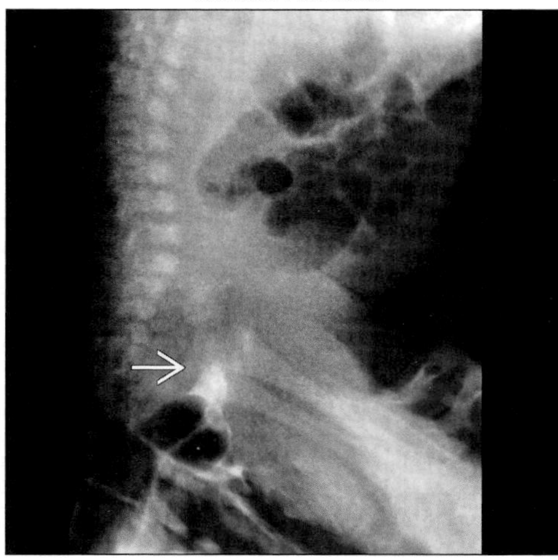

Colonic Atresia

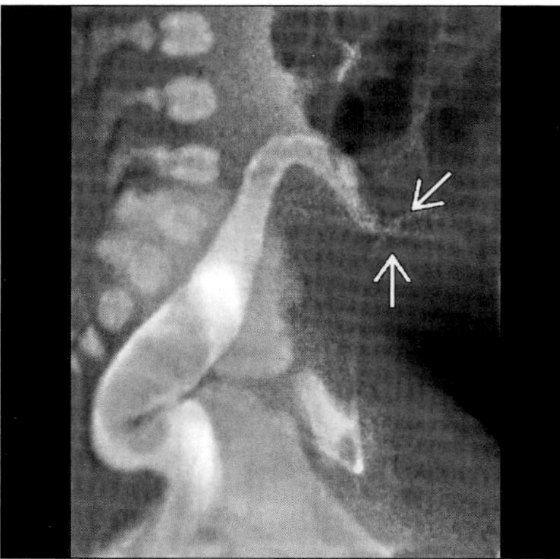

*(**Left**) Lateral contrast enema shows complete obstruction of the contrast head in the region of the rectum ➔, consistent with rectal atresia. (**Right**) Lateral contrast enema in a 1-day-old patient with failure to pass meconium shows filling of the rectum and sigmoid with abrupt termination of the contrast head at the junction of the sigmoid and descending colon ➔, consistent with colonic atresia.*

MICROCOLON

DIFFERENTIAL DIAGNOSIS

Common
- Meconium Ileus (MI)
- Jejunoileal Atresia
- Defunctionalized Colon
- Immature Colon

Less Common
- Total Colonic Hirschsprung Disease
- Omphalomesenteric Duct Remnant Obstruction
- Ileal Duplication Cyst
- Colon Atresia

Rare but Important
- Megacystis Microcolon Intestinal Hypoperistalsis Syndrome

ESSENTIAL INFORMATION

Key Differential Diagnosis Issues
- Patient age (including gestational age)
- History of ileostomy
- Family history of bowel disease
- Caliber of diffusely small colon on contrast enema
- Appearance of contrast-filled ileum refluxed from enema

Helpful Clues for Common Diagnoses
- **Meconium Ileus (MI)**
  - Almost always associated with cystic fibrosis (CF)
  - 1/2 of cases are complicated by perforation, pseudocyst formation, or segmental volvulus
  - 15% of CF patients born with MI
  - Findings of simple meconium ileus
    - Multiple dilated air-filled bowel loops
    - "Soap bubble" densities mid-right lower abdomen
    - Little or no air-fluid levels due to thick meconium
  - Findings of complicated meconium ileus
    - Curvilinear abdominal calcifications (peritoneal, pseudocyst) = meconium peritonitis
    - Soft tissue mass
    - Paucity of bowel gas
  - Contrast enema
    - Microcolon; some say MI causes smallest unused colon
    - Meconium pellets fill small terminal ileum (TI) like "pearls on a string"
    - Dilated ileum proximal to obstructing meconium
    - Rectosigmoid ratio usually normal (> 1)
    - Initially, very little meconium in colon
  - Ultrasound
    - Echogenic bowel loops
    - Meconium pseudocyst ± curvilinear calcifications of wall
    - Peritoneal calcifications
- **Jejunoileal Atresia**
  - Microcolon with little or no meconium in distal small bowel, which ends abruptly on neonatal enema
  - Due to in utero ischemic event
  - Multiple dilated air-filled bowel loops
  - Air-fluid levels within bowel loops
  - Gasless abdomen suggests bowel perforation
  - Peritoneal calcifications suggests meconium peritonitis
  - Contrast enema
    - Rectosigmoid ratio > 1
    - Microcolon: More distal the atresia = smaller the microcolon
    - Normal caliber terminal ileum without significant meconium
    - Abrupt termination of refluxed contrast within ileum
  - Proximal jejunal atresia; almost normal-sized colon
    - Succus entericus produced by remaining small bowel flows to colon; therefore, colon becomes normal caliber
- **Defunctionalized Colon**
  - Usually clinical history of prior disease requires colostomy
    - Necrotizing enterocolitis (NEC)
    - Bowel perforation
    - Gastroschisis
    - Omphalocele
    - Midgut volvulus with ischemic bowel resection due to malrotation
    - Inflammatory bowel disease (IBD): Crohn or ulcerative colitis
  - Small diameter of colon segment distal to created ostomy on contrast enema or colostogram
    - Caused by disuse; normal diameter usually regained after ostomy takedown

- Rectosigmoid ratio usually > 1
- **Immature Colon**
  - Similar in functional etiology to meconium plug syndrome (MPS), a.k.a. small left colon syndrome
  - Premature infant
  - Normal rectosigmoid ratio
  - Slightly small colon
  - No pathologic diagnosis
  - Sometimes meconium plugs scattered in colon

Helpful Clues for Less Common Diagnoses

- **Total Colonic Hirschsprung Disease**
  - a.k.a. total colonic aganglionosis
  - Often involves segment of distal small bowel
  - Rarely aganglionosis involves entire intestine (total intestinal Hirschsprung)
  - Neonatal bowel obstruction
  - Multiple dilated loops of bowel on radiography
  - ± distal ileal small bowel intraluminal calcifications
  - Contrast enema
    - Rectosigmoid ratio ≤ 1
    - Small colon throughout on neonatal contrast enema
    - Findings can sometimes mimic high-transition HD or MPS
    - Colon often shorter than normal
    - Sometimes squared-off flexures
    - Delayed spontaneous evacuation of contrast from colon
- **Ileal Duplication Cyst**
  - Small colon due to partial ileal obstruction
  - Normal rectosigmoid ratio (> 1)
  - Well-circumscribed, right lower quadrant fluid collection on US with gut signature
- **Colon Atresia**
  - Ischemic event similar to other nonduodenal atresias of small bowel or colon
  - Neonatal bowel obstruction
  - Dilated loop or several loops out of proportion to rest of obstructive pattern on radiograph
  - Microcolon at enema, which terminates at level of colonic atresia

Helpful Clues for Rare Diagnoses

- **Megacystis Microcolon Intestinal Hypoperistalsis Syndrome**
  - Rare, often fatal condition
  - M:F = 1:4
  - Similar features to prune belly syndrome
  - Autosomal recessive
  - Findings at presentation
    - Distal intestinal obstruction, multiple dilated bowel loops
    - Frequent malrotation
    - Lack of bowel peristalsis
    - Microcolon on neonatal enema
    - Large, nonobstructed urinary bladder ± hydronephrosis
  - Abdominal wall laxity
  - Survival prolonged by TPN, bowel transplant

Meconium Ileus (MI)

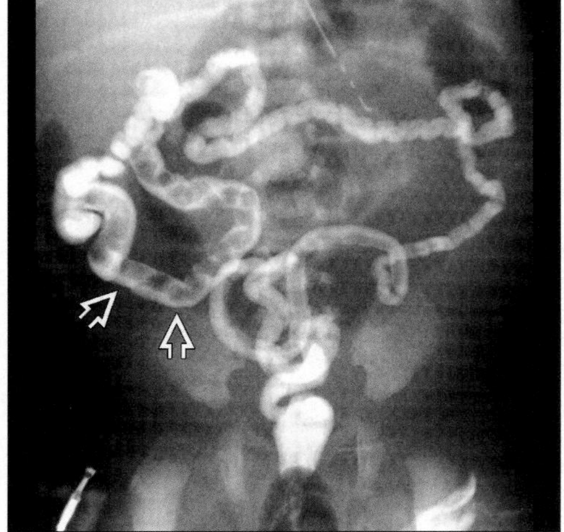

Anteroposterior contrast enema shows a microcolon, normal rectosigmoid, normal terminal ileum filled with meconium ("pearls on a string") ➡, and distal small bowel obstruction.

Meconium Ileus (MI)

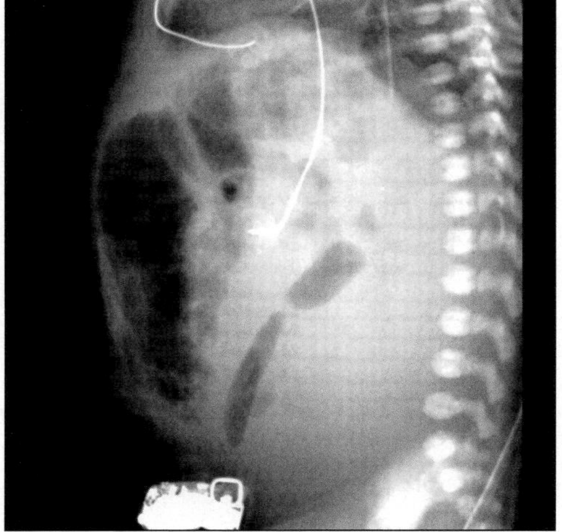

Lateral contrast enema x-table lateral scout view shows dilated loops of bowel but a paucity of air-fluid levels and no free air.

MICROCOLON

(**Left**) *Lateral contrast enema shows a rectosigmoid ratio > 1 with a tiny caliber of sigmoid colon.* (**Right**) *Anteroposterior contrast enema shows a microcolon with minimal if any meconium. There is reflux of contrast into the terminal ileum, which is filled with plugs of meconium →. This constellation of findings is most characteristic of meconium ileus, which should prompt further clinical evaluation for a definitive diagnosis of cystic fibrosis.*

Meconium Ileus (MI)

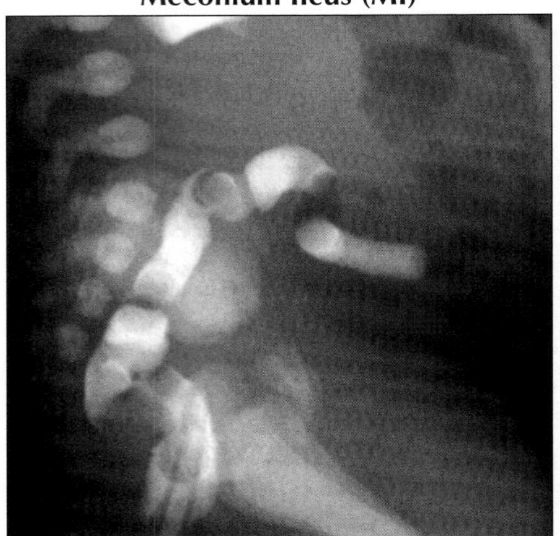

Meconium Ileus (MI)

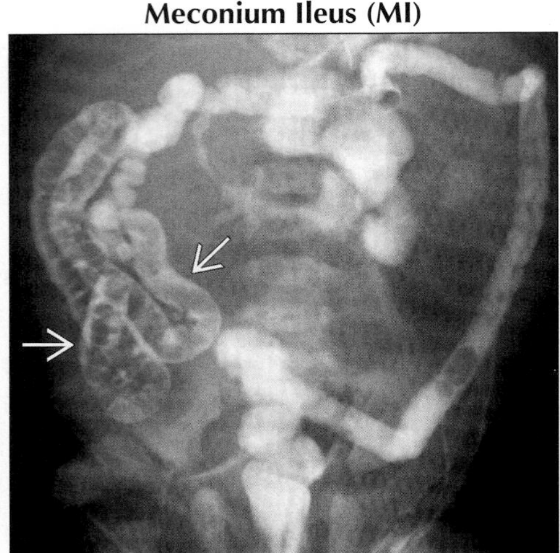

(**Left**) *Anteroposterior contrast enema scout image shows multiple dilated bowel loops, suggestive of distal bowel obstruction. "Soap bubble" density → is seen in the left abdomen. There is no definite pneumatosis intestinalis or free air.* (**Right**) *Anteroposterior contrast enema shows a normal rectosigmoid but a diffusely small colon with reflux into the normal terminal ileal loops that terminate abruptly within the ileum, consistent with ileal atresia.*

Meconium Ileus (MI)

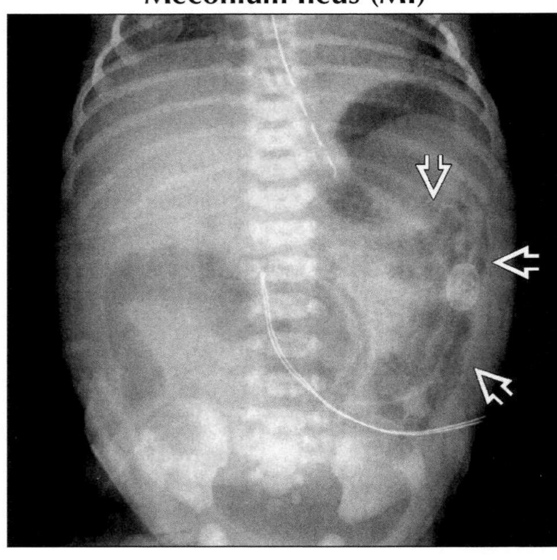

Jejunoileal Atresia

(**Left**) *Anteroposterior radiograph scout at 36 hours of age shows dilated bowel loops consistent with a distal intestinal obstruction. Soft tissue density → in the RLQ is likely fluid-filled bowel loops. No bowel thickening/pneumatosis is seen.* (**Right**) *Anteroposterior contrast enema shows a normal rectosigmoid ratio, a microcolon with no significant meconium in it, and abrupt termination of contrast in the terminal ileum →, consistent with ileal atresia.*

Jejunoileal Atresia

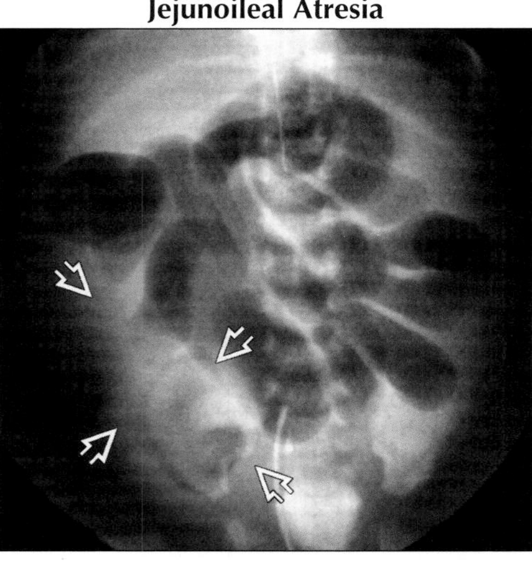

Jejunoileal Atresia

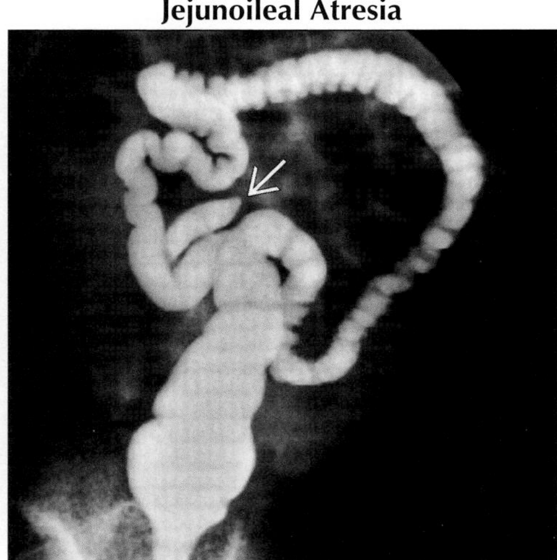

Defunctionalized Colon

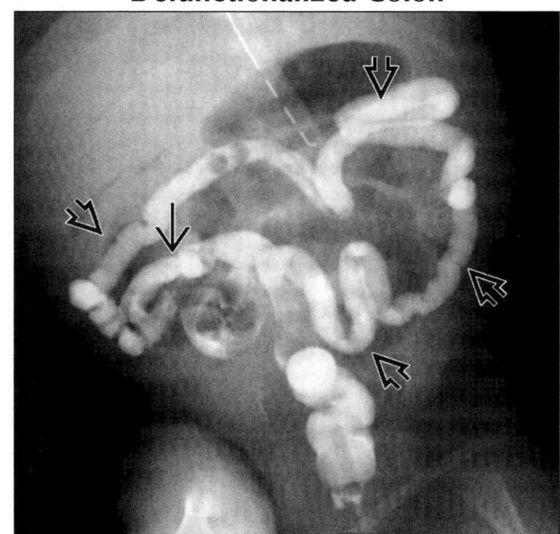

Immature Colon

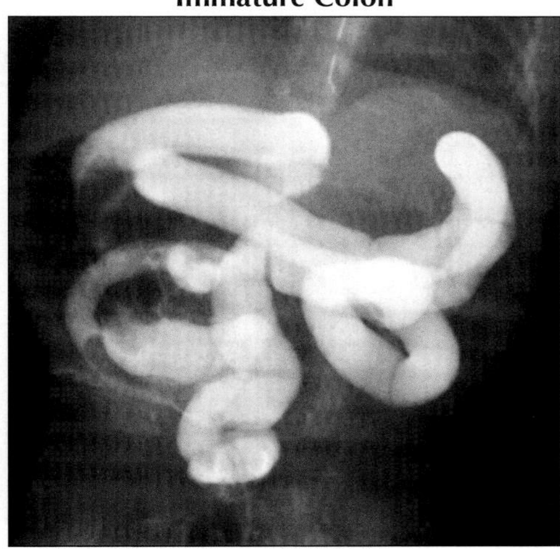

(Left) *Anteroposterior contrast enema shows a normal rectosigmoid, tiny colon ⇨, and normal terminal ileum →, in a patient with ileostomy for perforated NEC. Enema was performed prior to ileostomy takedown to exclude colonic NEC stricture.* ***(Right)*** *Anteroposterior contrast enema shows a smallish but otherwise normal colon in a premature infant. No pathologic diagnosis. Rectal biopsy showed ganglion cells. With time, small bowel dilation resolved.*

Total Colonic Hirschsprung Disease

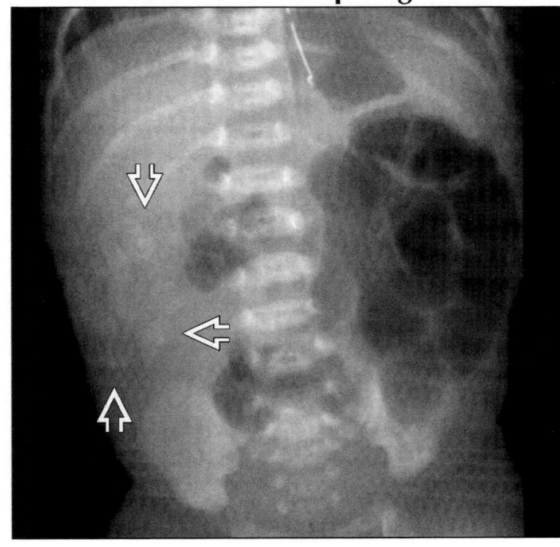

Total Colonic Hirschsprung Disease

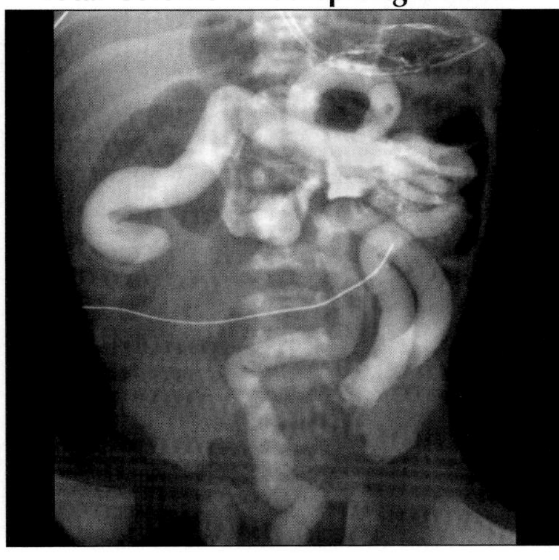

(Left) *AP radiograph shows dilated bowel loops and round intraluminal calcifications ⇨. Differential considerations of these intraluminal calcifications and bowel obstruction include anorectal malformation (mixing of meconium and urine), small bowel atresia, and total colonic Hirschsprung.* ***(Right)*** *AP contrast enema in same patient shows small rectosigmoid and microcolon. Total colonic Hirschsprung was the most likely diagnosis.*

Omphalomesenteric Duct Remnant Obstruction

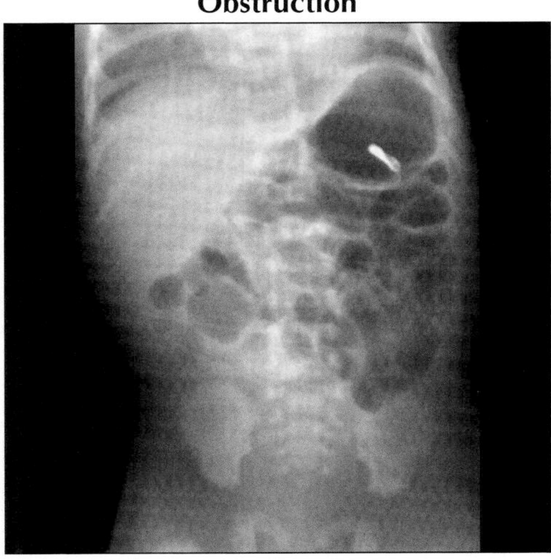

Omphalomesenteric Duct Remnant Obstruction

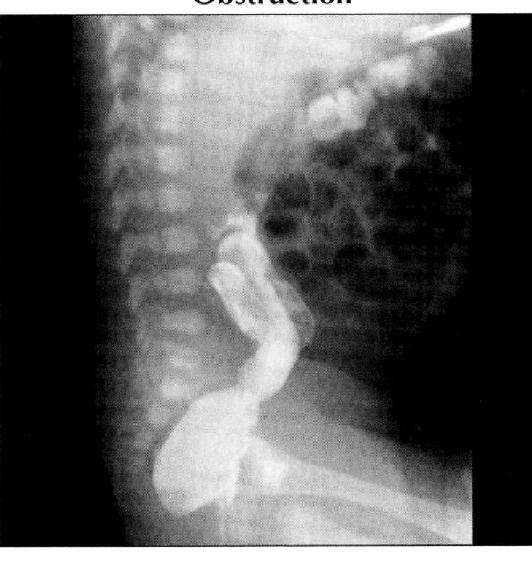

(Left) *AP radiograph in a 2 day old with no meconium per rectum shows dilated bowel loops suggestive of distal obstruction. No abnormal calcific densities or bowel thickening is seen.* ***(Right)*** *Lateral contrast enema shows a normal rectosigmoid with a normal to smallish caliber of the remaining colon. Upper GI (not shown) revealed normal rotation and no proximal bowel obstruction. Twisting of the omphalomesenteric duct remnant around ileum was found at operation.*

Omphalomesenteric Duct Remnant Obstruction

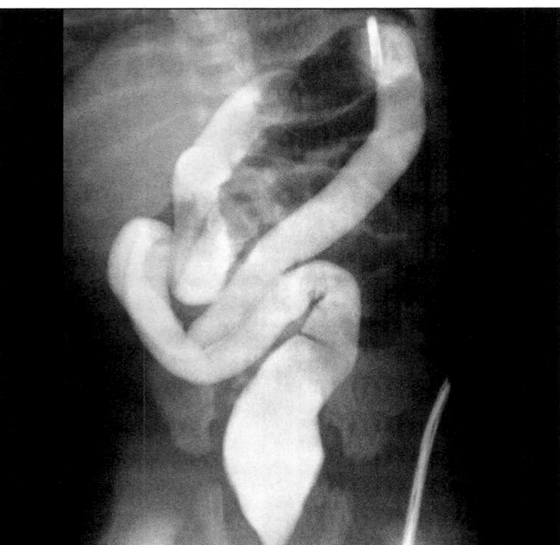

Ileal Duplication Cyst

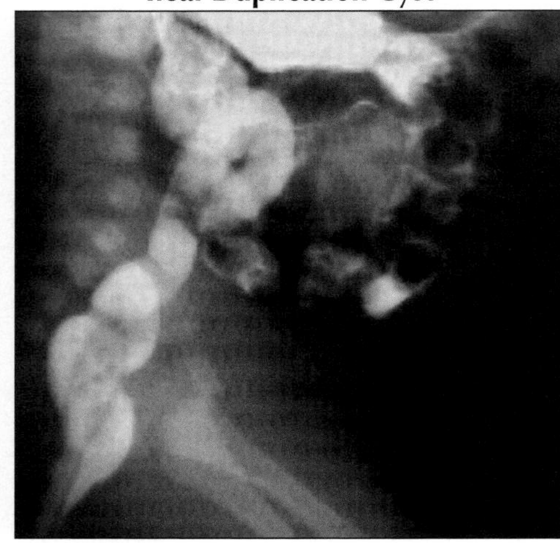

*(**Left**) AP contrast enema shows the normal to smallish caliber of the remainder of the colon, normal in configuration. In the face of distal bowel obstruction and a normal or near-normal enema, other causes of distal obstruction, including omphalomesenteric duct remnant obstruction, and distal obstruction due to ileal duplication cyst, should be considered. (**Right**) Lateral contrast enema in a 2 day old shows a normal rectosigmoid but a borderline small colon.*

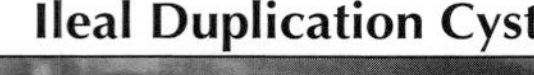

Ileal Duplication Cyst

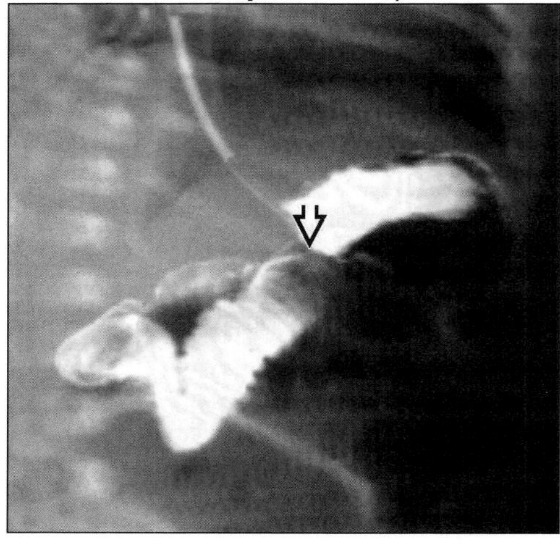

Ileal Duplication Cyst

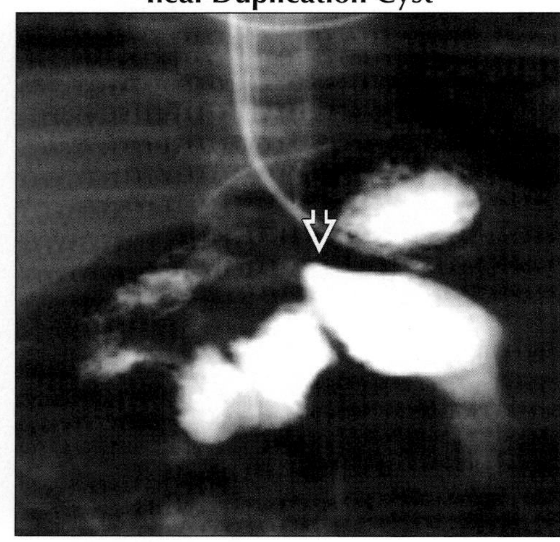

*(**Left**) Oblique upper GI through the nasogastric tube in the same patient shows a retroperitoneal duodenum with DJJ up to the level of the duodenal bulb. (**Right**) AP upper GI in the same patient shows DJJ at or left of the left vertebral pedicle with dilation of the contrast-filled proximal jejunum and dilated, air-filled distal loops, findings suggestive of distal intestinal bowel obstruction.*

Ileal Duplication Cyst

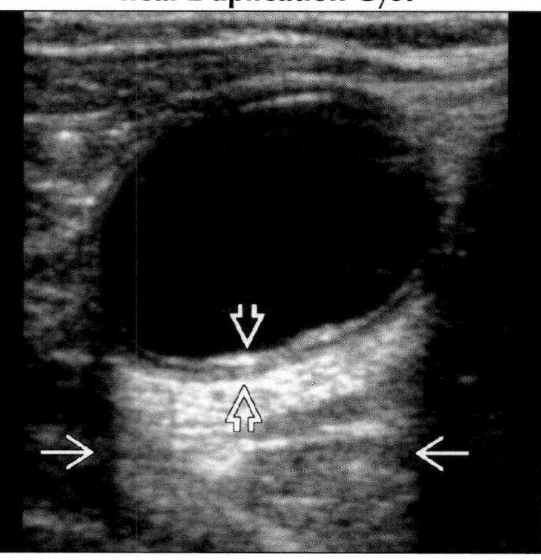

Ileal Duplication Cyst

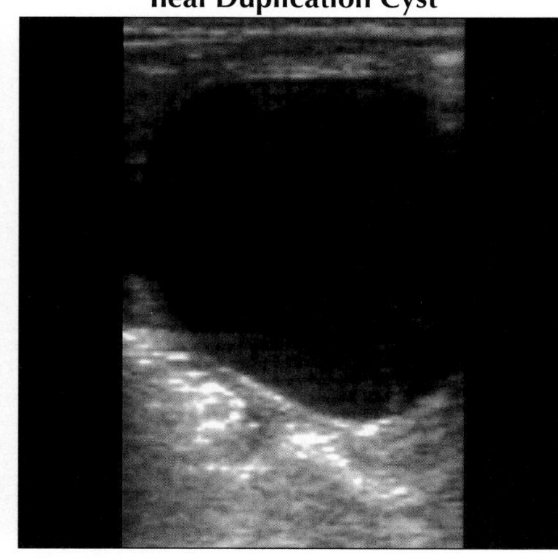

*(**Left**) Transverse harmonic ultrasound in the right lower quadrant of the abdomen shows a well-circumscribed, anechoic cyst with posterior acoustic enhancement and gut signature, characteristic sonographic findings of an intestinal duplication cyst. In this location, this is likely an ileal duplication cyst. (**Right**) Longitudinal harmonic ultrasound of the right lower quadrant shows findings of a probable ileal duplication cyst.*

Colon Atresia

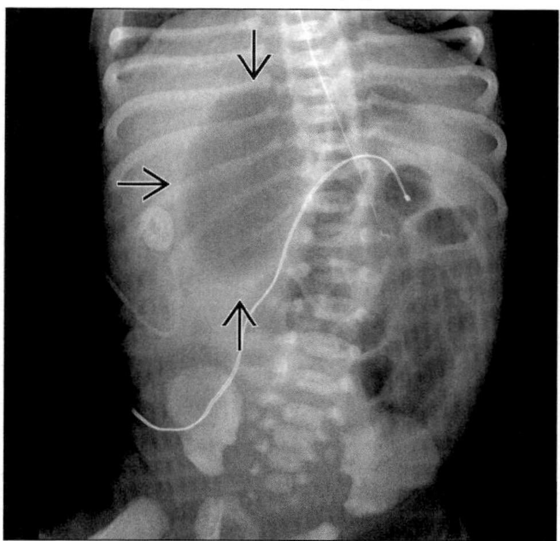

Colon Atresia

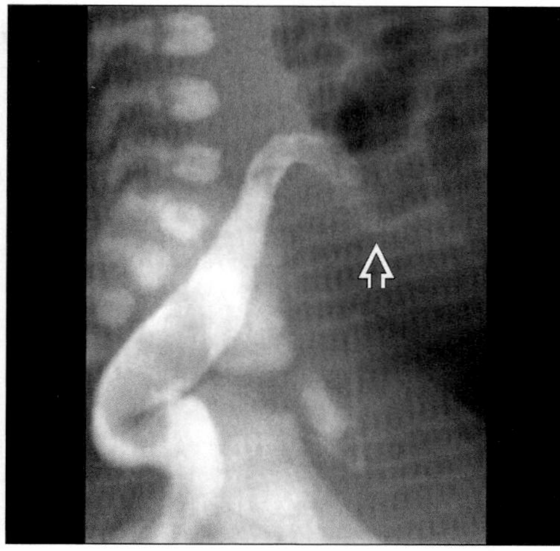

(Left) *AP radiograph in a 2 day old with failure to pass meconium shows multiple dilated bowel loops of a distal bowel obstruction. There is a large dilated loop ⇨ in the right upper abdomen, out of proportion to the other smaller distended loops in the left abdomen. This is not uncommon in colon atresia.* ***(Right)*** *Lateral contrast enema in the same patient shows a microcolon, which ends abruptly ➡ in this patient with colon atresia.*

Megacystis Microcolon Intestinal Hypoperistalsis Syndrome

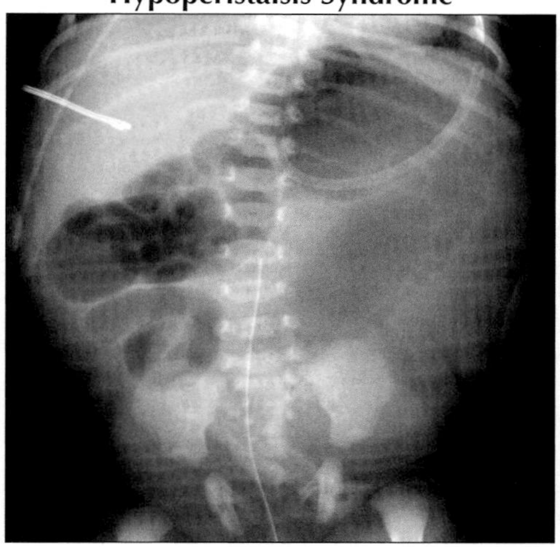

Megacystis Microcolon Intestinal Hypoperistalsis Syndrome

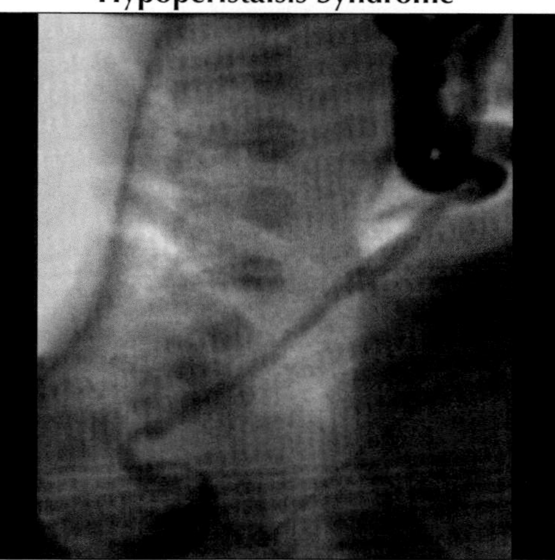

(Left) *AP radiograph of a 2 day old with failure to pass meconium and vomiting shows dilated bowel loops, suggestive of distal bowel obstruction.* ***(Right)*** *Lateral contrast enema in the same patient shows a tiny colon.*

Megacystis Microcolon Intestinal Hypoperistalsis Syndrome

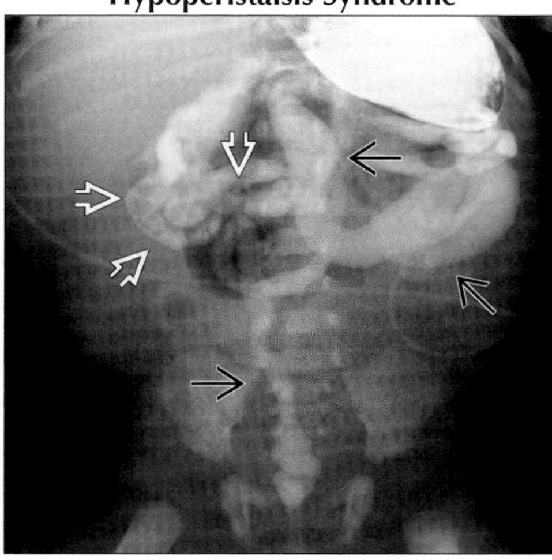

Megacystis Microcolon Intestinal Hypoperistalsis Syndrome

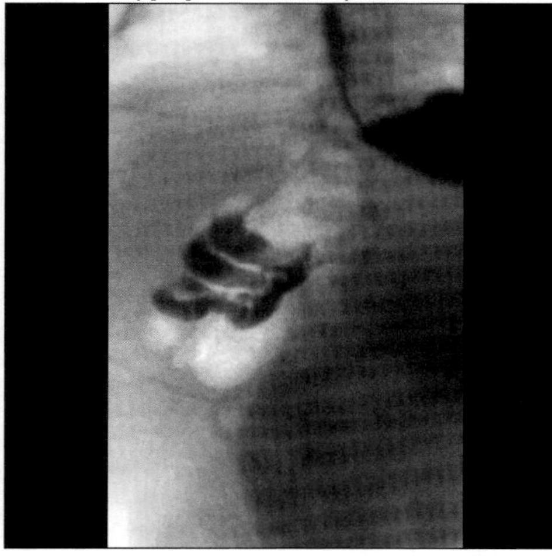

(Left) *AP contrast enema shows a microcolon on the left ⇨ and multiple proximal jejunal loops on the right ➡, suggestive of nonrotation. Abdominal ultrasound (not shown) revealed bilateral hydronephrosis and a large urinary bladder, which did not empty spontaneously, characteristic of MMIHS.* ***(Right)*** *AP upper GI in the same patient shows malrotation, not an uncommon finding in patients with MMIHS.*

CYSTIC ABDOMINAL MASS

DIFFERENTIAL DIAGNOSIS

Common
- Hydronephrosis
- Ovarian Cyst
- Multicystic Dysplastic Kidney
- Pancreatic Pseudocyst
- Appendiceal Abscess
- Duplication Cyst

Less Common
- Splenic Cyst
- Urachal Cyst
- Hydrometrocolpos
- Choledochal Cyst
- Cystic Wilms Tumor

Rare but Important
- Meconium Pseudocyst
- Multilocular Cystic Nephroma
- Mesenchymal Hamartoma
- Caroli Disease

ESSENTIAL INFORMATION

Key Differential Diagnosis Issues
- Organ of origin can be difficult to identify for large cystic masses
  - Most cystic masses have renal origin
- Patient age and mass location can focus differential diagnosis

Helpful Clues for Common Diagnoses
- **Hydronephrosis**
  - Most common pediatric abdominal mass
  - Diagnosed in 1-5% of pregnancies
    - Up to 30% are bilateral
    - Resolves on postnatal US in ~ 50%
    - 10% have ureteropelvic junction (UPJ) obstruction
    - Vesicoureteral reflux in 10%
  - Postnatal US should be 1st imaging test
  - **Hint**: Consider posterior urethral valves in males with bilateral hydronephrosis
- **Ovarian Cyst**
  - Most common during infancy and adolescence
  - Fetal cysts more common with maternal diabetes, toxemia, and Rh isoimmunization
  - At birth, up to 98% of girls have small ovarian cysts
    - 20% of neonatal cysts > 9 mm
    - Neonatal cysts resolve spontaneously
    - Cysts resolve as maternal hormones subside
  - In prepubertal girls, large cysts can cause precocious puberty
  - In adolescents, ovarian cysts are very common
    - Usually due to dysfunctional ovulation
    - Cysts often spontaneously resolve
    - Large cysts take longer to resolve
- **Multicystic Dysplastic Kidney**
  - More common in males
  - Left kidney more commonly affected
  - Distinguished from hydronephrosis as cysts do not connect with renal pelvis
  - Natural history is involution of kidney
- **Pancreatic Pseudocyst**
  - Most common cystic lesion of pediatric pancreas
    - Can occur after blunt abdominal trauma or pancreatitis
    - Usually has thin, well-defined wall
- **Appendiceal Abscess**
  - Seen after ruptured appendix
    - Occurs in ~ 4% of appendicitis cases
    - More common in children < 4 years old
  - Patients have symptoms more than 3 days
- **Duplication Cyst**
  - Can occur anywhere along GI tract
  - Located adjacent to GI wall
    - Usually spherical or tubular in shape
  - Lined with GI tract mucosa
    - Can have gastric mucosa in lining
    - Usually along mesenteric side
  - Ileum is most common site
    - Esophagus, duodenum next most common
  - Can create obstruction, bleeding, or intussusception

Helpful Clues for Less Common Diagnoses
- **Splenic Cyst**
  - Can be congenital or acquired
    - Acquired cysts are due to trauma or infection
    - Congenital cysts are more common in girls
  - Has well-defined, thin walls
  - Calcifications can be seen within cyst wall
- **Urachal Cyst**
  - Urachus remains patent between umbilicus and bladder

- Can become infected
  - US shows thick-walled cyst above bladder
  - CT shows thick-walled cyst with surrounding inflammation
- **Hydrometrocolpos**
  - Fluid-filled vagina + uterus
  - Can be caused by imperforate hymen, cervical stenosis, or atresia
  - Associated with anorectal malformations
    - Can lead to obstructive uropathy in neonate
- **Choledochal Cyst**
  - Cystic or fusiform dilation of biliary tree
  - Todani classification with 5 types
    - Type 1 (cystic dilation of extrahepatic bile duct) is most common
  - Associated with ductal and vascular anomalies
    - Anomalous hepatic arteries, accessory ducts, and primary duct strictures
  - US is best screening test
  - HIDA scan can be used to prove connection to biliary system
- **Cystic Wilms Tumor**
  - Most common abdominal neoplasm
  - Peak age is 3 years
  - Usually heterogeneous solid mass
    - Occasionally cystic mass

Helpful Clues for Rare Diagnoses

- **Meconium Pseudocyst**
  - After meconium peritonitis
  - Underlying condition may be meconium ileus, volvulus, or atresia
  - Calcifications often present
  - On US, cyst is thick walled and echogenic
- **Multilocular Cystic Nephroma**
  - a.k.a. multilocular cystic mass
  - Septae are only solid component
  - 2 age peaks with differing pathology
    - Boys ages 3 months to 4 years: Cystic, partially differentiated nephroblastoma
    - Adult women: Cystic nephroma
  - Must be differentiated from cystic Wilms tumor
- **Mesenchymal Hamartoma**
  - 2nd most common benign hepatic tumor in children
    - 85% present before age 3 years
  - Often presents as large RUQ mass
    - 75% in right lobe of liver
    - α-fetoprotein can be elevated
  - Multiloculated cystic mass
    - Tiny cysts can appear solid
    - On US, septae of cysts can be mobile
    - Large portal vein branch may feed mass
    - Calcification is uncommon
  - Reports of malignant degeneration to undifferentiated embryonal sarcoma
- **Caroli Disease**
  - a.k.a. type 5 choledochal cyst
    - May be associated with autosomal recessive polycystic kidney disease
  - Congenital cystic dilation of intrahepatic bile ducts
  - Presents with recurrent cholangitis or portal hypertension

Hydronephrosis

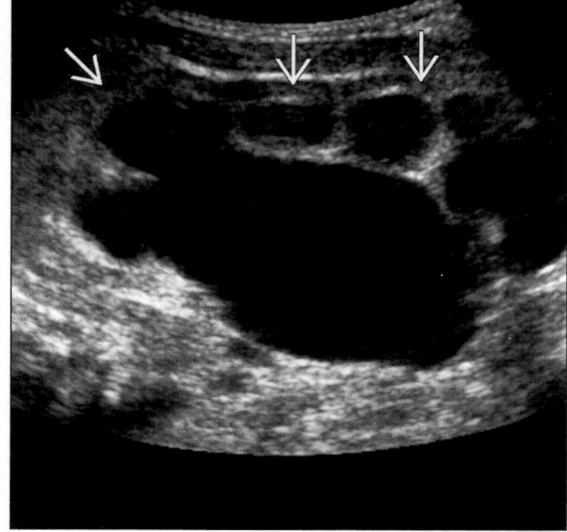

Longitudinal ultrasound shows marked hydronephrosis of the kidney ➡. Hydronephrosis is the most common abdominal mass in children and is most commonly caused by an obstruction of the ureteropelvic junction.

Hydronephrosis

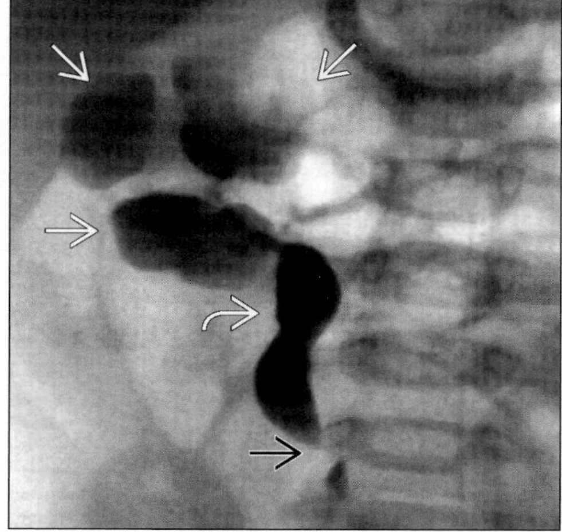

Anteroposterior retrograde pyelogram shows marked hydronephrosis with dilation of the renal calyces ➡. The ureter is dilated ➡ proximal to a focal area of narrowing near the ureteropelvic junction ➡.

CYSTIC ABDOMINAL MASS

*(**Left**) Transverse ultrasound in a 6-day-old girl shows an anechoic lesion ➡ arising from the ovary. There is a thin claw of normal ovarian tissue ➡ surrounding the cyst. Ovarian cysts are present in 98% of girls at birth due to maternal hormones. (**Right**) Axial CECT shows a large cystic mass ➡ extending from the pelvis to the mid-abdomen. The mass had simple characteristics on CT and ultrasound (not shown). Giant ovarian cysts such as this are uncommon.*

Ovarian Cyst

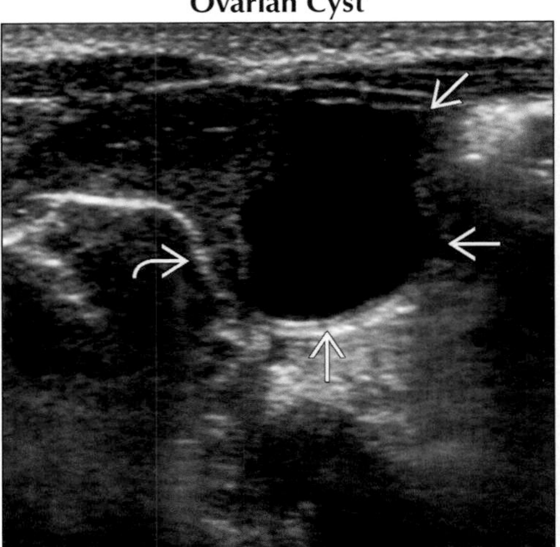

Ovarian Cyst

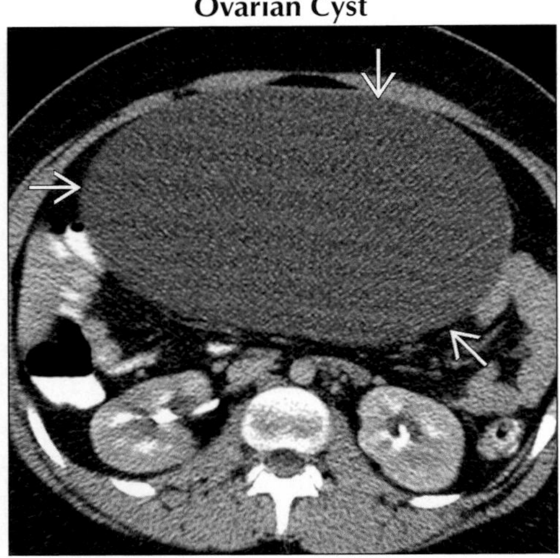

*(**Left**) Longitudinal US shows multiple cysts of various sizes ➡ replacing the right kidney. The cysts do not connect to the renal pelvis, and no normal renal parenchyma is seen. Multicystic dysplastic kidneys typically regress with age. (**Right**) Posterior renal scan in the same patient shows normal uptake of radiotracer in the left kidney ➡ and an absence of uptake in the right kidney. Multicystic dysplastic kidneys lack significant radionuclide uptake.*

Multicystic Dysplastic Kidney

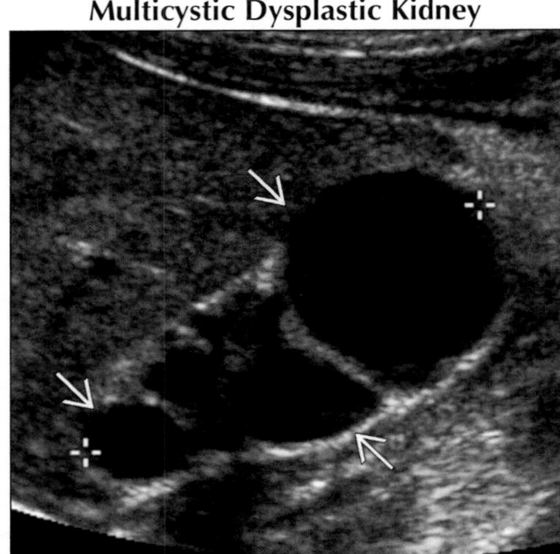

Multicystic Dysplastic Kidney

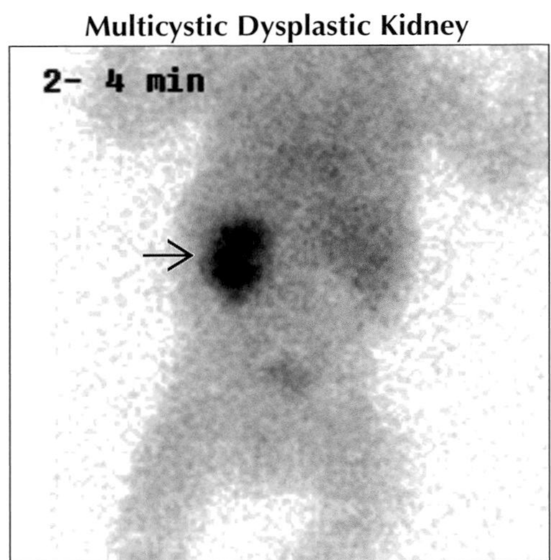

*(**Left**) Transverse ultrasound shows a cystic mass ➡ arising from the body of the pancreas ➡ in a patient 2 weeks after a known bout of pancreatitis. Pancreatic pseudocysts are the most common cystic lesion of the pediatric pancreas. (**Right**) Axial CECT shows a cystic mass arising from the body of the pancreas ➡. Little residual pancreatic tissue is present ➡. Pancreatic pseudocysts usually have a thin, well-defined wall.*

Pancreatic Pseudocyst

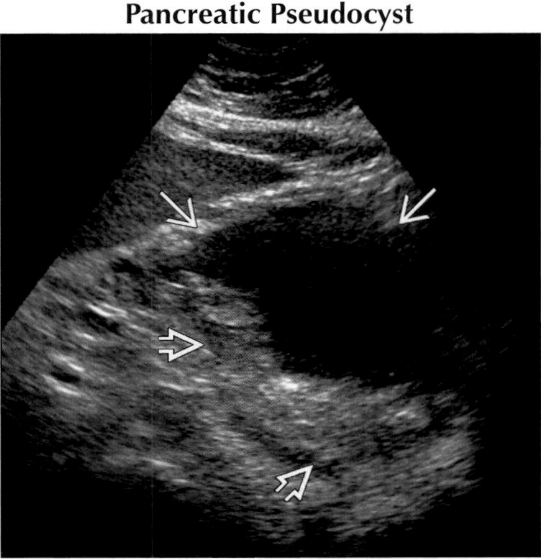

Pancreatic Pseudocyst

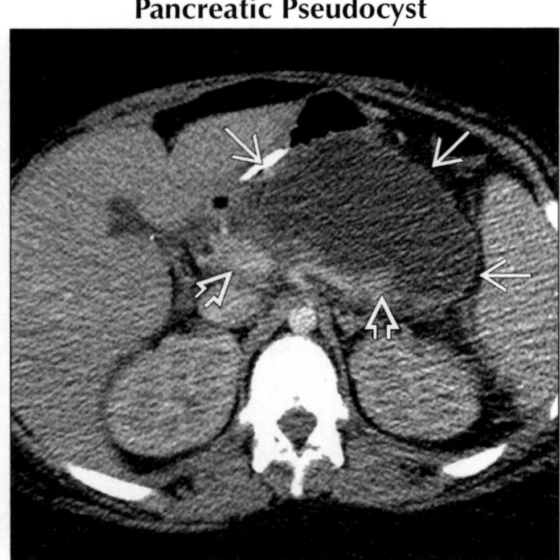

Appendiceal Abscess

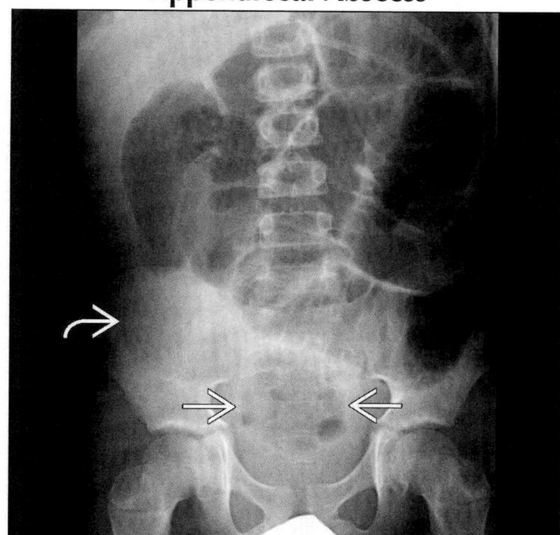

Appendiceal Abscess

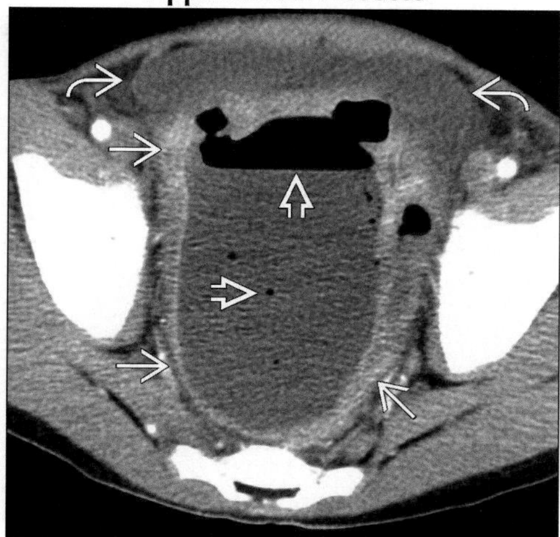

(Left) *Anteroposterior radiograph shows multiple dilated and distended air-filled loops of bowel, except in the right lower quadrant ➦. A faint ovoid area of lucency ➡ is present overlying the pelvis.* ***(Right)*** *Axial CECT in the same patient shows an irregular ovoid collection in the pelvis containing fluid density and locules of air ⇨. The collection has a thick wall ➡ and displaces the bladder anteriorly ➦.*

Duplication Cyst

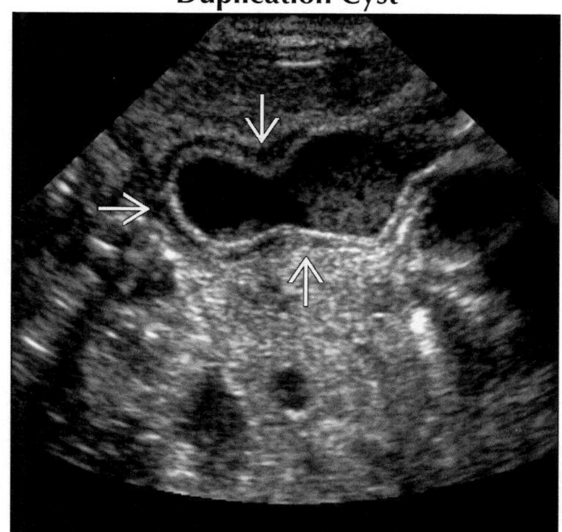

Duplication Cyst

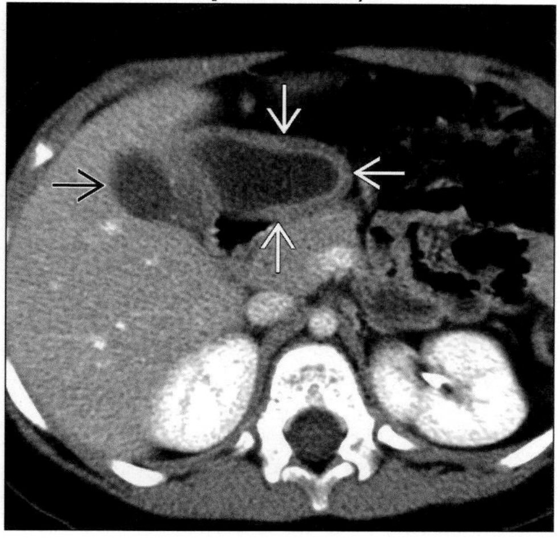

(Left) *Transverse ultrasound shows a cystic mass ➡ in the upper abdomen adjacent to the liver. The wall of the mass has a "bowel signature" with alternating hypoechoic and hyperechoic portions.* ***(Right)*** *Axial CECT shows a thick-walled cystic mass ➡ adjacent to the gallbladder ⇒. Although duplication cysts can arise anywhere along the GI tract, they are most common at the ileum. Gastric mucosa can be present in their lining and lead to GI bleeding.*

Splenic Cyst

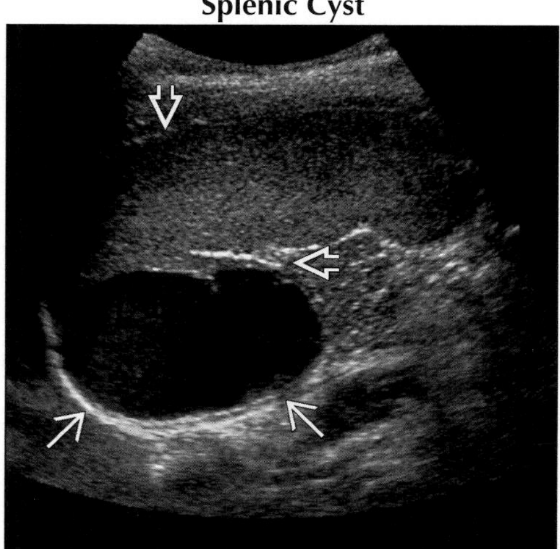

Splenic Cyst

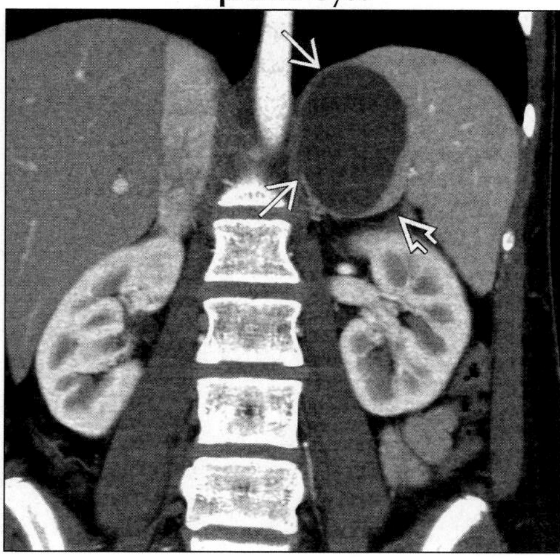

(Left) *Longitudinal ultrasound shows a simple cystic lesion ➡ arising from the superomedial aspect of the spleen ⇨. Splenic cysts may be congenital or acquired. Trauma is the most common cause of acquired splenic cysts.* ***(Right)*** *Coronal CECT shows a cystic mass ➡ arising from the superomedial aspect of the spleen. There is a thin rim of splenic tissue around the cyst's lateral border ⇨. Splenic cysts can have calcifications in their wall (not shown).*

Urachal Cyst

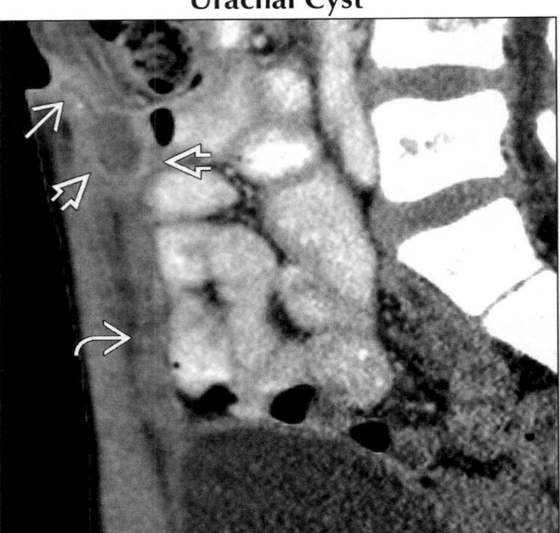

Urachal Cyst

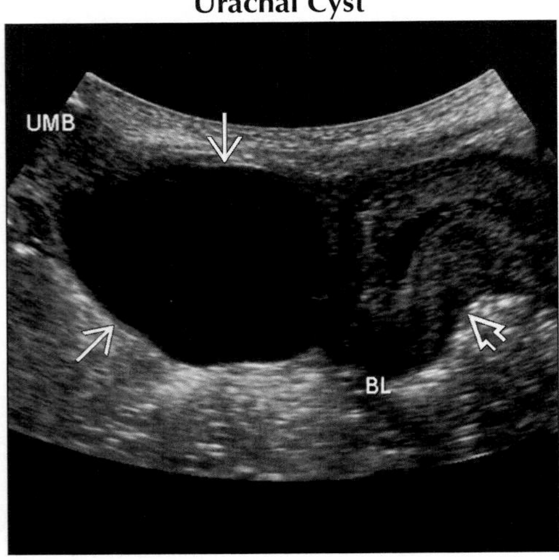

(Left) *Sagittal CECT shows a small cystic mass → just inferior to the umbilicus. The mass has a thick, enhancing wall with some surrounding fat stranding. There is a small sinus tract → extending from the mass to the umbilicus. Another sinus tract → connects the cystic mass to the bladder dome.* ***(Right)*** *Longitudinal ultrasound in a neonate with posterior urethral valves shows a large cystic mass → adjacent to the dome of the decompressed bladder →.*

Hydrometrocolpos

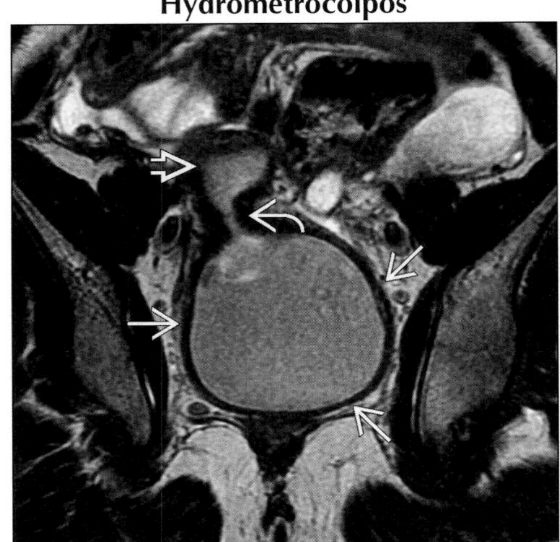

Hydrometrocolpos

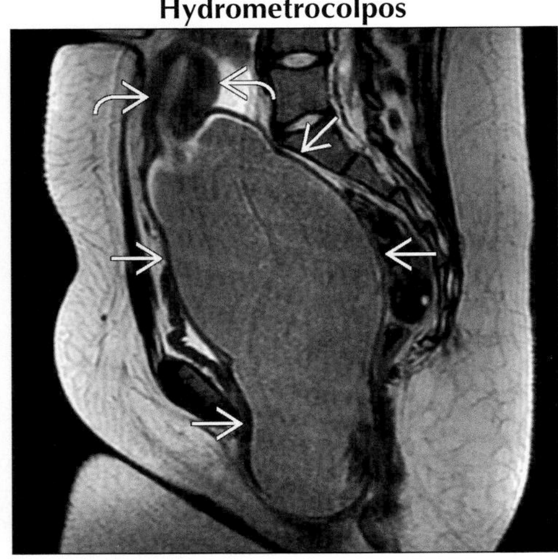

(Left) *Coronal T1WI MR shows a cystic mass filling the vagina →. The contents of the mass continue through the cervix → and into the uterus →. Hydrometrocolpos often does not present until adolescence. It can be caused by an imperforate hymen.* ***(Right)*** *Sagittal T2WI MR shows the vagina appearing as a large tubular cystic mass →. The contents of the vagina have a slightly different signal intensity than the uterine lining →.*

Choledochal Cyst

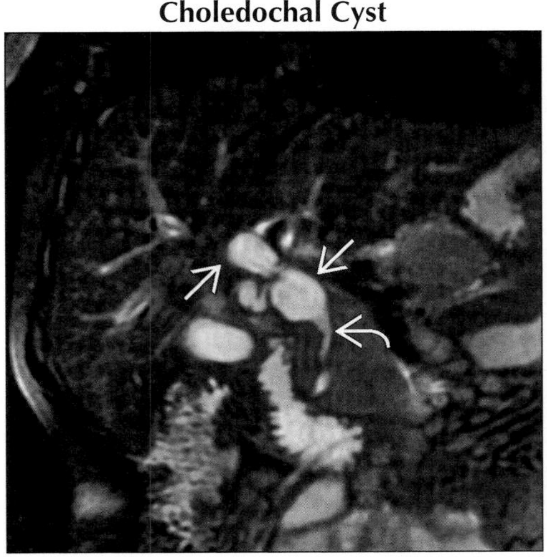

Choledochal Cyst

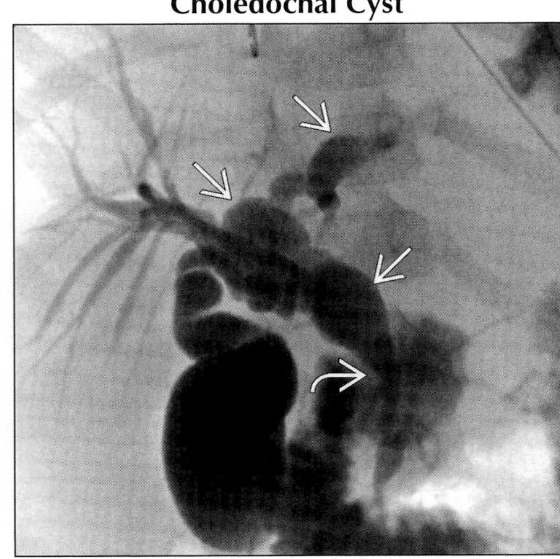

(Left) *Coronal MRCP shows cystic dilation of the common bile duct →. There is a focal transition to a normal caliber within the mid-common bile duct →.* ***(Right)*** *Anteroposterior ERCP in the same patient shows cystic dilation of the proximal common bile duct and the central intrahepatic bile ducts →. There is a focal tapering of the mid-common bile duct →. This is a type 4a choledochal cyst according to the Todani classification.*

Meconium Pseudocyst

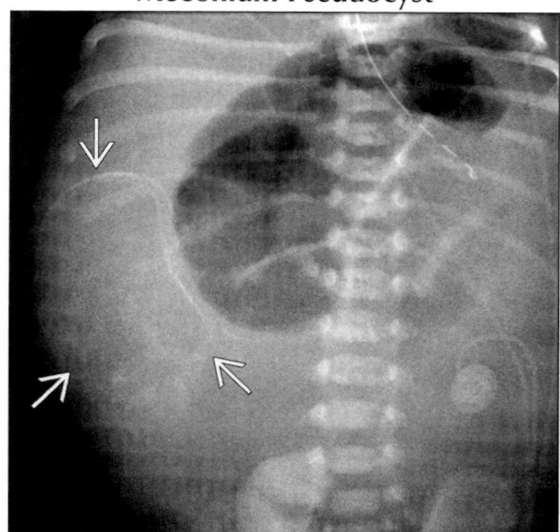

Meconium Pseudocyst

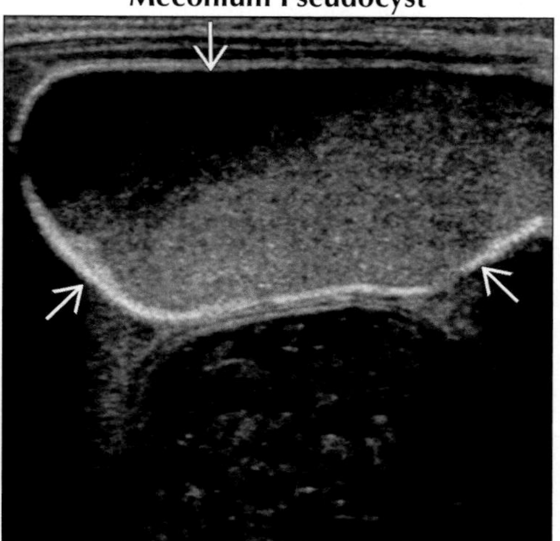

*(**Left**) Anteroposterior radiograph shows a faintly calcified mass ➡ in the right abdomen, displacing the bowel to the left. In neonates, meconium peritonitis can lead to abdominal calcifications. (**Right**) Longitudinal ultrasound shows a well-defined abdominal mass with a hyperechoic wall ➡. Note the debris layers within the mass. Meconium pseudocysts occur after perinatal perforation of the bowel due to meconium ileus, volvulus, or atresias.*

Multilocular Cystic Nephroma

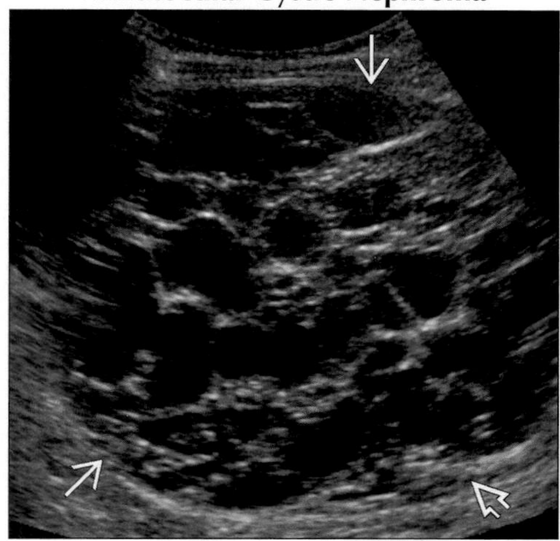

Multilocular Cystic Nephroma

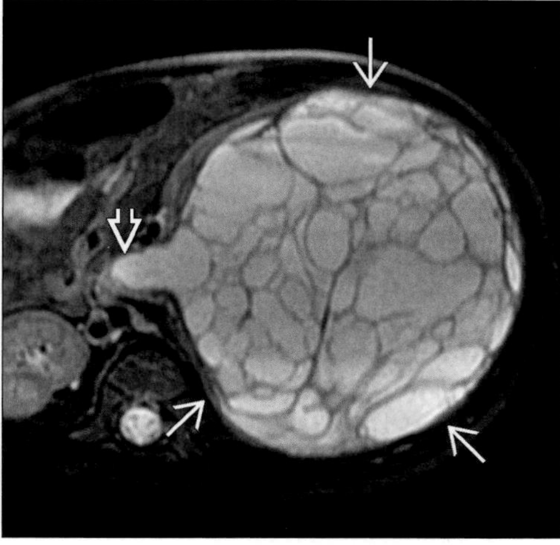

*(**Left**) Transverse ultrasound shows a multiloculated mass ➡ arising from the kidney. A thin rim of renal tissue is seen posteriorly ➡. In the pediatric population, multilocular cystic nephroma is more common in males. (**Right**) Axial T2WI MR shows a multiloculated cystic mass ➡ extending into the renal pelvis ➡, typical of multilocular cystic nephroma. Even though benign, the mass should be excised in order to exclude cystic Wilms tumor.*

Caroli Disease

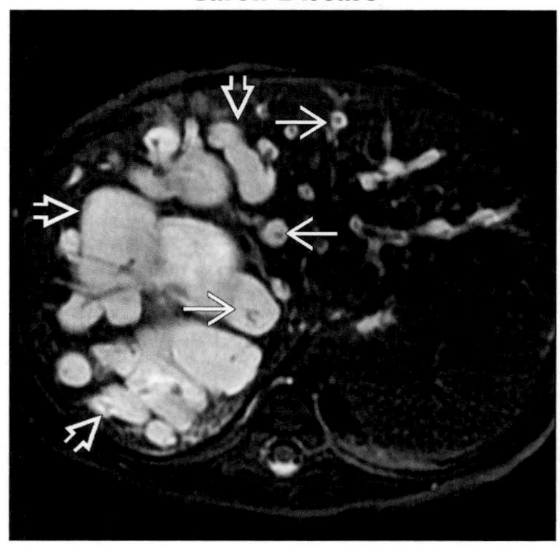

Caroli Disease

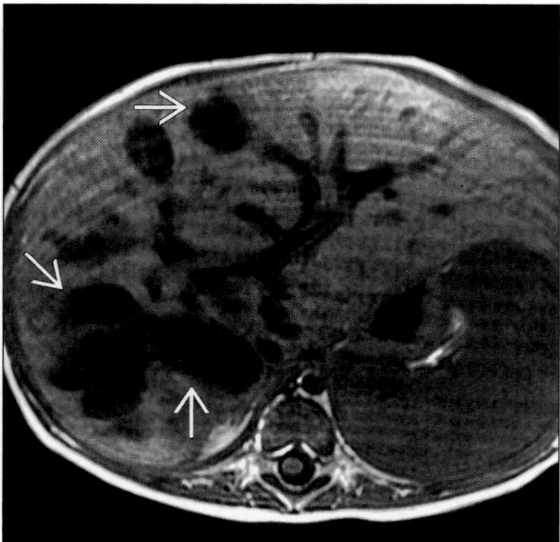

*(**Left**) Axial T2WI MR shows cystic dilation of multiple intrahepatic bile ducts ➡. Each duct has a central dot ➡ of hypointense signal, typical of Caroli disease. (**Right**) Axial T1WI MR shows cystic dilation of multiple intrahepatic bile ducts ➡. Caroli disease is associated with autosomal recessive polycystic kidney disease. Patients present with recurrent cholangitis or portal hypertension.*

ABDOMINAL MASS IN NEONATE

DIFFERENTIAL DIAGNOSIS

Common
- Urinary Tract Obstruction
  - Ureteropelvic Junction Obstruction
  - Ureteropelvic Duplications
- Multicystic Dysplastic Kidney
- Neuroblastoma, Congenital
- Adrenal Hemorrhage
- Gastrointestinal Duplication Cyst
- Mesenteric Lymphatic Malformations
- Mesoblastic Nephroma
- Teratoma

Less Common
- Ovarian Torsion
- Hepatoblastoma
- Meconium Pseudocyst
- Hemangioendothelioma
- Vascular Malformation
- Pulmonary Sequestration

Rare but Important
- Hydrocolpos/Hydrometrocolpos
- Wilms Tumor (Congenital)

ESSENTIAL INFORMATION

Key Differential Diagnosis Issues
- Male vs. female
- Other clinical findings: Skin lesions, urinary output, meconium passage
- Cystic, solid, or mixed cystic/solid
- Presence or absence of calcifications

Helpful Clues for Common Diagnoses
- **Urinary Tract Obstruction**
  - Ureteropelvic junction obstruction: Larger cystic, anechoic renal pelvis surrounded by smaller cystic, anechoic calyces
    - Most common congenital obstruction of urinary tract
    - Hydronephrosis without hydroureter
    - Sometimes difficult to differentiate from multicystic dysplastic kidney (MCDK)
    - Abnormalities common in contralateral kidney: Reflux or ureteropelvic junction obstruction
  - Duplication with obstructed upper pole appear as complex or simple cystic structure
    - Reflux common in lower pole ureter
    - Diagnosis is often bilateral but **asymmetric** in severity
- **Multicystic Dysplastic Kidney**
  - Most common appearance is noncommunicating cysts of varying sizes; usually spontaneously involute over time
  - Variable appearance depending on stage
    - May be massive and bizarre
    - Large enough to cause respiratory distress in rare cases
    - May have residual intervening dysplastic renal parenchyma
    - ± identifiable ureter
    - Timing to complete involution varies from prenatal period to late teens
  - Higher incidence of other genitourinary abnormalities
- **Neuroblastoma, Congenital**
  - Origin in sympathetic chain ganglia
    - Occurs anywhere from coccyx to skull base
    - Vast majority arise in adrenal gland
  - Often heterogeneous, mixed cystic and solid
  - Coarse calcifications are common
  - Assess for vertebral involvement, spinal canal invasion, rib splaying
  - Engulfs large vessels
    - Mass often elevates aorta from spine
- **Adrenal Hemorrhage**
  - May be large and difficult to differentiate from neuroblastoma
  - No internal blood flow detected on US
  - Involutes over time
  - Usually circumscribed, heterogeneous, often with cystic components
- **Gastrointestinal Duplication Cyst**
  - Usually round structure
    - ± bowel "wall signature" of hypoechoic wall/mucosa layers
    - Hypoechoic or echogenic contents
    - Usually does not communicate with GI lumen
  - Most common locations are terminal ileum and esophagus
    - Other GI locations are uncommon
- **Mesenteric Lymphatic Malformations**
  - Nonspecific hypoechoic/anechoic structure
    - May have irregular or lobulated borders
    - May have septations

- **Mesoblastic Nephroma**
  - Most common neonatal renal neoplasm
  - Encapsulated calcifications rare
  - Solid, may be heterogeneous
    - US: Whorled, heterogeneous, compared to uterine fibroid
    - CT: Solid, with mild enhancement
    - MR: Intermediate on T1, bright on T2
  - Usually benign; however, beware small subset that may recur or metastasize

Helpful Clues for Less Common Diagnoses

- **Ovarian Torsion**
  - May be suspected if only 1 ovary can be identified
  - Circumscribed, heterogeneous pelvic mass; may see peripheral follicles
  - May be precipitated by dominant cyst or underlying mass, such as teratoma
  - Pitfall: Demonstration of blood flow by US may confound diagnosis due to intermittent torsion or multiplicity of blood supply to ovaries
- **Meconium Pseudocyst**
  - Radiographically, large soft tissue density with mass effect
    - Lesional or peritoneal calcifications may have wispy or "eggshell" appearance
  - Distal bowel obstruction pattern typical
- **Hemangioendothelioma**
  - Variable appearance; most commonly multiple focal, round, target-like lesions within liver
  - May present as large solitary lesion
  - Highly vascular lesion
    - Great vessels distal to lesion (aorta, superior mesenteric artery) may be attenuated
    - Look for signs of congestive heart failure
- **Vascular Malformation**
  - Highly variable appearance, depending on histology, presence of necrosis, stage of involution

Helpful Clues for Rare Diagnoses

- **Hydrocolpos/Hydrometrocolpos**
  - Often associated with other anomalies
    - Cloaca, urogenital sinus, renal agenesis, cystic kidneys, esophageal/duodenal atresia, anorectal malformation
  - Occasionally seen in intersex conditions
- **Wilms Tumor (Congenital)**
  - Cannot be differentiated from mesoblastic nephroma by imaging
  - Associated with other conditions
    - Beckwith-Wiedemann: Hypertrophy
    - WAGR: **W**ilms, **a**niridia, **g**enitourinary anomalies, mental **r**etardation
    - Drash: Pseudohermaphroditism, renal failure
  - Tends to invade vessel lumen (renal vein, IVC) rather than surround/engulf vessels (as seen with neuroblastoma)
  - Contralateral kidney risks: Bilateral Wilms, nephroblastomatosis
  - Wilms tumor nearly always occurs **after** 1st year of life; congenital/neonatal presentation extremely uncommon

Ureteropelvic Junction Obstruction

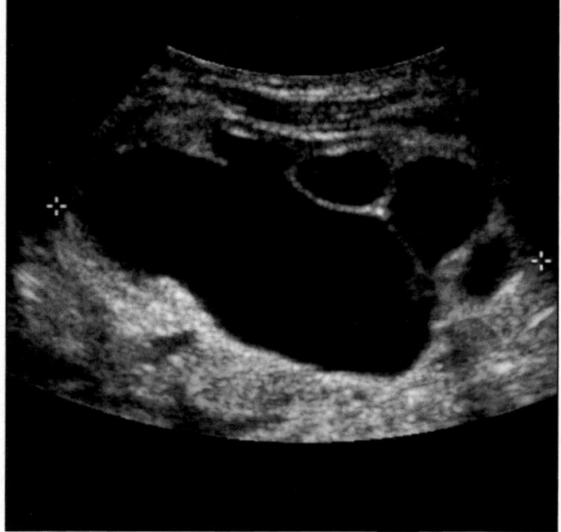

Longitudinal ultrasound shows massive and somewhat disproportionate dilatation of the renal pelvis with concomitant dilation of the calyces. Severe UPJ may be difficult to distinguish from MCDK in some patients.

Ureteropelvic Duplications

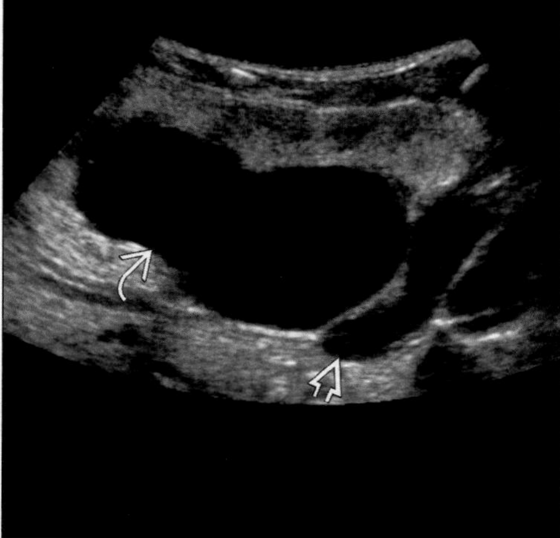

Longitudinal ultrasound shows a markedly dilated upper pole ➔ with portions of the dilated, tortuous upper pole ureter ➔ also visualized. A ureterocele was the cause of the upper pole obstruction.

ABDOMINAL MASS IN NEONATE

Multicystic Dysplastic Kidney

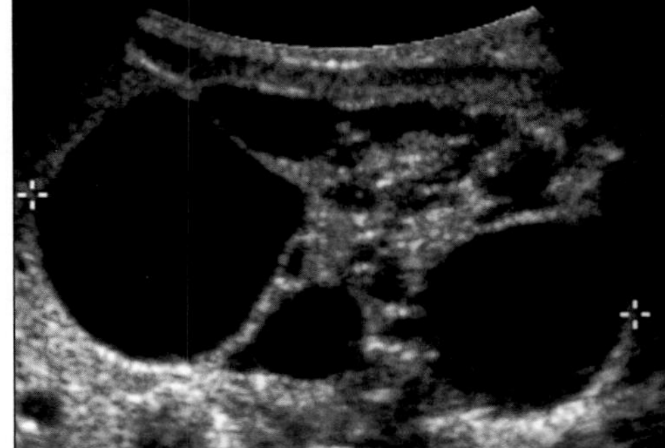

Multicystic Dysplastic Kidney

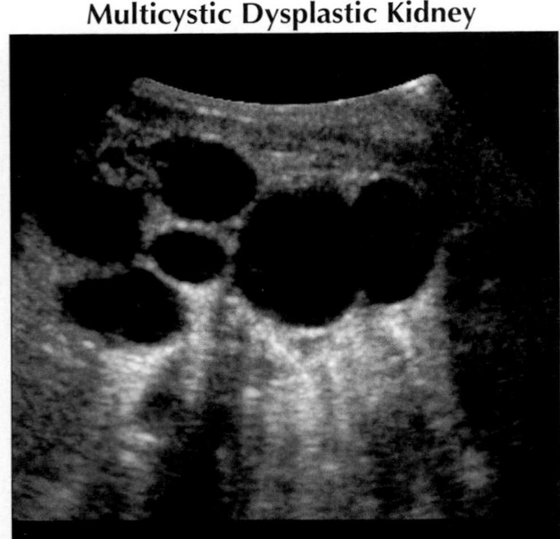

*(**Left**) Longitudinal ultrasound shows a predominantly cystic lesion with interspersed areas of echogenic tissue in the renal fossa. Depending on the stage of involution, a multicystic dysplastic kidney (MCDK) may have a variable appearance. (**Right**) Longitudinal ultrasound shows a different portion of the same MCDK, demonstrating the more typical appearance of noncommunicating cysts of varying sizes.*

Neuroblastoma, Congenital

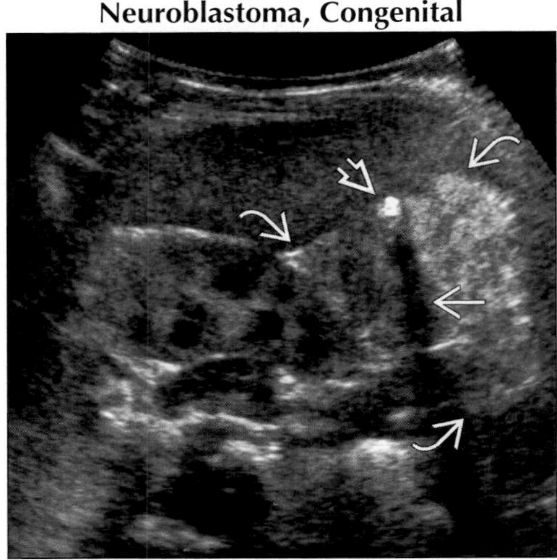

Neuroblastoma, Congenital

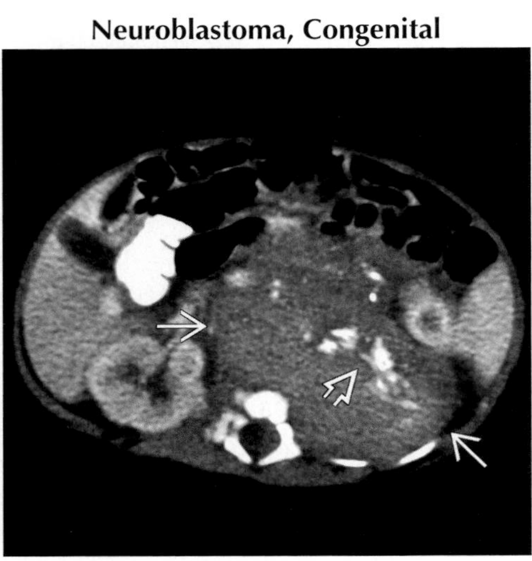

*(**Left**) Longitudinal ultrasound shows a solid echogenic mass ➔. A conspicuous area of calcification ➔ with posterior acoustic shadowing ➔ is a helpful observation in the differential diagnosis. Portions of the left kidney and spleen are seen. (**Right**) Axial CECT shows the same lesion ➔ with coarse chunky calcifications ➔. Intraspinal extension is noted.*

Neuroblastoma, Congenital

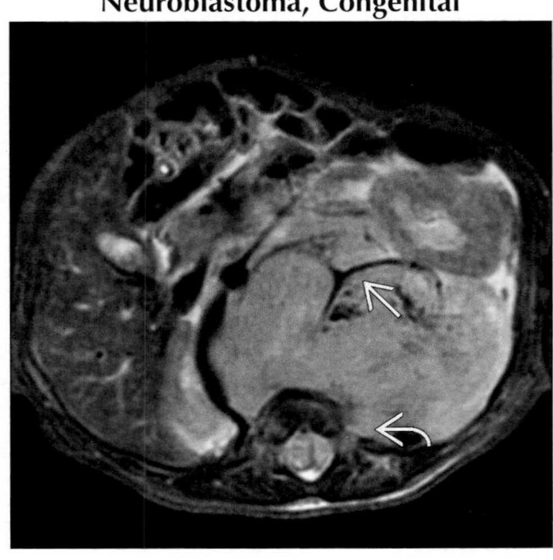

Neuroblastoma, Congenital

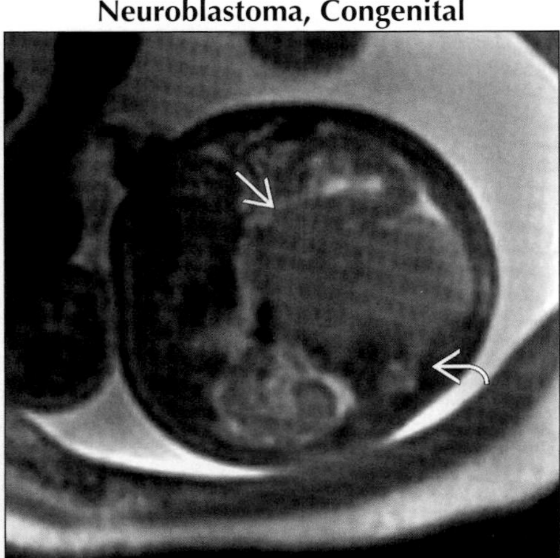

*(**Left**) Axial T2WI MR shows vascular encasement ➔ and displacement by the large hyperintense retroperitoneal mass. Notice the extension into the adjacent neural foramen ➔ with displacement of the spinal cord to the right. (**Right**) Axial T2WI MR shows the same lesion ➔ imaged prenatally. At that time, the neural foramen invasion ➔ was already visible.*

Gastrointestinal Duplication Cyst

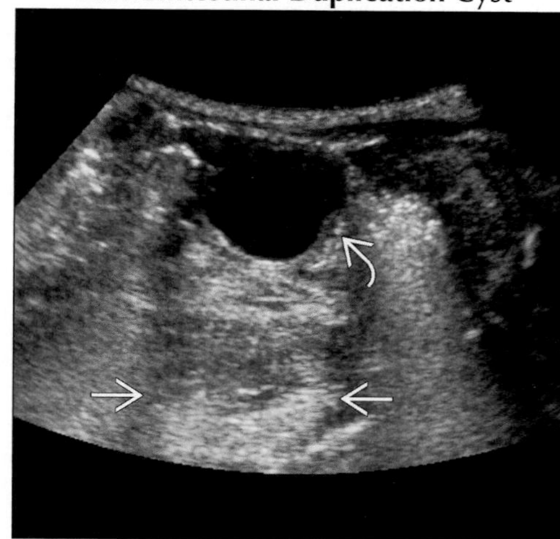

Gastrointestinal Duplication Cyst

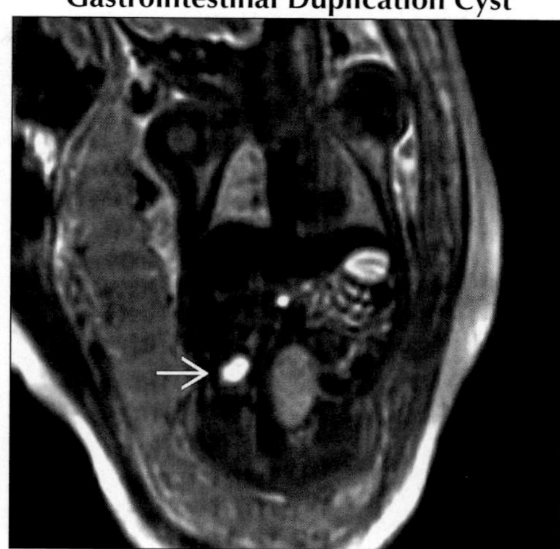

(Left) *Transverse ultrasound shows a cystic lesion. The bowel wall* ➡ *is seen but lacks the "bowel wall signature." Posterior increased through-transmission* ➡ *is typical of fluid-filled structures. This was an ileal duplication cyst.* ***(Right)*** *Coronal T2WI MR shows the prenatal appearance of the same right lower quadrant ileal duplication cyst* ➡.

Mesenteric Lymphatic Malformations

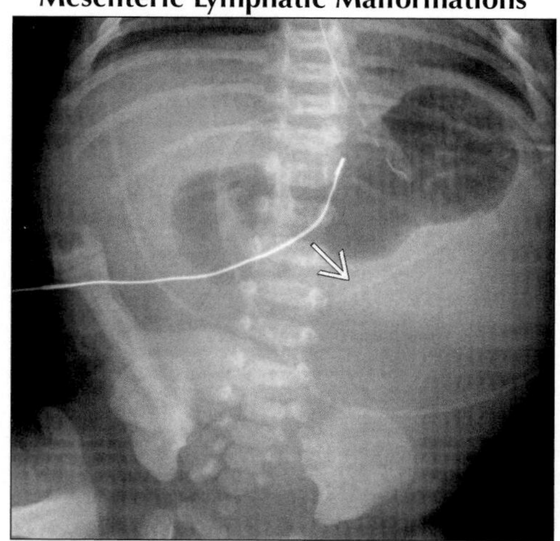

Mesenteric Lymphatic Malformations

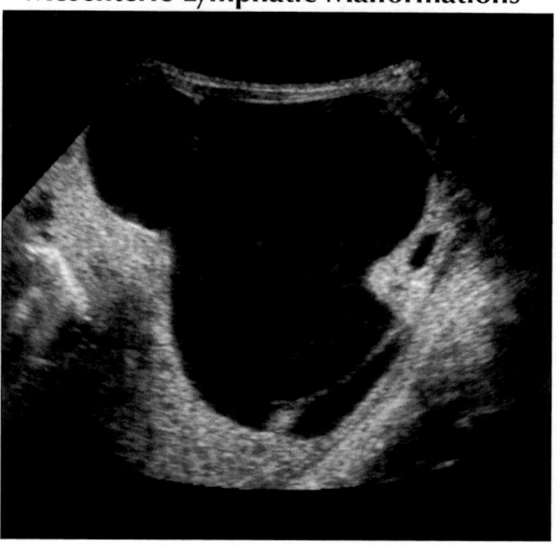

(Left) *Frontal radiograph shows a left mid-abdominal soft tissue density* ➡ *in this newborn, caused by a mesenteric cyst, resulting in a mildly bulging appearance of that side. Note that the mass effect results in duodenal obstruction.* ***(Right)*** *Transverse ultrasound shows the large, septated cystic mesenteric lymphatic malformation causing the soft tissue density seen on the x-ray. Note the contents are more echogenic than simple fluid, possibly from hemorrhage.*

Mesoblastic Nephroma

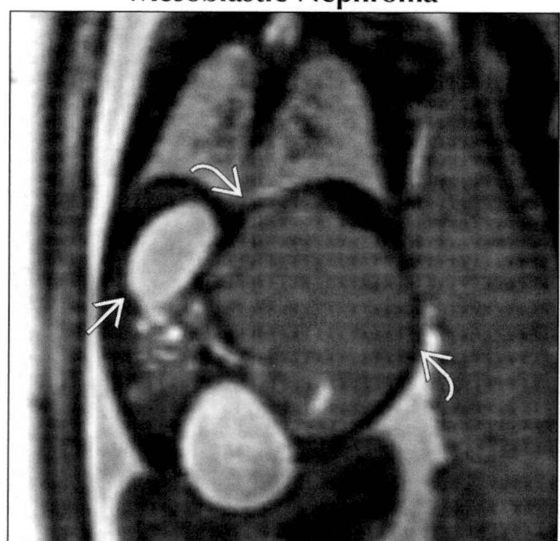

Mesoblastic Nephroma

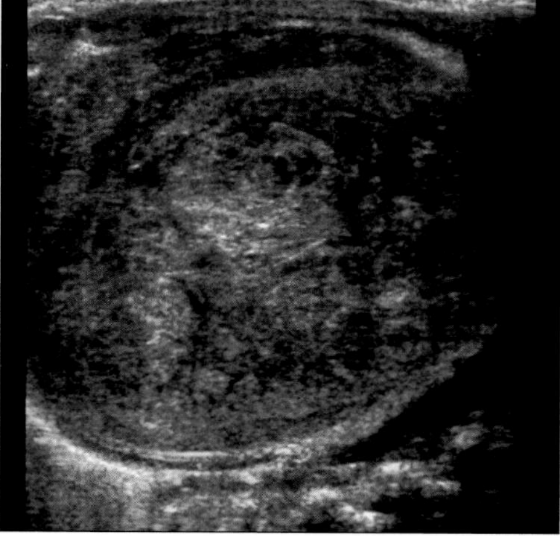

(Left) *Coronal T2WI MR shows the fetal MR appearance of a large mesoblastic nephroma* ➡*, surgically removed soon after birth. This is a posterior view of the fetus. Note the stomach* ➡. ***(Right)*** *Longitudinal ultrasound shows the whorled, solid, encapsulated, moderately heterogeneous appearance of the same mesoblastic nephroma as imaged in the immediate postnatal period. The appearance has been compared to a uterine fibroid.*

ABDOMINAL MASS IN NEONATE

(Left) *Longitudinal ultrasound shows a right suprarenal mass →, which is predominantly cystic with solid components, with calcification → along the edge. The calcification is a clue to the diagnosis of retroperitoneal teratoma.* **(Right)** *Longitudinal ultrasound shows a heterogeneous, circumscribed pelvic mass. No blood flow was detected. A chronically torsed right ovary was surgically removed.*

Teratoma

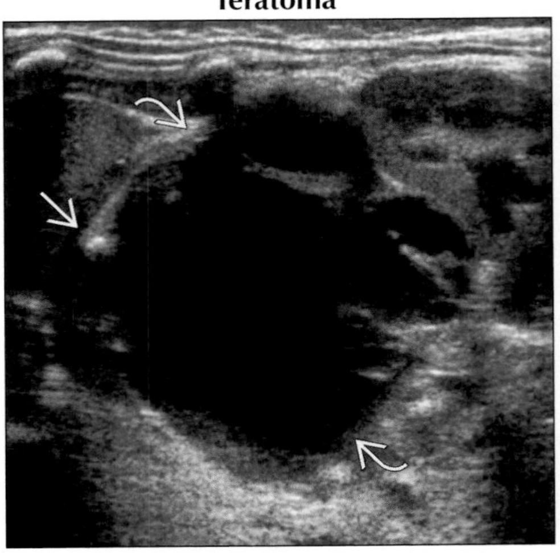

Ovarian Torsion

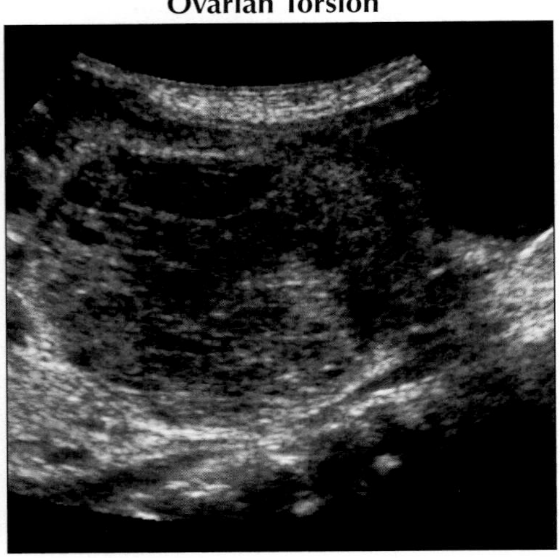

(Left) *Axial CECT shows a newborn with anterior abdominal wall bowing from this hepatoblastoma. Relatively well-defined margins and low attenuation relative to hepatic parenchyma are typical findings. Calcification may be present. These lesions are commonly hypervascular.* **(Right)** *Frontal radiograph shows abdominal distension and paucity of bowel gas. Note the wispy, linear calcifications outlining the pseudocyst →, reflecting meconium peritonitis.*

Hepatoblastoma

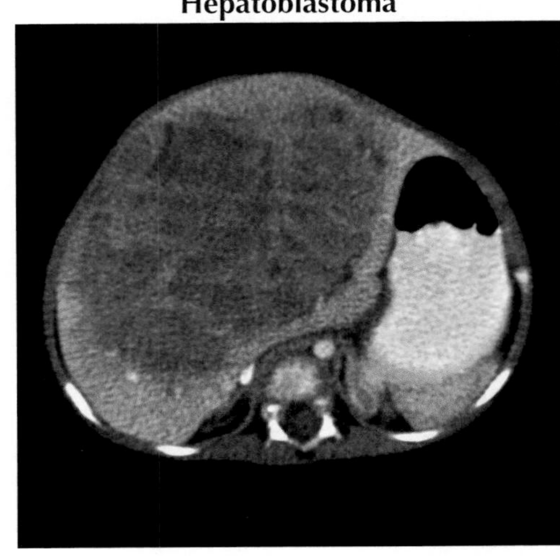

Meconium Pseudocyst

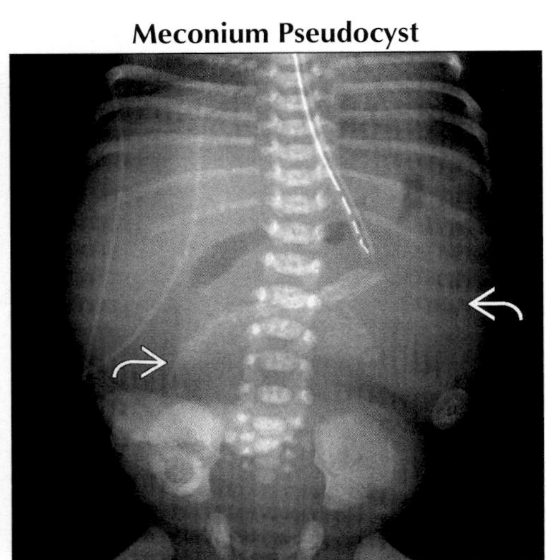

(Left) *Transverse ultrasound shows a cystic structure → with echogenic debris, some of which is dependently layering or adherent. Note the fluid-filled loops of bowel with thickened walls →.* **(Right)** *Axial CECT shows innumerable doughnut-shaped, peripherally enhancing lesions → scattered throughout the liver, consistent with diffusely distributed hemangioendotheliomas. These can also present as a large solitary lesion.*

Meconium Pseudocyst

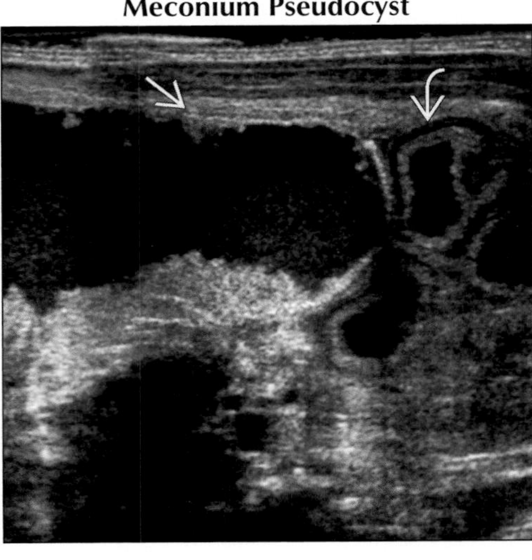

Hemangioendothelioma

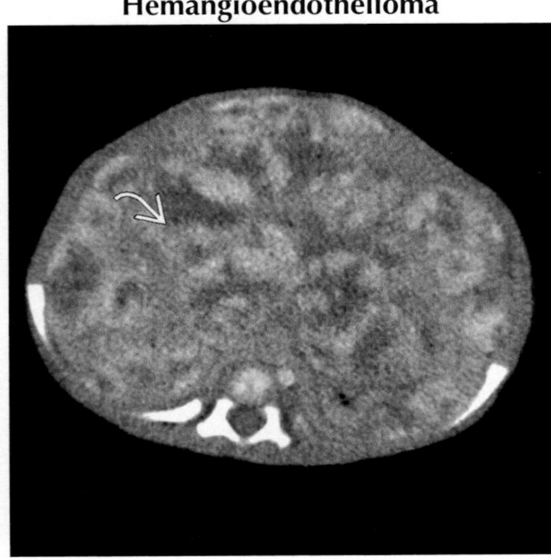

Pulmonary Sequestration

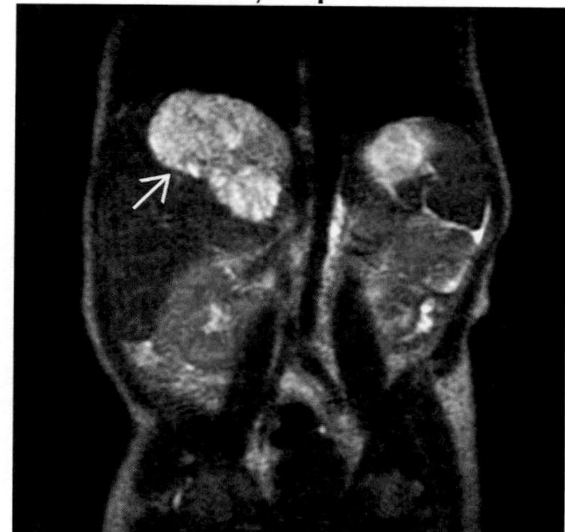

Pulmonary Sequestration

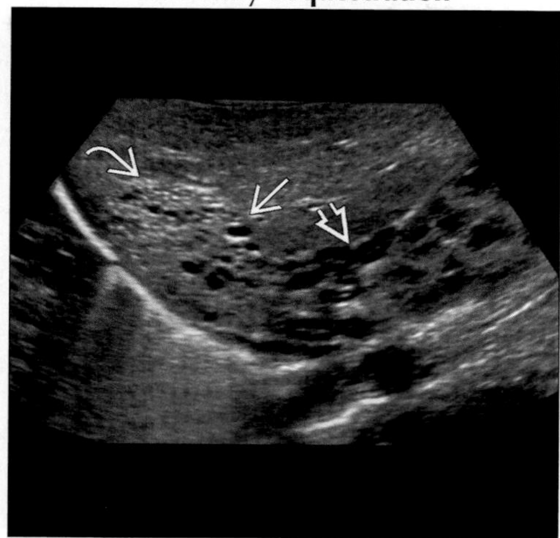

*(**Left**) Coronal T2WI MR shows a well-defined multicystic right suprarenal mass ➔ imposing upon the liver. This was an infradiaphragmatic pulmonary sequestration. (**Right**) Longitudinal ultrasound shows the lesion pressing into the liver ➔. The cystic structures ➔ correspond to the bronchiolar structures seen histologically. Portions of the normal adrenal gland are seen ➔.*

Pulmonary Sequestration

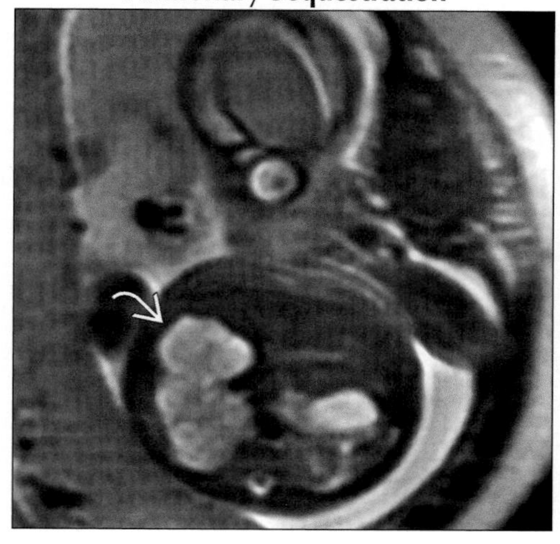

Hydrocolpos/Hydrometrocolpos

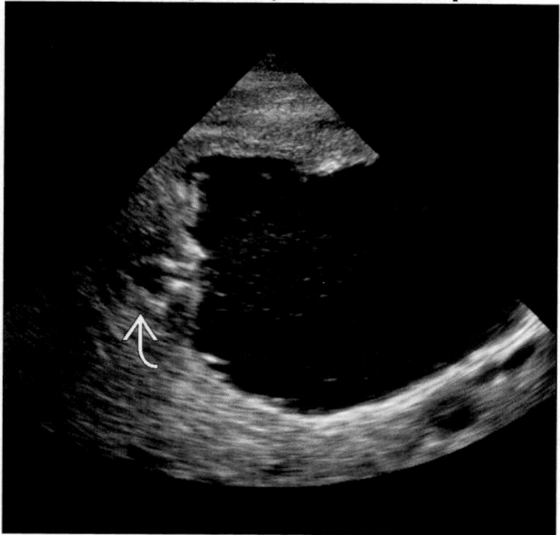

*(**Left**) Axial T2WI MR shows the infradiaphragmatic sequestration ➔ by fetal MR. The lobulated contour and possible liver invasion raised concern for an aggressive lesion. This lesion was easily removed, and the liver was unaffected. (**Right**) Longitudinal ultrasound shows a large midline pelvic fluid- and debris-filled lesion in this newborn with 2 hemivaginas, 2 uterine horns, and hydronephrosis. Note the small amount of fluid in the uterus ➔.*

Wilms Tumor (Congenital)

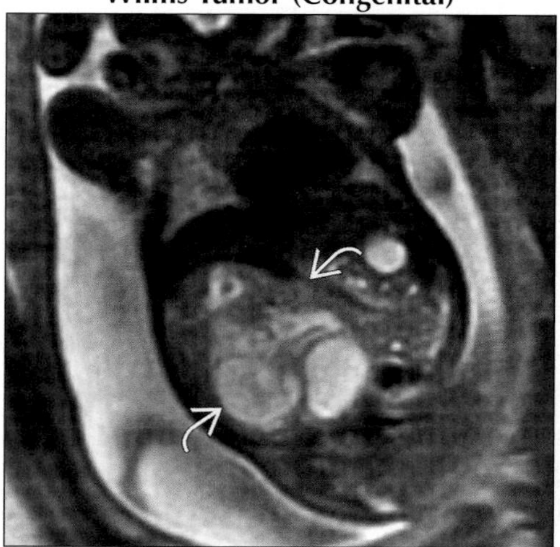

Wilms Tumor (Congenital)

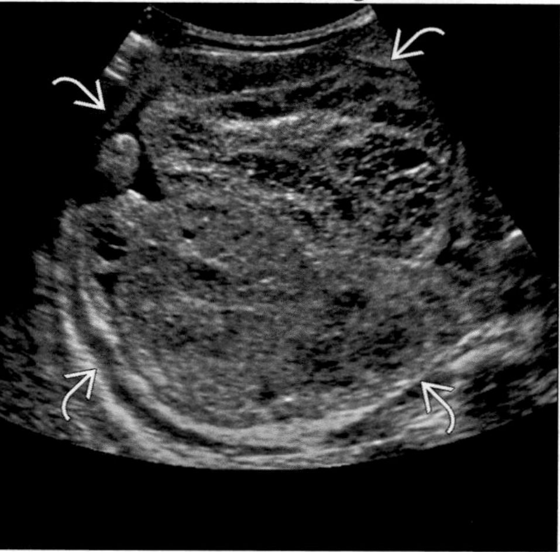

*(**Left**) Coronal T2WI MR shows a prenatal cystic and solid mass (congenital Wilms) ➔ replacing the right kidney. Subtle high signal foci were also seen in the left kidney (not shown). Those were rests of nephroblastomatosis and are followed closely. (**Right**) Longitudinal US shows an encapsulated, heterogeneous mass ➔ in the renal fossa, imaged in the immediate postnatal period. The lesion cannot be distinguished from a mesoblastic nephroma by imaging.*

ABDOMINAL MASS IN A CHILD

DIFFERENTIAL DIAGNOSIS

Common
- Hydronephrosis
- Splenomegaly
- Appendiceal Abscess
- Wilms Tumor
- Neuroblastoma

Less Common
- Rhabdomyosarcoma
- Ovarian Tumors
- Multicystic Dysplastic Kidney
- Hemangioendothelioma/Hemangioma
- Hepatoblastoma
- Mesoblastic Nephroma
- Hepatocellular Carcinoma

Rare but Important
- Renal Cell Carcinoma
- Pancreatoblastoma

ESSENTIAL INFORMATION

Key Differential Diagnosis Issues
- > 50% of abdominal masses are renal
    - Hydronephrosis and multicystic dysplastic kidney are most common in neonates
    - Hydronephrosis and Wilms tumor are most common in infants and children
- Neuroblastoma and Wilms tumor account for majority of abdominal malignancies

Helpful Clues for Common Diagnoses
- **Hydronephrosis**
    - Most common abdominal mass
    - Diagnosed in 1-5% of pregnancies
        - Up to 30% are bilateral
        - Resolves on postnatal US in ~ 50%
        - 10% have UPJ obstruction
        - Vesicoureteral reflux in 10%
    - Postnatal US should be 1st imaging test
    - **Hint**: In males with bilateral hydronephrosis, consider posterior urethral valves
- **Splenomegaly**
    - Many causes of splenomegaly in children
        - Common causes include infection, right heart failure, and leukemia/lymphoma
    - May appear as mass on radiograph with displacement of bowel and stomach
- **Appendiceal Abscess**
    - Seen after ruptured appendix
        - Occurs in ~ 4% of cases
        - More common in children < 4 years
    - Often have symptoms more than 3 days
- **Wilms Tumor**
    - Most common abdominal neoplasm
    - 2nd most common pediatric solid tumor
    - Occurs in children < 15 years of age with peak at 3 years
    - May be bilateral
    - Associated with WAGR, Denys-Drash syndrome, and Beckwith-Wiedemann
        - 2x more common with horseshoe kidney
    - Appears as heterogeneous renal mass
        - Calcifications in 15-20%
        - Typically displaces vessels ± inferior vena cava invasion
- **Neuroblastoma**
    - Most common pediatric solid tumor
        - 6-10% of all childhood cancers
        - ~ 15% of cancer-related deaths in children
        - ~ 30% occur in 1st year of life with peak at 0-4 years
    - 2nd most common abdominal tumor
        - ~ 65% arise in abdomen
    - Usually arise from adrenal medulla
        - Can arise anywhere along sympathetic chain
    - Usually presents as asymptomatic abdominal mass
    - Metastases present in 70% at diagnosis
        - Bone and bone marrow
        - Liver metastases can be focal or diffuse
    - Urine catecholamines are elevated in 90%
    - I-123 MIBG positive in 90%
    - Calcifications present in ~ 85% on CT
    - Typically encases vessels

Helpful Clues for Less Common Diagnoses
- **Rhabdomyosarcoma**
    - Most common pediatric soft tissue sarcoma
        - Accounts for 5% of pediatric cancers
    - GU origin common for abdominal tumors
        - Bladder is most common organ of origin
        - Usually presents before age 5
    - Metastases to lung and marrow
- **Ovarian Tumors**
    - Teratomas are most common tumor
        - Majority are benign
    - Malignant ovarian tumors account for 1% of pediatric cancers

        - 75-80% are germ cell tumors
    - Can become very large and extend to abdomen
- **Multicystic Dysplastic Kidney**
    - More common in males
    - Left kidney more commonly affected
    - Natural history is involution of kidney
    - Distinguished from hydronephrosis as cysts do not connect with renal pelvis
- **Hemangioendothelioma/Hemangioma**
    - a.k.a. infantile hepatic hemangioma
    - Most common benign hepatic tumor
    - 85% diagnosed in 1st 6 months
    - Skin hemangiomas present in ~ 50%
    - Can present with high-output heart failure
- **Hepatoblastoma**
    - Most common pediatric liver malignancy
        - 1% of all pediatric malignancies
        - 79% of liver malignancies < 15 years
        - Most diagnosed under 18 months of age
    - Associated with low birth weight, hemihypertrophy, Beckwith-Wiedemann, familial adenomatous polyposis, trisomy 18, and fetal alcohol syndrome
    - 90% have increased serum AFP
    - Most common in right lobe of liver
    - Calcifications in 40-55%
    - Distant metastases in 20% at diagnosis
        - Lung, brain, and bone
- **Mesoblastic Nephroma**
    - 3-10% of pediatric renal tumors
    - Most common renal tumor in infants, 90% diagnosed in 1st year
    - 2x more common in males
    - Predominantly solid with variable cystic areas
- **Hepatocellular Carcinoma**
    - 2nd most common pediatric liver malignancy
        - Rare before age 5
    - ~ 75% are not associated with liver disease
        - Risks: Preexisting cirrhosis due to biliary atresia, Fanconi syndrome, viral hepatitis, hereditary tyrosinemia, or glycogen storage disease
        - Other risks: Androgen steroids, oral contraceptives, methotrexate
    - Metastases common at diagnosis
        - Regional lymph nodes, lungs, bone
    - Elevated AFP in 60-80%

Helpful Clues for Rare Diagnoses

- **Renal Cell Carcinoma**
    - Accounts for 2-5% of pediatric renal tumors
    - Mean age 9-15 years
    - Metastases in 20% at diagnosis
    - Associated with von Hippel-Lindau disease
- **Pancreatoblastoma**
    - Most common pediatric pancreatic neoplasm
    - Neoplasm of acinar cells
    - Most common in 1st decade of life
    - Associated with Beckwith-Wiedemann
    - AFP elevated in up to 55%
    - Usually large solitary pancreatic mass
        - Well defined with lobulated margins
        - ~ 50% in pancreatic head

Hydronephrosis

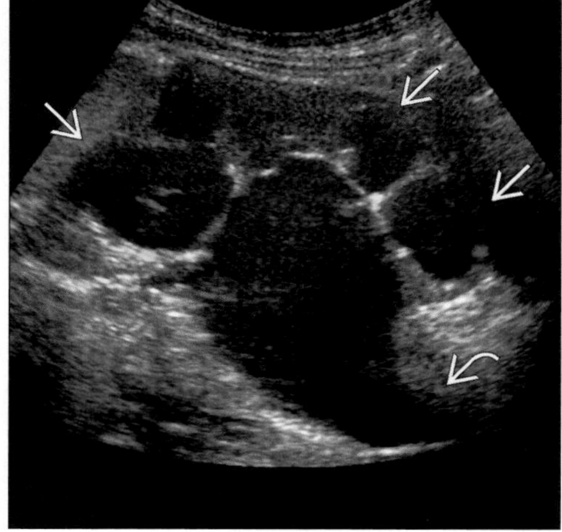

Longitudinal ultrasound shows marked hydronephrosis ➔ and a dilated proximal ureter ➔. The more distal ureter was not seen. Obstruction of the ureteropelvic junction is a common cause of hydronephrosis.

Hydronephrosis

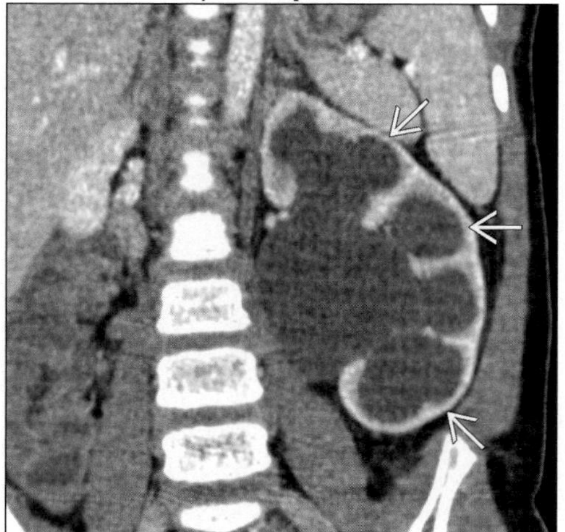

Coronal CECT shows marked hydronephrosis of the left kidney and associated cortical thinning ➔. The distal ureter was not seen. The patient was asymptomatic despite this congenital abnormality.

ABDOMINAL MASS IN A CHILD

*(**Left**) AP scout image from a CECT shows marked enlargement of the spleen in a patient with Alagille syndrome. (**Right**) Coronal CECT shows marked enlargement of the spleen. There is a focal area of decreased attenuation within the middle of the spleen that was due to splenic infarction. Common causes of splenomegaly in children include infection, right heart failure, portal hypertension, glycogen storage diseases, and leukemia/lymphoma.*

Splenomegaly

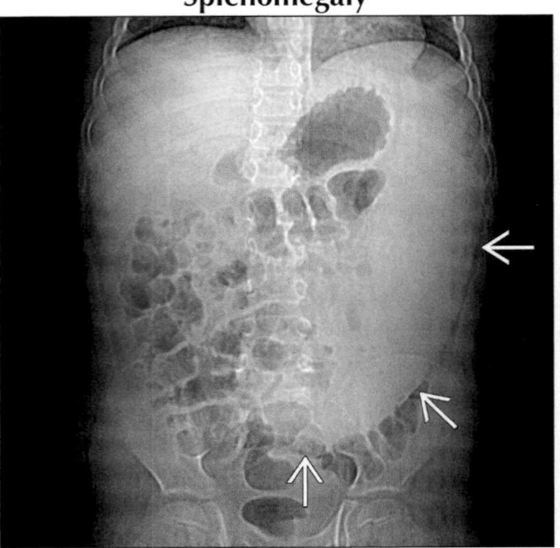

Splenomegaly

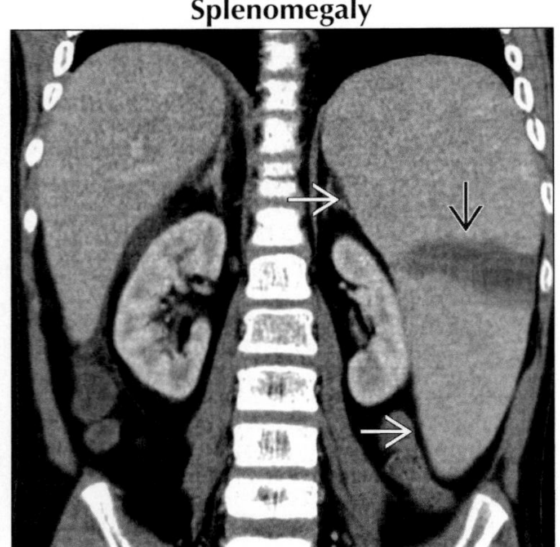

*(**Left**) Anteroposterior radiograph shows a mass in the right lower quadrant with a central area of air density. (**Right**) Axial CECT shows the right lower quadrant mass to have a thick wall and internal air. There is a circular area within the mass that represented the appendix. Appendiceal abscess occurs in up to 4% of cases of appendicitis. Patients often have symptoms for more than 3 days before the appendix ruptures.*

Appendiceal Abscess

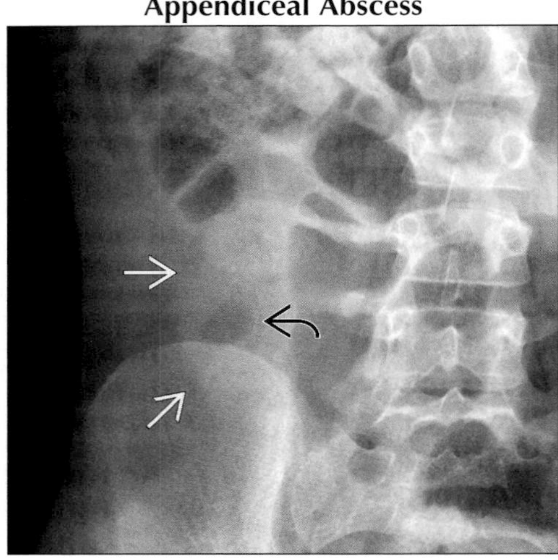

Appendiceal Abscess

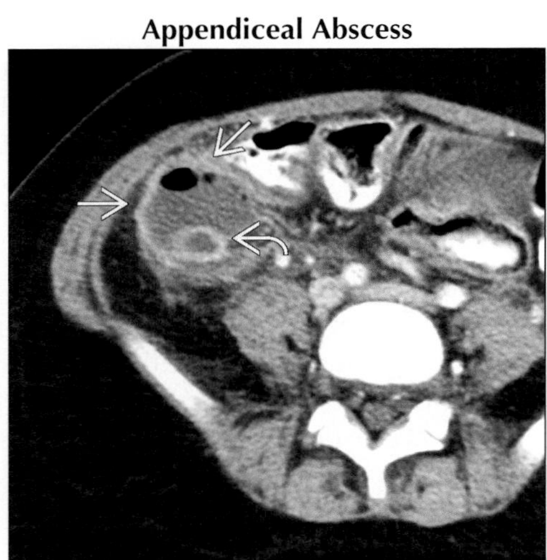

*(**Left**) Transverse ultrasound shows a large solid mass replacing most of the right kidney. There is a claw of residual renal tissue surrounding the posterior aspect of the mass. (**Right**) Axial CECT in the same patient confirms the ultrasound findings of a large solid mass replacing most of the right kidney. There is renal tissue surrounding the posterior and medial aspect of the mass. Wilms tumor is the most common abdominal neoplasm.*

Wilms Tumor

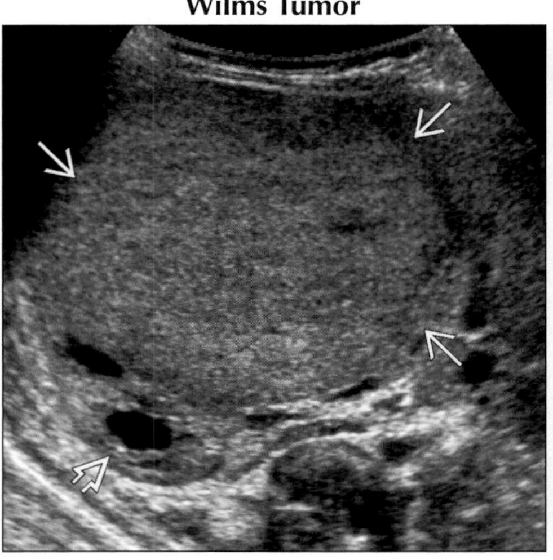

Wilms Tumor

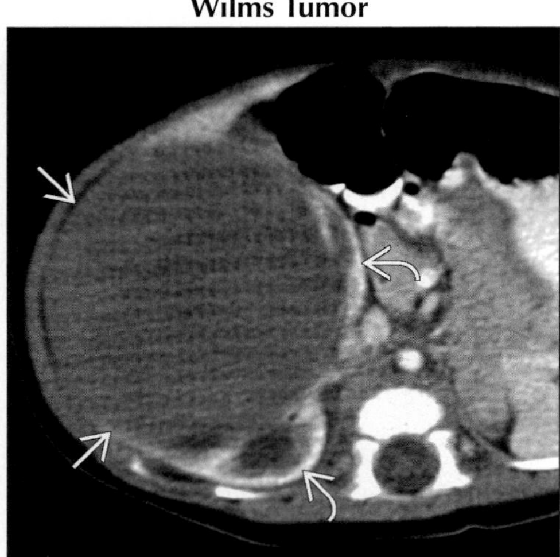

Neuroblastoma

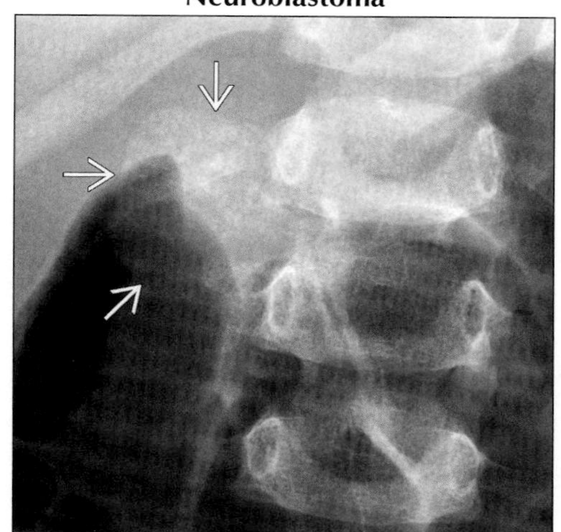

Neuroblastoma

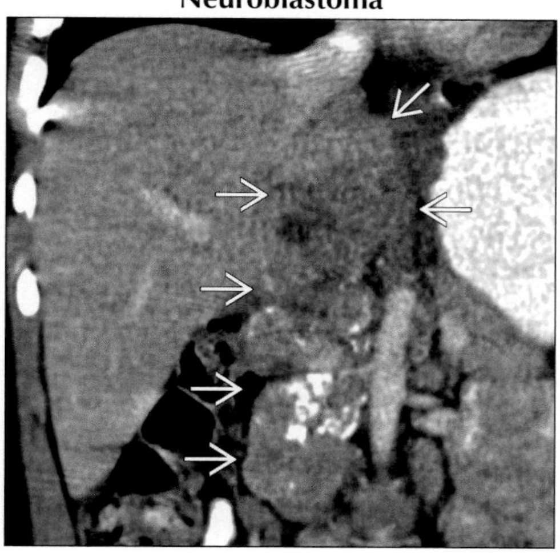

(Left) *Anteroposterior radiograph shows a speckled mass with calcifications ➔ in the right paraspinal region. A calcified paraspinal mass should raise suspicion for neuroblastoma.* ***(Right)*** *Coronal CECT shows an elongated, partially calcified mass ➔ in the right paraspinal region. This mass was not confined to a specific organ. Neuroblastoma most commonly arises from the adrenal medulla but can arise anywhere along the sympathetic chain.*

Rhabdomyosarcoma

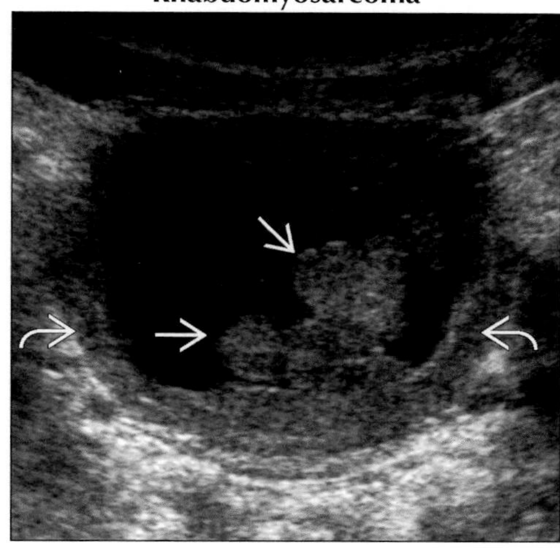

Rhabdomyosarcoma

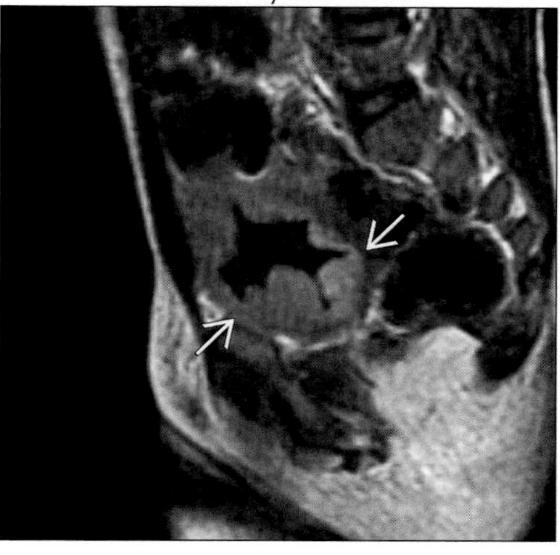

(Left) *Transverse ultrasound shows a lobulated mass ➔ in the base of the bladder. The bladder wall is also mildly thickened ➔. Rhabdomyosarcoma commonly affects the pelvis, and the bladder and prostate are common organs of origin.* ***(Right)*** *Sagittal FLAIR MR shows irregular wall thickening of the urinary bladder ➔. Rhabdomyosarcoma usually presents before age 5. Metastases can occur to the lungs and marrow.*

Ovarian Tumors

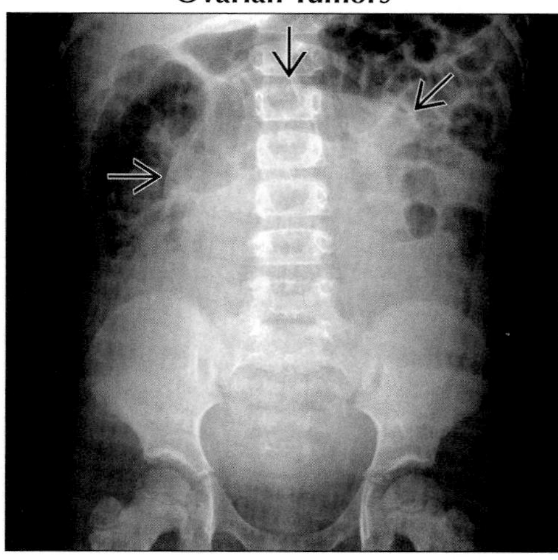

Ovarian Tumors

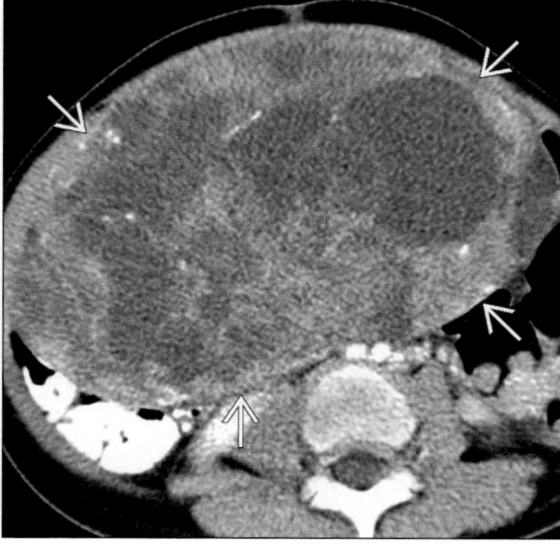

(Left) *Anteroposterior radiograph shows a large mass ➔ displacing the bowel superiorly.* ***(Right)*** *Axial CECT shows a large heterogeneous mass ➔ occupying the abdomen. In the pediatric population, most ovarian tumors are benign. At resection, this tumor was diagnosed as a granulosa cell tumor.*

*(**Left**) Coronal T2WI MR of a fetus shows a multicystic mass of the left kidney ➔. Multicystic dysplastic kidney is more common in males and occurs more frequently on the left side. (**Right**) Longitudinal ultrasound shows a multicystic mass replacing the left kidney ➔. Multicystic dysplastic kidney can be distinguished from hydronephrosis as the cysts of the multicystic dysplastic kidney do not connect with the renal pelvis. Multicystic dysplastic kidneys involute with age (not shown).*

Multicystic Dysplastic Kidney

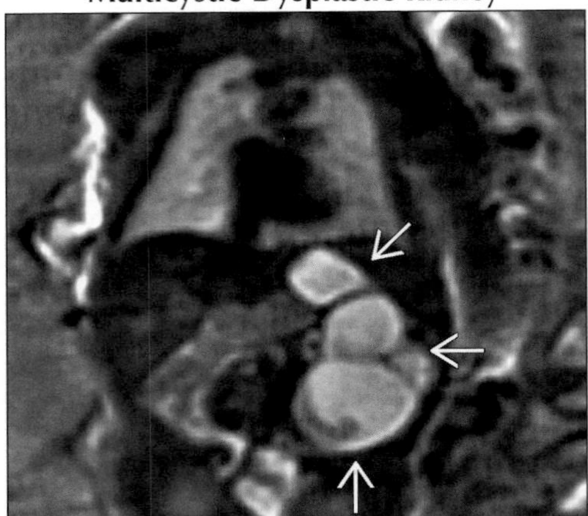

Multicystic Dysplastic Kidney

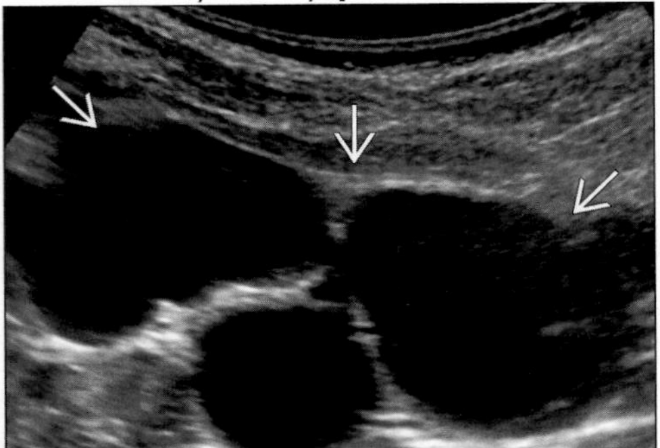

*(**Left**) Transverse ultrasound shows multiple hypoechoic lesions ➔ scattered throughout the liver. These lesions had increased color Doppler flow (not shown). Hepatic hemangiomas are often associated with cutaneous lesions. (**Right**) Axial T2WI MR shows multiple hyperintense lesions ➔ scattered throughout the liver. Patients with multiple or large lesions can present with high-output heart failure or hypothyroidism.*

Hemangioendothelioma/Hemangioma

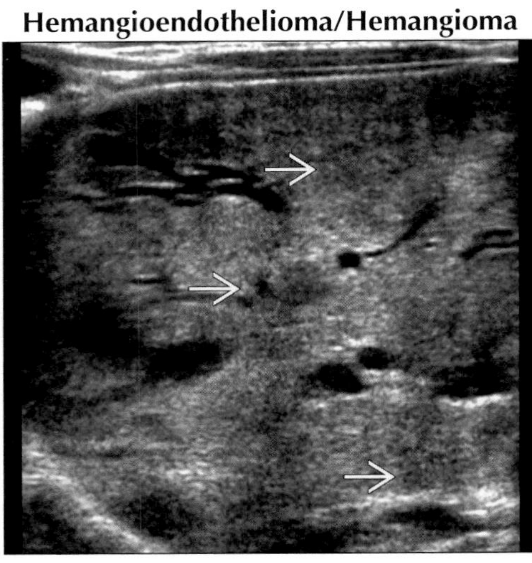

Hemangioendothelioma/Hemangioma

*(**Left**) Transverse ultrasound shows a heterogeneous mass ➔ arising from the inferior aspect of the liver. The mass has some hyperechoic areas representing calcifications ➔. Hepatoblastoma is the most common hepatic mass in children. (**Right**) Sagittal CECT shows a large heterogeneous mass ➔ with internal calcifications ➔ arising from the inferior aspect of the liver. Calcifications are present in 40-55% of hepatoblastomas.*

Hepatoblastoma

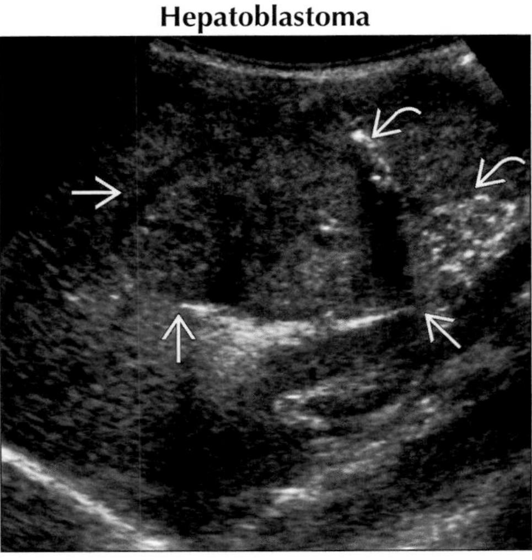

Hepatoblastoma

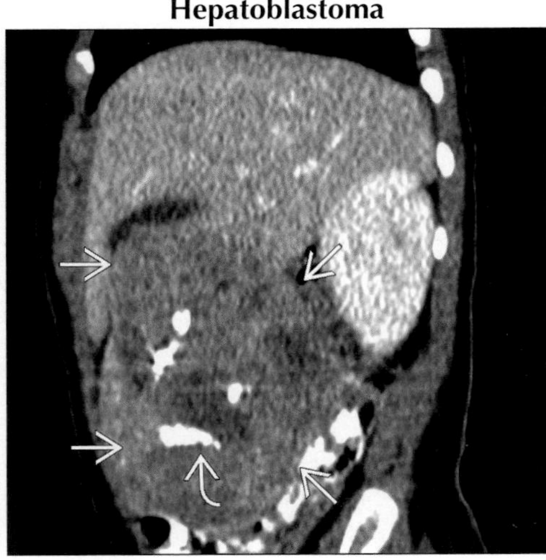

Mesoblastic Nephroma

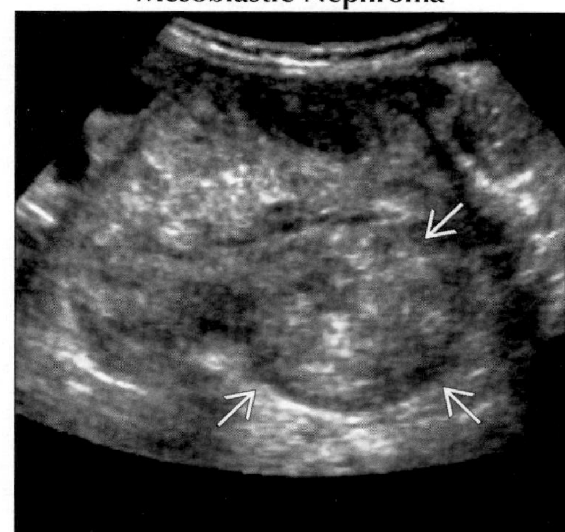

Mesoblastic Nephroma

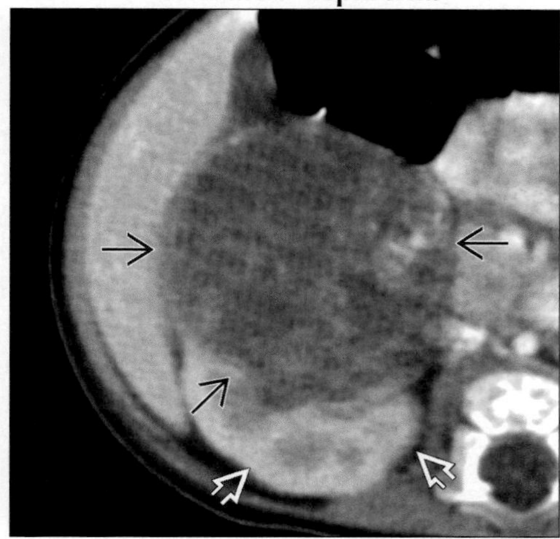

*(**Left**) Transverse ultrasound shows a heterogeneous solid mass ➡ arising from the left kidney. Mesoblastic nephroma is the most common renal tumor in infants. (**Right**) Axial CECT shows a heterogeneous solid mass ➡ arising form the right kidney. There is a claw of renal tissue ➡ surrounding the mass. Mesoblastic nephroma is predominantly a solid tumor, although it can have cystic areas.*

Hepatocellular Carcinoma

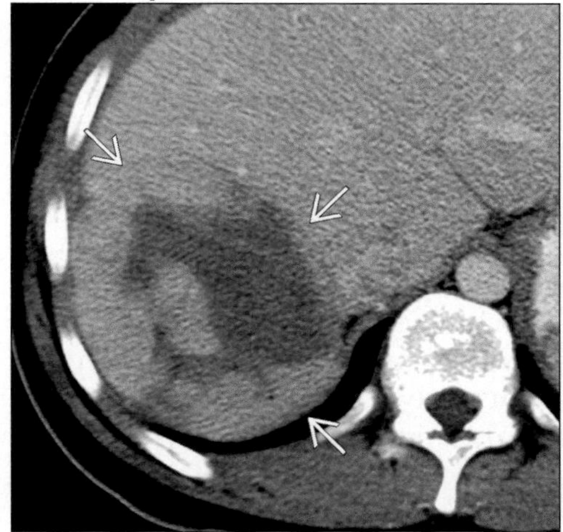

Renal Cell Carcinoma

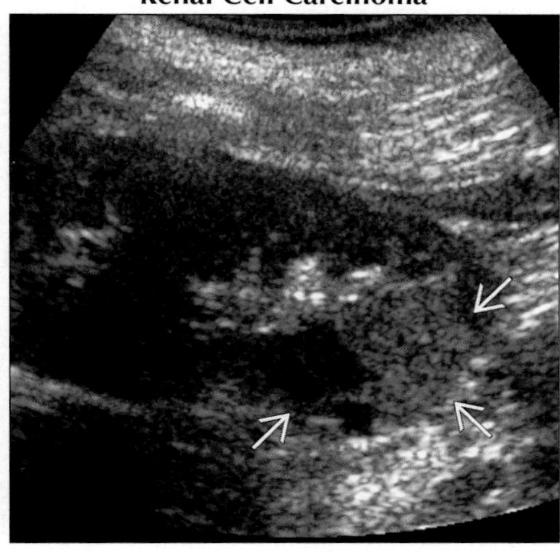

*(**Left**) Axial CECT shows a heterogeneous mass ➡ in the right lobe of the liver. Hepatocellular carcinoma is the 2nd most common hepatic tumor in children but is much less common than hepatoblastoma. It typically occurs in older children. (**Right**) Longitudinal ultrasound shows a mixed cystic and solid mass ➡ arising from the lower pole of the kidney. The mass is hyperechoic compared to the renal cortex. Renal cell carcinoma is an uncommon renal tumor in children.*

Renal Cell Carcinoma

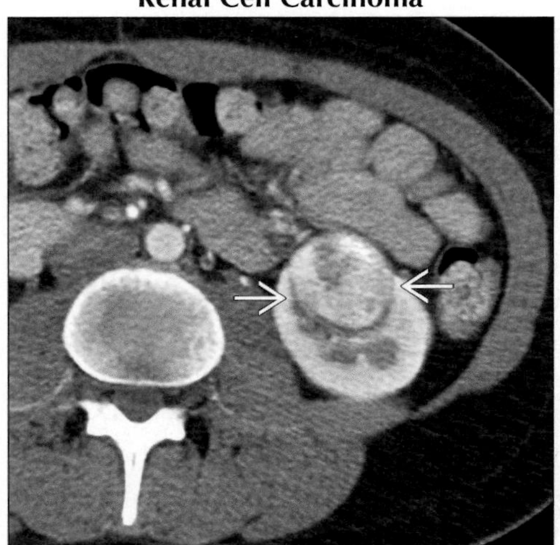

Pancreatoblastoma

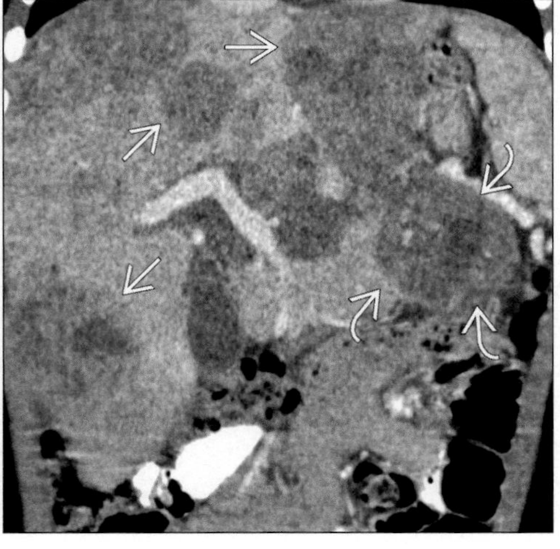

*(**Left**) Axial CECT shows a heterogeneous mass ➡ in the lower pole of the left kidney. There is a claw of normal renal tissue surrounding the mass. Renal cell carcinoma has a mean age of occurrence between 9 and 15 years. (**Right**) Coronal CECT shows a large mass ➡ arising from the tail of the pancreas. There is a claw of normal pancreatic tissue surrounding the mass. In addition, there are multiple hepatic metastases ➡.*

HEPATIC MASS IN A NEONATE

DIFFERENTIAL DIAGNOSIS

Common
- Hemangioendothelioma/Hemangioma
- Metastases
  - Neuroblastoma
  - Wilms Tumor
- Hepatoblastoma
- Mesenchymal Hamartoma

Less Common
- Unilocular Cyst
- Choledochal Cyst

Rare but Important
- Abscess
- Angiosarcoma

ESSENTIAL INFORMATION

Key Differential Diagnosis Issues
- Hepatic tumors uncommon in perinatal period
  - Account for ~ 5% of perinatal tumors
  - 6x more likely to be benign
- Most masses identified during antenatal US or neonatal physical exam
- Lab tests can help to differentiate masses
  - CBC, α-fetoprotein (AFP), β-HCG, are markers for neuroblastoma
- Biopsy or resection provide final diagnosis
  - Overlap of imaging and clinical finding

Helpful Clues for Common Diagnoses
- **Hemangioendothelioma/Hemangioma**
  - a.k.a. infantile hepatic hemangioma
  - Vascular neoplasms most common liver tumor in neonates
    - Account for ~ 60% of neonatal liver tumors
  - Hemangioendothelioma more often symptomatic than cavernous hemangioma
    - Symptoms include abdominal distension, hepatomegaly, congestive heart failure, and respiratory distress
    - Other symptoms: Consumptive coagulopathy (Kasabach-Merritt syndrome) and rupture with intraperitoneal hemorrhage
    - Can be associated with hypothyroidism
    - ~ 50% have cutaneous hemangiomas
  - Large lesions have peripheral nodular enhancement on CT and MR
  - Multiple lesions may be present
  - Celiac and hepatic arteries often enlarged
  - Angiosarcoma and choriocarcinoma can have similar appearance
    - Tumor markers (AFP and β-HCG) and follow-up imaging help confirm diagnosis
  - Lesions should regress with age
    - Symptomatic lesions treated with medical or surgical therapy
  - **Hint**: High-output heart failure with liver mass
- **Metastases**
  - More common than primary hepatic malignancies
  - Neuroblastoma most common primary tumor to metastasize to liver
    - Stage 4S neuroblastoma can have diffuse hepatic infiltration
  - Leukemia and Wilms tumor are next most common
  - Rare metastases include yolk sac tumor, rhabdomyosarcoma, and rhabdoid tumor
  - **Hint**: Known malignancy (i.e., neuroblastoma or Wilms tumor) with solitary or multiple liver masses
- **Hepatoblastoma**
  - < 10% occur in neonatal period
  - Associated with hemihypertrophy, Beckwith-Wiedemann, trisomy 18, familial adenomatous polyposis coli, fetal alcohol syndrome, and extreme prematurity
  - Differences in neonates compared to typical age range (0.5-3 years)
    - Worse prognosis
    - Metastases occur earlier and are often systemic
    - Fetal circulation allows metastases to bypass lungs
    - Do not produce excessive AFP
    - Tumor rupture can occur during labor/birth
  - **Hint**: Liver mass in patient < 2 years old containing internal calcification
- **Mesenchymal Hamartoma**
  - 2nd most common benign hepatic mass
  - Typically diagnosed in 1st 2 years of life
  - Usually presents as palpable right upper quadrant mass
    - Most common in right lobe (75%)
    - AFP may be moderately elevated

- Multiloculated cystic mass
  - Mixed cystic and solid
  - Multiple tiny cysts may appear solid
  - On US, septae of cysts may be mobile
  - Large portal vein branch may feed mass
  - Calcification uncommon
- May ↑ in size over 1st few months
- Reports of malignant transformation to undifferentiated embryonal sarcoma
  - Treatment is complete excision

Helpful Clues for Less Common Diagnoses

- **Unilocular Cyst**
  - Usually simple cyst
    - No connection to biliary system
    - Hepatic scintigraphy (DISIDA) can prove cyst does not contain bile
  - Often asymptomatic and requires no intervention
- **Choledochal Cyst**
  - Infantile type (patients < 1 year old)
    - Thought to have different etiology than childhood type
    - Presents with jaundice, vomiting, acholic stool, and hepatomegaly
    - Associated with biliary atresia in 44%
  - Todani type 1 cyst most common
  - Associated with ductal and vascular anomalies
    - Anomalous hepatic arteries, accessory hepatic ducts, and primary duct strictures
  - US is good screening test
    - Cyst usually in subhepatic region or porta hepatis
    - Distinct from gallbladder
    - Anechoic, thin walled, with round, tubular, or teardrop shape
  - MRCP or cholangiogram
    - Useful for showing connection of cyst to biliary system
    - Can see intra- or extrahepatic ductal abnormalities
  - Treated with excision
    - ↓ risk of malignant degeneration if diagnosed before age 10

Helpful Clues for Rare Diagnoses

- **Abscess**
  - In neonates, most small and multiple
    - Solitary abscess accounts for 30%
  - Risks include umbilical venous catheter, sepsis, and necrotizing enterocolitis requiring surgery
  - Other risks: Immunodeficiencies, long-term parenteral nutrition, and prematurity
  - *S. aureus* and gram-negative enteric bacteria most common organisms
- **Angiosarcoma**
  - a.k.a. hemangioendothelioma, type 2
  - Few cases of diagnosis before age 1
  - Looks like hemangioendothelioma
    - Continued growth after treatment should raise suspicion

Hemangioendothelioma/Hemangioma

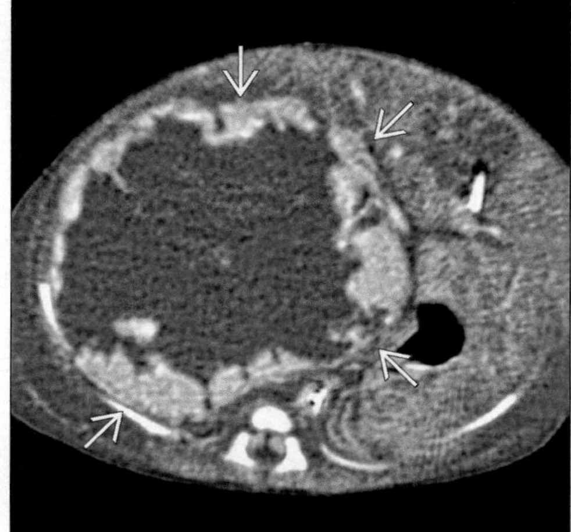

Axial CECT shows a large heterogeneous mass ➔ with peripheral nodular enhancement arising from the inferior aspect of the liver. This mass was later confirmed to be a cavernous hemangioma.

Hemangioendothelioma/Hemangioma

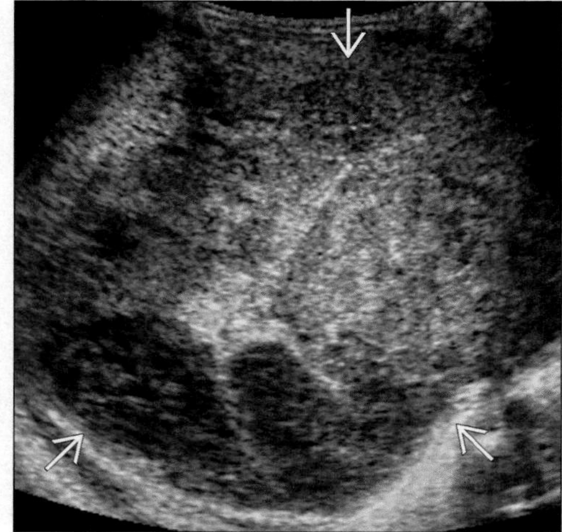

Transverse ultrasound in the same patient shows a heterogeneous mass ➔ occupying the entire visualized liver. Vascular neoplasms are the most common hepatic tumor in neonates.

HEPATIC MASS IN A NEONATE

*(**Left**) Transverse ultrasound shows marked enlargement of the left hepatic vein ➔. Posterior to the hepatic vein is a heterogeneous mass ➔ with focal areas of increased echogenicity ➔. (**Right**) Axial CECT in the same patient shows a large mass ➔ occupying the left hepatic lobe. This mass has peripheral nodular enhancement and a central area that is hypodense. The hepatic artery is enlarged → as is often the case with a hemangioendothelioma.*

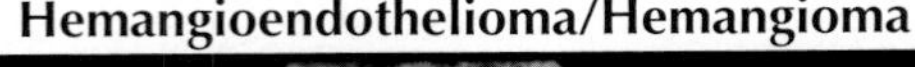

Hemangioendothelioma/Hemangioma

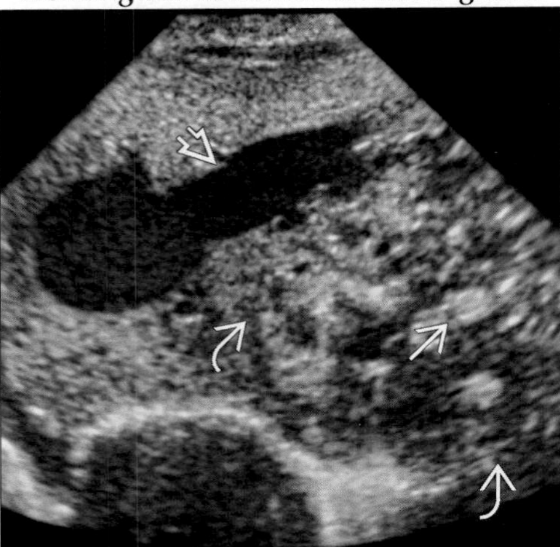

Hemangioendothelioma/Hemangioma

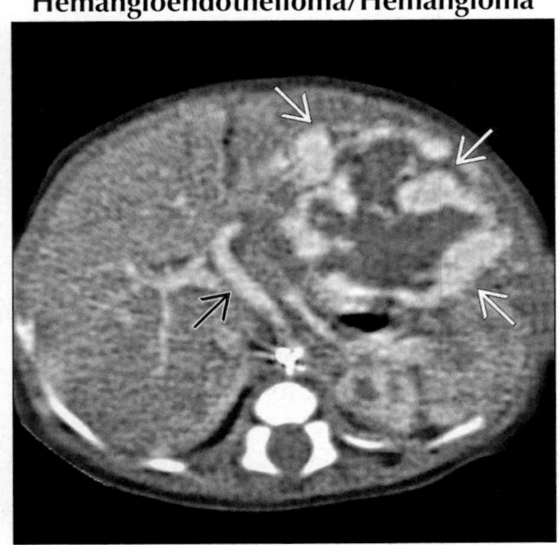

*(**Left**) Transverse ultrasound shows multiple hypoechoic lesions in the liver surrounded by an echogenic rim ➔. (**Right**) Axial T2WI MR in the same patient shows hyperintense lesions throughout both lobes of the liver. The liver is almost entirely replaced by the multiple vascular tumors. Patients with large or multiple hemangioendotheliomas can present with high-output heart failure or consumptive coagulopathy, among other symptoms.*

Hemangioendothelioma/Hemangioma

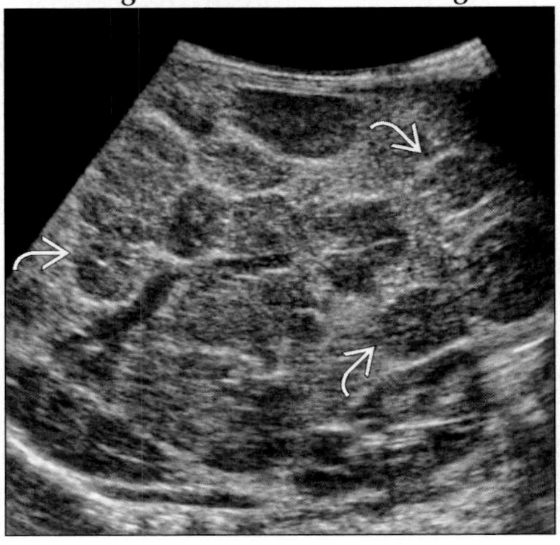

Hemangioendothelioma/Hemangioma

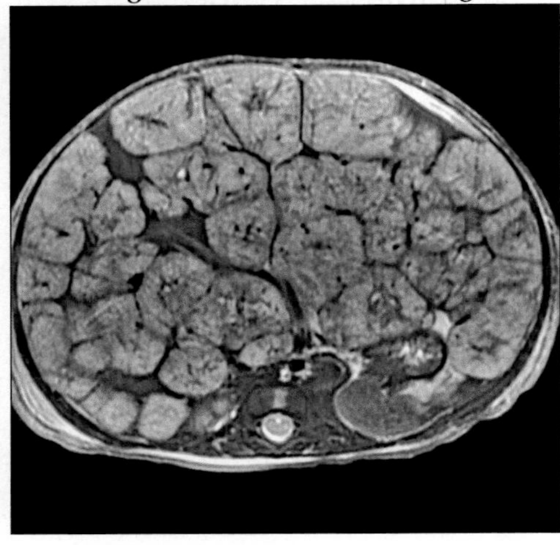

*(**Left**) Coronal T1WI MR LAVA sequence in the 1st pass shows innumerable lesions throughout both lobes of the liver. Each lesion has peripheral nodular enhancement that fills in with time. (**Right**) Coronal T1WI MR LAVA sequence in the 2nd pass after contrast administration also shows multiple lesions. Hemangioendotheliomas often regress with age, although in patients with such extensive disease, medical therapy is typically required.*

Hemangioendothelioma/Hemangioma

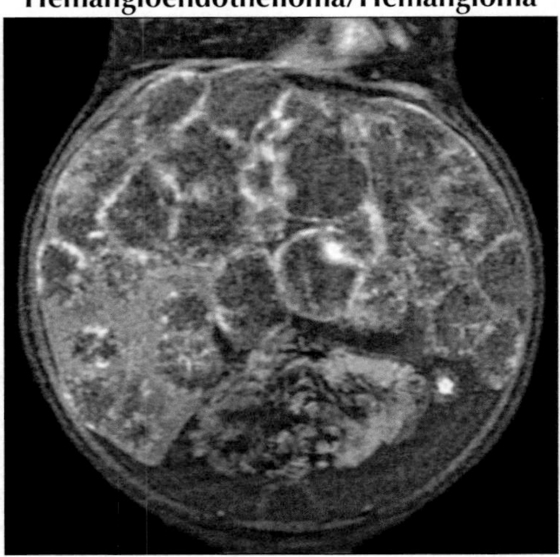

Hemangioendothelioma/Hemangioma

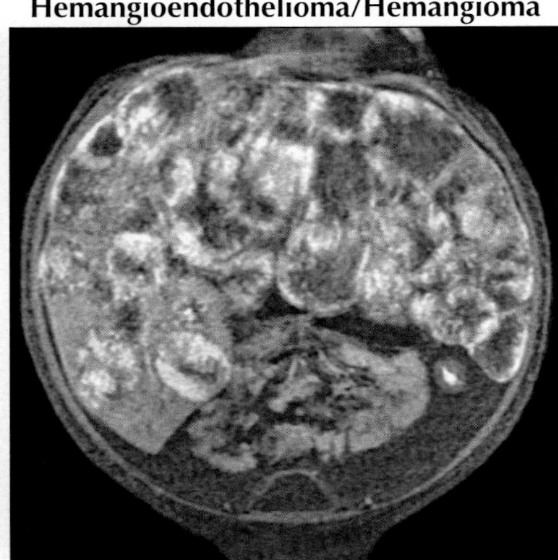

Metastases

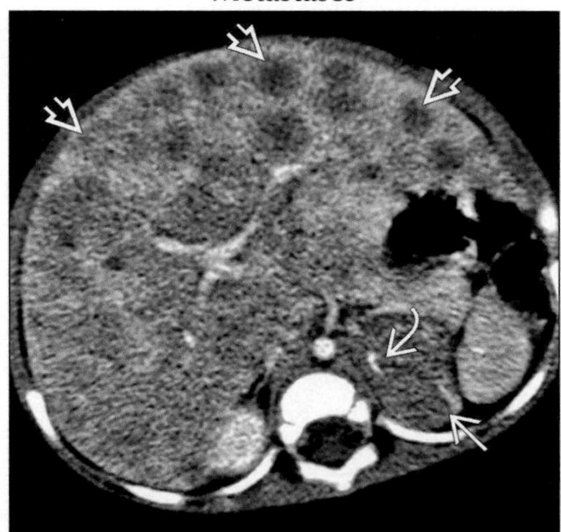

Metastases

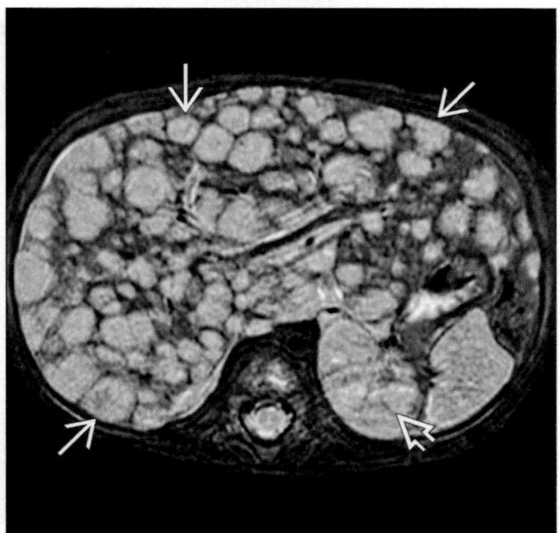

(Left) *Axial CECT shows hepatomegaly with multiple hypodense lesions ➩ throughout both lobes of the liver. There is a hypodense mass ➡ in the left suprarenal fossa with calcification ➩.* ***(Right)*** *Axial T2WI MR shows hepatomegaly and innumerable hyperintense lesions ➡ in both lobes of the liver. The primary tumor ➩ in the left suprarenal fossa is also hyperintense. Neuroblastomas are the most common metastatic tumors to the liver in children.*

Hepatoblastoma

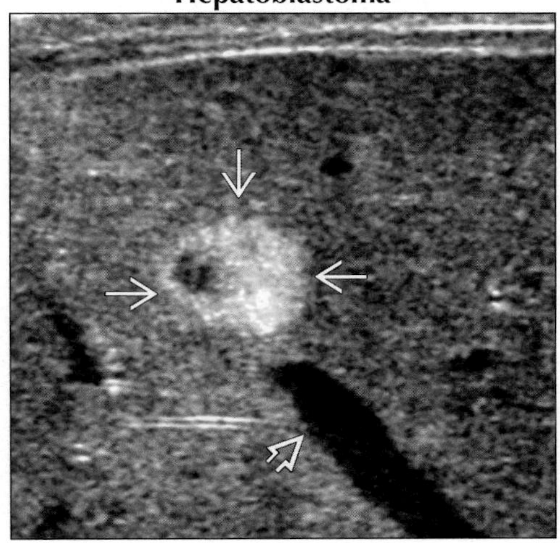

Hepatoblastoma

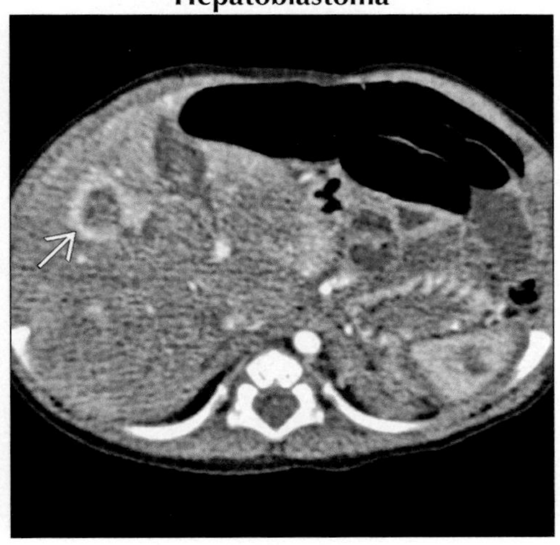

(Left) *Transverse ultrasound in a patient with Beckwith-Wiedemann syndrome shows a mostly hyperechoic lesion ➡ in the right lobe of the liver near the right hepatic vein ➩.* ***(Right)*** *Axial CECT in the same patient shows a hypodense lesion with a surrounding area of enhancement ➡. Patients with Beckwith-Wiedemann have a genetic predisposition to hepatoblastoma. Overall, less than 10% of hepatoblastomas occur in the neonatal period.*

Hepatoblastoma

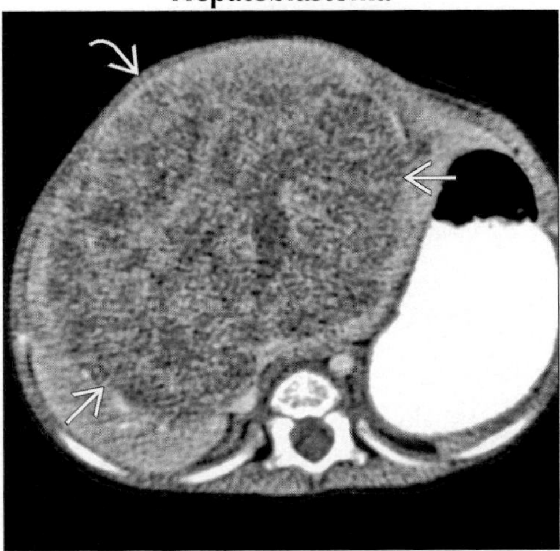

Hepatoblastoma

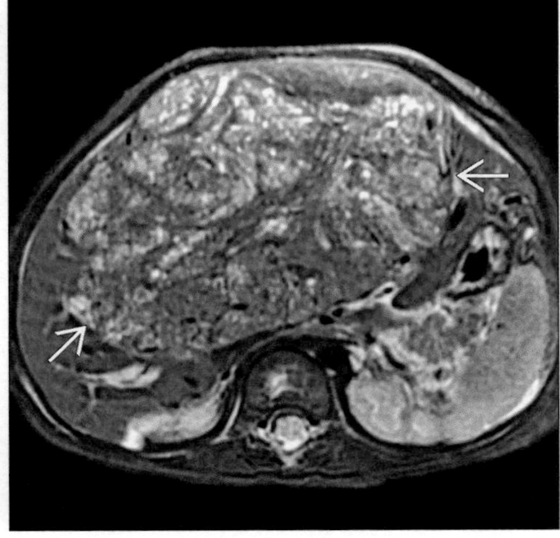

(Left) *Axial CECT shows a large heterogeneous mass ➡ of both the right and left lobe of the liver. This mass expands the liver capsule and deforms the anterior abdominal wall ➩.* ***(Right)*** *Axial T2WI MR in the same patient shows a mostly hyperintense mass ➡ occupying both the right and left lobe of the liver. Hepatoblastoma has a worse prognosis in neonates than in other patients, and metastases occur earlier and are often systemic.*

HEPATIC MASS IN A NEONATE

(**Left**) Transverse ultrasound shows a mixed multicystic and solid mass of the right lobe of the liver. No normal hepatic tissue is present on this image. This is the 1st of 4 images from the same patient. (**Right**) Coronal T1WI MR shows marked hepatomegaly. There is a mixed cystic and solid mass ➡ expanding the right lobe of the liver. Mesenchymal hamartoma is the 2nd most common benign hepatic mass. It is typically diagnosed before age 2.

Mesenchymal Hamartoma

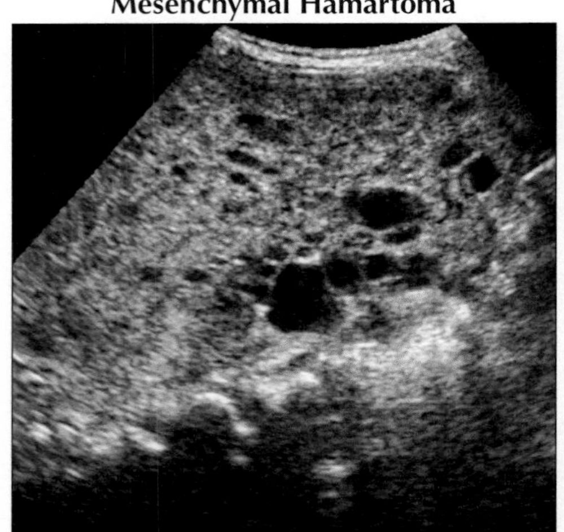

Mesenchymal Hamartoma

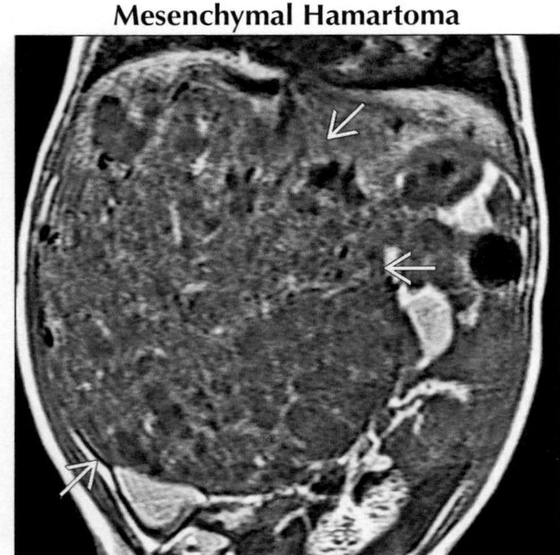

(**Left**) Coronal T2WI MR shows a multicystic and solid mass ➡ of the right lobe. The cysts vary in size from micro- to macrocystic. Mesenchymal hamartoma usually appears as a multicystic mass; if composed entirely of microcysts, however, it can appear solid. (**Right**) Axial T1WI C+ MR shows a mixed multicystic and solid mass ➡. The solid portion of the mass enhances. A small portion of normal liver is also present. Calcification is uncommon with this lesion.

Mesenchymal Hamartoma

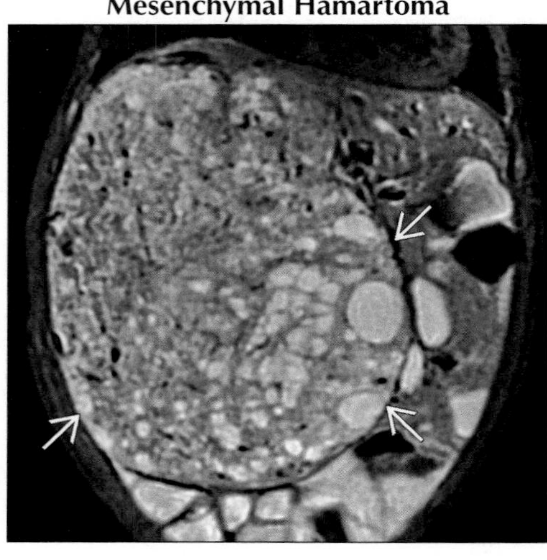

Mesenchymal Hamartoma

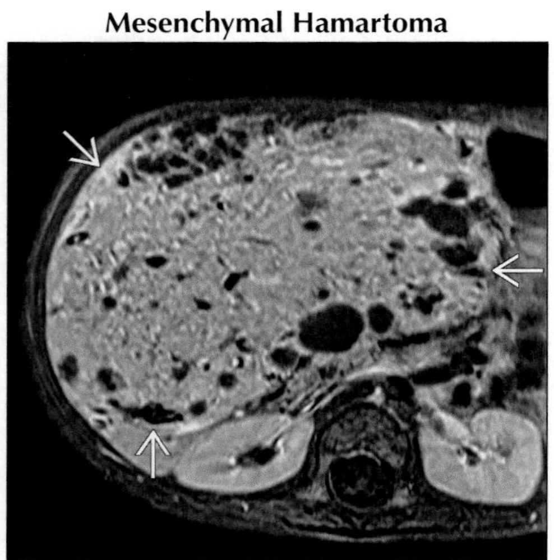

(**Left**) Radiograph of the chest and abdomen in a different patient shows a soft tissue mass in the left upper quadrant. The air-filled bowel is displaced to the right. (**Right**) Transverse ultrasound shows an anechoic mass ➡ arising from the left lobe of the liver. This mass had no internal color Doppler flow although there were multiple septations. The rim of the lesion is thin and uniform. Unilocular cysts such as this do not connect to the biliary system.

Unilocular Cyst

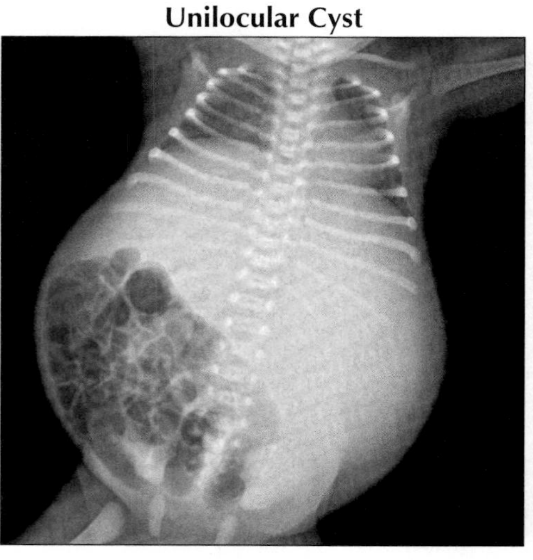

Unilocular Cyst

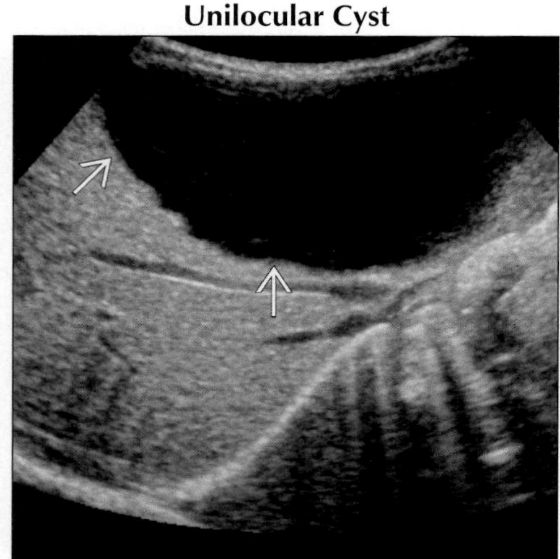

HEPATIC MASS IN A NEONATE

Unilocular Cyst

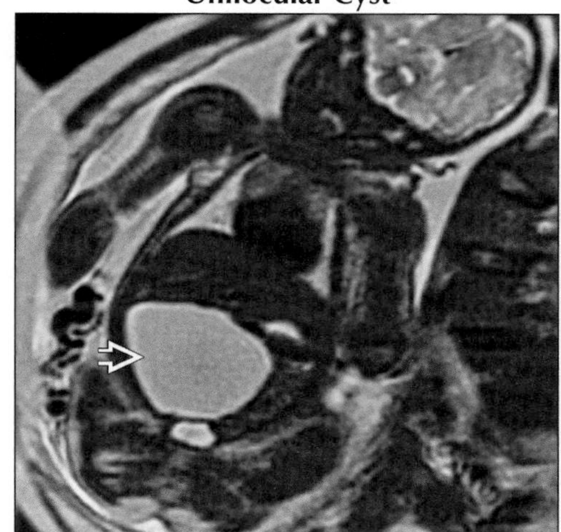

Unilocular Cyst

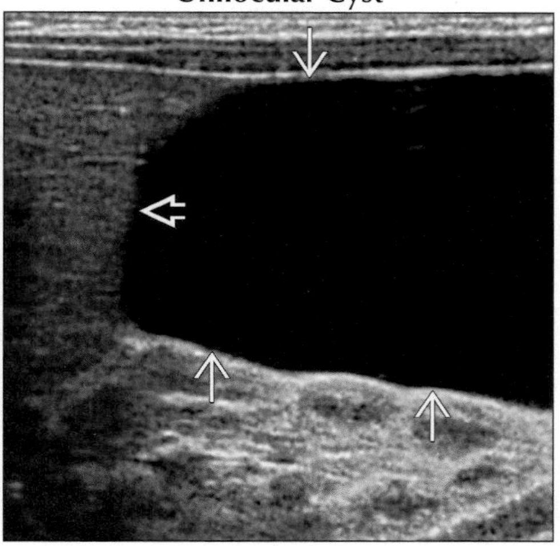

*(**Left**) Coronal T2WI MR of a fetus shows a large hyperintense mass ➡ along the inferior edge of the liver. (**Right**) Transverse ultrasound postnatally in the same patient shows a large anechoic lesion ➡ arising from the inferior aspect of the liver ➡. This mass has a simple appearance with no internal color Doppler flow, no septations, & a thin rim. At resection, it was confirmed to be a simple hepatic cyst. Unilocular cysts are often asymptomatic.*

Choledochal Cyst

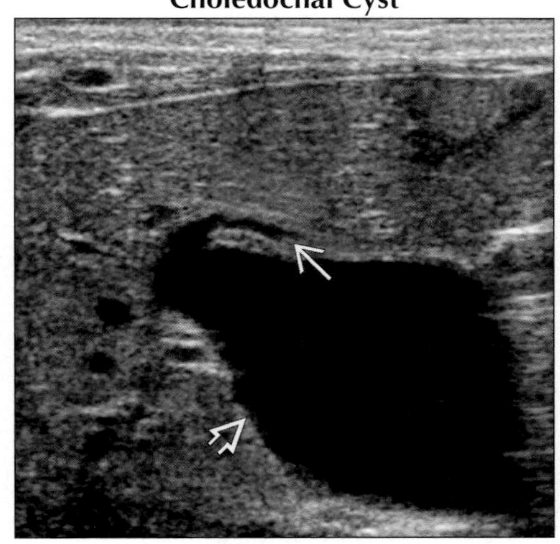

Choledochal Cyst

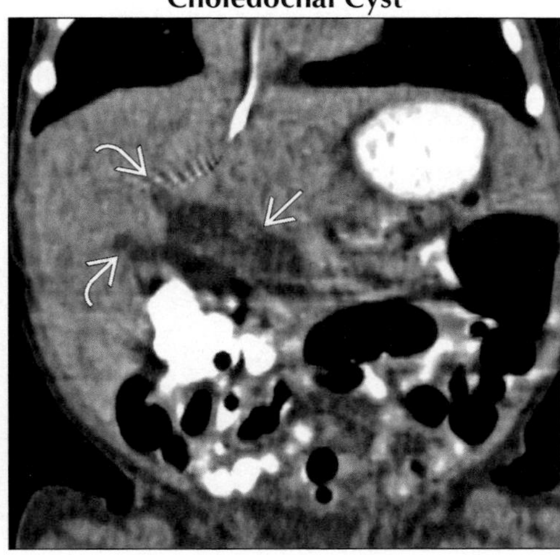

*(**Left**) Transverse ultrasound shows a pear-shaped cystic lesion ➡ extending from the common hepatic duct ➡. At real-time examination, this was consistent with fusiform dilation of the common bile duct. (**Right**) Coronal CECT in the same patient shows cystic dilatation of the common bile duct ➡. There is extension of the fusiform dilation into the intrahepatic bile ducts ➡. Choledochal cysts connect to the biliary system.*

Abscess

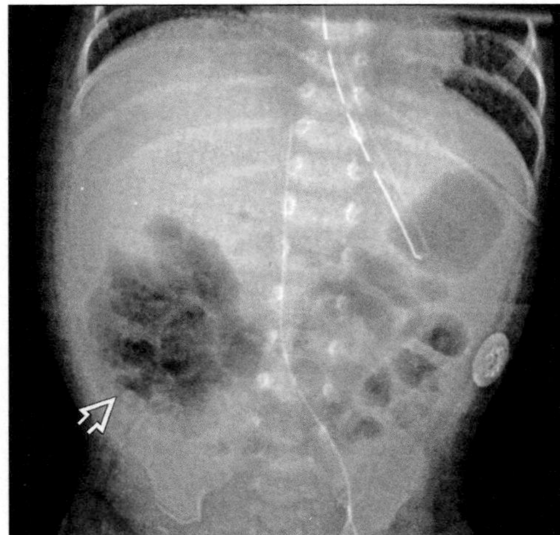

Abscess

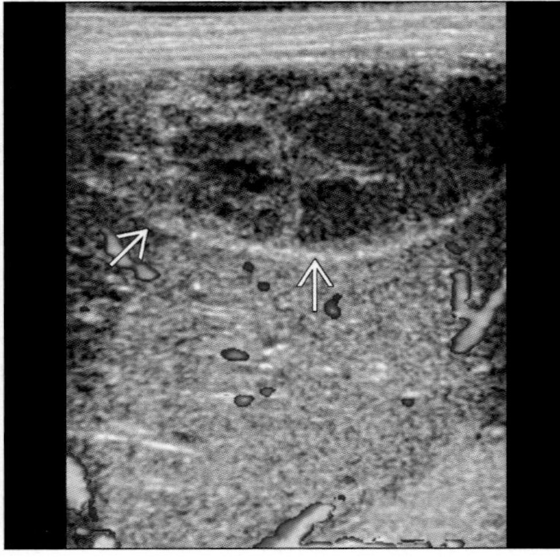

*(**Left**) Anteroposterior radiograph of the abdomen shows mottled lucency ➡ in the right lower quadrant, consistent with pneumatosis intestinalis in a child with necrotizing enterocolitis. (**Right**) Transverse color Doppler ultrasound shows a well-defined heterogeneous-appearing multiseptated mass ➡ arising from the liver without internal color Doppler flow. Bowel perforation and indwelling catheters are the most common cause of abscess in neonates.*

HEPATIC MASS IN A CHILD

DIFFERENTIAL DIAGNOSIS

Common
- Hepatoblastoma
- Hepatocellular Carcinoma
- Hemangioendothelioma

Less Common
- Abscess
- Focal Nodular Hyperplasia
- Metastases

Rare but Important
- Choledochal Cyst
- Mesenchymal Hamartoma
- Embryonal Sarcoma
- Hepatic Adenoma
- Angiomyolipoma (AML)
- Nodular Regenerative Hyperplasia
- Fibrolamellar Hepatocellular Carcinoma
- Biliary Rhabdomyosarcoma
- Angiosarcoma

ESSENTIAL INFORMATION

Key Differential Diagnosis Issues
- Primary hepatic neoplasms uncommon in children
  - 0.5-2% of all pediatric neoplasms
  - 2/3 malignant
- Differential diagnosis can be focused by age
- Biopsy often needed for diagnosis

Helpful Clues for Common Diagnoses
- **Hepatoblastoma**
  - Most common pediatric liver malignancy
    - 1% of all pediatric malignancies
    - 79% of all liver malignancies < 15 years of age
    - Majority diagnosed under 18 months
  - More common in boys
  - Associated with low birth weight, hemihypertrophy, Beckwith-Wiedemann, familial adenomatous polyposis, trisomy 18, and fetal alcohol syndrome
  - Often presents as asymptomatic mass
  - 90% have increased serum AFP
  - Most common in right lobe of liver, bilateral in 35%
  - Calcifications occur in 40-55%
  - Distant metastases in 20% at diagnosis
    - Lung most common, followed by brain and bone
  - Staged via PRETEXT staging system
  - Treatment via resection
    - Contraindications: Extensive bilateral disease, vascular invasion, or distant metastases
  - 75% 5-year survival rate
- **Hepatocellular Carcinoma**
  - 2nd most common liver malignancy in children
    - Rare before age 5
    - More common in males
  - ~ 75% not associated with liver disease
  - Risk factors: Preexisting cirrhosis due to biliary atresia, Fanconi syndrome, viral hepatitis, or glycogen storage disease
    - Other risks: Androgen steroids, oral contraceptives, methotrexate
  - Metastases common at diagnosis
    - Regional lymph nodes, lungs, bone
  - Elevated AFP in 60-80%
  - Staged via PRETEXT system
  - Poor long-term survival
- **Hemangioendothelioma**
  - a.k.a. infantile hemangioendothelioma
  - Most common benign hepatic tumor
  - 85% diagnosed in 1st 6 months
  - Often asymptomatic in childhood
  - Skin hemangiomas present in ~ 50%
  - **Hint**: High-output heart failure + liver tumor

Helpful Clues for Less Common Diagnoses
- **Abscess**
  - Associated with bacteremia, parasites, and chronic granulomatous disease
  - Can be seen with inflammatory process involving bowel
- **Focal Nodular Hyperplasia**
  - Occurs in all age groups
  - Well-circumscribed lobulated lesion with central stellate scar
  - More common in females and in patients who have received chemotherapy
- **Metastases**
  - Neuroblastoma and Wilms most common

Helpful Clues for Rare Diagnoses
- **Choledochal Cyst**
  - Cystic or fusiform dilation of biliary tree
  - Todani classification with 5 types
    - Type 1 most common
  - Associated with ductal and vascular anomalies

- Anomalous hepatic arteries, accessory ducts, and primary duct strictures
  - Ultrasound is best screening test
  - Treated with excision due to risk of malignant degeneration
- **Mesenchymal Hamartoma**
  - 2nd most common benign hepatic tumor of childhood
    - 6-8% of pediatric hepatic neoplasms
    - 85% present before age 3
  - Often present as large RUQ mass
    - 75% in right lobe
    - AFP can be elevated
  - Multiloculated cystic mass
    - Tiny cysts can give solid appearance
    - On US, septae of cysts may be mobile
    - Large portal vein branch may feed mass
    - Calcification uncommon
  - Associated with congenital heart disease, malrotation, esophageal atresia, annular pancreas, biliary atresia, and exomphalos
    - Also associated with myelomeningocele and Beckwith-Wiedemann syndrome
  - Rare malignant degeneration to undifferentiated embryonal sarcoma
  - Treatment via excision
- **Embryonal Sarcoma**
  - a.k.a. undifferentiated sarcoma
  - Accounts for 9-15% of all hepatic tumors
    - 3rd most common malignant hepatic tumor in children
  - Usually occurs between 6-10 years of age
  - On US, appears as solid mass with cystic areas
  - On CT, appears hypodense with septations and fibrous pseudocapsule
  - Case reports of spontaneous rupture
  - 4-year survival: 70-83%
- **Hepatic Adenoma**
  - Most common in young women
  - ↑ risk with oral contraceptive or anabolic steroid use
- **Angiomyolipoma (AML)**
  - Associated with tuberous sclerosis
  - Less common than renal AML
- **Nodular Regenerative Hyperplasia**
  - Multi-acinar regenerative lesion of liver
  - Associated with systemic diseases
  - 1/2 of patients have portal hypertension
- **Fibrolamellar Hepatocellular Carcinoma**
  - Occurs in adolescents, young adults
  - Calcifications seen in 35-68%
  - Central scar present in 20-71%
    - Low signal on all MR pulse sequences
  - Dismal prognosis if not resectable
- **Biliary Rhabdomyosarcoma**
  - Accounts for 0.5% of rhabdomyosarcomas
  - Intraductal mass on CT or MR
- **Angiosarcoma**
  - a.k.a. hemangioendothelioma, type 2
    - M:F = 1:2
    - Mean age: 3-4 years
  - Resembles hemangioendothelioma
  - Tumor usually involves both lobes
  - Metastases to lungs, nodes, pleura, bones, and adrenals

Hepatoblastoma

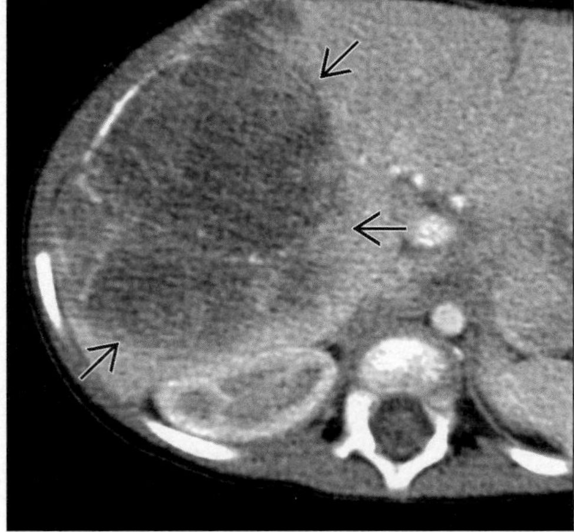

Axial CECT shows a large hypodense mass ➡ in the right lobe of the liver. This mass has some internal enhancement. Hepatoblastoma is the most common hepatic neoplasm in children.

Hepatoblastoma

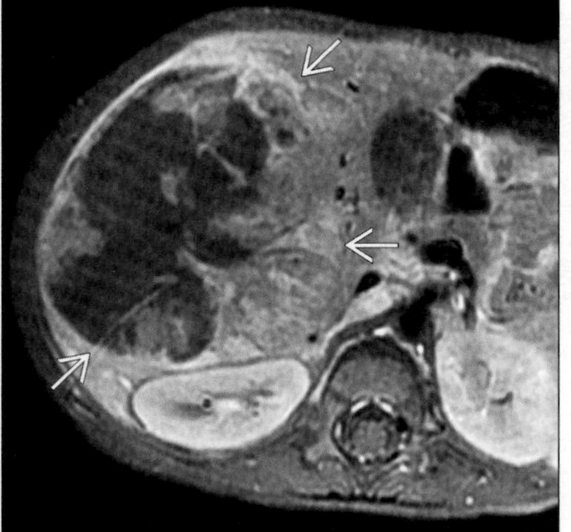

Axial T1WI C+ FS MR in the same patient shows a large mass ➡ in the right lobe of the liver. The mass is heterogeneous with a large central area that is hypointense to the rest of the liver.

HEPATIC MASS IN A CHILD

*(**Left**) Axial CECT shows a well-defined mass → in the liver. The mass has a heterogeneous appearance with areas of internal calcification →. Calcifications are present in 40-55% of cases. (**Right**) Axial T1WI C+ FS MR in the same patient shows a heterogeneous mass → of the liver. The calcifications seen on CT are hypointense on MR.*

Hepatoblastoma

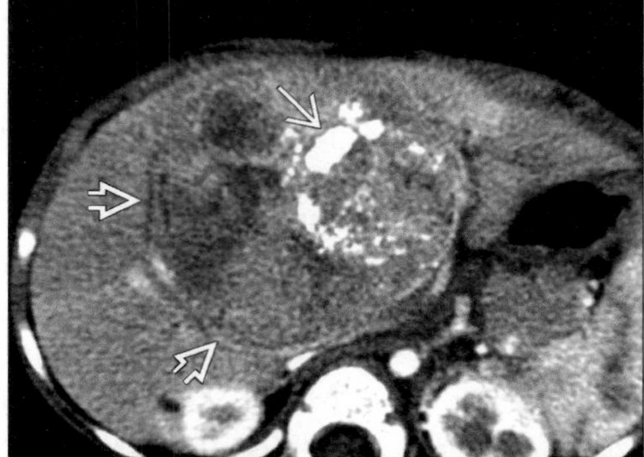

Hepatoblastoma

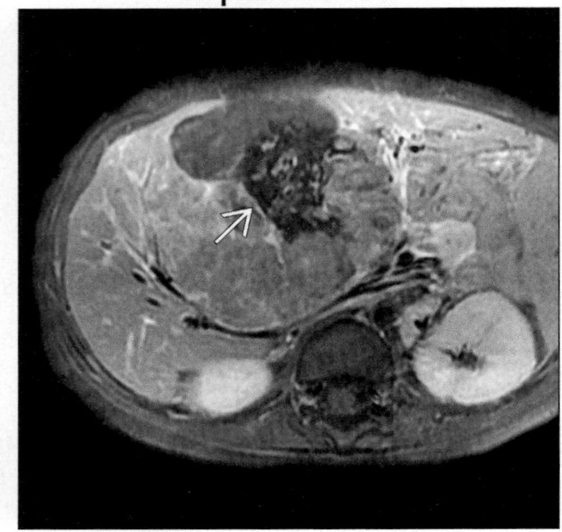

*(**Left**) Axial CECT shows a well-defined mass → in the left lobe of the liver. The mass has a heterogeneous appearance with a central area of hypodensity. (**Right**) Axial T1 C+ FS MR shows heterogeneous early enhancement of the liver mass →. There is a triangular area of early enhancement adjacent to the mass consistent with a transient hepatic intensity difference (THID) →. The THID occurs as a result of the dual blood supply to the liver.*

Hepatocellular Carcinoma

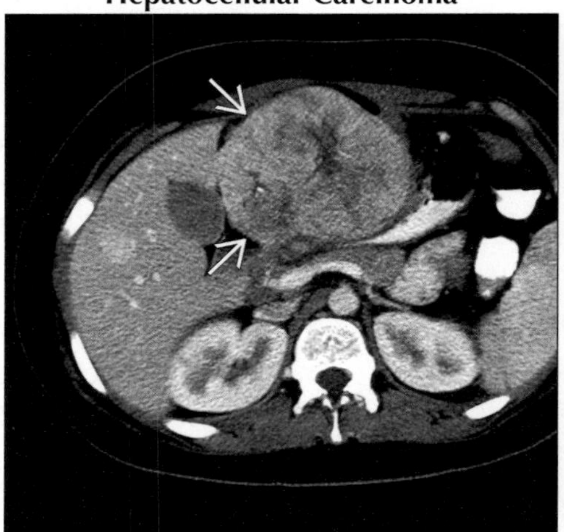

Hepatocellular Carcinoma

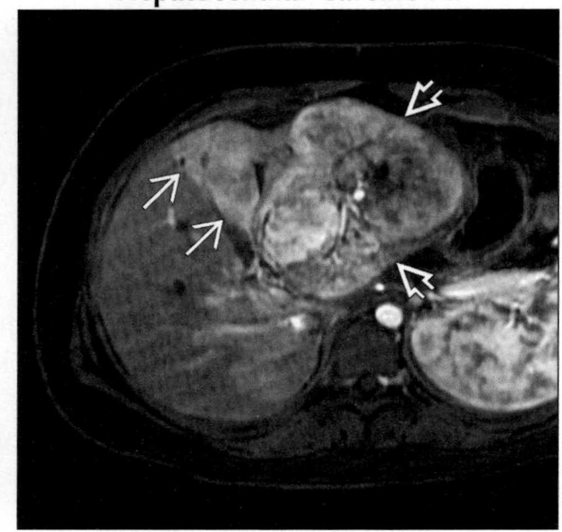

*(**Left**) Axial CECT shows a mostly hypodense lesion → at the dome of the liver with a peripheral rim of increased enhancement →. The center of the lesion has a heterogeneous appearance. (**Right**) Coronal T1WI C+ FS MR shows a hypointense lesion → at the dome of the liver with a surrounding area of increased enhancement →. This patient was later diagnosed with chronic granulomatous disease.*

Abscess

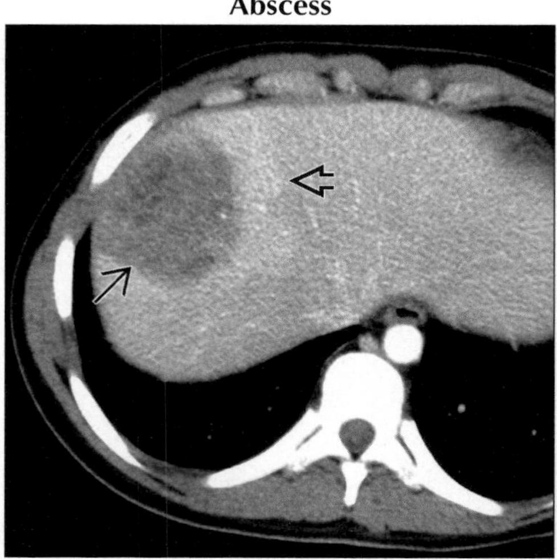

Abscess

Focal Nodular Hyperplasia

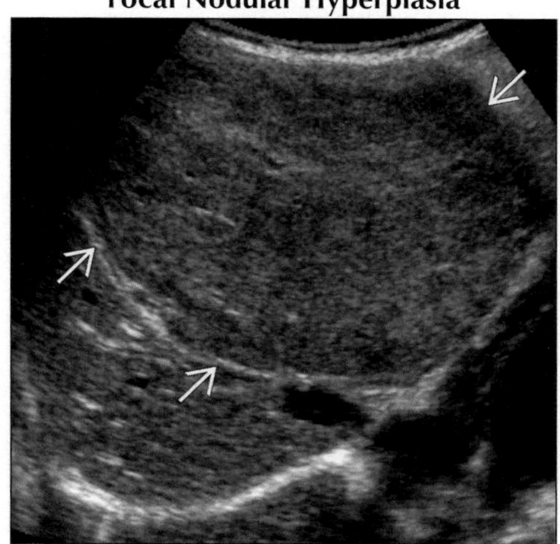

Focal Nodular Hyperplasia

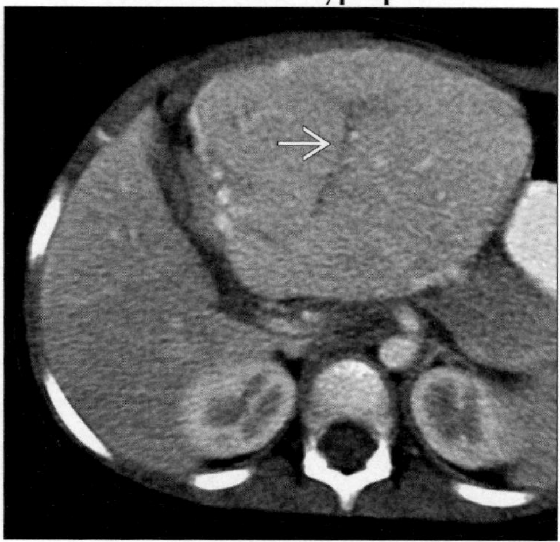

*(**Left**) Transverse ultrasound shows a well-defined isoechoic mass ➡ of the left lobe of the liver. (**Right**) Axial CECT shows a slightly hyperdense mass of the left lobe of the liver. There is a central stellate area of hypodensity representing a central scar ➡. Focal nodular hyperplasia is more common in females and in children who have received chemotherapy.*

Metastases

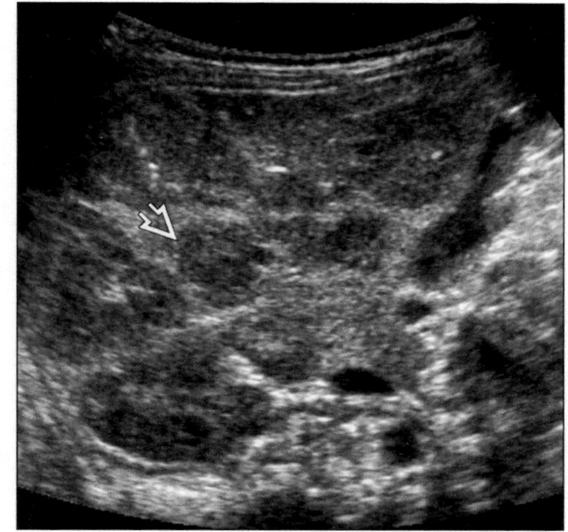

Metastases

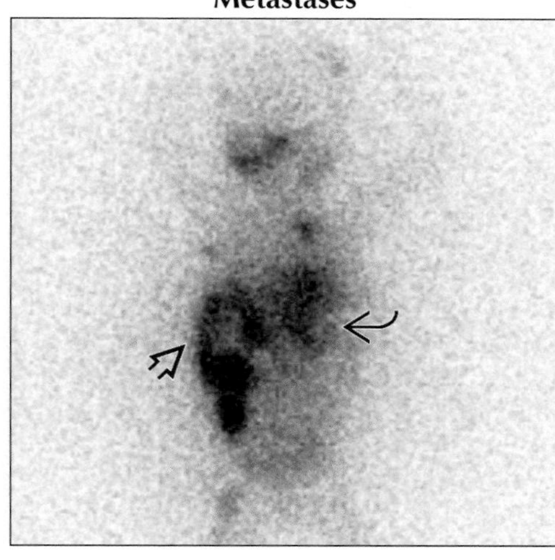

*(**Left**) Transverse ultrasound of the liver shows multiple hypoechoic lesions ➡ replacing most of the liver parenchyma. (**Right**) Anteroposterior MIBG scintigraphy shows abnormal uptake within the liver ⇨. This patient was known to have metastatic neuroblastoma. The primary tumor originated in the left adrenal gland ⇨. Neuroblastoma is the most common neoplasm to metastasize to the liver in children.*

Choledochal Cyst

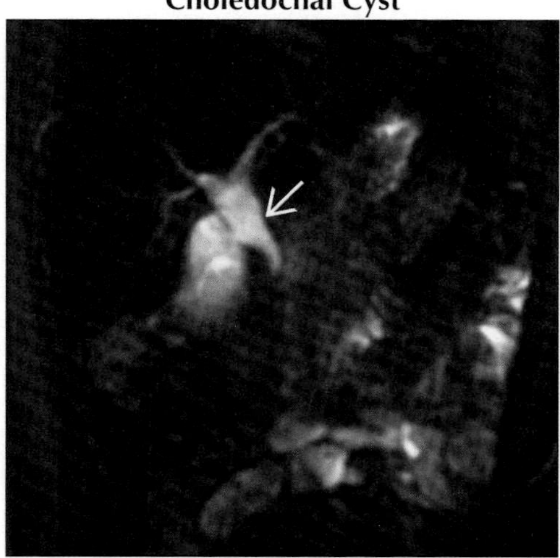

Choledochal Cyst

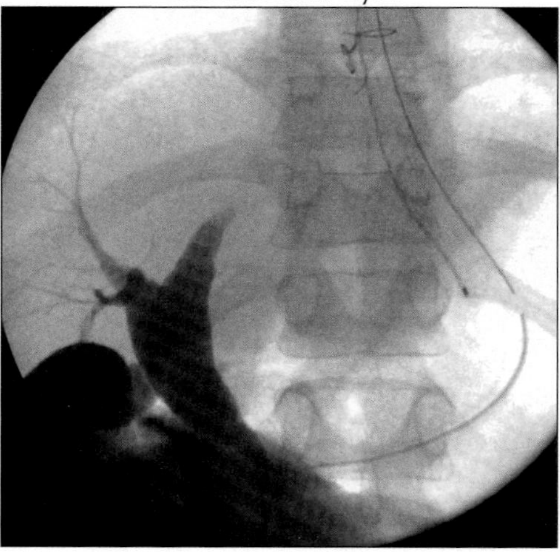

*(**Left**) Coronal MRCP shows cystic dilation of the common bile duct ➡. The proximal right and left intrahepatic bile ducts are also dilated. Connection with intrahepatic bile ducts confirms this as a choledochal cyst. (**Right**) AP ERCP shows findings similar to the MRCP with cystic dilation of the common bile duct as well as the proximal portions of the right and left intrahepatic bile ducts. The findings are consistent with a type 1 choledochal cyst.*

HEPATIC MASS IN A CHILD

Mesenchymal Hamartoma

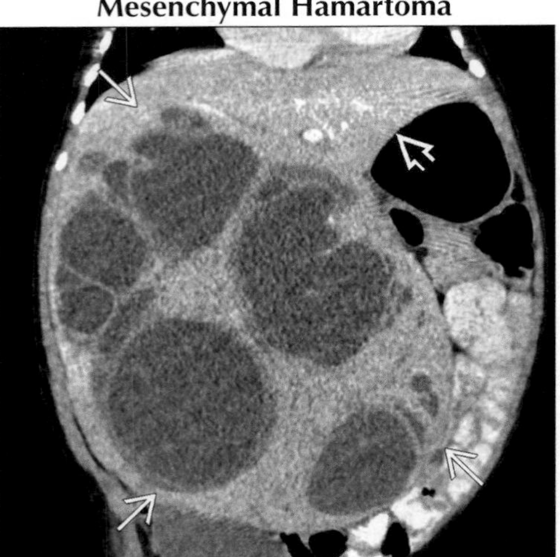

Mesenchymal Hamartoma

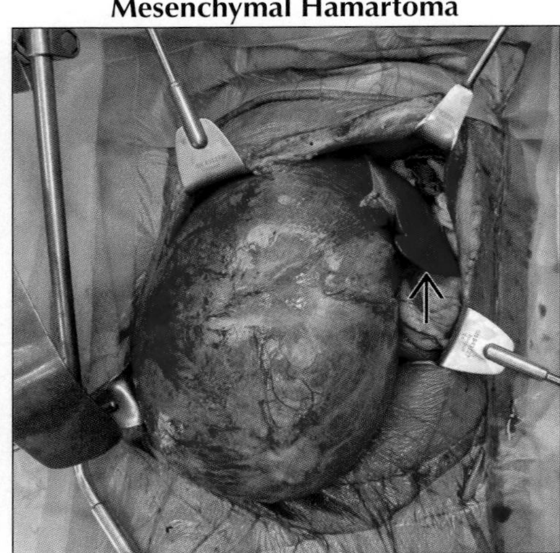

(Left) *Coronal CECT shows a large multicystic solid mass ➡ arising from the liver. Normal liver ➡ is present superior to the mass. Mesenchymal hamartoma is the most common benign cystic mass of the liver.* ***(Right)*** *Surgical photograph shows a large mass arising from the liver. The normal left lobe ➡ of the liver is seen medial to the mass.*

Embryonal Sarcoma

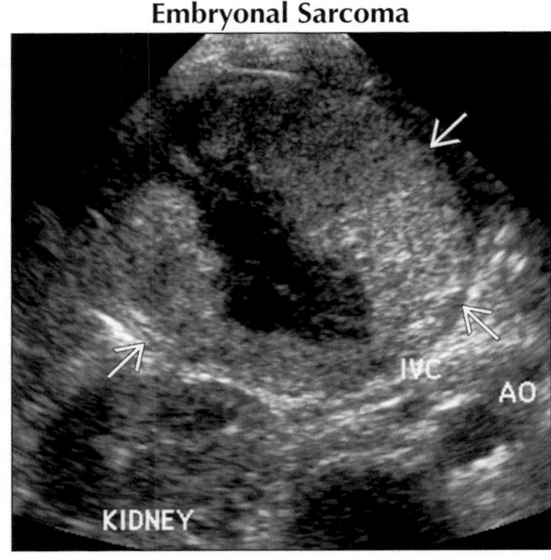

Embryonal Sarcoma

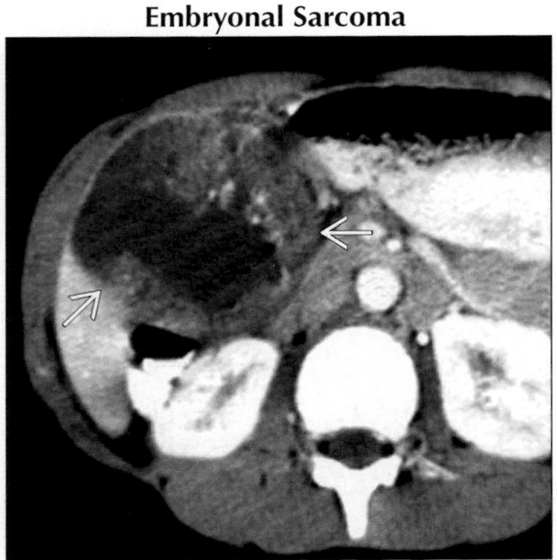

(Left) *Transverse ultrasound shows a large mass ➡ along the inferior aspect of the liver. The mass has a central anechoic area. On ultrasound, embryonal sarcoma often has a mixed cystic and solid appearance. Aorta (AO), inferior vena cava (IVC).* ***(Right)*** *Axial CECT shows a mostly hypodense mass ➡ along the inferior aspect of the liver. The mass has a central area that does not enhance.*

Hepatic Adenoma

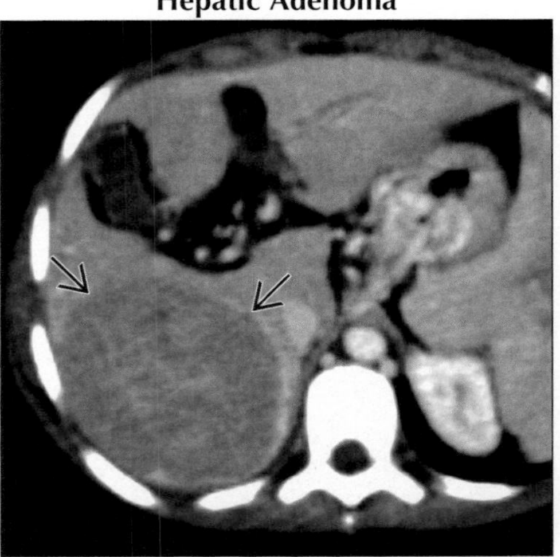

Hepatic Adenoma

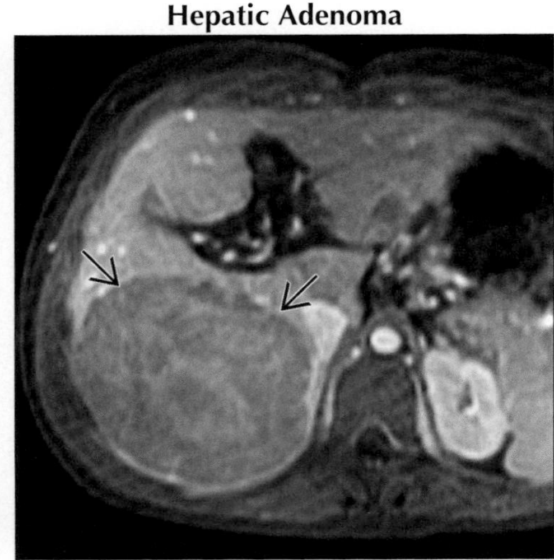

(Left) *Axial CECT shows a well-defined, heterogeneously enhancing, hypodense mass ➡ of the right lobe of the liver. Hepatic adenomas often have heterogeneous enhancement in the arterial phase.* ***(Right)*** *Axial T1WI C+ FS MR shows a heterogeneously enhancing, hypointense mass ➡ of the right lobe of the liver. Hepatic adenomas are much more common in females.*

Angiomyolipoma (AML)

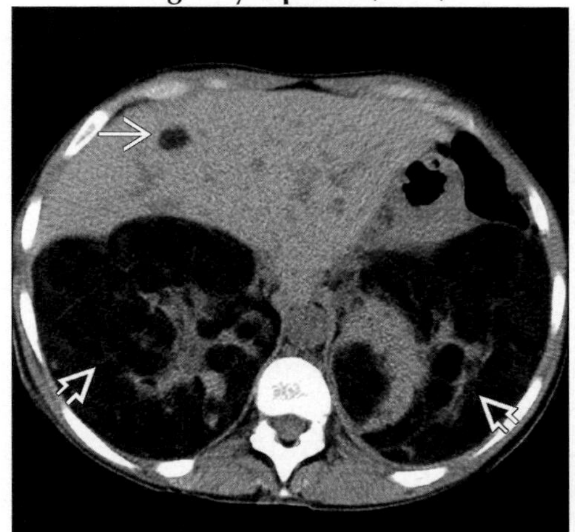

Angiomyolipoma (AML)

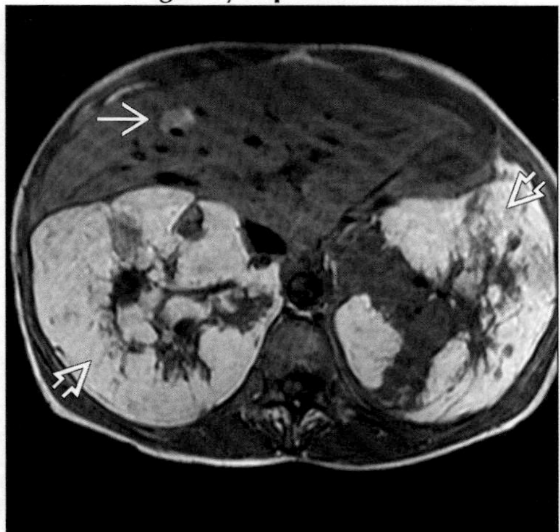

(Left) *Axial NECT shows a fat-density mass ➡ in the liver. The kidneys are enlarged, and the renal parenchyma is almost completely replaced with fat ➡.* ***(Right)*** *Axial T1WI MR shows a hyperintense mass ➡ within the liver. This mass followed fat signal on all pulse sequences. The kidneys are enlarged and almost completely replaced with fat ➡. This patient had known tuberous sclerosis. Hepatic AMLs are much less common than renal AMLs.*

Nodular Regenerative Hyperplasia

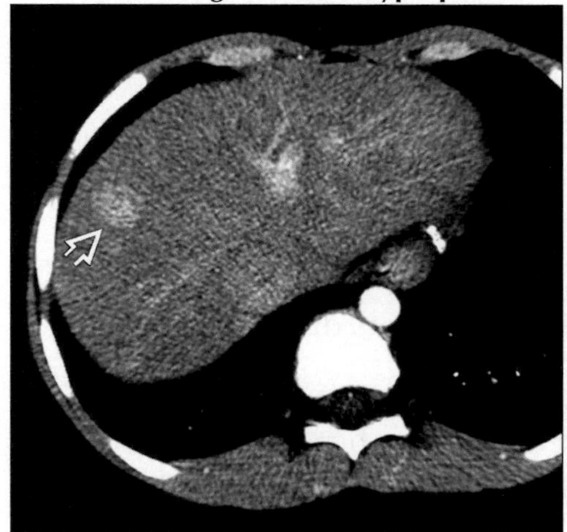

Nodular Regenerative Hyperplasia

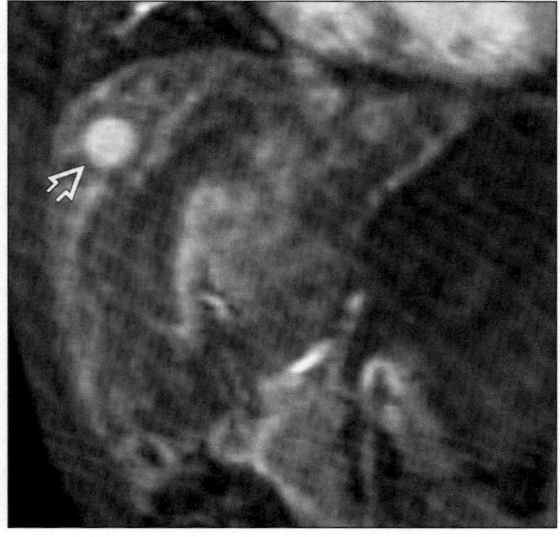

(Left) *Axial CECT in a patient with a long-term history of spontaneous portal vein thrombosis shows an enhancing mass ➡ near the dome of the liver. Overall, the liver had a heterogeneous appearance with multiple enhancing nodules.* ***(Right)*** *Coronal T1WI FS MR C+ in the same patient shows a circular enhancing mass ➡ near the dome of the liver. This patient is presumed to have multiple large regenerative nodules or nodular regenerative hyperplasia.*

Biliary Rhabdomyosarcoma

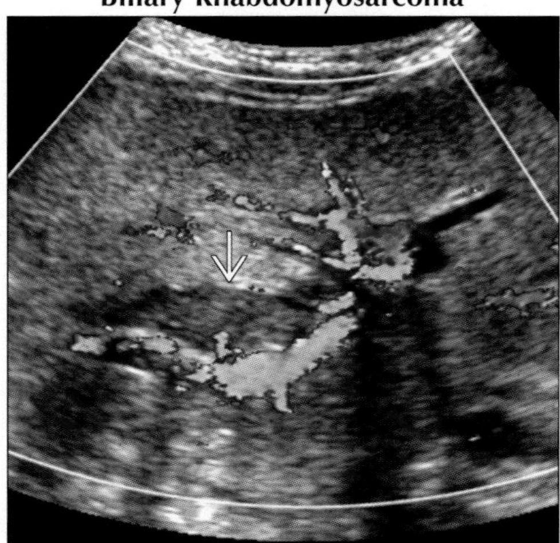

Biliary Rhabdomyosarcoma

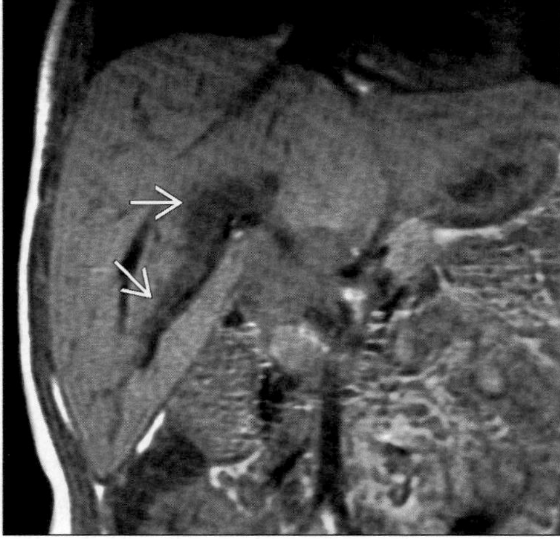

(Left) *Transverse ultrasound shows a hypoechoic solid mass ➡ within a dilated bile duct. Other bile ducts were dilated and fluid filled.* ***(Right)*** *Coronal T1WI MR shows a hypointense mass ➡ filling an expanded right-side bile duct. Central bile ducts were also filled by the soft tissue mass. Biliary rhabdomyosarcoma is a rare intraductal tumor.*

MULTIPLE LIVER LESIONS

DIFFERENTIAL DIAGNOSIS

Common
- Hemangioendothelioma/Hemangioma
- Hepatic Pyogenic Abscess
- Metastases
  - Neuroblastoma
  - Wilms Tumor
  - Lymphoma/Leukemia
- Hepatoblastoma

Less Common
- Mesenchymal Hamartoma
- Nodular Regenerative Hyperplasia

Rare but Important
- Caroli Disease
- Peliosis Hepatis
- Angiomyolipoma
- Echinococcosis
- Hepatocellular Carcinoma

ESSENTIAL INFORMATION

Key Differential Diagnosis Issues
- Various causes of multiple liver lesions
  - Benign and malignant
- Primary hepatic neoplasms are uncommon
  - 0.5-2% of all pediatric neoplasms
  - 2/3 are malignant
- Overlap in imaging appearance
  - Biopsy often required
- Differential diagnosis can be focused by age
- Lab tests may be helpful in forming differential diagnosis

Helpful Clues for Common Diagnoses
- **Hemangioendothelioma/Hemangioma**
  - a.k.a. infantile hepatic hemangioma
  - Most common benign hepatic tumor
  - 85% diagnosed in 1st 6 months
  - Skin hemangiomas present in ~ 50%
  - Single, multiple, or diffuse lesions
  - Diffuse lesions often have severe clinical course
    - Can cause massive hepatomegaly leading to compression of inferior vena cava and thoracic cavity
    - Mass effect can lead to abdominal compartment syndrome and multiorgan failure
    - Can be associated with severe hypothyroidism
- **Hepatic Pyogenic Abscess**
  - Associated with immunodeficiency, systemic infection, abdominal inflammatory processes, and chronic granulomatous disease
    - *S. aureus* most common organism
    - Fungal infections and *B. henselae* associated with microabscesses
  - Can be solitary or multiple
    - Multiple in 20-25% of children and up to 70% in neonates
  - Risks in neonate include necrotizing enterocolitis and umbilical vein catheterization
  - US useful for diagnosis and follow-up
- **Metastases**
  - Neuroblastoma and Wilms tumor most common
    - Neuroblastoma metastasizes to liver (15%)
    - Wilms tumor metastasizes to liver (12%)
  - Hepatic metastases more common overall than primary hepatic tumors
  - Can appear as discrete nodules or diffuse hepatic involvement
- **Hepatoblastoma**
  - Most common pediatric hepatic malignancy
    - Majority of patients diagnosed are < 18 months of age
  - More common in boys
  - Associated with low birth weight, hemihypertrophy, Beckwith-Wiedemann, familial adenomatous polyposis, trisomy 18, and fetal alcohol syndrome
  - 90% have increased serum α-fetoprotein
  - Most common in right lobe of liver
    - Bilateral disease in 35%
  - Calcifications in 40-55%
  - Usually solitary solid mass
    - Can be multifocal although there is usually 1 dominant mass

Helpful Clues for Less Common Diagnoses
- **Mesenchymal Hamartoma**
  - 2nd most common benign hepatic mass
  - Typically diagnosed in 1st 2 years of life
  - Often presents as large RUQ mass
    - 75% in right lobe
    - α-fetoprotein may be moderately elevated
  - Multiloculated cystic mass

- Mixed cystic and solid
- May be small or large
- Multiple tiny cysts may appear solid
- On US, septae of cysts may be mobile

- Rare malignant transformation to undifferentiated embryonal sarcoma
- Treatment via excision

- **Nodular Regenerative Hyperplasia**
  - Multiacinar regenerative lesion of liver in noncirrhotic liver
  - Associated with systemic diseases, such as vasculitis, collagen disorders, cardiovascular disorders, and neoplasms
  - Can cause portal hypertension
  - Can occur after spontaneous portal vein thrombosis
  - Radiologic findings not specific

Helpful Clues for Rare Diagnoses

- **Caroli Disease**
  - a.k.a. type 5 choledochal cyst
    - May be associated with autosomal recessive polycystic kidney disease
  - Congenital cystic dilation of intrahepatic bile ducts
  - Patients present with recurrent cholangitis or portal hypertension
- **Peliosis Hepatis**
  - Multiple blood-filled cavities
  - Rare in children
    - Associated with underlying chronic conditions, such as cystic fibrosis, malnutrition, Fanconi anemia, Marfan syndrome, and adrenal tumors
- **Angiomyolipoma**
  - Associated with tuberous sclerosis
  - Less common than renal angiomyolipoma
  - Often multiple when present
  - Lesions have imaging characteristics of fat
- **Echinococcosis**
  - a.k.a. hydatid disease
  - Most common in Mediterranean, Middle East, eastern Europe, Africa, South America, China, and Australia
  - Generally asymptomatic
  - Appears as single or multiple cysts
    - Daughter cysts present in 75%
    - Cysts slowly expand over years
- **Hepatocellular Carcinoma**
  - 2nd most common hepatic malignancy in children
  - Rare before age 5
  - More common in males
  - Most pediatric cases not associated with prior liver disease (> 60%)
    - Can be associated with preexisting cirrhosis due to biliary atresia, Fanconi syndrome, viral hepatitis, hereditary tyrosinemia, or glycogen storage disease
    - Other risk factors: Prior androgen steroid treatment, oral contraceptives, methotrexate
  - Metastases common at diagnosis
    - Regional lymph nodes, lungs, bone
  - Disease is multifocal in > 50%
    - Multifocal tumors influence overall survival and possibility of surgical resection

Hemangioendothelioma/Hemangioma

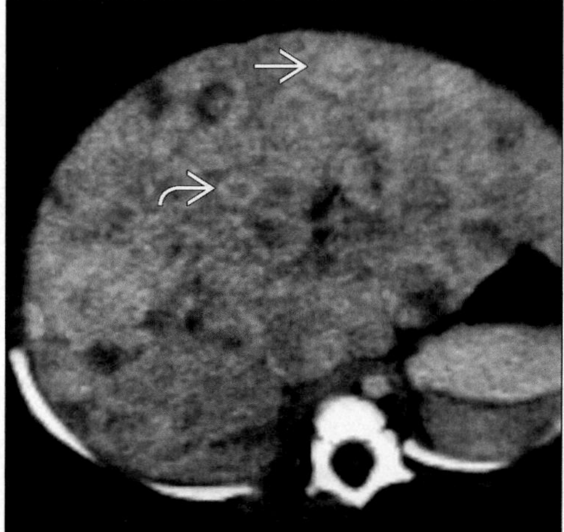

Axial CECT in a delayed phase of enhancement shows innumerable lesions throughout the liver. Some lesions have a ring of peripheral enhancement ➔ while others are completely enhancing ➔.

Hemangioendothelioma/Hemangioma

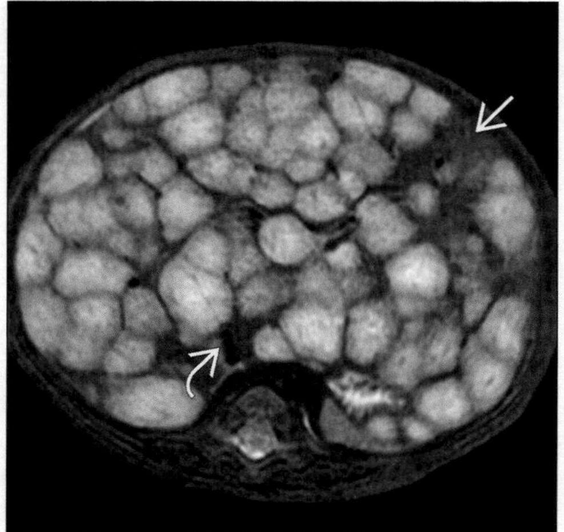

Axial T2WI MR shows innumerable hyperintense lesions throughout the liver. Only a small area of normal liver remains ➔. The inferior vena cava ➔ is compressed by multiple masses.

MULTIPLE LIVER LESIONS

Hemangioendothelioma/Hemangioma

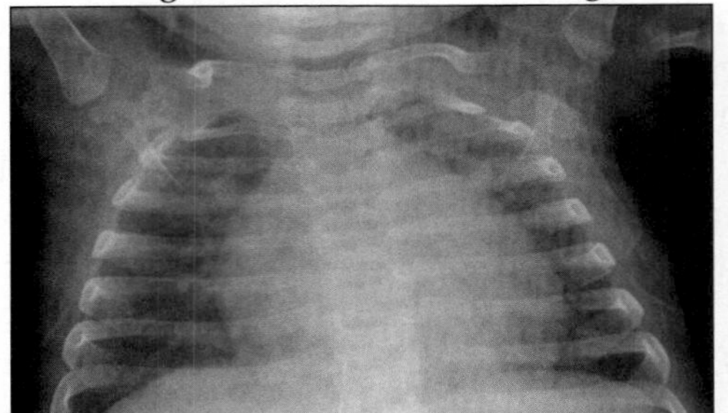

Hemangioendothelioma/Hemangioma

*(**Left**) Anteroposterior radiograph of the chest shows pulmonary vascular congestion and cardiomegaly. While not imaged completely, the abdomen is also enlarged. Hepatic hemangioendothelioma is part of the differential diagnosis for a neonate with high-output heart failure. (**Right**) Transverse ultrasound shows multiple hypoechoic lesions → replacing most of the liver parenchyma.*

Hemangioendothelioma/Hemangioma

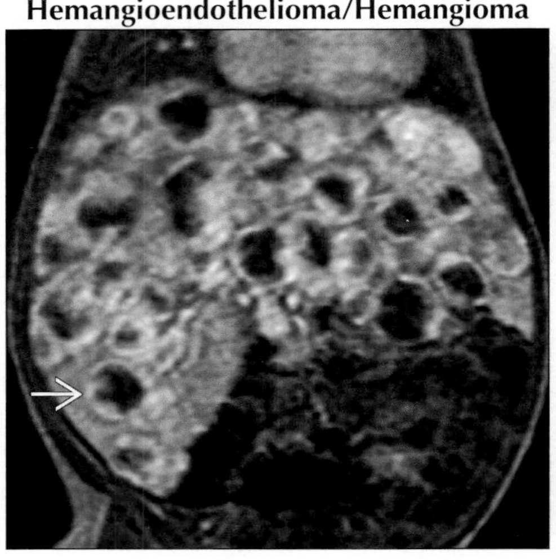

Hemangioendothelioma/Hemangioma

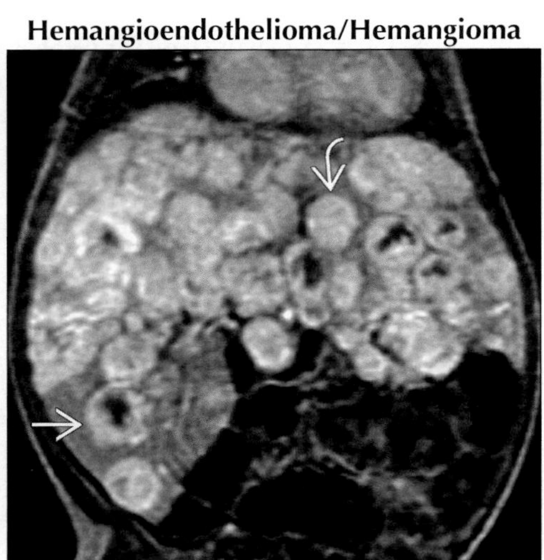

*(**Left**) Coronal T1WI FS MR C+ in an early phase of enhancement shows innumerable lesions throughout the liver. The lesions all have peripheral nodular enhancement →. (**Right**) Coronal T1WI C+ FS MR in the same patient in a more delayed phase of enhancement shows that the lesions have filled in with contrast. Most of the lesions now have a homogeneous enhancement pattern ↪, although some still have a targetoid appearance →.*

Hepatic Pyogenic Abscess

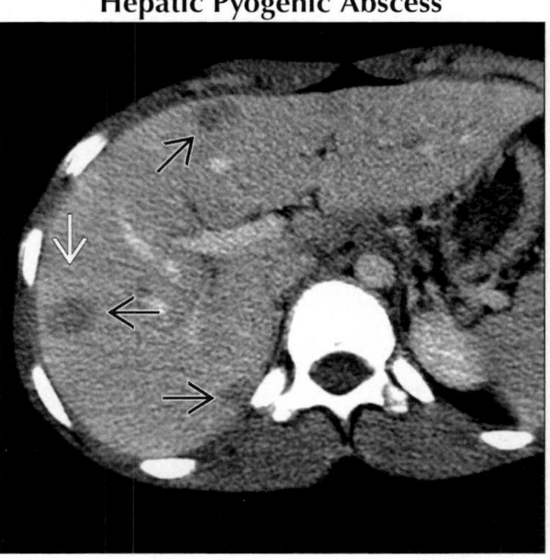

Hepatic Pyogenic Abscess

*(**Left**) Axial CECT shows multiple hypodense lesions → in the liver with a faint surrounding area of enhancement →. The patient had multiple cats, and Bartonella henselae was later isolated. (**Right**) Coronal CECT in a patient with a history of acute myelogenous leukemia shows multiple hypodense lesions → in the liver. The more inferior and peripheral lesion has a surrounding area of increased enhancement ⇒. On biopsy, Candida tropicalis was present.*

Metastases

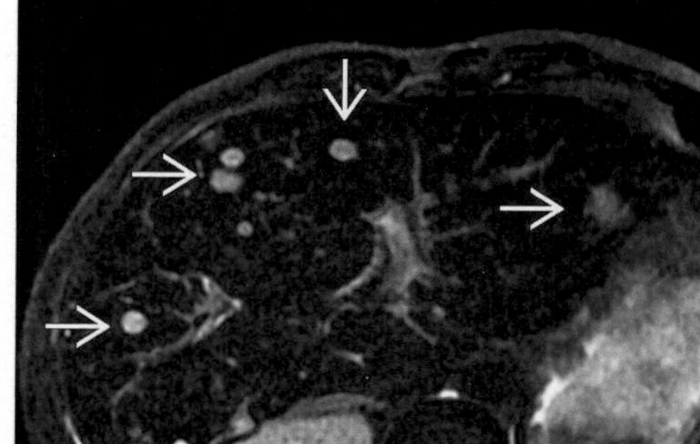

Metastases

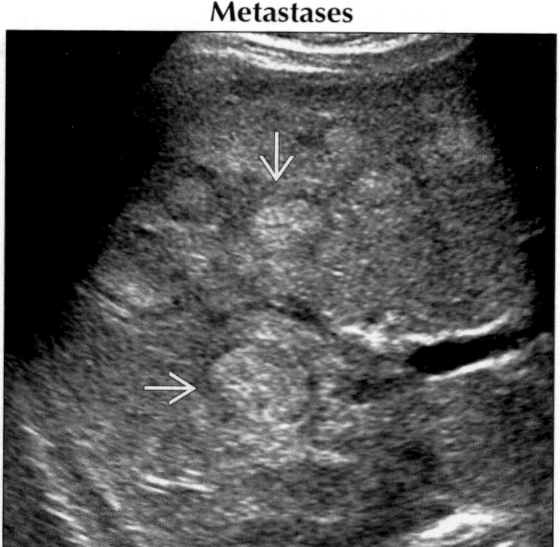

*(**Left**) Axial T2WI MR in a patient with a remote history of Wilms tumor shows multiple hyperintense nodules → within both lobes of the liver. These metastases continued to grow with time. (**Right**) Transverse ultrasound shows multiple hyperechoic lesions → in the liver. The lesions are well defined with a peripheral hypoechoic rim. Wilms tumor is the 2nd most common tumor to metastasize to the liver in children.*

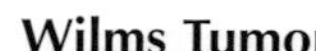

Wilms Tumor

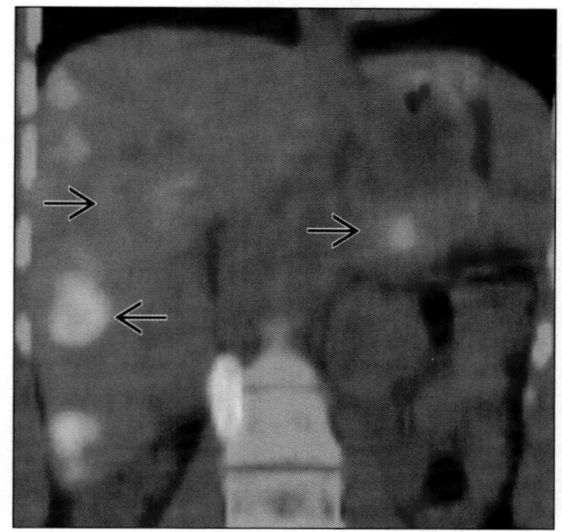

Hepatoblastoma

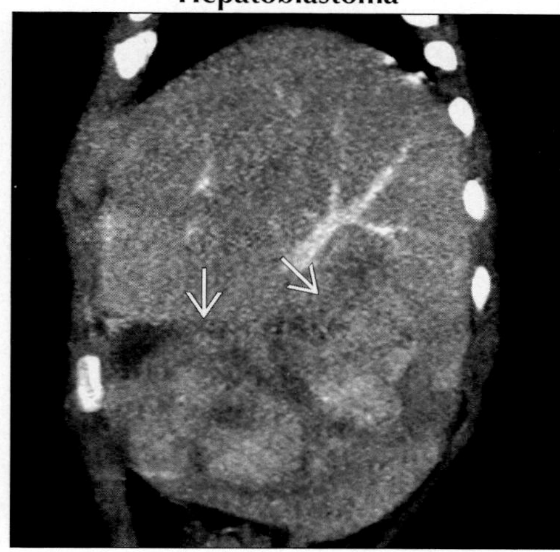

*(**Left**) Coronal fused PET/CT shows multiple lesions → with increased FDG uptake in the liver. Most of the lesions also have a peripheral area of increased FDG uptake. Wilms tumor metastasizes to the liver in 12% of patients. (**Right**) Sagittal CECT shows 2 distinct masses → within the liver. A 3rd mass was present more superiorly (not shown). Hepatoblastoma is the most common primary hepatic malignancy.*

Hepatoblastoma

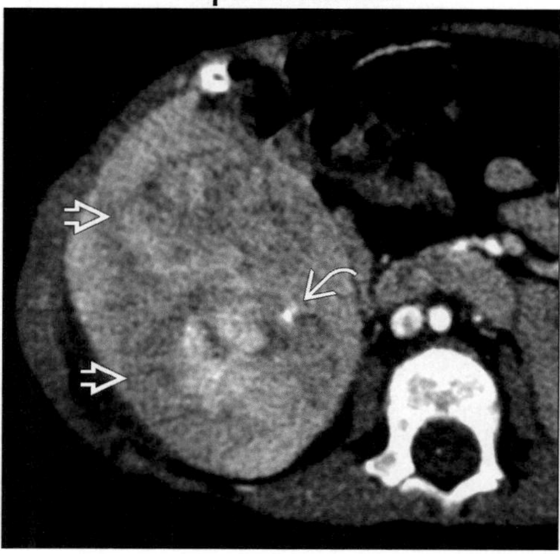

Hepatoblastoma

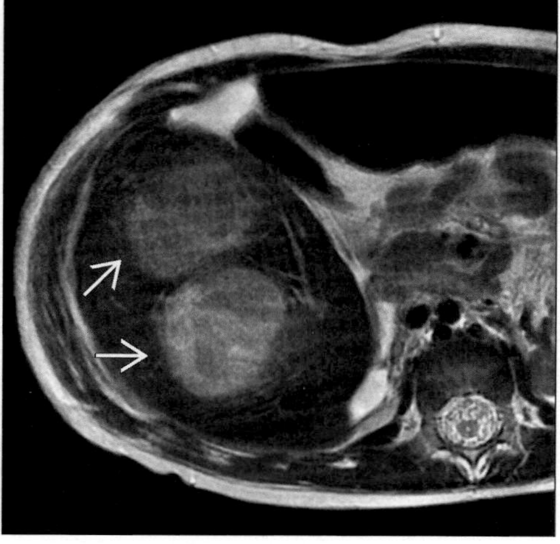

*(**Left**) Axial CECT shows 2 distinct lesions ⇨ abutting each other in the inferior liver. The masses have a heterogeneous appearance with a central area of increased enhancement. There is a focal calcification ↪ in the more posterior mass. Calcifications are present in up to 55% of hepatoblastomas. (**Right**) Axial T2WI MR shows 2 distinct hyperintense masses → in the inferior liver. Although hepatoblastoma is usually a solitary mass, it can be multifocal.*

MULTIPLE LIVER LESIONS

(Left) *Axial T2WI MR shows a large mass containing multiple cystic areas. Mesenchymal hamartomas are the 2nd most common benign hepatic mass in children. While mesenchymal hamartomas are solitary masses, they often are multicystic.* **(Right)** *Transverse ultrasound shows multiple small cystic areas* → *within the liver. On ultrasound, the septae of cyst may be mobile (not shown).*

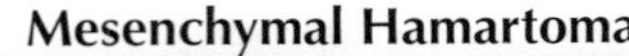

Mesenchymal Hamartoma

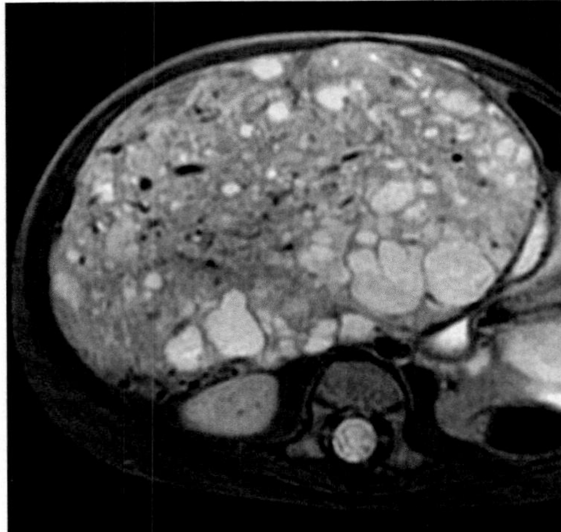

Mesenchymal Hamartoma

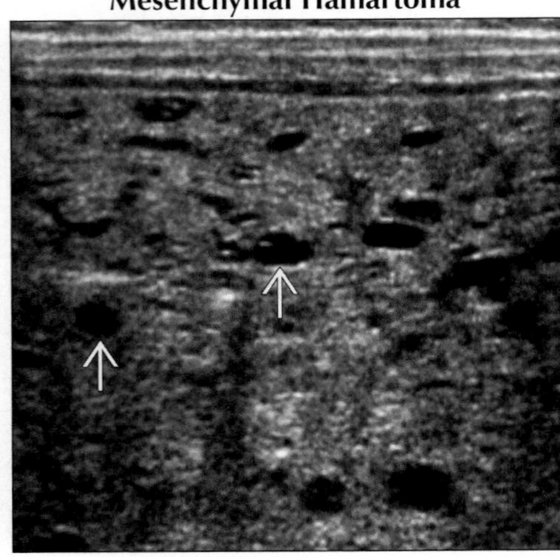

(Left) *Axial CECT in a patient with a history of spontaneous portal vein thrombosis shows a heterogeneous appearance of the liver. There are multiple enhancing nodules* → *throughout the liver. Nodular regenerative hyperplasia is associated with noncirrhotic portal vein thrombosis.* **(Right)** *Coronal T1WI FS MR + C in the same patient shows multiple enhancing nodules* → *within the liver. This patient is presumed to have nodular regenerative hyperplasia.*

Nodular Regenerative Hyperplasia

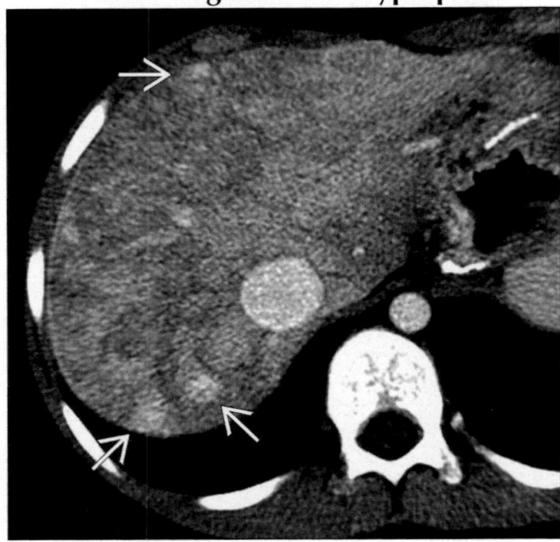

Nodular Regenerative Hyperplasia

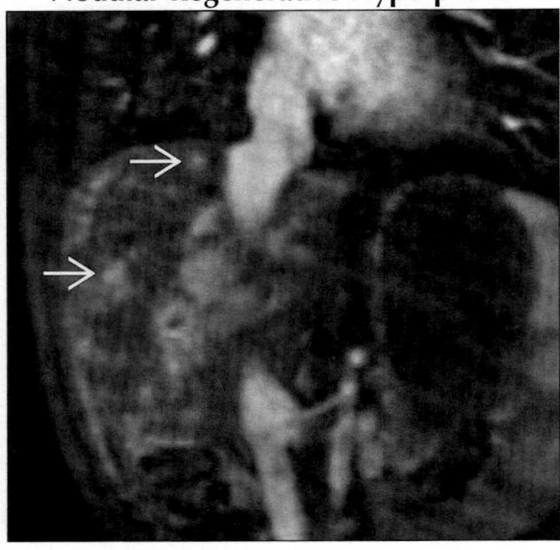

(Left) *Axial CECT shows multiple hypodense lesions throughout the liver. Each lesion has a branching tubular pattern and follows ductal anatomy. A central dot* → *is present within each lesion.* **(Right)** *Coronal T2WI MR shows multiple circular lesions with fluid signal* → *and a central hypointense dot* ↪. *In spanning the left lobe of the liver, the intrahepatic ducts have a branching pattern* ⇨.

Caroli Disease

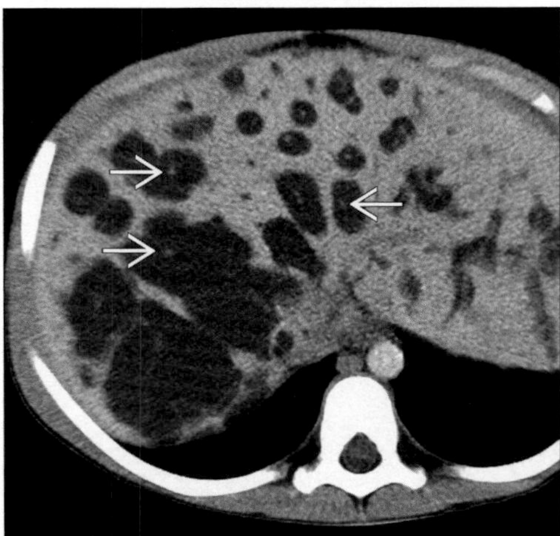

Caroli Disease

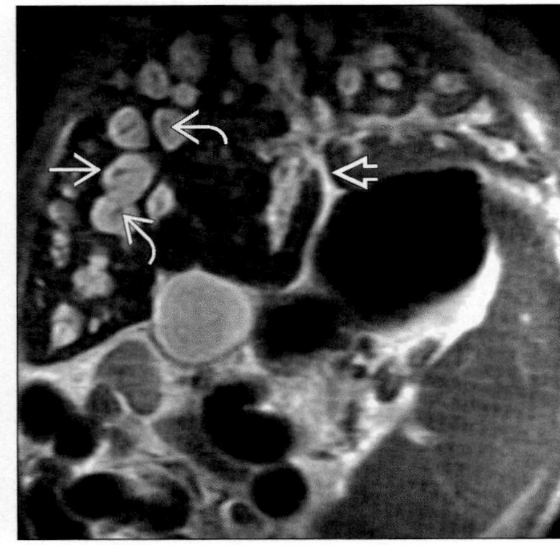

Peliosis Hepatis

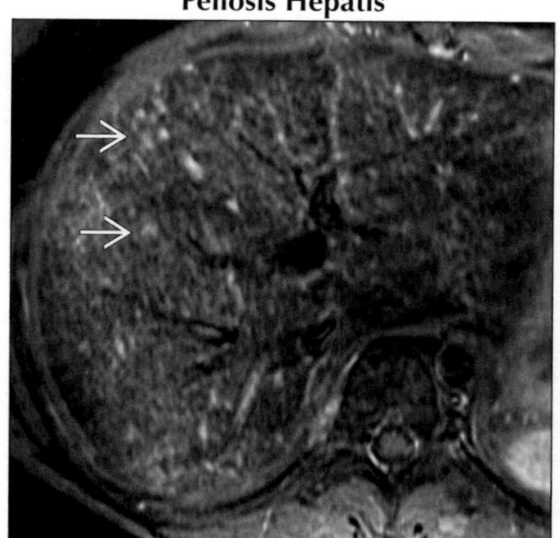

Peliosis Hepatis

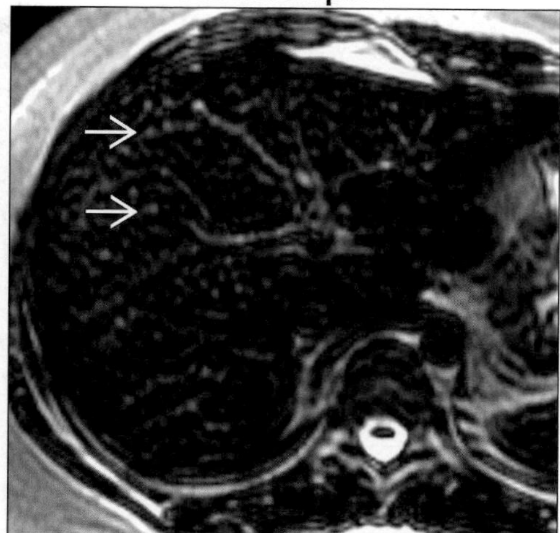

(Left) *Axial T1WI FS MR C+ in a patient with Fanconi anemia shows multiple tiny enhancing nodules → in the the liver. This gives the liver a heterogeneous appearance. Lesions in peliosis hepatis represent blood-filled cavities and typically enhance.* ***(Right)*** *Axial T2WI FSE MR shows multiple tiny hyperintense nodules → in the liver. Peliosis hepatis is associated with underlying chronic conditions such as Fanconi anemia.*

Angiomyolipoma

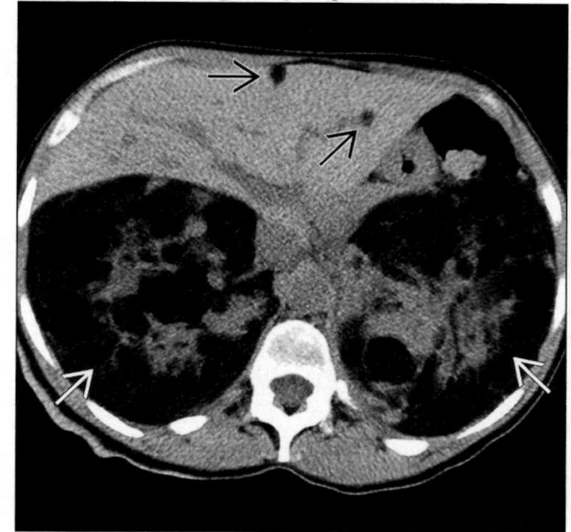

Angiomyolipoma

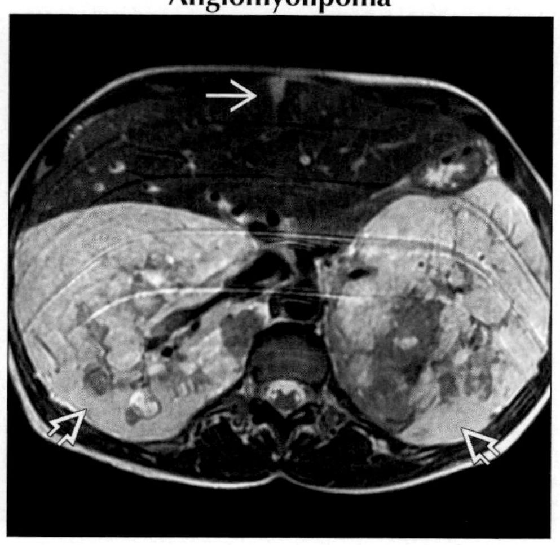

(Left) *Axial NECT shows 2 small lesions → with fat density in the liver. The kidneys are enlarged and almost completely replaced with fat →. When hepatic angiomyolipomas are present, they are often multiple.* ***(Right)*** *Axial T2WI MR shows a hyperintense lesion → in the anterior liver. The kidneys are almost completely replaced with fat →. Hepatic angiomyolipomas (AMLs) are associated with tuberous sclerosis but are less common than renal AMLs.*

Hepatocellular Carcinoma

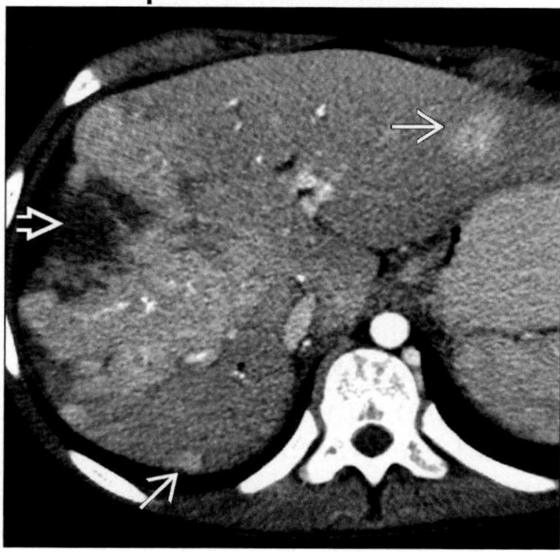

Hepatocellular Carcinoma

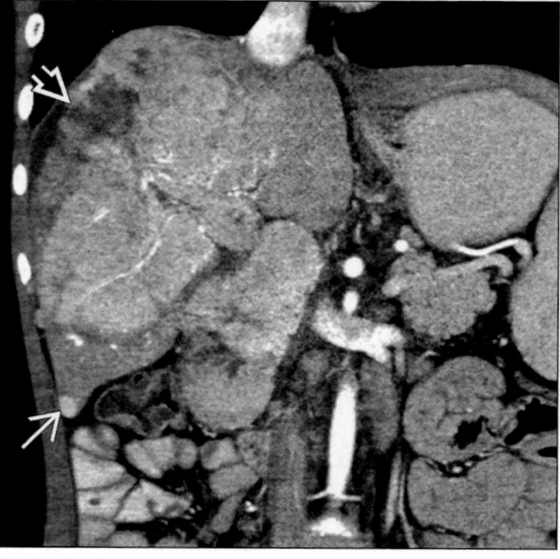

(Left) *Axial CECT shows a large hypodense lesion → in the periphery of the liver. There is associated capsular retraction and surrounding increased enhancement. At least 2 other distinct lesions are also present →. Hepatocellular carcinoma is multifocal in more than 50% of patients.* ***(Right)*** *Coronal CECT shows a large hypodense mass → with a larger surrounding area of increased enhancement. A smaller distinct lesion → is also present at the inferior liver margin.*

PANCREATIC MASS

DIFFERENTIAL DIAGNOSIS

Common
- Pancreatitis
- Pancreatic Pseudocyst
- Congenital Pancreatic Cysts

Less Common
- Annular Pancreas
- Metastases

Rare but Important
- Pancreatoblastoma
- Solid-Cystic Pancreatic Tumor
- Islet Cell Tumors
- Agenesis of Dorsal Pancreas
- Adenocarcinoma

ESSENTIAL INFORMATION

Key Differential Diagnosis Issues
- Pancreatic tumors are rare in children
  - Account for < 0.2% of all pediatric deaths due to malignancy
- DDx for pancreatic mass in children is different from DDx in adults
  - Adenocarcinoma is very rare
- Most tumors are well circumscribed
- Tumors can be divided into epithelial and nonepithelial
  - Epithelial tumors can arise from duct, acinar cells, or endocrine cells
  - Nonepithelial tumors are rare
    - Lymphoma is most common

Helpful Clues for Common Diagnoses
- **Pancreatitis**
  - Causes more varied than in adults
    - Accidental and nonaccidental trauma can cause pancreatitis
    - Other causes include infection, medications, gallstones, choledochal cysts, and pancreas divisum
    - Less common causes include metabolic disorders, hemolytic uremic syndrome, and hereditary pancreatitis
  - Pancreas can be focally or diffusely enlarged
    - Focal pancreatitis can appear mass-like
- **Pancreatic Pseudocyst**
  - Most common cystic lesion of pancreas in children
    - Occurs after blunt abdominal trauma or pancreatitis
  - Usually has thin, well-defined wall
- **Congenital Pancreatic Cysts**
  - Can be solitary or multiple
  - Usually asymptomatic
  - Associated with von Hippel-Lindau disease, Beckwith-Wiedemann syndrome, autosomal dominant polycystic kidney disease, and Meckel-Gruber syndrome

Helpful Clues for Less Common Diagnoses
- **Annular Pancreas**
  - Congenital anomaly
    - Pancreatic tissue surrounds 2nd portion of duodenum
    - Duodenum within pancreatic tissue may mimic mass
  - ~ 50% of patients present in neonatal period with duodenal obstruction
    - Can give "double bubble" appearance
  - Associated with other anomalies (70%)
    - Duodenal stenosis or atresia, Down syndrome, tracheoesophageal fistula, and congenital heart disease
- **Metastases**
  - Usually due to direct extension of tumor
    - Neuroblastoma is most common cause
  - Lymphoma can arise within pancreas or peripancreatic nodes
    - More common in large cell lymphoma and Burkitt lymphoma

Helpful Clues for Rare Diagnoses
- **Pancreatoblastoma**
  - Most common pancreatic neoplasm in young children
  - Neoplasm of acinar cells
  - Most common in 1st decade of life
  - Associated with Beckwith-Wiedemann syndrome
    - When congenital, tumor may be cystic
  - Slightly more common in males
    - > 50% of cases reported in Asians
  - Most commonly presents as asymptomatic abdominal mass
    - Mass is often large at presentation; may be difficult to identify organ of origin
    - ~ 50% arise from pancreatic head
    - α-fetoprotein is elevated in up to 55%
  - Usually large solitary pancreatic mass
    - Well-defined with lobulated margins

- Compresses surrounding structures without invasion
- Dilation of biliary tree is uncommon
- Metastasizes to liver and lymph nodes in 35% of patients

- **Solid-Cystic Pancreatic Tumor**
  - a.k.a. solid-pseudopapillary tumor, Frantz tumor, solid and papillary tumor, papillary cystic tumor, etc.
  - Up to 50% of cases are in children but also seen in elderly
  - 80-98.5% occur in females
    - Most commonly diagnosed in adolescent girls and young women
  - May be more common in African-Americans and Asians
  - Presents with abdominal pain and mass
  - Mass is well circumscribed and often exophytic
    - May appear solid or cystic
    - Internal hemorrhage can be present
    - Capsule may have calcifications
  - Slow-growing tumor with benign course
    - Most are cured with resection
- **Islet Cell Tumors**
  - Endocrine cell tumors
  - Most common in middle age but can be seen in children
    - Account for up to 20% of malignant pancreatic tumors in children
    - Patients with multiple endocrine neoplasms (MEN) present younger
    - Associated with von Hippel-Lindau disease
  - Insulinomas are most common, followed by gastrinomas
  - May be functioning or nonfunctioning
    - Functioning tumors produce symptoms related to hormonal release and typically present earlier and with smaller tumors
  - Insulinomas are usually in body or tail of pancreas
    - Gastrinomas are usually in pancreatic head
  - Sporadic islet cell tumors are usually solitary
    - Multiple islet cell tumors occur in MEN 1
  - Somatostatin receptor scintigraphy can be useful to identify tumor or metastases
- **Agenesis of Dorsal Pancreas**
  - a.k.a. congenitally short pancreas
  - Associated with polysplenia
  - Risk of diabetes mellitus as most islet cells are in pancreatic tail
  - Pancreas appears rounded and short
    - May mimic mass
- **Adenocarcinoma**
  - Most common neoplasm of pancreas but rare in patients under age 40
  - Most pediatric cases have familial predisposition
    - Associated with hereditary pancreatitis, hereditary pancreatic cancer syndrome, hereditary nonpolyposis colon carcinoma, Peutz-Jeghers syndrome, and *BRCA2*
  - Prognosis is dismal

Pancreatitis

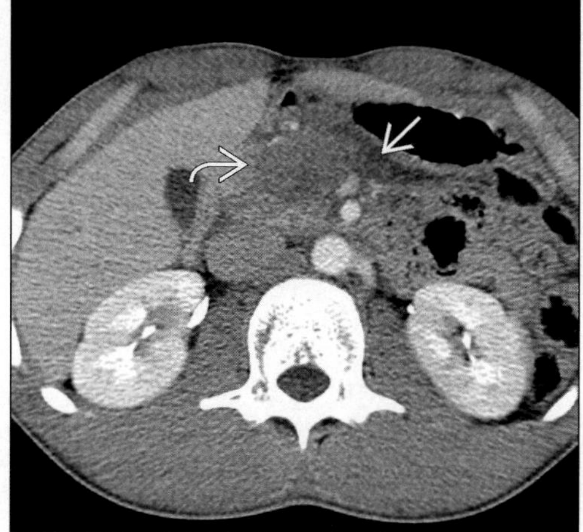

Axial CECT in a patient presenting after blunt abdominal trauma shows a hypodense mass ➔ in the head of the pancreas. There is some stranding of the peripancreatic mesentery ➔.

Pancreatitis

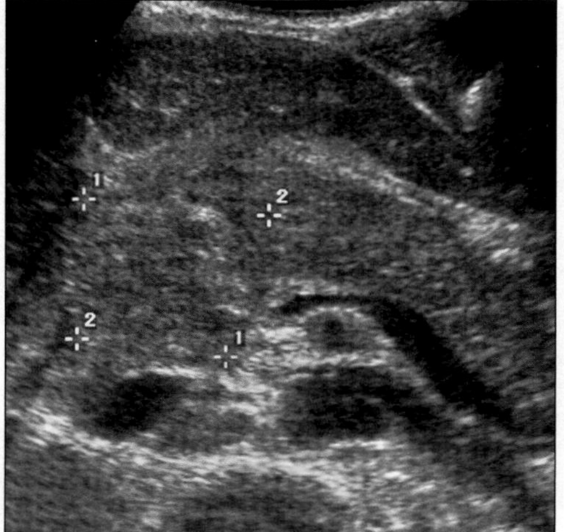

Transverse ultrasound in the same patient shows a hyperechoic mass (calipers) in the head of the pancreas. Trauma is a common cause of pancreatitis in children.

PANCREATIC MASS

Pancreatitis

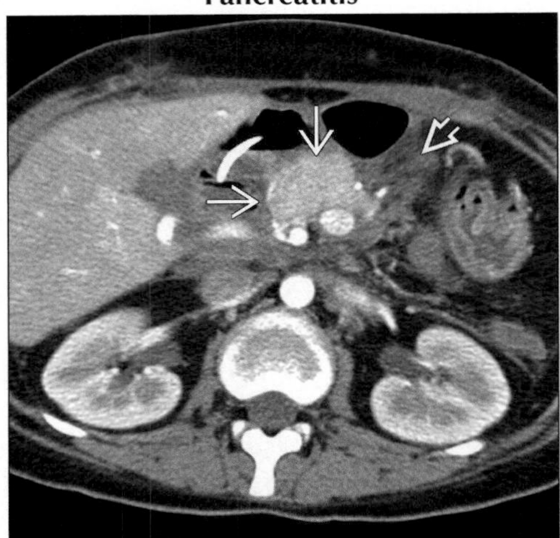

Pancreatitis

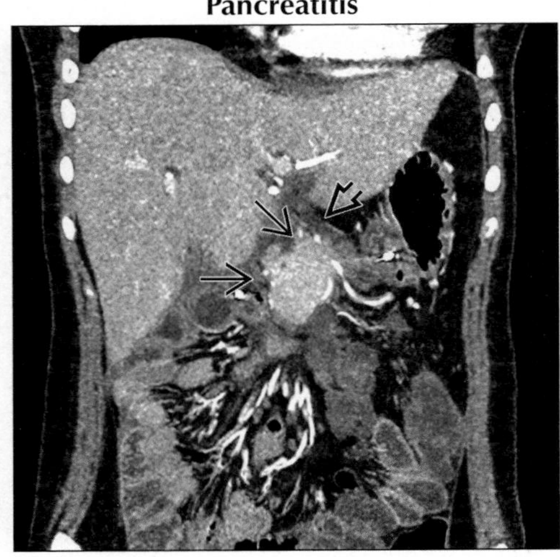

(Left) *Axial CECT shows focal enlargement of the pancreatic head ➔. There is stranding in the peripancreatic mesentery ➔. Focal pancreatitis can appear mass-like.* ***(Right)*** *Coronal CECT shows mass-like enlargement of the pancreatic head ➔ compared to the body and tail (not shown). Peripancreatic edema is also present ➔. The causes of pancreatitis are more varied in children than adults and include gallstones, infection, and medications.*

Pancreatic Pseudocyst

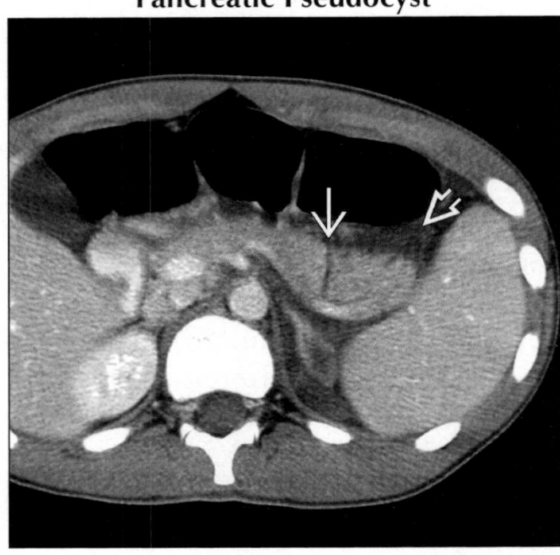

Pancreatic Pseudocyst

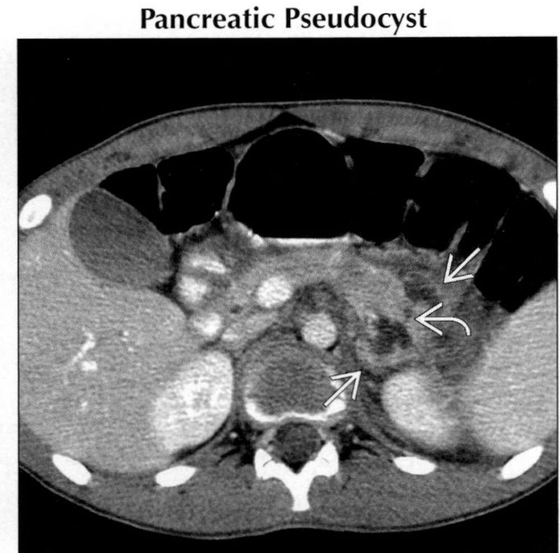

(Left) *Axial CECT in a patient involved in a motor vehicle crash shows a linear hypodensity band ➔ in the tail of the pancreas with surrounding peripancreatic edema ➔. Isolated pancreatic injury (in this case, pancreatic transection) is more common in children than in adults.* ***(Right)*** *Axial CECT in the same patient 8 days later shows the development of a well-defined bilobed cystic collection with an enhancing wall ➔ at the site of transection ➔.*

Pancreatic Pseudocyst

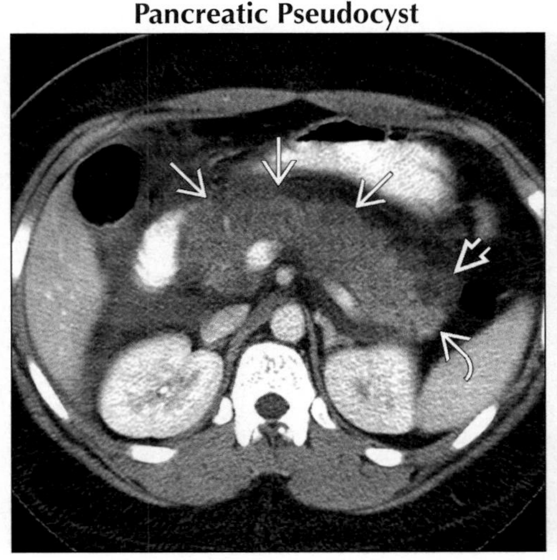

Pancreatic Pseudocyst

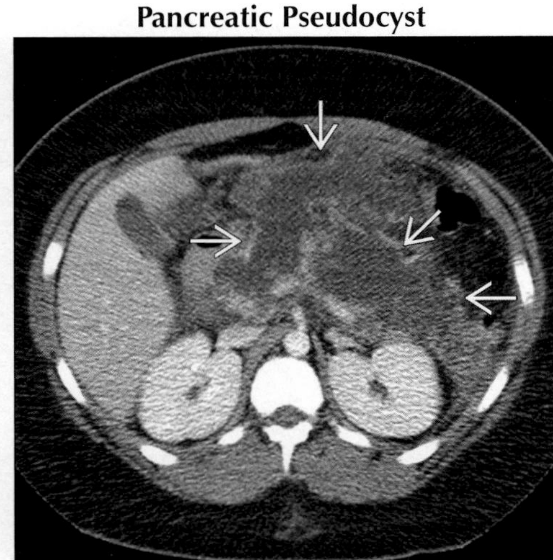

(Left) *Axial CECT shows a markedly abnormal pancreas. The pancreas is diffusely edematous and hypodense ➔; only a small portion enhances normally ➔. There is moderate peripancreatic edema ➔. The findings are typical of necrotic pancreatitis.* ***(Right)*** *Axial CECT in the same patient 8 days later shows an irregular cystic collection in place of the pancreas. This collection has thin well-defined walls ➔, typical of a pancreatic pseudocyst.*

Congenital Pancreatic Cysts

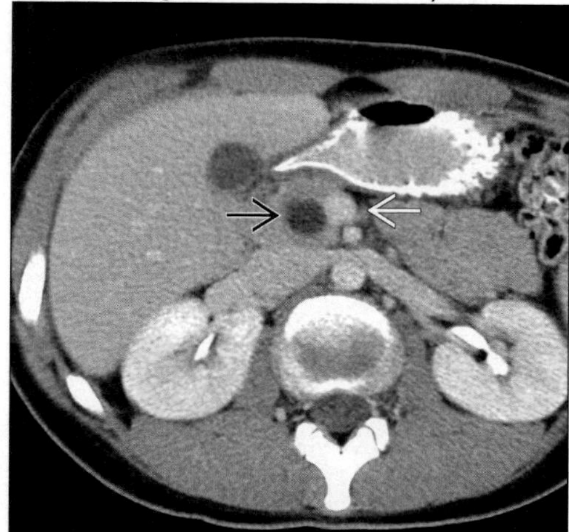

Congenital Pancreatic Cysts

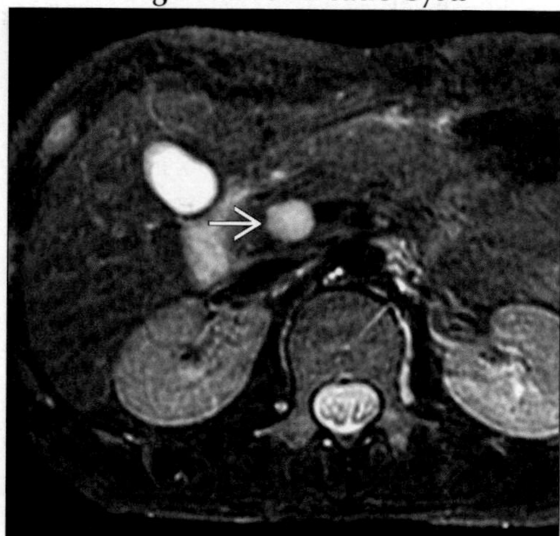

(Left) *Axial CECT shows a well-defined circular lesion ➔ in the uncinate process of the pancreas. This lesion has no appreciable wall and abuts the superior mesenteric vein ➔.* ***(Right)*** *Axial T2WI FS MR shows a well-defined fluid intensity structure ➔ in the uncinate process of the pancreas. This lesion did not connect to the pancreatic duct or common bile duct. Congenital pancreatic cysts are usually asymptomatic and are often found incidentally.*

Annular Pancreas

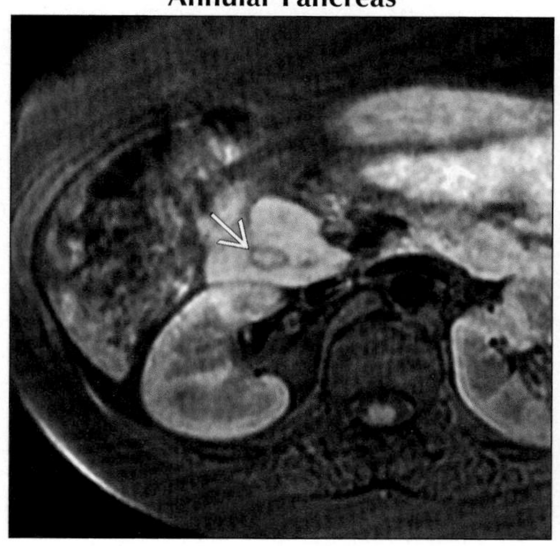

Annular Pancreas

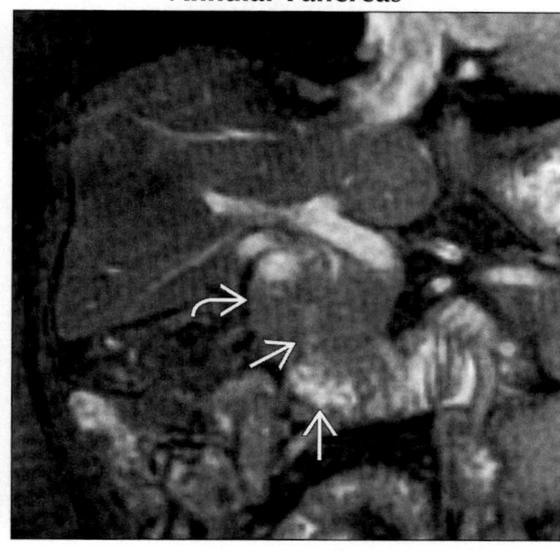

(Left) *Axial T1WI FS MR shows a hypointense "lesion" ➔ in the head of the pancreas with a central area of increased signal. Annular pancreas is a congenital lesion in which the 2nd portion of the duodenum is surrounded by pancreatic tissue. As the duodenum passes through the pancreas, it can mimic a mass.* ***(Right)*** *Coronal T2WI FSE MR shows the hyperintense duodenum ➔ passing through the hypointense pancreas ➔.*

Metastases

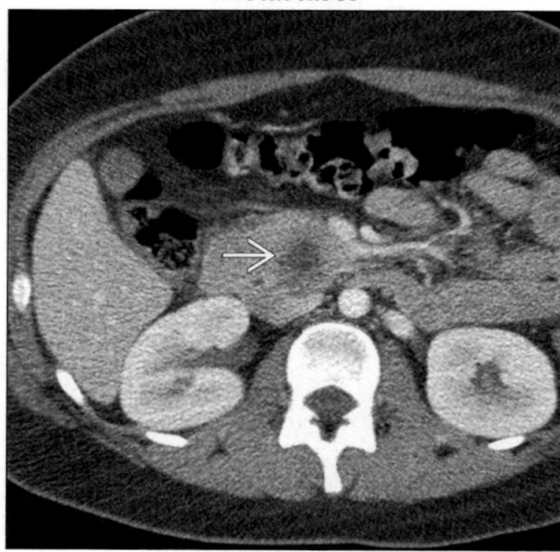

Metastases

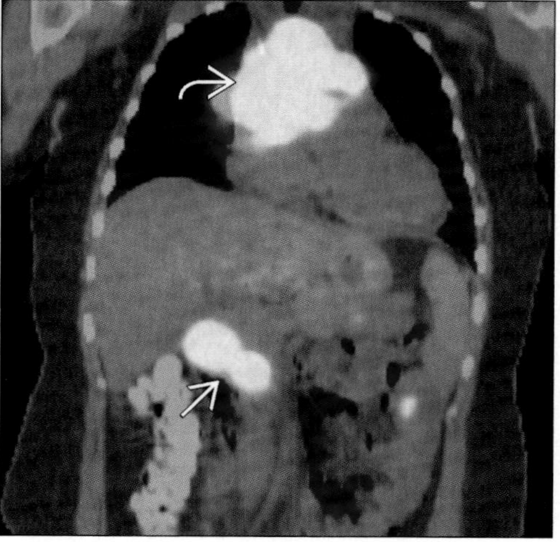

(Left) *Axial CECT shows a hypodense mass ➔ in the head of the pancreas in a patient with a large mediastinal mass and known large cell lymphoma. Pancreatic involvement in lymphoma can be primary or secondary. Peripancreatic lymph nodes may be involved.* ***(Right)*** *Coronal fused PET/CT shows intense FDG uptake in both the pancreatic head ➔ and anterior mediastinum ➔. Lymphoma is the most common nonepithelial tumor of the pancreas.*

PANCREATIC MASS

(Left) *Axial T1WI FS MR C+ in a patient with a metastatic Wilms tumor shows a well-defined mass ➡ in the tail of the pancreas. The mass is mostly hypointense and nonenhancing. Small liver metastases ➦ are also present.* **(Right)** *Axial CECT in the same patient shows a hypodense mass ➡ in the tail of the pancreas, as well as small hypodense liver metastases ➦. Most secondary tumor involvement of the pancreas occurs by direct extension.*

Metastases

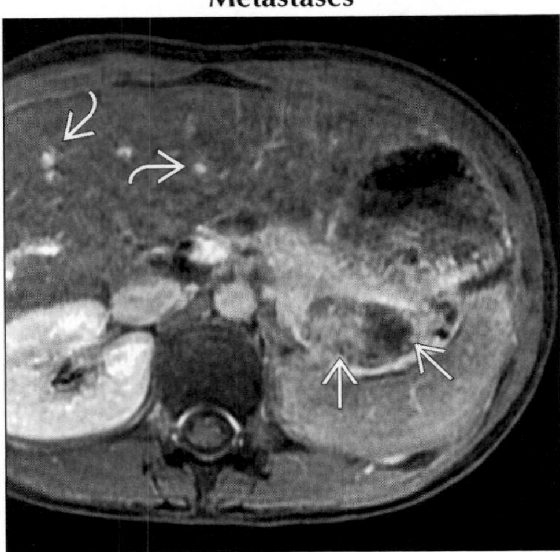

Metastases

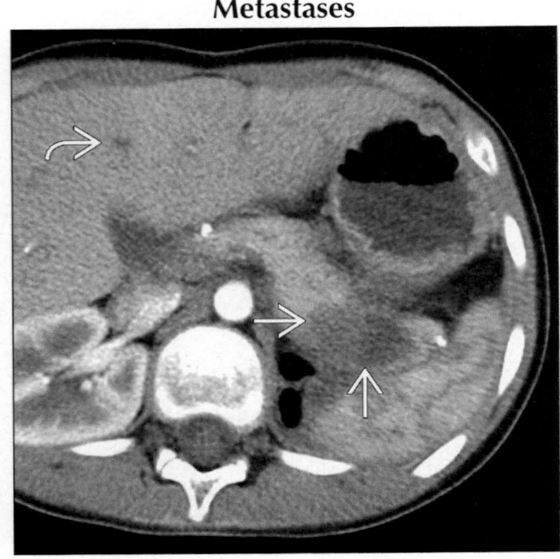

(Left) *Axial CECT shows a hypodense mass ➡ of the pancreatic tail. The mass has some internal enhancement and a thin rim of pancreatic tissue ➦ along the medial margin of the mass. Note multiple liver metastases ⇨.* **(Right)** *Gross photograph shows the large mass ➦ of the pancreatic tail and the resected spleen ➡ after excision. Pancreatoblastoma is the most common pancreatic neoplasm of children and is associated with Beckwith-Wiedemann syndrome.*

Pancreatoblastoma

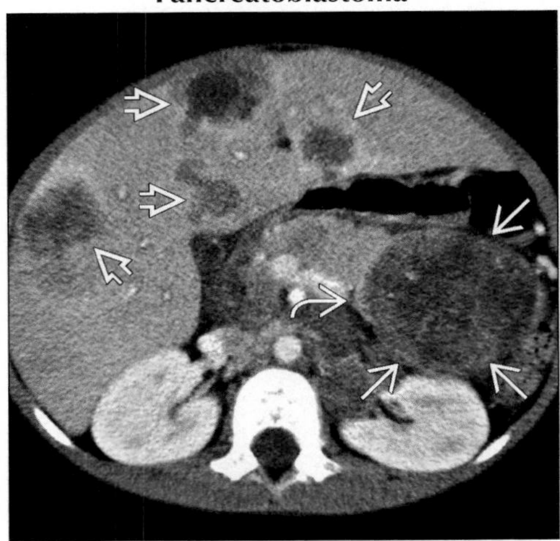

Pancreatoblastoma

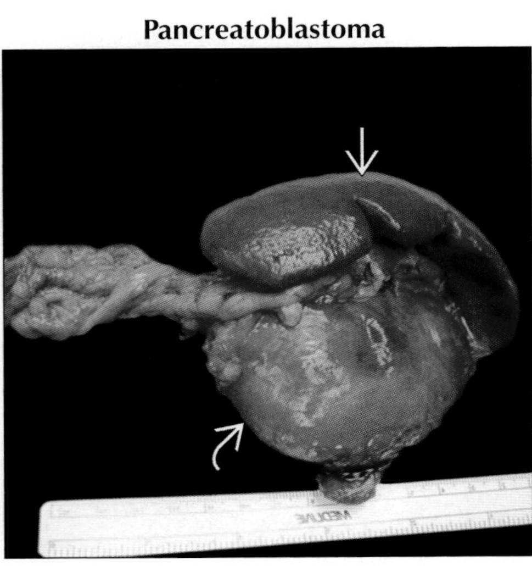

(Left) *Axial CECT shows a hypodense mass ➡ arising from the pancreatic tail. Some normal pancreatic tissue is present ➡. The mass is well defined, and the peripancreatic fat is normal.* **(Right)** *Axial T1WI FS MR C+ shows a well-defined hypointense mass ➡ of the pancreatic tail. Solid-cystic pancreatic tumor is most common in adolescent girls and young women.*

Solid-Cystic Pancreatic Tumor

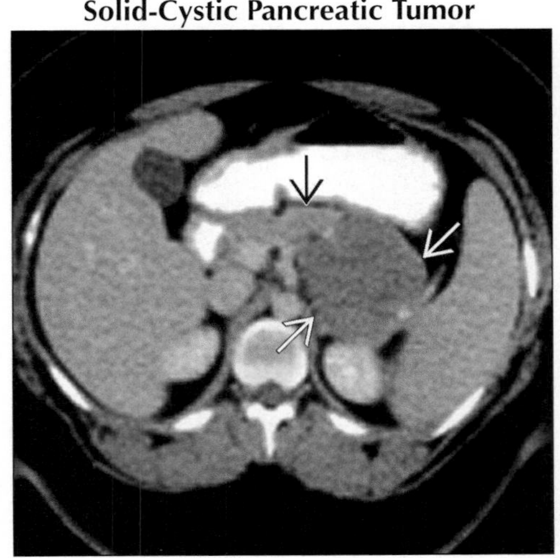

Solid-Cystic Pancreatic Tumor

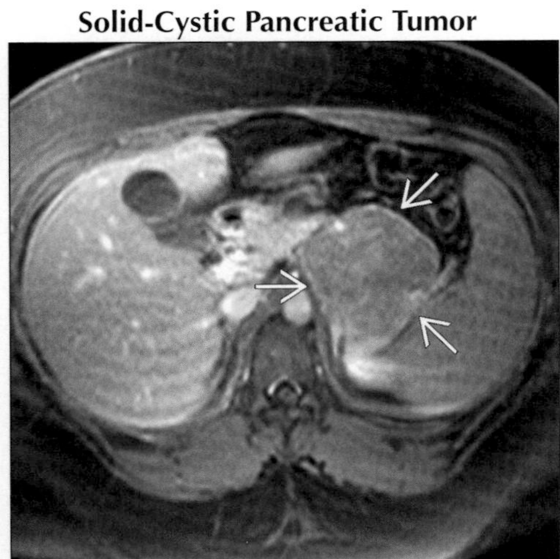

Solid-Cystic Pancreatic Tumor

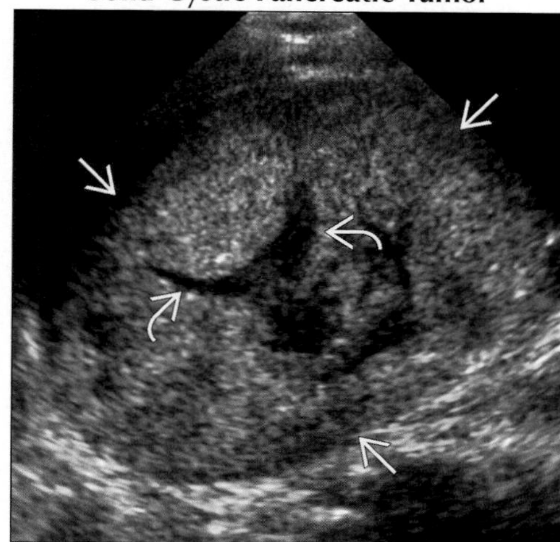

Solid-Cystic Pancreatic Tumor

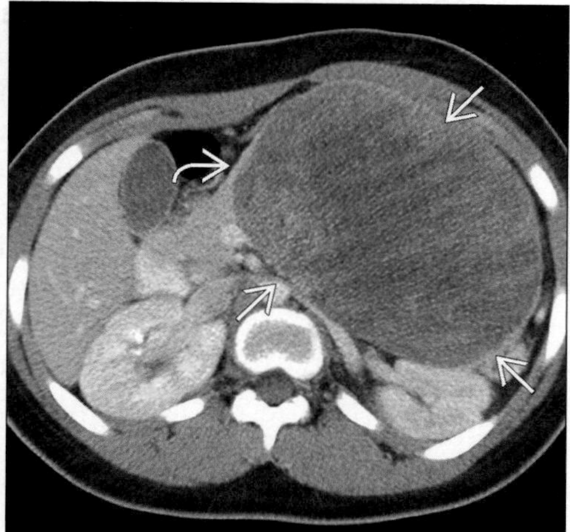

(Left) *Transverse ultrasound shows a mostly solid mass ➡ of the pancreas. There is a central irregular anechoic area ↪ within the mass.* ***(Right)*** *Axial CECT in the same patient shows a large heterogeneous but hypodense mass ➡ in the tail of the pancreas. There is a thin rim of pancreatic tissue along the medial border ↪. Solid-cystic tumors may appear completely cystic or solid. Internal hemorrhage may be present, giving the mass a heterogeneous appearance.*

Islet Cell Tumors

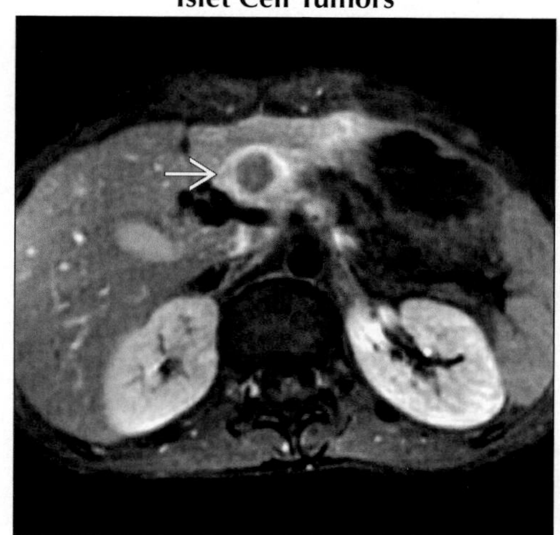

Agenesis of Dorsal Pancreas

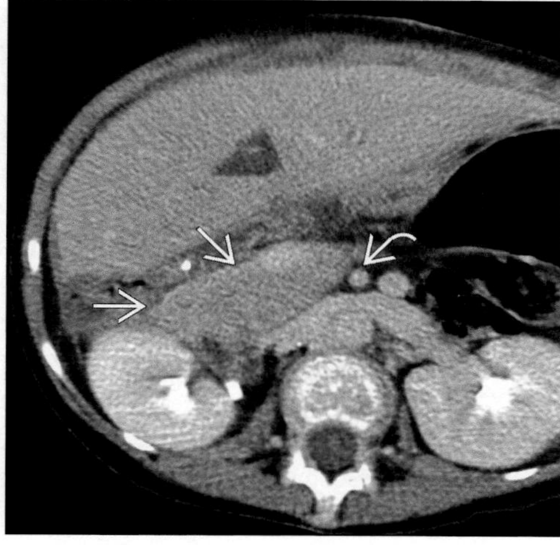

(Left) *Axial T1WI FS MR C+ shows a circular mass ➡ with peripheral enhancement in the neck of the pancreas. At resection, this mass was a poorly functioning insulinoma. Insulinomas are the most common islet cell tumors and are often in the pancreatic body or tail.* ***(Right)*** *Axial CECT shows a triangular-shaped pancreas ➡ in the right abdomen. No pancreatic tissue was present to the left of the superior mesenteric artery ↪.*

Agenesis of Dorsal Pancreas

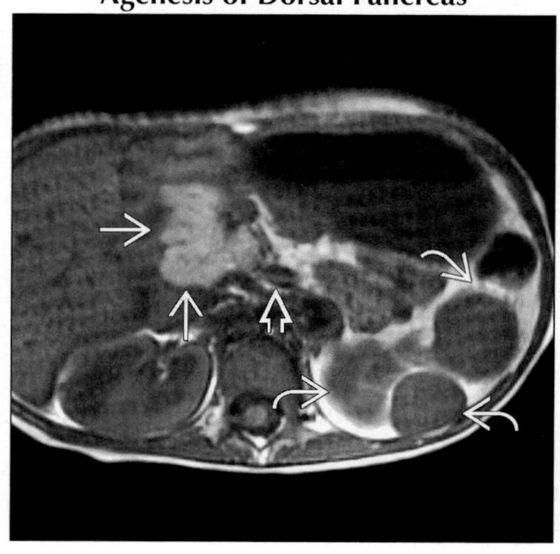

Agenesis of Dorsal Pancreas

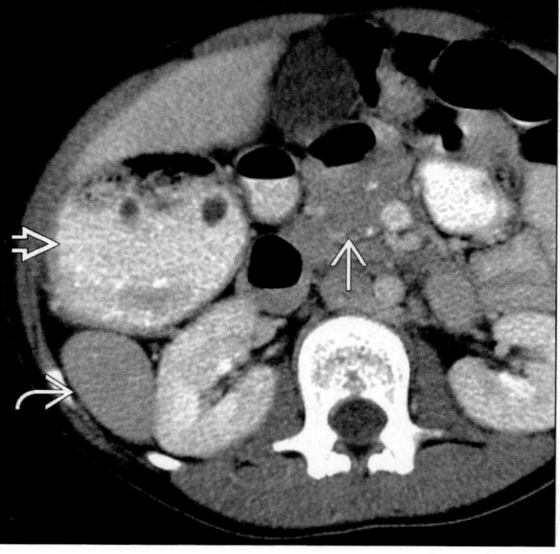

(Left) *Axial T1WI MR shows a relatively hyperintense pancreas ➡. The pancreas does not extend to the left of the mesenteric vessels ⇨. Multiple spleens are present ↪. Dorsal agenesis of the pancreas is associated with polysplenia.* ***(Right)*** *Axial CECT shows a mildly hypodense appearance to the pancreas ➡ in a patient with polysplenia. The pancreas has an amorphous shape and can mimic a mass. One spleen ↪ and the stomach ⇨ are in the right upper quadrant.*

SPLENIC MASS

DIFFERENTIAL DIAGNOSIS

Common
- Perfusion Artifact
- Trauma
- Granulomatous Disease
- Lymphoma
- Acquired Cyst
- Hematoma
- Infarction
- Infection and Abscess

Less Common
- Congenital Cyst
- Metastases
- Primary Tumor

Rare but Important
- Post-Transplant Lymphoproliferative Disease
- Lymphatic Malformation

ESSENTIAL INFORMATION

Key Differential Diagnosis Issues
- Primary and metastatic splenic malignancies are rare in children, except for lymphoma and leukemia
- Clinical history is crucial as many splenic lesions have similar imaging characteristics
  - Is child immunocompromised?
  - Is there known primary neoplasm?
  - Does patient have sickle cell disease or other hemoglobinopathy?
  - Is there history of trauma?

Helpful Clues for Common Diagnoses
- **Perfusion Artifact**
  - Seen during arterial phase of CT and MR
  - Patterns include striped, focal, and diffuse heterogeneity
  - Ultrasound helpful in difficult cases
  - **Hint**: Resolves on delayed phase imaging (> 70 sec)
- **Trauma**
  - Trauma history is helpful
  - Laceration, fracture, rupture all possible
  - Splenic injury more common when spleen is enlarged, i.e., with infectious mononucleosis
  - Active bleeding manifests as foci of high attenuation
  - American Association for the Surgery of Trauma grading system
    - Grade 1: Subcapsular hematoma, < 10% surface area OR < 1 cm deep laceration
    - Grade 2: Subcapsular hematoma, 10-50% surface area OR 1-3 cm laceration not involving parenchymal vessel
    - Grade 3: Subcapsular hematoma, > 50% surface area or expanding/ruptured, OR parenchymal hematoma > 5 cm OR laceration > 3 cm
    - Grade 4: Laceration of vessel producing devascularization of > 25% of spleen
    - Grade 5: Shattered spleen OR hilar vascular injury
- **Granulomatous Disease**
  - Old granulomatous disease (such as histoplasmosis) frequently demonstrates small calcified splenic lesions
  - Wegener granulomatosis may involve spleen
  - Sarcoidosis may involve spleen
- **Lymphoma**
  - Hodgkin or non-Hodgkin lymphoma can involve spleen
  - Focal lesions or diffuse involvement
  - Typically hypoattenuating on CT and hypoechoic on US
  - **Hint**: Look for associated lymphadenopathy
- **Acquired Cyst**
  - Pseudocysts (lack epithelial lining)
  - Typically result from prior trauma, infarct, or infection
  - Differentiation by imaging from congenital cyst not reliable
- **Hematoma**
  - Typically secondary to trauma
  - May be parenchymal or subcapsular
  - May lead to acquired splenic cyst
- **Infarction**
  - Secondary to occlusion of noncommunicating end arteries of spleen
  - Commonly seen in children with hemoglobinopathies, such as sickle cell disease, and malignancies
  - Variable appearance depending on stage
    - Early: Ill-defined mottled changes in density on CT or echogenicity on US
    - Late: Well-defined peripheral hypoechoic or hypodense wedge-shaped regions
  - May resolve completely or evolve into acquired cyst

- **Infection and Abscess**
  - Fungal and bacterial infections occur most frequently in immunocompromised patients
  - Fungal splenic abscesses are hypodense and typically small
    - **Hint**: Look for lesions in liver, kidneys, and lungs as well
  - Hydatid abscesses are rare

Helpful Clues for Less Common Diagnoses

- **Congenital Cyst**
  - True cyst (epithelial lining)
  - Includes epidermoid cysts and mesothelial cysts
  - Differentiation by imaging from acquired cyst not reliable
- **Metastases**
  - Splenic metastases are rare
    - **Hint**: Look for metastases in other visceral organs
  - Melanoma
  - Variable imaging appearance
    - Typically hypoechoic/hypodense relative to normal spleen
    - Can see cystic splenic metastases
- **Primary Tumor**
  - Malignant
    - Majority lymphoma and leukemia
  - Benign hamartoma
    - Nonneoplastic mixture of normal splenic components
    - Can be seen in tuberous sclerosis patients with hamartomas in other organs
    - Nonspecific imaging appearance, occasionally with calcifications
  - Benign hemangioma
    - Most common primary splenic neoplasm
    - Can be solitary or multiple
    - Can cause Kasabach-Merritt syndrome (thrombocytopenia and consumptive coagulopathy)
    - Variable imaging appearance

Helpful Clues for Rare Diagnoses

- **Post-Transplant Lymphoproliferative Disease**
  - Complication of solid organ transplant and allogeneic bone marrow transplant
  - Associated with EBV infection
  - Spleen involved in ~ 20% of cases
  - Similar imaging appearance to lymphoma
  - **Hint**: Look for involvement of other organs
    - Lymph nodes
    - Liver
    - Lung
    - CNS
- **Lymphatic Malformation**
  - Nonneoplastic endothelial-lined lymph channels
  - Septate cystic lesions most commonly
  - May contain debris or fluid-fluid levels
  - Septa and rim typically enhance

Perfusion Artifact

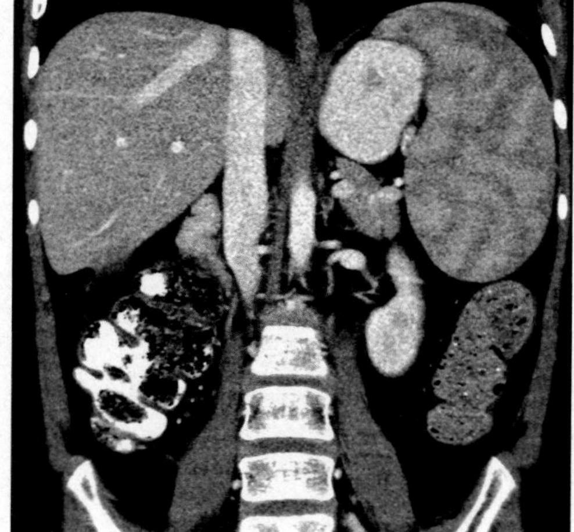

Coronal CECT shows heterogeneous stripes of low attenuation in the spleen, a common normal variant seen during arterial phase imaging. This pattern has been referred to as "tiger" or "zebra" striped.

Perfusion Artifact

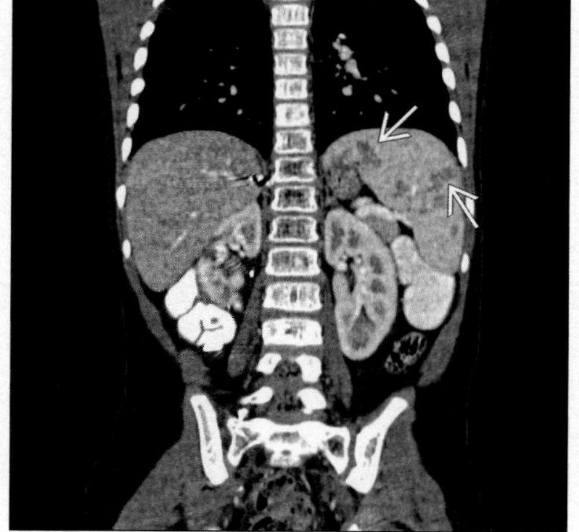

Axial CECT shows multifocal areas of decreased attenuation of the spleen ➔ that proved to be normal variant heterogeneous enhancement. This appearance resolved on portal venous phase imaging.

SPLENIC MASS

(Left) Axial CECT shows multifocal mass-like areas of decreased attenuation of the spleen ➡ that proved to be normal variant heterogeneous enhancement. The spleen was normal on a follow-up ultrasound. **(Right)** Axial CECT shows a splenic rupture ➡ in a 9 year old with infectious mononucleosis. There was no active contrast extravasation. This is a grade 3 splenic injury.

Perfusion Artifact

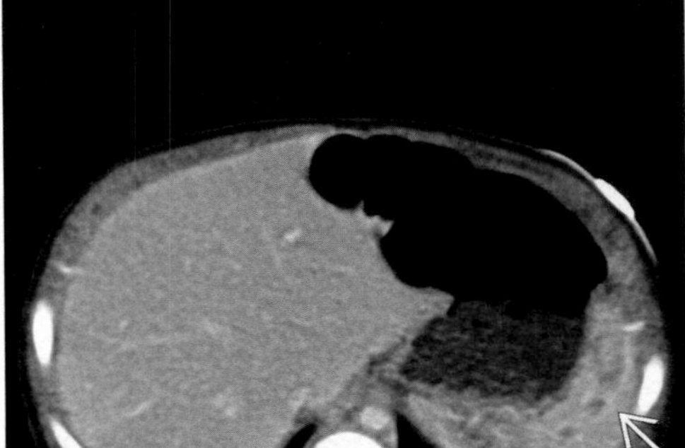

Trauma

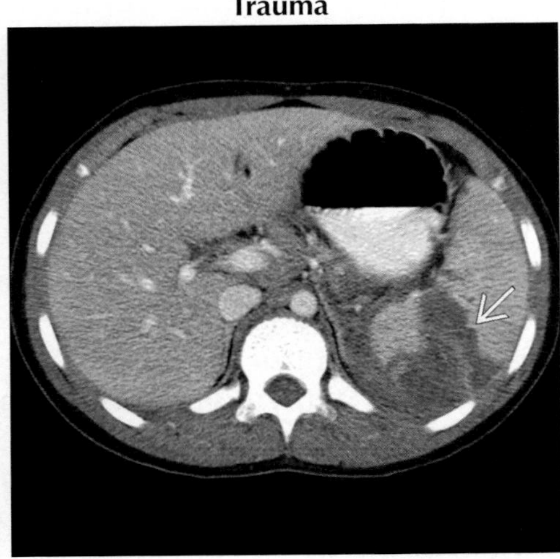

(Left) Axial CECT shows a traumatic laceration of the spleen with active contrast extravasation ➡ and large hemoperitoneum ➡ in this 16 year old who suffered a football-related injury. This is a grade 5 splenic injury as the hilar vessels of the spleen were involved (not shown). **(Right)** Axial CECT in this 12-year-old patient shows multiple punctate calcified foci scattered throughout the spleen, findings consistent with prior granulomatous infection.

Trauma

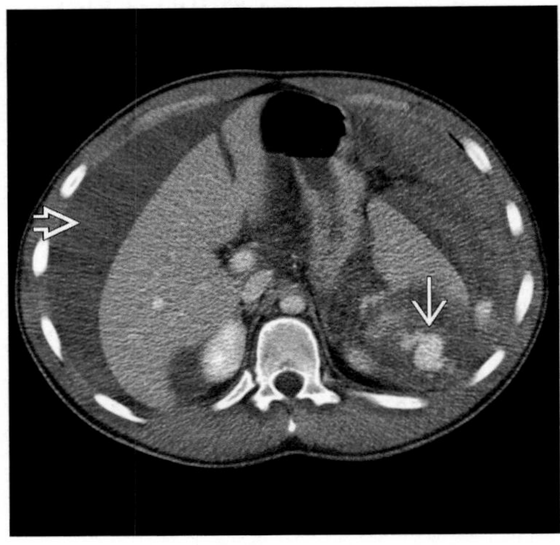

Granulomatous Disease

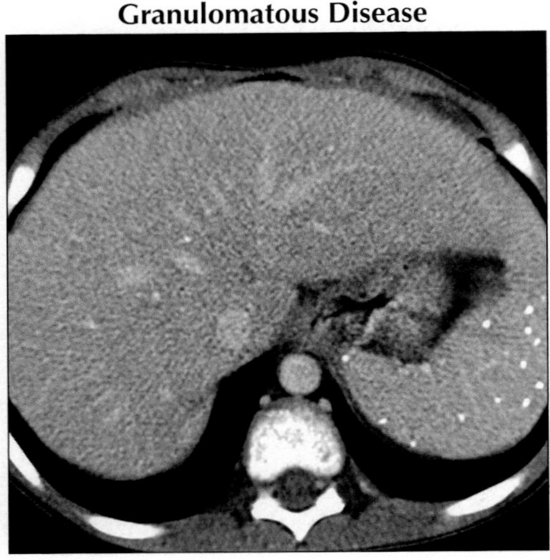

(Left) Longitudinal ultrasound shows multiple scattered punctate echogenic foci ➡ in an otherwise normal-appearing spleen, findings consistent with calcifications secondary to prior granulomatous infection. **(Right)** Coronal CECT shows a markedly heterogeneous enhancement pattern of the spleen with ill-defined scattered areas of decreased attenuation in a child with known Wegener granulomatosis.

Granulomatous Disease

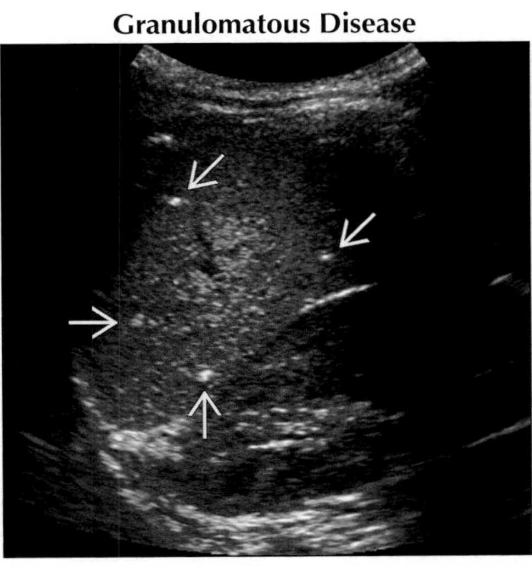

Granulomatous Disease

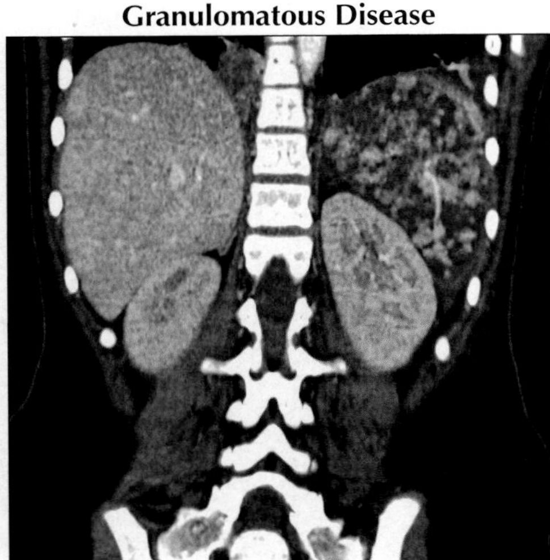

SPLENIC MASS

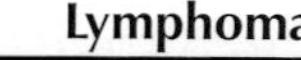

Lymphoma

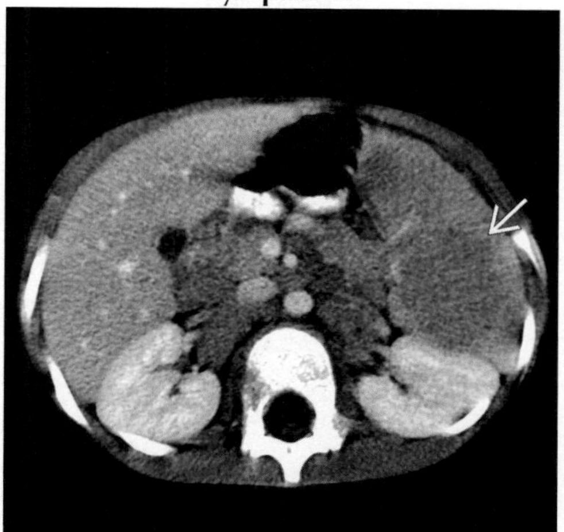

Acquired Cyst

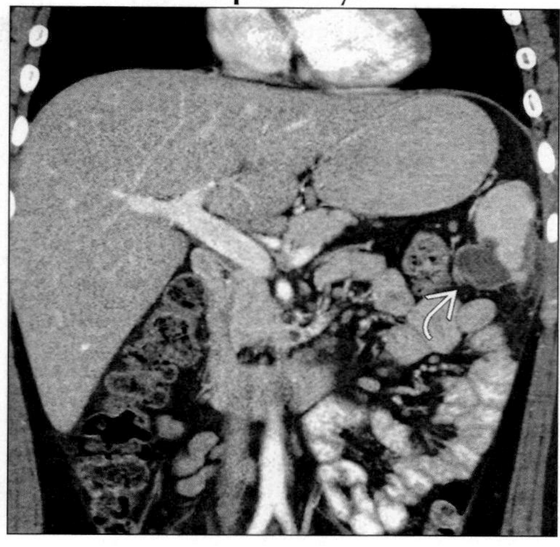

(Left) *Axial CECT shows a large hypodense splenic mass ➔ in a 6 year old that proved to be Hodgkin lymphoma. The presence of multiple enlarged lymph nodes (not shown) aided in the diagnosis, though ultimately the diagnosis was proven by biopsy.* ***(Right)*** *Coronal CECT shows a well-circumscribed cyst ➔ arising from the inferior tip of the spleen in this 11 year old following trauma and a prior splenic laceration in this location.*

Hematoma

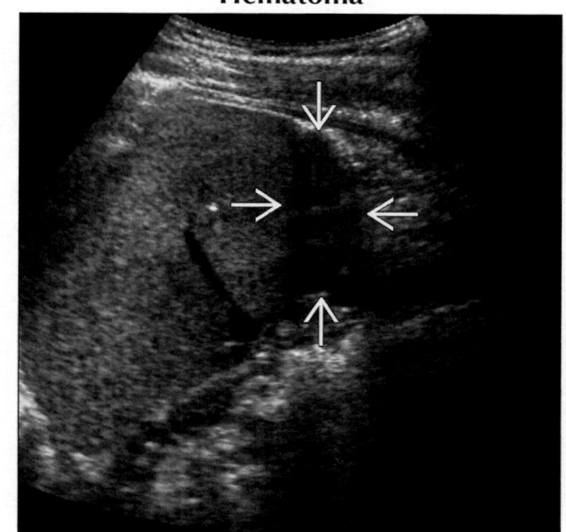

Infarction

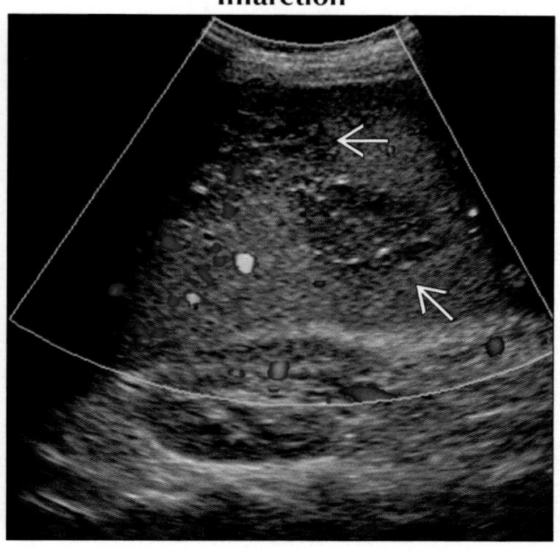

(Left) *Longitudinal ultrasound shows a well-circumscribed area of decreased echogenicity ➔ involving the inferior aspect of the spleen. This 15 year old was being monitored for a splenic subcapsular hematoma following a motor vehicle crash.* ***(Right)*** *Longitudinal ultrasound shows wedge-shaped and peripheral well-demarcated areas of hypoechogenicity ➔ relative to a normal spleen without internal color flow, findings consistent with splenic infarcts.*

Infarction

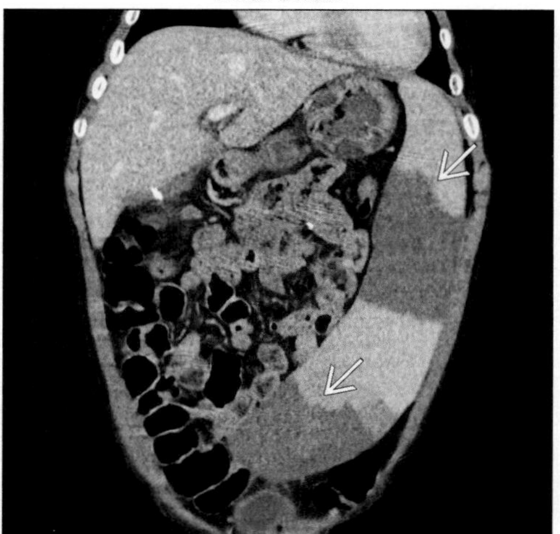

Infection and Abscess

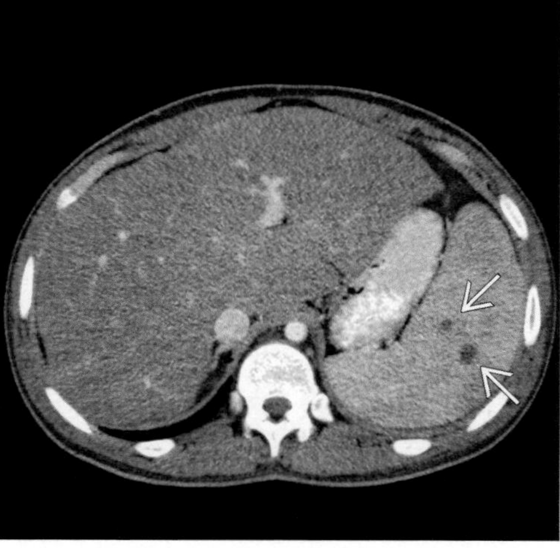

(Left) *Coronal CECT in a 9-year-old liver transplant recipient shows splenomegaly and well-demarcated areas of decreased enhancement ➔ within the spleen, findings consistent with infarcts.* ***(Right)*** *Axial CECT shows 2 of several small round hypodense foci ➔ within the spleen in this adolescent with congenital heart disease and bacteremia. The findings are consistent with septic emboli in this patient.*

SPLENIC MASS

(Left) Axial CECT shows multiple small, round, hypodense foci throughout the spleen, and 1 ⇒ in the liver, consistent with fungal abscesses in this febrile, immunocompromised 11 year old with a history of acute lymphocytic leukemia. (Right) Coronal CECT shows a homogeneous hypodense mass ⇒ arising from the inferior aspect of the spleen. The mass is nonspecific on CECT and was pathologically proven to be a congential mesothelial cyst following excision.

Infection and Abscess

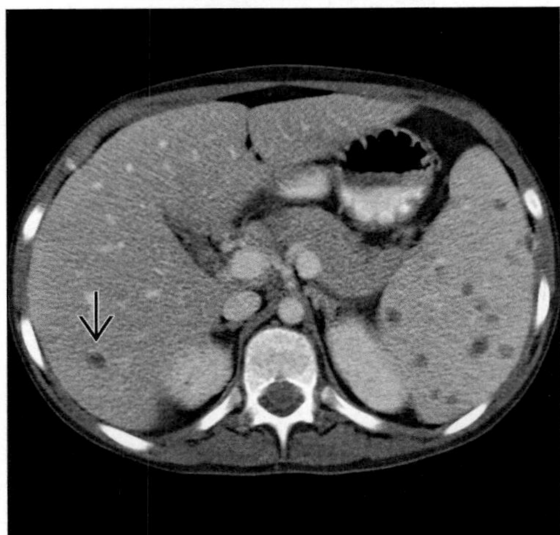

Congenital Cyst

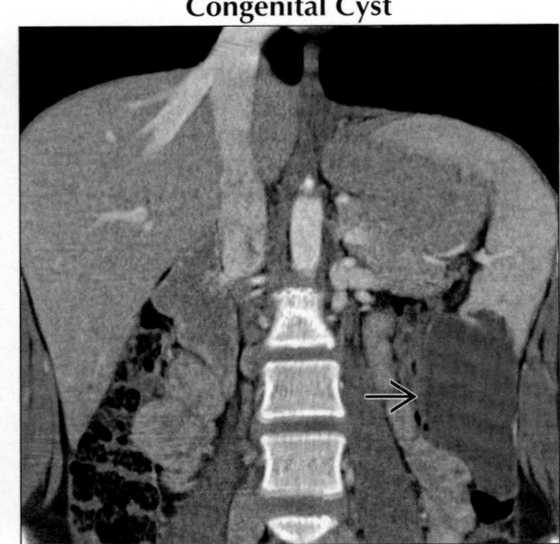

(Left) Coronal T2WI MR shows a well-circumscribed round hyperintense mass ⇒ arising from the inferior aspect of the spleen. The mass did not show any enhancement (not shown). (Right) Longitudinal and transverse ultrasound images of the same patient show a complex cystic mass ➡ within the spleen. The mass is nonspecific on MR and ultrasound and was pathologically proven to be a congential mesothelial cyst following excision.

Congenital Cyst

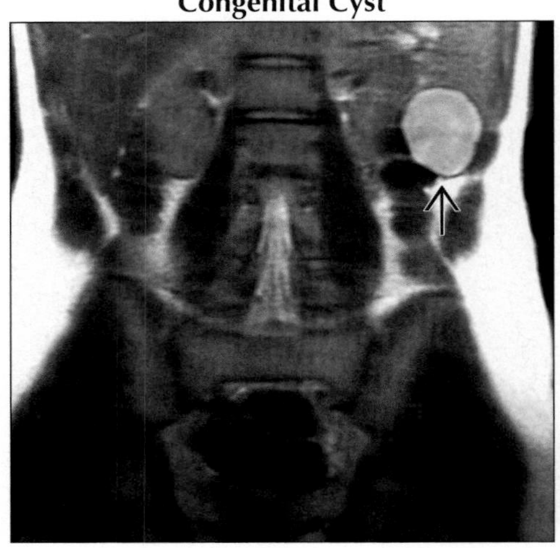

Congenital Cyst

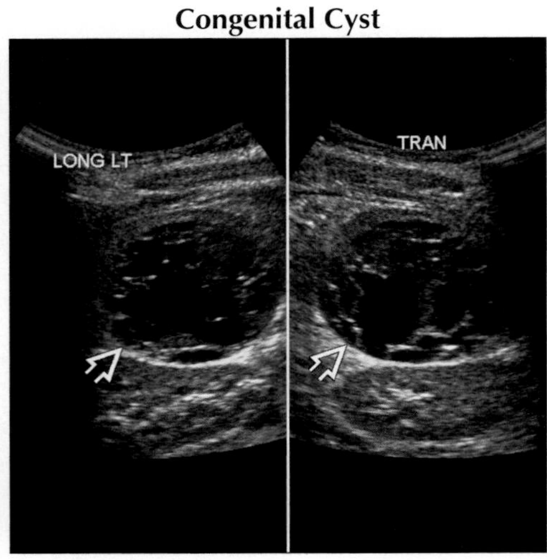

(Left) Axial CECT shows a well-circumscribed homogeneous cystic mass ➡ with a single septation within the spleen. There is no enhancement. The mass is nonspecific on CECT and was biopsy-proven to be a congential epidermoid cyst. (Right) Transverse ultrasound shows a round hypoechoic splenic mass ➡ with increased through-transmission. The mass is nonspecific and was proven to be a congential epidermoid cyst after excision.

Congenital Cyst

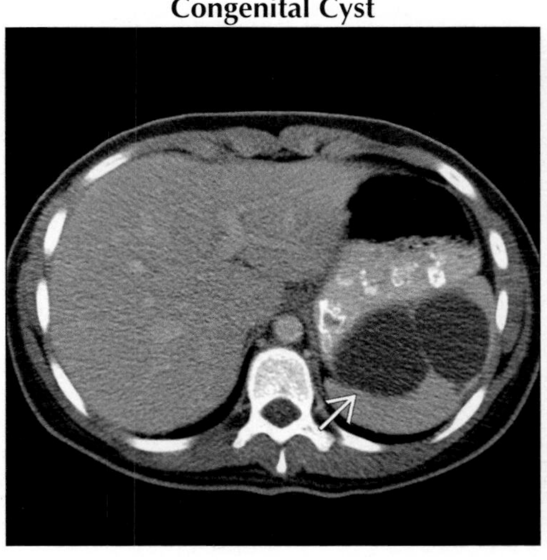

Congenital Cyst

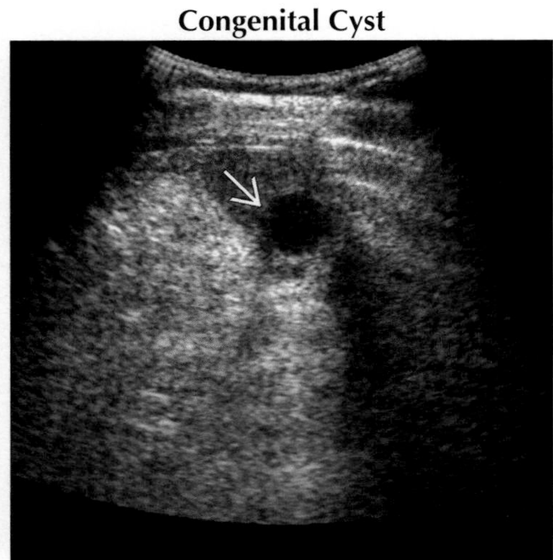

Metastases

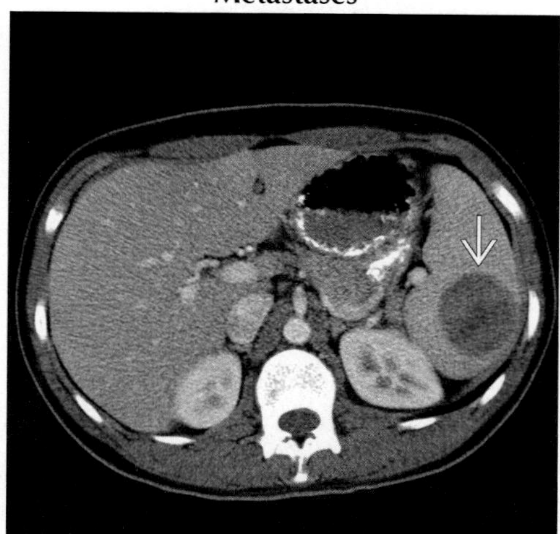

Primary Tumor

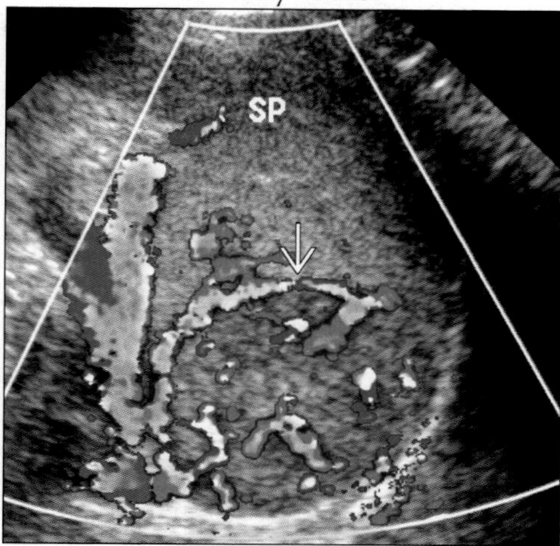

*(**Left**) Axial CECT shows a well-defined hypodense mass ➡ in the spleen. The mass is nonspecific on CECT but is consistent with metastatic disease in this 18-year-old patient with known metastatic melanoma. (**Right**) Transverse ultrasound shows a well-defined relatively hypoechoic mass ➡ with internal hypervascular flow presumed to be a splenic hemangioma in this 13-year-old patient.*

Primary Tumor

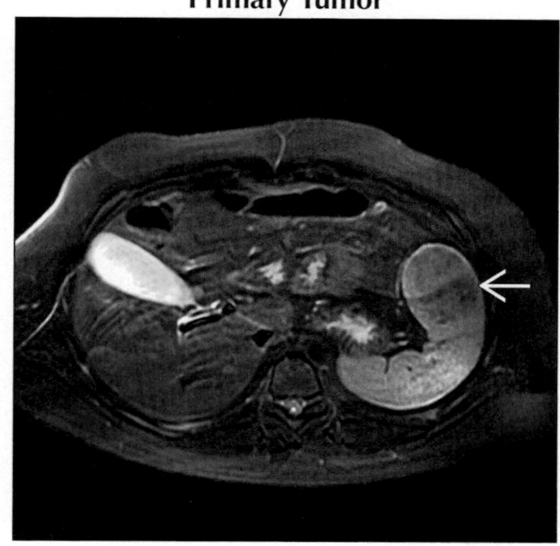

Post-Transplant Lymphoproliferative Disease

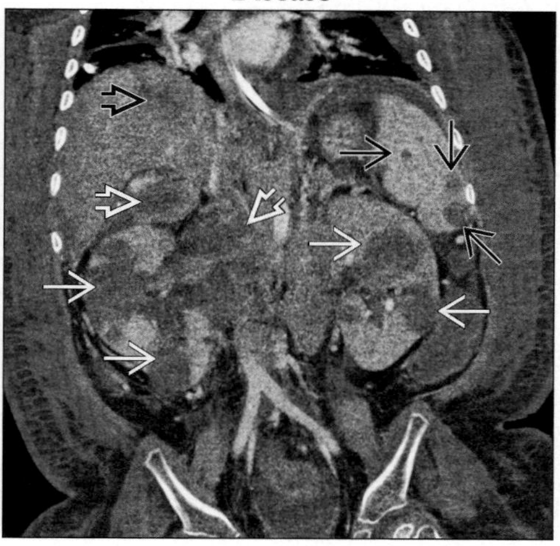

*(**Left**) Axial T2WI FSE MR shows a hypointense splenic mass ➡ presumed to be a splenic hamartoma in this 15 year old with tuberous sclerosis and multiple renal hamartomatous lesions (not shown). (**Right**) Coronal CECT shows multiple hypodense masses ➡ within the spleen in a 2-year-old liver transplant recipient. Note the adenopathy ➡, as well as additional masses in the liver ➡ and kidneys ➡. Biopsy demonstrated post-transplant lymphoproliferative disease.*

Lymphatic Malformation

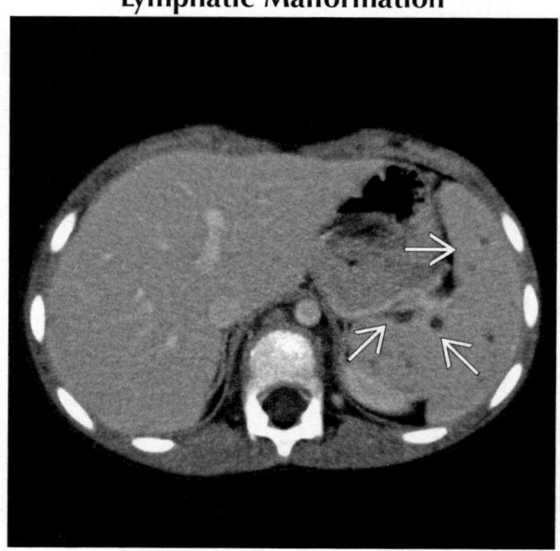

Lymphatic Malformation

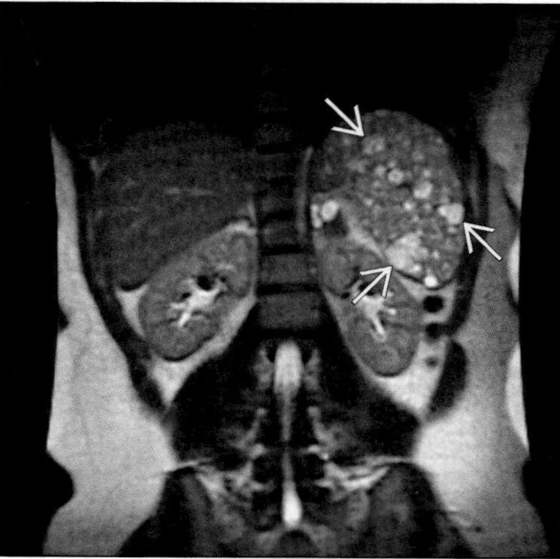

*(**Left**) Axial CECT shows multiple small hypodense foci ➡ throughout the spleen in this 5 year old. The lesions are nonspecific on CECT but were proven to represent small lymphatic malformations. (**Right**) Coronal T2WI MR shows multiple small hyperintense lesions ➡ throughout the spleen in this 18 year old with Klippel-Trenaunay-Weber syndrome. These lesions are nonspecific and consistent with lymphatic malformations.*

ABDOMINAL CALCIFICATIONS

DIFFERENTIAL DIAGNOSIS

Common
- Nephrolithiasis
- Cholelithiasis
- Hepatic and Splenic Granulomas
- Neuroblastoma
- Hepatoblastoma
- Teratoma (Ovarian)
- Appendicolith

Less Common
- Remote Adrenal Hemorrhage
- Meconium Peritonitis

ESSENTIAL INFORMATION

Key Differential Diagnosis Issues
- Age of patient
- Location of calcification
- Morphology of calcifications: Coarse, punctate, or curvilinear

Helpful Clues for Common Diagnoses
- **Nephrolithiasis**
  - Conventional radiographs show punctate or coarse calcification that projects over
    - Renal shadow
    - Course of ureters
    - Expected location of bladder
  - Renal calculi are echogenic with posterior shadowing on ultrasound
    - Color Doppler may be used to look for "twinkling" artifact or "comet tail" artifact posterior to small renal stones
- **Cholelithiasis**
  - ~ 30% of gallstones are detectable by plain film
  - Look for calcification projecting over medial aspect of hepatic silhouette on conventional radiographs
  - US is preferred modality for evaluation
    - Gallstones are echogenic with posterior shadowing
- **Hepatic and Splenic Granulomas**
  - Multiple, punctate, round , or ovoid-shaped calcifications projecting over spleen &/or liver on plain film
  - Appear as multiple, punctate, echogenic foci on ultrasound that may or may not have posterior shadowing
- **Neuroblastoma**
  - Can arise anywhere along sympathetic chain from skull base to pelvis
  - Median age at diagnosis is 2 years old
  - Involvement of adrenal glands and extraadrenal retroperitoneum make up more than 60% of cases
  - Conventional radiographic findings
    - Paraspinal soft tissue mass
    - 30% will have associated calcifications
    - May have lytic, sclerotic, or mixed metastatic bone lesions
  - CT findings
    - Soft tissue mass with heterogeneous attenuation (necrosis &/or hemorrhage)
    - Associated calcifications in up to 85% of cases
    - Engulfs adjacent vascular structures, such as celiac and superior mesenteric artery
    - Metastasis most common to liver & bone
    - Bone metastasis may be lytic, sclerotic, or mixed pattern
    - Look for involvement of neuroforamina
  - MR findings: Best for detecting intraspinal extension of tumor
- **Hepatoblastoma**
  - Majority occur in children < 3 years old
  - Painless abdominal mass
  - Elevated α-fetoprotein levels
  - Conventional radiographic findings
    - Large, soft tissue mass in right upper quadrant of abdomen
    - May displace bowel
    - Roughly 1/2 will have visible calcifications, usually coarse
  - CT findings
    - Usually large at presentation
    - Well-defined lesion
    - > 60% located in right lobe of liver
    - Heterogeneous in attenuation due to necrosis and hemorrhage
    - Heterogeneous enhancement
    - Roughly 50% have coarse calcifications
    - CT of chest is performed for metastatic workup
- **Teratoma (Ovarian)**
  - Conventional radiographic findings
    - Punctate or coarse calcifications projecting over pelvis
    - May see associated "teeth" within pelvis
    - Mass effect upon adjacent structures
  - Ultrasound findings

- Heterogeneous echogenicity
- Solid and cystic components
- Fat and hair are echogenic
- Calcifications are echogenic with posterior shadowing
- May contain fat-fluid levels
- Ovarian torsion may be a complication

- CT findings
  - Solid and cystic components
  - May have fluid levels
  - May contain fat
  - May contain coarse calcifications
  - May be bilateral in up to 15% of cases

- **Appendicolith**
  - 10-15% of acute appendicitis associated with appendicolith
    - Appendicolith may be round or oval-shaped
  - Usually in right lower abdomen/pelvis
  - May be in right upper abdomen in retrocecal appendix
  - Conventional radiographic findings
    - Appendicolith (10-15%)
    - Air-fluid levels localized to right lower abdomen
    - Splinting (levocurvature of lower spine)
  - CT findings
    - Appendicolith
    - Appendiceal diameter > 6 mm
    - Fluid-filled appendix with enhancement of appendiceal wall
    - Periappendiceal soft tissue infiltration
    - Look for abscess and extraluminal appendicolith with perforation

Helpful Clues for Less Common Diagnoses

- **Remote Adrenal Hemorrhage**
  - Resolving adrenal hemorrhage may calcify
  - Secondary to any stress in perinatal period
  - Bilateral in 10% of cases
  - Punctate calcification may be seen on conventional radiographs projecting over suprarenal region
  - Noncontrast abdominal CT to confirm intra-adrenal location
  - Ultrasound with Doppler helpful to show lack of flow vs. flow in neuroblastoma
- **Meconium Peritonitis**
  - Sterile chemical reaction resulting from bowel perforation in utero
  - 1 in 35,000 live births
  - Conventional radiographic findings
    - Diffuse calcification
    - Sometimes pseudocyst formation (peripheral calcifications)
    - May displace bowel
  - Ultrasound findings
    - May be diagnosed in utero during 2nd or 3rd trimester
    - Diffuse hyperechoic punctate echoes with or without acoustic shadowing
    - Especially along hepatic surface & in scrotum
    - May have ascites, polyhydramnios &/or bowel distention
    - If pseudocyst formation: Cystic heterogeneous mass with an irregular, calcified wall

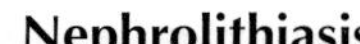

Nephrolithiasis

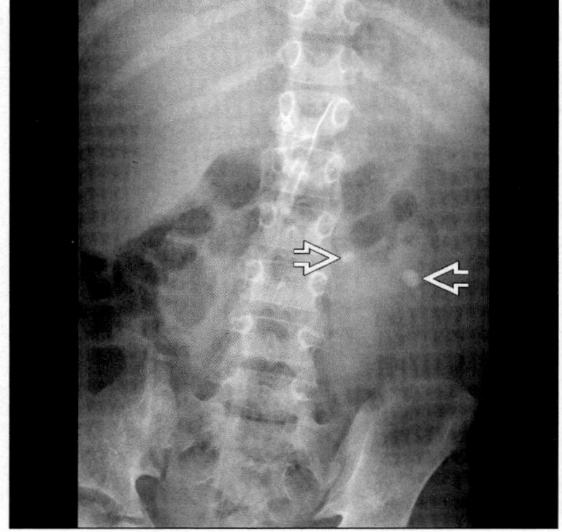

Frontal radiograph shows 2 rounded calcifications projecting over the left renal shadow. An upright or decubitus view will help to show that the calcifications move with the renal silhouette.

Nephrolithiasis

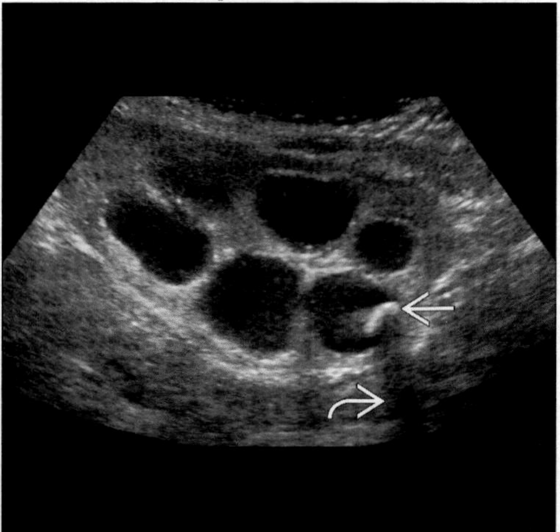

Longitudinal ultrasound shows an echogenic, shadowing renal stone. The associated hydronephrosis of the kidney suggests that there is an obstructing renal stone distally in the collecting system.

ABDOMINAL CALCIFICATIONS

(**Left**) *Longitudinal ultrasound shows an echogenic renal stone with "comet tail" artifact ➔ on color Doppler. The "comet tail" artifact is useful to identify small renal stones that demonstrate poor acoustic shadowing. More than 80% of renal stones have this artifact.* (**Right**) *Transverse ultrasound demonstrates an echogenic renal stone ➔ lodged at the right ureterovesicular junction.*

Nephrolithiasis

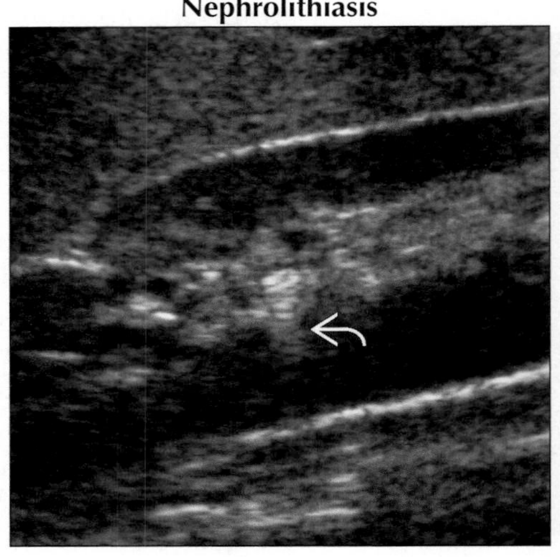

Nephrolithiasis

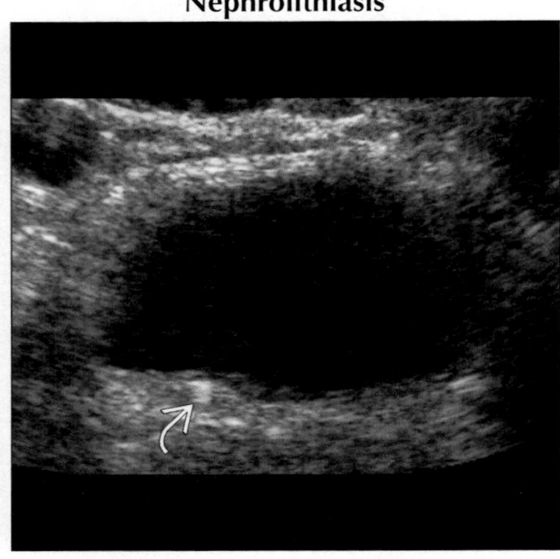

(**Left**) *Frontal radiograph shows an oval calcification ➔ projecting medial to the right lobe of the liver. Gallstones are visible in approximately 30% of patients on conventional radiographs.* (**Right**) *Transverse ultrasound shows an oval-shaped echogenic foci ➔ in the dependent portion of the gallbladder. There was no gallbladder wall thickening, hyperemia on color Doppler, or fluid in the gallbladder fossa to suggest acute cholecystitis.*

Cholelithiasis

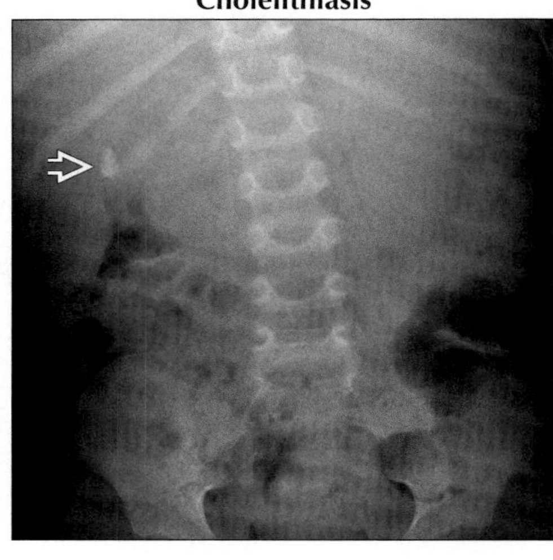

Cholelithiasis

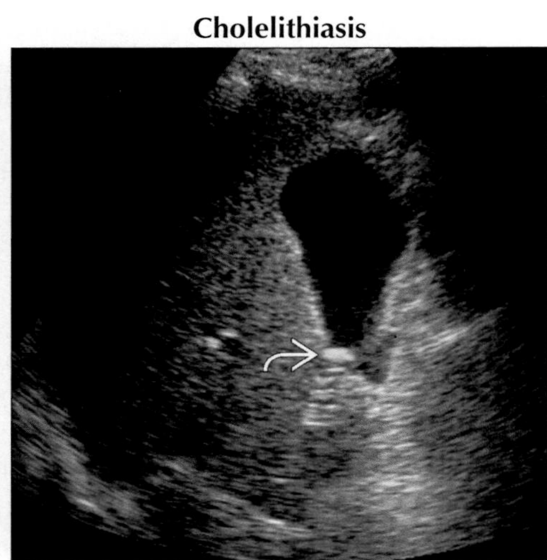

(**Left**) *Longitudinal ultrasound demonstrates the classic wall ➔ echo ➔ shadow ➔ (WES) complex of a collapsed gallbladder around multiple gallstones.* (**Right**) *Frontal radiograph shows numerous punctate calcifications ➔ projecting over the liver silhouette. The number of calcifications and distribution pattern help to narrow the differential diagnosis.*

Cholelithiasis

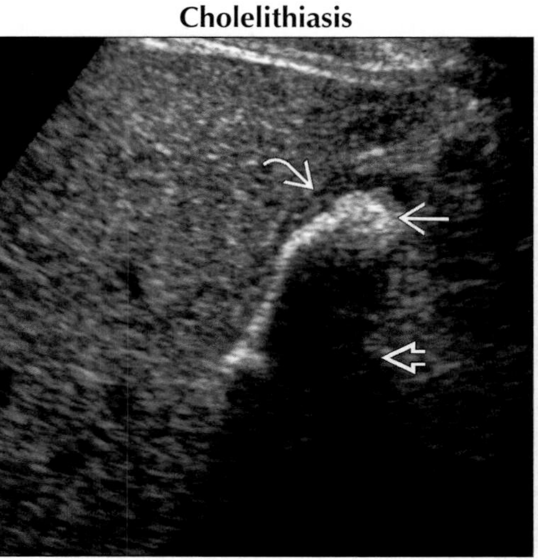

Hepatic and Splenic Granulomas

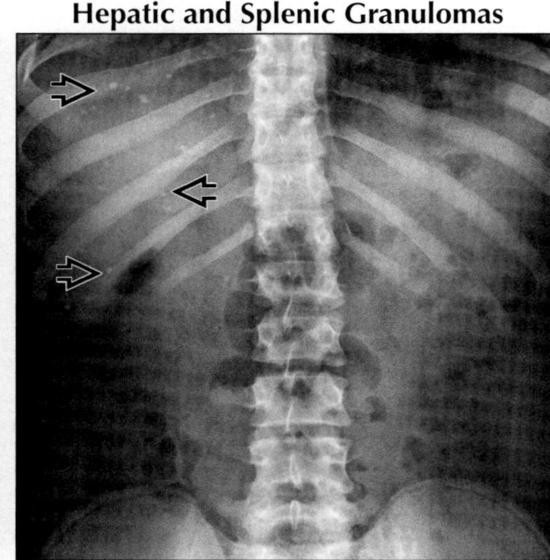

Hepatic and Splenic Granulomas

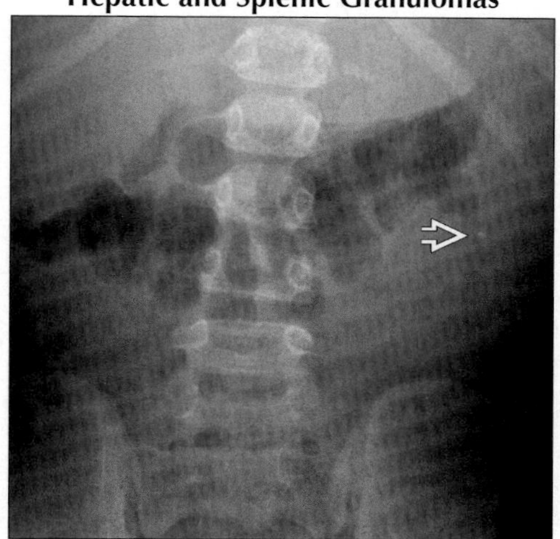

Hepatic and Splenic Granulomas

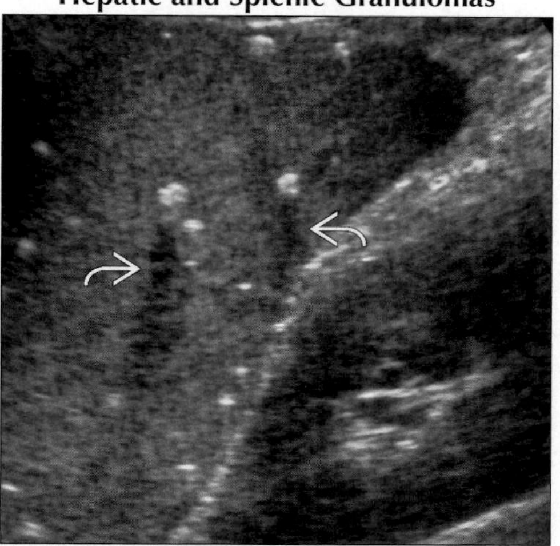

*(**Left**) Frontal radiograph shows an incidental punctate calcification ➡ projecting over the lower pole of the splenic silhouette. This was determined to be a splenic granuloma in this asymptomatic patient. (**Right**) Longitudinal ultrasound demonstrates numerous scattered echogenic foci. Only 2 of these echogenic foci demonstrate posterior acoustic shadowing ➡.*

Neuroblastoma

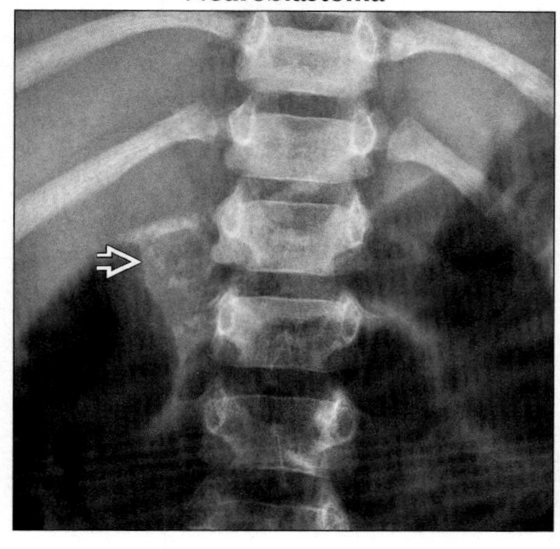

Neuroblastoma

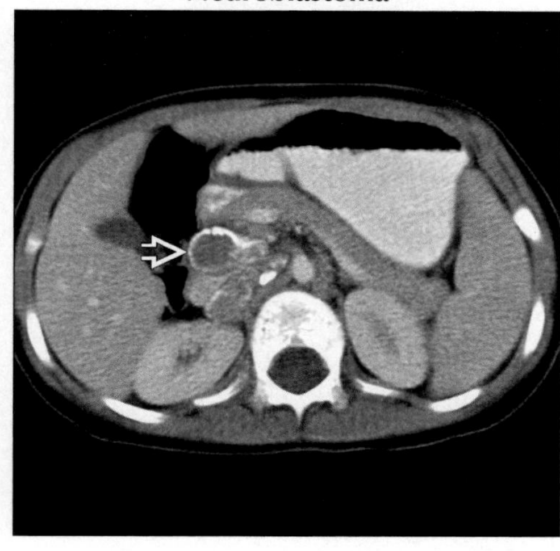

*(**Left**) Frontal radiograph shows a tight cluster of curvilinear calcifications ➡ to the right of the proximal lumbar spine. In a paraspinal location, one should scrutinize the CT or MR findings to exclude intraspinal extension. (**Right**) Axial CECT demonstrates curvilinear calcifications ➡ associated with a solid mass in a right paraspinal location. No intraspinal extension was identified. Look for a neuroblastoma to encase instead of displace vascular structures.*

Neuroblastoma

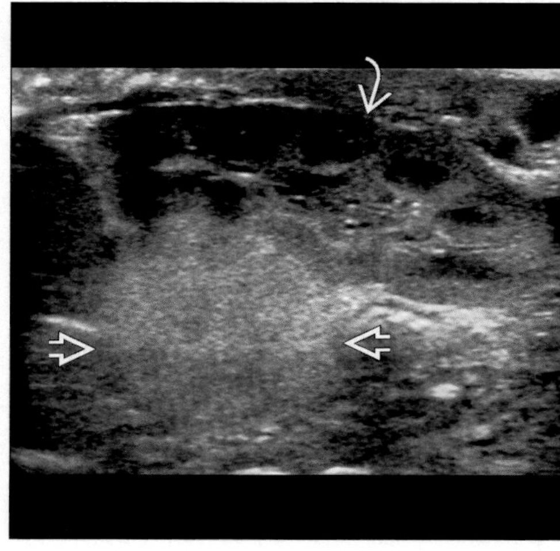

Hepatoblastoma

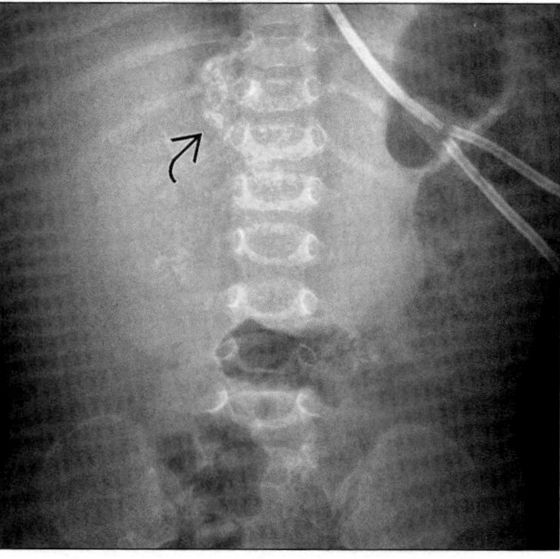

*(**Left**) Longitudinal oblique ultrasound demonstrates a solid paraspinal mass ➡ that is displacing the left kidney ➡ laterally and inferiorly. This mass proved to be MIBG avid, consistent with a neuroblastoma. (**Right**) Frontal radiograph shows a cluster of coarse calcifications ➡ projecting over the left lobe of the liver. With this paraspinal location, both a neuroblastoma and hepatoblastoma should be considered.*

ABDOMINAL CALCIFICATIONS

Hepatoblastoma

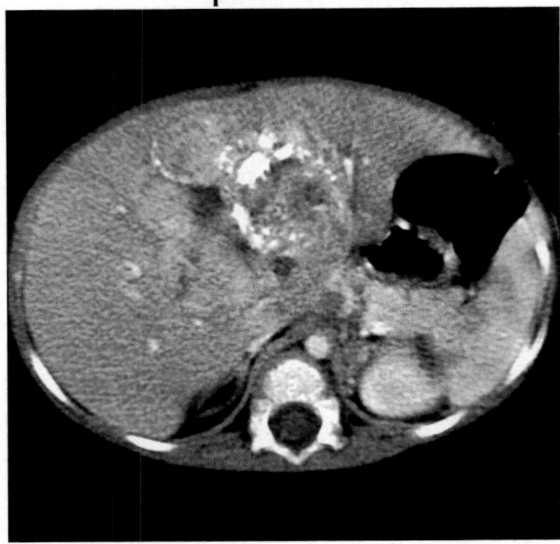

Hepatoblastoma

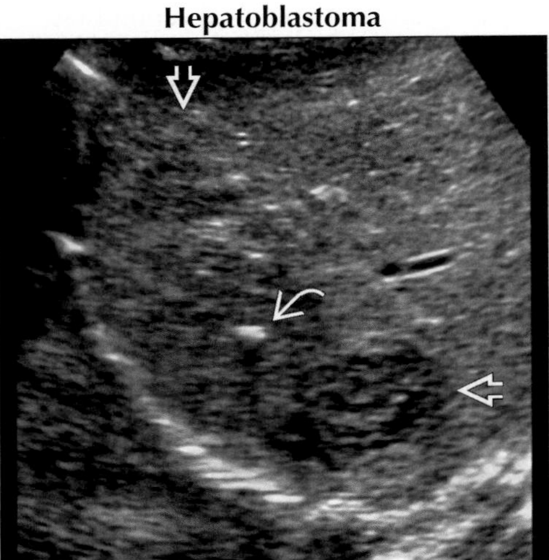

(Left) *Axial CECT in the same patient shows numerous coarse calcifications associated with a solid left hepatic mass. This mass was confined to the left lobe of the liver, which is unusual, as the majority of hepatoblastomas are located within the right lobe of the liver.* ***(Right)*** *Longitudinal ultrasound demonstrates a permeative hypoechoic solid lesion ➡ in the right lobe of the liver. Note the shadowing calcifications ➡ associated with this lesion.*

Teratoma (Ovarian)

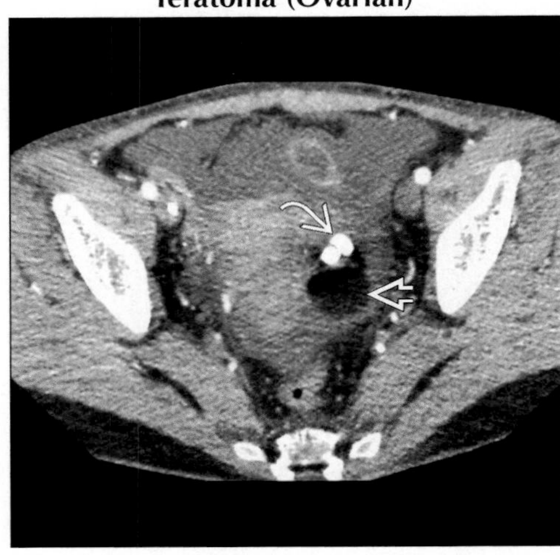

Teratoma (Ovarian)

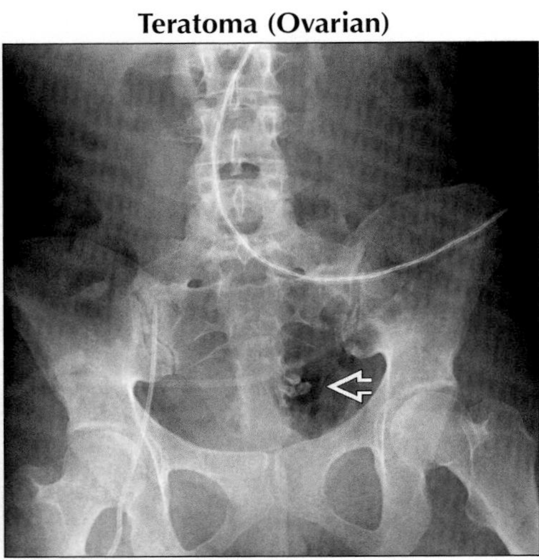

(Left) *Axial CECT demonstrates a left adnexal teratoma with 2 rounded calcifications ➡ and a fat-fluid level ➡. Ovarian torsion may be a complication; however, that was not the case with this patient.* ***(Right)*** *Frontal radiograph shows a cluster of rounded calcifications ➡ projecting over the left lower pelvis. In this location, teratoma as well as bladder stones may be in the differential diagnosis.*

Teratoma (Ovarian)

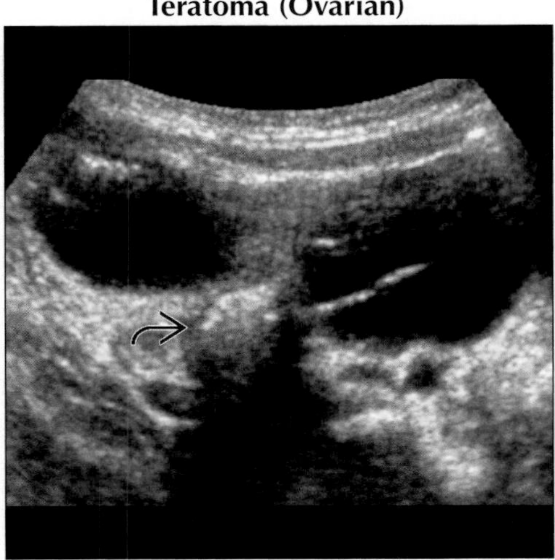

Appendicolith

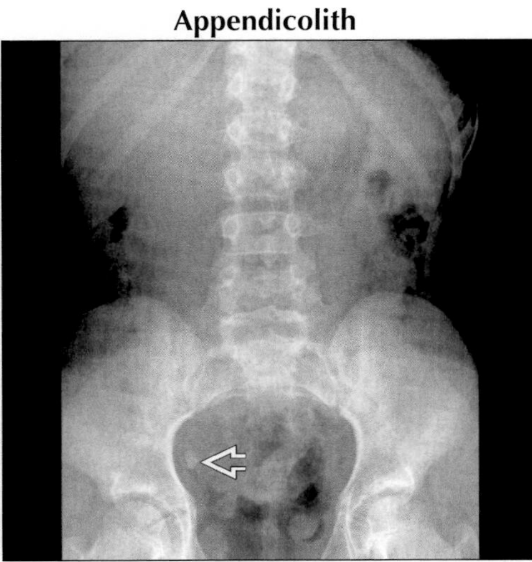

(Left) *Transverse ultrasound demonstrates a mixed cystic and solid lesion in the left adnexa. There are numerous shadowing calcifications ➡ associated with this lesion.* ***(Right)*** *Frontal radiograph demonstrates a calcification in the right lower pelvis ➡. Appendicolith are identified on conventional radiographs in 10-15% of patients. The patient had a positive McBurney sign.*

Appendicolith

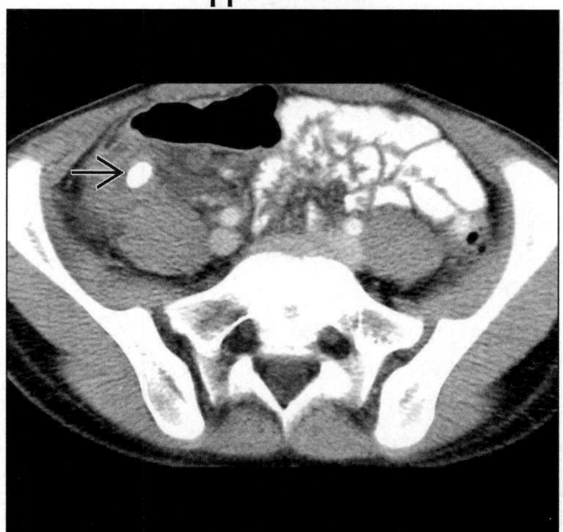

Appendicolith

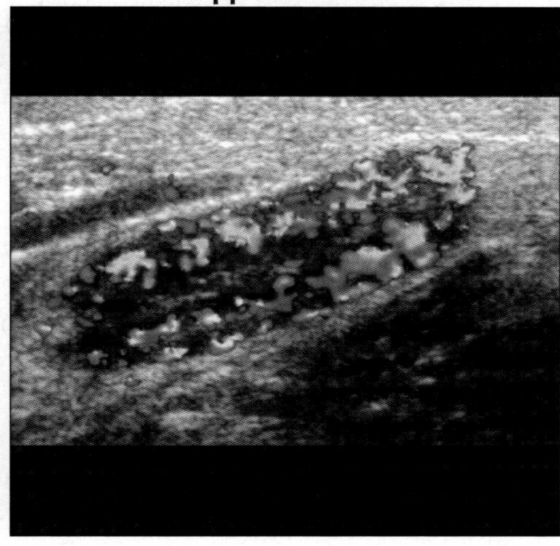

(Left) *Axial CECT demonstrates an extraluminal appendicolith ⇒ in a perforated appendix. The signs of perforation include the surrounding pelvic fluid, mesenteric induration, and phlegmon. There was no drainable abscess present.* ***(Right)*** *Longitudinal oblique color Doppler ultrasound demonstrates diffuse hyperemia of the acutely inflamed appendix.*

Remote Adrenal Hemorrhage

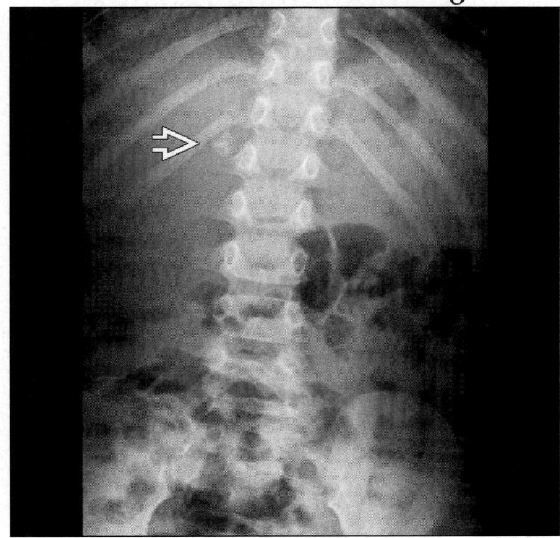

Remote Adrenal Hemorrhage

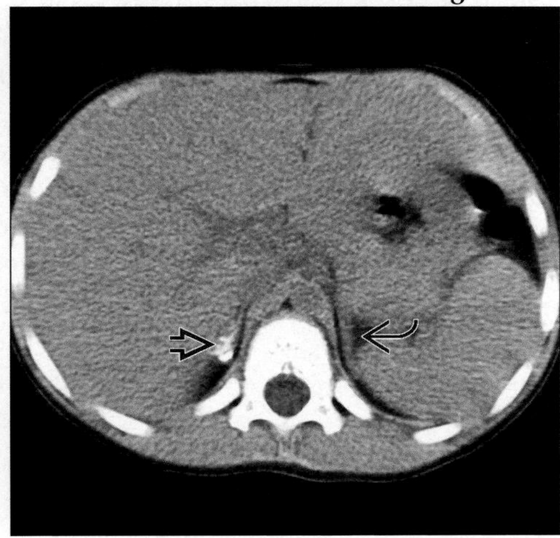

(Left) *Frontal radiograph shows an incidental cluster of punctate calcifications ⇨ located to the right of the lumbar spine. This collection of calcifications is situated cranial to the right renal silhouette.* ***(Right)*** *Axial NECT shows a small cluster of calcifications associated with the right adrenal gland ⇨. The left adrenal gland ↪ is not calcified. Bilateral adrenal calcifications related to prior hemorrhage occur in approximately 10% of cases.*

Remote Adrenal Hemorrhage

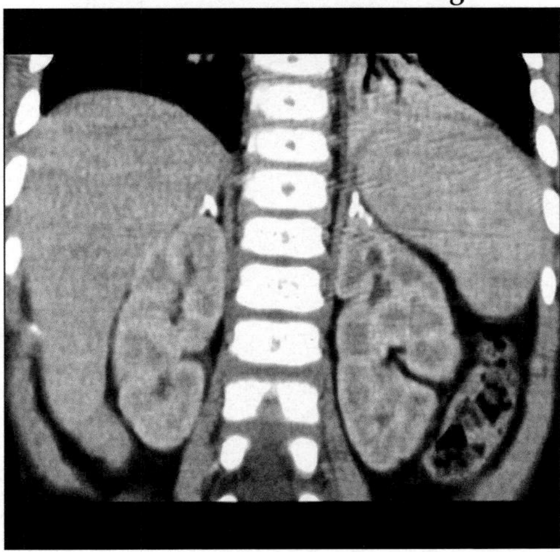

Meconium Peritonitis

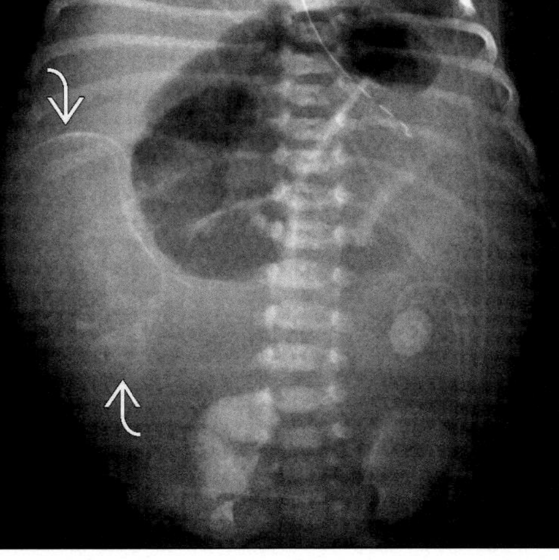

(Left) *Coronal CECT demonstrates bilateral adrenal gland calcifications. Notice that the calcifications conform to the expected contour of the adrenal gland. The primary diagnosis would be resolved adrenal hemorrhage.* ***(Right)*** *Frontal radiograph demonstrates a large space-occupying lesion with a thin calcified rim ↪. Notice the mass effect with displacement of bowel to the left. This was a 1 day old neonate with an in utero diagnosed meconium pseudocyst.*

PNEUMATOSIS

DIFFERENTIAL DIAGNOSIS

Common
- Necrotizing Enterocolitis
- Neutropenic Colitis

Less Common
- Steroid Use
- Rotavirus, Other Infection
- High Intrathoracic Pressures
  - Asthma
  - Cystic Fibrosis, Lung
  - High Ventilator Pressures
- Post-Surgery/Post-Endoscopy
- Idiopathic

ESSENTIAL INFORMATION

Key Differential Diagnosis Issues
- Does the child appear toxic or well?
- Concurrent medical/surgical history

Helpful Clues for Common Diagnoses
- **Necrotizing Enterocolitis**
  - Most common in premature infants
    - Others at risk include those with congenital heart disease, indomethacin therapy, perinatal asphyxia
  - Progresses over short period of time
  - Normal bowel gas pattern → elongated distended loops → pneumatosis ± portal venous gas &/or pneumoperitoneum
  - Radiographs
    - Fine linear arrays of air within wall when seen on edge
    - Foamy appearance when seen en face, sometimes difficult to distinguish from normal stool
  - Ultrasound
    - Thickened walls, poor peristalsis
    - Intramural air may be seen
- **Neutropenic Colitis**
  - High risk groups include those with acute lymphocytic leukemia, acute myelogenous leukemia, bone marrow transplant recipients
  - Can involve any segment of small bowel or colon: Proclivity for right colon; cecum most commonly involved
  - Commonly accepted etiology: Breakdown of bowel mucosa with bacterial infiltration
  - CT findings
    - Bowel wall thickening with pneumatosis
    - Inflammatory stranding, ascites

Helpful Clues for Less Common Diagnoses
- **Steroid Use**
  - Used by patients with asthma, cystic fibrosis, inflammatory/autoimmune disorders; ask clinician
- **Rotavirus, Other Infection**
  - None of above comorbidities; positive stool culture
- **High Ventilator Pressures**
  - May be either benign pneumatosis intestinalis or incipient bowel necrosis in ICU patients

Necrotizing Enterocolitis

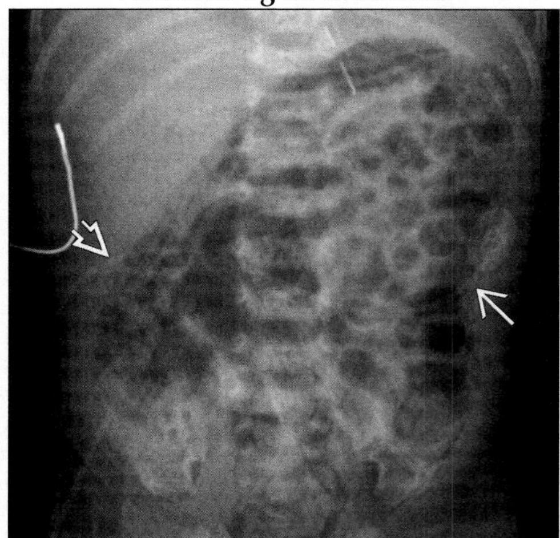

Frontal radiograph in an infant shows extensive pneumatosis. Note the linear bubbly arrays seen on edge ➔ and the foamy areas seen en face ➔. The pneumatosis resolved in this patient.

Necrotizing Enterocolitis

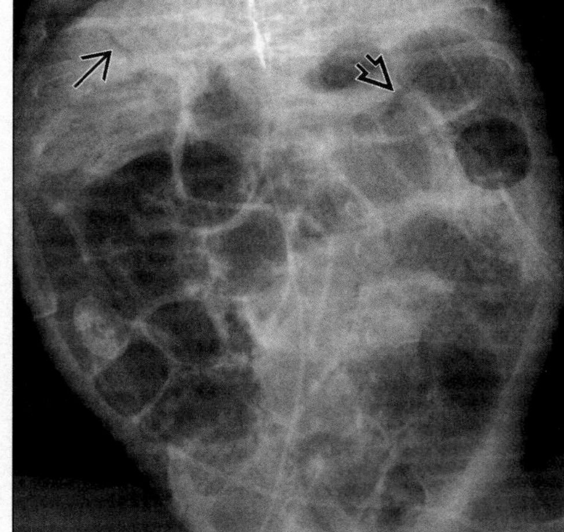

Frontal radiograph shows striking portal venous gas ➔, bowel distension, and pneumatosis ➔. Branches of portal venous gas typically extend to the periphery of the liver. This patient died.

PNEUMATOSIS

Neutropenic Colitis

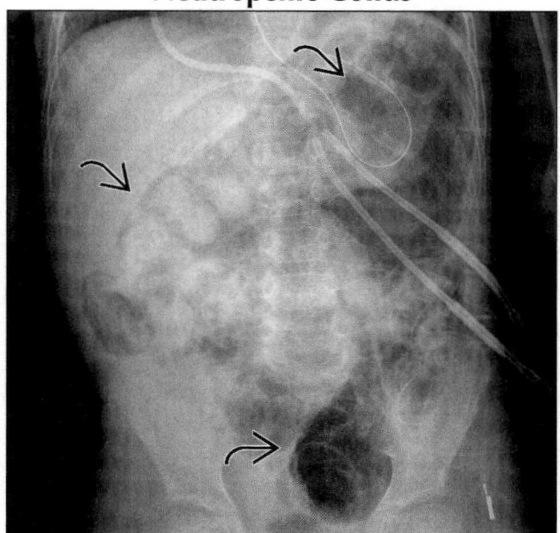

Neutropenic Colitis

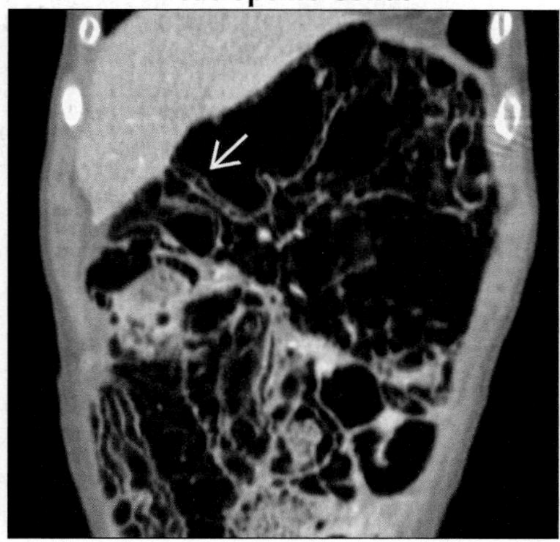

(Left) *Frontal radiograph shows such widespread pneumatosis → that the normal bowel wall is difficult to identify. Other clues such as accompanying pneumoperitoneum or portal venous gas are helpful, if they are present.* ***(Right)*** *Coronal CECT in the same patient shows the extensive pneumatosis in greater detail. Compare the right hepatic flexure appearance of pneumatosis → with the same region on the previous radiograph.*

Steroid Use

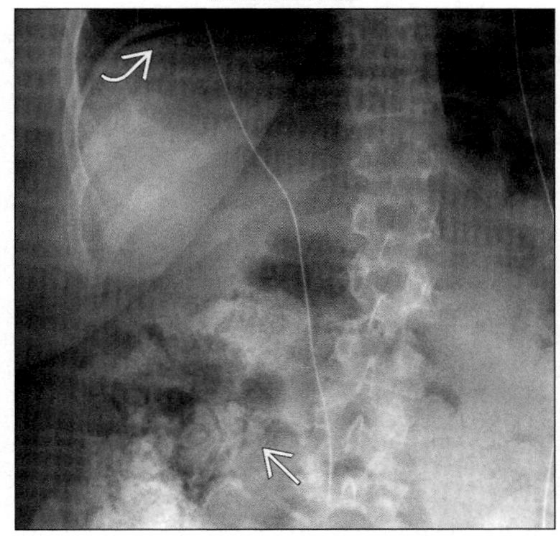

Rotavirus, Other Infection

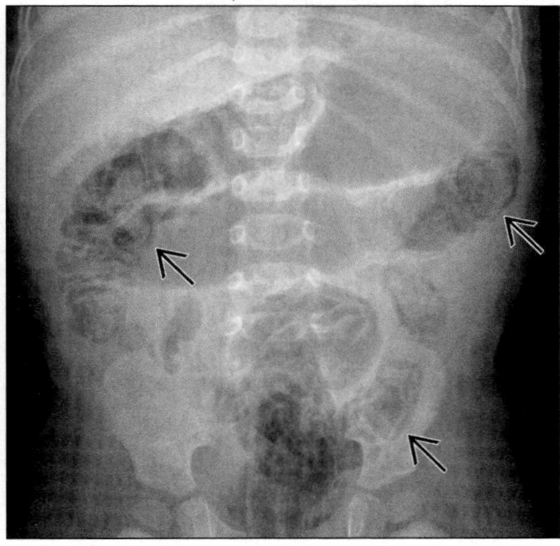

(Left) *Frontal radiograph shows subtle linear lucencies → representing mild pneumatosis at the hepatic flexure in this female teenager requiring steroids for dermatomyositis. This was confirmed with CT. Note the small amount of pneumoperitoneum → under the diaphragm.* ***(Right)*** *Frontal radiograph → shows pan-colonic pneumatosis in this child with a stool culture positive for rotavirus. The child recovered, and the pneumatosis resolved within a week.*

Post-Surgery/Post-Endoscopy

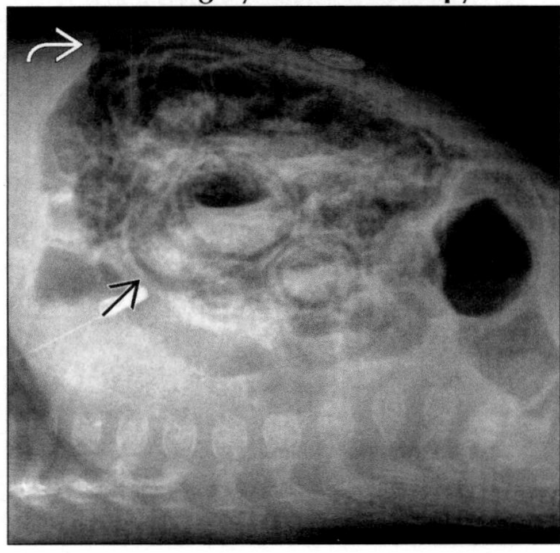

Post-Surgery/Post-Endoscopy

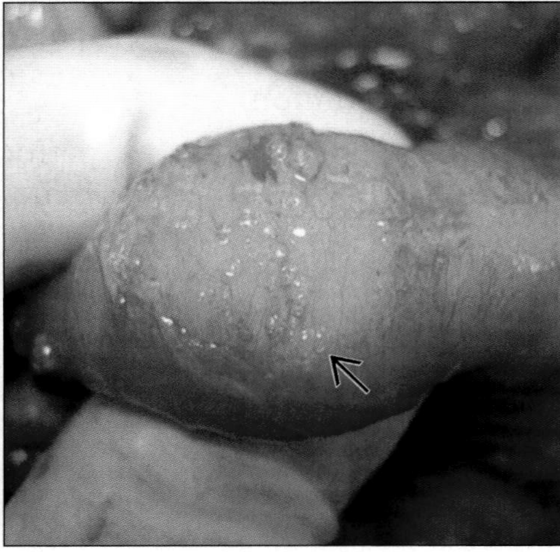

(Left) *Tangential radiograph shows unexpected extensive ring-like lucencies representing pneumatosis → and a small amount pneumoperitoneum → in this patient with prior gastroschisis repair.* ***(Right)*** *Surgical photograph in the same patient shows a pink healthy bowel wall discovered at surgery (post-gastroschisis repair). Note the grossly visible air bubbles → on the serosal surface. This was benign idiopathic pneumatosis.*

PNEUMOPERITONEUM

DIFFERENTIAL DIAGNOSIS

Common
- Postoperative
- Necrotizing Enterocolitis (NEC)

Less Common
- Traumatic Bowel Injury
- Dissection from Pneumothorax or Pneumomediastinum
- Medications
- Appendicitis
- Iatrogenic
- Infection

Rare but Important
- Spontaneous Gastric Perforation
- Distal Intestinal Obstruction
- Lymphoma
- Perforated Peptic Ulcer
- Ehlers-Danlos Syndrome

ESSENTIAL INFORMATION

Key Differential Diagnosis Issues
- CT is most sensitive modality
  - Air rises to nondependent location
- Left lateral decubitus and cross table lateral views are most sensitive radiographic views
- In neonates, "football" sign may be present
  - Falciform ligament appears as laces of football due to massive pneumoperitoneum
  - Less common in older children and adults
- Other radiographic signs
  - Air under diaphragm
  - Triangular lucencies
  - Air outlining both sides of bowel wall

Helpful Clues for Common Diagnoses
- **Postoperative**
  - Residual pneumoperitoneum is common after abdominal surgery
    - Duration of free air is determined by its initial volume and absorption rate
    - Usually resolves within 1 week
    - May last as long as 10-24 days
  - Laparoscopy uses carbon dioxide to distend abdomen during surgery
    - CO_2 is absorbed faster than room air
  - Amount and duration of postoperative air is proportional to age in pediatric patients
    - Older children have larger volume of free air → lasts longer
  - If greater than expected air is present, evaluate for perforation or dehiscence
- **Necrotizing Enterocolitis (NEC)**
  - 1 of most common surgical emergencies in infants
  - Disease of prematurity
    - > 90% occur in children born < 36 weeks
    - Occurs in 3-7% of NICU patients
  - Rate is inversely related to birth weight
  - ↑ incidence in African-Americans and males
  - May present with feeding intolerance, bilious aspirates, or abdominal distension
  - Radiographic findings include fixed dilated loops of bowel, pneumatosis, portal venous gas, and free air
    - If clinical suspicion for NEC exists, abdominal radiographs should be performed every 6 hours
  - Treatment can be medical or surgical
    - Indications for surgical treatment include pneumoperitoneum or other signs of bowel perforation
    - 20-40% with NEC require surgery

Helpful Clues for Less Common Diagnoses
- **Traumatic Bowel Injury**
  - Incidence of small bowel injury has increased with increased seat belt use
  - ~ 5% of patients admitted with major trauma suffer small bowel injury
  - Jejunal injuries may be most common
  - Delay in diagnosis of bowel injury can lead to ↑ morbidity and mortality
  - Often associated with other injuries
  - Radiologic findings of bowel injury include free fluid, bowel wall thickening, and pneumoperitoneum
  - CT can be useful to predict site of perforation
    - Findings include concentration of extraluminal gas, segmental bowel wall thickening, and focal defect
  - In infants and neonates, penetrating trauma can be caused by thermometer placement
  - Sexual abuse can cause colonic perforation
- **Dissection from Pneumothorax or Pneumomediastinum**

- Free air from pneumothorax or pneumomediastinum can dissect into abdomen
- Air enters through diaphragmatic crus or rents in diaphragm

- **Medications**
  - Indomethacin
    - Used to help close patent ductus arteriosus
    - Also can ↓ GI blood flow and lead to intestinal perforation
- **Appendicitis**
  - Pneumoperitoneum is rare with perforated appendicitis
  - If present, usually only a few locules of air
- **Iatrogenic**
  - Bowel perforation can be caused by tube placement or endoscopy
  - Air enema for intussusception reduction
    - Incidence of perforation is very low
    - With air enema, perforation can lead to tension pneumoperitoneum
    - Tension pneumoperitoneum should be treated with needle decompression
- **Infection**
  - Most common cause of nontraumatic colonic perforation
    - *Salmonella* is most common bacteria that causes perforation

Helpful Clues for Rare Diagnoses

- **Spontaneous Gastric Perforation**
  - Usually occurs at 2-7 days of life in term infants
  - More common in African-Americans and males
  - Prenatal risk factors
    - Premature rupture of membranes, toxemia, breech delivery, diabetic mother, group B *Streptococcus* positive mother, placenta previa, abruption, and emergent cesarean delivery
  - Postnatal risk factors
    - Prematurity, low birth weight, small for gestational age, low Apgar scores, respiratory distress, exchange transfusion, and indomethacin treatment
  - Presents with sudden onset of abdominal distension
  - Large volume of pneumoperitoneum
    - Most common cause of "football" sign
- **Distal Intestinal Obstruction**
  - In neonate, causes can include Hirschsprung disease, meconium ileus, atresias, or malrotation with midgut volvulus
- **Lymphoma**
  - Primary bowel lymphoma manifests as focal bowel wall thickening
  - With chemotherapy, perforation can occur
- **Perforated Peptic Ulcer**
  - Now rare with treatment of *H. pylori*
- **Ehlers-Danlos Syndrome**
  - Connective tissue disorder
  - Spontaneous colonic perforation is seen in Ehlers-Danlos type 4

Postoperative

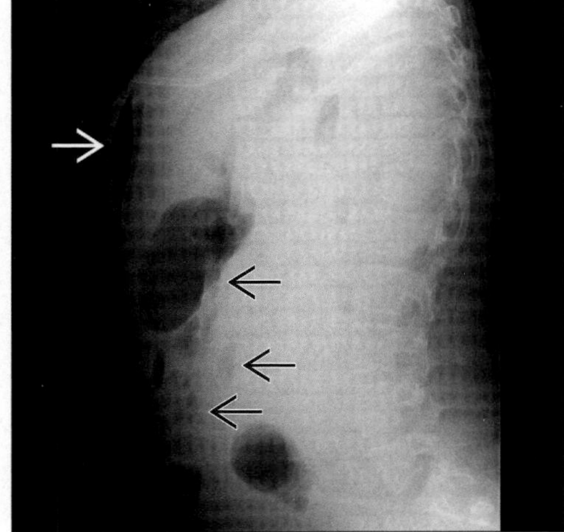

Cross table lateral radiograph in a patient 12 days status post Nissen fundoplication shows pneumoperitoneum ➡ within the upper abdomen. Multiple air-fluid levels are also present ➡.

Postoperative

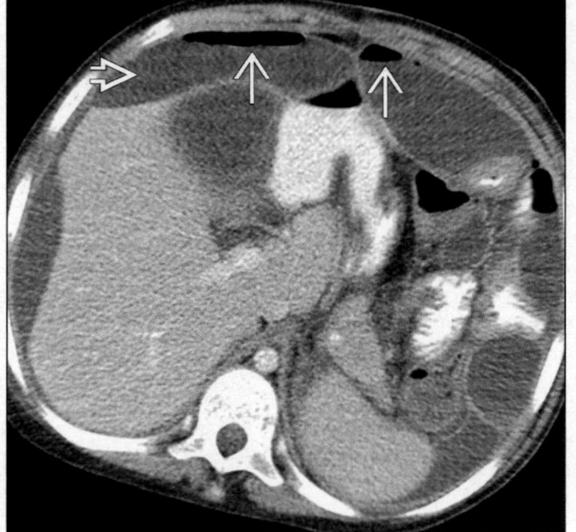

Axial CECT in the same patient shows locules of free air ➡ within a moderate amount of ascites ➡. Residual pneumoperitoneum is common after surgery and may last as long as 10-24 days.

PNEUMOPERITONEUM

(Left) Anteroposterior radiograph in a patient post cholecystectomy shows a small amount of pneumoperitoneum → just below the right hemidiaphragm. Amount & duration of postoperative pneumoperitoneum is proportional to age. (Right) Anteroposterior radiograph shows multiple dilated & distended air-filled loops of the bowel →. Note the bubbly lucencies of pneumatosis → in the LLQ & branching lucencies of portal venous gas →.

Postoperative

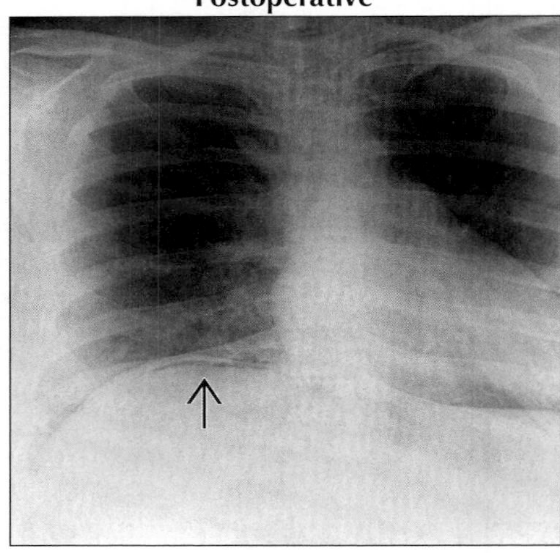

Necrotizing Enterocolitis (NEC)

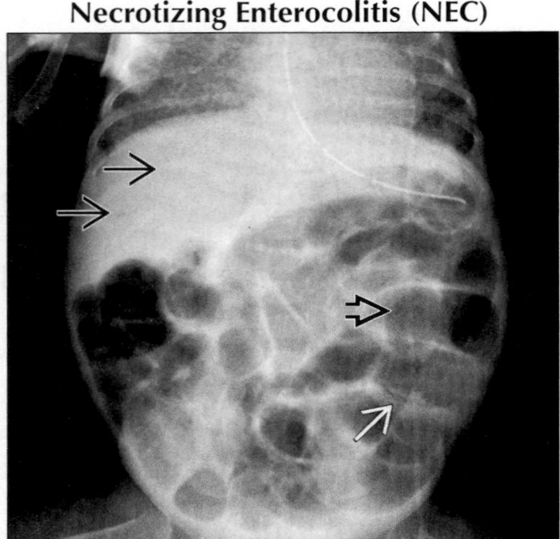

(Left) Anteroposterior radiograph shows a large volume of free air. Air is seen underneath the right hemidiaphragm → and throughout the lower abdomen. Air outlines both sides of the bowel wall (Rigler sign) →. (Right) Cross table lateral radiograph shows a large volume of free air outlining the anterior liver edge → and multiple loops of the bowel →. Necrotizing enterocolitis is a disease of prematurity with its incidence inversely related to birth weight.

Necrotizing Enterocolitis (NEC)

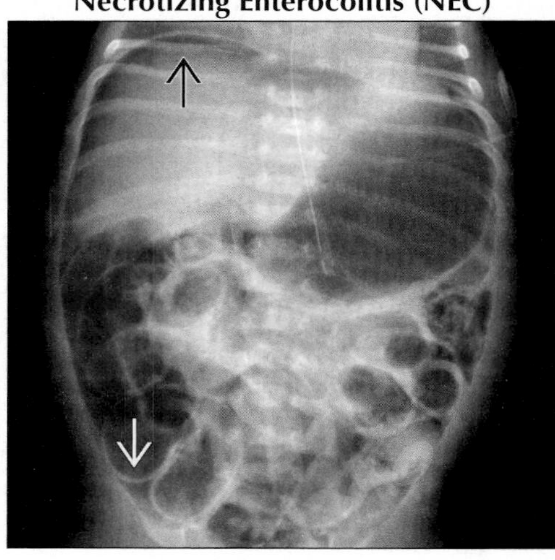

Necrotizing Enterocolitis (NEC)

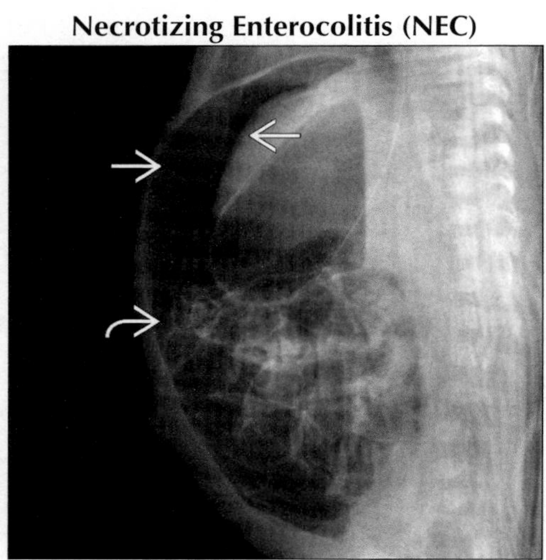

(Left) Anteroposterior radiograph shows extensive pneumatosis intestinalis →. Note the triangular lucency → in the right upper quadrant, consistent with a small amount of pneumoperitoneum. NEC is 1 of the most common surgical emergencies in children. (Right) Cross table lateral radiograph in the same patient shows extensive pneumatosis → and a small triangular lucency → of pneumoperitoneum.

Necrotizing Enterocolitis (NEC)

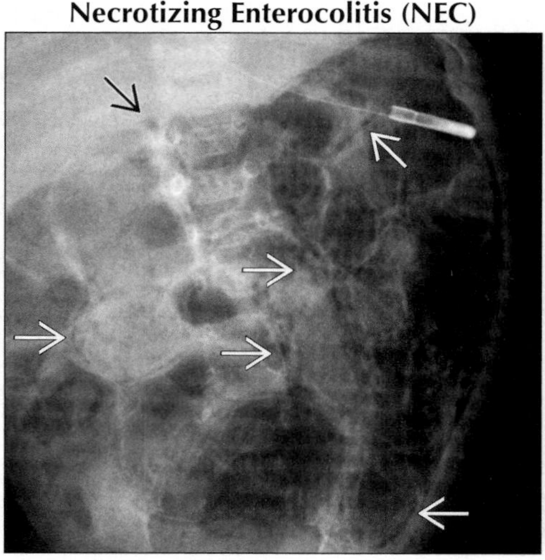

Necrotizing Enterocolitis (NEC)

Traumatic Bowel Injury

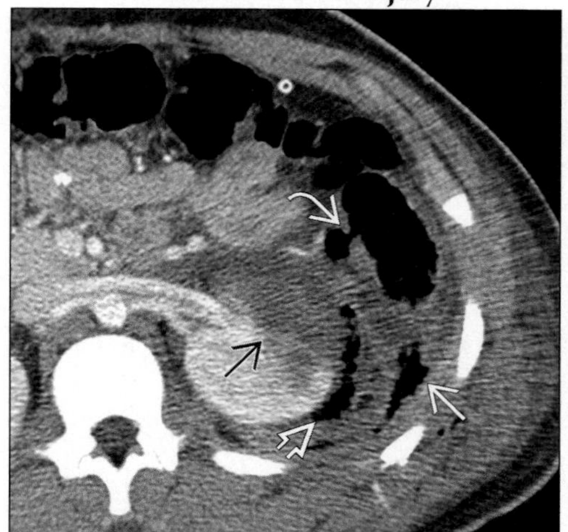

Dissection from Pneumothorax or Pneumomediastinum

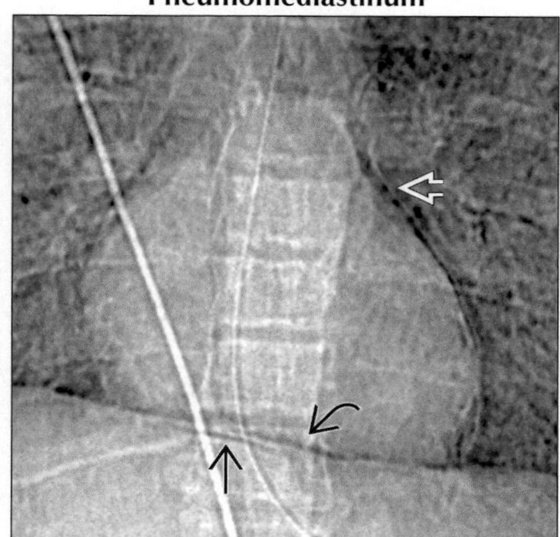

(Left) *Axial CECT in a patient with a gunshot wound shows a colonic perforation ➦ and pneumoperitoneum ➡. The anterior half of the left kidney was injured and does not enhance ➔. Air is present in the left perirenal space ➡.* ***(Right)*** *Anteroposterior scout image from CECT shows air both above ➦ and below ➔ the diaphragm. Pneumomediastinum is present ➡. Earlier studies (not shown) revealed a large tension pneumothorax.*

Medications

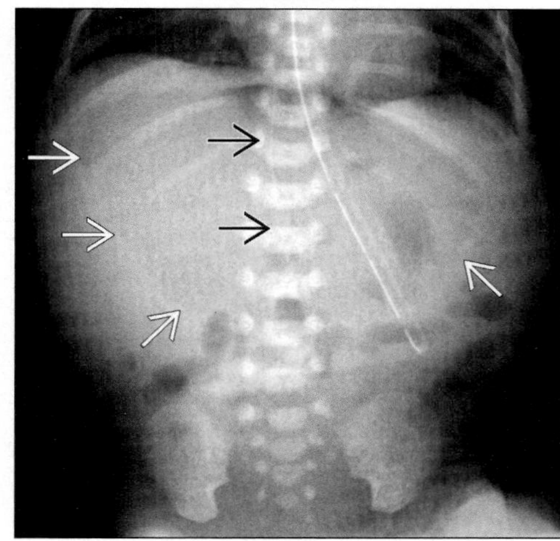

Iatrogenic

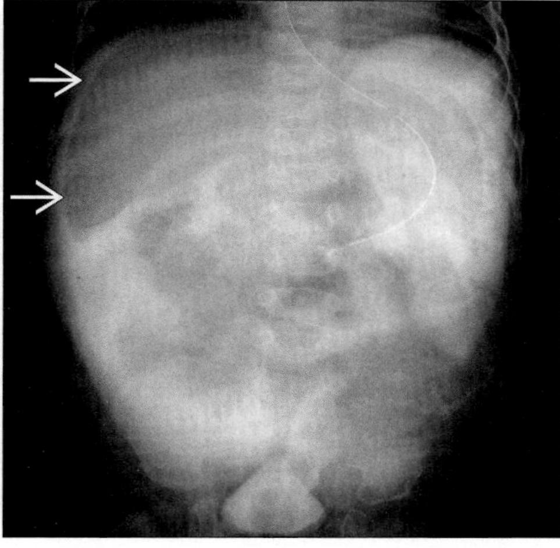

(Left) *Anteroposterior radiograph shows a large volume of pneumoperitoneum ➡ in a premature infant treated with indomethacin. The falciform ligament ➔ is seen overlying the spine, giving the "football" sign.* ***(Right)*** *Anteroposterior radiograph in a patient with bowel perforation during colostogram shows a dense intraperitoneal contrast. The lucency ➡ that corresponds to the liver mimics pneumoperitoneum.*

Spontaneous Gastric Perforation

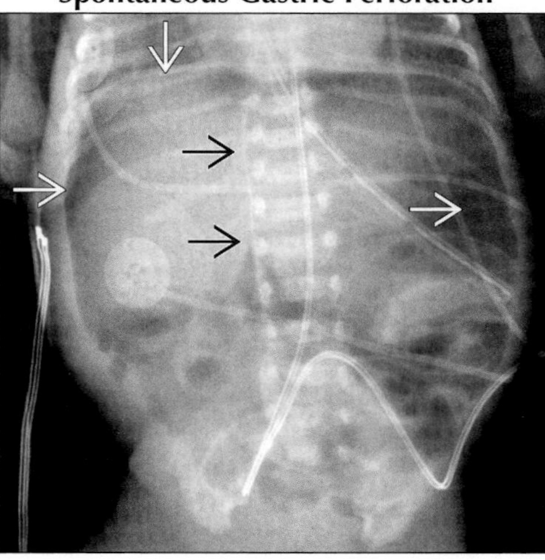

Spontaneous Gastric Perforation

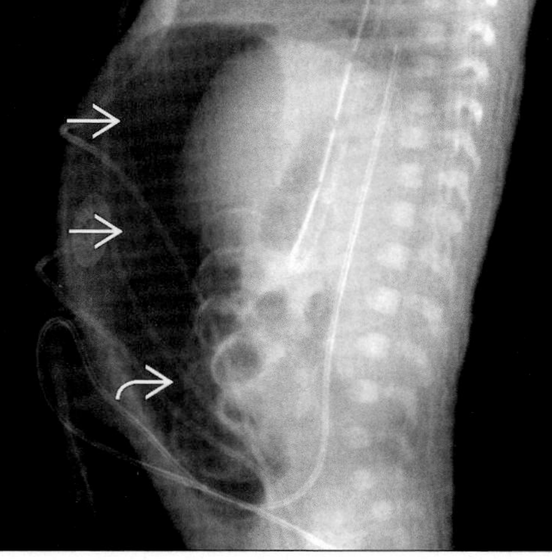

(Left) *Anteroposterior radiograph shows massive pneumoperitoneum ➡. The falciform ligament ➔ is outlined adjacent to the spine. Spontaneous gastric perforation is the most common cause of "football" sign.* ***(Right)*** *Cross table lateral radiograph shows massive pneumoperitoneum ➡. This, along with intraluminal bowel gas, outlines both sides of the bowel wall ➦. Spontaneous gastric perforation usually occurs at 2-7 days of life in term infants.*

SECTION 4
Genitourinary

RETROPERITONEAL MASS

DIFFERENTIAL DIAGNOSIS

Common
- Lymphoma
- Neuroblastoma

Less Common
- Abscess
- Lymphatic Malformation
- Metastases
- Retroperitoneal Hematoma
- Duodenal Hematoma

Rare but Important
- Neurofibromatosis Type 1
- Extraadrenal Pheochromocytoma
- Lipoblastoma
- Retroperitoneal Fibrosis

ESSENTIAL INFORMATION

Key Differential Diagnosis Issues
- Most retroperitoneal masses are malignant
  - Lymphoma and neuroblastoma most common
- US is useful screening modality

Helpful Clues for Common Diagnoses
- **Lymphoma**
  - 3rd most common pediatric malignancy after leukemia and CNS tumors
  - 10-15% of all childhood cancers
  - Incidence increases with age
  - Non-Hodgkin lymphoma is more common than Hodgkin lymphoma in children younger than 10 years old
  - More common in males
  - Burkitt and diffuse large B-cell lymphoma most common types to affect retroperitoneum
- **Neuroblastoma**
  - Most common solid extracranial malignancy
    - 6-10% of all childhood cancers
    - 15% of pediatric cancer deaths
  - 4th most common pediatric malignancy (leukemia, CNS tumors, and lymphoma)
  - 2nd most common abdominal neoplasm (Wilms tumor)
  - > 90% of patients diagnosed before age 5
    - Median age at diagnosis is 22 months
    - Peak incidence in 1st year of life (30%)
  - Can arise anywhere along sympathetic chain
  - ~ 70% originate in retroperitoneum
    - 35% in adrenal medulla
    - 30-35% in extraadrenal paraspinal ganglia
  - Mediastinum is 3rd most common location (20%)
  - Patients < 1 year old have better prognosis
  - Abdominal mass is most common presentation
    - Can present with bruising around eyes
    - Paraneoplastic syndromes in ~ 2%
  - 50% have metastases at diagnosis
    - Most common to liver, bone, and bone marrow
    - Hepatic metastases can be diffuse or nodular
  - Calcifications are present in ~ 85%
  - I-123 MIBG uptake in 90-95% of patients
  - MR is useful to see intraspinal involvement
  - Prognosis varies depending on stage
    - Staged by International Neuroblastoma Staging System

Helpful Clues for Less Common Diagnoses
- **Abscess**
  - Can be due to ruptured appendix, surgery, Crohn disease, and osteomyelitis
  - Most infections are polymicrobial
  - Can cross boundaries
  - Consider tuberculosis if vertebral osteomyelitis extends to retroperitoneal soft tissues
- **Lymphatic Malformation**
  - a.k.a. mesenteric cyst
  - Congenital benign tumor
  - Can be found at all anatomic locations
    - Most common in head and neck
    - ~ 20% in abdomen
    - ~ 5% in retroperitoneum
  - Can cross anatomic compartments
  - Large, thin-walled, multiseptated cystic mass
  - Rare calcifications in wall
- **Metastases**
  - Testicular metastases are most common
    - Spreads to retroperitoneal lymph nodes
- **Retroperitoneal Hematoma**
  - Can be seen after trauma or in hypocoagulable state

- Appearance depends on time between hemorrhage and imaging
- **Duodenal Hematoma**
  - Unusual finding in setting of trauma
    - Accounts for < 5% of intraabdominal injuries
  - Due to forces that compress duodenum between spine and fixed object
    - Seatbelt, handlebars, and abuse are most common causes
    - Iatrogenic trauma from instrumentation can also occur
  - Associated with pancreatic injuries

Helpful Clues for Rare Diagnoses

- **Neurofibromatosis Type 1**
  - Autosomal dominant disorder
  - Classical clinical findings include café-au-lait spots, axillary freckling, and dermal and plexiform neurofibromas
  - Plexiform neurofibromas can occur in abdomen
    - Most common in abdominal wall and retroperitoneum
  - Retroperitoneal neurofibromas can cause mass effect on spinal cord, bowel obstruction, and ureteric obstruction
  - Plexiform neurofibromas have targetoid appearance on MR
    - Loss of targetoid appearance should raise concern for degeneration into malignant peripheral nerve sheath tumor
- **Extraadrenal Pheochromocytoma**
  - a.k.a. paraganglioma
  - ~ 30% of all pediatric pheochromocytomas are extraadrenal
  - 85% of extraadrenal pheochromocytomas are retroperitoneal
    - Organ of Zuckerkandl is most common site of origin
  - Most common in 2nd-3rd decade
  - Associated with von Hippel Lindau, MEN type 2, and neurofibromatosis type 1
  - 20-50% are malignant
    - Most commonly metastasize to bone, liver, and lungs
  - Often presents with hypertension
    - Cause of hypertension in ~ 1% of children
  - Appear hyperintense on T2WIs
  - I-123 MIBG both sensitive and specific for detection
  - No proven risk of hypertensive crisis with iodinated contrast
- **Lipoblastoma**
  - Most common in children under age 3
  - Most commonly occurs in trunk and extremities
- **Retroperitoneal Fibrosis**
  - Rare disorder in children
  - In children, 50% are related to systemic process or autoimmune disorder
  - Insidious onset with nonspecific signs and symptoms
  - Appears as misty mesentery on CT early in disease process

Lymphoma

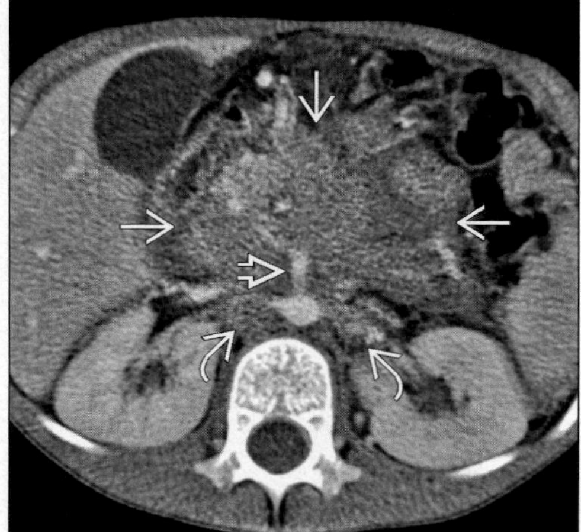

Axial CECT shows a conglomerate nodal mass ➔ surrounding the superior mesenteric artery ⇨. Nodes are also present in the periaortic and aortocaval region ↷.

Lymphoma

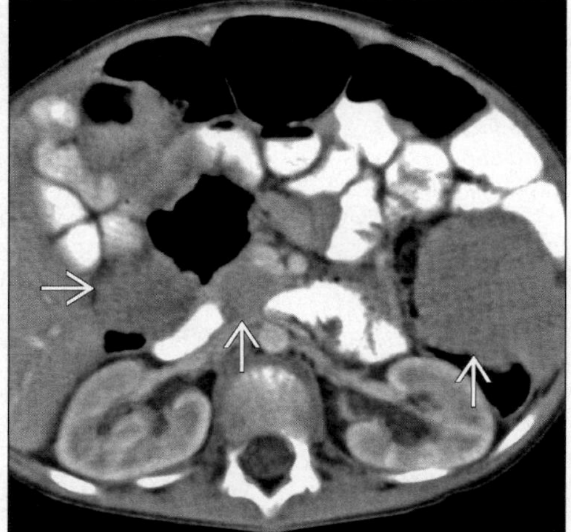

Axial CECT shows multiple enlarged lymph nodes ➔. Lymphoma is the 3rd most common malignancy in children, though more common in males than in females.

RETROPERITONEAL MASS

Lymphoma

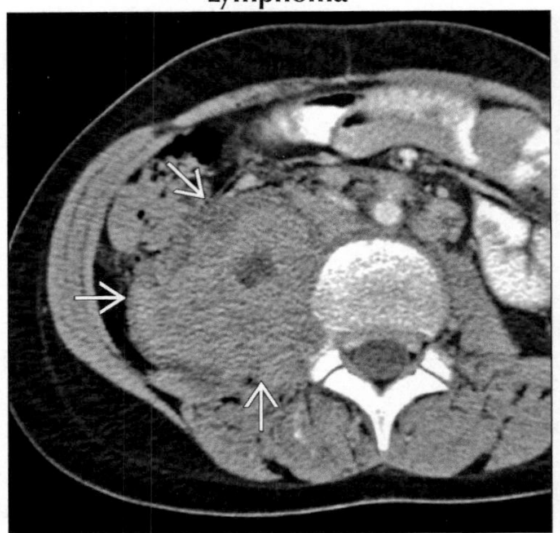

Lymphoma

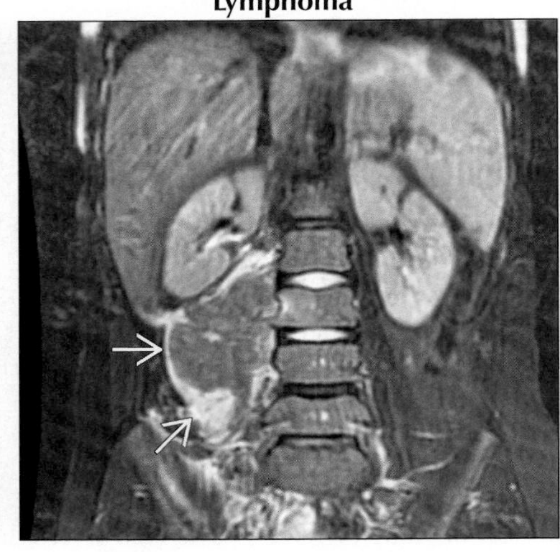

(Left) *Axial CECT shows a heterogeneous enhancing mass of the right psoas muscle ➡. The mass has a central area that does not enhance. Lymphoma accounts for 10-15% of all childhood cancers; its incidence increases with age.* ***(Right)*** *Coronal T2WI MR shows a large right paraspinal mass ➡ inferior to the kidney. The most common types of lymphoma to affect the retroperitoneum are Burkitt and diffuse large B-cell lymphoma.*

Neuroblastoma

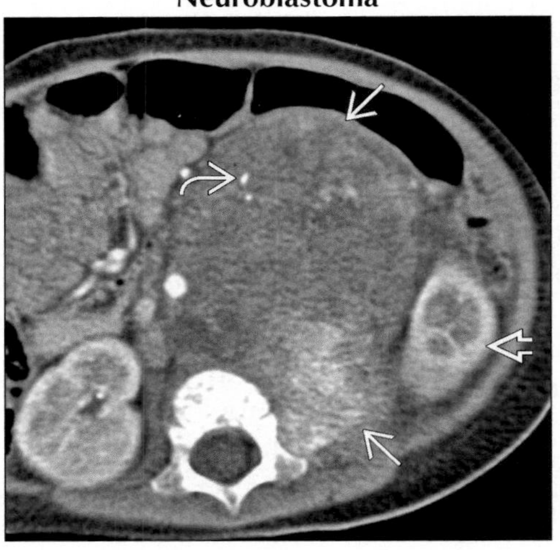

Neuroblastoma

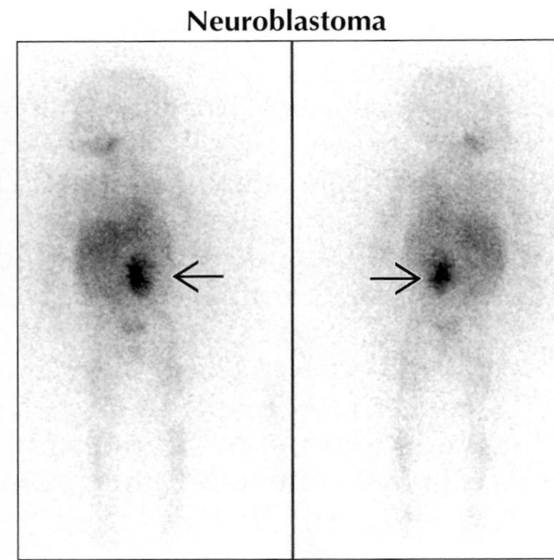

(Left) *Axial CECT shows a large left paraspinal mass ➡. There are several foci of increased attenuation ➡ within the mass that represents calcifications. The mass displaces the kidney ➡ laterally. In the paraspinal location, a neuroblastoma can extend through the neural foramina and compress the spinal cord (not shown).* ***(Right)*** *MIBG scintigraphy in the same patient in the anterior and posterior projection shows uptake confined to the left paraspinal mass ➡.*

Neuroblastoma

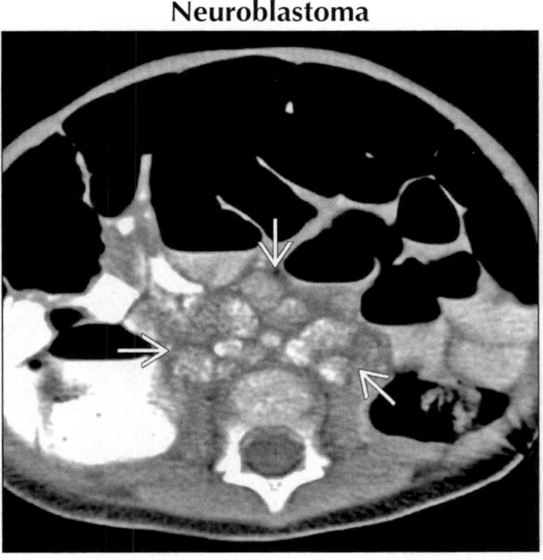

Neuroblastoma

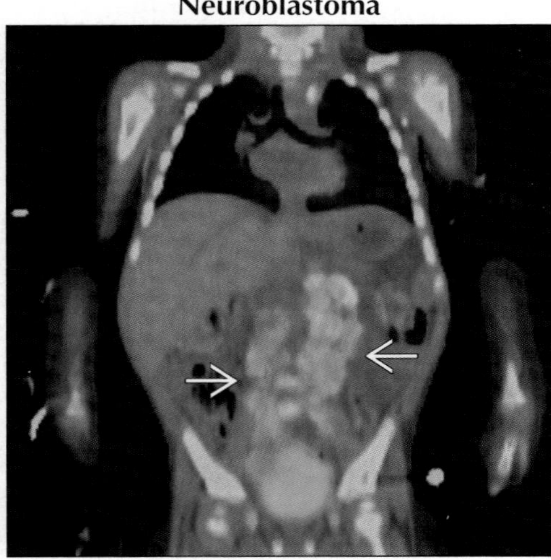

(Left) *Axial CECT shows a partially calcified paraspinal mass ➡. Neuroblastomas originate in the retroperitoneum in 70% of patients, and 85% of tumors have calcifications.* ***(Right)*** *Coronal PET CT shows FDG uptake in the paraspinal mass ➡. Neuroblastomas can arise anywhere along the sympathetic chain. It most commonly metastasizes to the liver, bone marrow, or cortex. MIBG shows uptake in 90-95% of cases when there is no MIBG uptake, FDG PET is useful.*

Abscess

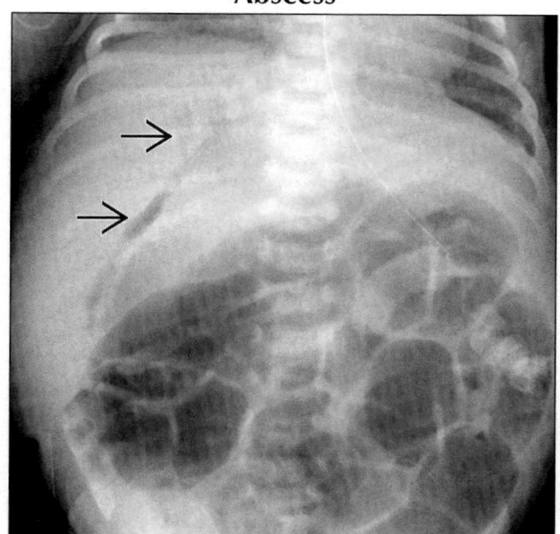

Abscess

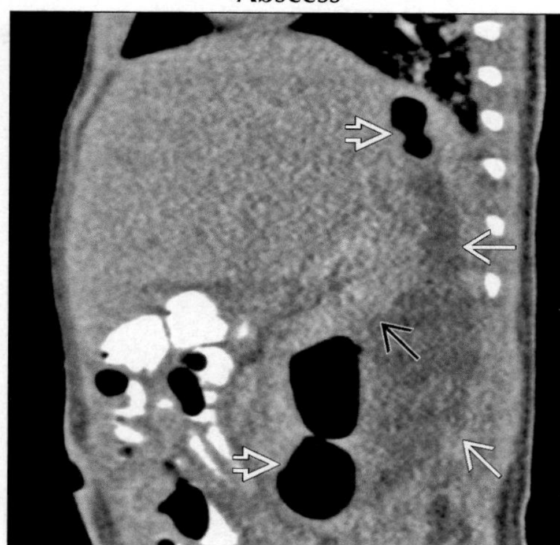

*(**Left**) Anteroposterior radiograph shows an irregular lucency → overlying the liver. A retroperitoneal abscess is most often due to an acute appendicitis with rupture. Other causes of abscess include surgery, Crohn disease, and osteomyelitis. (**Right**) Sagittal CECT shows an irregularly shaped, fluid collection ➔ extending posterior to the right kidney → and liver. Air is present in both the superior and anteroinferior aspect of the abscess ➔.*

Lymphatic Malformation

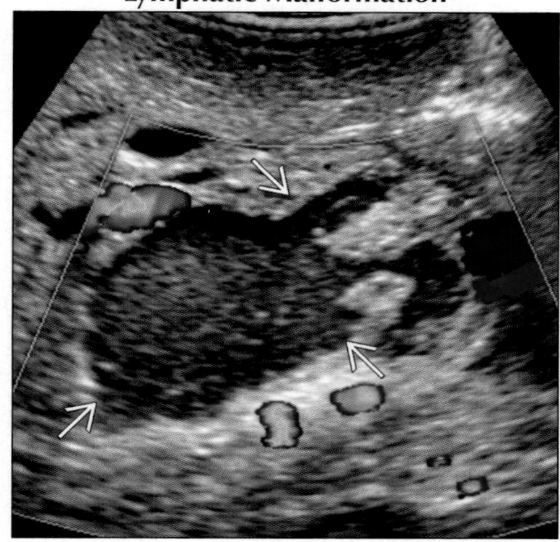

Lymphatic Malformation

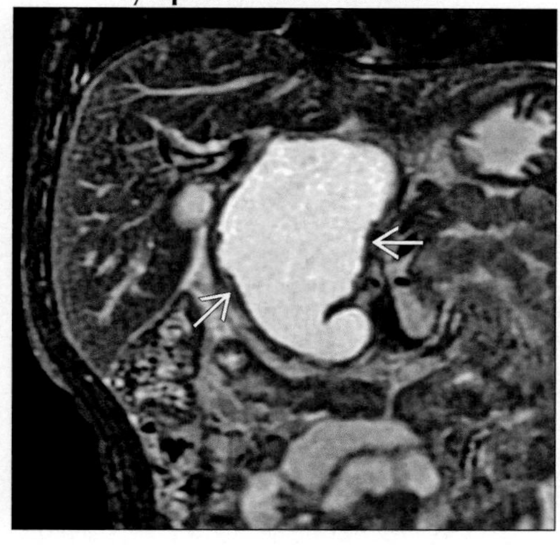

*(**Left**) Transverse ultrasound shows an irregular, hypoechoic collection ➔ adjacent to the liver. There is no color Doppler flow within the collection. Lymphatic malformations are most common in the head and neck; only about 5% occur in the retroperitoneum. (**Right**) Coronal T2WI MR shows an irregularly shaped lesion ➔ with fluid signal intensity and a thin, smooth wall. Lymphatic malformations rarely have calcifications in their wall.*

Lymphatic Malformation

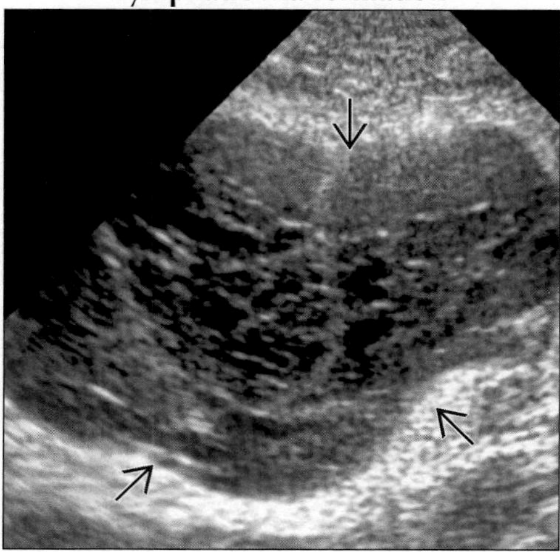

Lymphatic Malformation

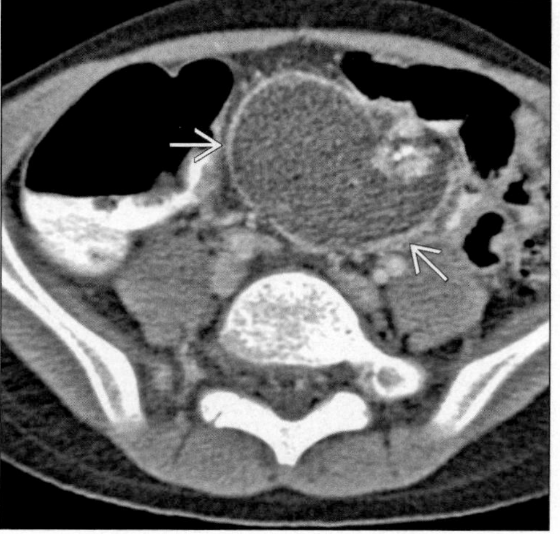

*(**Left**) Transverse ultrasound shows a hypoechoic lesion → with internal septations. Lymphatic malformations are known to frequently cross anatomic compartments. (**Right**) Axial CECT in the same patient shows a cystic collection ➔ anterior to the lower lumbar spine. The lesion has a thin enhancing wall. The septations visible on ultrasound are not seen on CT.*

RETROPERITONEAL MASS

Metastases

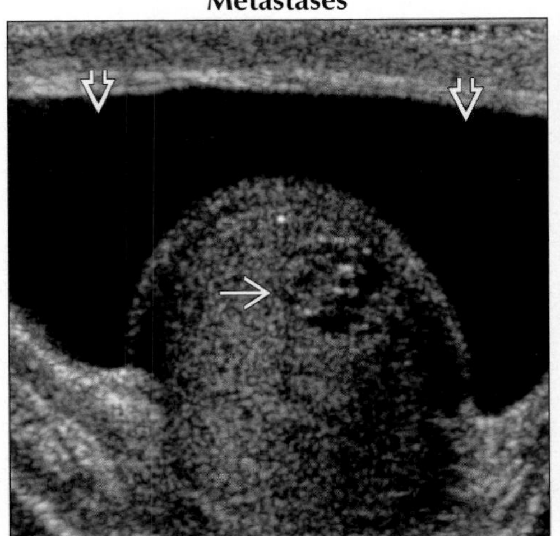

Metastases

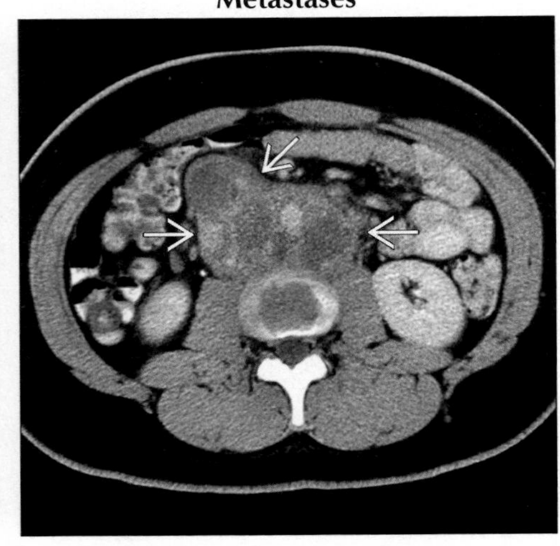

(Left) *Transverse ultrasound shows a heterogeneous mass → of the testis. In addition, there is a moderate hydrocele ⇨.* ***(Right)*** *Axial CECT in the same patient shows a conglomerate nodal mass → surrounding the aorta at the level of the kidneys. Testicular germ cell tumors frequently metastasize to retroperitoneal lymph nodes; in fact, 25-50% of patients will have metastases at presentation.*

Retroperitoneal Hematoma

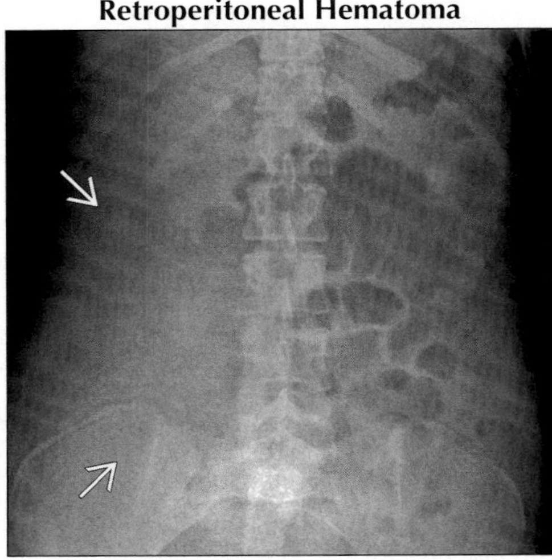

Retroperitoneal Hematoma

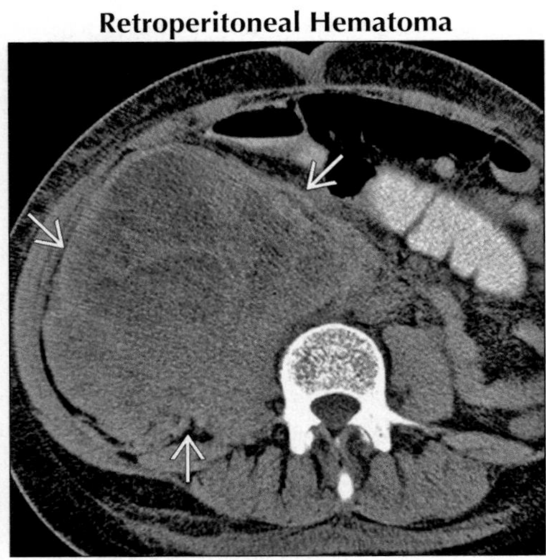

(Left) *Anteroposterior radiograph shows a paucity of bowel gas on the right side of the abdomen →.* ***(Right)*** *Axial NECT shows a hyperdense mass arising from the right psoas muscle →. Retroperitoneal hematomas occur after trauma or in hypocoagulable states. In the latter, fluid levels may be present, representing coagulated and uncoagulated blood. The appearance of the hematoma depends on the length of time between hemorrhage and imaging.*

Duodenal Hematoma

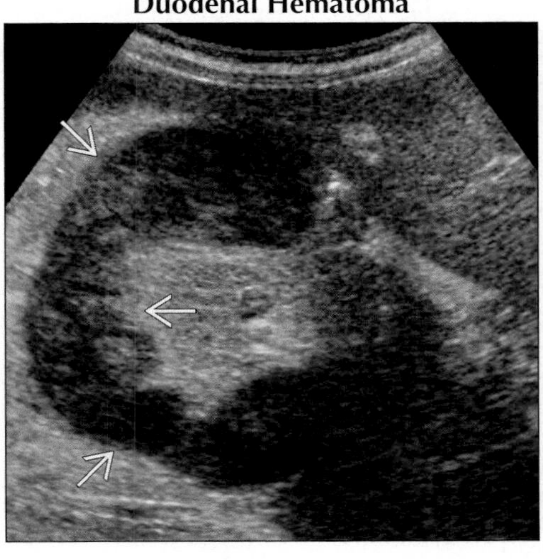

Duodenal Hematoma

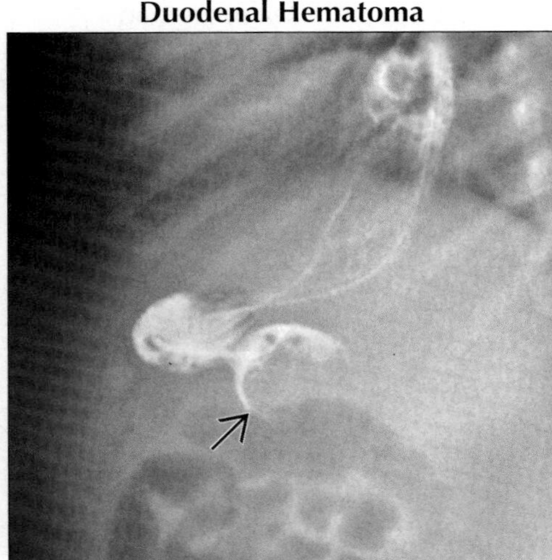

(Left) *Longitudinal ultrasound of the upper abdomen shows a C-shaped area of hypodensity →. On real-time imaging, there was no peristalsis. Duodenal hematomas are due to trauma, and the most common mechanisms of injury are handlebars, seatbelts, and abuse.* ***(Right)*** *Lateral upper GI shows a filling defect in the 1st portion of the duodenum →. Contrast does not easily pass this point. Duodenal hematomas are associated with pancreatic injury.*

Neurofibromatosis Type 1

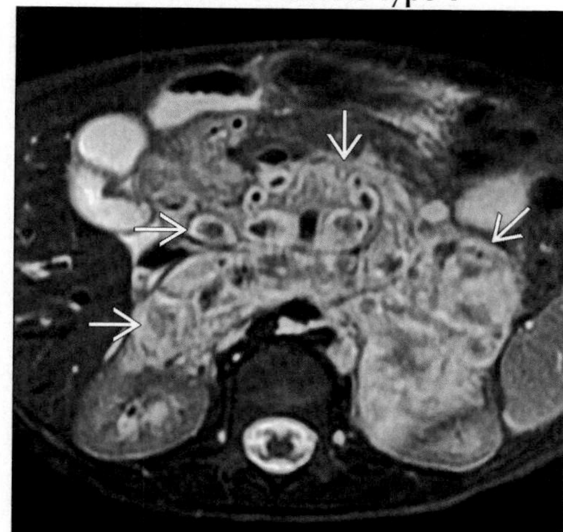

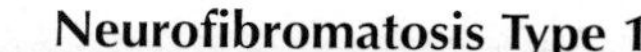

Neurofibromatosis Type 1

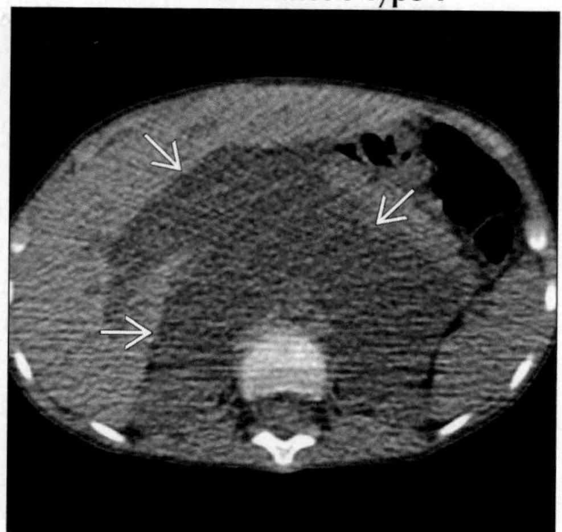

*(**Left**) Axial T2WI MR shows a large paraspinal mass ➔. The mass is composed of multiple small lesions, each with the targetoid appearance characteristic of plexiform neurofibromas on MR. Plexiform neurofibromas are a hallmark of neurofibromatosis type 1. If a plexiform neurofibroma degenerates to a malignant peripheral nerve sheath tumor, it will often lose the target appearance. (**Right**) Axial NECT shows a hypodense paraspinal mass ➔.*

Extraadrenal Pheochromocytoma

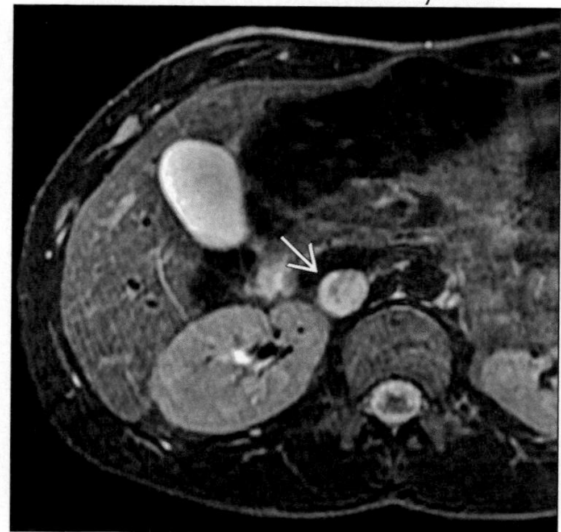

Extraadrenal Pheochromocytoma

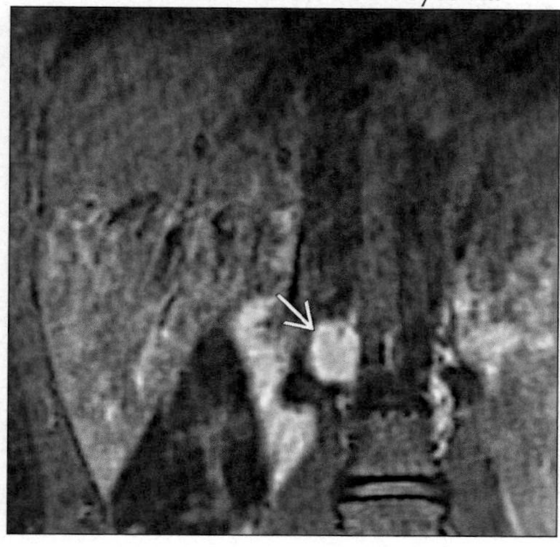

*(**Left**) Axial T2WI MR shows a hyperintense paraspinal mass ➔ distinct from the right adrenal gland. Pheochromocytoma is associated with von Hippel-Lindau, MEN type 2, and neurofibromatosis type 1. About 30% of all pediatric pheochromocytomas are extraadrenal. (**Right**) Coronal T2WI MR shows a hyperintense paraspinal mass ➔ distinct from the right adrenal gland. The majority of extraadrenal pheochromocytomas are retroperitoneal (85%).*

Extraadrenal Pheochromocytoma

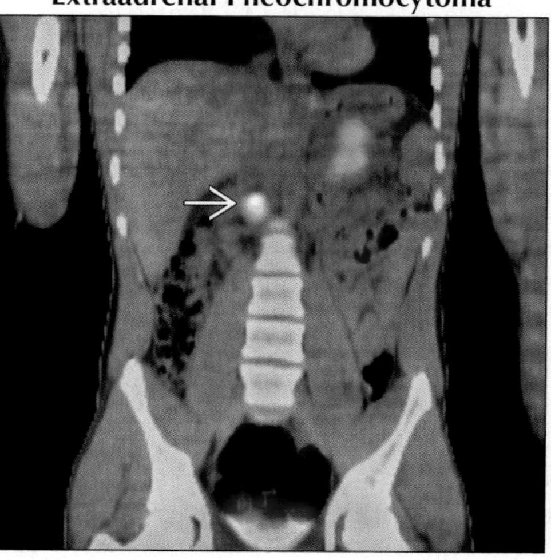

Retroperitoneal Fibrosis

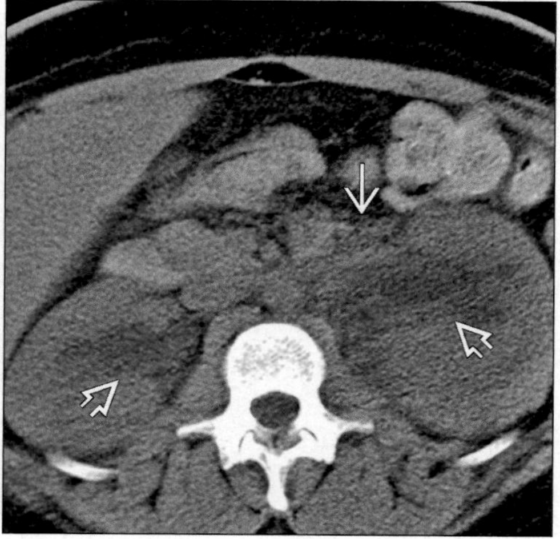

*(**Left**) Coronal PET CT in the same patient shows intense FDG uptake in the right paraspinal mass ➔. 20-50% of extraadrenal pheochromocytomas are malignant. (**Right**) Axial NECT shows a soft tissue density ➔ surrounding the left renal pelvis. Note the hydronephrosis of both kidneys ⇨. In 50% of children, retroperitoneal fibrosis is related to a systemic process or autoimmune disorder. It has an insidious onset with nonspecific symptoms.*

SUPRARENAL MASS

DIFFERENTIAL DIAGNOSIS

Common
- Normal Adrenal Hypertrophy of Neonate
- Neuroblastoma

Less Common
- Adrenal Hemorrhage
- Pulmonary Sequestration
- Ganglioneuroma
- Ganglioneuroblastoma

Rare but Important
- Adrenal Carcinoma
- Adrenal Adenoma
- Congenital Adrenal Hyperplasia
- Pheochromocytoma

ESSENTIAL INFORMATION

Key Differential Diagnosis Issues
- Adrenal masses are usually malignant
- DDx for suprarenal mass in fetus or neonate
  - Neuroblastoma, adrenal hemorrhage, or pulmonary sequestration

Helpful Clues for Common Diagnoses
- **Normal Adrenal Hypertrophy of Neonate**
  - At birth, normal adrenal is 10-20x larger than adult gland relative to body weight
    - ~ 1/3 size of neonatal kidney
  - Consists mostly of cortical tissue
  - Gland decreases in size over 1st 2 weeks
  - Thick hypoechoic outer layer and echogenic core on US
- **Neuroblastoma**
  - Most common solid extracranial malignancy
    - 6-10% of all childhood cancers
    - 15% of pediatric cancer deaths
  - 4th most common pediatric malignancy after leukemia, CNS tumors, and lymphoma
  - 2nd most common abdominal neoplasm after Wilms tumor
  - > 90% of patients diagnosed before age 5
    - Median age at diagnosis is 22 months
    - Peak incidence in 1st year of life (30%)
  - Most common malignancy in 1st month of life
    - Almost always adrenal in origin (90%)
    - Metastases to liver, bone marrow, and skin present at diagnosis (50%)
    - Good prognosis: > 90% survival rate
  - Can arise anywhere along sympathetic chain
  - ~ 70% originate in retroperitoneum
    - 35% in adrenal medulla
    - 30-35% in extraadrenal paraspinal ganglia
  - Mediastinum is 3rd most common location (20%)
  - Patients < 1 year have better prognosis
  - Abdominal mass is most common presentation
    - Can present with bruising around eyes
    - Paraneoplastic syndromes in ~ 2%
  - 50% have metastases at diagnosis
    - Most common to liver, bone, and bone marrow
    - Hepatic metastases can be diffuse or nodular
  - Calcifications present in ~ 85% of tumors
  - I-123 MIBG uptake in 90-95% of patients
  - MR is useful to see intraspinal involvement
  - Prognosis varies depending on stage
    - Staged by International Neuroblastoma Staging System

Helpful Clues for Less Common Diagnoses
- **Adrenal Hemorrhage**
  - Multiple causes, including neonatal asphyxia, perinatal stress, trauma, septicemia, coagulopathies, and Henoch-Schönlein purpura
  - Bilateral hemorrhage in 10%
  - When unilateral, R > L
  - Can be asymptomatic or life-threatening
  - US: Initially appears as hyperechoic mass
    - Liquefies by 2-3 days; becomes anechoic
  - CT: Usually seen in setting of trauma
    - Associated with ipsilateral abdominal and thoracic injuries
  - Can eventually calcify
- **Pulmonary Sequestration**
  - Congenital anomaly
  - Nonfunctioning pulmonary tissue
    - No connection to tracheobronchial tree
    - Systemic arterial supply
  - Intralobar: Sequestered lung adjacent to normal lung
  - Extralobar: Sequestered lung with separate pleural covering
    - More common on left side
    - Can be subdiaphragmatic and suprarenal

    - Intraabdominal in 10-15%
    - Associated with congenital heart disease, congenital diaphragmatic hernia, skeletal malformations, and foregut anomalies
- **Ganglioneuroma**
  - Well-differentiated, benign form of neuroblastoma
  - Neuroblastoma or ganglioneuroblastoma can mature to ganglioneuroma
    - Most common in stage 4S tumors
  - Median age at diagnosis is 7 years
  - Most common in mediastinum, retroperitoneum, and adrenal gland
- **Ganglioneuroblastoma**
  - Intermediate-grade tumor between ganglioneuroma and neuroblastoma
  - Seen in similar locations as neuroblastoma
  - Has malignant potential

Helpful Clues for Rare Diagnoses

- **Adrenal Carcinoma**
  - < 1% of pediatric malignancies
  - More common in females
  - Usually occurs before age 6
  - Most are hormonally active
    - Usually present with virilization in girls and pseudoprecocious puberty in boys
  - Associated with hemihypertrophy, brain neoplasms, and hamartomas
  - Tumors are usually large at presentation
  - Difficult to differentiate from adenoma
    - Helpful criteria include size > 5 cm, invasion of inferior vena cava, and metastases
  - Metastasizes to lung, liver, lymph nodes, and inferior vena cava
- **Adrenal Adenoma**
  - Rare in children
  - 3x less common than adrenal carcinomas
  - Most are hormonally active
    - Cushing syndrome most common
  - Often have high lipid content and lose signal on out-of-phase MR imaging
- **Congenital Adrenal Hyperplasia**
  - Autosomal recessive error of metabolism
  - Infants present with salt-wasting
    - Can be virilization of females
  - On US, adrenal measures > 20 mm in length or 4 mm in width
  - Adrenals may have wrinkled or cerebriform contour
- **Pheochromocytoma**
  - 10-20% of pheochromocytomas occur in children
  - Presents with sustained hypertension
    - Accounts for ~ 1% of hypertension in children
  - Associated with von Hippel-Lindau, MEN type 2, and neurofibromatosis type 1
  - 50-85% arise in adrenal medulla
  - Bilateral pheochromocytomas in 18-38%
  - Appear extremely hyperintense on T2
  - Malignant pheochromocytomas are less common than in adults
    - Metastasize to bone, liver, lymph nodes, and lungs
  - I-123 MIBG is sensitive and specific

Normal Adrenal Hypertrophy of Neonate

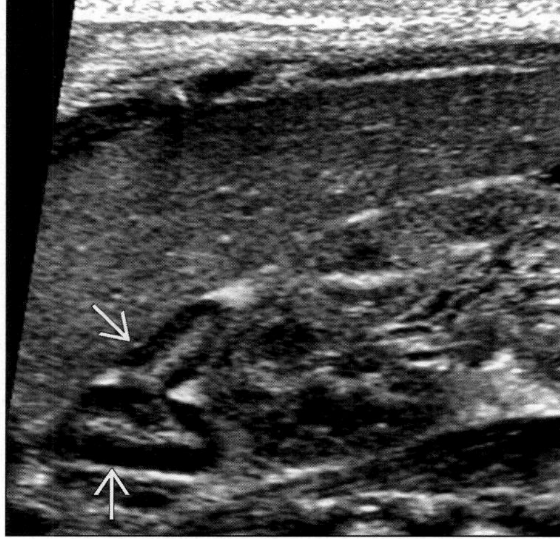

Longitudinal ultrasound shows a prominent but normal right adrenal gland ➡ in a neonate. It is enlarged with a hypoechoic cortex and echogenic core. Normal neonatal adrenal glands can be 1/3 the size of the kidney.

Normal Adrenal Hypertrophy of Neonate

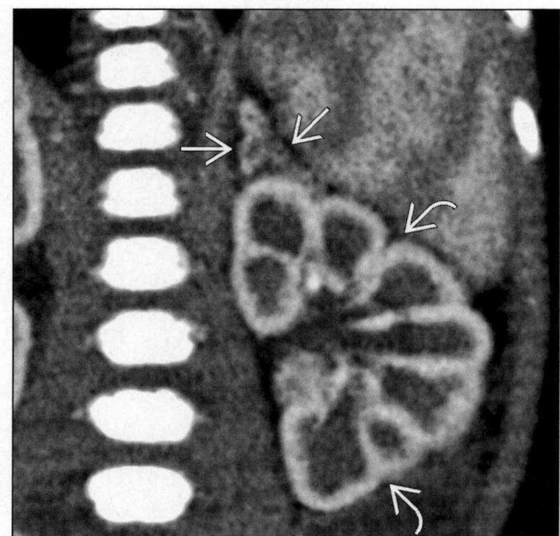

Coronal CECT shows a prominent left adrenal gland ➡ with an enhancing cortex and hypodense core. There is fetal lobulation of the left kidney ➡.

SUPRARENAL MASS

(Left) *Anteroposterior radiograph shows a partially calcified right suprarenal mass ➡. Neuroblastoma is the most common extracranial solid malignancy. It can occur anywhere along the sympathetic chain but is most commonly retroperitoneal.* **(Right)** *Axial CECT shows a partially calcified mass → arising from the right adrenal gland. Neuroblastoma has calcifications in 85% of cases and accounts for 15% of pediatric cancer deaths.*

Neuroblastoma

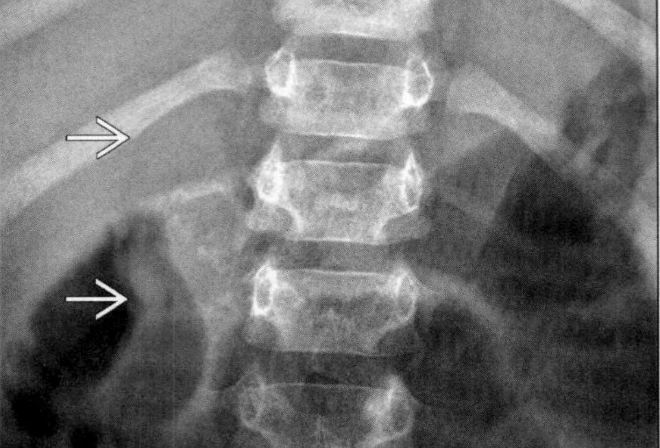

Neuroblastoma

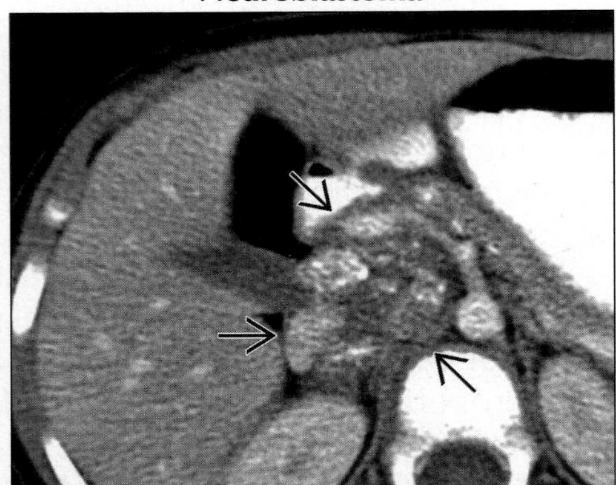

(Left) *Sagittal T2WI MR of a fetus shows a heterogeneous left suprarenal mass ➡ displacing the kidney inferiorly ➥. The differential diagnosis for a suprarenal mass in a fetus is neuroblastoma, adrenal hemorrhage, and pulmonary sequestration.* **(Right)** *Longitudinal ultrasound in the same patient after birth shows a large suprarenal mass ➡, which is hyperechoic compared to the renal cortex. The mass still displaces the kidney inferiorly ➥.*

Neuroblastoma

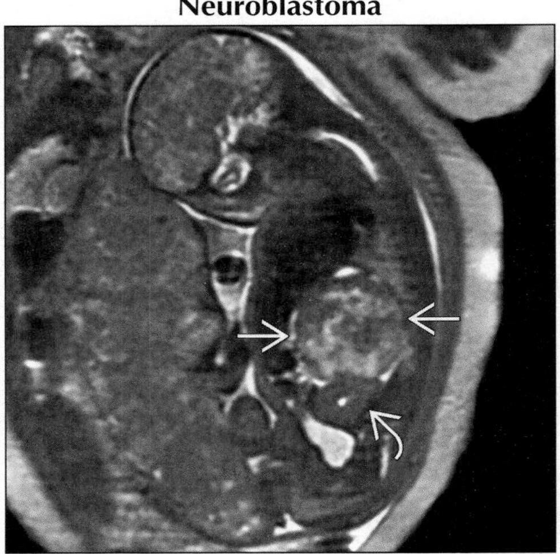

Neuroblastoma

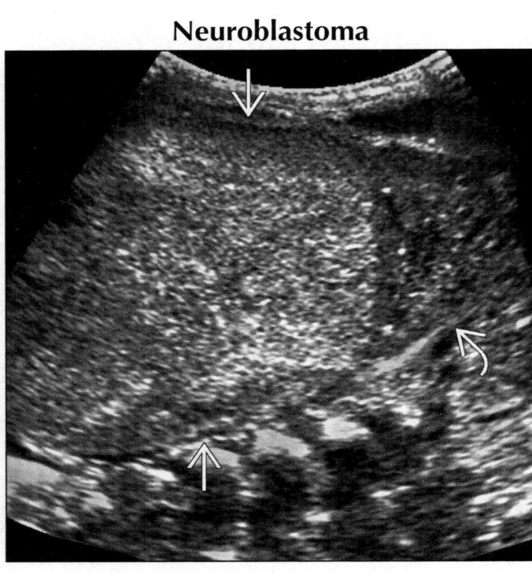

(Left) *Coronal T2WI MR in the same patient shows a large heterogeneous mass ➡ displacing the left kidney inferiorly ➥. Neuroblastoma is the most common malignancy in the 1st month of life.* **(Right)** *Coronal PET shows FDG uptake in the periphery of the large suprarenal mass →. There is considerable uptake in the brown fat in the upper thorax ↷. Neonatal neuroblastoma has a good prognosis and is almost always adrenal in origin.*

Neuroblastoma

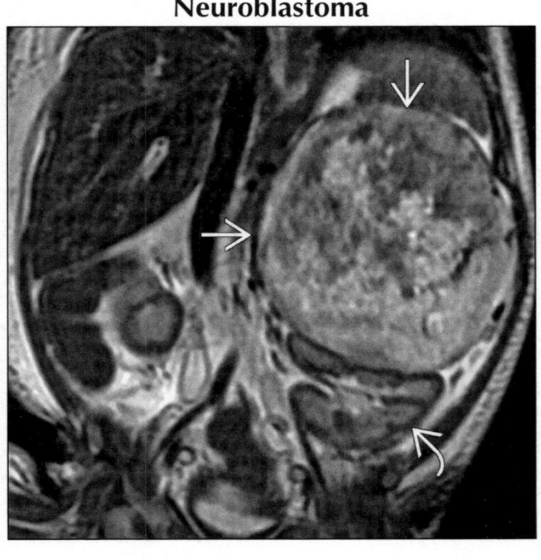

Neuroblastoma

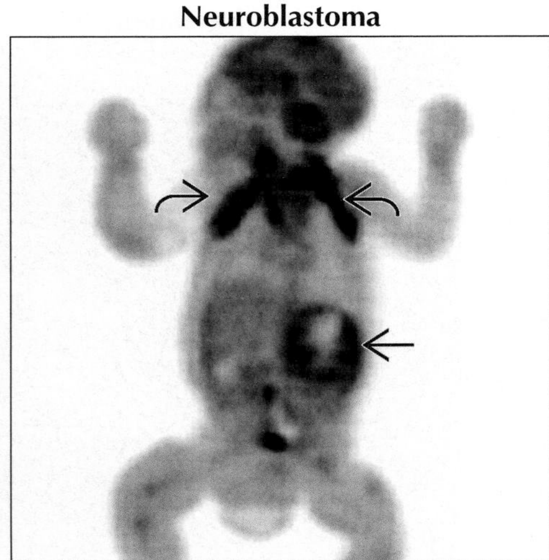

SUPRARENAL MASS

Adrenal Hemorrhage

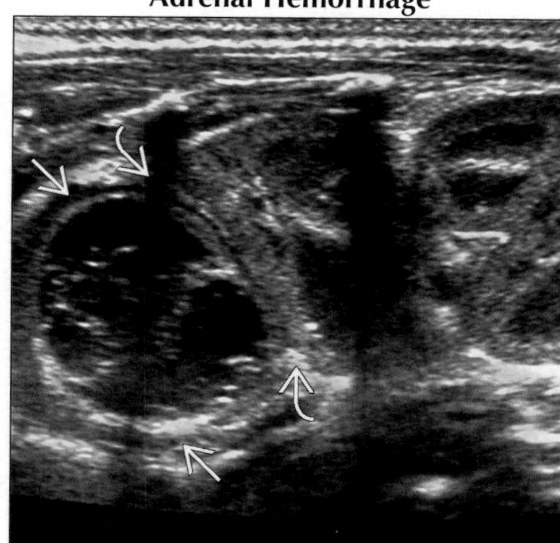

Adrenal Hemorrhage

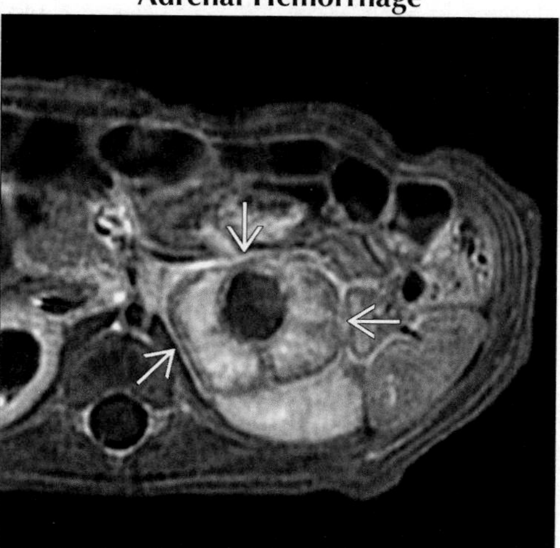

(Left) *Longitudinal ultrasound shows a hypoechoic suprarenal mass with an echogenic rim and internal septations. The mass distorts the upper pole of the kidney. Adrenal hemorrhage liquefies in 2-3 days.* ***(Right)*** *Axial T1WI C+ FS MR in a different patient shows a left suprarenal mass with a central area that is hypointense and a peripheral area that is enhancing. In a neonate, adrenal hemorrhage is most commonly due to perinatal stress.*

Adrenal Hemorrhage

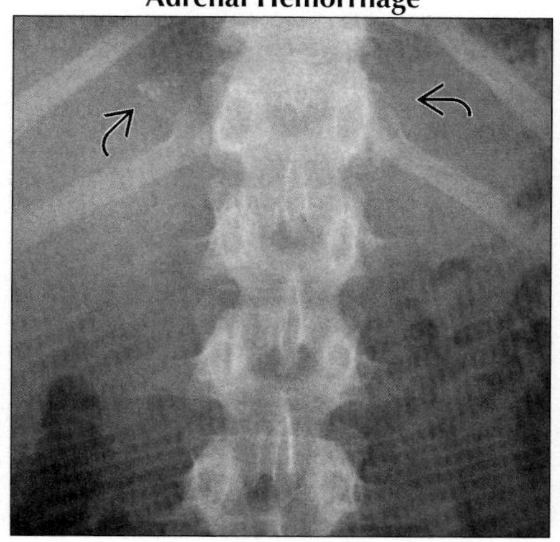

Adrenal Hemorrhage

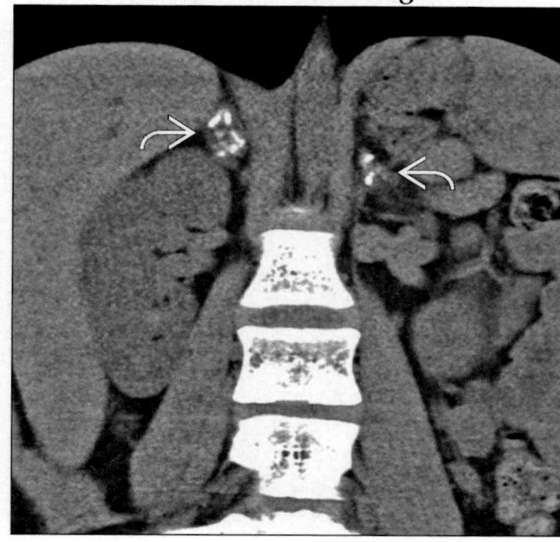

(Left) *Anteroposterior radiograph shows faint calcifications in the suprarenal region bilaterally. Suprarenal calcifications are most commonly due to neuroblastoma or sequela of adrenal hemorrhage. US or limited CT can be used to distinguish between these 2 causes.* ***(Right)*** *Coronal NECT shows bilateral adrenal calcifications. The adrenal glands maintain their adeniform shape. Adrenal hemorrhage is bilateral in 10% of patients.*

Pulmonary Sequestration

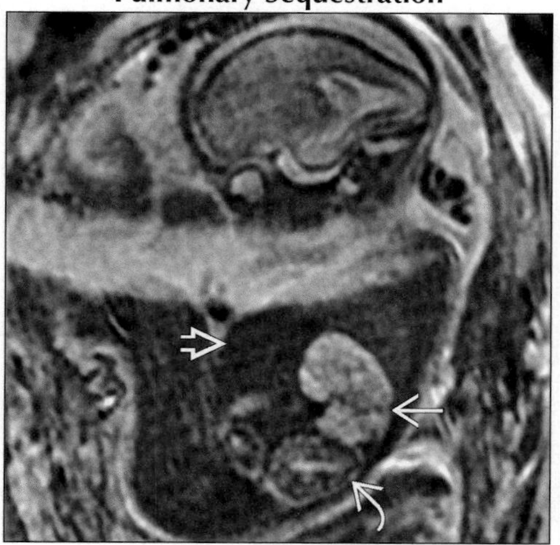

Pulmonary Sequestration

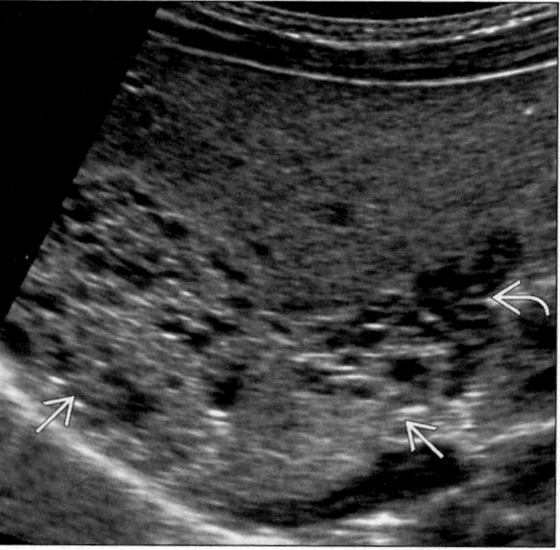

(Left) *Sagittal T2WI MR of a fetus shows a hyperintense bilobed right suprarenal mass. The mass deforms the adjacent liver and kidney. Extralobar pulmonary sequestration is extraabdominal in 10-15% of patients.* ***(Right)*** *Longitudinal ultrasound shows an echogenic mass with multiple anechoic regions. The normal adrenal gland is present and is distinct from the mass. Pulmonary sequestration is characterized by a systemic arterial supply.*

SUPRARENAL MASS

Ganglioneuroma

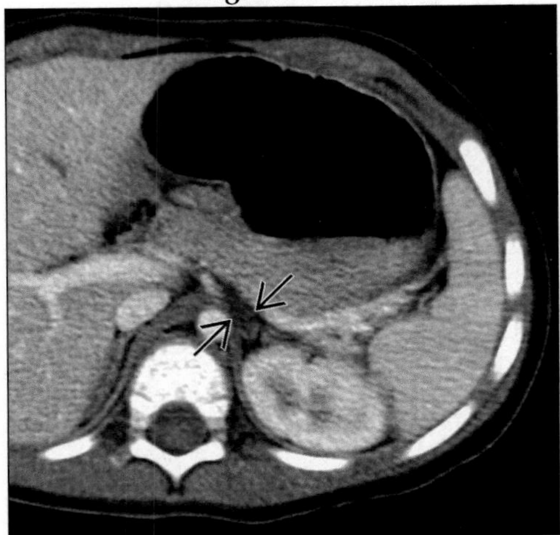

Ganglioneuroma

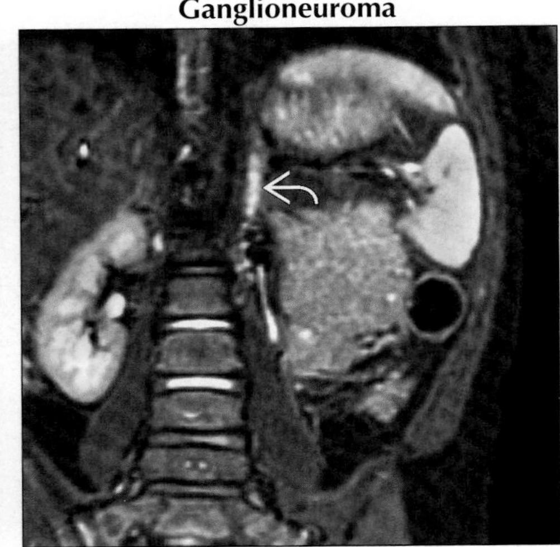

(Left) *Axial CECT shows a small hypodense lesion of the left adrenal gland →. Ganglioneuromas are composed of ganglion cells and Schwannian stroma and can arise independently or represent maturation of neuroblastoma or ganglioneuroblastoma.* ***(Right)*** *Coronal T2WI MR shows a linear hyperintense lesion in the left suprarenal region ➦. Ganglioneuromas present later in life than neuroblastomas with a median age of 7 years at diagnosis.*

Ganglioneuroblastoma

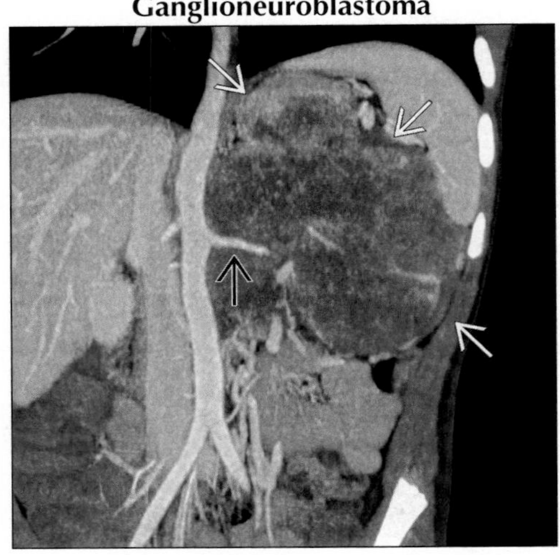

Ganglioneuroblastoma

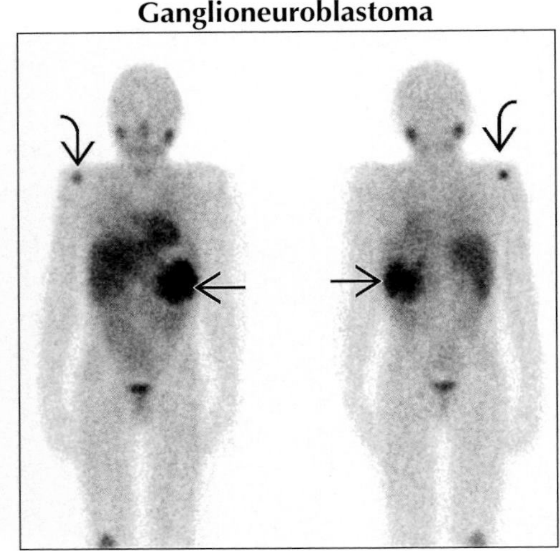

(Left) *Coronal CECT shows a large heterogeneous mass ➡ surrounding the left renal artery →. Ganglioneuroblastoma has malignant potential and is an intermediate-grade tumor between neuroblastoma and ganglioneuroma.* ***(Right)*** *MIBG scintigraphy in the anterior and posterior projection shows uptake in the left suprarenal mass → and at the site of injection ➦ in the right shoulder. Ganglioneuroblastoma occurs at the same locations as neuroblastoma.*

Adrenal Carcinoma

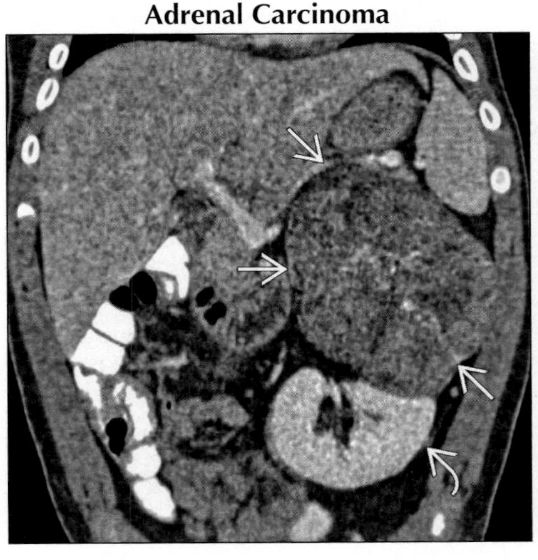

Adrenal Carcinoma

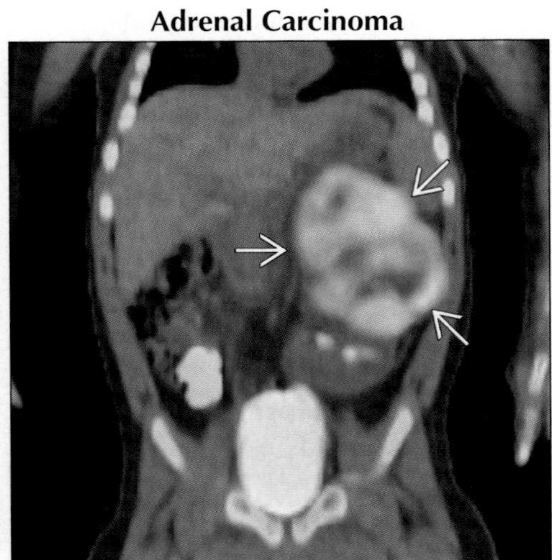

(Left) *Coronal CECT shows a large hypodense mass with minimal enhancement ➡. The mass displaces the left kidney inferiorly ➦. Adrenal carcinomas are often hormonally active. They metastasize to the lung, liver, lymph nodes, and inferior vena cava.* ***(Right)*** *Coronal PET CT shows FDG uptake in the large left suprarenal mass ➡. Adrenal carcinomas are difficult to differentiate from adenoma. Clues to diagnosis include size > 5 cm, metastases, and vascular invasion.*

Adrenal Adenoma

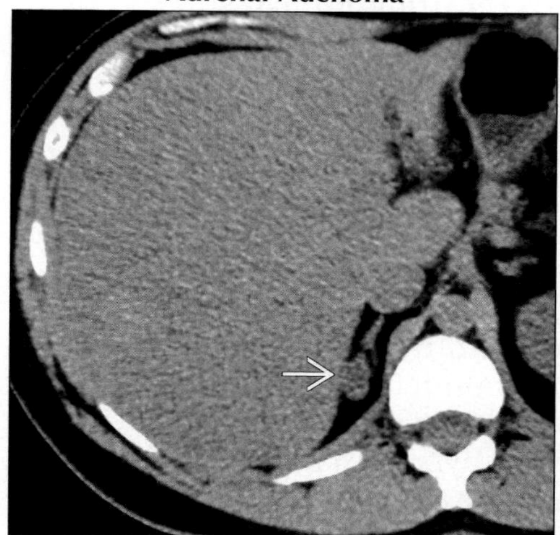

Adrenal Adenoma

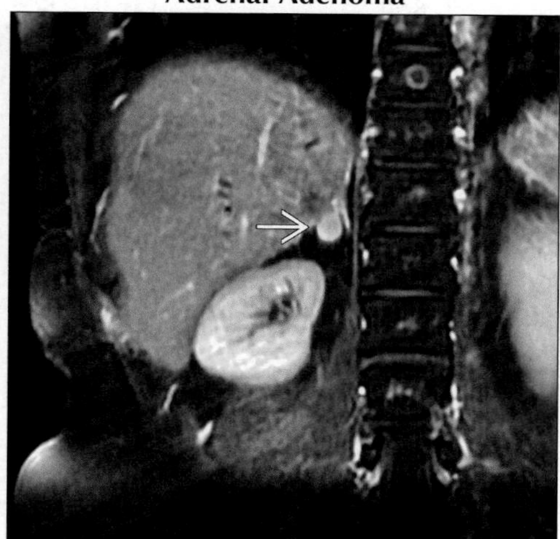

(Left) *Axial NECT shows a slightly hypodense mass ➡ arising from the right adrenal gland. This mass was stable in size over several years. Adrenal adenomas are rare in children and 3x less common than adrenal carcinomas.* ***(Right)*** *Coronal T1WI C+ FS MR shows an enhancing nodule ➡ arising from the lateral arm of the right adrenal gland. Adrenal adenomas are often hormonally active in children. Cushing syndrome is the most frequent presentation.*

Congenital Adrenal Hyperplasia

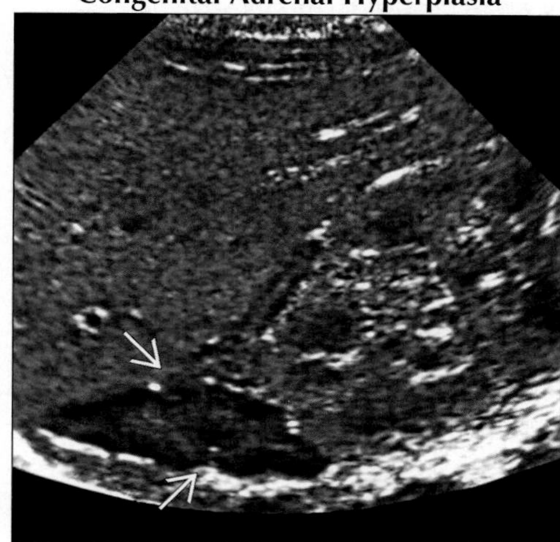

Congenital Adrenal Hyperplasia

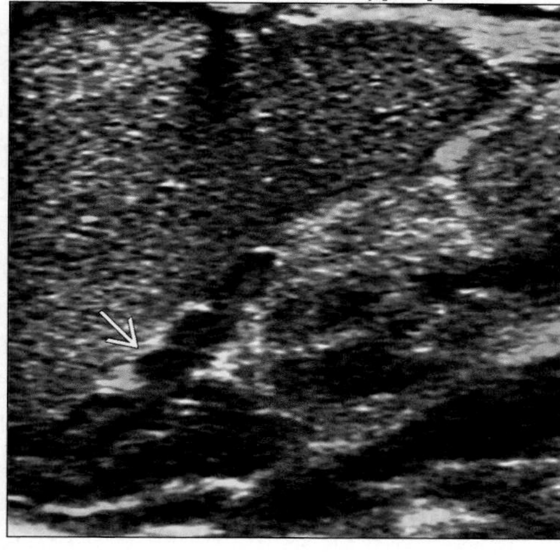

(Left) *Longitudinal ultrasound shows an enlarged adrenal gland with a wrinkled or cerebriform contour ➡. Although the adrenal gland is enlarged, it has a different appearance from normal neonatal adrenal hypertrophy, in which the cortex is thicker and more hypoechoic.* ***(Right)*** *Longitudinal ultrasound in a different patient shows the adrenal gland to have a wrinkled contour ➡. Infants may present with salt-wasting.*

Pheochromocytoma

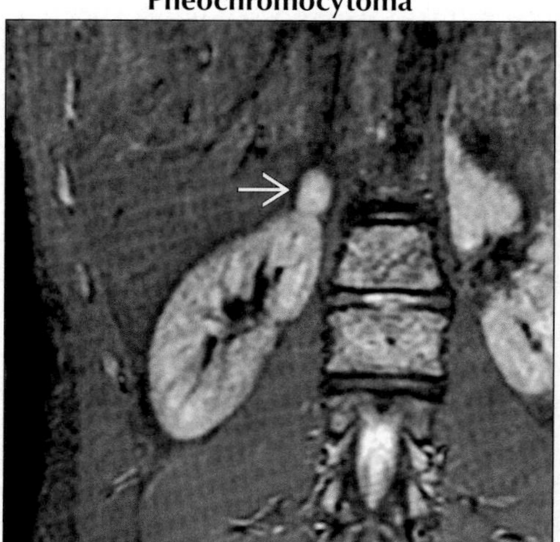

Pheochromocytoma

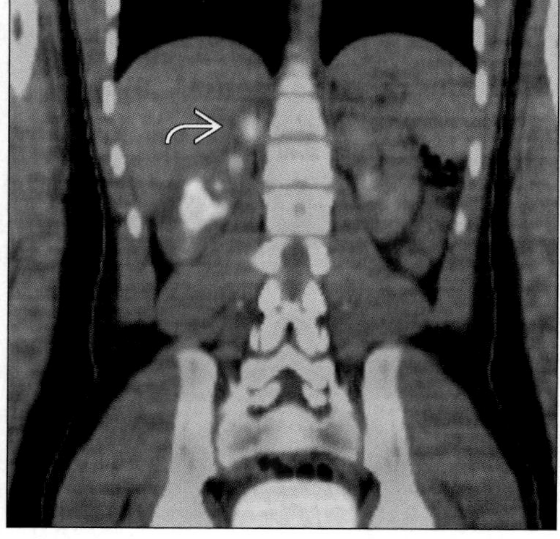

(Left) *Coronal T2WI MR shows a hyperintense right suprarenal mass ➡. Pheochromocytomas usually present in children with sustained hypertension and are associated with von Hippel-Lindau, MEN type 2, and neurofibromatosis type 1.* ***(Right)*** *Coronal PET CT shows uptake within the right suprarenal mass ↪. Malignant pheochromocytomas are less common in children than in adults. When malignant, they metastasize to bone, liver, lymph nodes, and lungs.*

UNILATERAL SMALL KIDNEY

DIFFERENTIAL DIAGNOSIS

Common
- Congenital Hypoplasia/Dysplasia
- Scarring
  - Postinfectious Scarring
  - Postinflammatory Scarring
  - Obstructive Scarring
  - Vesicoureteral Reflux (VUR) Scarring
- Post-Traumatic
- Multicystic Dysplastic Kidney (MCDK)

Less Common
- Page Kidney
- Renal Vein Thrombosis, Chronic
- Other Vascular Insult

Rare but Important
- Partial Resection

ESSENTIAL INFORMATION

Key Differential Diagnosis Issues
- Hypoplasia, dysplasia, and scarring are all different from aplasia
  - Aplasia is congenital absence of renal tissue
  - Associated ureteral agenesis with absence of ipsilateral trigone and ureteral orifice
  - Contralateral hypertrophy
    - Seen commonly with aplasia
    - Less common with hypoplasia/dysplasia
    - Also seen following early surgical removal of 1 kidney
  - Hypoplastic kidney < 1/2 size of contralateral kidney
    - Calyces and parenchyma are normal in proportion
    - Architecture should be normal, not scarred or dysplastic
    - Just smaller version of opposite kidney
  - Dysplasia: Congenitally malformed parenchyma
    - Chronic scarring and fibrosis also sometimes called "dysplasia"
- All other diagnoses are acquired, typically chronic or recurrent
- Differential by location
  - Prerenal: Arterial stenosis, shock, infarction
  - Renal: Postinfectious, hypoplasia, dysplasia, MCDK, radiation
  - Postrenal: Obstructive or vesicoureteral reflux (VUR) atrophy

Helpful Clues for Common Diagnoses
- **Congenital Hypoplasia/Dysplasia**
  - Hypoplasia results from insufficient branching of ureteric bud
  - Nephrons formed are normal but deficient in number
  - Renal parenchymal volume is diminished but does function
  - Segmental hypoplasia more often associated with hypertension
    - Hypertension refractory to medical Rx, may require surgical/ablative Rx
    - Segmental hypoplasia (a.k.a. Ask-Upmark kidney) may actually be segmental scar
    - Patients are typically female and present with hypertension
  - Dysplasia results from faulty formation of nephrons &/or collecting system
  - Renal volume may be normal or decreased initially but tends to decrease with age
  - Nephrons are poorly functioning or malfunctioning → salt wasting
- **Postinfectious Scarring**
  - After pyelonephritis, renal abscess, sepsis
  - Patchy or global, affecting entire kidney
  - Xanthogranulomatous pyelonephritis
    - Chronic pyelonephritis with granulomatous abscess formation and severe kidney destruction
  - Controversy exists regarding
    - Increased scarring in infants and young children compared with older children
    - Increased scarring when antibiotic therapy is delayed
    - Prospective, randomized trials on subject are lacking
  - Imaging
    - Ultrasound: Cortical thinning, volume loss, increased echogenicity
    - DMSA: Absent radiotracer in areas of scar and fibrosis, often crescentic
    - CT & MR: Poorly enhancing, thinned cortex, lobulated contour
    - IVP: Seldom performed in children
- **Postinflammatory Scarring**
  - May be seen after any "nephritis"
    - Glomerulonephritis
    - Radiation nephritis
    - Autoimmune

- Henoch-Schönlein purpura
- Hemolytic uremic syndrome
- Scarring can affect 1 kidney asymmetrically, even when both kidneys have nephritis
- Imaging shows smaller kidney, typically with global scarring

- **Obstructive Scarring**
  - Scarring and nephron damage from any downstream obstruction
    - Ureteropelvic junction obstruction
    - Ureterovesical junction obstruction
    - Urinary calculi
    - Bladder outlet obstruction, posterior urethral valves
    - Neurogenic bladder and other voiding dysfunction
    - Pelvic mass or inflammation
- **Vesicoureteral Reflux (VUR) Scarring**
  - Scarring has been shown with reflux, even in absence of infection
  - Higher grades of reflux are more likely to cause scarring
  - Higher grades of reflux are less likely to spontaneously resolve with age/somatic growth
- **Post-Traumatic**
  - Underlying causes vary
    - Vascular insult, infarction, emboli, venous infarct
    - Obstruction to urine flow, superimposed infection
    - Perinephric hematoma with compressive injury
- **Multicystic Dysplastic Kidney (MCDK)**
  - Severely dysplastic, nonfunctional tissue
  - Enlarged, normal size, or small in newborn
  - Over years, tissue involutes and atrophies
  - Recognizable only by location in teenagers

Helpful Clues for Less Common Diagnoses

- **Page Kidney**
  - Hypertension and renal insufficiency caused by compression of kidney
  - Typically due to subcapsular hematoma, though other perinephric masses (tumor or urinoma) also possible
  - In 1939, Dr. Irvine H. Page (1901-89) demonstrated that wrapping cellophane tightly around animal kidneys can cause hypertension
- **Renal Vein Thrombosis, Chronic**
  - Initially causes renal enlargement
  - Kidney atrophies over weeks to months
  - Seen in thrombotic conditions, premature infants with umbilical catheters, sepsis
- **Other Vascular Insult**
  - Numerous other vasculitides can cause chronic scarring or atrophy of 1 kidney

Helpful Clues for Rare Diagnoses

- **Partial Resection**
  - Nephron-sparing surgery continues to gain popularity
  - Any surgery done to remove segment of kidney results in remaining tissue being "small"
  - Consider partial resection when 1 renal pole appears flattened or truncated

Congenital Hypoplasia/Dysplasia

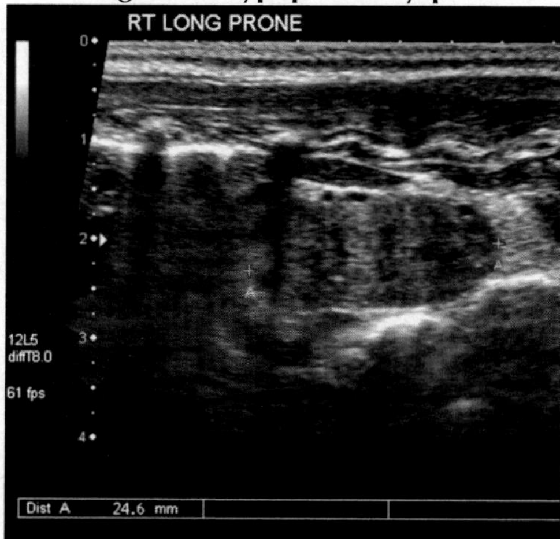

Longitudinal harmonic ultrasound shows a small, echogenic right kidney with poor corticomedullary differentiation in a newborn with a prenatal history of suspected right renal aplasia/hypoplasia.

Congenital Hypoplasia/Dysplasia

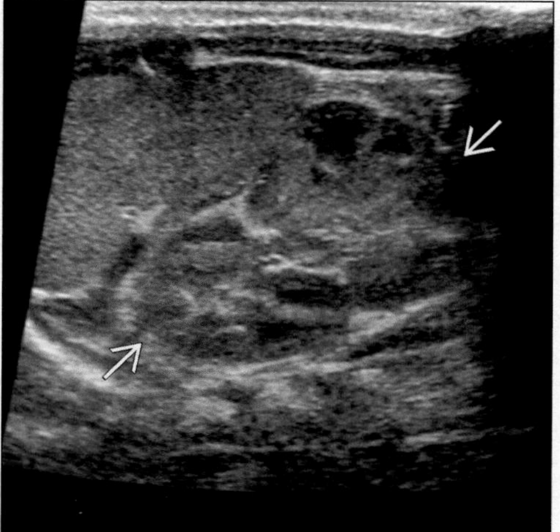

Longitudinal harmonic ultrasound shows a normal left kidney ➔ in the same infant. There is no compensatory hypertrophy of the left kidney at this point.

UNILATERAL SMALL KIDNEY

Scarring

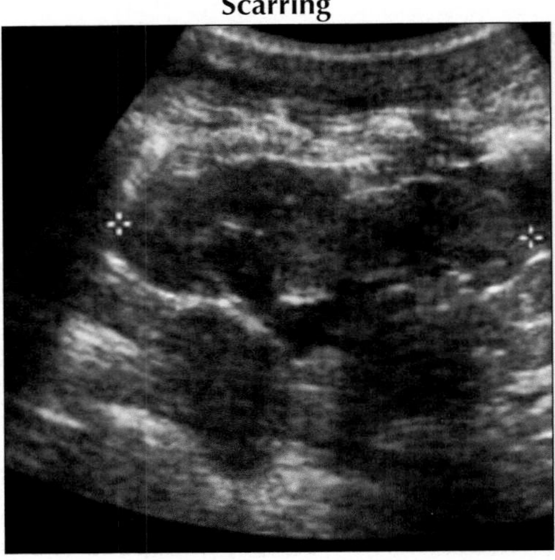

Scarring

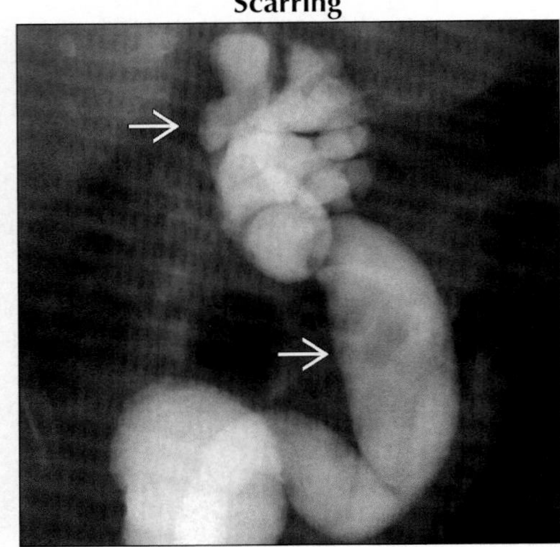

(Left) *Longitudinal oblique ultrasound shows a globally scarred left kidney (calipers) from a posterior prone imaging approach. This patient had recurrent urinary tract infections and vesicoureteral reflux.* ***(Right)*** *AP voiding cystourethrogram shows high-grade reflux ➡ into the left kidney, contributing to scarring. This patient is unlikely to outgrow the reflux and would be a good candidate for surgical intervention.*

Scarring

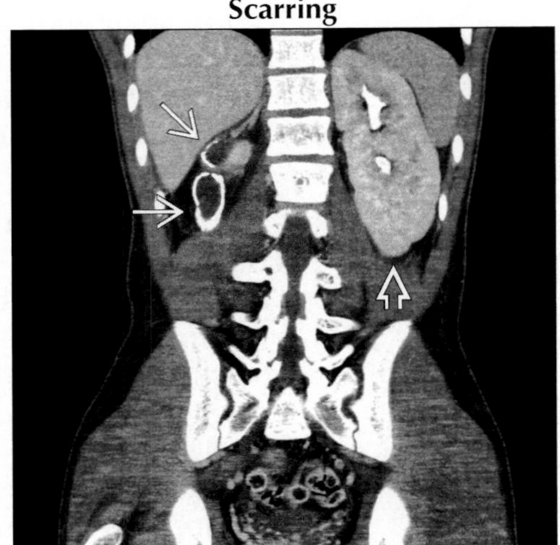

Scarring

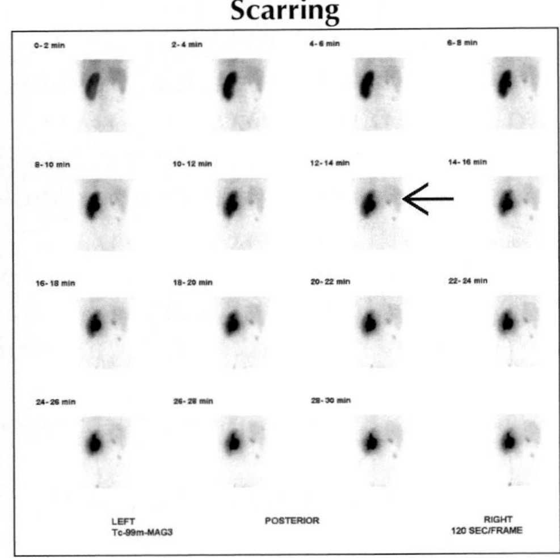

(Left) *Coronal CECT shows a calcified rim ➡ in the right renal fossa, found incidentally in this teenager. Right renal atrophy may be post-traumatic, postinfectious, or vascular in origin. Note the compensatory hypertrophy of the left kidney ⇨, measuring over 15 cm in length.* ***(Right)*** *Posteroanterior renal scan in the same patient shows absent function on the right side →.*

Scarring

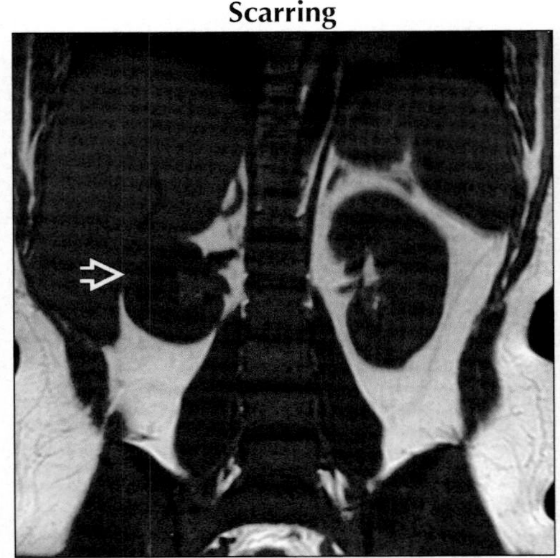

Scarring

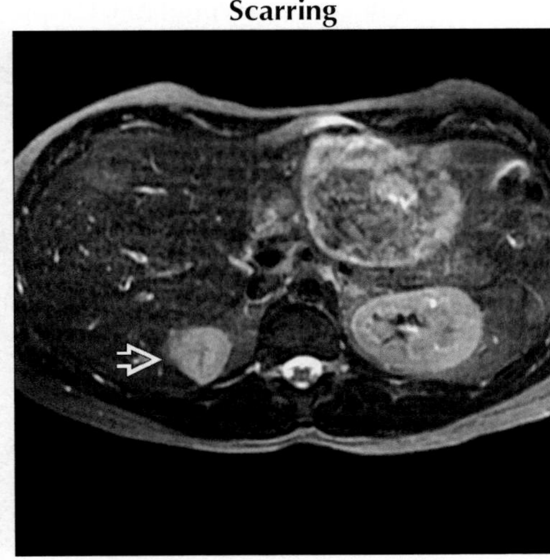

(Left) *Coronal T1WI MR shows a small right kidney ⇨ in this teenager with a history of a neuroblastoma, which was resected at 2 years of age and treated with radiation to the surgical bed. Right renal growth has lagged behind the nonradiated left kidney.* ***(Right)*** *Axial T2WI MR in the same patient shows global scarring in the smaller right kidney ⇨. There was no evidence of recurrent neuroblastoma.*

Scarring

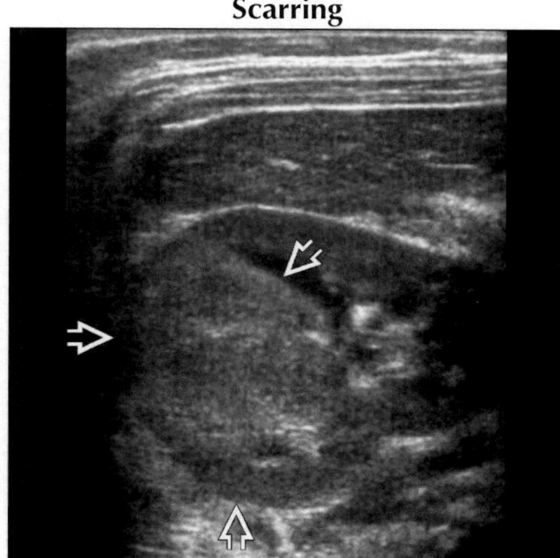

Scarring

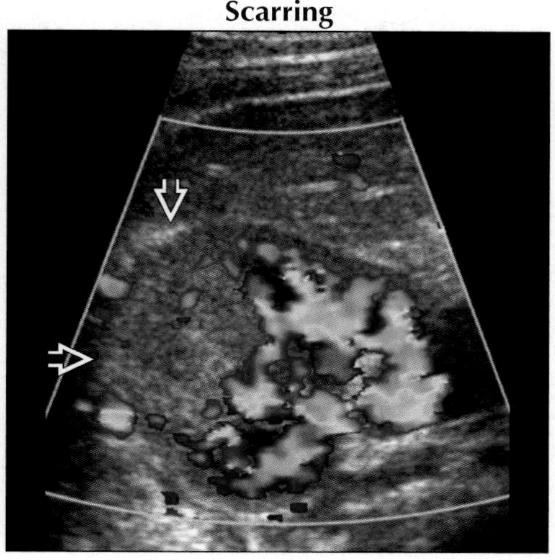

*(**Left**) Transverse ultrasound shows a rounded area of increased echoes ➡ in the lower pole of the right kidney in this 2-year-old boy with fever and flank pain. Urinalysis confirmed acute pyelonephritis. (**Right**) Transverse color Doppler ultrasound in the same child shows a rounded area of decreased perfusion ➡ in the lateral aspect of the right kidney, consistent with acute pyelonephritis.*

Scarring

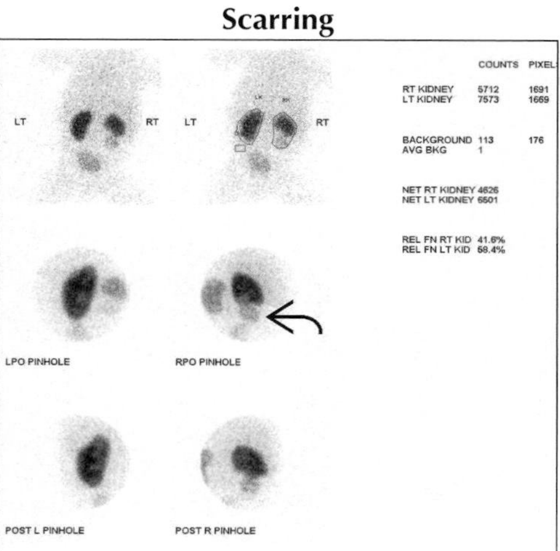

Scarring

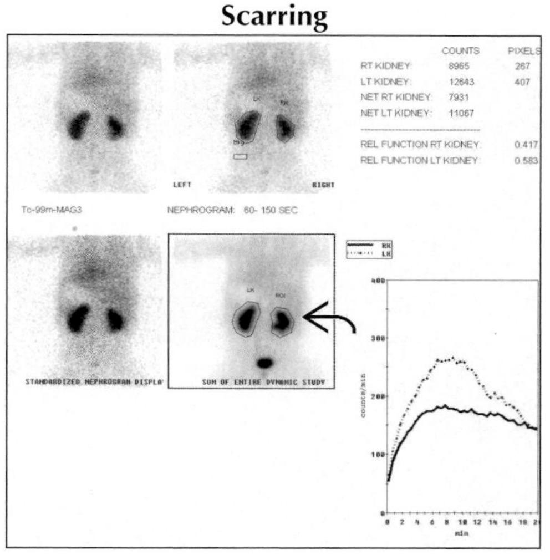

*(**Left**) Posteroanterior renal cortical scan in the same patient performed during the acute phase of his illness shows decreased radiotracer in the lower 1/2 of the right kidney ↩, again consistent with acute pyelonephritis. Patient was found to have a duplicated right kidney and VUR. (**Right**) Posteroanterior renal scan performed 1 year later shows decreased function in the right kidney ↩ compared to the left (42% vs. 58%). The right kidney is smaller than the left and has lower pole scarring.*

Scarring

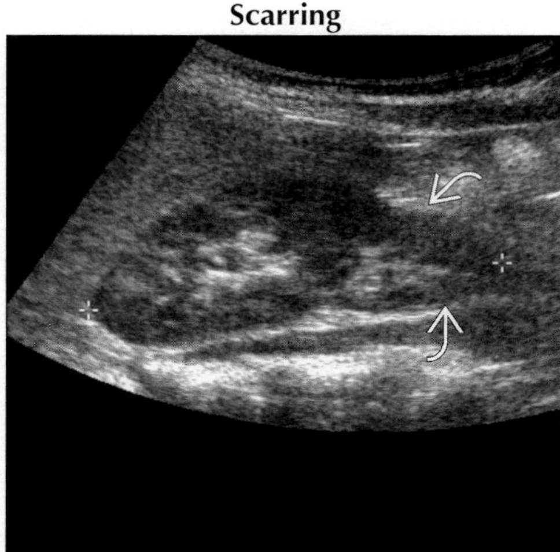

Scarring

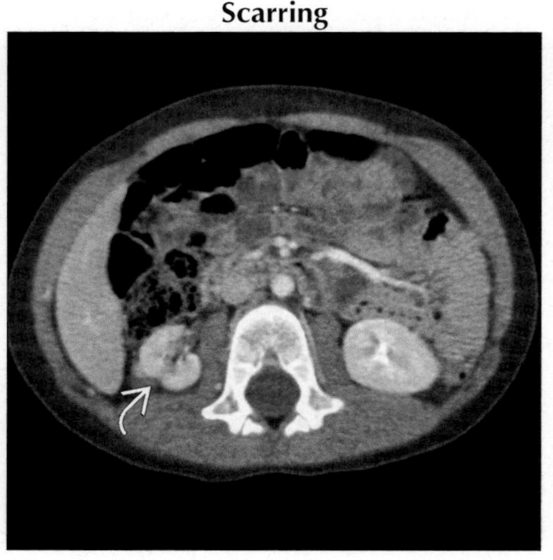

*(**Left**) Longitudinal ultrasound 3 years following the initial episode of pyelonephritis shows focal cortical thinning ↩ in the lower pole of the right kidney. (**Right**) Axial CECT 4 years after initial presentation shows scarring in the lower pole of the right kidney ↩. The scan was performed for symptoms of appendicitis.*

UNILATERAL SMALL KIDNEY

*(**Left**) Axial CECT shows only patchy enhancement of the left kidney ➡, which is smaller than the right kidney, in this patient with sports-related flank trauma several weeks prior. (**Right**) Coronal CECT in the same patient shows the smaller left kidney ➡ with essentially no contrast enhancement or excretion. The nonfunctioning portion of this kidney is likely to continue to atrophy and shrink in size.*

Post-Traumatic

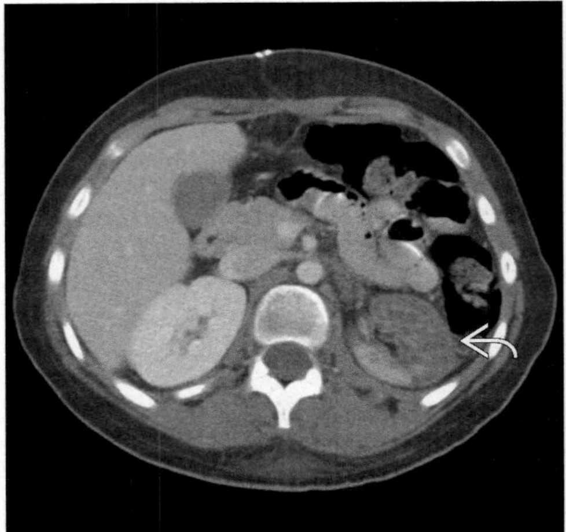

Post-Traumatic

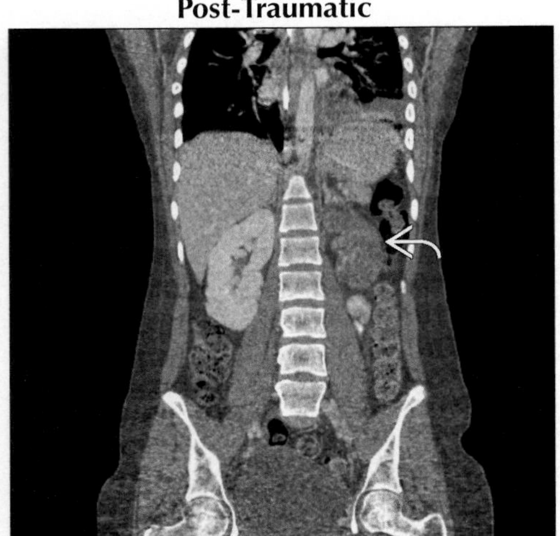

*(**Left**) Longitudinal harmonic ultrasound shows numerous cystic spaces and intervening echogenic parenchyma in this involuting multicystic dysplastic kidney (calipers). (**Right**) Coronal CECT shows the left kidney ➡ displaced cephalad by a large perinephric hematoma ➡ related to pancreatitis and thrombotic disorder. This patient's blood pressure was elevated despite the blood loss.*

Multicystic Dysplastic Kidney (MCDK)

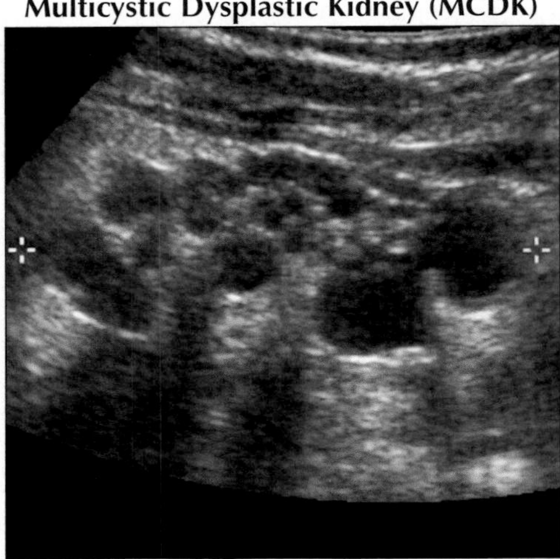

Page Kidney

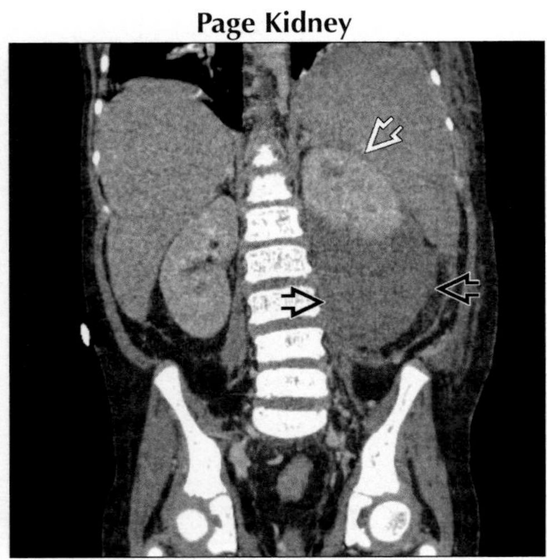

*(**Left**) Longitudinal ultrasound shows a swollen right kidney (calipers) in a neonate with acute renal vein thrombosis. Note the poor corticomedullary differentiation and lack of expected fetal lobulation. (**Right**) Longitudinal ultrasound in the same patient shows a change to a more hypoechoic parenchyma ➡ just a few days later, suggesting renal infarction and necrosis.*

Renal Vein Thrombosis, Chronic

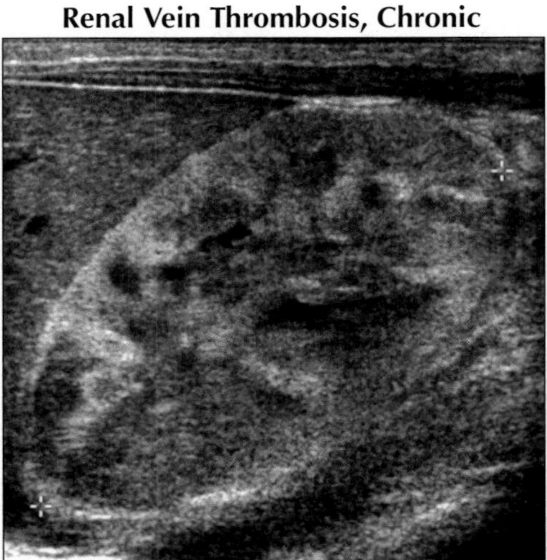

Renal Vein Thrombosis, Chronic

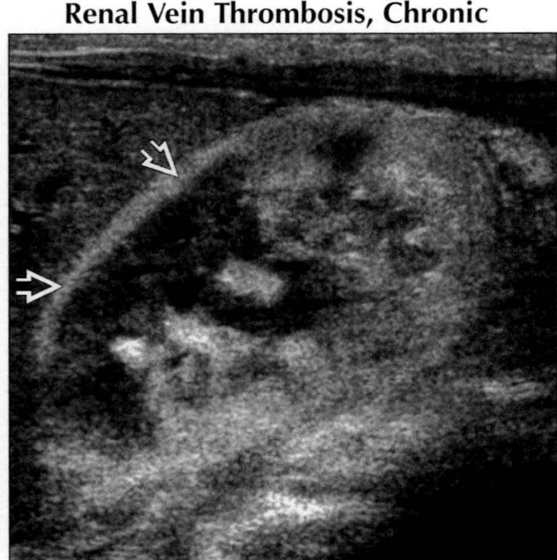

Renal Vein Thrombosis, Chronic

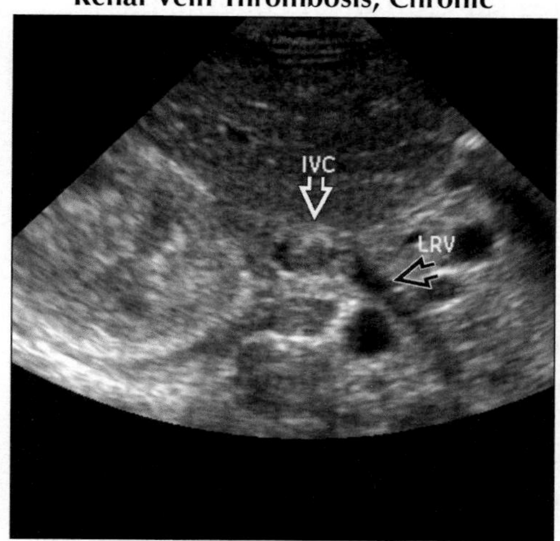

Renal Vein Thrombosis, Chronic

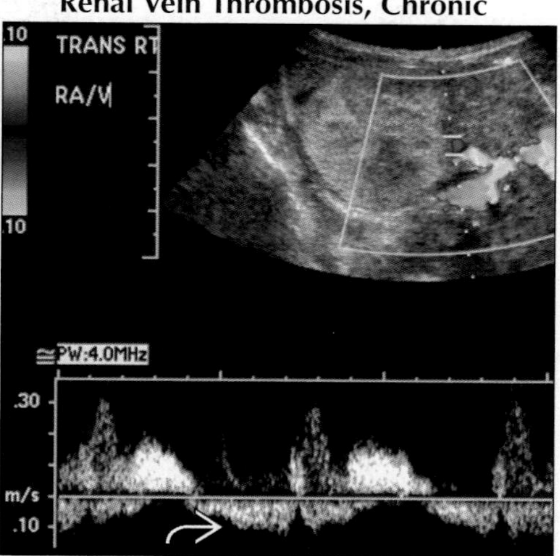

(Left) *Transverse ultrasound shows echogenic nonocclusive thrombus extending into the inferior vena cava from the right renal vein (not shown). The left renal vein remained patent, and the left kidney was working well.* ***(Right)*** *Transverse pulsed Doppler ultrasound shows highly pulsatile arterial flow in the main right renal artery in the acute phase of renal vein thrombosis. Note the reversal of diastolic flow below the baseline due to high intrarenal pressure.*

Renal Vein Thrombosis, Chronic

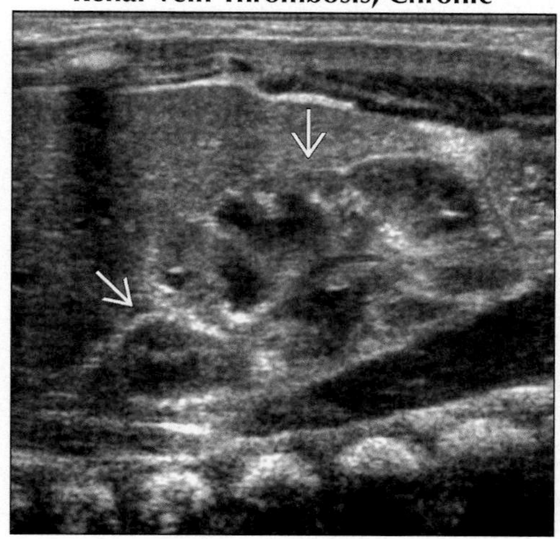

Renal Vein Thrombosis, Chronic

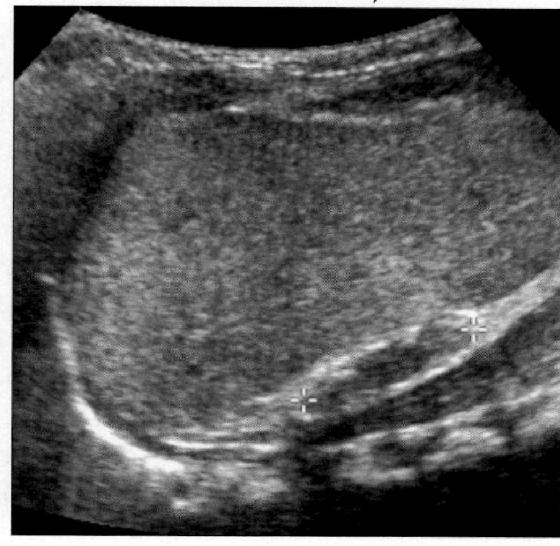

(Left) *Longitudinal ultrasound shows early scarring and atrophy of the affected right kidney, just 2 weeks after renal vein thrombosis was diagnosed.* ***(Right)*** *Longitudinal ultrasound in the same patient 8 months later shows that the right kidney (calipers) measures only 2 cm in length. This residual tissue is difficult to recognize as renal in origin; the series of exams and history of renal vein thrombosis explain the dramatic atrophy.*

Partial Resection

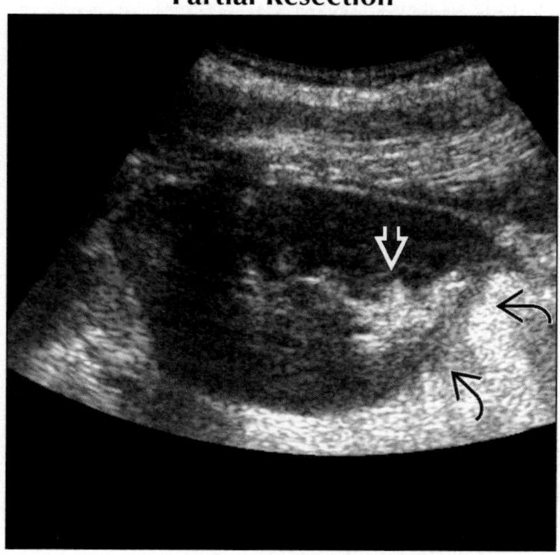

Partial Resection

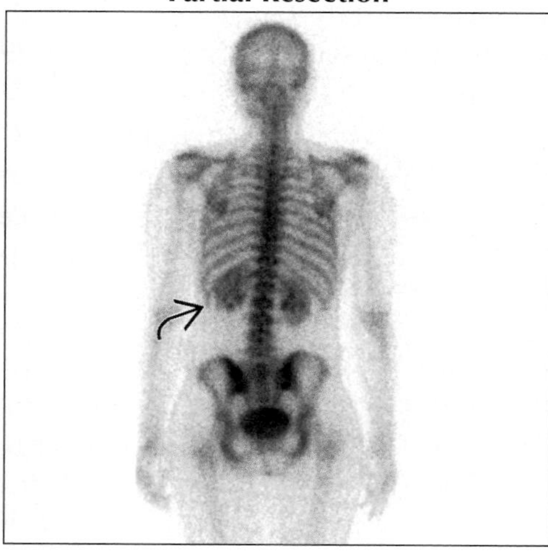

(Left) *Longitudinal ultrasound shows the truncated lower pole of the left kidney in a patient who had a partial nephrectomy for a renal tumor. Note the echogenic fat in the lower renal bed and proximity of the central sinus fat to the lower margin of the kidney.* ***(Right)*** *Bone scan (posterior view) performed to evaluate for metastatic disease shows a normal skeleton but smaller left kidney than right, following partial lower pole nephrectomy.*

BILATERAL SMALL KIDNEYS

DIFFERENTIAL DIAGNOSIS

Common

- End-Stage Renal Disease (ESRD)
  - Cystic/Hereditary/Congenital Causes
  - Glomerulonephritis
  - Vasculitis
- Scarring
  - Recurrent Infections
  - Vesicoureteral Reflux

Less Common

- Congenital Hypoplasia/Dysplasia
- Medically Induced/Iatrogenic
  - Radiation Nephritis
  - Chemotherapy Induced
  - Organ Transplant Induced
- Shock/Trauma/Cortical Necrosis
- Arterial Insufficiency
  - Fibromuscular Dysplasia
  - Renal Artery Stenosis
  - Polyarteritis Nodosa
  - Mid Aortic Syndrome

Rare but Important

- Tuberculosis
- Medullary Cystic Disease and Nephronophthisis
- Alport Syndrome

ESSENTIAL INFORMATION

Key Differential Diagnosis Issues

- Imaging appearance of ESRD is same regardless of cause
  - Bilaterally small kidneys
  - Poor corticomedullary differentiation
  - Poor contrast excretion
  - Contours may be smooth or lobulated
- Imaging without contrast preferred when renal function is compromised
  - Ultrasound often 1st modality
  - Doppler useful to assess renal vascular state
  - CT, MR, VCUG, and nuclear scans all complimentary modalities
- Medical history helpful in narrowing differential causes
- Biopsy for histologic diagnosis often needed as imaging cannot differentiate causes
- Refer to pediatric renal size charts to determine if kidneys are small
  - Rule of thumb for renal length
    - Newborn: 3.5-5 cm
    - 7-year-old child: 7-10 cm
    - Teenager: 10-12 cm

Helpful Clues for Common Diagnoses

- **End-Stage Renal Disease (ESRD)**
  - Causes
    - Cystic/hereditary/congenital (33%)
    - Glomerulonephritis (25%)
    - Vasculitis (11%)
  - Patients on peritoneal or hemodialysis or with renal transplant
  - > 6,000 new cases diagnosed yearly
  - 5-year survival rates
    - With renal transplant (93%)
    - On hemodialysis (77%)
    - On peritoneal dialysis (82%)
  - Deaths most often related to
    - Cardiovascular complications, likely due to prolonged hypertension and fluid overload, &/or lipid abnormalities
    - Infections
  - Other systemic signs
    - Growth retardation
    - Anemia
    - Oliguria/polyuria
    - Hypertension
    - Renal osteodystrophy
    - Lipid/triglyceride abnormalities
- **Scarring**
  - Most often caused by recurrent infections or vesicoureteral reflux
  - Ultrasound and DMSA renal scans most often used to follow progression
  - Scars also seen on CT, MR, and angiography
  - Differentiate scars from fetal lobation and junctional defects
    - Scar = cortical loss over pyramid
    - Fetal lobation or junctional defect = divot between pyramids

Helpful Clues for Less Common Diagnoses

- **Congenital Hypoplasia/Dysplasia**
  - Typically diagnosed in infancy
  - May present with renal insufficiency, edema, failure to thrive
  - Search family history for inherited disorders
- **Medically Induced/Iatrogenic**
  - Past medical history makes this diagnosis
  - Children with history of prior malignancy
    - Radiation and chemotherapy can cause renal enlargement acutely

- Long-term effect is global scarring and atrophy
- Radiation-induced findings can be unilateral, based on XRT port
- Organ transplant recipients
  - Develop gradual nephropathy likely related to medications/immune modulation
  - High incidence of cystic changes in this population
  - Renal cysts seen in 30% of liver transplant patients at 10-year follow-up
- **Shock/Trauma/Cortical Necrosis**
  - Acute insult causes renal enlargement but leads to scarring
  - Cortical necrosis may develop dystrophic calcification
- **Arterial Insufficiency**
  - Not necessarily symmetric or even bilateral
  - Appearance dependent on artery involved
  - Hypertension often symptom
  - Pediatric etiologies in decreasing order
    - Fibromuscular dysplasia
    - Renal artery stenosis
    - Polyarteritis nodosa
    - Mid-aortic syndrome
    - Other vasculitides
  - Iatrogenic causes
    - Following grafting or stenting
    - Following trauma

Helpful Clues for Rare Diagnoses

- **Tuberculosis**
  - Rarely seen in developed countries
  - Consider travel history and TB exposure in setting of suppurative pyelonephritis
- **Medullary Cystic Disease and Nephronophthisis**
  - Rare, inherited diseases
    - *MCKD1* and *MCKD2* autosomal dominant gene mutations
    - *NPH1*, *NPH2*, and *NPH3* are recessive gene traits
  - Similar pathophysiology
    - Bilateral small corticomedullary cysts
    - Tubulointerstitial sclerosis
  - Kidneys of normal or reduced size
  - Symptoms: Salt wasting, polyuria, anemia, growth retardation
  - End-stage renal disease by age 20-60
    - Earlier in familial nephronophthisis
- **Alport Syndrome**
  - Hereditary disorder
  - Family history often prompts initial evaluation
  - Mutations in *COL4A3*, *COL4A4*, and *COL4A5* (collagen biosynthesis genes)
  - Faulty type 4 collagen network
  - Leads to abnormal basement membranes in kidney, inner ear, and eye
  - Progressive nephritis and deafness
  - Hematuria and proteinuria
  - Renal insufficiency & ESRD by age 30-50

SELECTED REFERENCES

1. 2008 Annual Report of USRDS, Section 8: Pediatric ESRD, published on US Renal Data System website, www.usrds.org/adr.htm

Cystic/Hereditary/Congenital Causes

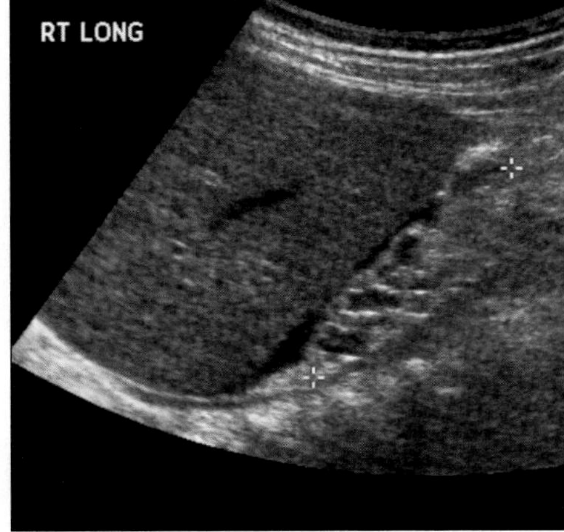

Longitudinal harmonic ultrasound shows cystic dysplastic right renal tissue (calipers) in this 8-day-old girl with renal insufficiency on routine laboratory testing.

Cystic/Hereditary/Congenital Causes

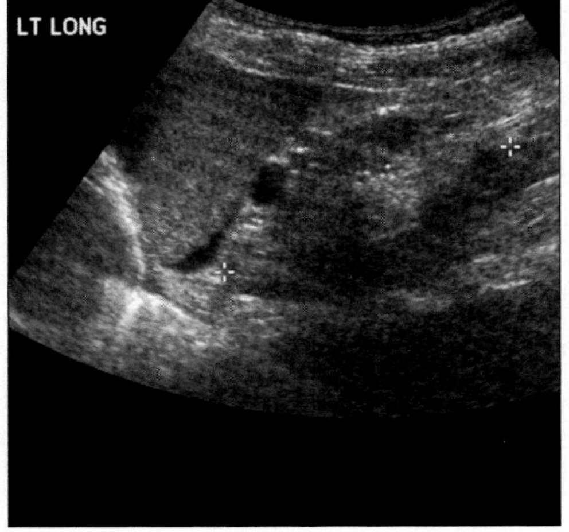

Longitudinal harmonic ultrasound in the same girl shows similar cystic and dysplastic changes in left kidney (calipers). Note a small amount of free fluid in the abdomen related to poor renal function.

BILATERAL SMALL KIDNEYS

Cystic/Hereditary/Congenital Causes

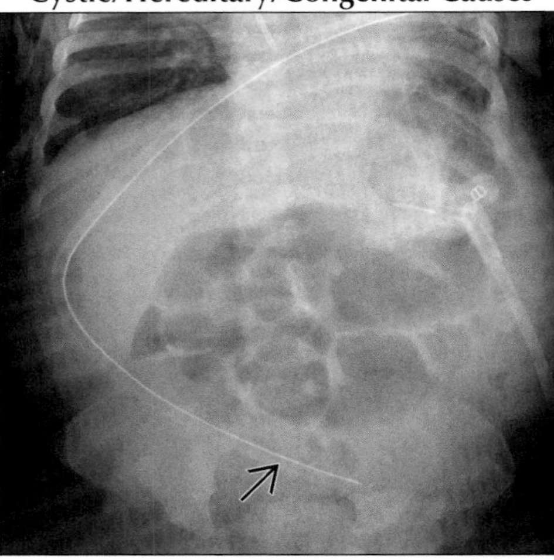

Cystic/Hereditary/Congenital Causes

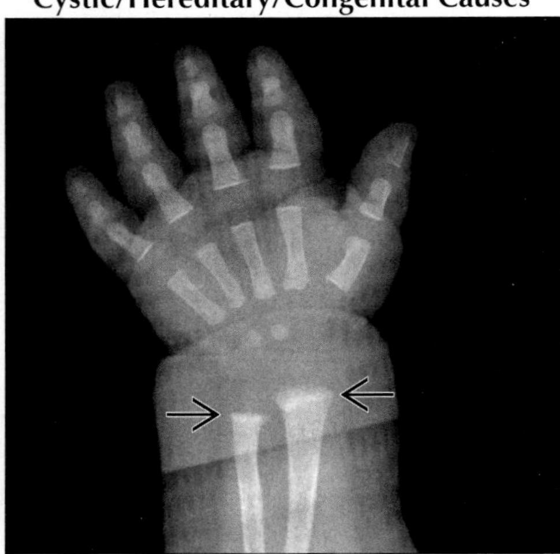

(Left) *AP radiograph shows a large bore catheter ⇒ placed for peritoneal dialysis in the pelvis of this neonate with renal failure due to posterior urethral valves. Although the valve tissue was ablated in the 1st days of life, renal damage had already occurred.* ***(Right)*** *Radiograph shows changes of renal osteodystrophy in the same patient 2 years later. Note the fraying and cupping of the distal radial and ulnar metaphyses ⇒.*

Cystic/Hereditary/Congenital Causes

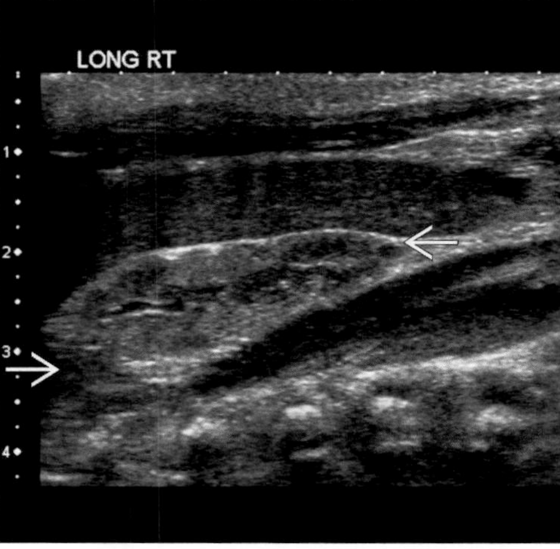

Cystic/Hereditary/Congenital Causes

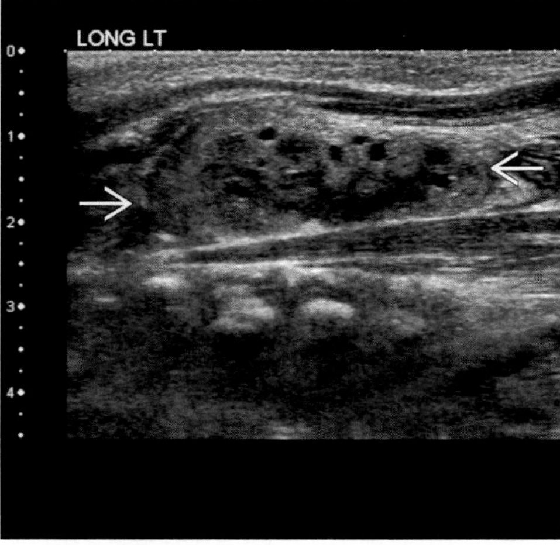

(Left) *Longitudinal harmonic ultrasound shows a very echogenic right kidney ➡ with small peripheral cysts. This boy had bilateral renal dysplasia related to posterior urethral valves.* ***(Right)*** *Longitudinal harmonic ultrasound shows similar increased echotexture in the left kidney ➡ of the same boy. Note the cortical cysts in the near field. The trace-free fluid seen around the kidney is peritoneal dialysis fluid.*

Glomerulonephritis

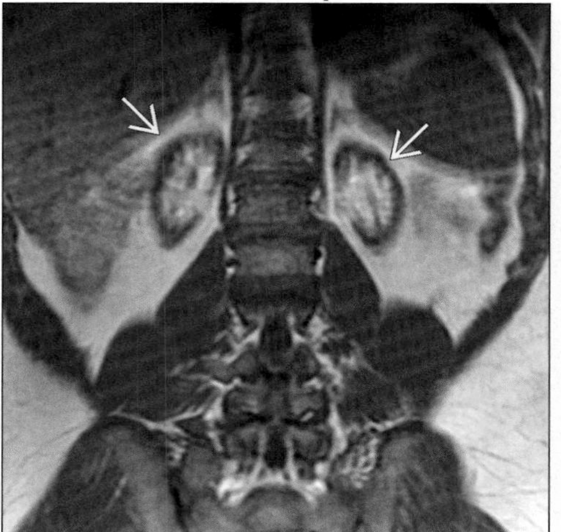

Glomerulonephritis

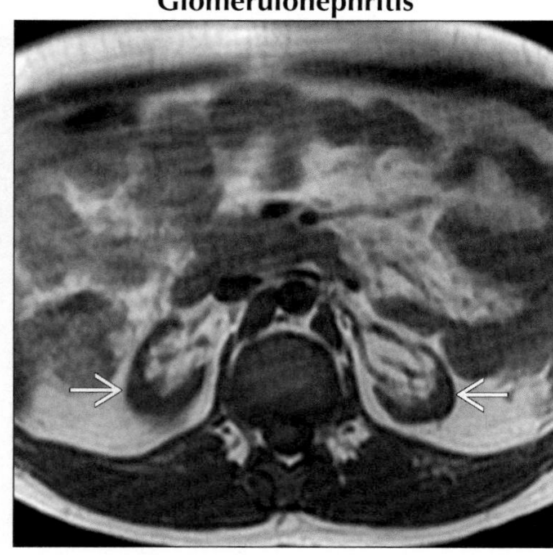

(Left) *Coronal T1WI MR shows very small, atrophic kidneys ➡ bilaterally in this adolescent with chronic glomerulonephritis.* ***(Right)*** *Axial T1WI MR shows bilaterally small, globally scarred kidneys ➡ in the same teenager, who was being evaluated for renal transplantation. Note that the kidneys are smaller than the adjacent vertebral body.*

BILATERAL SMALL KIDNEYS

Vesicoureteral Reflux

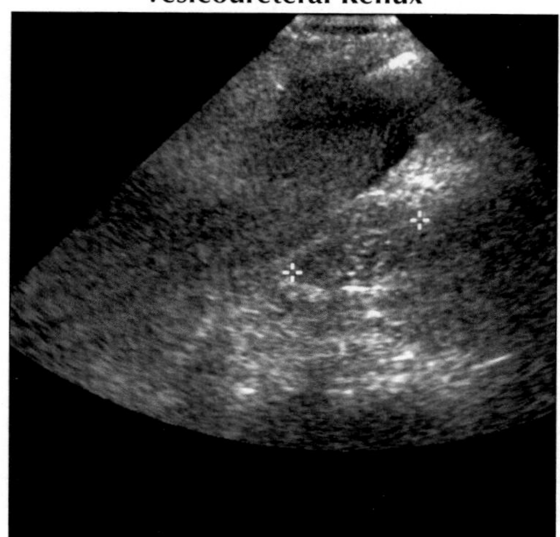

Vesicoureteral Reflux

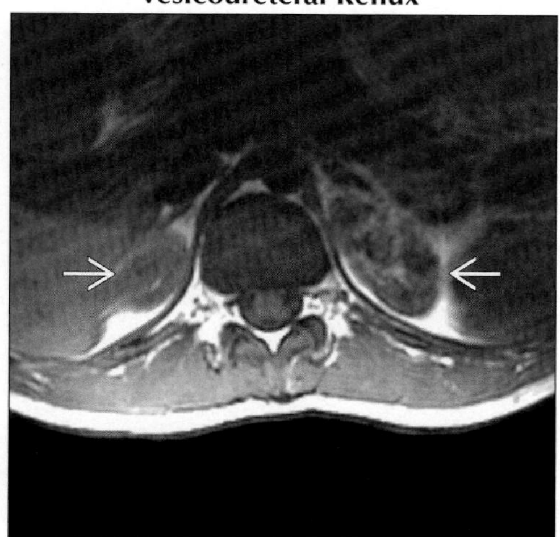

(Left) *Longitudinal ultrasound shows a chronically scarred left kidney (calipers), which is difficult to recognize as renal tissue. This teenage patient with chronic vesicoureteral reflux was poorly compliant with medical recommendations.* ***(Right)*** *Axial T1WI MR shows bilateral renal scarring* ➔ *related to chronic vesicoureteral reflux. The MR exam was performed for back symptoms and was not a dedicated renal exam.*

Vesicoureteral Reflux

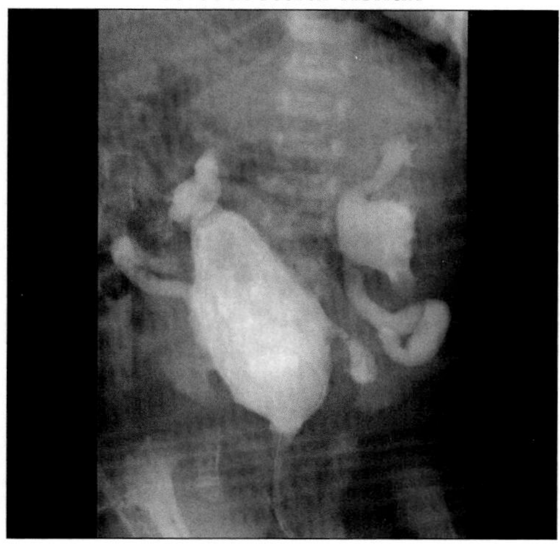

Vesicoureteral Reflux

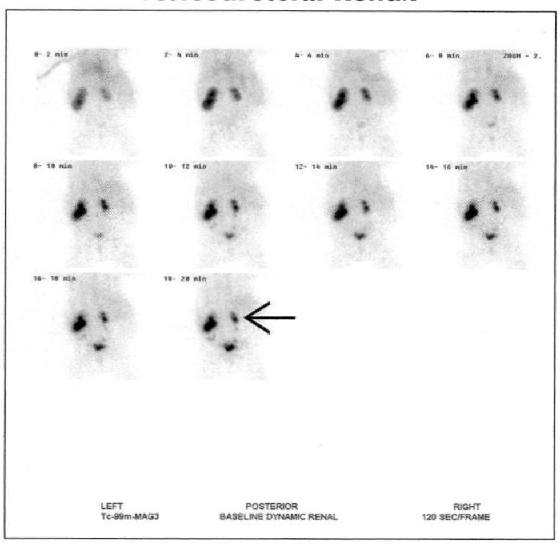

(Left) *Voiding cystourethrogram shows high-grade reflux in another patient who eventually developed small, globally scarred kidneys, this time due to prune belly syndrome.* ***(Right)*** *Posteroanterior renal scan shows a poorly functioning right kidney* ⇨ *in the same patient with prune belly. Renal deterioration may be asymmetric initially. Note the high background counts throughout the scan, reflecting renal insufficiency.*

Vesicoureteral Reflux

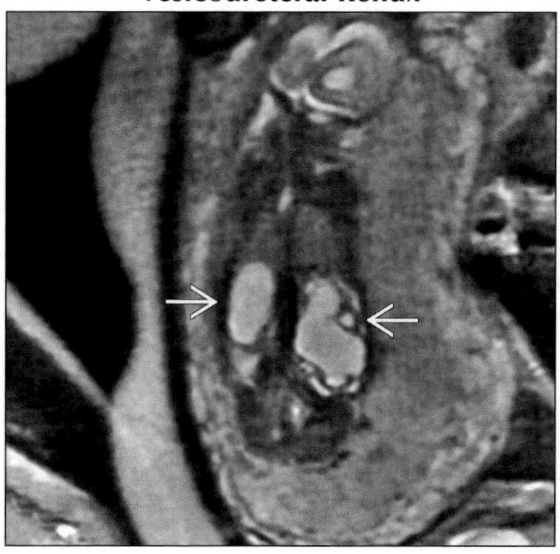

Vesicoureteral Reflux

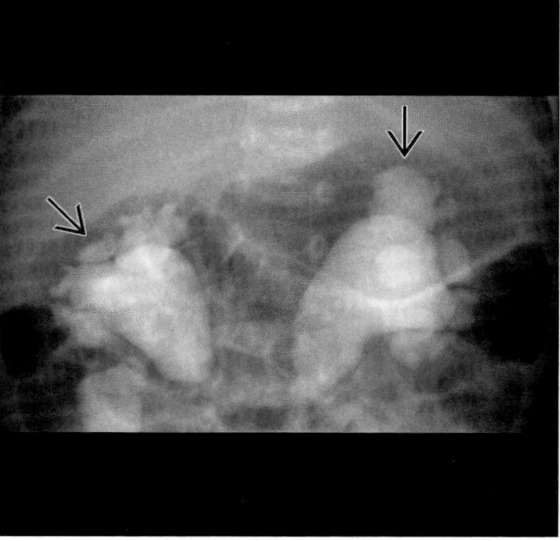

(Left) *Coronal T2WI MR shows bilateral hydronephrosis* ➔ *in utero in a patient with posterior urethral valves. Initially the kidneys are enlarged, but over time they scar down and shrink.* ***(Right)*** *Voiding cystourethrogram shows high-grade reflux bilaterally into massively dilated calyces* ⇨*. Chronic reflux, even without infection, will cause progressive renal scarring.*

BILATERAL SMALL KIDNEYS

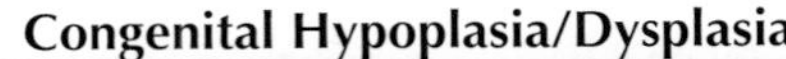

Congenital Hypoplasia/Dysplasia | **Congenital Hypoplasia/Dysplasia**

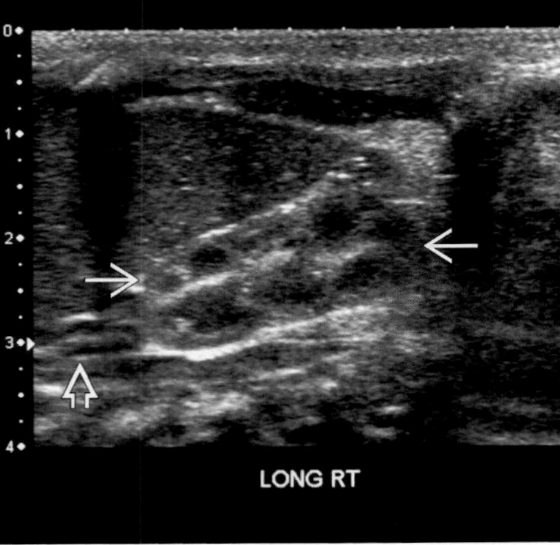

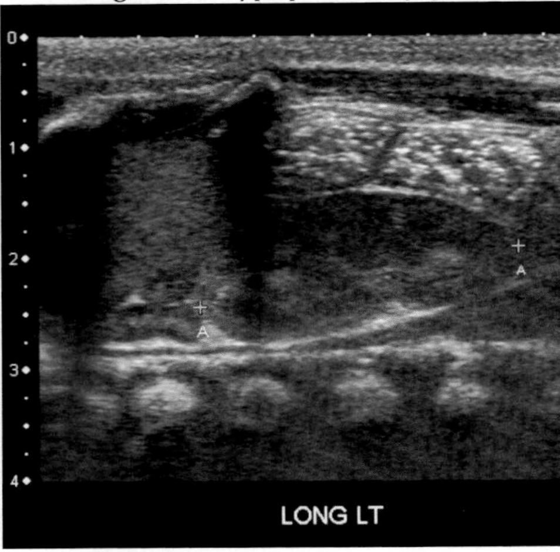

(Left) *Longitudinal ultrasound shows a small right kidney ➔ with good corticomedullary differentiation in a full-term newborn. Note the adjacent normal newborn adrenal gland ➔, almost half the size of the kidney.* ***(Right)*** *Longitudinal ultrasound in the same infant shows a small left kidney (calipers), below the 2nd standard deviation in length. Biopsy is needed to determine the cause of hypo-/dysplasia.*

Chemotherapy Induced | **Chemotherapy Induced**

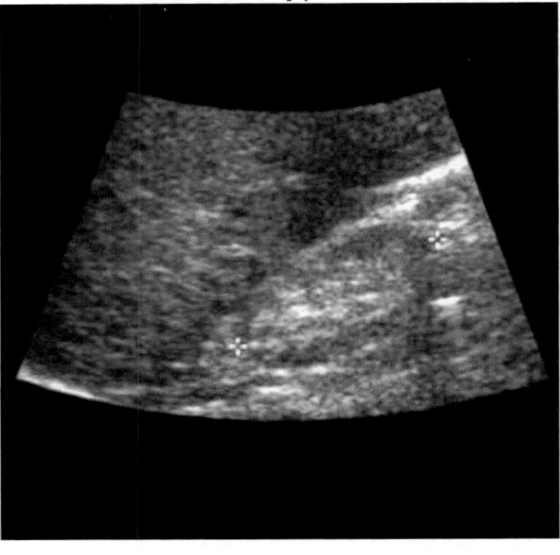

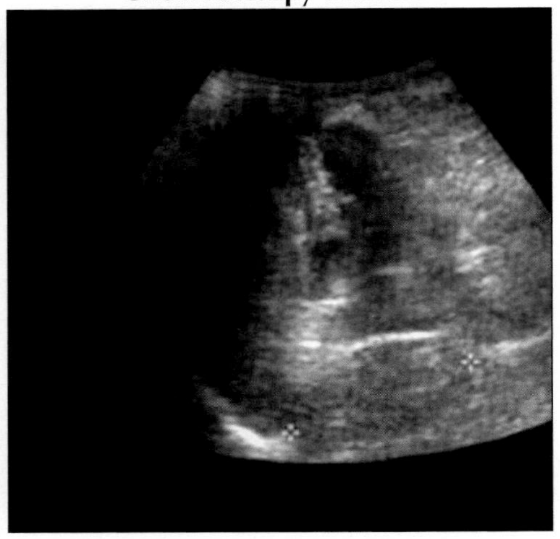

(Left) *Longitudinal ultrasound shows a small right kidney (calipers) with no corticomedullary differentiation in a patient with renal failure following chemotherapy and a bone marrow transplant for leukemia.* ***(Right)*** *Longitudinal ultrasound shows a small left kidney (calipers) with no corticomedullary differentiation in this patient post chemotherapy and bone marrow transplant for leukemia.*

Shock/Trauma/Cortical Necrosis | **Shock/Trauma/Cortical Necrosis**

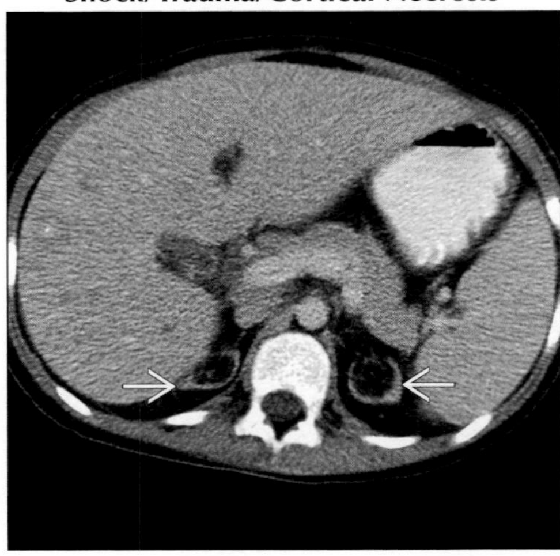

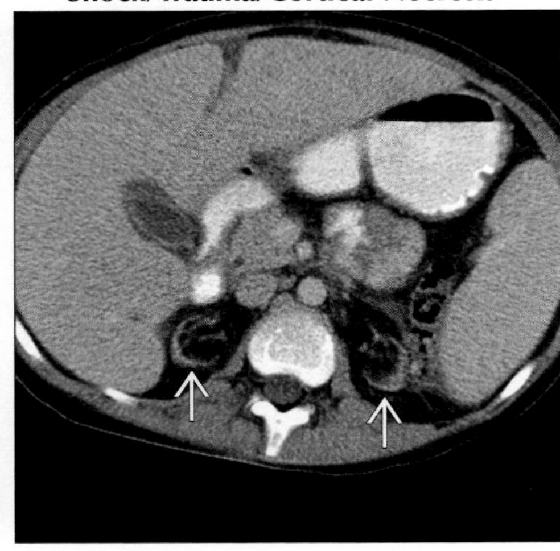

(Left) *Axial CECT shows only a thin rim of remaining renal cortex ➔ in this young patient who had bilateral renal cortical necrosis as a complication of meningococcemia.* ***(Right)*** *Axial CECT shows a thin rim of scarred renal cortex ➔ and fatty hilum in the same patient who required a renal transplant due to cortical necrosis and end-stage renal disease.*

Mid Aortic Syndrome

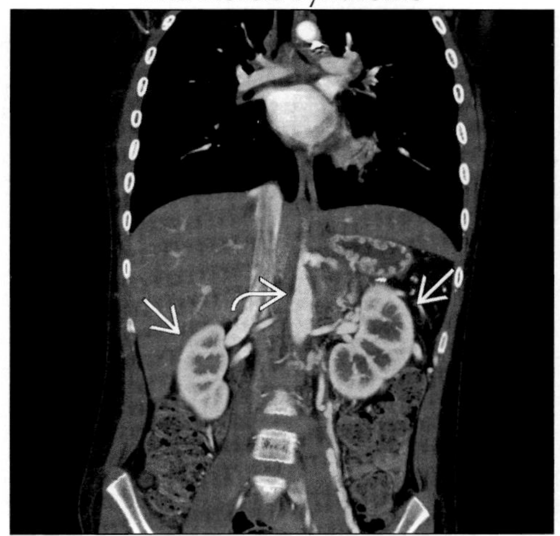

Mid Aortic Syndrome

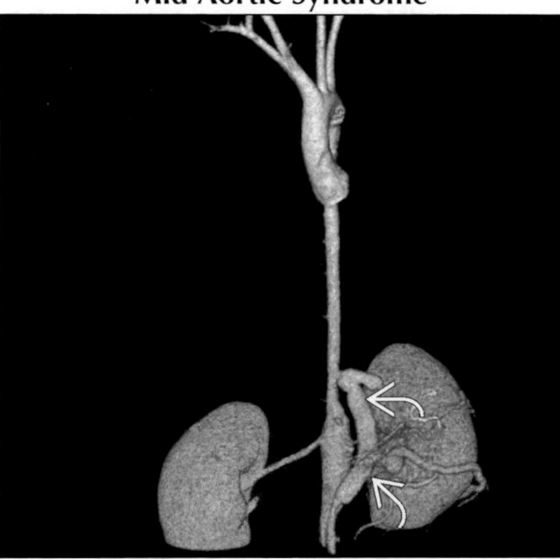

(Left) *Coronal reformat CECT shows small kidneys ➡ after a jump graft ➡ for mid aortic syndrome in a 7-year-old boy who presented with lower extremity paresthesias and chronic abdominal pain related to ischemia.* ***(Right)*** *3D reconstruction of a CTA shows the small kidneys and jump graft ➡ in the same patient with mid aortic syndrome. The patient had numerous re-stenoses and vascular complications contributing to renal ischemia.*

Medullary Cystic Disease and Nephronophthisis

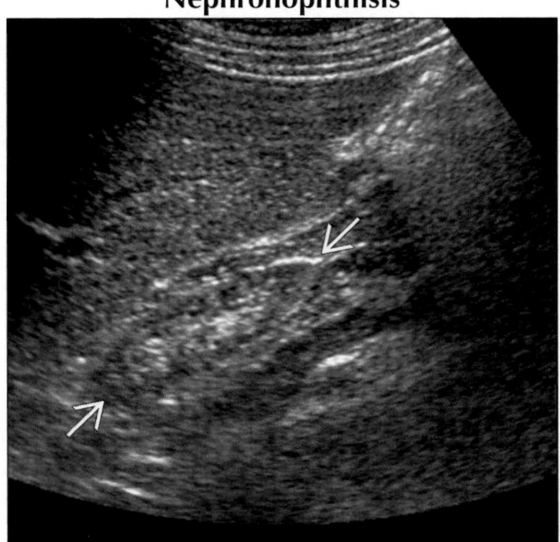

Medullary Cystic Disease and Nephronophthisis

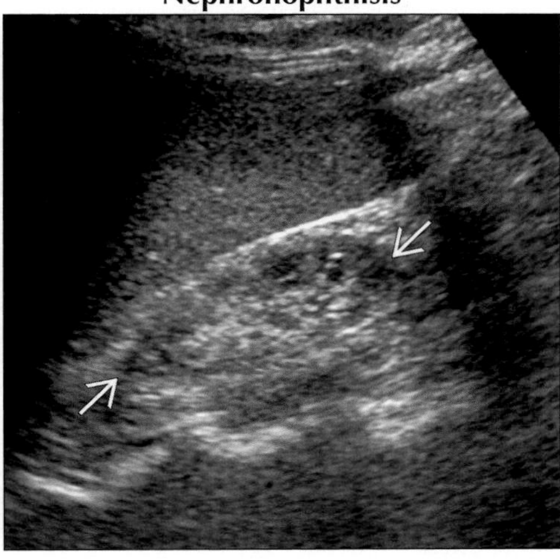

(Left) *Longitudinal harmonic ultrasound shows a very echogenic right kidney ➡ with poor corticomedullary differentiation and a few tiny cysts in this teenage girl with medullary cystic disease.* ***(Right)*** *Longitudinal harmonic ultrasound shows a similar appearance of the left kidney ➡ in the same girl. The patient eventually needed a renal transplant, as did her 2 sisters, both with medullary cystic disease.*

Alport Syndrome

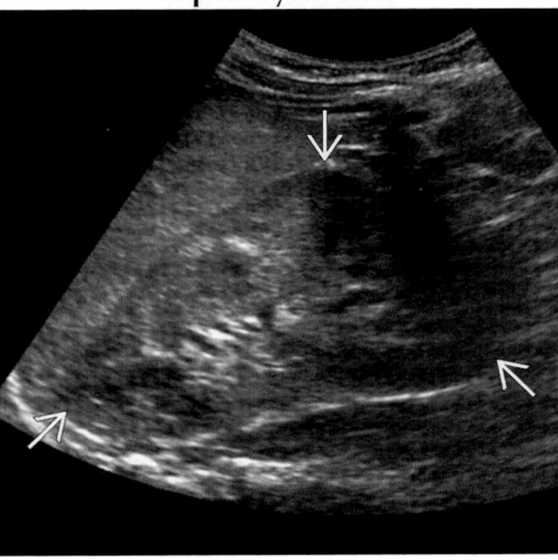

Alport Syndrome

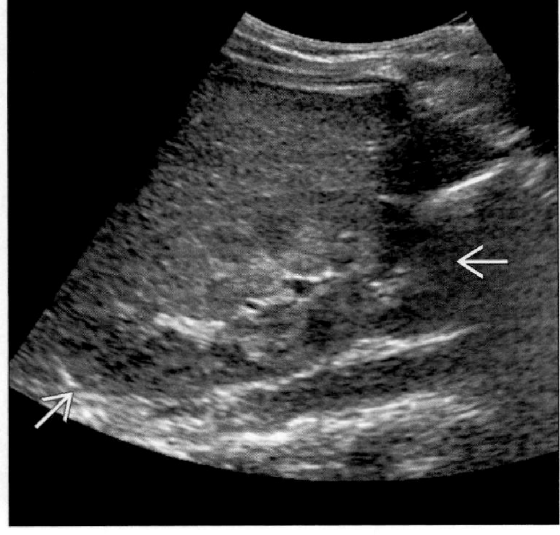

(Left) *Longitudinal harmonic ultrasound shows increased echoes ➡ and poor corticomedullary differentiation. This 4-year-old boy had sensorineural hearing loss, proteinuria, hematuria, and a maternal grandfather with Alport syndrome.* ***(Right)*** *Longitudinal harmonic ultrasound shows a similar appearance of the right kidney ➡ in the same boy. His kidneys will continue to shrink in size and deteriorate in function over the years.*

UNILATERAL LARGE KIDNEY

DIFFERENTIAL DIAGNOSIS

Common
- Hydronephrosis
- Duplication
- Crossed Fused Ectopia
- Compensatory Hypertrophy
- Multicystic Dysplastic Kidney (MCDK)
- Pyelonephritis
- Wilms Tumor

Less Common
- Multilocular Cystic Nephroma
- Mesoblastic Nephroma
- Renal Vein Thrombosis, Acute Phase
- Trauma

Rare but Important
- Infarction
- Venolymphatic Malformations
- Renal Medullary Carcinoma
- Unusual Renal Tumors

ESSENTIAL INFORMATION

Key Differential Diagnosis Issues
- Comparison to contralateral kidney is key
- Look up renal length when side of abnormality is not apparent
- Assess
  - Renal contour
  - Corticomedullary differentiation
  - Contrast enhancement pattern
  - Presence of cysts or masses
  - Vascular compromise: Abnormal supply, compression, tumor thrombus
  - Adjacent spaces and nodes

Helpful Clues for Common Diagnoses
- **Duplication**
  - Look for band of cortex separating upper and lower poles
  - Look for 2nd renal pelvis and ureter
- **Crossed Fused Ectopia**
  - Contralateral kidney will be absent
  - Occasionally lower renal tissue lies in midline, "J" shape
  - Part of spectrum of renal ascent and rotation abnormalities
  - Lower renal moiety ureter will cross to contralateral trigone
- **Compensatory Hypertrophy**
  - Seen most commonly with contralateral aplasia or MCDK
  - Also seen following early surgical removal of kidney
  - Less common with hypoplasia/dysplasia
- **Multicystic Dysplastic Kidney (MCDK)**
  - Classic type: Conglomerate cysts without discernible renal pelvis
  - Hydronephrotic type: Central cyst thought to be remnant of obstructed pelvis
  - High incidence of contralateral renal abnormalities
    - Ureteropelvic junction obstruction
    - Vesicoureteral reflux
  - MCDK initially large, but vast majority shrink over course of years
  - 1/2 of all MCDK have involuted by age 5
  - 12 reported cases of Wilms and renal cell carcinoma occurring in MCDK
    - National MCDK Registry tracks incidence and behavior
  - Imaging: Ultrasound and nuclear scan to confirm nonfunction
- **Pyelonephritis**
  - May have normal echotexture on ultrasound
  - Look for
    - Altered corticomedullary interface
    - Focal hypoechoic area
    - Decreased perfusion on Doppler exam
    - Bulge in cortex from focal swelling
    - Striated nephrogram on CT, MR, or IVP
    - Poorly enhancing areas on contrast studies
    - Wedge-shaped photopenic area on DMSA
  - Imaging
    - DMSA most sensitive exam
    - CT & MR next most sensitive
    - Ultrasound least sensitive but does exclude complications of abscess, perinephric collection, obstruction
- **Wilms Tumor**
  - Malignant tumor of primitive metanephric blastema
  - Most common renal tumor in children
  - Peak incidence ages 2-5
  - Typically heterogeneous soft tissue
  - Vascular extension and tumor thrombus common

- 5-10% are bilateral, associated with nephroblastomatosis
- Large tumors grow into perinephric space, periaortic nodes
- Metastasize to lung
- Cure rate is 90% or better with chemotherapy
- Imaging: Ultrasound, CT, MR, nucs (per treatment protocol)

Helpful Clues for Less Common Diagnoses

- **Multilocular Cystic Nephroma**
  - a.k.a. cystic nephroma
  - Rare, benign tumor
  - Bimodal age distribution
    - Childhood: M:F = 2:1, 3 months to 2 years
    - Adulthood: M:F = 1:8, 30 years or older
  - Can mimic cystic Wilms tumor; always removed
  - Imaging: Ultrasound, CT, MR, nucs (per treatment protocol)
- **Mesoblastic Nephroma**
  - Most common renal tumor in neonate
  - Peak age 3 months
  - Typically solid but can also be cystic
  - Predominantly benign but can be locally invasive or recur
  - Imaging: Ultrasound, CT, MR, nucs (per treatment protocol)
- **Renal Vein Thrombosis, Acute Phase**
  - Obstruction to venous outflow causes renal engorgement, ischemia, and eventually infarction if not relieved
  - Chronically, kidney scars and atrophies
  - Imaging: Ultrasound with Doppler, CT angiography, conventional angiography (rarely)
- **Trauma**
  - Contusion of kidney with global swelling
  - Perinephric hematomas, urinomas, subcapsular hematomas, etc. can all mimic enlarged kidney
  - Imaging: CT best in acute setting, ultrasound to follow-up

Helpful Clues for Rare Diagnoses

- **Infarction**
  - Arterial compromise, particularly from emboli, can cause renal enlargement
- **Venolymphatic Malformations**
  - Rarely retroperitoneal vascular malformation may involve kidney
- **Renal Medullary Carcinoma**
  - Rare tumor
  - Young patients with sickle cell trait
  - Highly aggressive tumor
  - Central, infiltrating tumor with caliectasis and regional adenopathy
  - Metastases often seen at presentation
  - Poor prognosis
- **Unusual Renal Tumors**
  - Clear cell carcinoma
  - Rhabdoid tumor
  - Primitive neuroectoderm tumor (PNET)
  - Renal cell carcinoma

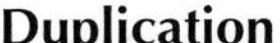

Duplication

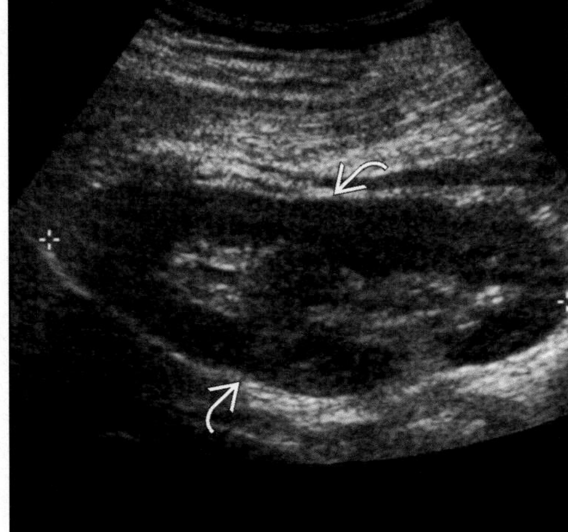

Longitudinal ultrasound shows a band of parenchyma crossing the central sinus fat and dividing the kidney into upper and lower moieties in this 14 year old with a 15 cm long right kidney.

Duplication

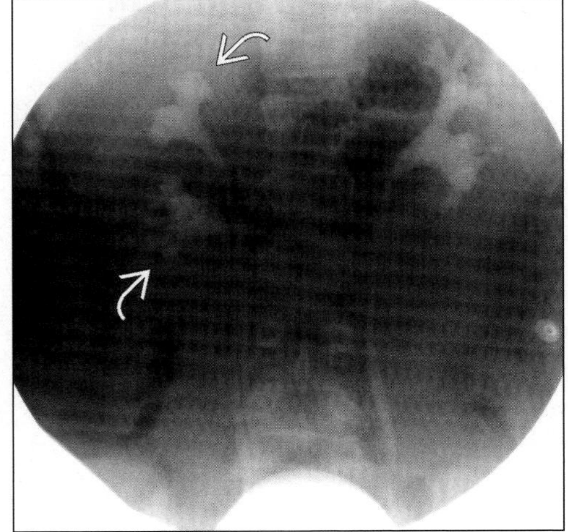

AP voiding cystourethrogram in the same patient shows bilateral vesicoureteral reflux and duplication of the right-sided collecting system, with mild caliectasis in the right upper pole.

UNILATERAL LARGE KIDNEY

(Left) *Longitudinal ultrasound shows what should have been the left kidney (calipers) attached to the lower pole of the right kidney ➡, which is located in the right flank in this patient with crossed fused renal ectopia.* *(Right)* *Coronal T2WI MR shows a left crossed fused ectopic kidney ➡ in a different child being evaluated for diastematomyelia and a split spinal cord. The upper pole of the left kidney is partially intrathoracic in location.*

Crossed Fused Ectopia

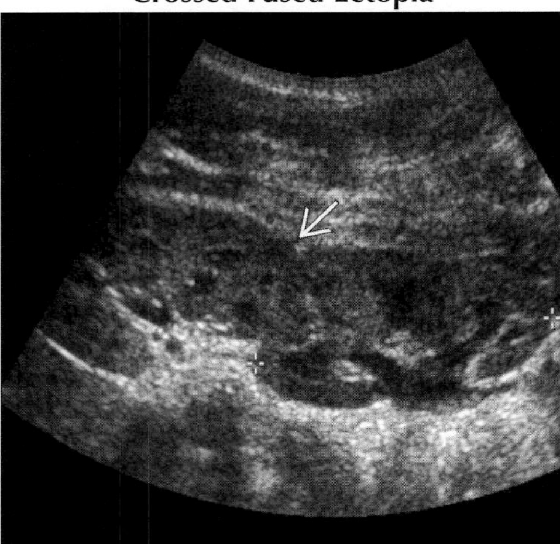

Crossed Fused Ectopia

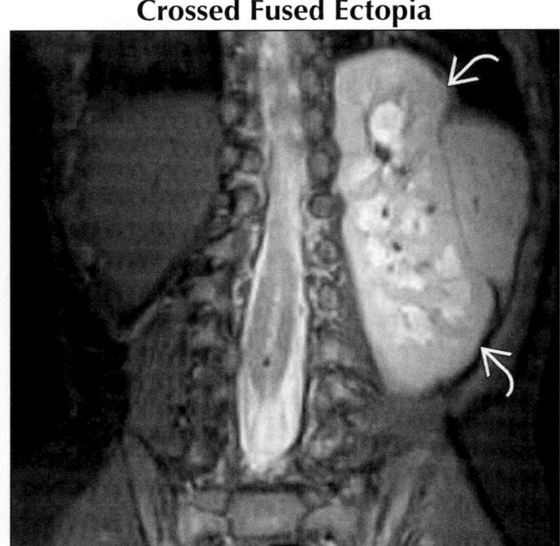

(Left) *Longitudinal harmonic ultrasound shows the left kidney measuring more than 17 cm in this teenager. There is no evidence of a duplication or parenchymal band crossing the central sinus fat in this patient with a solitary left kidney with compensatory hypertrophy.* *(Right)* *Longitudinal harmonic ultrasound shows bowel gas occupying the right renal fossa ➡ in this patient with agenesis of the right kidney and compensatory hypertrophy of the solitary left kidney.*

Compensatory Hypertrophy

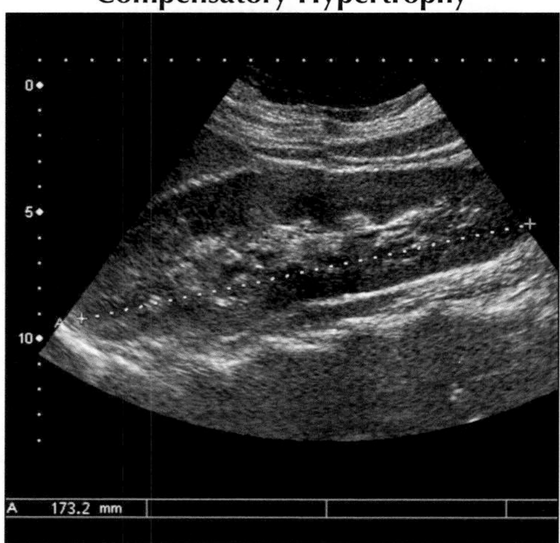

Compensatory Hypertrophy

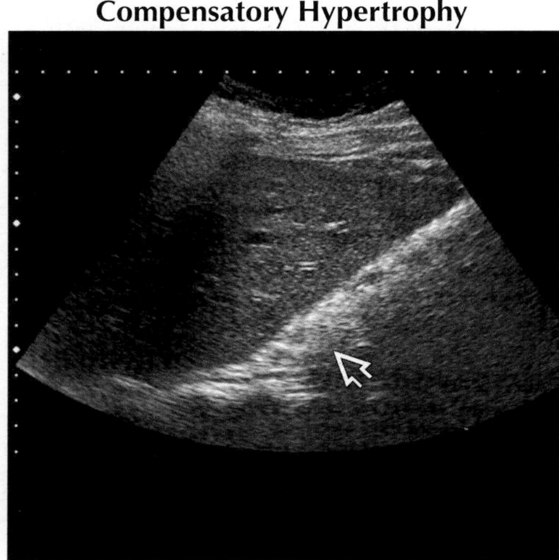

(Left) *Coronal oblique T2WI MR shows numerous cysts ➡ replacing the left kidney in this fetus with a renal anomaly on a screening ultrasound exam. The contralateral kidney was normal. A left-sided ureterocele (not shown) was seen at the bladder base, suggesting an obstructive etiology to this multicystic dysplastic kidney.* *(Right)* *Coronal oblique T2WI MR shows the left MCDK ➡ with high signal intensity fluid in the stomach ➡ just above the kidney.*

Multicystic Dysplastic Kidney (MCDK)

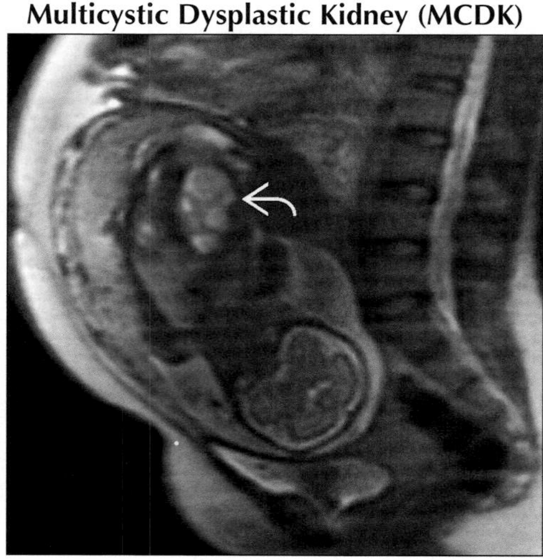

Multicystic Dysplastic Kidney (MCDK)

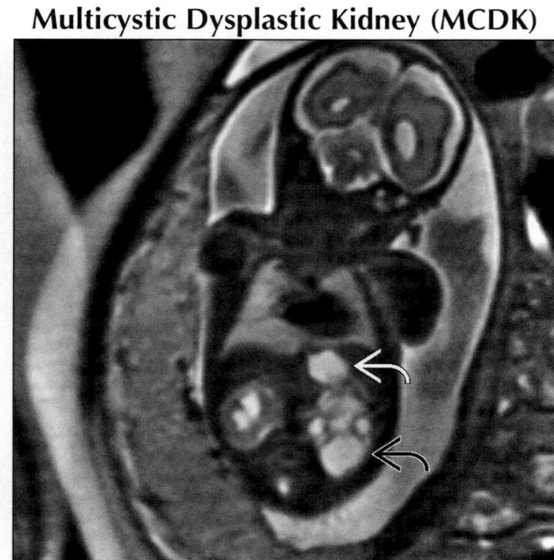

UNILATERAL LARGE KIDNEY

Multicystic Dysplastic Kidney (MCDK)

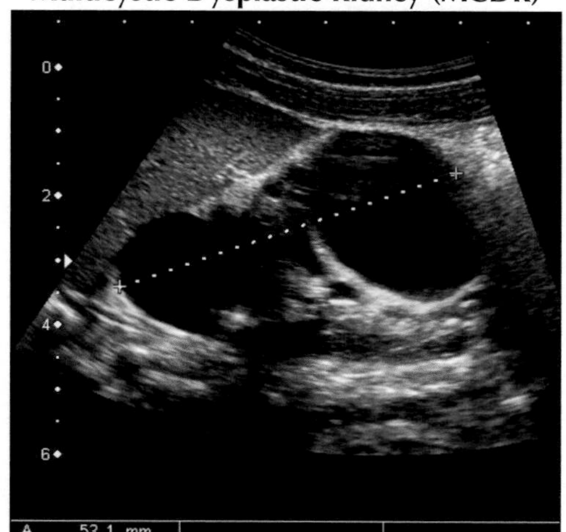

Multicystic Dysplastic Kidney (MCDK)

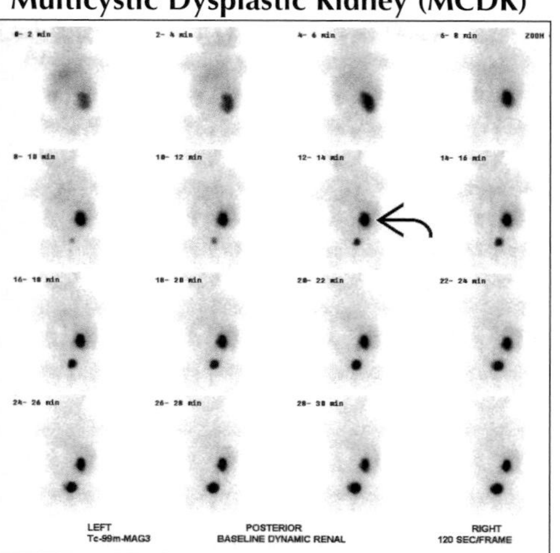

(Left) *Longitudinal harmonic ultrasound performed postnatally shows numerous cysts replacing the left kidney (calipers) with some echogenic intervening parenchyma.* ***(Right)*** *Posteroanterior renal scan in a newborn shows normal uptake and excretion in the right kidney → but no functional renal tissue on the left side, confirming the diagnosis of MCDK.*

Pyelonephritis

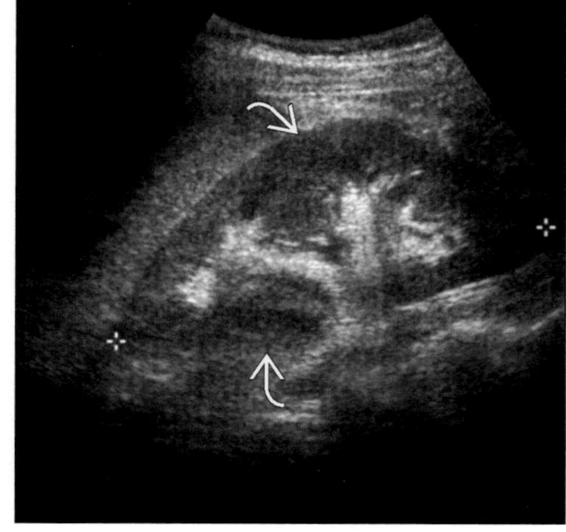

Pyelonephritis

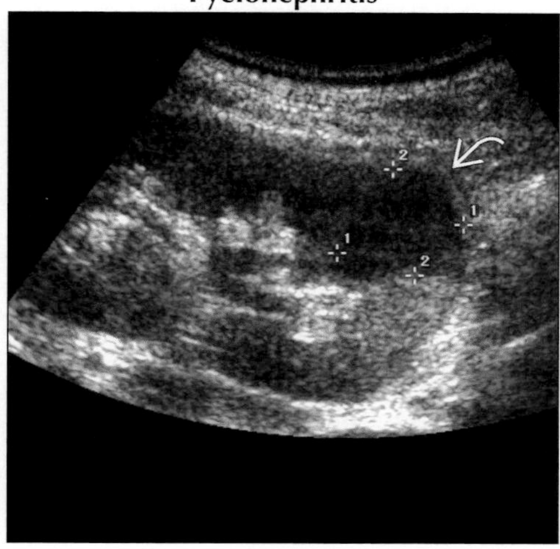

(Left) *Longitudinal ultrasound shows several areas of focal swelling with poor corticomedullary differentiation → within the left kidney, which was larger than the right. The patient complained of flank pain and dysuria.* ***(Right)*** *Longitudinal prone image in the same patient shows the margins of a focal abnormal area (calipers) in the lower pole of the left kidney. Note the focal bulge in the renal contour → and decreased echogenicity.*

Pyelonephritis

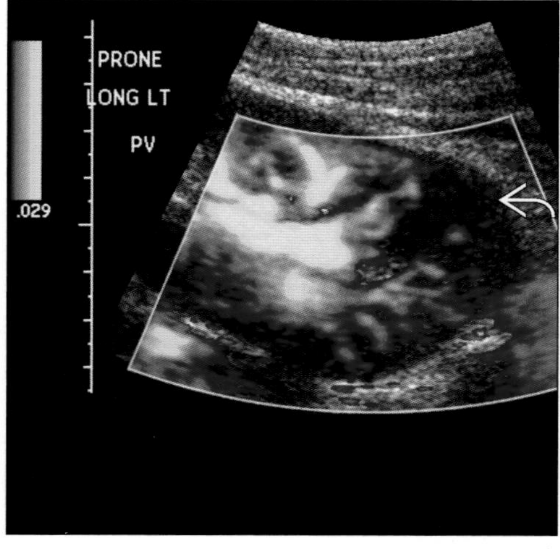

Pyelonephritis

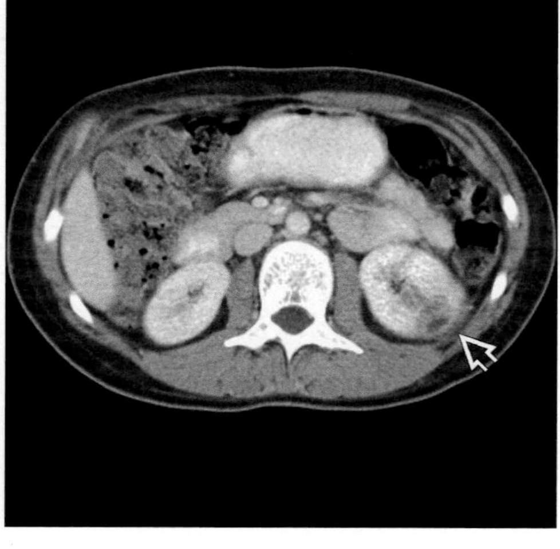

(Left) *Longitudinal power Doppler ultrasound shows decreased perfusion of this hypoechoic region in the left lower pole →, consistent with focal pyelonephritis. Note that there is no liquefaction or perinephric collection that would suggest an abscess.* ***(Right)*** *Axial CECT in the same patient shows focal abscess formation → in the same region 1 week later, when a CT scan was performed due to persistent fevers and flank pain.*

UNILATERAL LARGE KIDNEY

*(**Left**) AP radiograph shows a soft tissue mass ➔ in the left side of the abdomen displacing the bowel. This 3 year old was being evaluated for emesis and fatigue. (**Right**) Longitudinal ultrasound shows a very large soft tissue mass in the left abdomen (calipers). The mass was so large that it was difficult to determine the organ of origin.*

Wilms Tumor

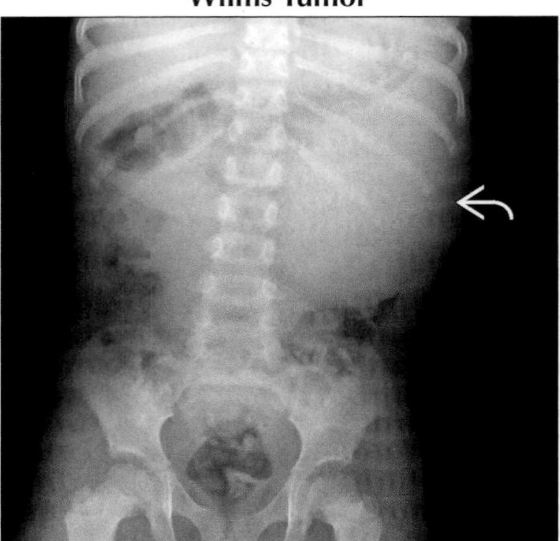

Wilms Tumor

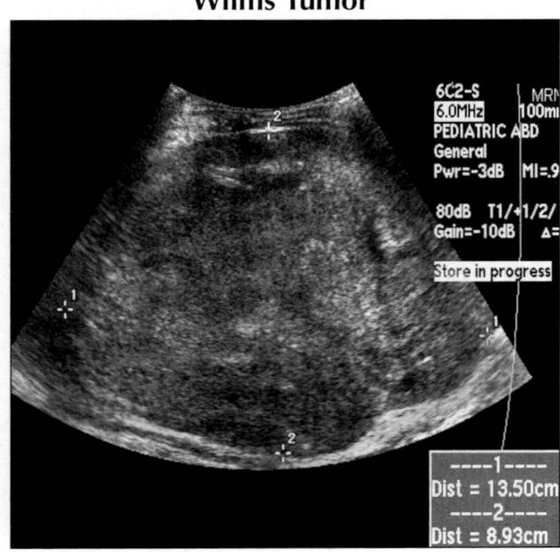

*(**Left**) Axial CECT shows a heterogeneous soft tissue mass filling the left abdomen and displacing the bowel anteriorly and rightward. Note the filling defect in the inferior vena cava (IVC) ➔ suggesting tumor thrombus in this patient with Wilms tumor. (**Right**) Axial CECT shows tumor thrombus extending cephalad to the junction of the intrahepatic IVC and the right atrium ➔. This patient was treated with chemotherapy before resection of his stage III Wilms tumor.*

Wilms Tumor

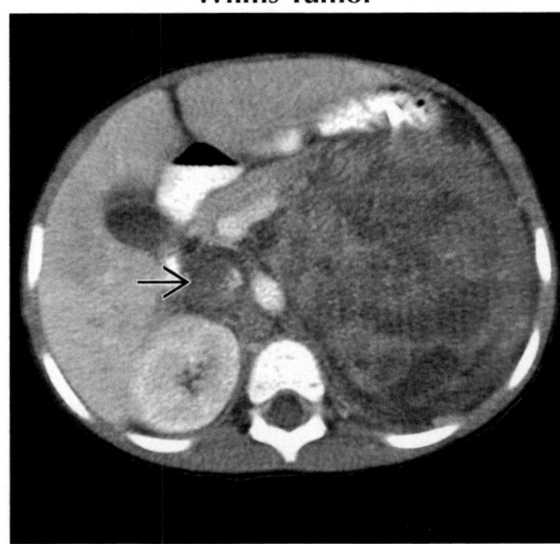

Wilms Tumor

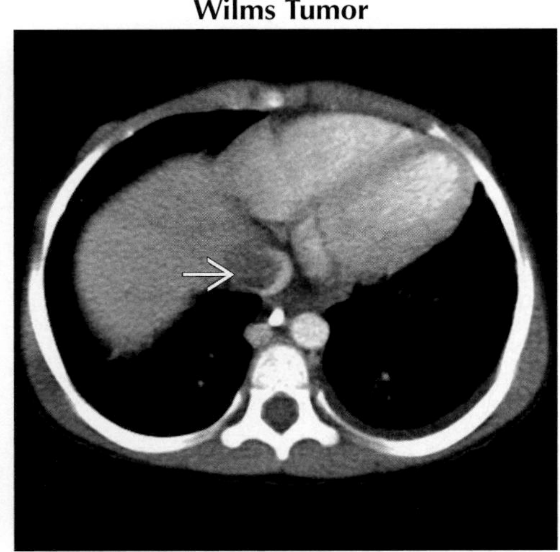

*(**Left**) Longitudinal ultrasound shows a large, multiseptated, cystic lesion (calipers) replacing the left kidney in this 1-year-old girl whose parents reported her having 2 months of abdominal distention. (**Right**) Coronal T2WI MR in the same patient shows the large cystic, septated mass ➔, a multilocular cystic nephroma, filling the left side of the abdomen. A thin crescent of residual renal parenchyma ➔ is seen along the medial border.*

Multilocular Cystic Nephroma

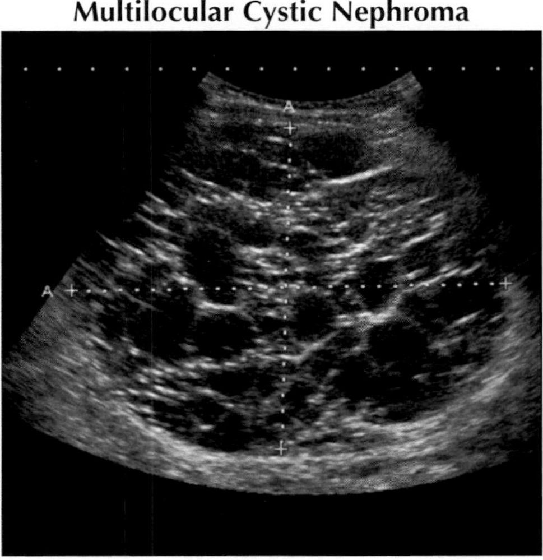

Multilocular Cystic Nephroma

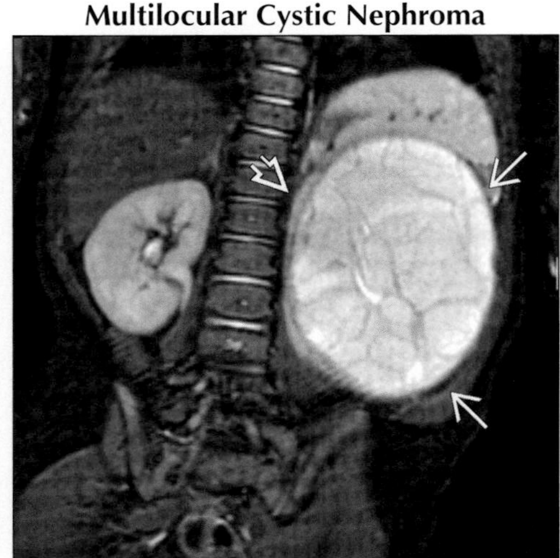

Mesoblastic Nephroma

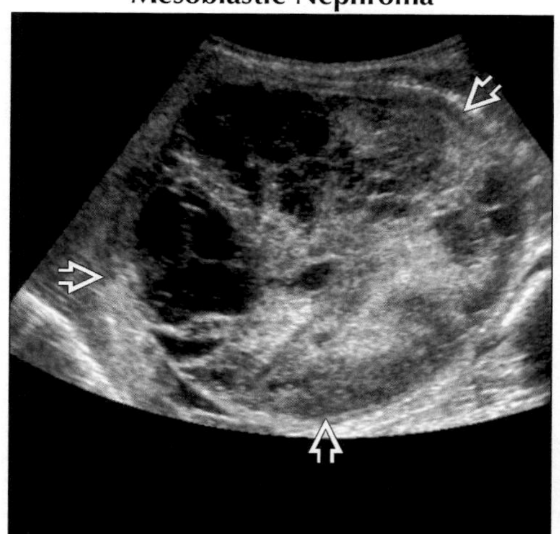

Mesoblastic Nephroma

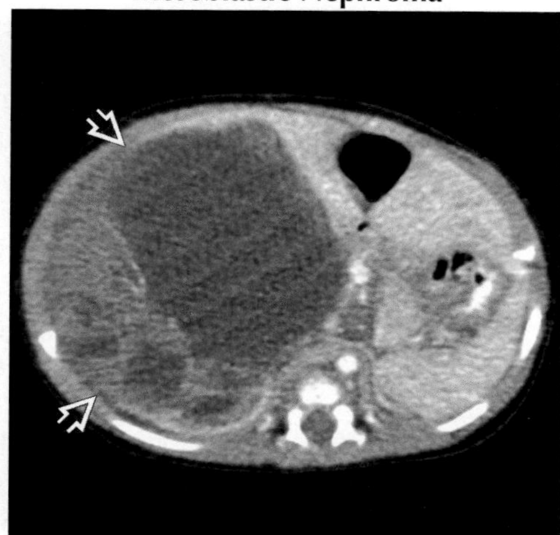

*(**Left**) Longitudinal ultrasound shows a heterogeneous solid and cystic mass ➡ in the right flank of this 1-month-old boy with a palpable mass. (**Right**) Axial CECT in the same patient shows the large, mixed solid and cystic mass ➡ replacing the right kidney. The differential included malignancy, so the mass was removed. Pathology showed a benign mesoblastic nephroma, which is typically more solid and not this large.*

Renal Vein Thrombosis, Acute Phase

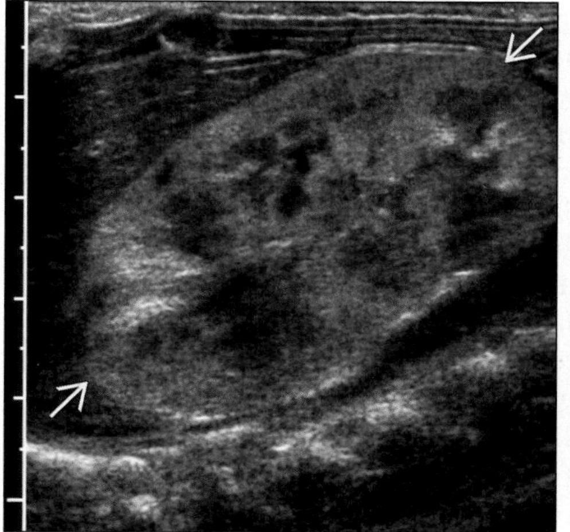

Renal Vein Thrombosis, Acute Phase

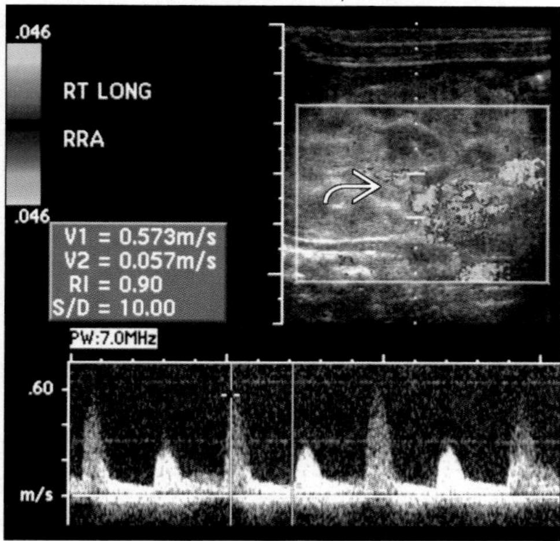

*(**Left**) Longitudinal ultrasound shows a plump kidney ➡ with increased echotexture in this premature infant with sepsis and deteriorating renal function. (**Right**) Pulsed Doppler ultrasound shows high resistance to intrarenal perfusion, though the main renal artery is patent. The Doppler gate ➡ is wide open, but no venous signal is detected in this infant with acute renal vein thrombosis and an enlarged right kidney.*

Trauma

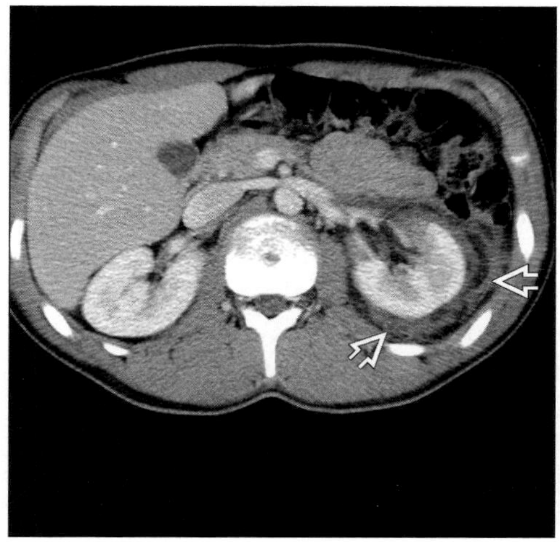

Trauma

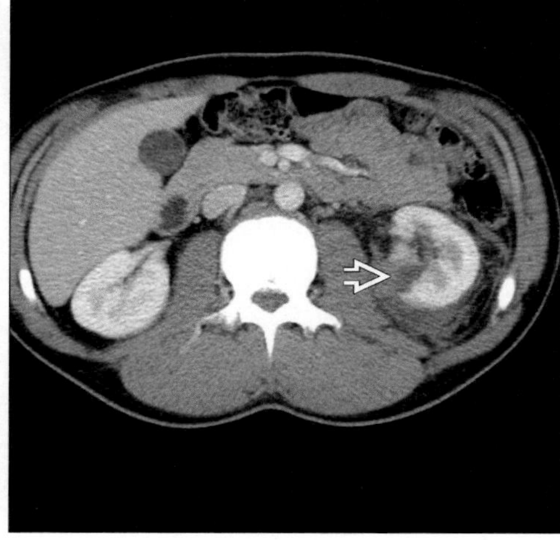

*(**Left**) Axial CECT shows hematoma ➡ surrounding the left kidney in this 15-year-old boy who hit his side while snowboarding. (**Right**) Axial CECT slightly more inferiorly shows frank laceration ➡ of the kidney extending to the central sinus. Although the kidney itself is not enlarged, the perinephric collection of blood and urine mimics unilateral renal enlargement.*

BILATERAL LARGE KIDNEYS

DIFFERENTIAL DIAGNOSIS

Common
- Hydronephrosis
- Duplicated Kidney
- Pyelonephritis
- Glomerulonephritis
- Nephrotic Syndrome
- Polycystic Kidney Disease
  - Autosomal Recessive
  - Autosomal Dominant
- Lymphoma/Leukemia

Less Common
- Lymphoproliferative Disorder
- Sickle Cell Disease
- Renal Vein Thrombosis
- Hemolytic Uremic Syndrome
- Henoch-Schönlein Purpura

Rare but Important
- Nephroblastomatosis
- Prune Belly Syndrome
- Angiomyolipomas
- Tuberous Sclerosis
- Glycogen Storage Disease
- Megacalycosis
- Caroli Polycystic Kidney Disease

ESSENTIAL INFORMATION

Key Differential Diagnosis Issues
- Bilaterally enlarged kidneys often abnormal in morphology
  - Hydronephrotic
  - Cystic
  - Mass lesions
  - Altered cortex or medulla
  - Duplicated kidney
  - Exceptions where kidneys may appear large but otherwise "normal"
    - Pyelonephritis
    - Glomerulonephritis
    - Nephrotic syndrome
- Refer to pediatric renal size charts to determine if kidneys are large
  - Rule of thumb for renal length range
    - Newborn: 3.5-5 cm
    - 7-year-old child: 7-10 cm
    - Teenager: 10-12 cm

Helpful Clues for Common Diagnoses
- **Hydronephrosis**
  - Look for site of obstruction
- **Duplicated Kidney**
  - Look for band of cortex separating upper and lower pole
  - Look for 2nd renal pelvis and ureter
- **Pyelonephritis**
  - May have normal echotexture on US
  - Look for
    - Altered corticomedullary interface
    - Focal hypoechoic area
    - Decreased perfusion on Doppler exam
    - Bulge in cortex from focal swelling
    - Striated nephrogram on CT, MR, or IVP
    - Poorly enhancing areas on contrast studies
    - Wedge-shaped photopenic area on DMSA scan
- **Glomerulonephritis**
  - Kidneys are enlarged in acute phase
  - Kidneys may atrophy over time if insult continues and develop into ESRD
- **Nephrotic Syndrome**
  - Classically enlarged with poor corticomedullary differentiation
  - Ascites and anasarca may be clue to diagnosis
- **Polycystic Kidney Disease**
  - **Autosomal Recessive**
    - ~ 10% of all polycystic kidney diseases
    - More common cause of bilateral large kidneys in pediatric patients than autosomal dominant
    - Mutation of *PKHD1* gene
    - Problems begin in utero
    - Many patients die within hours or days of birth
    - Some patients may live for years with chronic renal insufficiency
    - Imaging: Huge echogenic kidneys, tiny cysts, and dilated tubules visible with newer ultrasound machines
  - **Autosomal Dominant**
    - ~ 90% of polycystic kidney diseases
    - Variable penetrance and severity
    - Cysts replace functional nephrons and impair renal function
    - Cysts usually visible in 2nd and 3rd decade but can also be seen in infants and children
- **Lymphoma/Leukemia**

- Nonenhancing or hypoechoic rounded masses
  - Occasionally enlarged kidneys without discernible masses

Helpful Clues for Less Common Diagnoses

- **Lymphoproliferative Disorder**
  - Transplant history or altered immune status
  - Nonenhancing or hypoechoic rounded masses
  - Associated adenopathy often impressive
- **Sickle Cell Disease**
  - Renal medullary hyperechogenicity
  - RBCs sludging in vasa rectae
  - Papillary necrosis and hematuria
- **Renal Vein Thrombosis**
  - Bilateral cases often involve thrombus of inferior vena cava
  - Kidneys enlarge acutely → infarct and atrophy
- **Hemolytic Uremic Syndrome**
  - Disease of infants and children
  - Triad: Hemolytic anemia, thrombocytopenia, acute renal failure
  - Often follows GI, respiratory, or other febrile illness
  - Survival > 85% with early dialysis and supportive therapy
- **Henoch-Schönlein Purpura**
  - Vasculitis often follows respiratory illness
  - Purpuric rash, arthralgias, fever, glomerulonephritis, bowel wall thickening

Helpful Clues for Rare Diagnoses

- **Nephroblastomatosis**
  - Persistence of fetal metanephric blastema after 34 weeks gestation
  - Associated with
    - Beckwith-Wiedemann syndrome
    - Hemihypertrophy
    - Sporadic aniridia
  - Seen in 1% of infant autopsies
  - Increased risk of Wilms tumor
- **Prune Belly Syndrome**
  - Kidneys are enlarged due to marked hydroureteronephrosis
  - Patulous collecting system without obstruction
  - Triad: Undescended testes, absent abdominal wall musculature, dilated urinary tract
- **Angiomyolipomas**
  - Highly vascular tumors most often seen in tuberous sclerosis
- **Tuberous Sclerosis**
  - Variable severity of renal cysts and angiomyolipomas
- **Glycogen Storage Disease**
  - Metabolic products deposited in liver and kidneys cause enlargement
- **Megacalycosis**
  - Nonobstructive caliectasis
- **Caroli Polycystic Kidney Disease**
  - End of spectrum of autosomal recessive kidney disease with biliary ductal ectasia and hepatic fibrosis

Duplicated Kidney

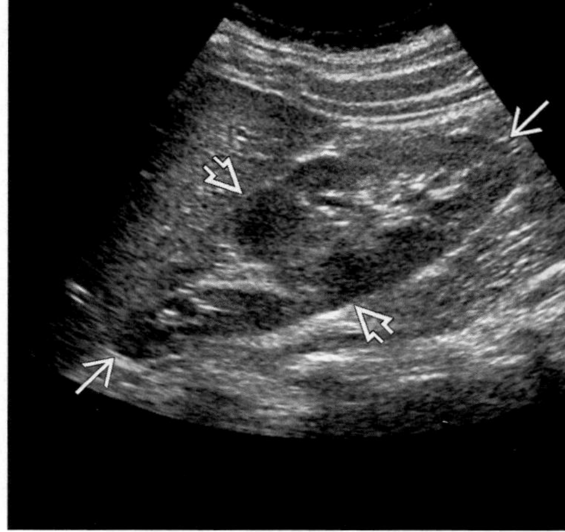

Longitudinal ultrasound shows a band of cortex ➲ crossing the central sinus fat, indicating a duplicated right kidney ➡ in this 9-year-old girl.

Duplicated Kidney

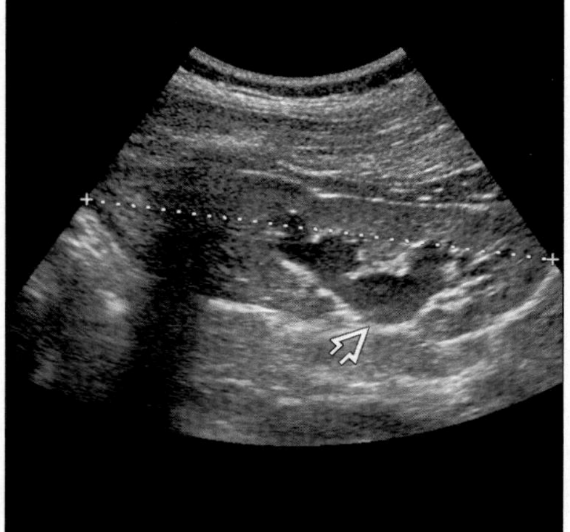

Longitudinal ultrasound in the same girl shows a 13.6 cm left kidney (calipers), which is also duplicated. Note the mild prominence of the lower pole collecting system ➲.

BILATERAL LARGE KIDNEYS

Duplicated Kidney

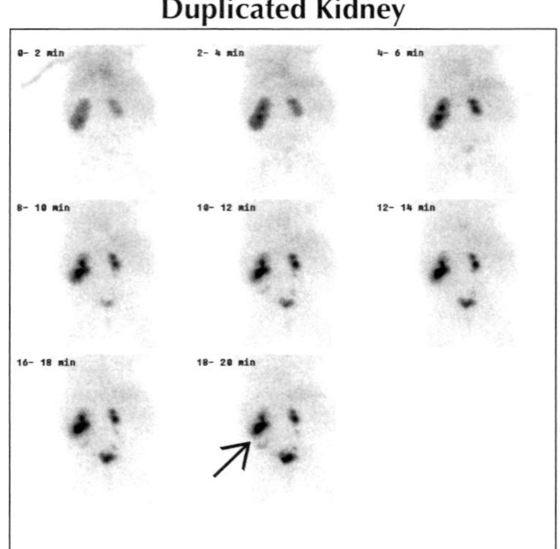

Duplicated Kidney

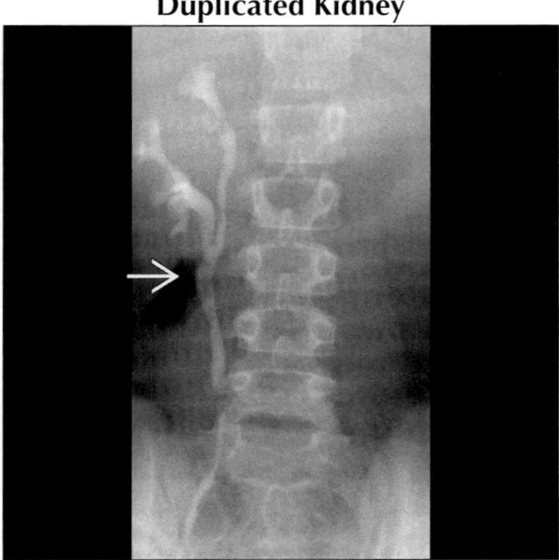

(Left) *Posteroanterior renal scan in a child shows altered uptake and excretion from the 4 components in these bilateral duplicated kidneys. There is some retention and delayed excretion from the lower pole moiety of the left kidney* ⇒. ***(Right)*** *Anteroposterior voiding cystourethrogram shows reflux into a partially duplicated right kidney. The 2 ureters fuse at the L3 level* ➔ *and enter the bladder in a single ureter at the trigone.*

Pyelonephritis

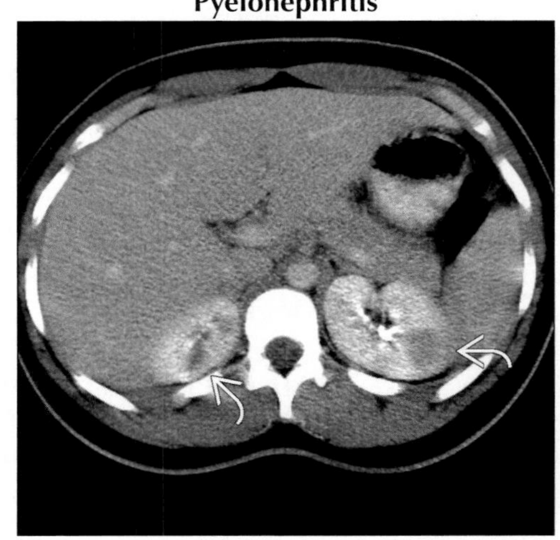

Pyelonephritis

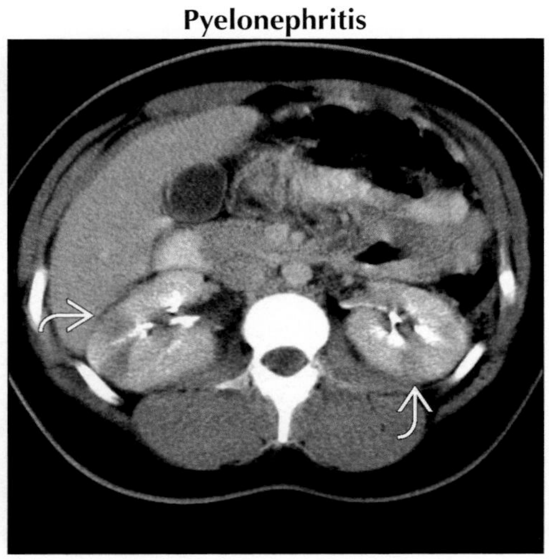

(Left) *Axial CECT shows triangular and striated areas of decreased renal enhancement* ➔ *in this teenager with bacteremia and bacteruria, consistent with bilateral pyelonephritis.* ***(Right)*** *Axial CECT shows similar findings* ➔ *in the more inferior aspect of both kidneys. The patient looked very ill and was scanned for suspected an intraabdominal abscess.*

Glomerulonephritis

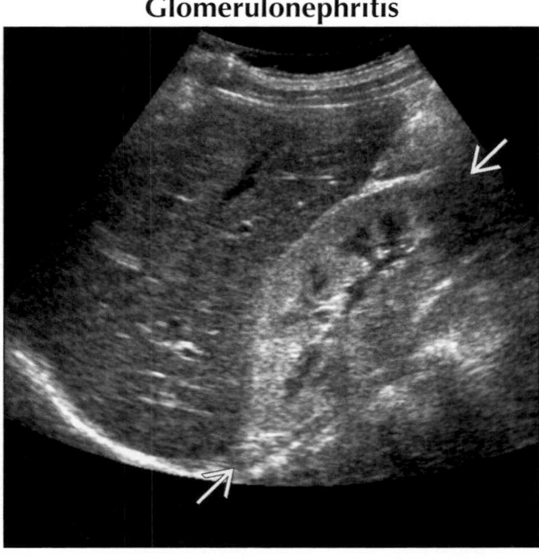

Glomerulonephritis

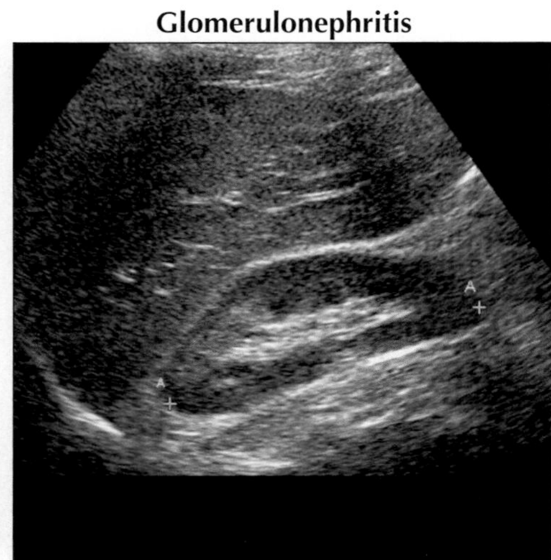

(Left) *Longitudinal US shows a very echogenic renal cortex* ➔ *in this 3-year-old boy with acute renal failure following an episode of febrile gastroenteritis. The renal length exceeds the 2nd upper standard deviation for age.* ***(Right)*** *Longitudinal US in the same patient several years later shows the kidneys with a normal appearance. The prior episode was caused by hemolytic uremic syndrome but could have been any glomerulonephritis/nephrotic syndrome.*

Polycystic Kidney Disease

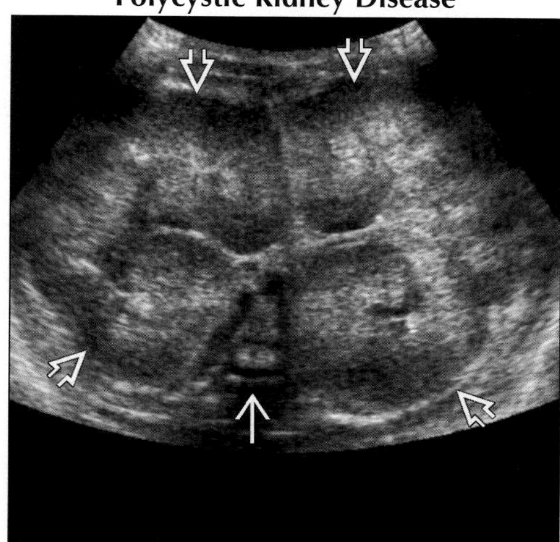

Polycystic Kidney Disease

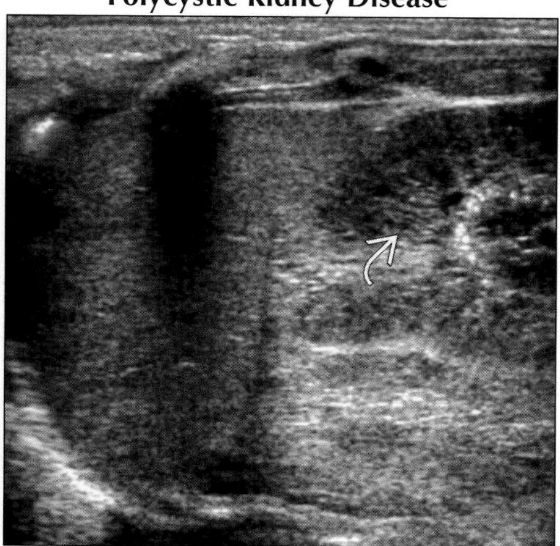

(Left) Transverse US shows massively enlarged, echogenic kidneys ➡ filling the lower abdomen & touching at the midline, anterior to the spine ➡ in a newborn with oligohydramnios. *(Right)* Longitudinal harmonic US with a high-frequency transducer shows tubular ectasia & tiny cysts ➡ throughout the left kidney upper pole. The interfaces created by the dilated tubules & cysts create the diffusely ↑ echotexture typical of ARPCKD.

Polycystic Kidney Disease

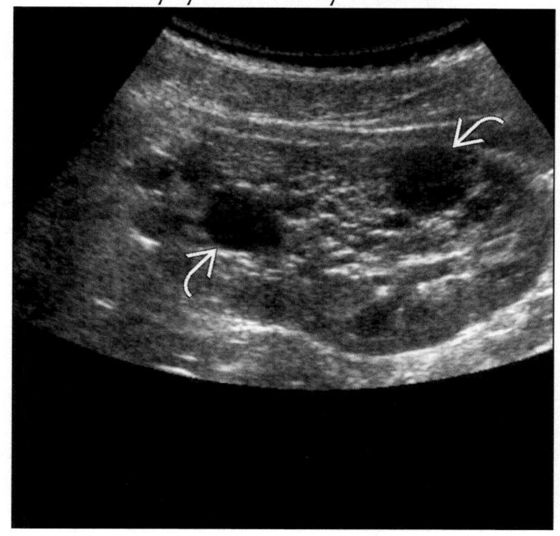

Autosomal Recessive

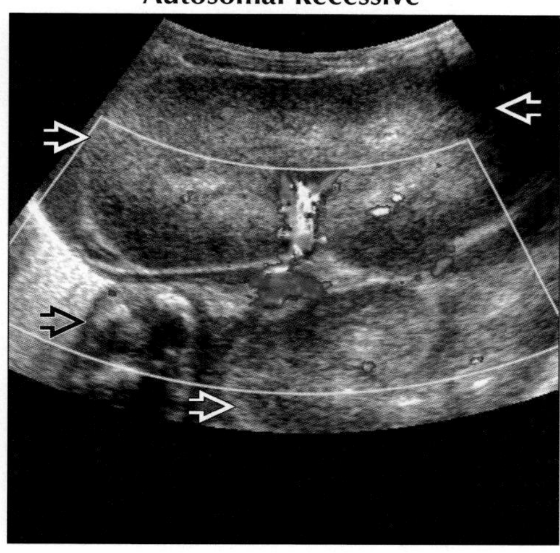

(Left) Longitudinal US shows numerous small cysts ➡ in the right kidney in this 6-year-old child with a family history of renal cystic disease. The kidney's length is within the upper 2nd deviation for age but above the mean. The renal function was normal at the time of the scan. *(Right)* Coronal color Doppler ultrasound from a lateral approach in the same patient shows echogenic renal tissue ➡ filling the upper abdomen. Note the stomach ➡.

Autosomal Recessive

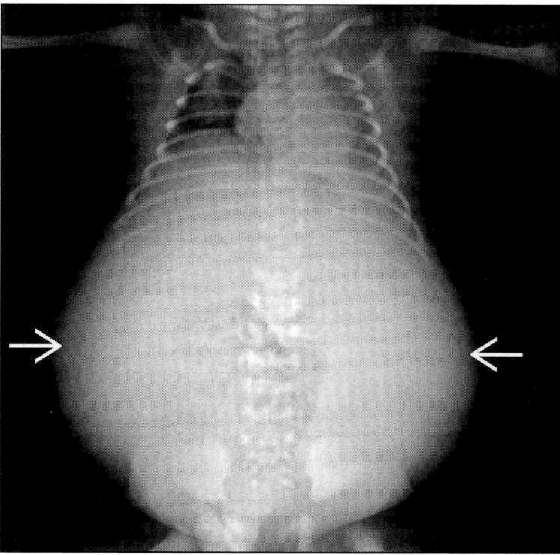

Autosomal Dominant

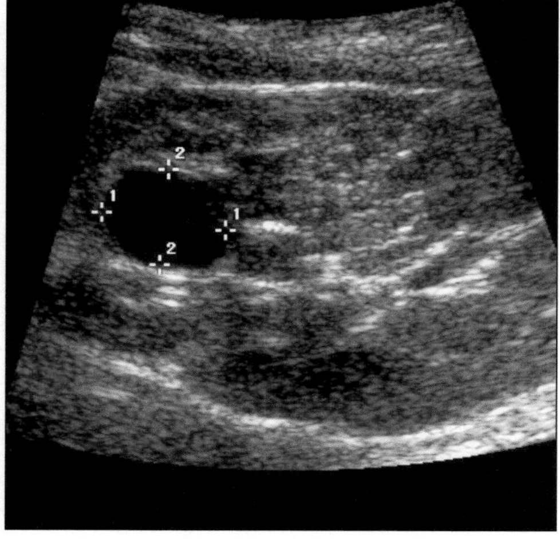

(Left) AP radiograph of the chest and abdomen shows a hypoplastic thoracic cavity and massive renal shadows ➡ filling the abdomen and displacing the bowel loops centrally. *(Right)* Longitudinal ultrasound in the same patient shows 1 of the cysts (calipers) in greater detail. The high-frequency linear transducer shows optimal detail of the cyst wall and its contents.

BILATERAL LARGE KIDNEYS

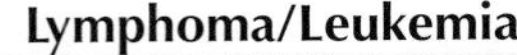

(**Left**) *PA radiograph shows marked soft tissue fullness in the mediastinum and right neck in a patient with fatigue, night sweats, and dyspnea on exertion. This 13 year old was subsequently diagnosed with T-cell lymphoma, which also involved the kidneys.* (**Right**) *Axial CECT shows poorly enhancing areas in both kidneys, which are mildly enlarged, and consistent with lymphomatous involvement.*

Lymphoma/Leukemia

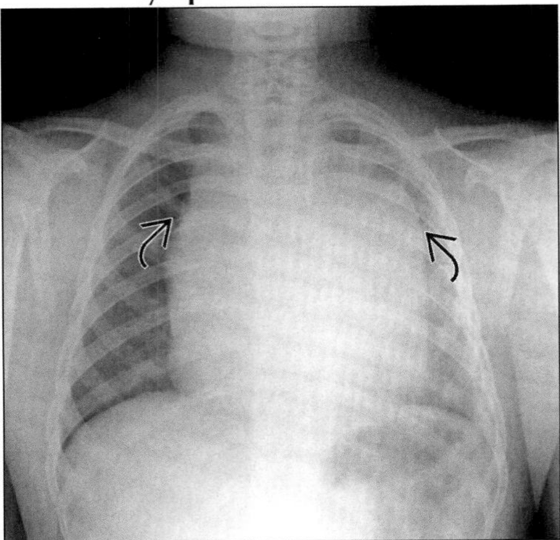

Lymphoma/Leukemia

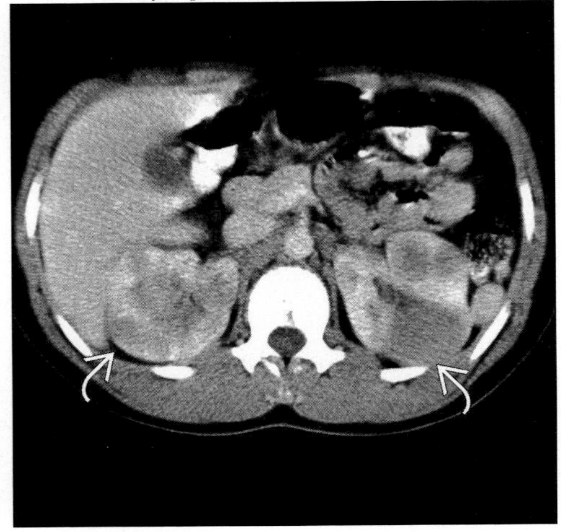

(**Left**) *Axial CECT shows poorly enhancing lesions in both kidneys, bulky periaortic adenopathy, and ascites in this 2-year-old liver transplant recipient with lymphoproliferative disorder.* (**Right**) *Coronal CECT in the same patient shows poorly enhancing renal lesions diffusely, periaortic adenopathy, ascites, and body wall anasarca.*

Lymphoproliferative Disorder

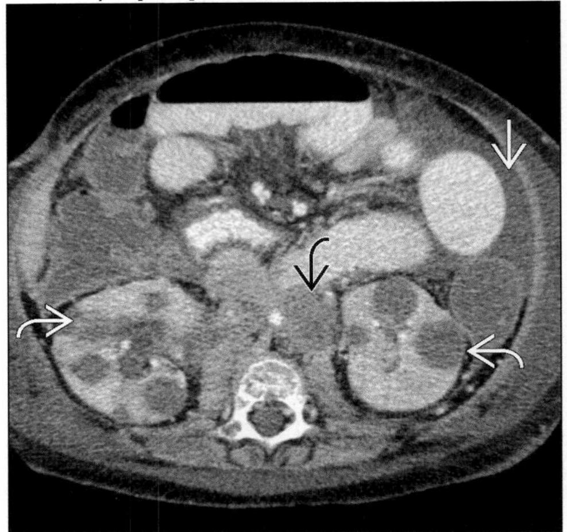

Lymphoproliferative Disorder

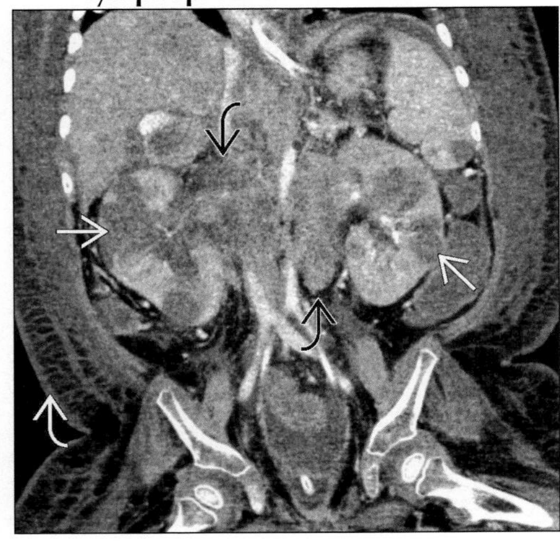

(**Left**) *Longitudinal ultrasound shows increased medullary echoes/echogenic pyramids. This teenager with sickle cell disease had microscopic hematuria, likely reflecting red-cell sludging in the vasa rectae &/or papillary necrosis.* (**Right**) *Bone scan in the same patient shows marked retention of radiotracer in both kidneys, which are mildly enlarged. No definite bone infarcts are seen, but the patient has some dental disease on the left.*

Sickle Cell Disease

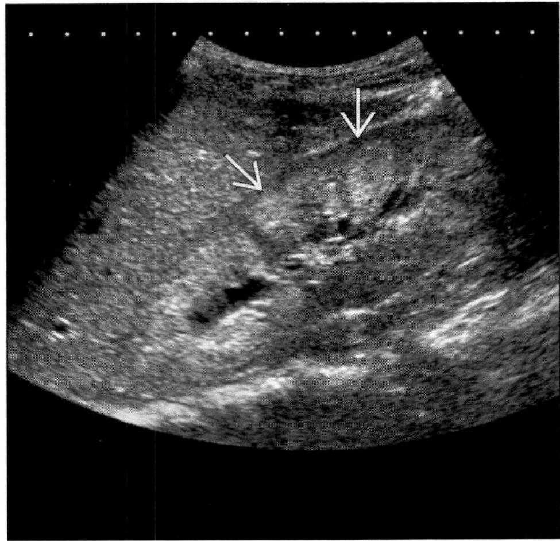

Sickle Cell Disease

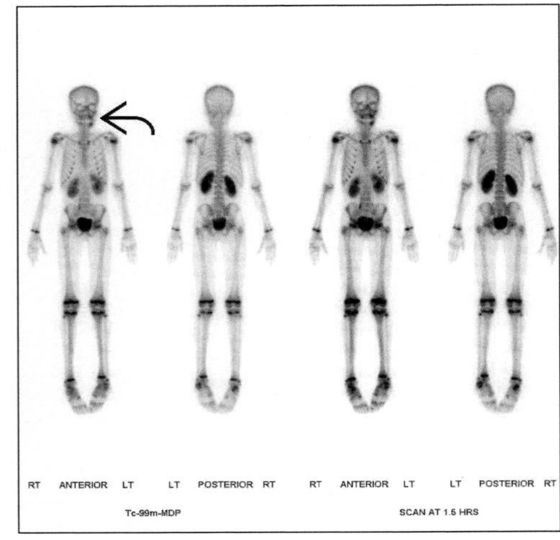

BILATERAL LARGE KIDNEYS

Nephroblastomatosis

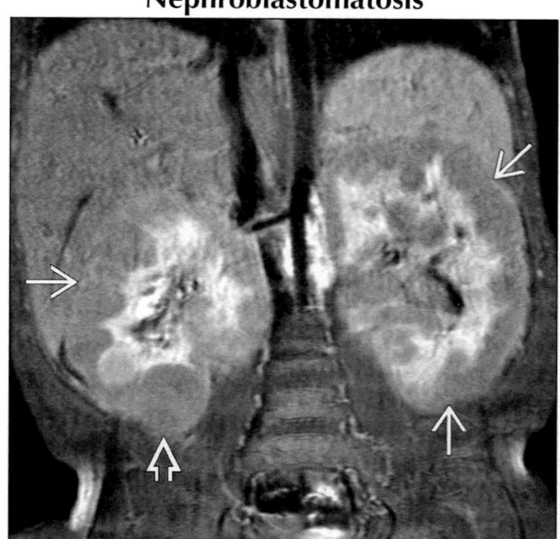

Nephroblastomatosis

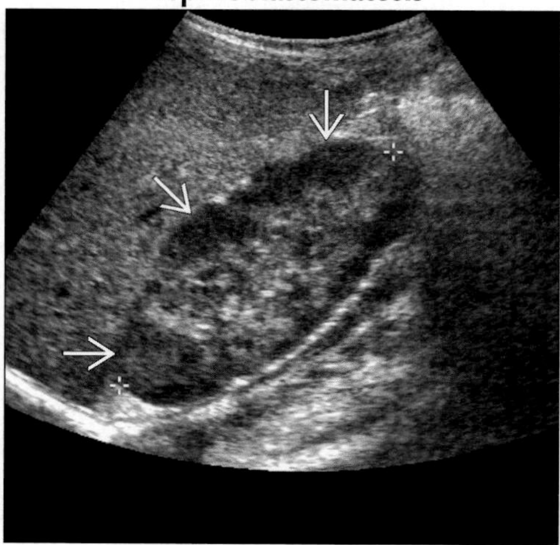

(Left) *Coronal T1WI FS MR C+ in a 1 year old with Beckwith-Wiedemann syndrome shows nonenhancing lesions and nephroblastomatosis ➡, in both kidneys. The lesions regressed over a few years, except for a focal right lower pole mass ➡, which was resected.* ***(Right)*** *Longitudinal US shows hypoechoic lesions ➡ in the kidney of the same patient, who was imaged by alternating US and MR exams to exclude malignant transformation.*

Tuberous Sclerosis

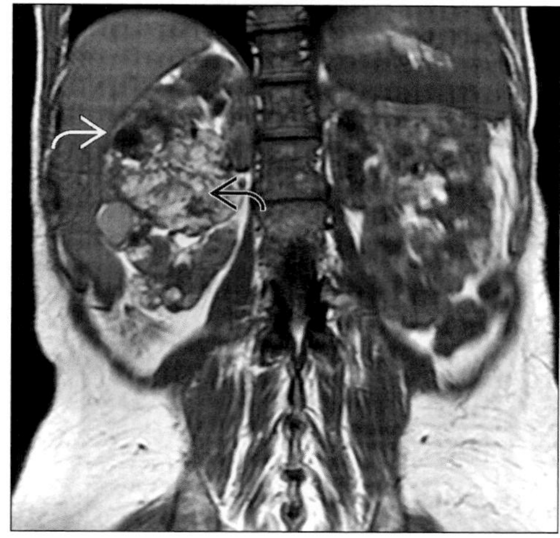

Tuberous Sclerosis

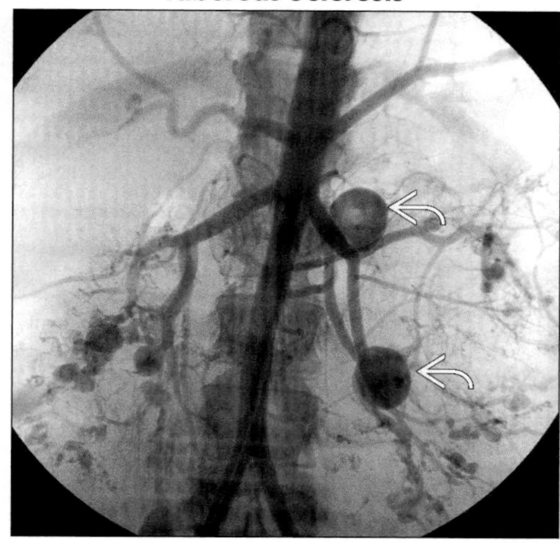

(Left) *Coronal T1WI MR shows numerous low signal intensity cysts ➡ and high signal intensity angiomyolipomas ➡ in the enlarged kidneys of this young woman with tuberous sclerosis.* ***(Right)*** *AP angiography in the same patient shows several large aneurysms ➡ and numerous small arterial abnormalities in association with the angiomyolipomas. Several of these aneurysms were embolized.*

Caroli Polycystic Kidney Disease

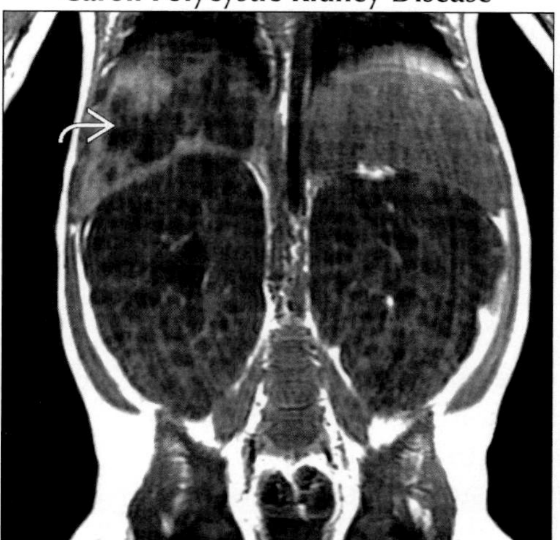

Caroli Polycystic Kidney Disease

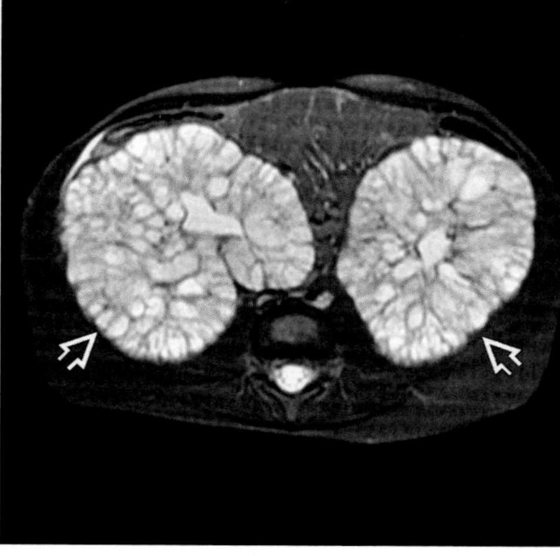

(Left) *Coronal T1WI MR shows marked enlargement of both kidneys, which are virtually replaced by cysts. Note the dilated biliary tree ➡ in the liver of this 19-month-old girl with liver and renal failure due to Caroli disease.* ***(Right)*** *Axial T2WI FSE MR in the same patient shows cystic replacement of the kidneys bilaterally ➡ with protuberant abdomen and jaundice clinically.*

UNILATERAL HYDRONEPHROSIS

DIFFERENTIAL DIAGNOSIS

Common

- Ureteropelvic Junction (UPJ) Obstruction
- Ureterovesical Junction (UVJ) Obstruction
- Ureterocele
- Posterior Urethral Valves
- Urolithiasis (Stones)
- Vesicoureteral Reflux

Less Common

- Megaureter
- Bladder Mass
- Iatrogenic
  - VUR Post Ureterocele Incision
  - Deflux Complications
  - Ureteral Re-Implant Complications
  - Stent Misplacement or Blockage
  - Ureteral Ligation During Pelvic Surgery

Rare but Important

- Ureteral Fibroepithelial Polyp

ESSENTIAL INFORMATION

Key Differential Diagnosis Issues

- Many cases are found prenatally and precisely diagnosed in newborn period
- Determining extent or level of dilation is key to narrowing differential
- Dilated calyces and disproportionately enlarged renal pelvis often indicate UPJ obstruction
- Dilation from top to bottom points to problems at UVJ
  - Intrinsic UVJ obstruction
  - UVJ stone
  - Ureterocele
  - Megaureter
  - Bladder mass
  - Compression from other pelvic mass
- Mid-ureteral transitions to normal caliber are unusual; if present, consider
  - Urolithiasis
  - Aberrant anatomy: Crossing vessel
  - Stricture: Postsurgical or radiation related
  - Compression by adjacent mass
  - Ureteral mass or polyp is very uncommon

Helpful Clues for Common Diagnoses

- **Ureteropelvic Junction (UPJ) Obstruction**
  - Most common cause of hydronephrosis in children
  - Focal narrowing at junction of renal pelvis and ureter
  - Degree of UPJ obstruction
    - Varies from mild to severely obstructed
    - May change with age and hydration state
  - Obstruction may be intrinsic or extrinsic
    - Intrinsic likely starts in fetal life
    - Fibrosis, abnormal innervation, failure of canalization are all suspected etiologies
    - By the time narrowing is resected, pathologically cannot determine cause
    - Extrinsic causes are typically crossing vessels, adenopathy, or mass
  - Imaging of UPJ obstruction
    - Ultrasound and diuretic renography are mainstays for degree of obstruction, scarring, renal growth, superimposed infection
  - Treatment of UPJ obstruction
    - Dismembered pyeloplasty
- **Ureterovesical Junction (UVJ) Obstruction**
  - 2nd most common cause of hydronephrosis in children
  - Megaureter is specific subtype of UVJ obstruction
    - Caused by distal adynamic segment
  - Other causes of UVJ obstruction
    - Stricture, fibrosis, aberrant anatomy
    - Compressed distal ureter: Bladder wall hypertrophy, mass, adenopathy, etc.
  - Imaging: Diuretic renogram, ultrasound, RUG, VCUG, MR urogram
- **Ureterocele**
  - Congenital cystic dilation of distal submucosal ureter
  - Location: Intra- or extravesical
  - Insertion site
    - Orthotopic at trigone ("simple")
    - Ectopic insertion anywhere else, typically medial and distal to trigone
  - Kidney being drained
    - Single system; typically simple, intravesicle variety
    - Duplex system; typically ectopic &/or extravesical
  - Imaging: VCUG, US, MR urography
- **Posterior Urethral Valves**
  - Congenital condition
  - Seen only in boys
  - Persistent tissue just distal to verumontanum partially obstructs urethra

- Unilateral VUR or urinoma protective to contralateral kidney
  - Better long-term prognosis
- Degree of obstruction varies
  - Severe obstruction seen in fetus and newborn
  - Secondary oligohydramnios, respiratory and renal insufficiency
  - Mild obstruction may go undetected for several years
  - Can present late with renal failure, bladder dysfunction
- Imaging: VCUG
  - Shows valve tissue &/or urethral caliber change
- Treatment: Endoscopic valve ablation

- **Urolithiasis (Stones)**
  - Much less common problem in pediatrics than in adults
  - Stone types in decreasing frequency
    - Calcium phosphate or oxalate
    - Struvite
    - Uric acid
    - Cystine
    - Mixed
  - Degree of obstruction varies with stone size and location
  - Imaging: Ultrasound, CT, IVP (rare)
  - Treatment: Hydration, diuretics, endoscopic basketing, lithotripsy
- **Vesicoureteral Reflux**
  - Retrograde flow of urine from bladder toward kidneys
  - Graded from 1 (mild) to 5 (severe)
  - 80% of children outgrow reflux by puberty
  - Associated infection and renal scarring
  - Imaging: VCUG, nuclear cystogram, sonocystogram (where ultrasound contrast is available)

Helpful Clues for Less Common Diagnoses

- **Megaureter**
  - Focal concentric narrowing of extravesical distal ureter 1-3 cm in length
  - Unknown etiology; theorized causes include
    - Paucity of ganglion cells
    - Hypoplasia/atrophy of muscle fibers in distal ureteral segment
  - Refluxing and nonrefluxing varieties
  - Imaging: Diuretic renogram, ultrasound, VCUG, MR urography
  - Treatment: Resection of narrowed segment and re-implantation
- **Bladder Mass**
  - Rhabdomyosarcoma most common
  - Inflammatory pseudotumor
  - Neuroblastoma and transitional cell rare
  - Imaging: Ultrasound, VCUG, CT, or MR for local extent
  - Treatment: Resection and ureteral re-implant or diversion
- **Iatrogenic**
  - Consider whenever there has been recent surgery or invasive procedure

Helpful Clues for Rare Diagnoses

- **Ureteral Fibroepithelial Polyp**
  - Benign, rare tumor of urothelium

Ureteropelvic Junction (UPJ) Obstruction

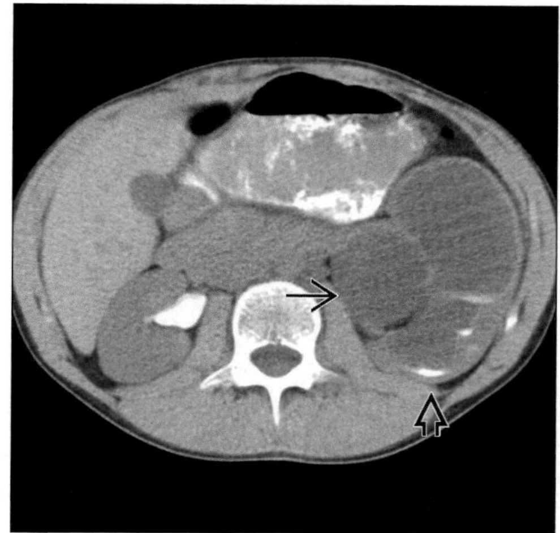

Axial CECT after 10-minute delay shows marked dilation of the left renal pelvis ➔ and calyces, with minimal contrast layering in the calyces ⇨. Excreted contrast is seen in the right renal pelvis with none in the left.

Ureteropelvic Junction (UPJ) Obstruction

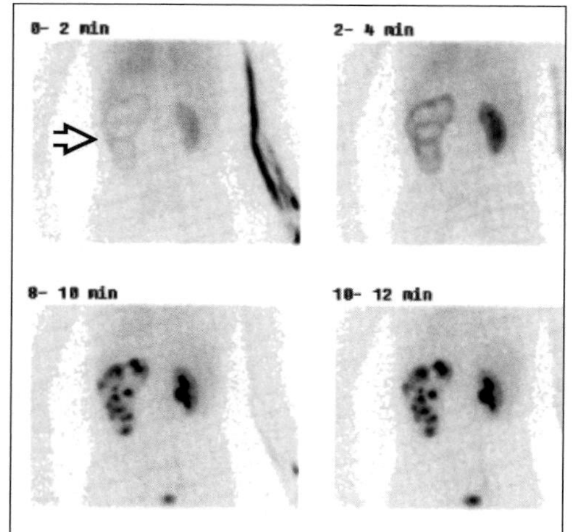

Posterior diuretic renography shows delayed function of the enlarged, hydronephrotic left kidney ⇨. The right kidney is normal.

UNILATERAL HYDRONEPHROSIS

(Left) *Posterior diuretic renography following diuretic challenge shows gradual filling of the dilated left renal pelvis ➡ but no visualization of the left ureter. The right kidney drains rapidly and is only faintly seen.* **(Right)** *Diuretic renography time-activity curves show prompt drainage and dropping counts in the normal right kidney but a flat curve with no washout in the left kidney. These findings are diagnostic of a left UPJ obstruction.*

Ureteropelvic Junction (UPJ) Obstruction

Ureteropelvic Junction (UPJ) Obstruction

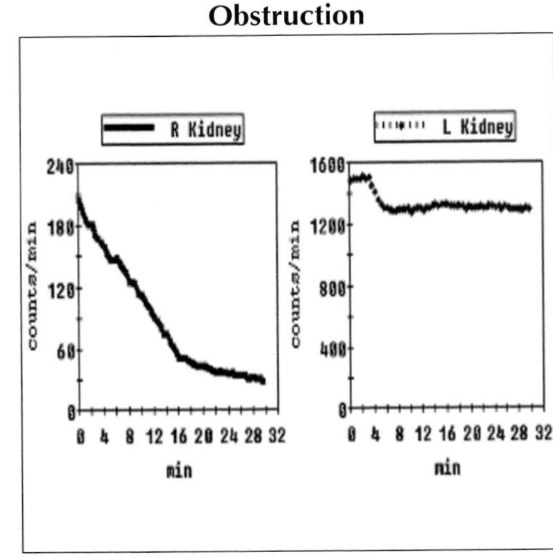

(Left) *Longitudinal harmonic ultrasound shows marked calyceal dilation and an enlarged renal pelvis, which could be followed into a dilated right ureter.* **(Right)** *Anteroposterior retrograde pyelogram shows contrast in dilated calyces and a dilated tortuous right ureter and rapid tapering at the bladder trigone ➡. A UVJ obstruction was found at surgery, and the ureter was re-implanted.*

Ureterovesical Junction (UVJ) Obstruction

Ureterovesical Junction (UVJ) Obstruction

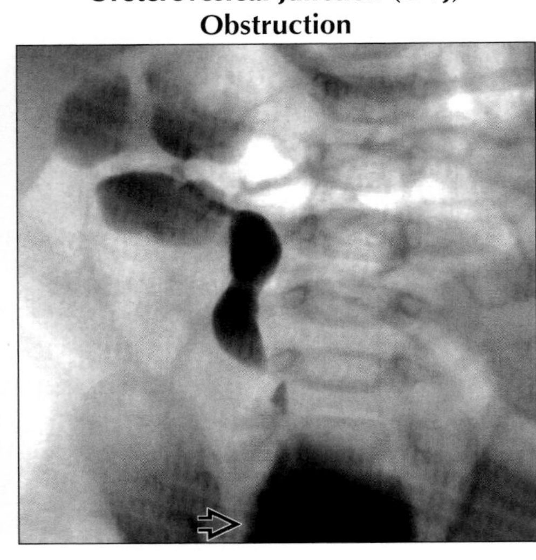

(Left) *Longitudinal harmonic ultrasound shows a round cystic lesion within the urinary bladder ➡. The distal left ureter ➡ is also dilated but peristalsed vigorously on real-time scanning.* **(Right)** *Posterior renal scan shows left-sided hydroureteronephrosis and a filling defect ➡ in the left side of the bladder base, representing the obstructed ureterocele.*

Ureterocele

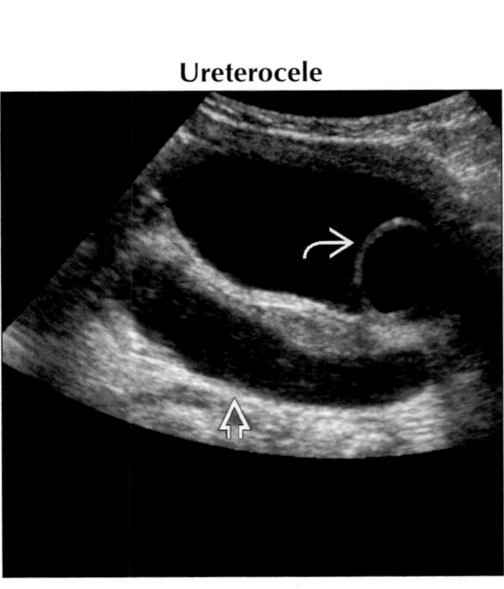

Ureterocele

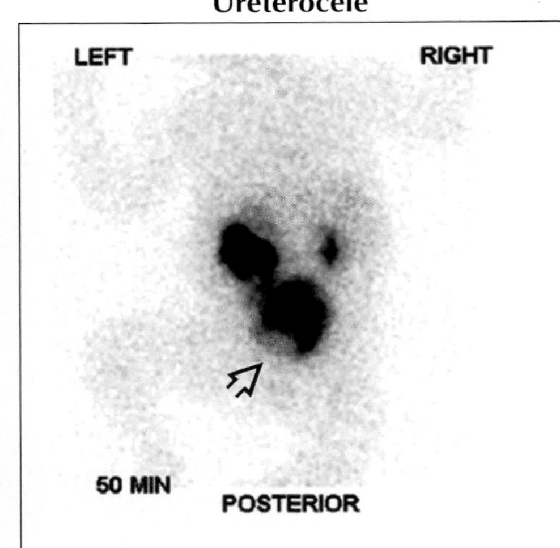

UNILATERAL HYDRONEPHROSIS

Posterior Urethral Valves

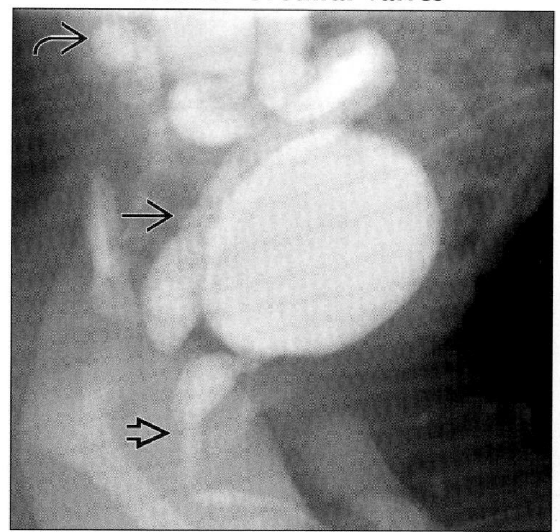

Posterior Urethral Valves

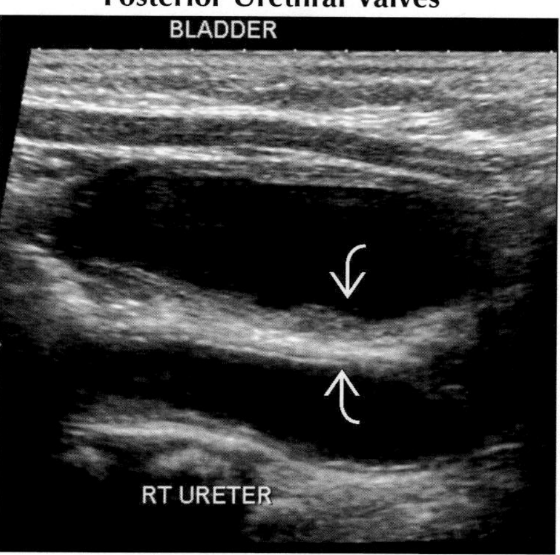

*(**Left**) Oblique voiding cystourethrogram shows high-grade vesicoureteral reflux into the right ureter → and intrarenal collecting system ↪ in this newborn with a prenatal diagnosis of bladder outlet obstruction and unilateral hydroureteronephrosis. Note the valve tissue in the posterior urethra ⇨. (**Right**) Longitudinal oblique harmonic ultrasound shows the same dilated ureter. Note the relatively thick-walled bladder ↪.*

Urolithiasis (Stones)

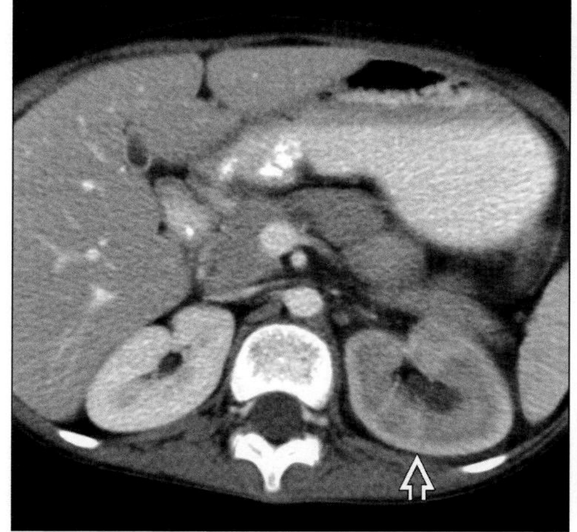

Urolithiasis (Stones)

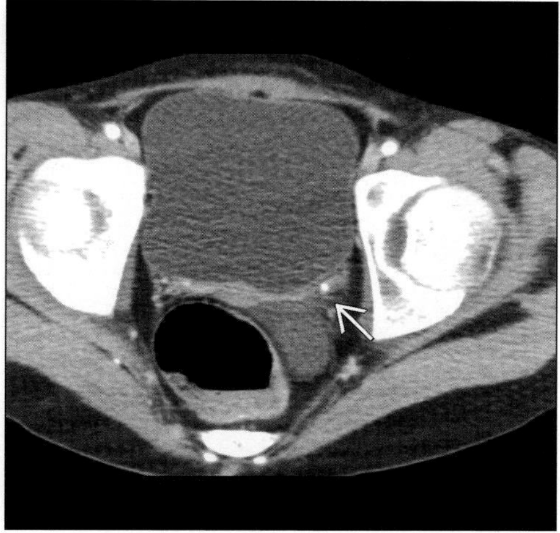

*(**Left**) Axial CECT shows delayed function of the left kidney ⇨ in this 9-year-old girl with acute flank pain. The left kidney is mildly swollen, and the intrarenal collecting system is mildly dilated. (**Right**) Axial CECT shows a calcific density in the left distal ureter → consistent with a partially obstructing distal ureteral calculus. Additional imaging in this patient failed to show any other stones.*

Urolithiasis (Stones)

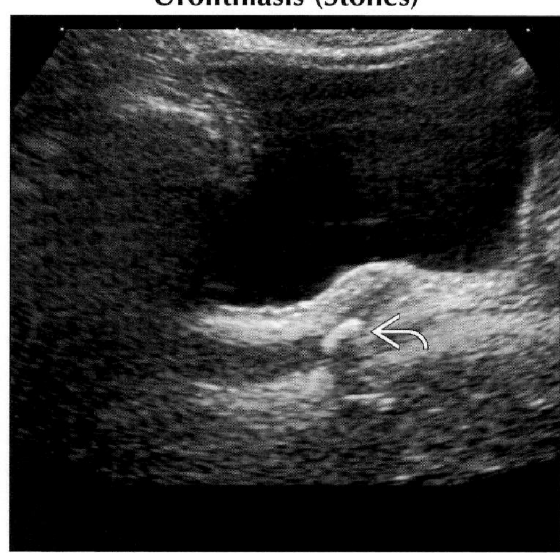

Vesicoureteral Reflux

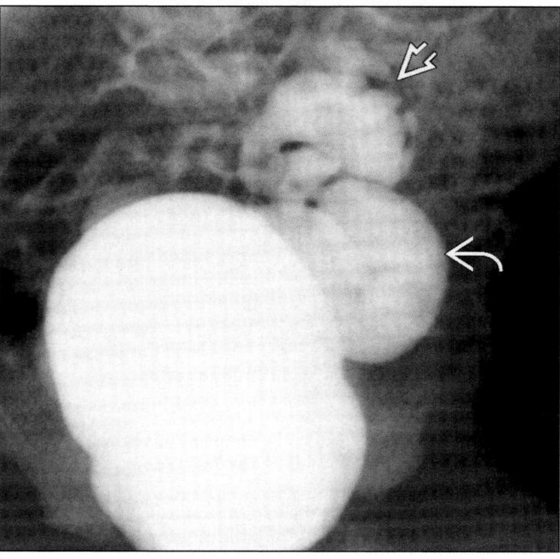

*(**Left**) Longitudinal oblique harmonic ultrasound shows an echogenic, shadowing calculus ↪ in a teenager with a history of urolithiasis, hematuria, and typical pain. Note the edema in the ureter distal to the stone. A ureteral jet could not be demonstrated on this side. (**Right**) Anteroposterior voiding cystourethrogram in this infant shows high-grade reflux into the left ureter ↪ and intrarenal collecting system ⇨.*

UNILATERAL HYDRONEPHROSIS

(Left) *Longitudinal harmonic ultrasound shows moderate to marked hydronephrosis of the left kidney in this infant with prenatally diagnosed unilateral hydroureteronephrosis.* **(Right)** *Longitudinal ultrasound shows the dilated distal left ureter, which is much larger than the adjacent bladder. No debris was seen in this dilated collecting system, an important finding to exclude in chronically obstructed patients.*

Megaureter

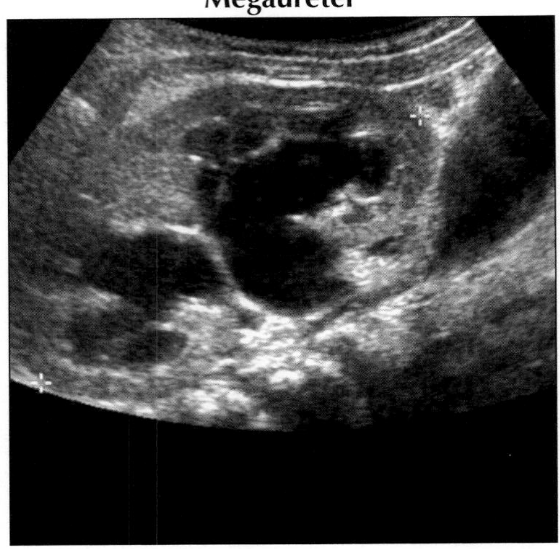

Megaureter

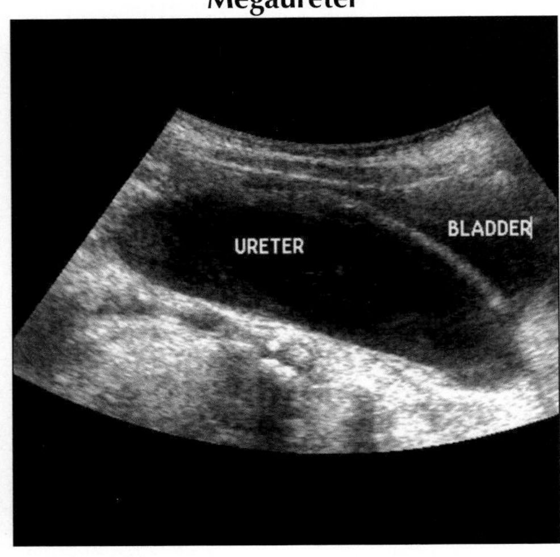

(Left) *Oblique voiding cystourethrogram shows a normal-caliber male urethra and impressive reflux into the dilated left ureter. Note the short segment of the narrowed distal ureter → in this patient with refluxing megaureter.* **(Right)** *Posterior diuretic renography shows poor drainage from the dilated left kidney and ureter in the same patient who has a refluxing and partially obstructed megaureter. The normal right kidney is not seen at the end of the exam.*

Megaureter

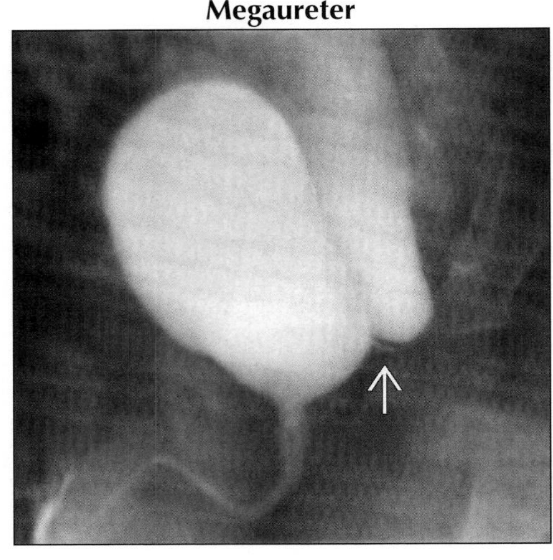

Megaureter

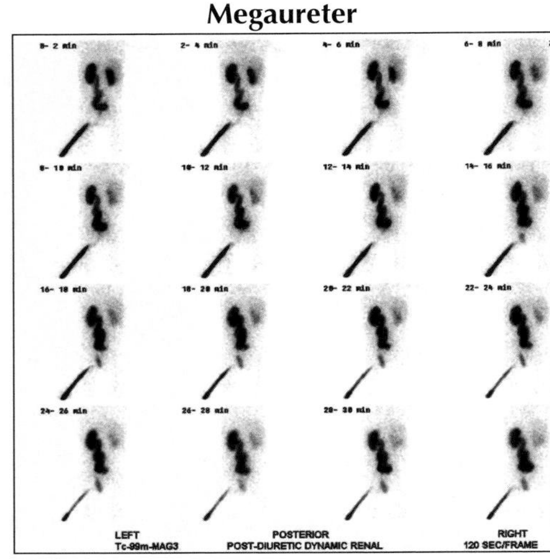

(Left) *Transverse harmonic ultrasound shows a lobulated soft tissue mass ↪ in the left side of the urinary bladder in a 20-month-old male with hematuria. The distal left ureter ⇨, seen in cross section, is also dilated.* **(Right)** *Longitudinal oblique color Doppler ultrasound shows blood vessels branching within the bladder mass, excluding a bladder clot or fungus ball. No flow is seen in the distal left ureter ⇨.*

Bladder Mass

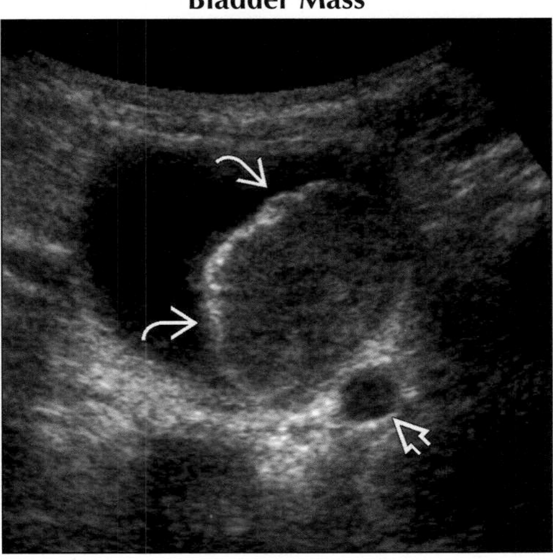

Bladder Mass

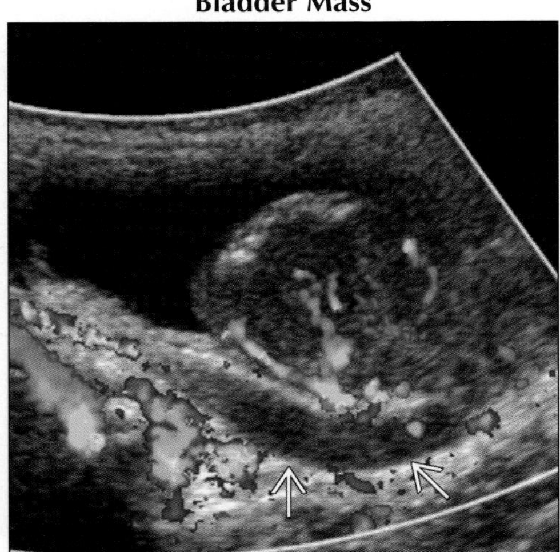

UNILATERAL HYDRONEPHROSIS

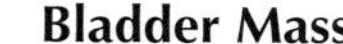

Bladder Mass

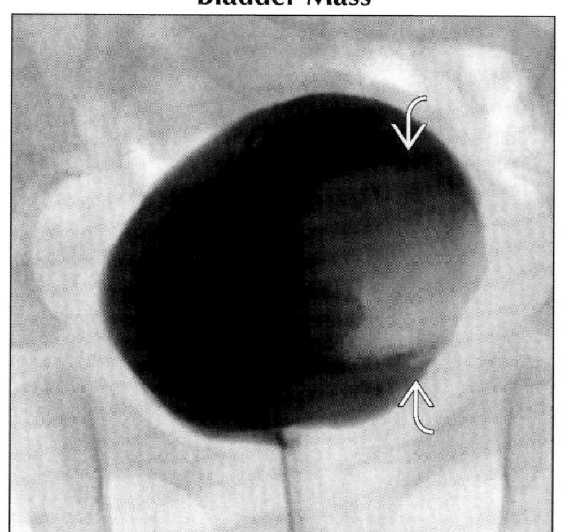

Bladder Mass

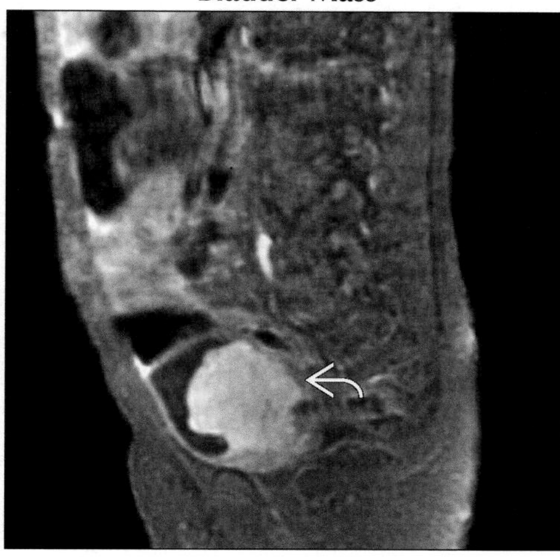

(Left) *Cystogram in the same patient shows a lobulated filling defect ➔ in the left side of the bladder base. It was difficult to know from either the ultrasound or VCUG if the mass had extended beyond the bladder wall into the surrounding pelvic tissues.* ***(Right)*** *Sagittal T1 C+ FS MR shows the enhancing lobulated mass ➔ in the bladder base. The mass was resected and pathologically proven to be an inflammatory pseudotumor (benign).*

VUR Post Ureterocele Incision

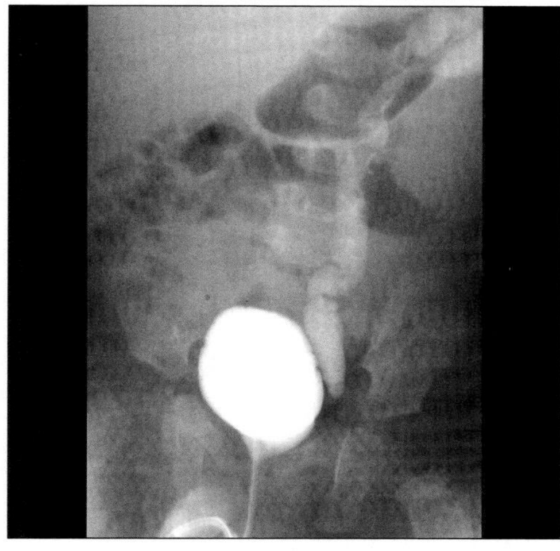

Deflux Complications

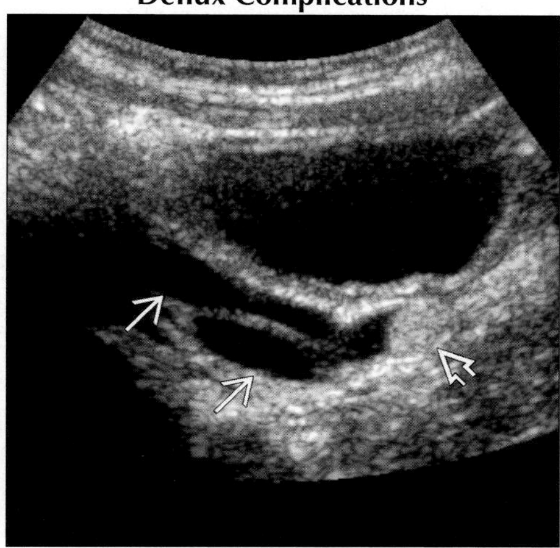

(Left) *AP voiding cystourethrogram shows new reflux into a left ureter in a patient who recently had a large, left-sided ureterocele incised through a cystoscope. Reflux after ureterocele incision is fairly common.* ***(Right)*** *Longitudinal oblique ultrasound shows dilated ureters ➔ joining above the bladder and an echogenic mound of deflux material ➔ just outside the bladder wall. This Y-shaped ureter was not dilated prior to the deflux procedure.*

Ureteral Fibroepithelial Polyp

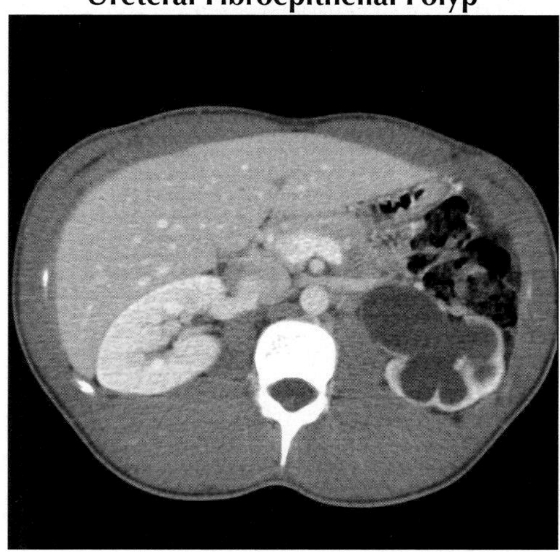

Ureteral Fibroepithelial Polyp

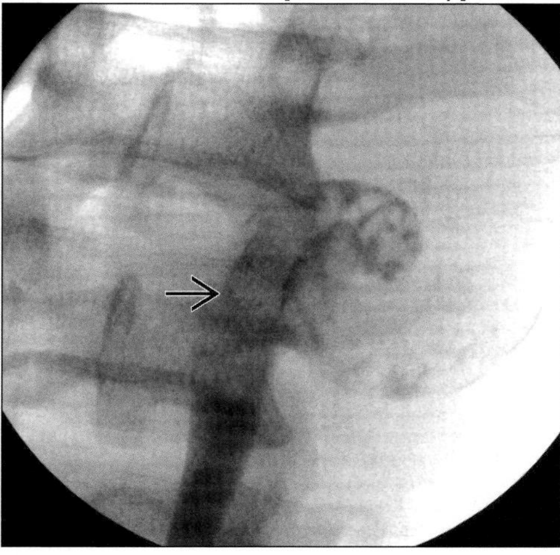

(Left) *Axial CECT shows marked hydronephrosis of the left kidney with global cortical thinning in this 17 year old with chronic, intermittent hematuria and flank pain. Images more inferiorly showed soft tissue in the dilated ureter initially felt to be a hematoma.* ***(Right)*** *AP retrograde pyelogram performed in the operating room shows a tubular filling defect → in the ureter and normal-caliber ureter distally. Biopsy of the intraluminal lesion showed a fibroepithelial polyp.*

BILATERAL HYDRONEPHROSIS

DIFFERENTIAL DIAGNOSIS

Common
- Vesicoureteral Reflux (VUR)
- Posterior Urethral Valves
- Neurogenic Bladder

Less Common
- Megaureter
- Crossed Fused Ectopia
- Horseshoe Kidney
- Megacystis Megaureter
- Bladder Outlet Obstruction
  - Cecoureterocele
  - Bladder Rhabdomyosarcoma
  - Pelvic Mass with Compression
  - Cloacal and Anorectal Malformations

Rare but Important
- Prune Belly
- Urethral Duplication
- Anterior Urethral Valves
- Megacalycosis

ESSENTIAL INFORMATION

Key Differential Diagnosis Issues
- Some potential diagnoses may occur unilaterally or bilaterally
- Severe cases typically noted on prenatal imaging and further evaluated in newborn
- Clinical history and associated anomalies narrow differential

Helpful Clues for Common Diagnoses
- **Vesicoureteral Reflux (VUR)**
  - Retrograde flow of urine from bladder toward kidneys
  - Graded from 1 (mild) to 5 (severe)
  - 80% of children outgrow reflux by puberty
  - Associated infection and renal scarring
  - Imaging: Voiding cystourethrography (VCUG), nuclear cystogram, sonocystogram (if US contrast available)
- **Posterior Urethral Valves**
  - Congenital condition found only in boys
  - Persistent or prominent plicae colliculi in urethra causes variable degree of obstruction
  - Unilateral VUR or urinoma decompresses system, protective of contralateral kidney
    - Better long-term prognosis
  - Degree of obstruction varies
    - Severe: Usually diagnosed in fetus/newborn with oligohydramnios, respiratory, and renal insufficiency
    - Mild: May go undetected for years; late symptoms include renal failure and bladder dysfunction
  - Imaging: VCUG
    - Shows valve tissue &/or urethral caliber change
  - Treatment: Endoscopic valve ablation
- **Neurogenic Bladder**
  - Malfunctioning bladder from any neurologic disorder
  - Upper tract compromised by
    - Poor bladder emptying and VUR
    - Urinary tract infections
    - Elevated bladder pressures
  - Highly compliant bladder in infancy common
    - Huge bladder capacity, poor emptying
  - Gradually develops muscular hypertrophy, which decreases compliance and capacity
  - End stage: Low capacity, noncompliant, noncontractile bladder
  - Imaging: VCUG, US, CT, MR
    - Shows bladder wall trabeculation, VUR, diverticula, capacity, emptying
  - Urodynamics very important to monitor
  - Treatment
    - Medications to improve bladder compliance
    - Catheterization to simulate normal bladder distention and emptying

Helpful Clues for Less Common Diagnoses
- **Megaureter**
  - a.k.a. primary megaureter
  - Focal concentric narrowing of extravesical distal ureter 1-3 cm in length
  - Unknown etiology but theorized to be
    - Paucity of ganglion cells or
    - Hypoplasia/atrophy of muscle fibers in distal ureteral segment
  - Refluxing and nonrefluxing varieties
  - Imaging: Diuretic renogram, US, VCUG, MR urography
  - Treatment
    - Resection of narrowed segment and re-implantation
- **Crossed Fused Ectopia**
  - Results from abnormal migration of kidney in utero

- Upper kidney is orthotopic; other kidney is on wrong side and in low position
- Lower pole of orthotopic kidney fused to upper pole of ectopic kidney
- Ureter from lower kidney crosses to contralateral trigone
- Associated aberrant and accessory vessels
- Hydroureteronephrosis may be segmental or involve whole kidney
- Imaging: Diuretic renogram, US, VCUG, MR urography

- **Horseshoe Kidney**
  - Results from abnormal migration of kidney in utero
  - Lower poles of kidney fused in midline
  - Upper poles are lower than usual
  - Aberrant and accessory vessels and ureters common
  - Hydroureteronephrosis may be segmental or involve whole kidney
  - Imaging: Diuretic renogram, US, VCUG, MR urography
- **Megacystis Megaureter**
  - Large, thin-walled, smooth bladder from constant recycling of refluxed urine
  - Bladder contracts normally but never empties completely due to reflux
  - Bladder capacity and function normalize when VUR is corrected
  - Imaging: VCUG
- **Bladder Outlet Obstruction**
  - Any cause of bladder outlet obstruction can lead to bilateral hydroureteronephrosis
  - **Cecoureterocele**
    - Prolapsed ureterocele
  - **Bladder Rhabdomyosarcoma**
    - Typically large with significant mass effect
  - **Pelvic Mass with Compression**
    - Sacrococcygeal teratoma, Burkitt, etc.
  - **Cloacal and Anorectal Malformations**
    - Look for associated genital anomalies, hematometrocolpos

Helpful Clues for Rare Diagnoses

- **Prune Belly**
  - Classic triad
    - Absent/hypoplastic abdominal wall muscles
    - Cryptorchidism
    - Patulous urinary collecting system
  - Males almost exclusively (97%)
  - Imaging: US, VCUG, diuretic renogram, MR urography
- **Urethral Duplication**
  - Duplications can occur anywhere from kidneys to urethra
  - Duplicated urethra may obstruct and cause hydroureteronephrosis
- **Anterior Urethral Valves**
  - Similar tissue as in posterior valves
  - Varying degree of obstruction
- **Megacalycosis**
  - Rare, congenital anomaly
  - Nonobstructive dilation of calyces due to hypoplastic renal pyramids

Vesicoureteral Reflux (VUR)

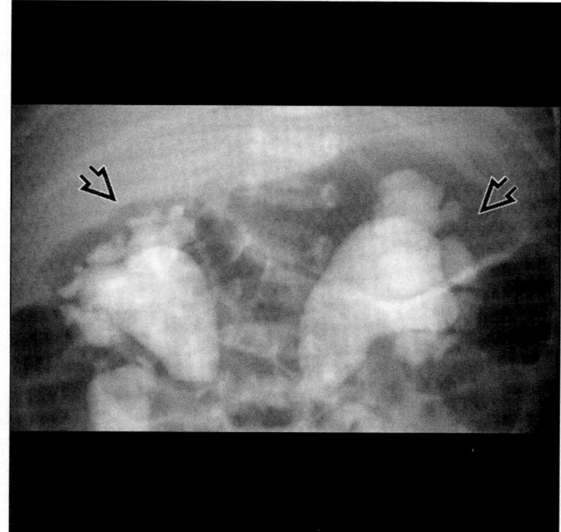

AP voiding cystourethrogram shows bilateral, high-grade (4-5) vesicoureteral reflux ⇒ in an infant with a history of prenatal hydroureteronephrosis.

Vesicoureteral Reflux (VUR)

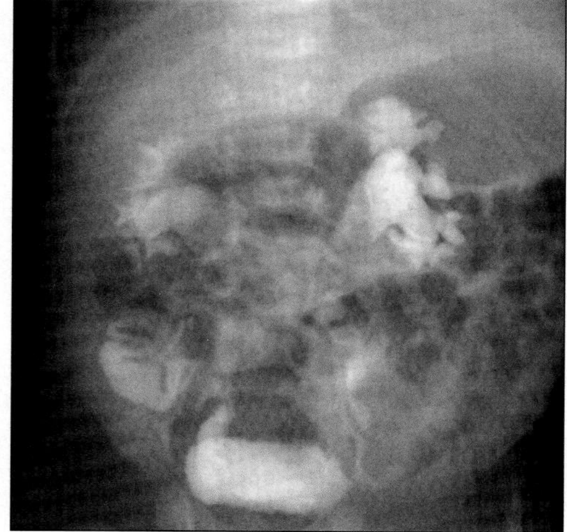

AP voiding cystourethrogram shows incomplete drainage of the upper urinary tracts after voiding. Though the infant voided completely, the bladder refilled with contrast that had refluxed into the kidneys.

BILATERAL HYDRONEPHROSIS

*(**Left**) Sagittal T2WI MR shows a very distended bladder with a prominent bladder neck in this fetus with bladder outlet obstruction. Several bladder aspirations had previously been performed. (**Right**) Coronal T2WI MR shows marked hydroureteronephrosis in the same fetus with bladder outlet obstruction in utero.*

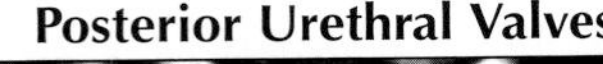

Posterior Urethral Valves

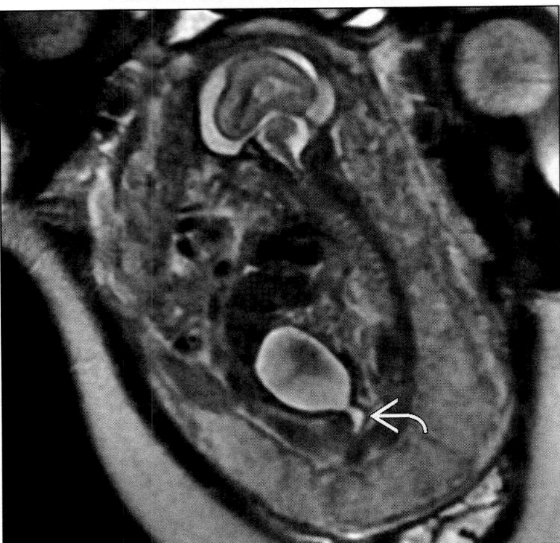

Posterior Urethral Valves

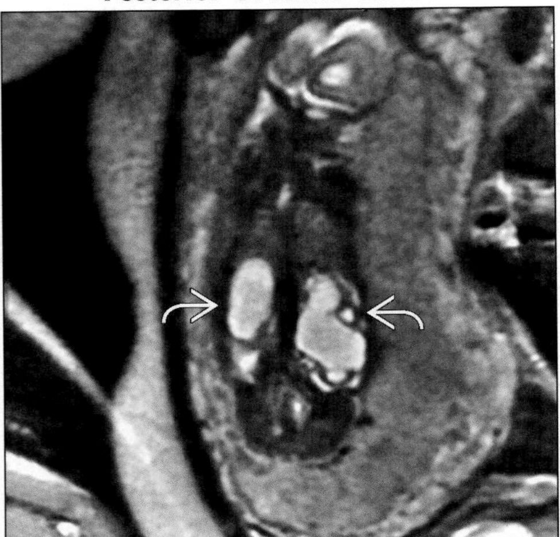

*(**Left**) Longitudinal ultrasound performed immediately postnatal shows bilateral hydroureteronephrosis with preserved cortical thickness and corticomedullary differentiation. (**Right**) Longitudinal ultrasound shows similar hydroureteronephrosis in the right kidney. Note the normal fetal lobation in this newborn.*

Posterior Urethral Valves

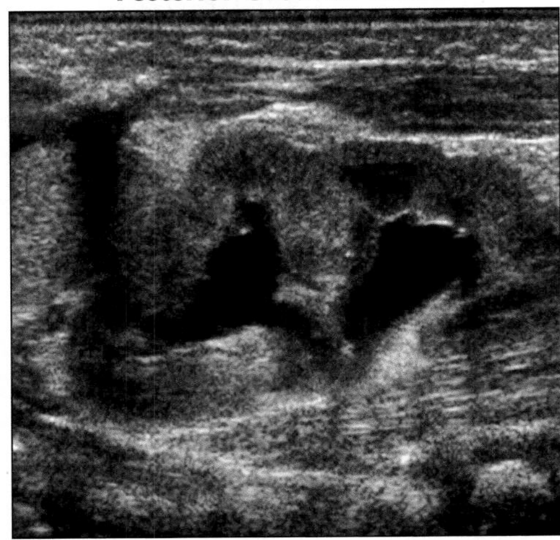

Posterior Urethral Valves

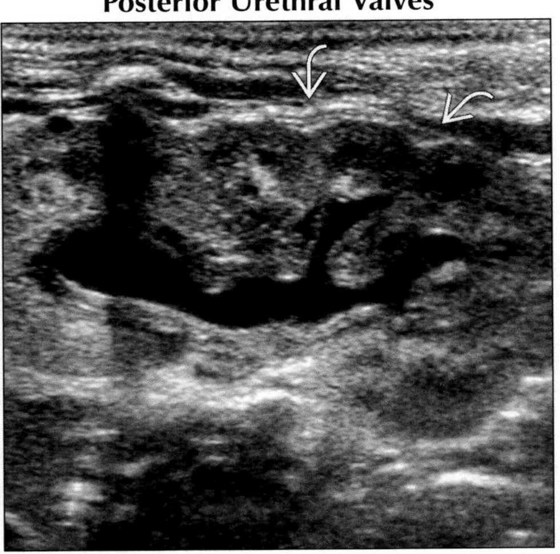

*(**Left**) Transverse ultrasound shows marked, concentric bladder wall thickening in the same newborn. Note the dilated distal ureters bilaterally. (**Right**) Oblique voiding cystourethrogram confirms posterior urethral valves as the cause of obstructive uropathy. Note the thin, linear filling defect created by the valve tissue. Urethral valves, though quite thin, typically cause significant obstruction.*

Posterior Urethral Valves

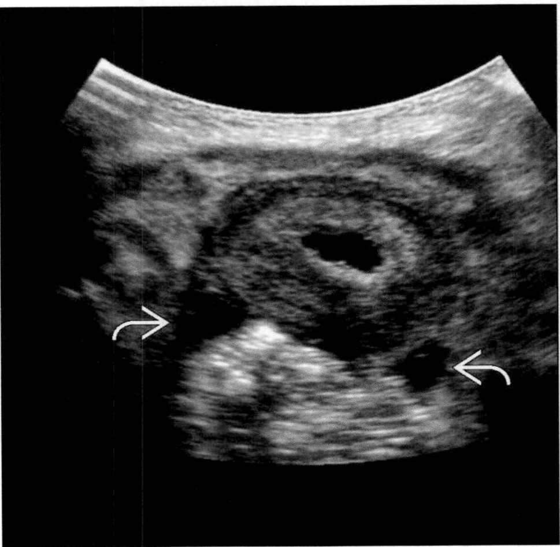

Posterior Urethral Valves

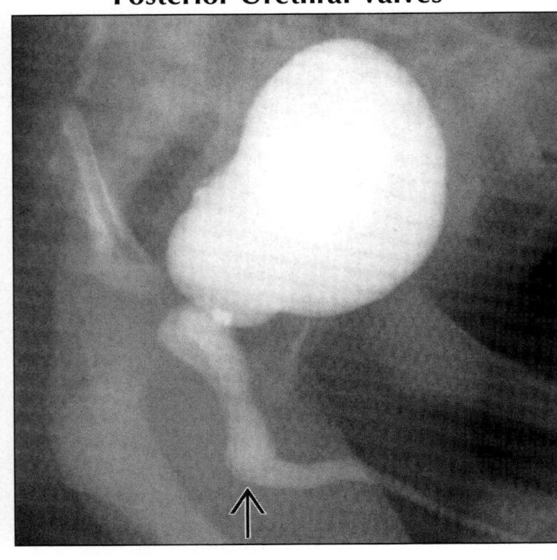

BILATERAL HYDRONEPHROSIS

Neurogenic Bladder

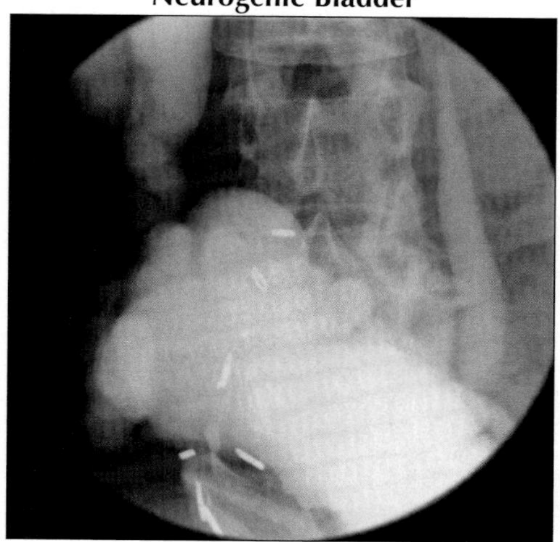

Neurogenic Bladder

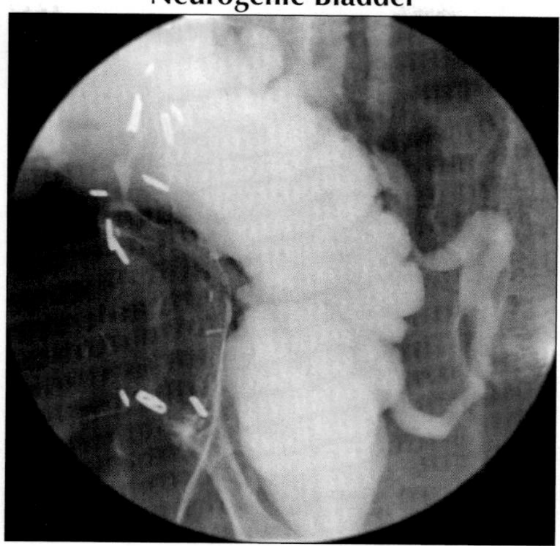

*(**Left**) AP voiding cystourethrogram shows numerous surgical clips from radical partial pelvic bone resection years ago for Ewing sarcoma. Contrast opacifies an irregularly shaped bladder with numerous diverticula and vertical orientation, consistent with a neurogenic bladder. Bilateral vesicoureteral reflux is also seen. (**Right**) Oblique voiding cystourethrogram in the same patient shows irregular bladder contour, elongation, and bladder diverticula.*

Megaureter

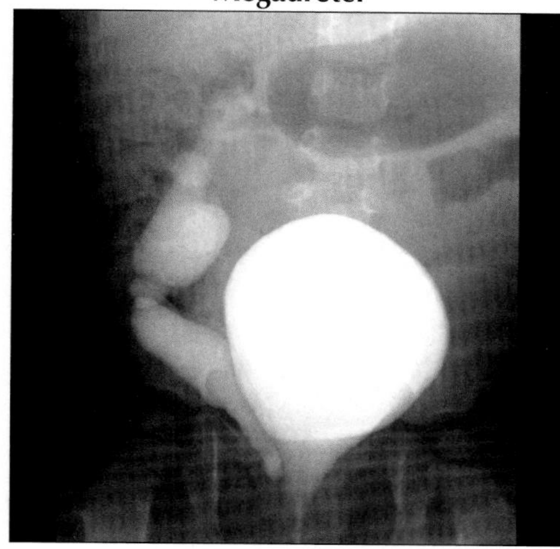

Crossed Fused Ectopia

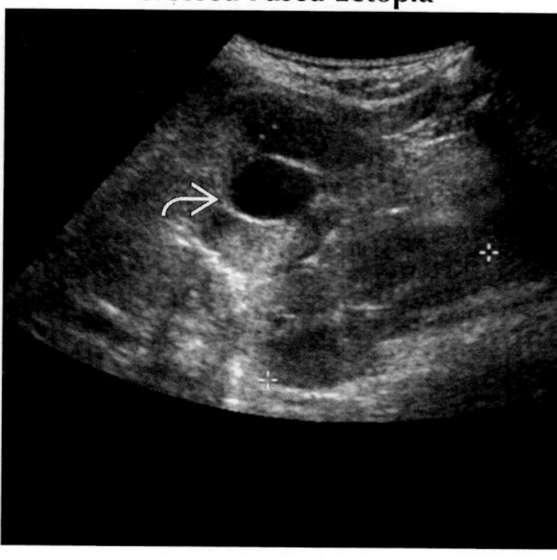

*(**Left**) AP voiding cystourethrogram shows vesicoureteral reflux into a dilated right ureter with a blunted intrarenal collecting system. (**Right**) Longitudinal oblique ultrasound shows hydronephrosis ➔ in the right kidney of the same patient, who also had crossed fused renal ectopia. The tissue that should have been in the left renal fossa (calipers) abuts the lower pole of the right kidney.*

Crossed Fused Ectopia

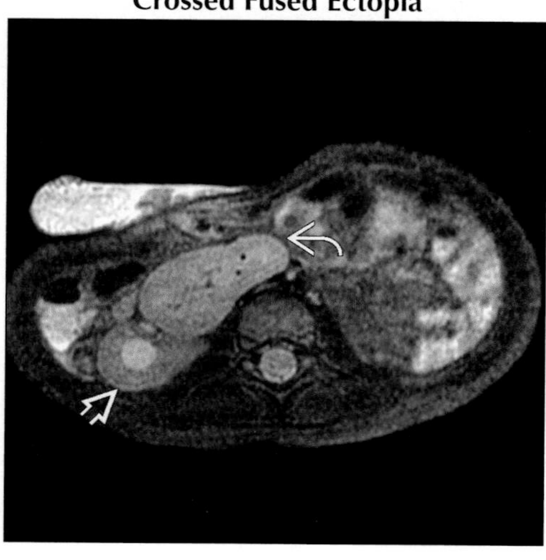

Crossed Fused Ectopia

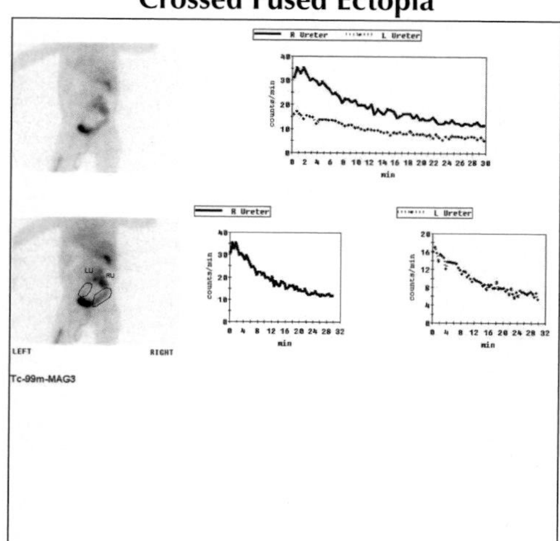

*(**Left**) Axial PDWI MR shows the left kidney ➔ anterior to the lower pole of the right kidney ➔. Note the hydroureteronephrosis of the right kidney. The patient has an ostomy bag on the right anterior abdomen. (**Right**) Posteroanterior renal scan shows both kidneys in the right side of the abdomen in this patient with refluxing megaureter and crossed fused ectopia. Time activity curves for the ureters show no obstruction.*

BILATERAL HYDRONEPHROSIS

(Left) Transverse US in the midline abdomen shows marked hydronephrosis to the left of the spine and renal tissue crossing the midline in this patient with horseshoe kidney. ***(Right)*** *Posteroanterior renal scan in the same patient shows bilateral prominence of the intrarenal collecting system, worse on the left side, and abnormal renal axis (lower poles directed medially). Hydronephrosis, stones, and stasis are common complications of horseshoe kidney.*

Horseshoe Kidney

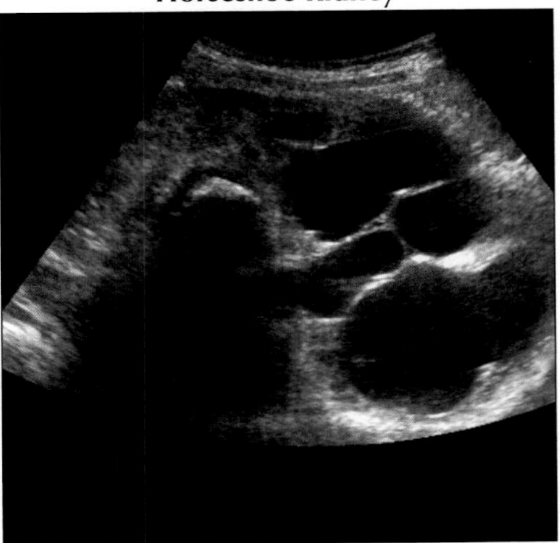

Horseshoe Kidney

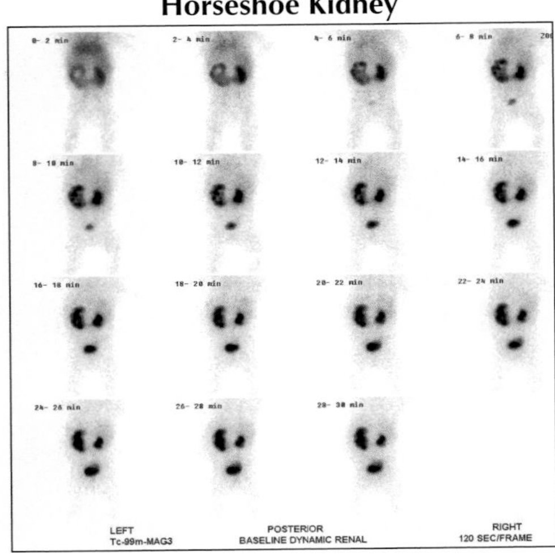

(Left) *Oblique voiding cystourethrogram shows bilateral, high-grade reflux but a thin-walled, smooth bladder, characteristic of megacystis megaureter. Refluxed urine constantly refills the bladder. This is not a neurogenic bladder.* ***(Right)*** *Oblique voiding cystourethrogram shows a filling defect in the bladder neck ⇒ below the Foley catheter balloon. The patient had just started to void when the ureterocele prolapsed into the urethra, stopping urine flow.*

Megacystis Megaureter

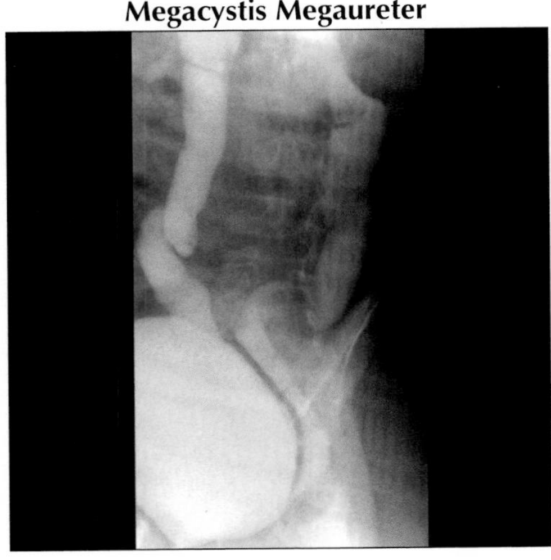

Cecoureterocele

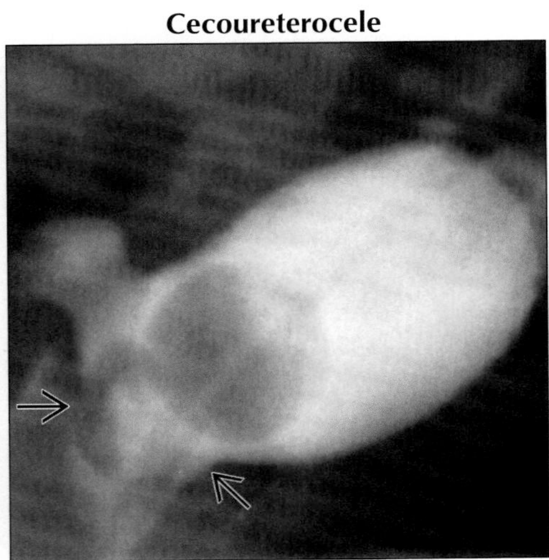

(Left) *Oblique voiding cystourethrogram shows an irregular filling defect ➡ at the bladder base in this child with hematuria. Subsequent biopsy showed rhabdomyosarcoma. Tumors that involve trigone or cause bladder outlet obstruction can cause secondary hydroureteronephrosis.* ***(Right)*** *Axial CECT in the same patient shows marked mural thickening of the bladder base with irregular enhancement. Note the Foley catheter in place.*

Bladder Rhabdomyosarcoma

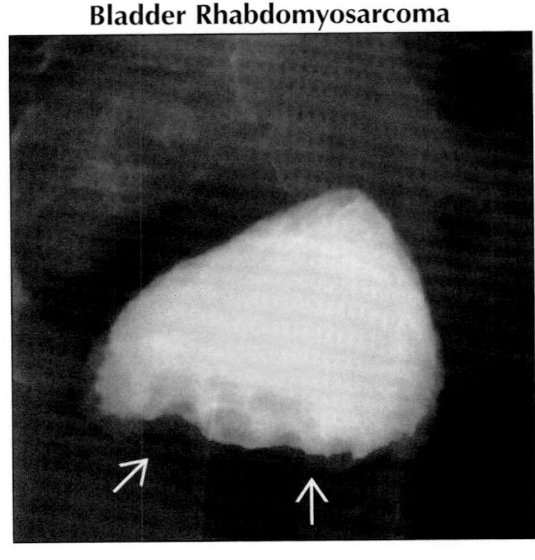

Bladder Rhabdomyosarcoma

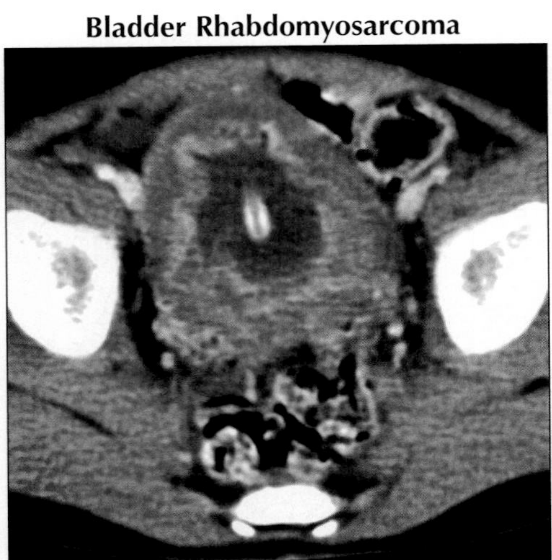

Pelvic Mass with Compression

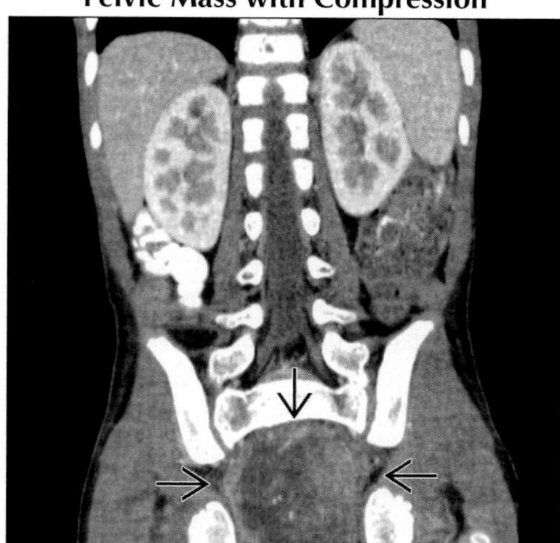

Cloacal and Anorectal Malformations

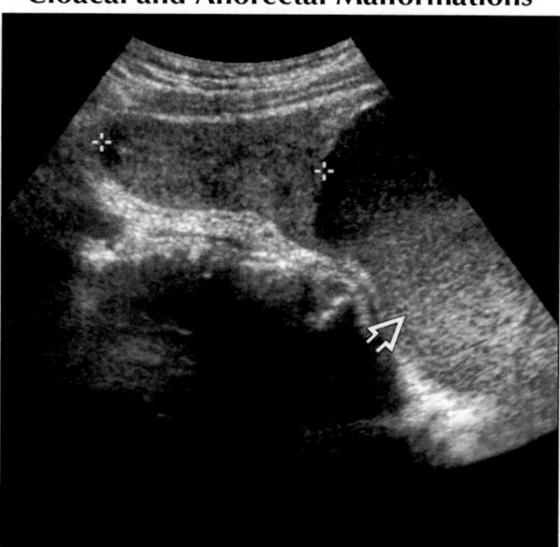

(Left) *Coronal CECT shows bilateral hydroureteronephrosis in a patient with a large pelvic tumor, a prostate rhabdomyosarcoma ⇒.* ***(Right)*** *Longitudinal harmonic ultrasound shows echogenic debris ➡ distending the vagina and uterus (calipers) in this patient with cloacal anomaly and hematometrocolpos.*

Prune Belly

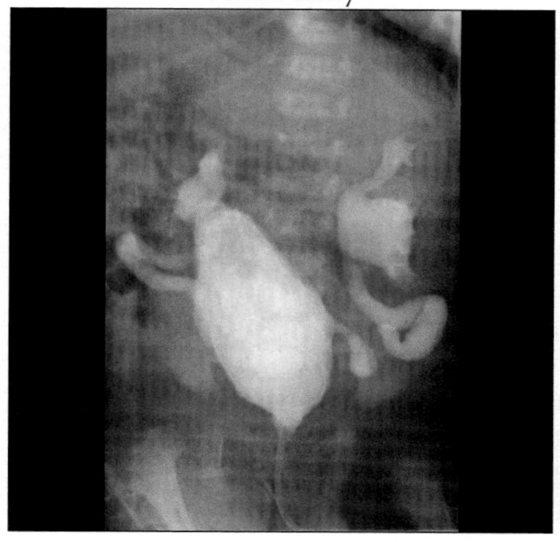

Urethral Duplication

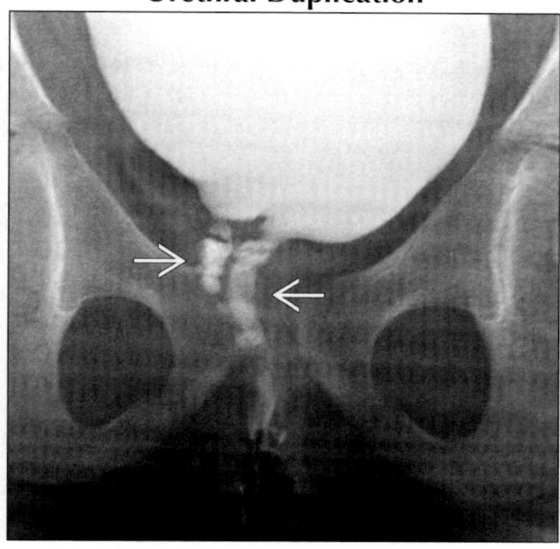

(Left) *Anteroposterior voiding cystourethrogram shows bilateral reflux and a vertically oriented bladder in a newborn with a flaccid anterior abdominal wall, consistent with prune belly.* ***(Right)*** *Anteroposterior voiding cystourethrogram shows 2 female urethras ➡ in this unusual congenital anomaly, which can be complicated by bladder outlet obstruction, meatal stenosis, and hydronephrosis.*

Anterior Urethral Valves

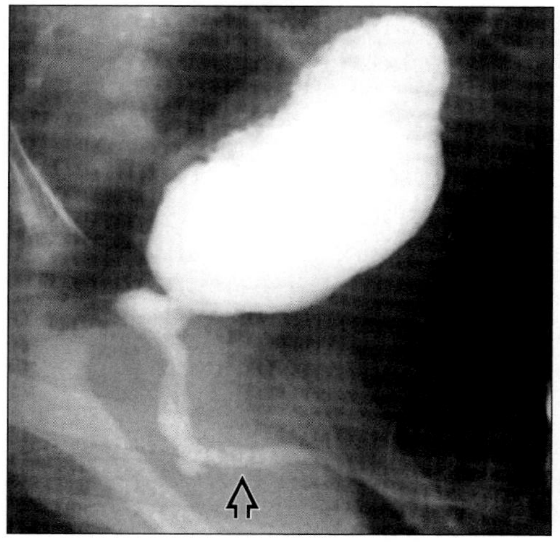

Megacalycosis

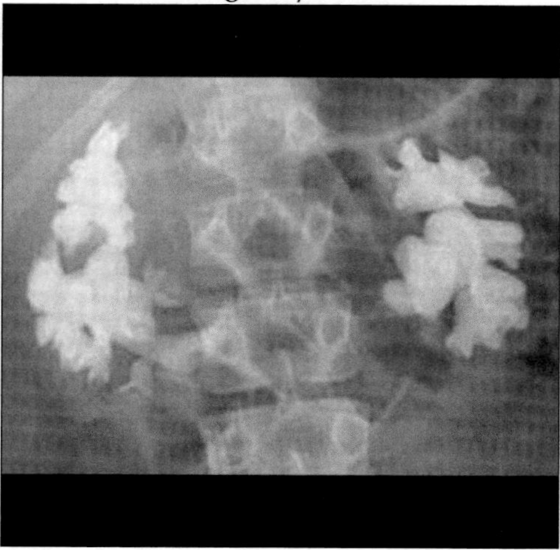

(Left) *Oblique voiding cystourethrogram shows valve tissue ⇒, more distal than is typically seen in the posterior urethral valves, and reflux into the Cowper gland just proximal to the anterior valve.* ***(Right)*** *Anteroposterior excretory urography shows bilateral dilated calyces in this teenager with hematuria.*

RENAL MASS

DIFFERENTIAL DIAGNOSIS

Common
- Wilms Tumor-Nephroblastoma
- Nephroblastomatosis
- Renal Cell Carcinoma
- Mesoblastic Nephroma
- Lymphoma

Less Common
- Multilocular Cystic Renal Tumor
- Abscess
- Xanthogranulomatous Pyelonephritis
- Clear Cell Sarcoma
- Angiomyolipoma

Rare but Important
- Rhabdoid Tumor
- Renal Medullary Carcinoma
- Ossifying Renal Tumor of Infancy
- Metanephric Adenoma

ESSENTIAL INFORMATION

Key Differential Diagnosis Issues
- DDx can be further limited by age, unique clinical or imaging features

Helpful Clues for Common Diagnoses
- **Wilms Tumor-Nephroblastoma**
  - Most common (87%) of pediatric solid renal masses, bilateral in 10%
  - Age of presentation peaks at 3-4 years old; earlier peak for bilateral Wilms at 15 mo.
  - Associations: Cryptorchidism, sporadic aniridia, hypospadias, & hemihypertrophy
    - WAGR syndrome: **W**ilms, **a**niridia, **G**U anomalies, mental **r**etardation
    - Drash syndrome: Male pseudohermaphroditism, glomerulonephritis
    - Beckwith-Wiedemann syndrome
  - Presents most commonly as palpable mass
    - Pain or hematuria are uncommon, hypertension in 1/4
  - Radiologically presents as large solid mass, often with vascular invasion
    - Spreads by direct extension; occasionally presents as cystic mass
    - Evaluate contralateral kidney for synchronous tumor or nephrogenic rests
    - Metastases most common to lungs (85%) and regional lymph nodes
  - Treatment (Tx): Nephrectomy followed by adjuvant chemotherapy
    - Presurgical treatment in bilateral disease with nephron-sparing surgery
    - 90% 5-year survival rate
- **Nephroblastomatosis**
  - Nephrogenic rests persisting to 36 weeks gestational age; rests seen in 1% of infants
  - Give rise to 30-40% of Wilms tumors
  - Found in 99% of bilateral Wilms tumors
  - CECT: Nephrogenic rests show relative ↓ enhancement to normal renal parenchyma
  - MR: Low signal intensity on T1 and T2
  - US: Hypoechoic compared with renal cortex, but US is less sensitive
    - Diffuse: Hypoechoic subcapsular layer
    - Nodular: Large hypoechoic masses
  - Natural history is regression but can transform to Wilms tumor
  - Syndromes associated with Wilms screened by US every 3 months to ~ 7 years old
- **Renal Cell Carcinoma**
  - Reported in ages 6 months to adulthood
    - 7% of pediatric renal masses
    - > 10 years old: Diagnostic probability of renal cell vs. Wilms is equal
  - von Hippel-Lindau (VHL) syndrome
    - Often bilateral tumors
  - Presentation: Pain and hematuria
  - Metastases to lungs, bones, liver, or brain are frequent (20%) at diagnosis
  - More likely than Wilms tumor to be calcified (25% vs. 9%)
  - Tx: Radical nephrectomy and is resistant to chemotherapy
- **Mesoblastic Nephroma**
  - a.k.a. fetal renal hamartoma and leiomyomatous hamartoma
  - Most common solid renal tumor in neonates
  - Majority present < 3 mo. as palpable mass
    - 90% are diagnosed before 1 year of age
  - Large solid mass with ill-defined transition, no capsule, and usually involving renal sinuses
  - Local infiltration of perinephric tissue
  - Behavior is usually benign and cured by nephrectomy with wide resection of perinephric tissue to prevent recurrence
    - Rare metastasis to lungs, brain, or bones
- **Lymphoma**

- Involvement is common at autopsy
  - Only 3-8% show involvement at CT, mostly non-Hodgkin lymphoma
- Primary involvement of kidney is rare
- Symptoms do not occur until late stage
- CT: Multiple hypoenhancing masses
- US: Generally hypoechoic and can show increase through transmission

Helpful Clues for Less Common Diagnoses

- **Multilocular Cystic Renal Tumor**
  - a.k.a. multilocular cystic nephroma
  - Cystic mass with scarce solid tissue
  - Age peaks of presentation: Up to 4 years old in boys or adult women
  - Appearance on imaging is multiple cysts
    - US is best at showing cystic nature
    - Multiple small cysts may give appearance of solid lesion on CT
  - Tx: Wide surgical resection; if recurrent, consider chemotherapy and radiation
- **Abscess**
  - Predisposing factors: Reflux, urinary tract obstruction or anomalies, and diabetes
  - US: Complex mass with hypoechoic regions of liquefaction
  - Main differentiating features from other renal masses are fever, leukocytosis, and pyuria
- **Xanthogranulomatous Pyelonephritis**
  - Diffuse type is unilateral with calcification and complex US appearance
  - Treatment is partial nephrectomy for focal type and nephrectomy for diffuse type
- **Clear Cell Sarcoma**
  - a.k.a. bone metastasizing renal tumor
  - Peak incidence is 1-4 years old
  - Metastasizes to bones, lymph nodes, brain, liver, and lung
  - Tx: Nephrectomy and chemotherapy
    - Long-term survival approaches 70%
- **Angiomyolipoma**
  - TS, neurofibromatosis type 1, and VHL syndrome
  - Lesions > 4 cm ↑ risk of hemorrhage
  - Fat on CT or MR is diagnostic

Helpful Clues for Rare Diagnoses

- **Rhabdoid Tumor**
  - Rare aggressive tumor that histologically resembles tumor of skeletal muscle
  - Synchronous or metachronous brain tumors (especially posterior fossa)
  - Subcapsular fluid collections and tumor lobules differentiate from Wilms tumor
- **Renal Medullary Carcinoma**
  - Adolescent with sickle cell trait or hemoglobin SC, not hemoglobin SS
  - Presents with gross hematuria and pain
  - Central, infiltrative causes caliectasis
  - Extremely aggressive with poor prognosis
- **Ossifying Renal Tumor of Infancy**
  - Benign lesion, 8 of 11 cases reported in boys, 9 of 11 in left kidney
  - Calcified mass in infant is suggestive
- **Metanephric Adenoma**
  - Benign tumor, no reports of bilateral cases, local resection can spare nephrons

Wilms Tumor-Nephroblastoma

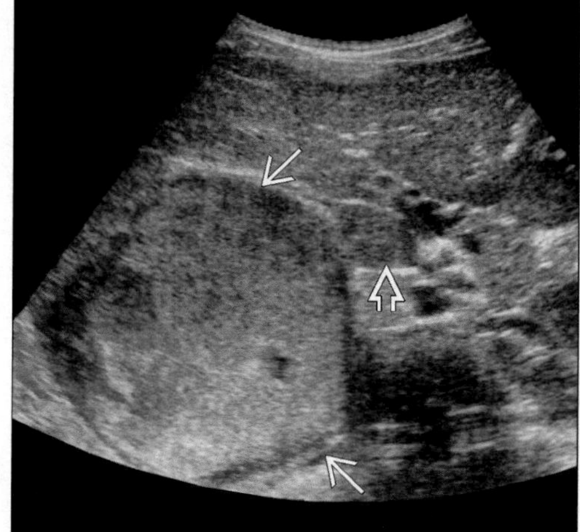

Transverse ultrasound shows a large heterogeneous mass ➡ in the kidney region of a young child. Attentive sonography revealed tumor thrombus extending into the inferior vena cava (IVC) ➡.

Wilms Tumor-Nephroblastoma

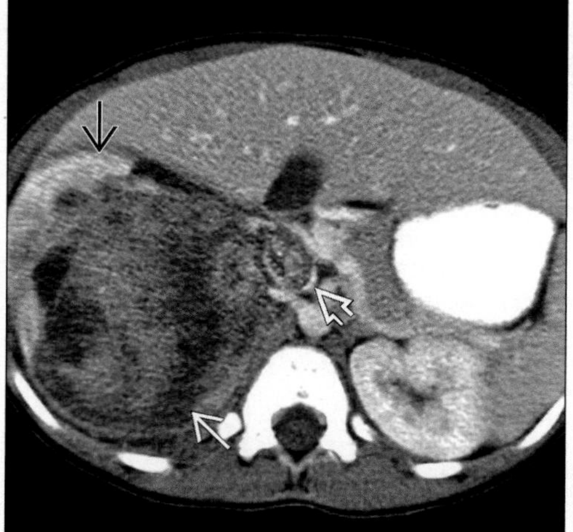

Axial CECT in the same patient shows a partially enhancing mass ➡ and a portion of a normally enhancing renal cortex ➡. The IVC tumor thrombus is surrounded by a crescent of contrast ➡.

RENAL MASS

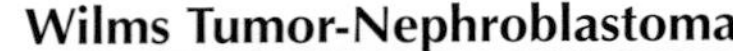

Wilms Tumor-Nephroblastoma

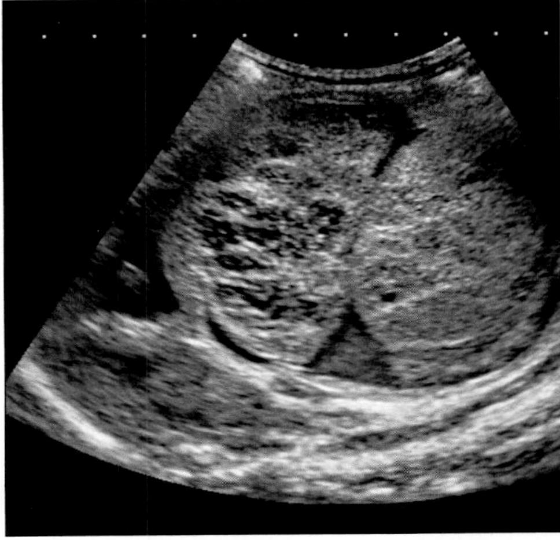

Wilms Tumor-Nephroblastoma

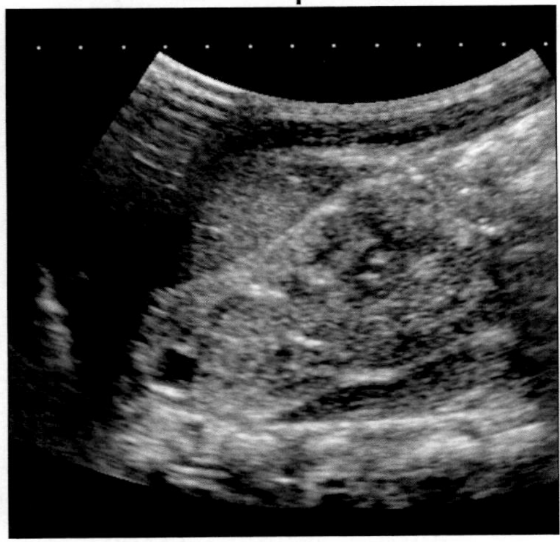

(Left) *Longitudinal ultrasound shows a heterogeneously echoic solid mass, replacing most of the right kidney in this infant. The most probable diagnosis is Wilms tumor.* ***(Right)*** *Longitudinal ultrasound in the same patient shows a poorly defined kidney with poor cortical medullary differentiation and focal hypoechoic areas. The mass was removed with a right nephrectomy. The left was biopsied, showing nephroblastomatosis followed with MR imaging.*

Nephroblastomatosis

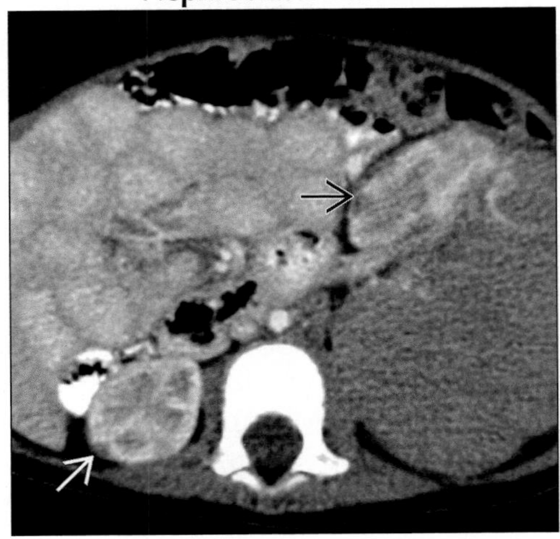

Nephroblastomatosis

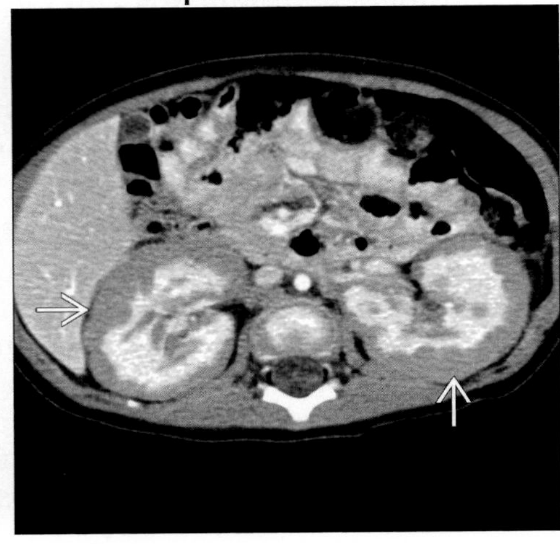

(Left) *Transverse CECT shows a large mass replacing the left kidney compatible with Wilms. Distorted renal cortex is present anteriorly* →. *Note the small area of hypoenhancement* ➡ *in the right kidney, compatible with nephrogenic rest.* ***(Right)*** *Axial CECT shows the renal parenchyma of both kidneys encased by soft tissue* ➡, *which enhances less than normal renal cortex would during cortical phase enhancement, in a patient with known Beckwith-Wiedemann.*

Nephroblastomatosis

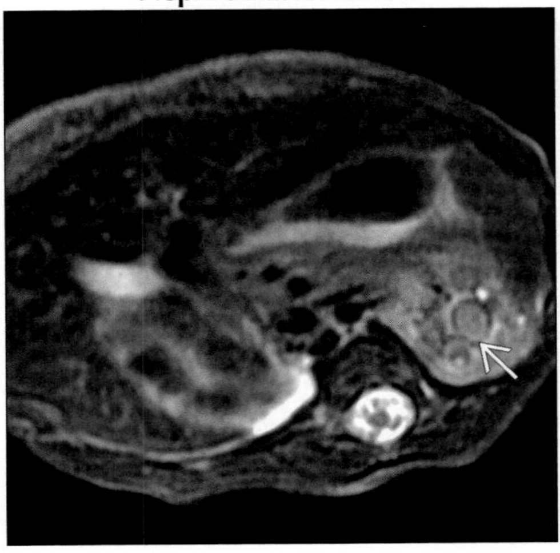

Nephroblastomatosis

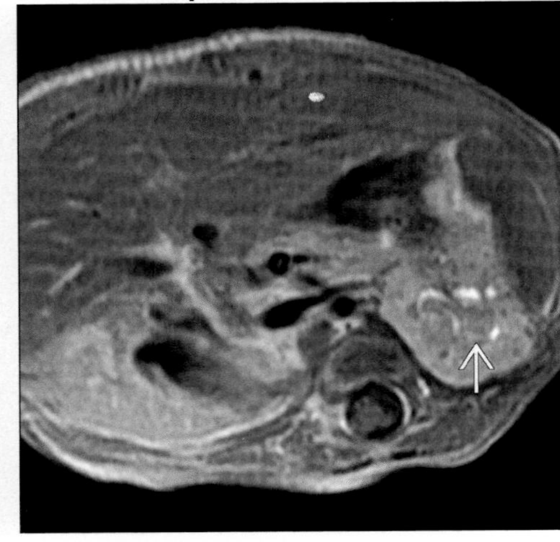

(Left) *Axial T2WI FS MR shows the nephroblastic mass* ➡ *in the upper pole of the left kidney after right nephrectomy. The mass is isointense to much of the kidney parenchyma on T2WI and enhanced to a similar degree post-contrast.* ***(Right)*** *Axial T1WI FS MR C+ shows the mass* ➡ *in the left kidney enhancing similarly to the renal cortex in this phase of enhancement. Follow-up showed progressively decreasing enhancement and size with some calyceal distortion.*

Nephroblastomatosis

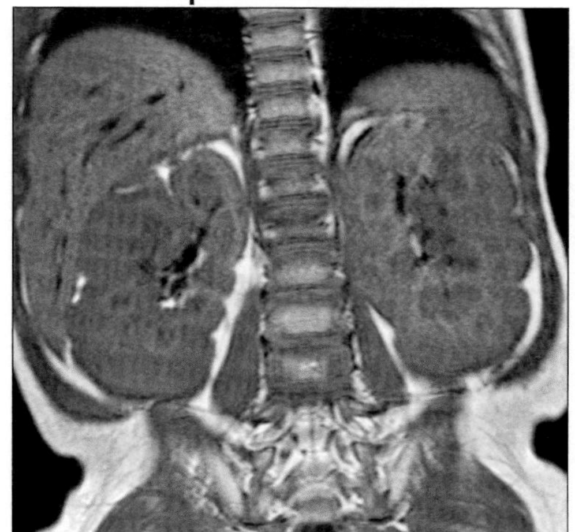

Nephroblastomatosis

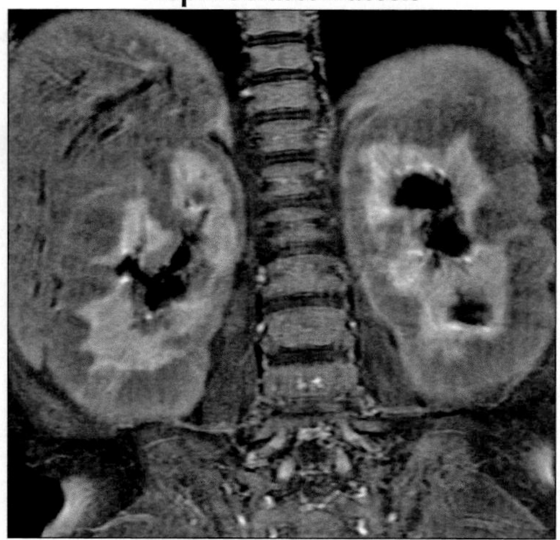

(Left) *Coronal T1WI FSE MR shows large kidneys, thick cortex, and a mantle of nephroblastema that is isointense to renal parenchyma. T1/T2 signal can be isointense, mildly hyperintense, or mildly hypointense to the renal parenchyma.* ***(Right)*** *Coronal T1WI FS MR C+ shows enhancement of renal tissue with nephroblastomatosis tissue showing enhancement to a lesser degree. The lesser degree of enhancement in the nephroblastema tissue is the most common pattern.*

Renal Cell Carcinoma

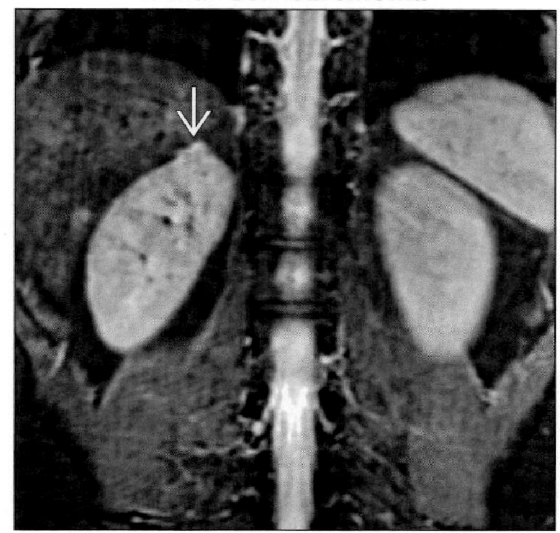

Renal Cell Carcinoma

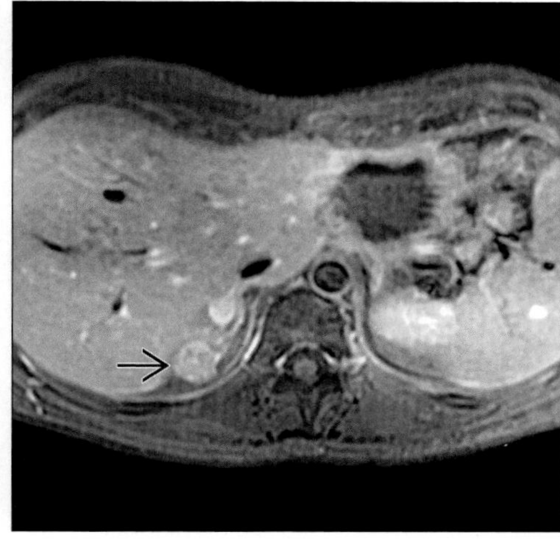

(Left) *Coronal STIR MR shows a small irregular lesion ➔ projecting from the superior pole of the right kidney in this patient with a remote history of neuroblastoma. The lesion is not as bright as a cyst.* ***(Right)*** *Axial T1 C+ FS MR shows a small irregular mass projecting from the superior pole of the right ➔ kidney. The mass enhances less than the renal parenchyma. A noncontrast CT showed no calcifications. This lesion was new from 1 year earlier.*

Renal Cell Carcinoma

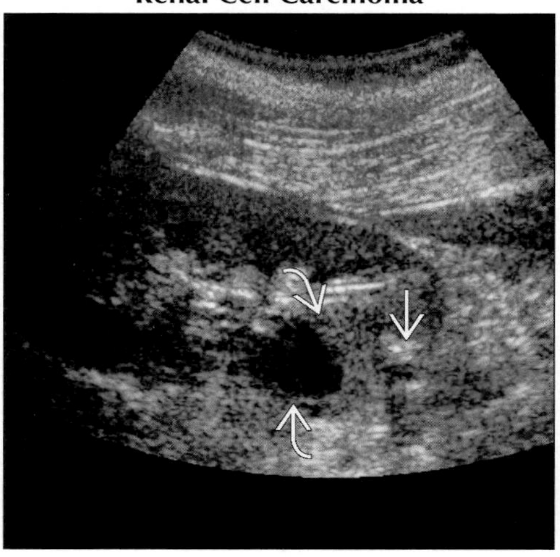

Mesoblastic Nephroma

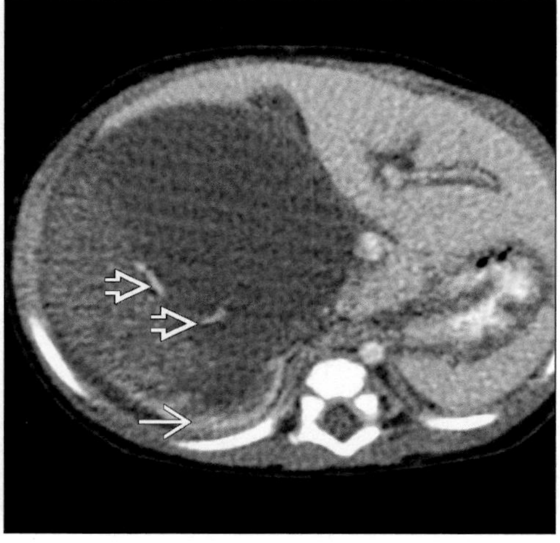

(Left) *Longitudinal ultrasound shows a cystic, solid lesion ➔ in the lower pole of the left kidney with an irregular echogenic area ➔ with posterior shadowing, indicating calcification. Resection showed renal cell carcinoma.* ***(Right)*** *Axial CECT shows a partially enhancing mass replacing the right renal parenchyma ➔ in a 1-month-old infant. Dense linear structures in the center of the mass ➔ are vessels, not calcifications.*

RENAL MASS

*(**Left**) Axial CECT shows multiple large masses in the kidneys in a patient with a large mediastinal mass, which was later diagnosed as a T-cell lymphoma. Renal involvement is often present but rarely causes significant renal dysfunction. (**Right**) AP radiograph shows a large gas-free area pushing air-filled bowel loops downward and toward the right lower quadrant. This is a relatively common appearance of large renal masses in young children.*

Lymphoma

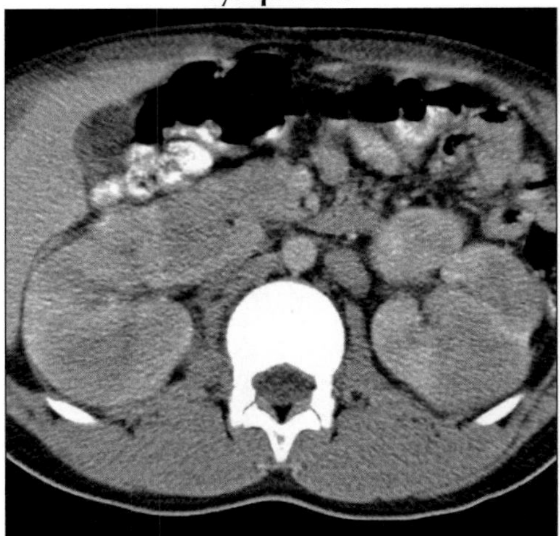

Multilocular Cystic Renal Tumor

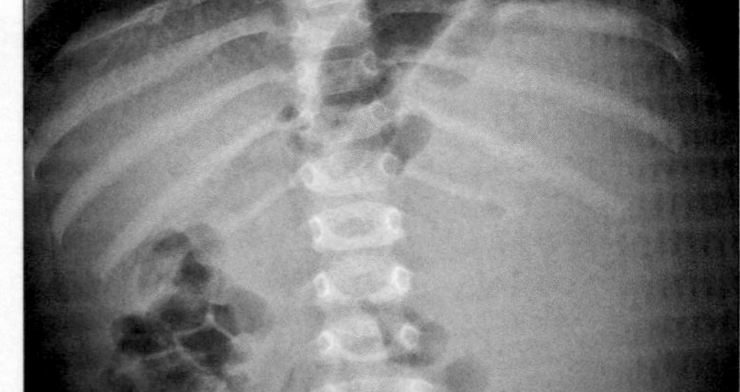

*(**Left**) Longitudinal ultrasound shows multiple anechoic cysts with scant solid tissue in this 15 month old with a palpable mass. US is best for defining the small cysts that can mimic a solid lesion on CT. (**Right**) Coronal FLAIR MR shows a well-defined mass with high water content and innumerable septations and cysts.The mass pouches into the renal collecting system ➡, which is fairly specific for multilocular cystic renal tumor.*

Multilocular Cystic Renal Tumor

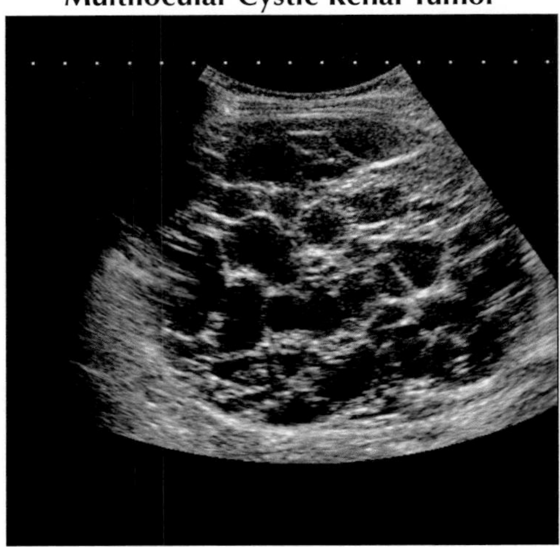

Multilocular Cystic Renal Tumor

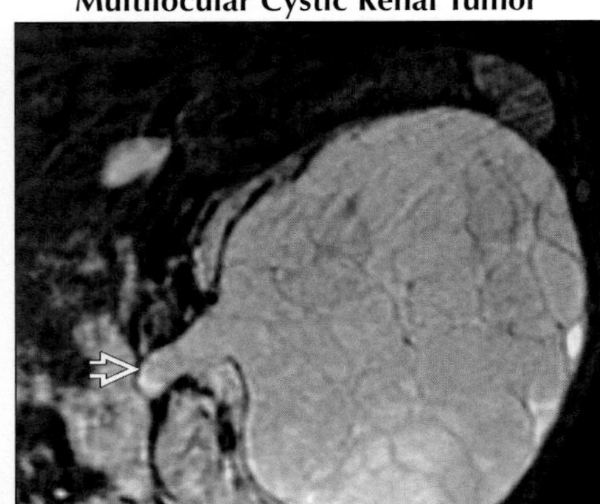

*(**Left**) Coronal T1WI FS MR C+ shows a mass with enhancing septations between the nonenhancing cysts with little solid tissue. The cortex of the lower pole of the kidney shows normal enhancement ➡. Note the herniation into the collecting system ➡. (**Right**) Coronal CECT shows a complex mass in the right kidney with fluid density areas separated by thick septation with irregular edges. US displayed a less well-defined and more solid appearance.*

Multilocular Cystic Renal Tumor

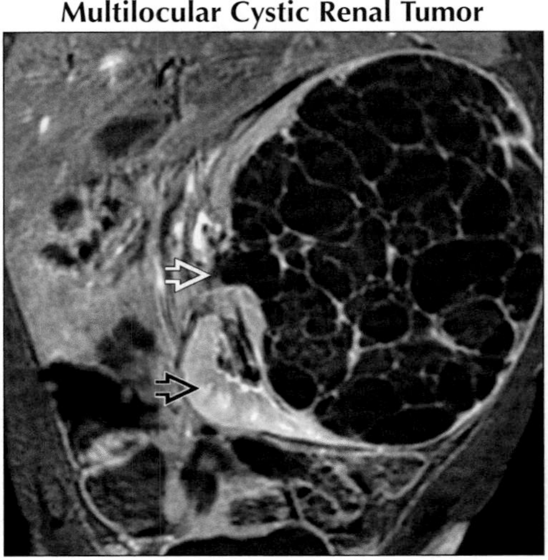

Abscess

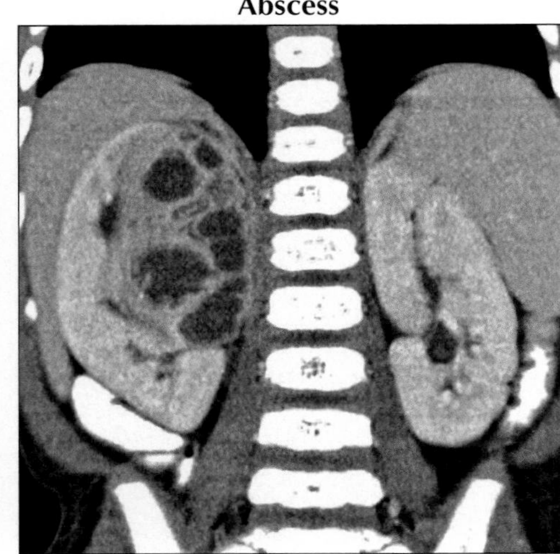

Clear Cell Sarcoma

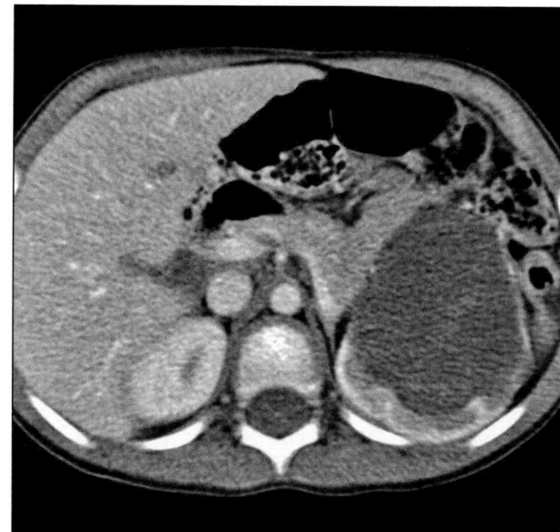

Angiomyolipoma

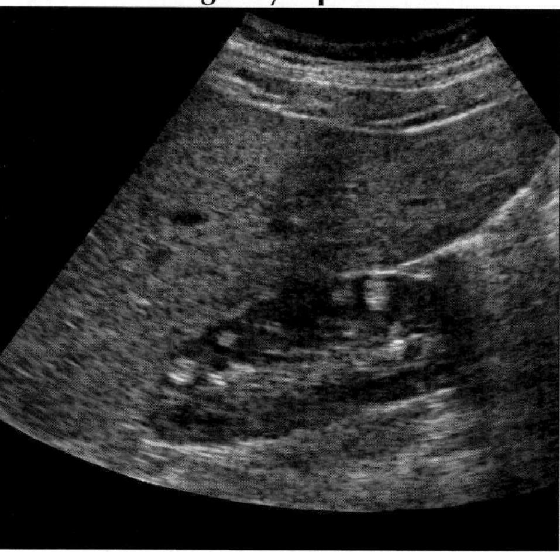

(Left) Axial CECT shows a large low-attenuation mass in the left kidney in a patient who presented with hematuria. Brain MR and bone radiographs showed no evidence of metastasis. The tumor is aggressive, but long-term survival is ~ 70%. (Right) Longitudinal US shows multiple, small, echogenic foci in a child with a history of tuberous sclerosis, the typical US appearance of small angiomyolipomas. There is increased risk of hemorrhage if the foci are > 4 cm.

Angiomyolipoma

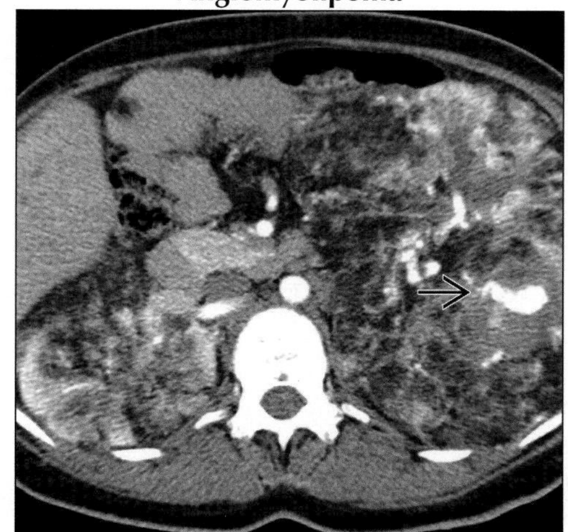

Angiomyolipoma

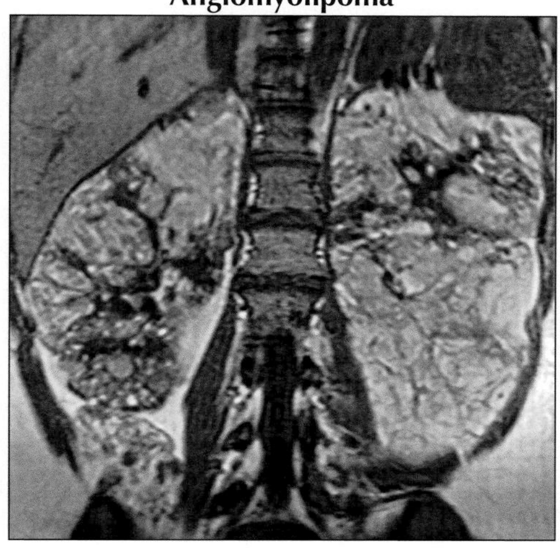

(Left) Axial CECT shows extensive renal fat density bilaterally in a teenager with tuberous sclerosis. CT is reserved to evaluate for aneurysms that can cause severe retroperitoneal hemorrhage. This aneurysm ⇒ was treated by an angiographic embolism. (Right) Coronal T1WI MR shows extensive infiltration of both kidneys by fat-containing tumors, which are diagnostic of AML. Lesions greater than 4 cm have ↑ risk of hemorrhage due to aneurysms.

Rhabdoid Tumor

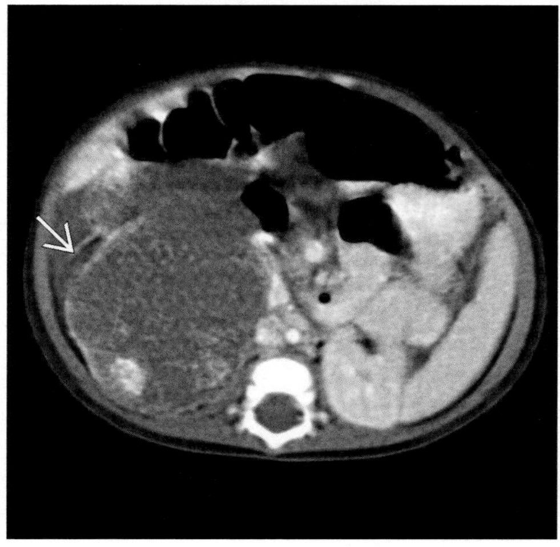

Renal Medullary Carcinoma

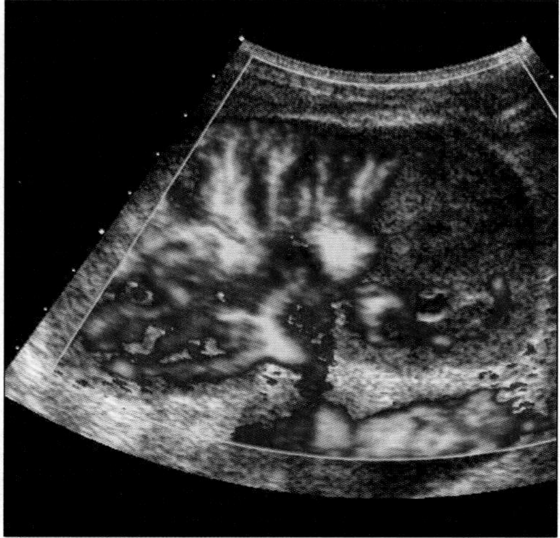

(Left) Axial CECT shows a large heterogeneous mass replacing the right kidney with areas of subcapsular fluid collection ➡, which can help distinguish rhabdoid tumor from Wilms. No brain tumors were found in this patient. (Right) Longitudinal power Doppler ultrasound shows a hypovascular mass in the lower pole with mild heterogeneous echotexture. The patient presented with back pain and was positive for sickle trait. (Courtesy V.J. Rooks, MD.)

RENAL CYSTS

DIFFERENTIAL DIAGNOSIS

Common
- Multicystic Dysplastic Kidney (MCDK)
- Ureteropelvic Duplications
- Simple Renal Cyst
- Autosomal Dominant Polycystic Renal Disease (ADPCKD)
- Calyceal Diverticulum
- Cystic Renal Dysplasia

Less Common
- Autosomal Recessive Polycystic Renal Disease (ARPCKD)
- Acquired Cystic Kidney Disease
- Renal Injury

Rare but Important
- Tuberous Sclerosis (TS) Complex
- Multilocular Cystic Nephroma (MLCN)

ESSENTIAL INFORMATION

Key Differential Diagnosis Issues
- Cystic lesions of kidney in pediatric populations are seldom malignant
  - Cystic forms of renal cell, clear cell, and Wilms tumors are exceptions
- Narrowing differentials
  - Unilateral
    - MCDK, duplication, simple renal cyst, calyceal diverticulum, trauma, MLCN
  - Bilateral
    - ADPCKD, ARPCKD, post-transplant acquired cystic disease, TS
  - Variable
    - Cystic dysplasia, duplications

Helpful Clues for Common Diagnoses
- **Multicystic Dysplastic Kidney (MCDK)**
  - Classic type: Conglomerate cysts without discernible renal pelvis
  - Hydronephrotic type: Central cyst thought to be remnant of obstructed pelvis
  - High incidence of contralateral renal abnormalities: UPJ obstruction and vesicoureteral reflux (VUR)
  - MCDK initially large, but vast majority shrink over course of years
  - 1/2 of all MCDK have involuted by age 5
  - 12 reported cases of Wilms and renal cell carcinoma occurring in MCDK
  - National MCDK Registry tracks incidence and behavior
  - Imaging: Confirm lack of function with nuclear renal scan
- **Ureteropelvic Duplications**
  - Upper poles of duplex kidneys tend to obstruct due to
    - Ectopic ureteral insertion
    - Ureterocele
    - Search bladder and pelvis carefully for ectopic ureter when evaluating upper pole cystic lesions
  - Lower poles have high incidence of VUR
    - **Note**: High-grade VUR may dilate calyces
  - Imaging: US, VCUG, diuretic renal scan
- **Simple Renal Cyst**
  - Smooth, sharply marginated, water-density lesions
  - Through transmission on ultrasound
  - Does not enhance on CT and MR
  - If positive family history of cystic kidneys, consider ADPCKD
  - Imaging: US, CT, MR
- **Autosomal Dominant Polycystic Renal Disease (ADPCKD)**
  - Hereditary disorder of renal cysts and other organ abnormalities
    - Renal cysts (100%)
    - Liver cysts (50%)
    - Pancreatic cysts (9%)
    - Brain/ovary/testis (1%)
    - Cardiac valvular disease (26%)
    - Cerebral aneurysms (5-10%)
  - Cyst visibility and prevalence increase with age
  - 1/2 of patients have cysts in 1st decade, 72% in 2nd
  - Prognosis
    - Excellent in childhood
    - Variable in adulthood: Based on degree of renal insufficiency and hypertension
  - Imaging: US, CT, MR, nuclear for function
- **Calyceal Diverticulum**
  - Urine-filled eventration of calyx into renal parenchyma connected by narrow channel
  - Smooth, round to ovoid, thin walled; abuts calyx
  - May contain stones or debris
  - Delayed contrast excretion into diverticulum is diagnostic but not always seen

- Imaging: US, CT, MR, nuclear renal scan
- **Cystic Renal Dysplasia**
  - Generally progressive scarring and nephron loss due to repetitive injury
    - Vesicoureteral reflux
    - Pyelonephritis
    - High bladder pressure
    - Vascular compromise
    - Toxins, medications, radiation, etc.
  - Corticomedullary differentiation lost, increased echotexture, cysts
  - Imaging: US, CT, MR, nuclear renal scan

Helpful Clues for Less Common Diagnoses

- **Autosomal Recessive Polycystic Renal Disease (ARPCKD)**
  - Single gene disorder (*PKHD1*)
  - Bilateral, enlarged, microcystic kidneys
  - Ectatic distal convoluted tubules and collecting ducts
  - Renal insufficiency/failure
  - Associated lung disease, oligohydramnios, MSK abnormalities
  - Prognosis is poor, but mild form may survive childhood
  - Imaging: US pre- and post-natally
- **Acquired Cystic Kidney Disease**
  - Seen in almost 1/2 of patients on dialysis and with post solid organ transplant
  - Increased incidence with cyclosporin immune suppression
  - Screening important: ESRD and renal transplant patients have increased incidence of renal cell carcinoma
  - Clinical history narrows differential
  - Imaging: US, CT, MR
- **Renal Injury**
  - Cystic change in kidney from trauma or infection
  - Cysts will not meet "simple" criteria
    - Have irregular walls, debris, septations
  - Without associated mass or enhancement, safe to follow with imaging
  - Imaging: US, CT, MR, nuclear renal scan

Helpful Clues for Rare Diagnoses

- **Tuberous Sclerosis (TS) Complex**
  - Neurocutaneous syndrome: Hamartomatosis
  - Classic triad: Adenoma sebaceum, seizures, and mental retardation
  - Organs involved: Cardiac rhabdomyoma, lung lymphangiomyomatosis, renal cysts and angiomyolipomas, nonrenal hamartomas
  - Imaging: US, CT, MR, nuclear renal scan
- **Multilocular Cystic Nephroma (MLCN)**
  - Benign cystic renal neoplasm
  - Bimodal age distribution
    - M > > F, 3 months to 2 years
    - M < < F, 5th and 6th decades
  - Imaging: US, CT, MR

Multicystic Dysplastic Kidney (MCDK)

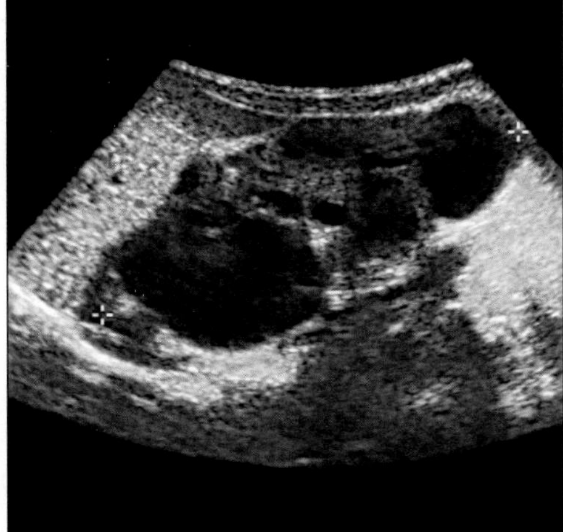

Longitudinal harmonic ultrasound shows an enlarged, but roughly reniform-shaped collection of cysts and echogenic soft tissue (calipers) in the right renal fossa in a newborn.

Multicystic Dysplastic Kidney (MCDK)

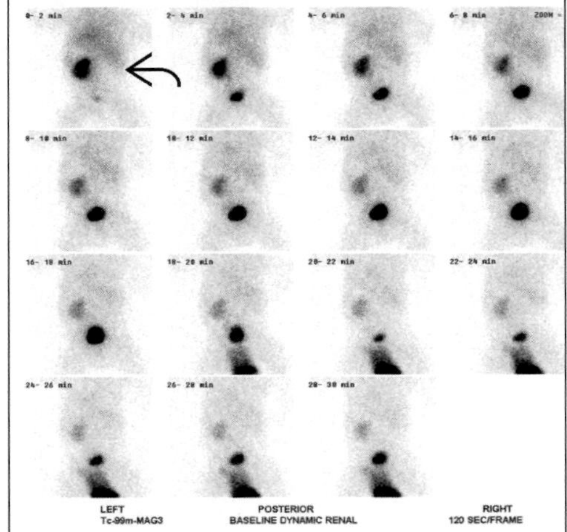

Posterior renal scan shows no functional renal tissue on the right side ➔ in this newborn with right multicystic dysplastic kidney. The solitary left kidney is working well.

RENAL CYSTS

(Left) Longitudinal ultrasound shows a large cyst ➡ in the upper pole of the left kidney and caliectasis in the lower pole of this infant who showed hydronephrosis on a prenatal scan. Ultrasound of the pelvis (not shown) revealed a ureterocele in the left side of the bladder. ***(Right)*** Posterior renal cortical scan shows poor function of the upper pole ➡. Regions of interest can be drawn to estimate the function of the upper vs. lower pole.

Ureteropelvic Duplications

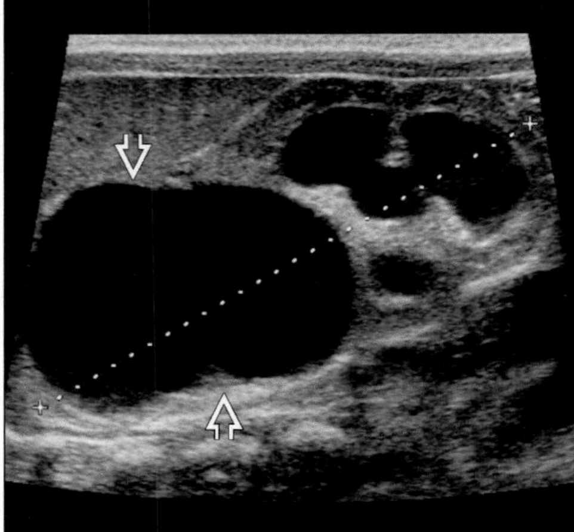

Ureteropelvic Duplications

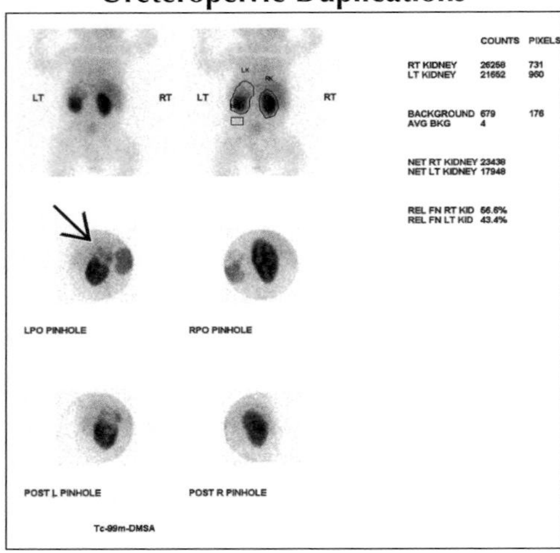

(Left) Longitudinal harmonic ultrasound shows a well-defined cyst ➡ in the lower pole of the kidney in a child with no family history of renal disease. No other cysts were seen in the contralateral kidney. ***(Right)*** Longitudinal harmonic ultrasound in a different patient shows a well-defined cyst ➡ with smooth walls and through transmission in the upper pole. Simple cysts may be peripheral, as in this case, or central in location.

Simple Renal Cyst

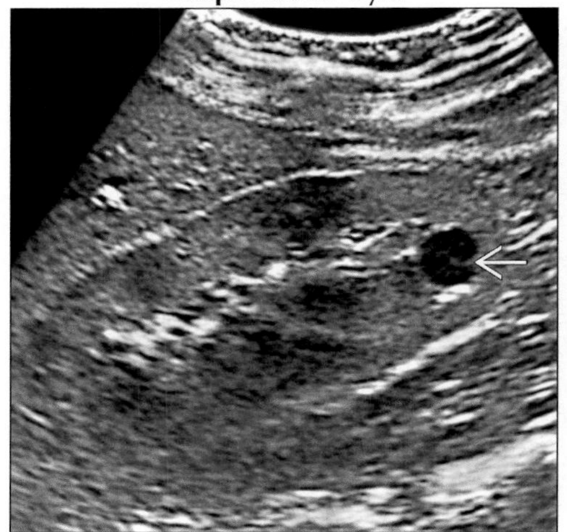

Simple Renal Cyst

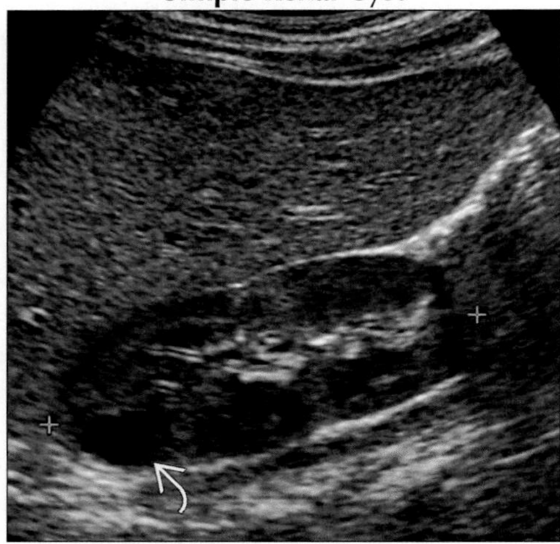

(Left) Longitudinal harmonic ultrasound shows numerous cysts ➡ in both the medulla and cortex of the left kidney in this male teenager with a family history of polycystic renal disease. The patient was asymptomatic but being screened for autosomal dominant polycystic disease. ***(Right)*** Longitudinal harmonic ultrasound in the same patient shows a cyst in the lower pole of the right kidney. The number of cysts and measurements of the largest cyst in each kidney are typically reported.

Autosomal Dominant Polycystic Renal Disease (ADPCKD)

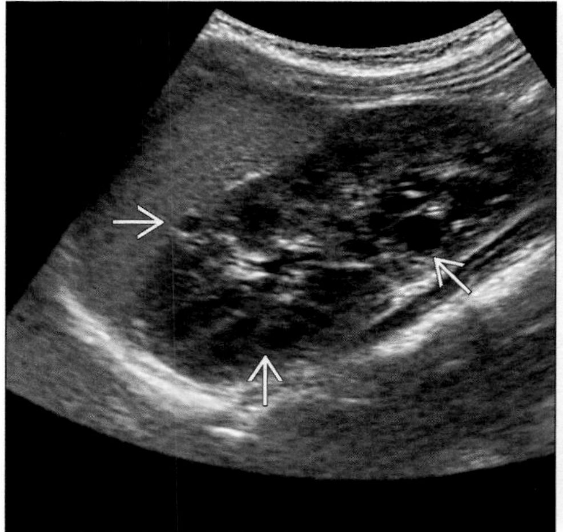

Autosomal Dominant Polycystic Renal Disease (ADPCKD)

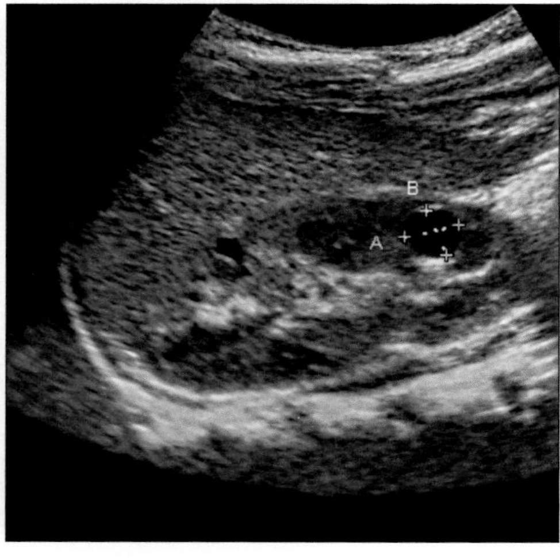

Calyceal Diverticulum

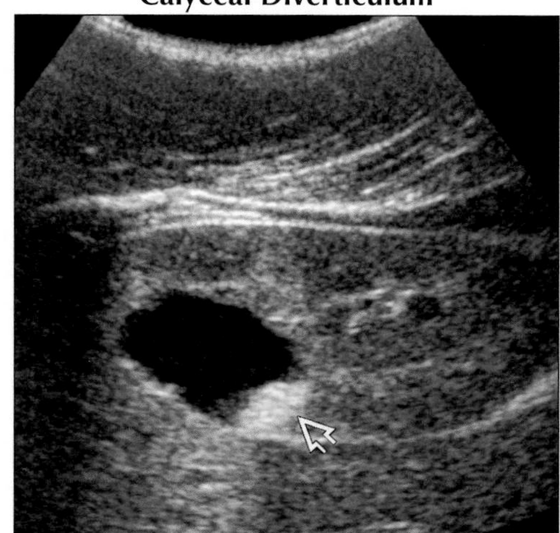

Calyceal Diverticulum

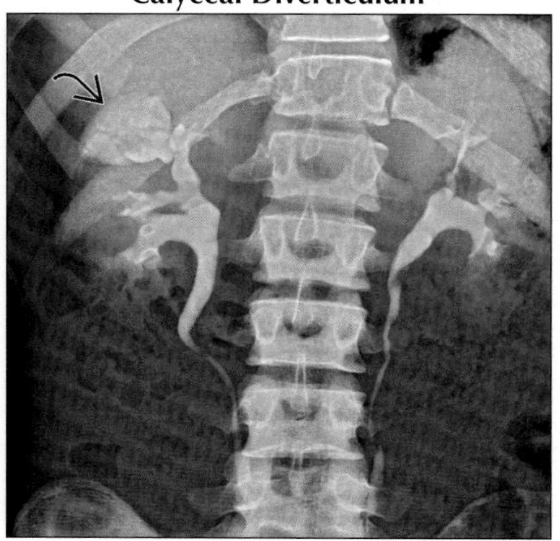

(Left) *Longitudinal harmonic ultrasound shows a large cyst in the upper pole of the right kidney in a 17-year-old boy with intermittent hematuria and flank pain. Note the dependent, layering echogenic material* ➡. ***(Right)*** *AP excretory urography in the same patient shows an ovoid contrast collection* ➡ *in the upper pole of the right kidney, corresponding to the region seen on ultrasound. Note the distortion of the calyx adjacent to the collection.*

Calyceal Diverticulum

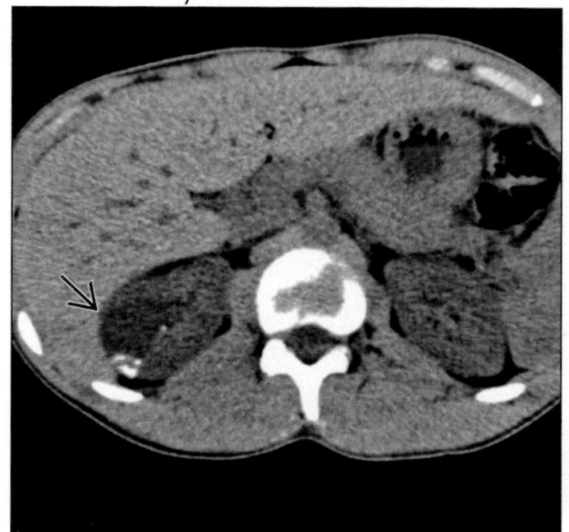

Calyceal Diverticulum

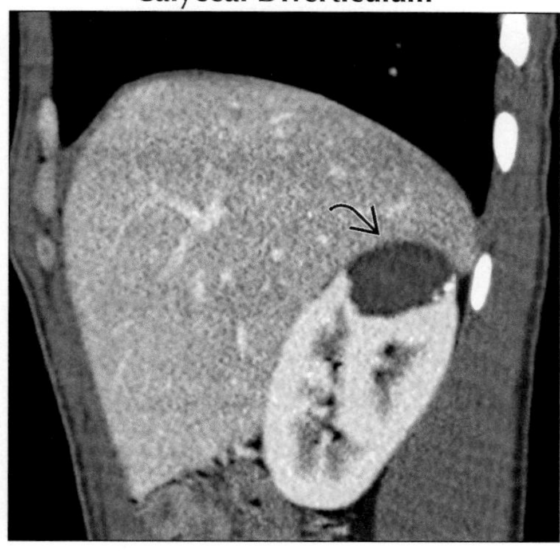

(Left) *Axial NECT in the same teenager shows calcifications layering dependently within the cystic area* ➡ *in the right kidney upper pole.* ***(Right)*** *Sagittal reformat CECT shows good perfusion of the rest of the right kidney but no early contrast within the cystic upper pole lesion* ➡. *Delayed filling or enhancement of a calyceal diverticulum is often seen but not required for the diagnosis.*

Cystic Renal Dysplasia

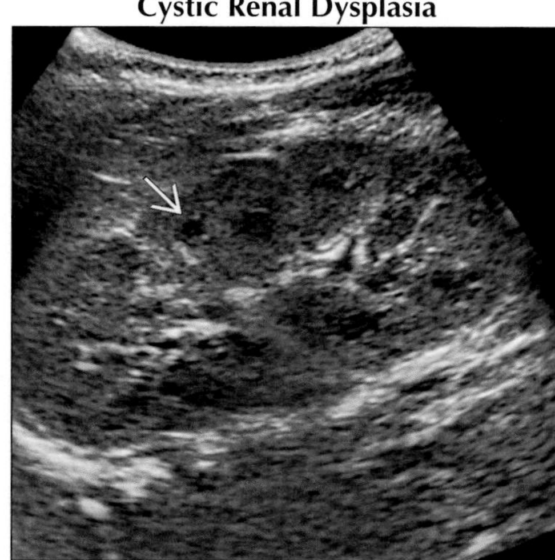

Cystic Renal Dysplasia

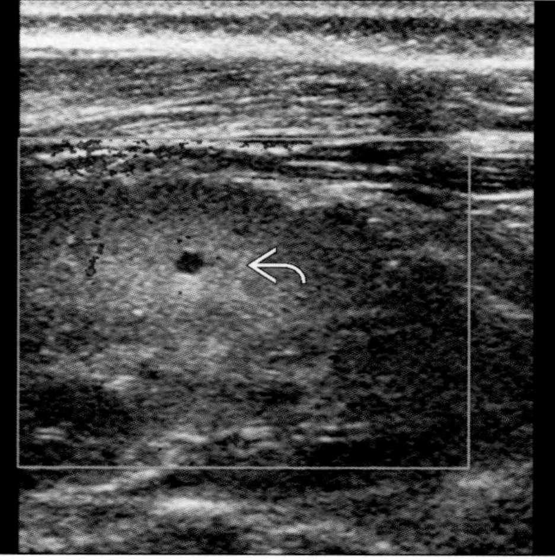

(Left) *Longitudinal harmonic ultrasound shows generalized increased echotexture of the kidney and at least 1 cyst* ➡ *in this follow-up for vesicoureteral reflux. Lagging renal growth, recurrent infections, and this US appearance prompted surgery to correct the reflux.* ***(Right)*** *Transverse harmonic ultrasound with a high frequency linear transducer shows a very small cortical cyst* ➡ *in this child with cystic renal dysplasia.*

RENAL CYSTS

(**Left**) *AP radiograph in a newborn with respiratory distress and a distended abdomen shows bulging flanks and central displacement of bowel loops. The lungs are poorly aerated in this anuric infant.* (**Right**) *Longitudinal harmonic ultrasound shows a dramatically enlarged, echogenic right kidney, spanning 8+ vertebral bodies. The renal echotexture is diffusely increased, and corticomedullary differentiation is lost.*

Autosomal Recessive Polycystic Renal Disease (ARPCKD)

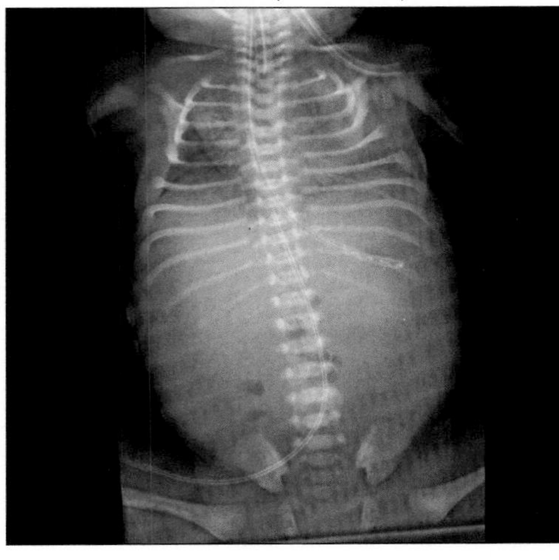

Autosomal Recessive Polycystic Renal Disease (ARPCKD)

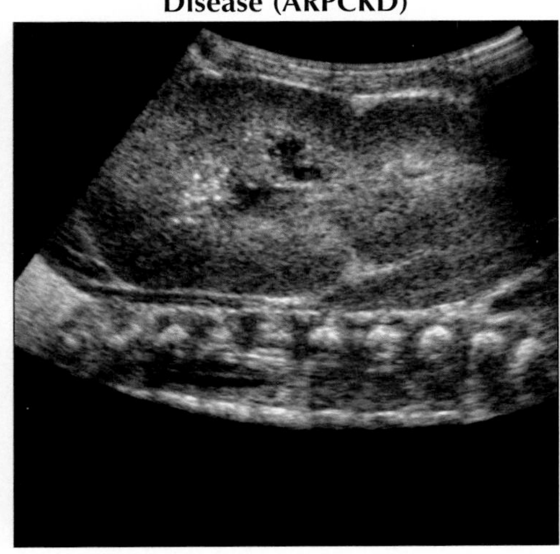

(**Left**) *Transverse harmonic ultrasound through the lower abdomen in the same newborn shows that both kidneys are involved and dramatically enlarged, touching in the midline ➡. Note the spine posteriorly ➡.* (**Right**) *Longitudinal spatial compounding ultrasound with a high frequency linear transducer shows the dilated tubules and innumerable cysts, whose interfaces create the generalized increased echoes on US. Macrocysts are also often seen.*

Autosomal Recessive Polycystic Renal Disease (ARPCKD)

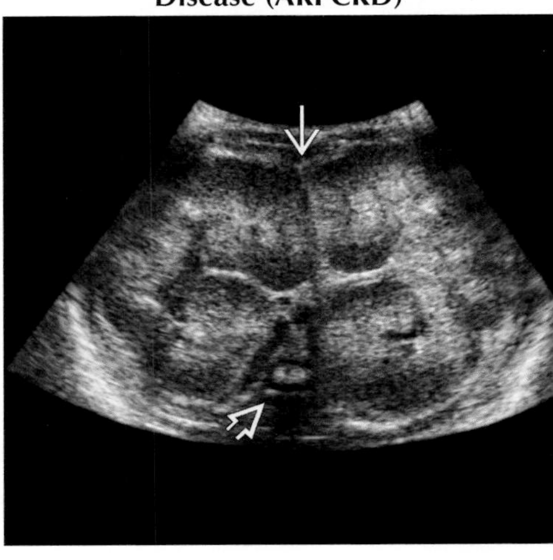

Autosomal Recessive Polycystic Renal Disease (ARPCKD)

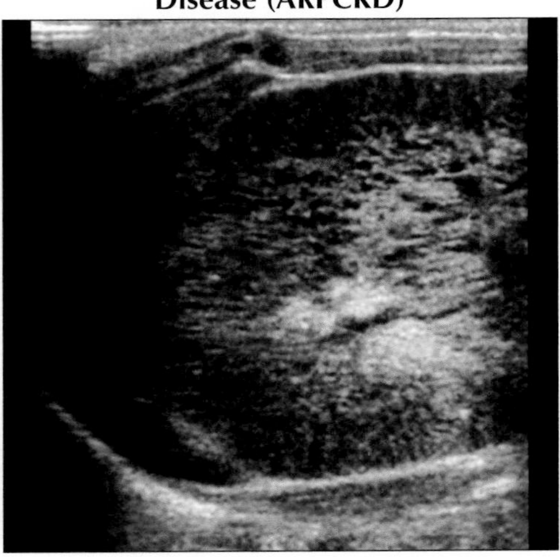

(**Left**) *Axial T2WI MR shows bright signal in a cyst ➡ along the posterior margin of a globally scarred left kidney in a young adult with a history of posterior urethral valves status post renal transplant. The native right kidney was removed years prior.* (**Right**) *Longitudinal ultrasound in a different renal transplant patient shows a globally scarred, dysplastic right kidney with a cyst ➡. Often the patients' native kidneys are difficult to see.*

Acquired Cystic Kidney Disease

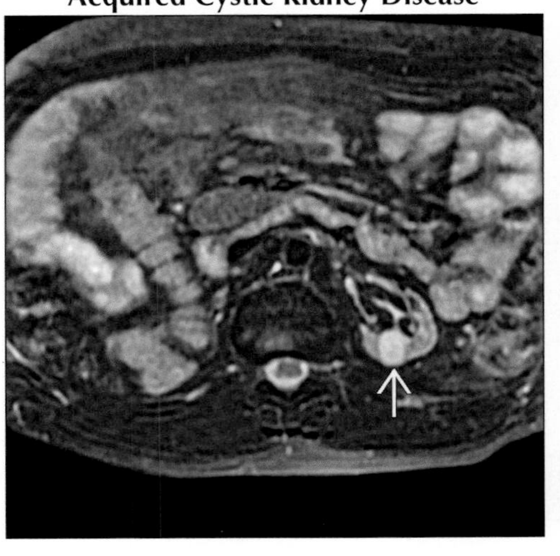

Acquired Cystic Kidney Disease

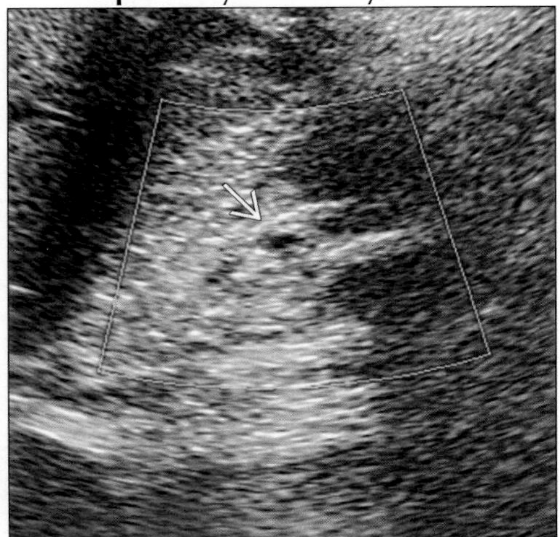

Renal Injury

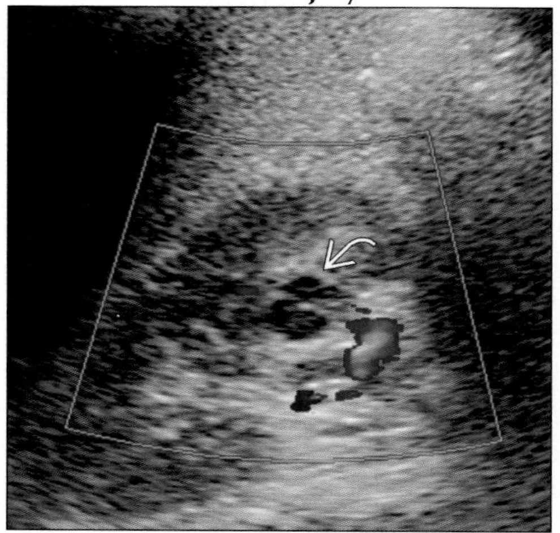

Renal Injury

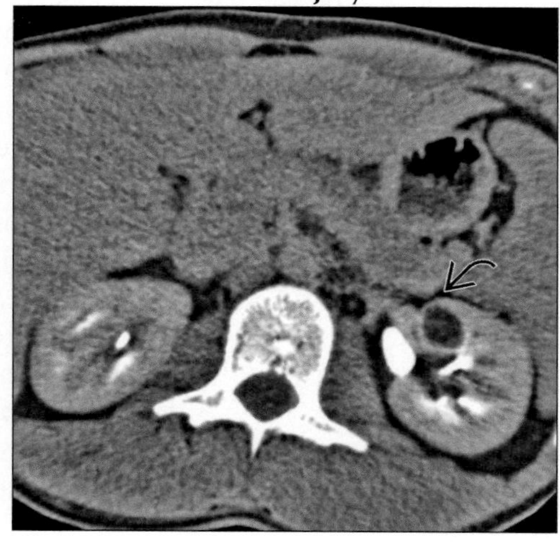

*(**Left**) Transverse ultrasound shows a complex, septated cyst ➡ in the midpole region of the left kidney. This teenager was active in contact sports and complained of rib pain. The cystic area was not seen on prior imaging. (**Right**) Axial CECT after a 10-minute delay shows no contrast in the cystic area ➡ and no associated mass or contour abnormality. These complex cysts are most likely post-traumatic or postinfectious and can be safely followed with imaging.*

Tuberous Sclerosis (TS) Complex

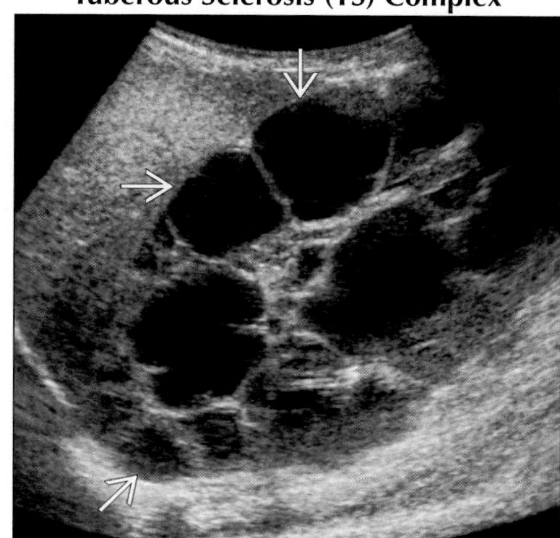

Tuberous Sclerosis (TS) Complex

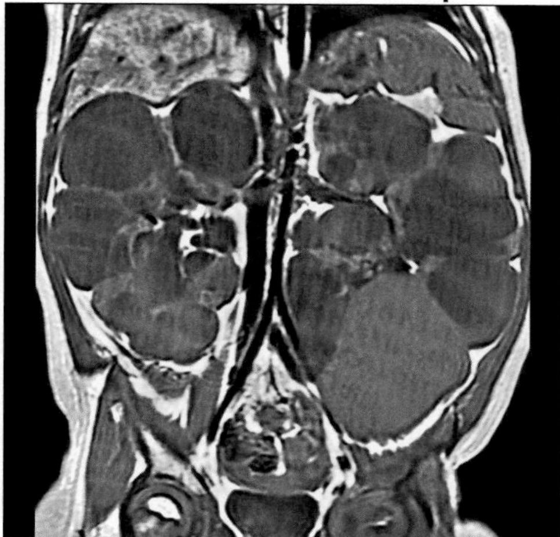

*(**Left**) Longitudinal ultrasound shows numerous cystic areas ➡ replacing the normal renal parenchyma. This child had seizures and a family history of tuberous sclerosis. The renal function was borderline. (**Right**) Coronal T1WI MR in the same patient shows massive kidneys essentially replaced by cysts. Some of the cysts contain higher signal intensity, which reflects hemorrhage, protein, or infection.*

Multilocular Cystic Nephroma (MLCN)

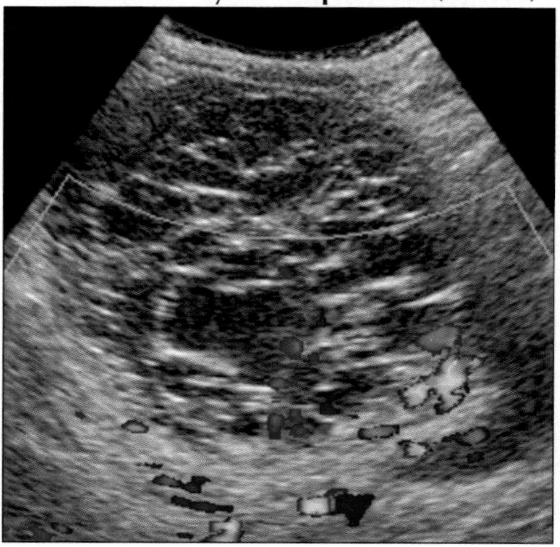

Multilocular Cystic Nephroma (MLCN)

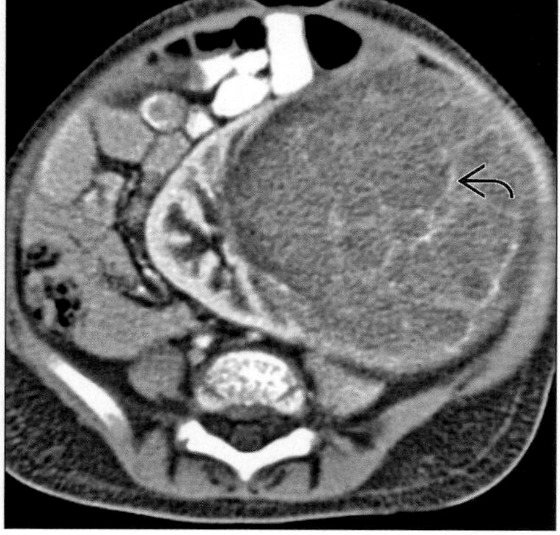

*(**Left**) Transverse color Doppler ultrasound shows a large, multiseptated mass replacing much of the left kidney in a 1 year old with a palpable mass. Blood flow is seen in some of the septations and surrounding tissues. (**Right**) Axial CECT shows fine septations ➡ within the primarily cystic mass in the left kidney. The kidney and mass are displaced inferiorly into the pelvis. The left kidney was removed, and multilocular cystic nephroma was found pathologically.*

RENAL CALCIFICATIONS

DIFFERENTIAL DIAGNOSIS

Common
- Miscellaneous Hypercalcemia/Hypercalciuria
- Chronic Diuretic Therapy
- Renal Tubular Acidosis
- Medullary Sponge Kidney
- Tamm-Horsfall Proteins (Mimic)

Less Common
- Chronic Glomerulonephritis
- Papillary Necrosis
- Infection/Infarction/Trauma
- Oxalosis/Hyperoxaluria
- Alport Syndrome

Rare but Important
- Salt-Wasting Nephropathies
  - Bartter, Gitelman Syndromes
- Malignancies
  - Wilms Tumor
  - Sarcoma
  - Renal Cell Carcinoma
- Poisoning/Toxicity
- Tuberculosis

ESSENTIAL INFORMATION

Key Differential Diagnosis Issues
- Distribution
  - Medullary nephrocalcinosis
    - Abnormal calcium deposition within renal medullary pyramids
    - Within interstitium or distal tubules
    - Represents between 85-95% of all cases of nephrocalcinosis
  - Cortical nephrocalcinosis
    - Abnormal calcium deposition within renal cortex
    - Represents minority of cases of nephrocalcinosis
- Basic definitions
  - Nephrocalcinosis: Abnormal calcium deposition within renal parenchyma
  - Nephrolithiasis: Formation/presence of calculi within upper renal collecting system (renal calyces or renal pelvis)
    - Often calcium compounds but not exclusively
    - Calculi may or may not obstruct
  - Urolithiasis: Presence of calculi in mid to lower urinary tract (ureters, urinary bladder); obstructing or nonobstructing

Helpful Clues for Common Diagnoses
- **Miscellaneous Hypercalcemia/Hypercalciuria**
  - Distribution: Medullary region
  - Numerous etiologies: Dietary, pharmaceutical, immobilization, metabolic, steroid use, familial, idiopathic, sarcoid, endocrine abnormalities
  - US more sensitive than radiographs
    - Calcifications on US have variable appearance: Punctate, coarse, granular, round, linear; ± shadowing
- **Chronic Diuretic Therapy**
  - Distribution: Medullary region
  - Results from use of loop diuretics, commonly furosemide (Lasix)
    - Associated with hypercalciuria
  - More common in premature infants; many cases will resolve several months after discontinuation
- **Renal Tubular Acidosis**
  - Distribution: Medullary region
    - Most reliably identified by US
    - Calcifications may be deposited at periphery of medulla or may occupy entire medullary pyramid
    - Small or sparse calcifications may not demonstrate posterior acoustic shadowing
  - Results from proximal tubule defect in bicarbonate resorption
    - Urine: May have hypercalciuria, urolithiasis
    - Blood: May have secondary hyperparathyroidism &/or hypophosphatemia
- **Medullary Sponge Kidney**
  - Distribution: Medullary region
  - Primary abnormality is cystic/patulous dilatation of distal tubules
    - Urinary stasis in tubules results in precipitation of urinary calcium crystals
    - Distribution of calcifications may be patchy/asymmetric
  - Intravenous pyelogram reveals linear opacities of accumulated contrast material within dilated distal tubules
- **Tamm-Horsfall Proteins (Mimic)**
  - Common mammalian urinary proteins; often conspicuous in newborn kidney

- Considered incidental finding; typically resolves within 2-3 weeks of birth
- Typically noted on US
  - Evenly distributed echogenicity of renal medullary pyramids; may be confused with renal medullary calcifications

Helpful Clues for Less Common Diagnoses

- **Chronic Glomerulonephritis**
  - Distribution: Nearly exclusively cortical
  - Granular, cortical intratubular
- **Papillary Necrosis**
  - Distribution: Medullary region, particularly papillae
  - Consider medical background
    - Analgesic use, sickle cell, dehydration, renal vein thrombosis, infection, liver disease
- **Infection/Infarction/Trauma**
  - Distribution: Predominantly cortical, unilateral or bilateral, depending on underlying etiology
    - Unilateral: Prior infection, focal vascular injury, trauma, renal vein thrombosis
    - Bilateral: Systemic vascular compromise, disseminated infection (TB), chronic glomerulonephritis, hemolytic uremic syndrome
- **Oxalosis/Hyperoxaluria**
  - Distribution: Predominantly medullary, may be cortical
  - Underlying cause may be genetic, enteric, dietary, or mild/idiopathic
- **Alport Syndrome**
  - Distribution: Classically cortical
  - Multiple genetic forms; associated with variable severity of deafness, hypertension, hematuria, ocular disease
  - More severe in males

Helpful Clues for Rare Diagnoses

- **Salt-Wasting Nephropathies**
  - Bartter, Gitelman syndromes
  - Distribution: Medullary region
  - Chloride channel disorder, associated with hypercalcuria
- **Malignancies**
  - **Wilms Tumor**
    - Calcifications less common, often wispy or punctate
    - Coarse calcifications may be associated with areas of necrosis
  - **Renal Cell Carcinoma**
    - Hematuria more common than in Wilms
    - Calcifications also more common
- **Poisoning/Toxicity**
  - Distribution: Medullary region
  - Common culprits: Heavy metals or ethylene glycol
- **Tuberculosis**
  - Distribution: Medullary/papillary > cortical
  - Usually bilateral but **asymmetric**
  - Calcifications punctate/granular/coarse
    - End-stage TB kidney is shrunken, diffusely/densely calcified ("autonephrectomy")

Miscellaneous Hypercalcemia/Hypercalciuria

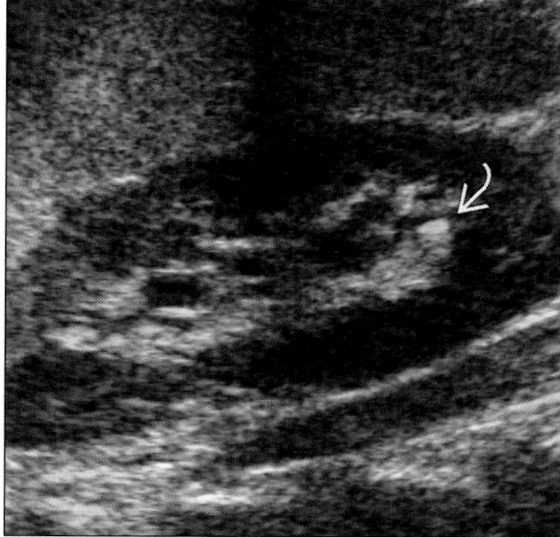

Longitudinal ultrasound shows an ovoid echogenic focus ➔ in the lower pole of the left kidney, consistent with a small calculus in this 11-year-old boy with recurrent stones of unknown etiology.

Miscellaneous Hypercalcemia/Hypercalciuria

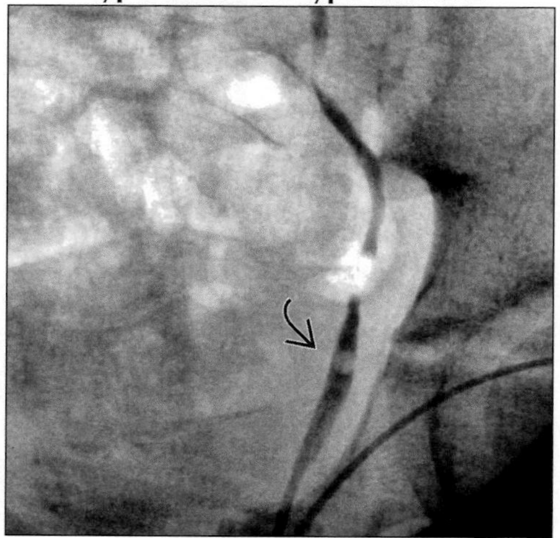

Anteroposterior fluoroscopic spot radiograph in the same patient shows 1 of the stones ➔ in the distal left ureter depicted during a retrograde pyelogram.

RENAL CALCIFICATIONS

*(**Left**) Longitudinal ultrasound shows echogenic medullary pyramids ➔ in a 9-year-old boy with idiopathic juvenile osteoporosis. Note that there is no posterior acoustic shadowing. Although the kidneys appear stable on US, the patient's renal function has slowly declined. (**Right**) Longitudinal ultrasound shows subtle, speckled, bright foci ➔ within echogenic medullary regions in a 3 year old with congenital adrenal hyperplasia.*

Miscellaneous Hypercalcemia/Hypercalciuria

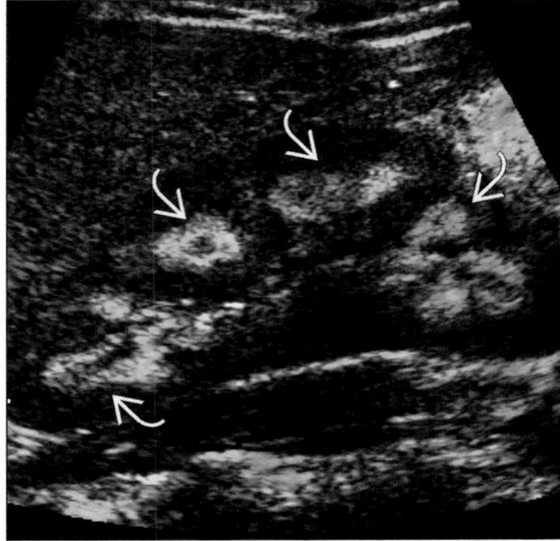

Miscellaneous Hypercalcemia/Hypercalciuria

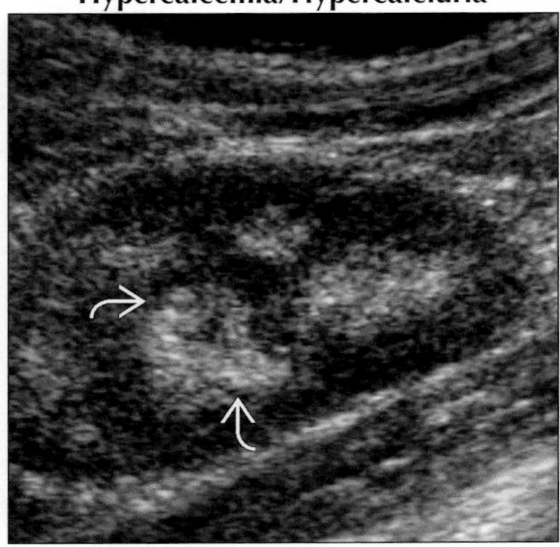

*(**Left**) Longitudinal ultrasound shows coarse calcium deposits at the tips of the medullary pyramids in this 5 month old on Lasix therapy for chronic lung disease that resulted from prematurity. The ultrasound obtained at 19 days of age was normal; changes related to loop diuretics take several weeks to appear. (**Right**) Longitudinal ultrasound shows numerous punctate echogenic foci ➔ in the medullary regions in this 5 year old on Lasix for contralateral UPJ.*

Chronic Diuretic Therapy

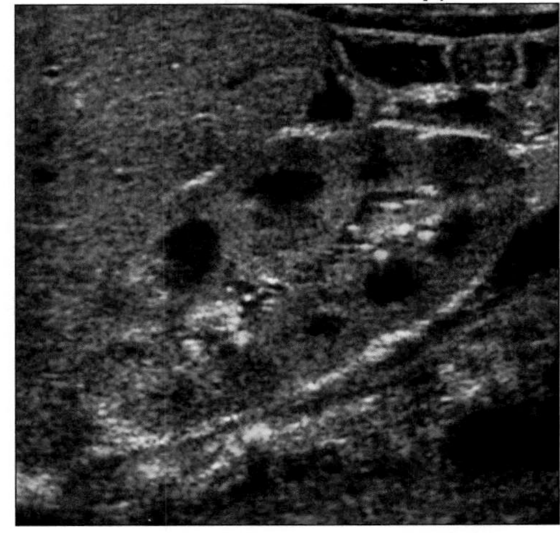

Chronic Diuretic Therapy

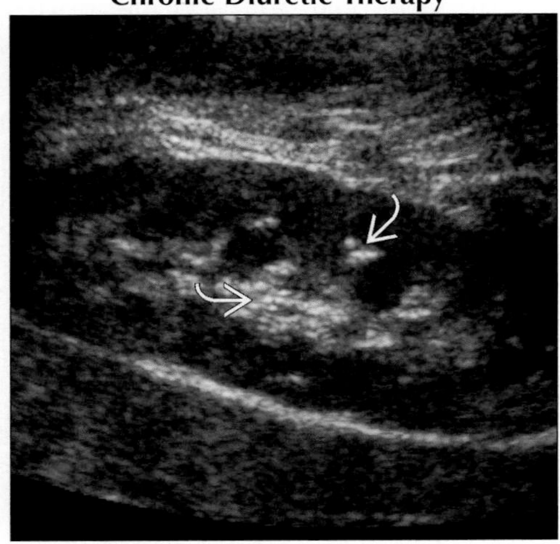

*(**Left**) Longitudinal ultrasound shows dense, echogenic, medullary pyramids ➔ in this 22-month-old child with medullary sponge kidney. There is posterior acoustic shadowing ➔, a finding not always observed with medullary nephrocalcinosis as the calcium particles may be small and dispersed. (**Right**) AP radiograph shows dense medullary calcifications ➔ in the right kidney of the same patient.*

Medullary Sponge Kidney

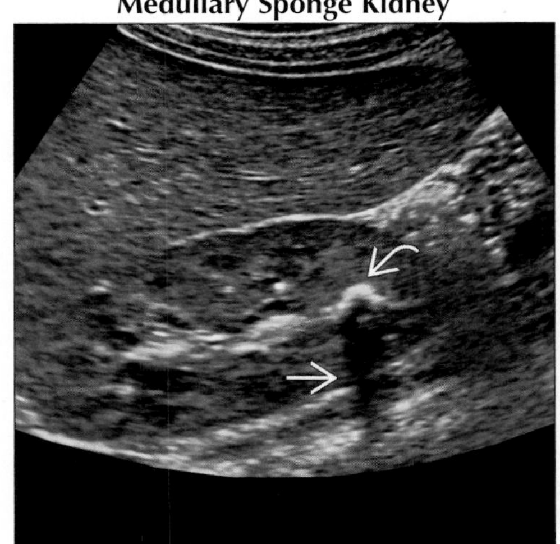

Medullary Sponge Kidney

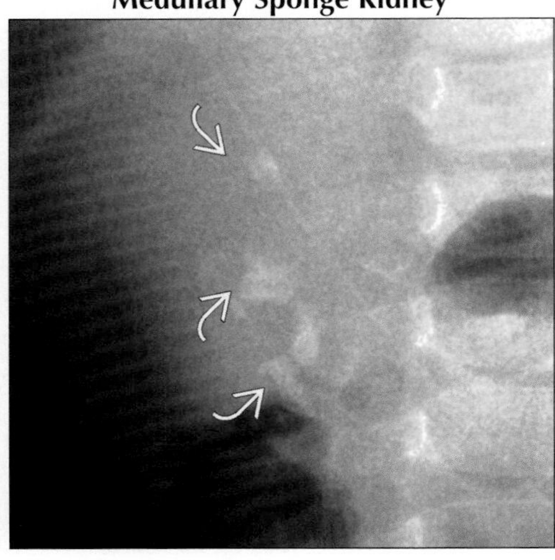

Tamm-Horsfall Proteins (Mimic)

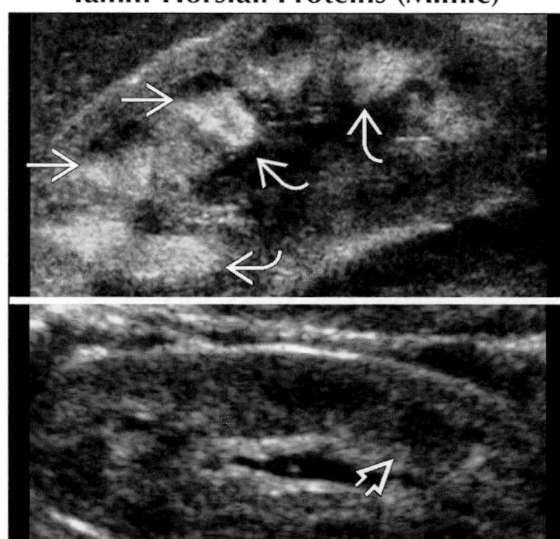

Infection/Infarction/Trauma

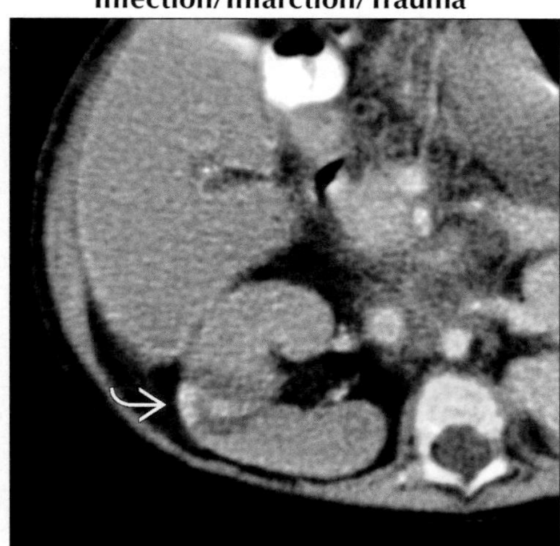

(Left) *Composite image shows softly layered, echogenic Tamm-Horsfall proteins ➡ in a 3-day-old infant with contralateral UPJ (top image). Note the debris levels ➡. Follow-up at 4 weeks of age (bottom image) demonstrates resolution and normal medullary pyramids ➡.* ***(Right)*** *Axial CECT shows a wedge-shaped area of cortical nephrocalcinosis ➡ in the right kidney. This is likely an infarct, given its distribution and the patient's complex medical history.*

Oxalosis/Hyperoxaluria

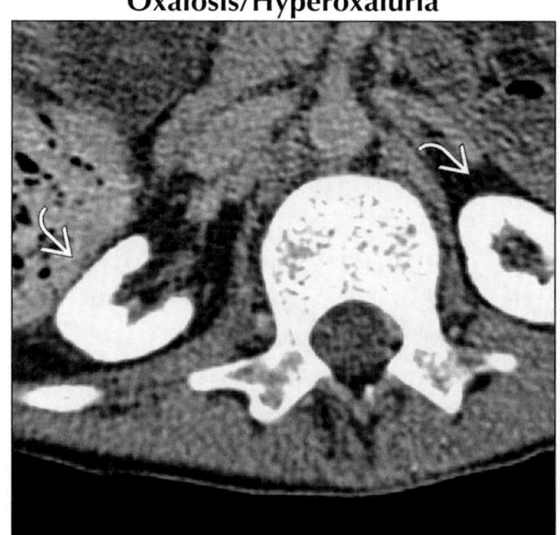

Wilms Tumor

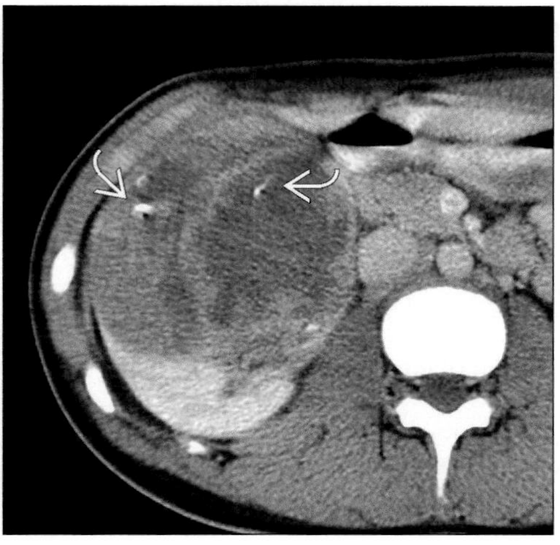

(Left) *Axial CECT shows dense corticomedullary calcifications ➡ symmetrically involving both kidneys in this 12 year old with primary oxalosis. The patient, who underwent a combined liver and kidney transplant, eventually died.* ***(Right)*** *Axial CECT shows a circumscribed, heterogeneous mass arising from the right kidney in this 17 year old who presented with an unusual sarcomatous variant of Wilms tumor. A few wispy and dystrophic calcifications ➡ are seen.*

Renal Cell Carcinoma

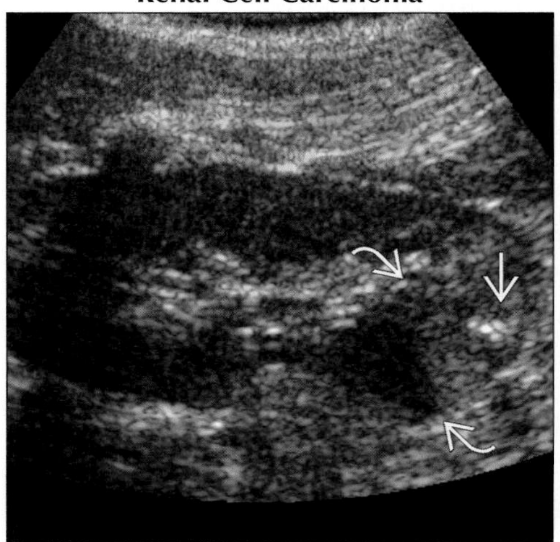

Renal Cell Carcinoma

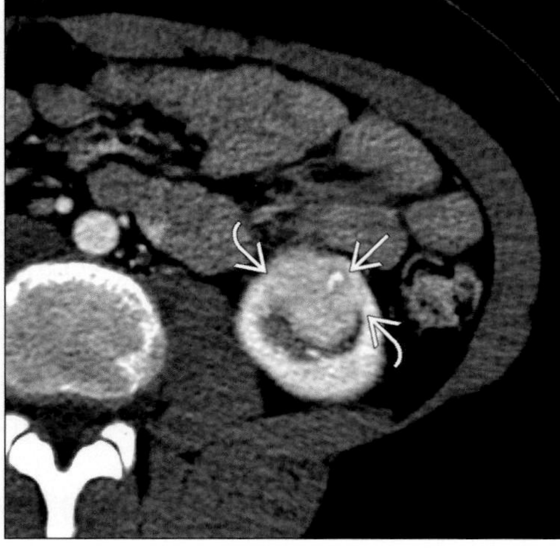

(Left) *Longitudinal ultrasound shows the incidental finding of an ill-defined mixed cystic and solid lesion ➡ with a focal area of dystrophic calcification ➡ in the inferior pole of the left kidney. This 17-year-old female presented with right-sided discomfort.* ***(Right)*** *Axial CECT shows the same heterogeneous lesion ➡. In the inferior aspect of the mass, the focal dystrophic calcification ➡ is again seen.*

PELVIS MASS

DIFFERENTIAL DIAGNOSIS

Common

- Ovarian Lesion, Nonneoplastic
  - Simple Cyst
  - Parovarian Cyst
  - Hemorrhagic Cyst
- Ovarian Lesion, Neoplastic
  - Germ Cell Tumors
  - Stromal Cell Tumors
  - Epithelial Cell Tumors
- Ovarian Torsion
- Duplication Cyst, GI Tract

Less Common

- Genitourinary Anomalies
  - Obstructed Urinary Bladder
  - Horseshoe Kidney
  - Cloaca
  - Hydrometrocolpos/Hematometrocolpos
- Lymphoma (Burkitt)
- Sacrococcygeal Teratoma
- Anterior Sacral Meningocele
- Neuroblastoma
- Desmoid
- Ewing Sarcoma
- Rhabdomyosarcoma, Genitourinary

ESSENTIAL INFORMATION

Key Differential Diagnosis Issues

- Gender and age of patient

Helpful Clues for Common Diagnoses

- **Ovarian Lesion, Nonneoplastic**
  - **Simple Cyst**
    - Anechoic, larger than 3-5 cm
    - If large, may cause torsion; occasionally large enough to extend into abdomen
  - **Parovarian Cyst**
    - Wolffian duct remnant; anechoic
    - Appearance/size will not change with time
  - **Hemorrhagic Cyst**
    - Appearance depends on chronicity
    - May be echogenic/solid, lacy/septated, or mixed with fluid-debris levels
- **Ovarian Lesion, Neoplastic**
  - **Germ Cell Tumors**
    - Various types: Teratoma, dysgerminoma, yolk sac tumor, embryonal cell carcinoma, choriocarcinoma
    - Most common teratoma features are
    - Mixed cystic, solid, calcified elements
    - Fat within lesion well seen on CT
    - Identifying teeth "clenches" diagnosis
    - May be bilateral
    - "Tip of iceberg" sign: Posterior acoustic shadows of teeth/bone/calcifications obscure full extent of mass
  - **Stromal Cell Tumors**
    - Granulosa cell tumor: Often solid; may cause sexual precocity
    - Leydig cell tumors: Cystic, solid, or mixed; often cause virilization
  - **Epithelial Cell Tumors**
    - e.g., cystadenoma, cystadenocarcinoma
    - Predominantly cystic appearance
    - Uncommon in children
- **Ovarian Torsion**
  - Marked asymmetry in ovarian volumes
  - Appearance varies with chronicity
    - Hypoechoic or heterogeneous
    - Peripheral follicles often seen
  - Presence of blood flow may reflect intermittent torsion or multiple vessels serving ovary
  - Underlying cyst or mass is common
- **Duplication Cyst, GI Tract**
  - Often round or tubular; may be multiple
  - Hypoechoic on US, low attenuation on CT
    - On US may see bowel wall layers (echogenic mucosa, serosa, intervening hypoechoic muscularis)

Helpful Clues for Less Common Diagnoses

- **Genitourinary Anomalies**
  - **Obstructed Urinary Bladder**
    - Must search for structural anomalies, i.e., posterior urethral valves, cloaca, spinal cord anomaly, obstructing mass
  - **Horseshoe Kidney**
    - May be partially obstructed or multicystic
    - Increased risk of infections, Wilms tumor, or injury (superficial location)
  - **Cloaca**
    - Large fluid-filled structure(s) often seen
    - Complex anatomic abnormalities associated with anorectal malformations, vaginal/uterine anomalies
    - Search for coexisting upper urinary tract anomalies or obstructive hydronephrosis
  - **Hydrometrocolpos/Hematometrocolpos**
    - Without cloacal anomaly

- More commonly seen in teenagers but occasionally seen in neonates
- Causes range from simple imperforate hymen to complex Müllerian duct anomalies
- Expect to see bulging structures filled with fluid, debris, &/or blood products

- **Lymphoma (Burkitt)**
  - Commonly involves abdominal/pelvic organs, especially distal bowel
  - Clinically causes obstruction or intussusception
  - Suggestive imaging findings
    - US: Hypoechoic, mildly heterogeneous
    - CT: Homogeneous, wall thickening, adenopathy
    - MR: Homogeneous, intermediate/bright signal
- **Sacrococcygeal Teratoma**
  - Heterogeneous, mixed cystic/solid mass
  - Calcifications common but not universal
  - Prognosis depends on prompt diagnosis; higher risk of malignancy after 2 months
    - Type 1 is extrapelvic
    - Type 2 is predominantly extrapelvic, small intrapelvic component
    - Type 3 is predominantly intrapelvic, small extrapelvic component
    - Type 4 is entirely intrapelvic, delayed diagnosis is therefore common
- **Anterior Sacral Meningocele**
  - Usually purely cystic in appearance
  - Few associated with Currarino triad
  - Other considerations: Neurofibromatosis, Marfan syndrome
- **Neuroblastoma**
  - Arises from neural crest cells in sympathetic chain ganglia or adrenal medulla
  - Poorly marginated, encases vessels
  - Typical CT/US/MR findings
    - Heterogeneous soft tissue mass with calcifications, necrosis, hemorrhage
    - Metastases typically to liver, skin (younger ages), and bones (older children)
- **Desmoid**
  - Benign tumor with well-marginated or infiltrating margins
  - CT and MR imaging characteristics depend upon histologic features, relative amounts of collagen, spindle cells
- **Ewing Sarcoma**
  - Pelvic origin not uncommon
  - Soft tissues: Large heterogeneous mass is commonly seen
  - Bone: May be lytic, sclerotic, or mixed, with periosteal reaction
- **Rhabdomyosarcoma, Genitourinary**
  - May arise from any pelvic structure: Bladder, vagina, uterus, or prostate
  - Polypoid appearance is typical but not universal
  - Hydronephrosis is common finding

Hemorrhagic Cyst

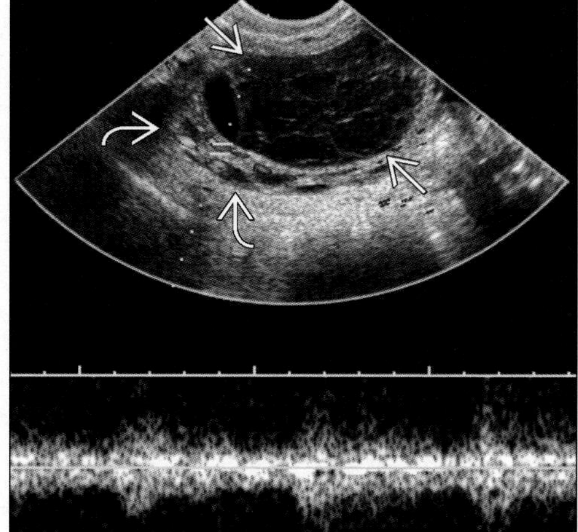

Longitudinal ultrasound shows a circumscribed, hypoechoic, septated, ovoid pelvic mass ➡. There is a crescent of normal ovarian tissue, seen with normal Doppler signal, stretched along its edge ➡.

Hemorrhagic Cyst

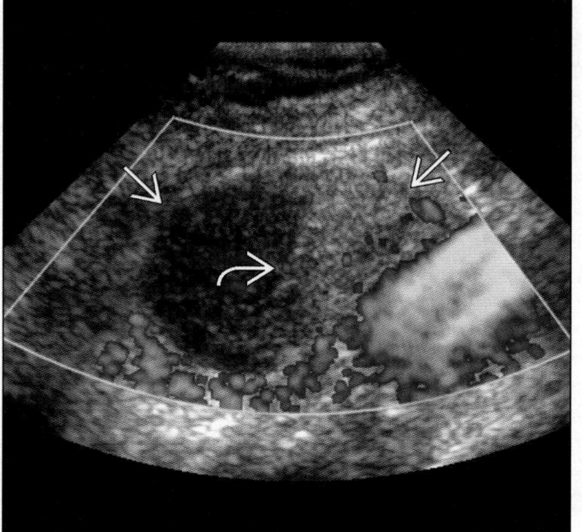

Longitudinal ultrasound shows a well-defined oval lesion ➡ with no blood flow (gain is turned up high). Note the fluid-debris level ➡. This hemorrhagic cyst involuted over time.

PELVIS MASS

(**Left**) *Axial CECT shows an ovoid pelvic lesion ➔ in the generally expected region of the left ovary. Note the classic components: Fluid-containing cyst ➔, low-attenuation fat ➔, and a tooth.* (**Right**) *Transverse ultrasound shows a round lesion ➔ posterior to the bladder ➔. The lesion is predominantly cystic with an ill-defined, linear, echogenic area that represents fat or hair ➔.*

Germ Cell Tumors

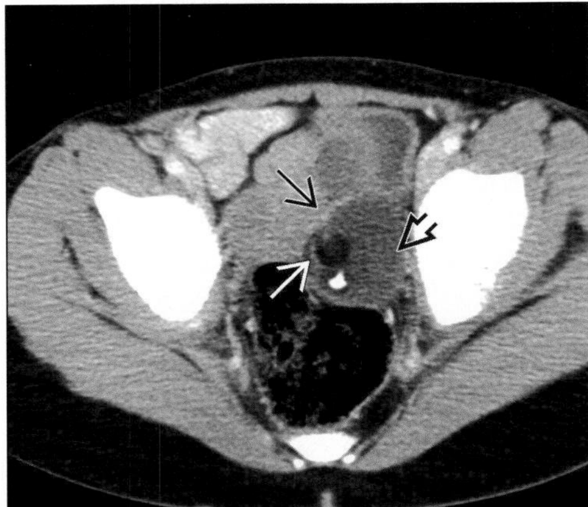

Germ Cell Tumors

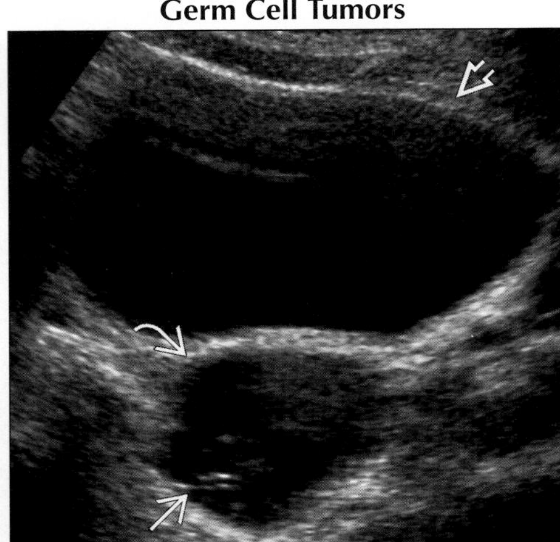

(**Left**) *Axial CECT shows a very large complex mass ➔ arising from the pelvis in this 3-year-old girl whose mother first palpated the abnormality. Low attenuation areas ➔ are pathologically proven cysts and areas of necrosis in this juvenile granulosa cell tumor.* (**Right**) *Axial CECT shows the chest of the same patient. There is abnormal breast development ➔, a clue to a hormonally active tumor.*

Germ Cell Tumors

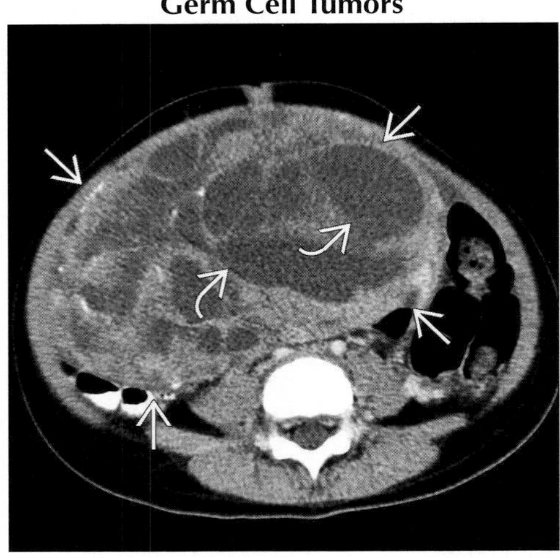

Germ Cell Tumors

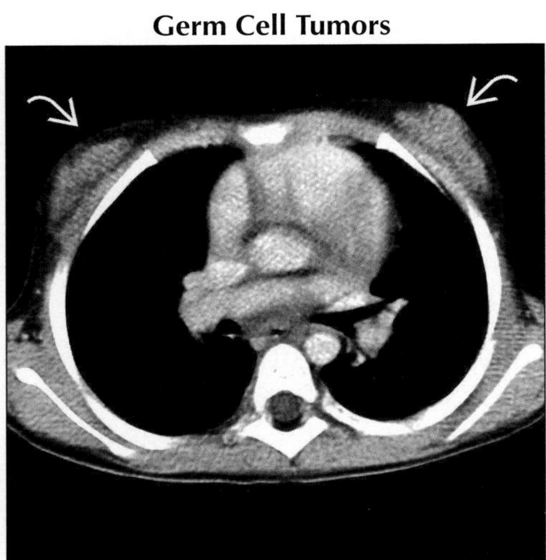

(**Left**) *Longitudinal ultrasound shows a large, heterogeneous, circumscribed lesion ➔ superior to the bladder. Note several peripheral follicles ➔. Only 1 (contralateral) ovary was seen, although not depicted here.* (**Right**) *Axial CECT shows a well-defined, oval, heterogeneous, soft tissue mass ➔ an unexpected finding in a patient with right lower quadrant pain. In retrospect, subtle low-attenuation peripheral follicles can be seen ➔.*

Ovarian Torsion

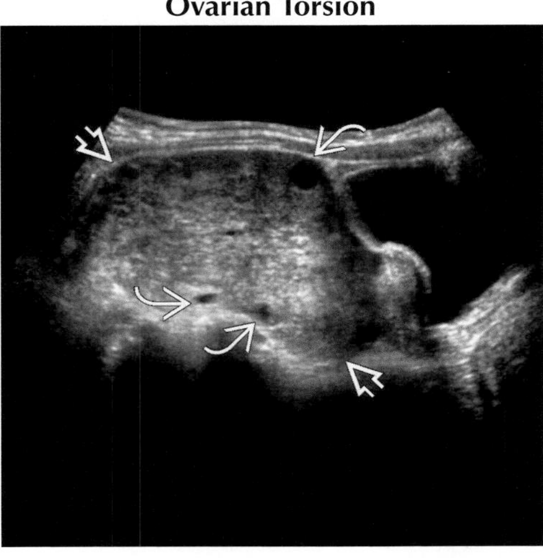

Ovarian Torsion

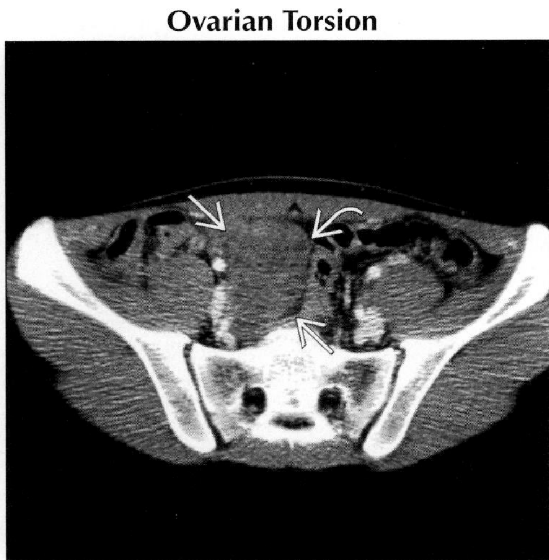

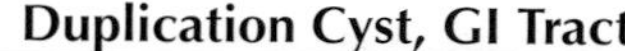

Duplication Cyst, GI Tract

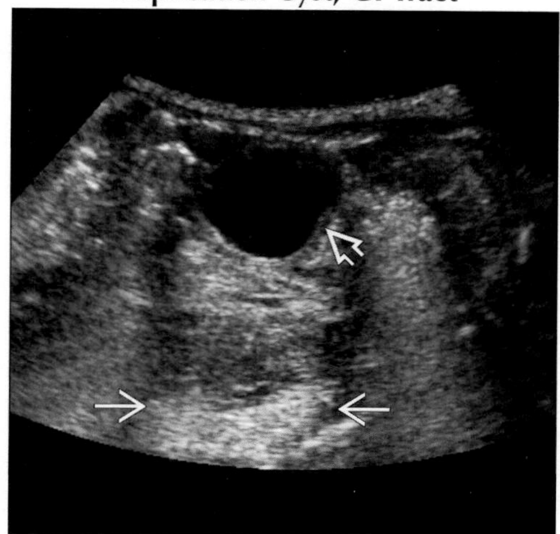

Obstructed Urinary Bladder

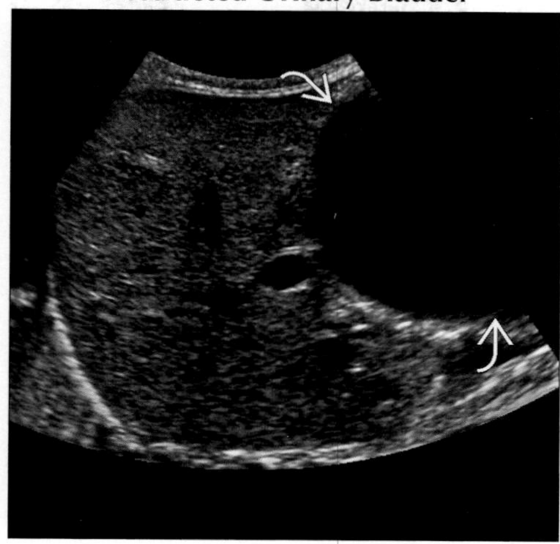

*(**Left**) Transverse ultrasound shows a cystic pelvic ➡ lesion. The bowel wall, though visible, lacks the "bowel wall signature." Brightened soft tissues of posterior increased through-transmission ➡ are typical of fluid-filled structures. This was an ileal duplication cyst. (**Right**) Longitudinal US shows a massively distended urinary bladder ➡ in an infant with a large soft tissue mass seen on a radiograph. Spinal cord abnormalities were also discovered.*

Horseshoe Kidney

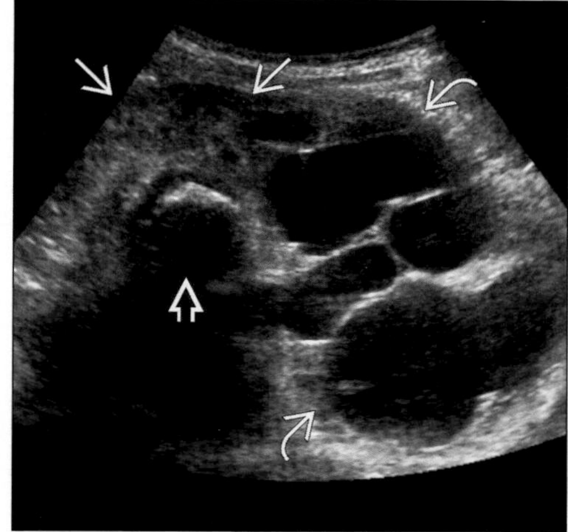

Cloaca

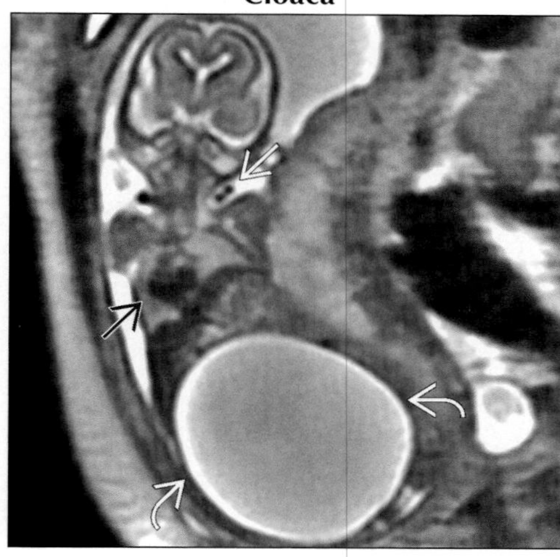

*(**Left**) Transverse ultrasound shows a pelvic horseshoe kidney with an enlarged obstructed left moiety ➡, which explains the "mass" incidentally noted on the radiograph of this 2 year old. Unobstructed renal parenchyma extends across midline ➡ anterior to the spine ➡. (**Right**) Coronal T2WI MR shows a 19-week fetus with a large, cystic cloaca ➡. Note the dextrocardia ➡ and a 2-vessel umbilical cord ➡. This child had all VACTERL manifestations.*

Hydrometrocolpos/Hematometrocolpos

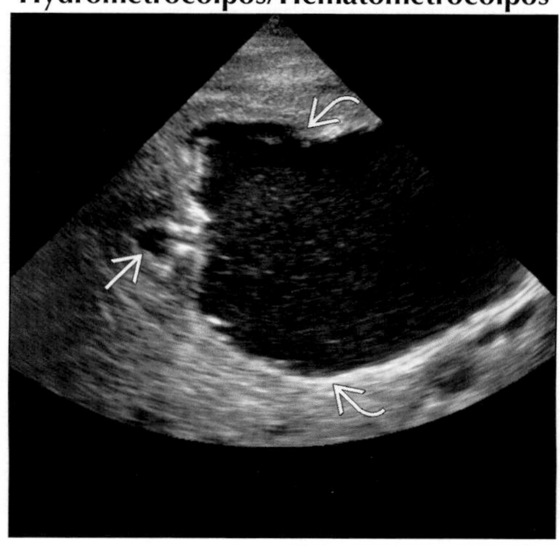

Hydrometrocolpos/Hematometrocolpos

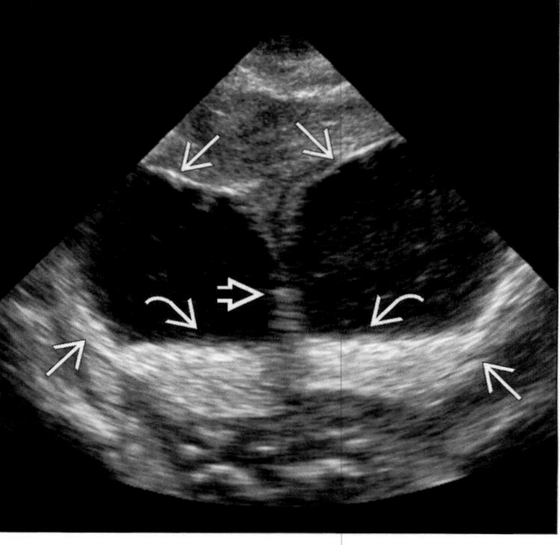

*(**Left**) Longitudinal ultrasound shows a large, midline, pelvic, fluid- and debris-filled lesion ➡ in this newborn with 2 hemivaginas, 2 uterine horns, and hydronephrosis. Note the small amount of fluid in the uterus ➡. (**Right**) Transverse ultrasound in the same supine patient shows the paired hemivaginas ➡ as massively distended tubular structures seen in cross-section, with apposed, adjacent walls ➡, and a fluid-debris level ➡ in each.*

PELVIS MASS

(**Left**) *Axial CECT shows a homogeneous soft tissue mass → deep in the pelvis in a patient who presented after 5 days of abdominal pain and distension. The mass displaces the bladder anteriorly →.* (**Right**) *Axial T2WI MR from the same patient shows a homogeneous soft tissue mass of Burkitt lymphoma → encircling the rectum → and causing high-grade partial obstruction. Note the urethra →.*

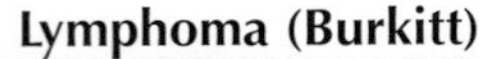

Lymphoma (Burkitt)

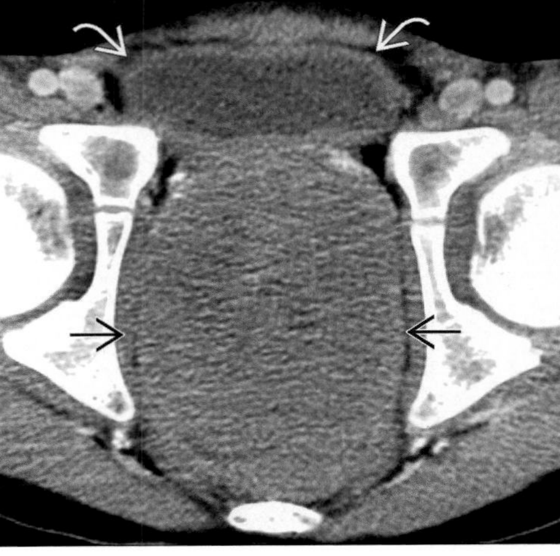

Lymphoma (Burkitt)

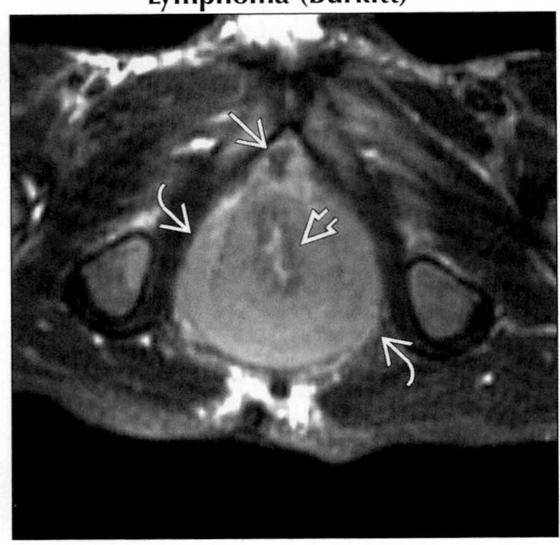

(**Left**) *Sagittal T2WI MR of a fetus demonstrates a very large, mixed cystic, solid lesion → with an extensive intrapelvic component, consistent with a type 3 sacrococcygeal teratoma. The bladder is compressed anteriorly →. There is also hydronephrosis →.* (**Right**) *Sagittal T2WI MR shows a lobular, high signal intensity mass encircling the coccyx →. The mass was discovered not by a physical exam but by a renal/bladder ultrasound after a urinary tract infection.*

Sacrococcygeal Teratoma

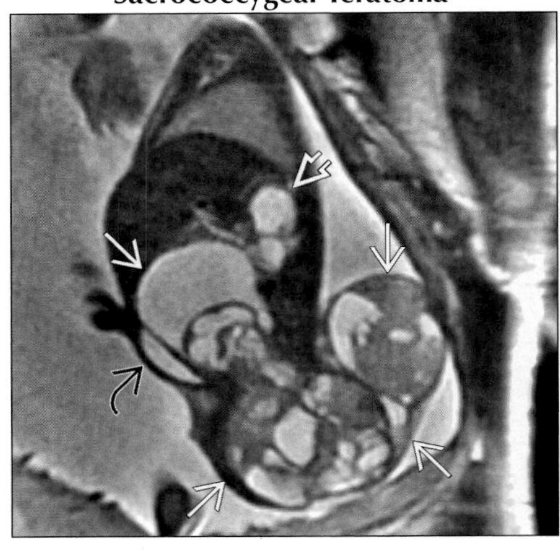

Sacrococcygeal Teratoma

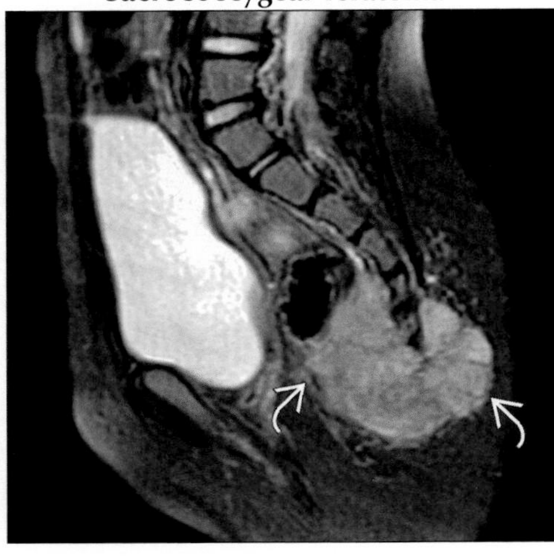

(**Left**) *Sagittal T2WI MR shows a lobular, cystic lesion → anterior and inferior to an abnormally truncated sacrum →. Note the tethered nerve roots clinging to the posterior spinal canal →.* (**Right**) *Frontal radiograph in the same patient shows an abnormally curved "scimitar" sacrum →. The 3 findings of a scimitar sacrum, any presacral mass and an anorectal malformation comprise Currarino triad.*

Anterior Sacral Meningocele

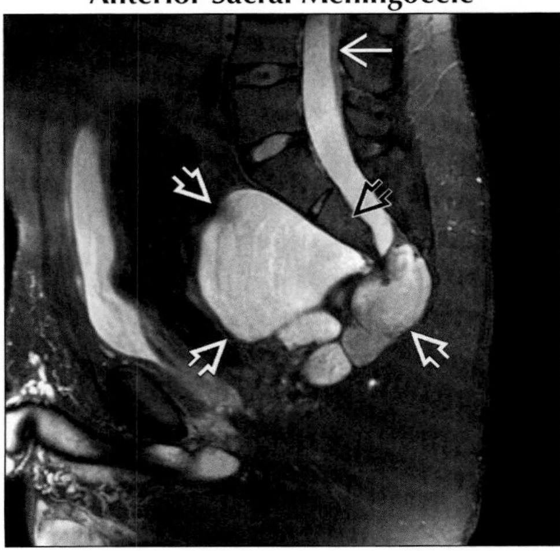

Anterior Sacral Meningocele

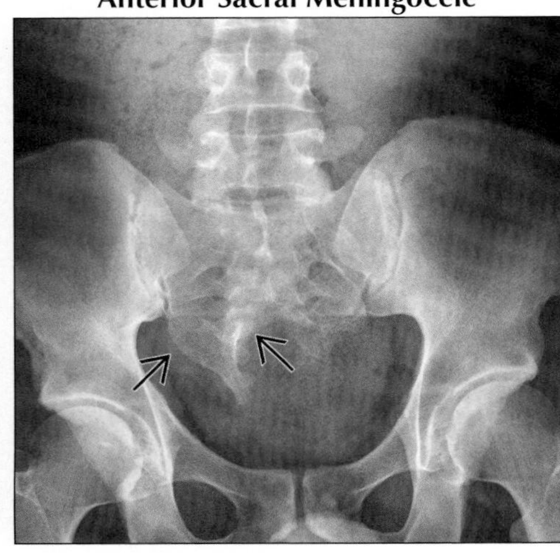

PELVIS MASS

Neuroblastoma

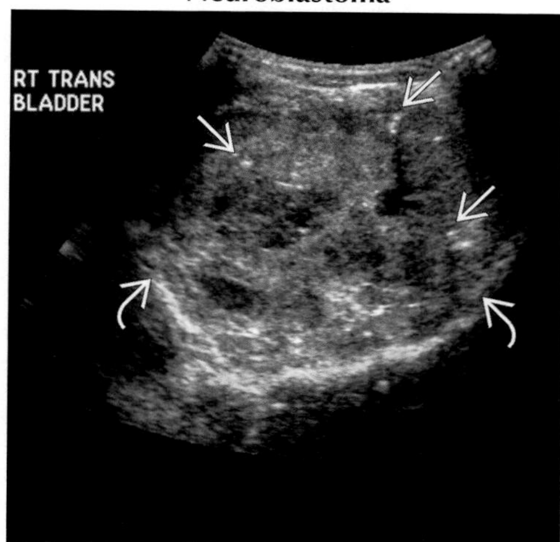

Neuroblastoma

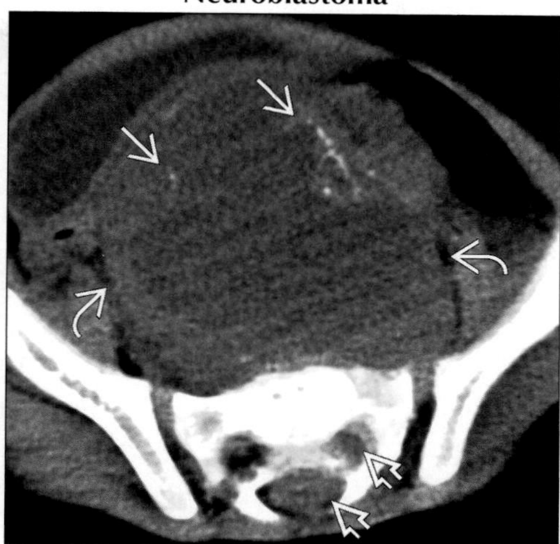

*(**Left**) Transverse ultrasound shows a heterogeneous pelvis mass ➔ with scattered flecks of calcification ➔, some with subtle posterior acoustic shadowing. This lesion was very low in the pelvis, a known but less common location for this entity. (**Right**) Axial CECT shows the same lesion ➔, though the mass now appears only mildly heterogeneous. Note the calcifications ➔ and extension into the sacral neural foramen and spinal canal ➔.*

Desmoid

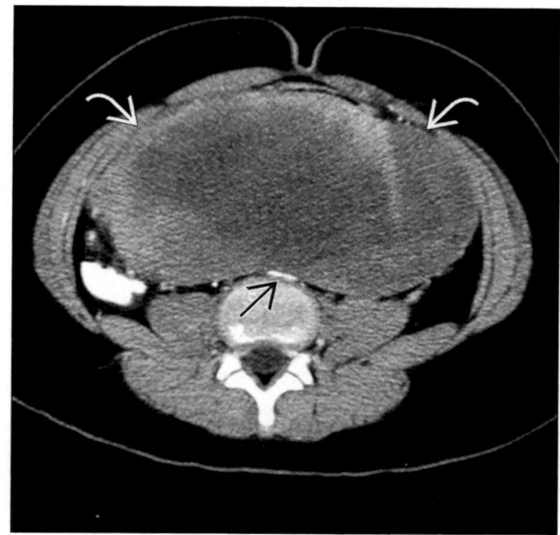

Ewing Sarcoma

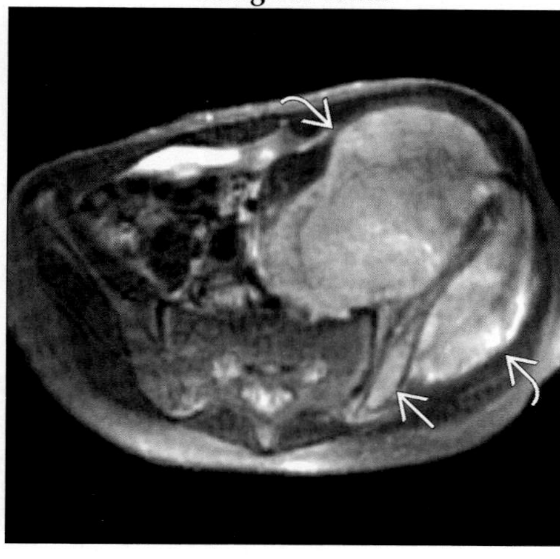

*(**Left**) Axial CECT shows a circumscribed, mildly heterogeneous, abdominopelvic mass ➔ in a 12 year old who presented with hypertension. Note the flattened aorta ➔. (**Right**) Axial T2WI MR shows a bulky high signal intensity lesion ➔ arising from the left iliac wing in this child with metastatic Ewing sarcoma, who initially presented with a 5-month history of intermittent hip pain. Note also the marrow signal abnormality of the iliac bone ➔.*

Rhabdomyosarcoma, Genitourinary

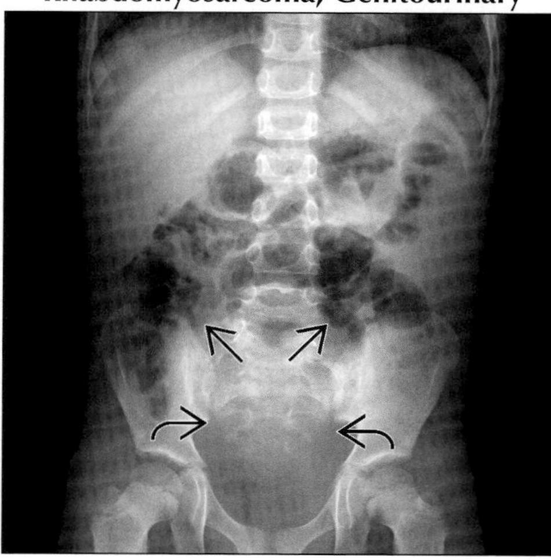

Rhabdomyosarcoma, Genitourinary

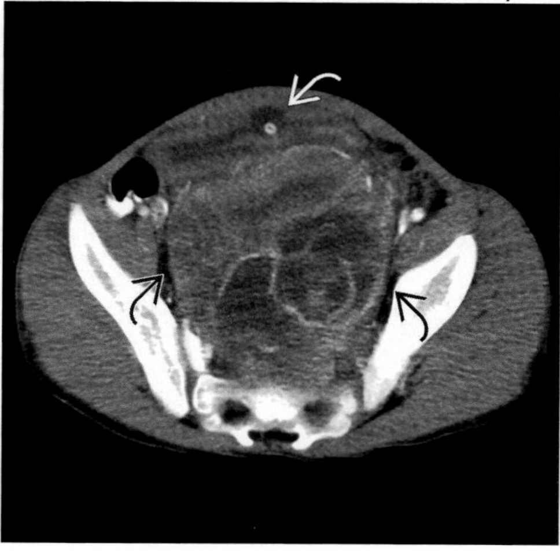

*(**Left**) AP radiograph shows symmetric pelvic soft tissue fullness ➔ in this patient who presented with constipation. There are no calcifications or bony destructive changes. Bowel loops are displaced superiorly ➔. (**Right**) Axial CECT shows the same lesion as a circumscribed, heterogeneous, pelvic mass ➔, now seen to emanate from the prostate. The urinary bladder is displaced superiorly and anteriorly. A Foley catheter ➔ is also visible.*

OVARIAN MASS

DIFFERENTIAL DIAGNOSIS

Common
- Functional Ovarian Cysts
- Hemorrhagic Cyst
- Endometrioma
- Ovarian Torsion
- Mature Teratoma
- Tuboovarian Abscess
- Polycystic Ovary Syndrome

Less Common
- Ectopic Pregnancy
- Dysgerminoma
- Yolk Sac Tumor
- Sertoli-Leydig Cell Tumor

Rare but Important
- Ovarian Fibroma
- Granulosa Cell Tumor, Juvenile

ESSENTIAL INFORMATION

Key Differential Diagnosis Issues
- Ovarian masses can be
  - Benign
  - Borderline (low malignant potential)
  - Malignant
- Benign
  - Functional cysts
  - Hemorrhagic cysts/endometriomas
  - Serous and mucinous cystadenomas
  - Mature teratomas
  - Fibromas
- Borderline (low malignant potential)
  - Serous tumors (65%)
  - Mucinous tumors (30%)
  - Endometrioid tumors
  - Clear cell, Brenner cell
  - Monodermal teratoma (struma ovarii, carcinoid, neural tumors)
  - Mixed neoplasms
- Malignant
  - Epithelial ovarian carcinoma
    - 70% of all ovarian tumors
    - Postmenopausal women
  - Germ cell tumors
    - 20% of all ovarian tumors
    - These cell types more common in adolescents/young adults
    - Dysgerminoma
    - Yolk sac/endodermal sinus
    - Embryonal carcinoma
    - Choriocarcinoma
    - Immature teratoma
    - Mixed
  - Sex cord stromal tumor, including
    - 8% of all ovarian tumors
    - Sertoli-Leydig cell
    - Granulosa theca cell
  - Metastatic spread to ovary
- Clues to malignancy on imaging
  - Persistent or growing mass
  - Solid tumors or mixed solid and cystic
  - Size > 8 cm
  - Local invasion
  - Peritoneal fluid
  - Nodular omentum (implants)
  - Adenopathy

Helpful Clues for Common Diagnoses
- **Functional Ovarian Cysts**
  - Most are "simple" cysts
  - Large cysts with diameter > 3 cm should be re-imaged
  - Physiologic cysts will involute in 6-8 weeks
- **Hemorrhagic Cyst**
  - Complex cysts containing debris ± echogenic free fluid
  - Should resolve with next menstrual cycle
- **Endometrioma**
  - Low-level, homogeneous echoes ("chocolate" cyst)
  - Endometriosis in childhood or adolescence associated with genital tract anomalies
- **Ovarian Torsion**
  - Excessive rotation of ovary, fallopian tube, or both
  - Causes ischemia and pain
  - Not typically associated with masses in pediatrics, unlike adult population
  - 1/2 of cases occur in premenarchal girls
  - ~ 10% occur neonatally
  - Ultrasound
    - Unilateral enlarged ovary; 5x volume highly predictive
    - Stromal edema: Peripheral follicles
    - Free pelvic fluid/blood
    - Areas of hemorrhage
    - Normal Doppler exam does not exclude torsion
  - Treatment: Urgent surgical detorsion, conservation of ovarian tissue
  - Salvage rates for ovarian torsion are much better than for testicular torsion

- Length of symptoms does not predict viability
- **Mature Teratoma**
  - Benign germ cell tumor
  - ~ 60% of ovarian neoplasms in women < 40 years old
  - Contains all 3 germ cell lines
  - Hair, fat, teeth, calcification seen on imaging
  - Cysts may contain oily, milky, or serous fluid
  - Generally have well-defined capsule
  - Bilateral in up to 15%
- **Tuboovarian Abscess**
  - Fever, cervical tenderness, vaginal discharge
  - Ultrasound shows inflammation and ill-defined structures
  - Focal fluid/pus collections in tubes and adnexal spaces with thick hyperemic rim
  - Generally treated medically, not surgically
- **Polycystic Ovary Syndrome**
  - Ovarian dysfunction, hyperandrogenism, polycystic ovary
  - ≥ 12 follicles per ovary
  - Ovarian volume > 10 mL

Helpful Clues for Less Common Diagnoses

- **Ectopic Pregnancy**
  - Check quantitative β-hCG level
  - Decidual reaction in uterus with no intrauterine gestational sac
  - Enlarged, hyperemic adnexa
  - Gestational sac may be visible in adnexa
    - Usually on same side as corpus luteum
  - Occasionally implant distant from uterus
- **Dysgerminoma**
  - ~ 50% of all germ cell tumors
  - 5% secrete β-hCG
  - Similar to male seminoma
  - Masses tend to be large and heterogeneous
  - 15% recur but are re-treated with good prognosis
- **Yolk Sac Tumor**
  - a.k.a. endodermal sinus tumor
  - ~ 25% of all germ cell tumors
  - May secrete α-fetoprotein
  - Poor prognosis without adjuvant chemotherapy
    - 5-20% survival with surgery alone
- **Sertoli-Leydig Cell Tumor**
  - Sex cord stromal tumor
  - ~ 75% occur in women < 40 years old
  - May cause virilization
  - Heterosexual precocious puberty
  - Recurrence and malignant behavior seen with poorly differentiated subtypes

Helpful Clues for Rare Diagnoses

- **Ovarian Fibroma**
  - ~ 4% of all ovarian tumors
  - Meigs syndrome with ascites and pleural effusions
- **Granulosa Cell Tumor, Juvenile**
  - ~ 2% of all ovarian tumors
  - < 5% of these are juvenile type
  - Often secrete estrogen

Functional Ovarian Cysts

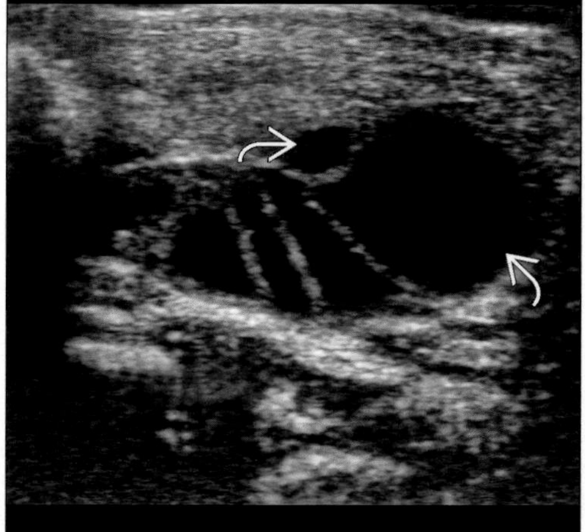

Longitudinal harmonic ultrasound shows several, small, functional, physiologic cysts ➔ in a newborn girl. Ovarian cysts are common in newborns due to the influence of maternal hormones.

Functional Ovarian Cysts

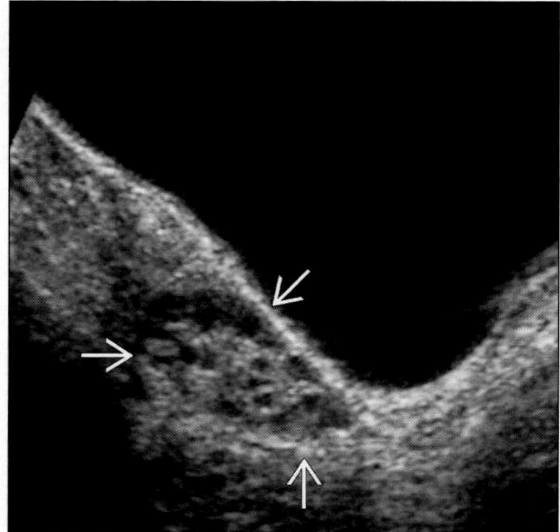

Longitudinal harmonic ultrasound shows several, small ovarian (< 1 cm diameter) follicles ➔ in a postpubertal girl.

OVARIAN MASS

(**Left**) *Transvaginal ultrasound shows a complex, cystic, septated lesion in the left ovary. Note the crescent of normal-appearing ovarian tissue ➔ along the deep margin of the lesion.* (**Right**) *Transvaginal ultrasound shows abundant color Doppler flow around the lesion but no significant flow within the lesion. Differential considerations include hemorrhagic cyst, endometrioma, and less likely, tuboovarian abscess (no inflammatory changes or free fluid seen).*

Hemorrhagic Cyst

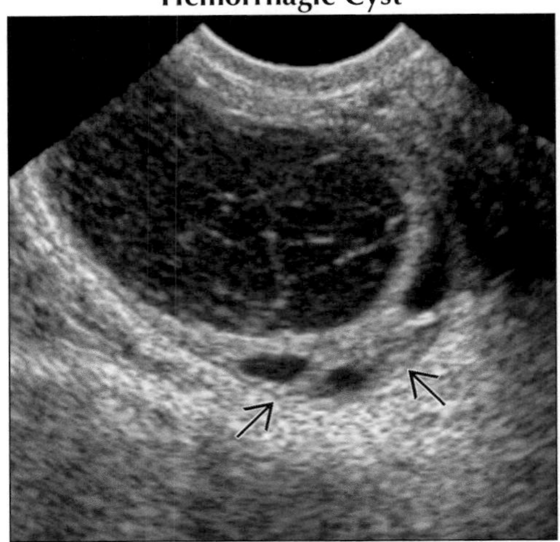

Hemorrhagic Cyst

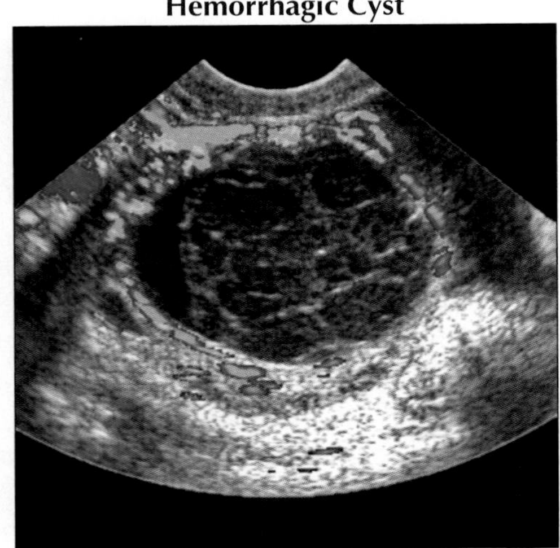

(**Left**) *Transverse transabdominal ultrasound shows the width of the uterus (calipers) and a heterogeneous soft tissue mass ➔ posterior to the uterus with small peripheral cysts.* (**Right**) *Transverse transabdominal ultrasound shows color Doppler flow to the uterus and broad ligaments but absent flow in the mass. The left ovary was normal; a normal right ovary could not be found. The mass was 5x the volume of the normal ovary in this patient with ovarian torsion.*

Ovarian Torsion

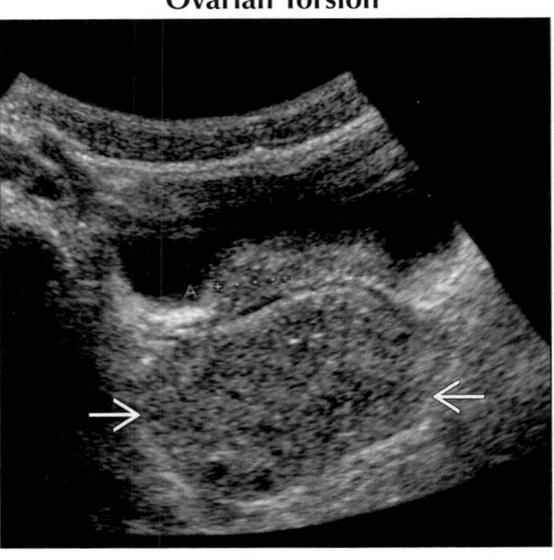

Ovarian Torsion

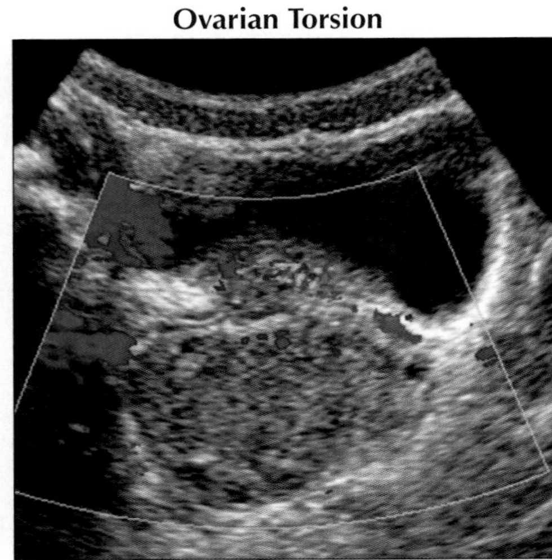

(**Left**) *Axial NECT performed for suspected urolithiasis shows an ovoid mass containing fat ➔ in the left adnexal region.* (**Right**) *Axial NECT shows a punctate calcification ➔ on the next caudal image, consistent with a mature teratoma or dermoid tumor. This benign tumor is an incidental finding in this case, though dermoids can predispose to ovarian torsion.*

Mature Teratoma

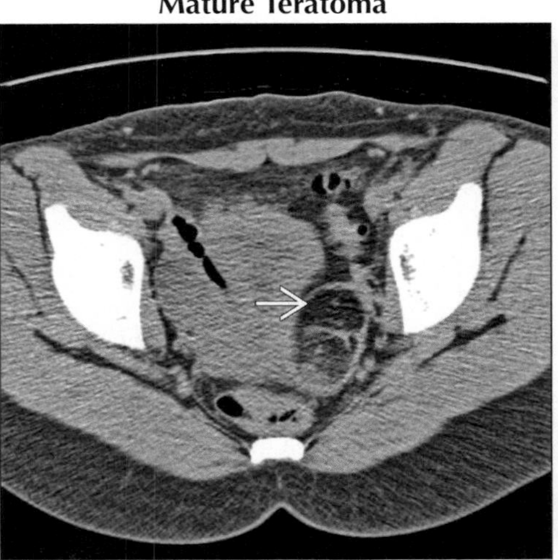

Mature Teratoma

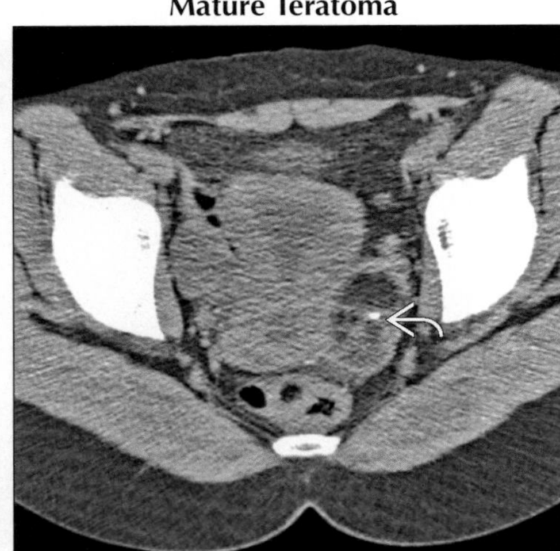

Tuboovarian Abscess

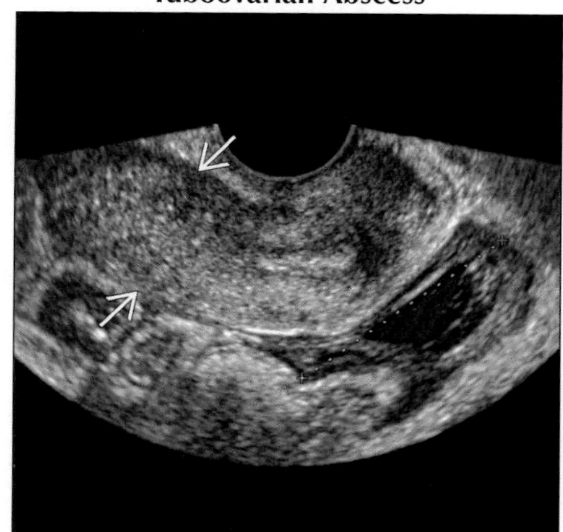

Tuboovarian Abscess

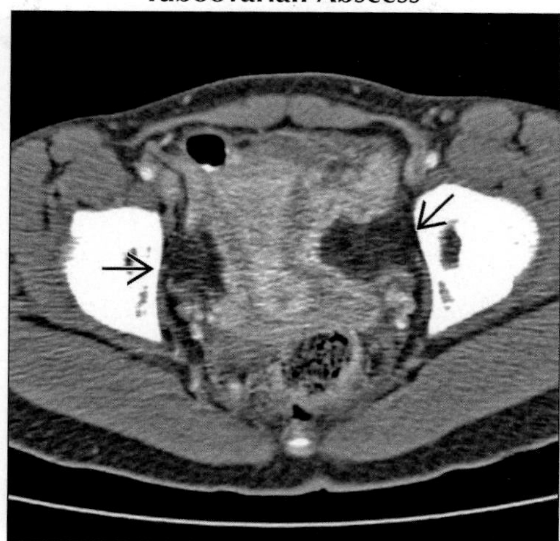

*(**Left**) Transvaginal ultrasound shows a poorly defined area of mixed echogenicity and some swirling debris (calipers) on real-time scanning. Uterine fundus ➔ is seen in this 17-year-old girl with pelvic pain, vaginal discharge, and tenderness on exam. (**Right**) Axial CECT to evaluate the appendix shows inflammatory changes throughout the pelvis with enhancement of the parametrial structures and fluid collections ➔ or cysts in both adnexal regions.*

Polycystic Ovary Syndrome

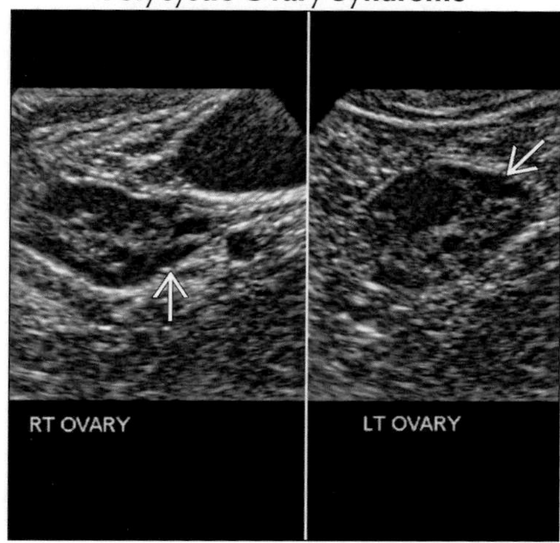

Polycystic Ovary Syndrome

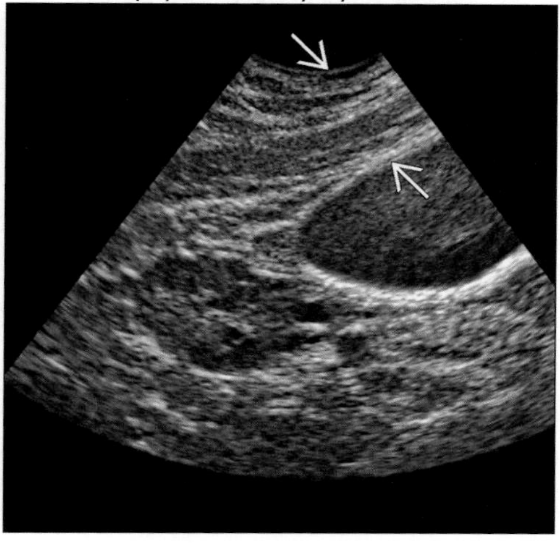

*(**Left**) Longitudinal harmonic ultrasound shows more than 12 follicles ➔ in each ovary in this teenager with irregular menses, weight gain, and acne. The ovarian volumes were greater than 10 mL. (**Right**) Longitudinal harmonic ultrasound shows another view of the right ovary and illustrates the prominence of the subcutaneous fat ➔ anterior to the bladder in this overweight girl with polycystic ovarian syndrome.*

Ectopic Pregnancy

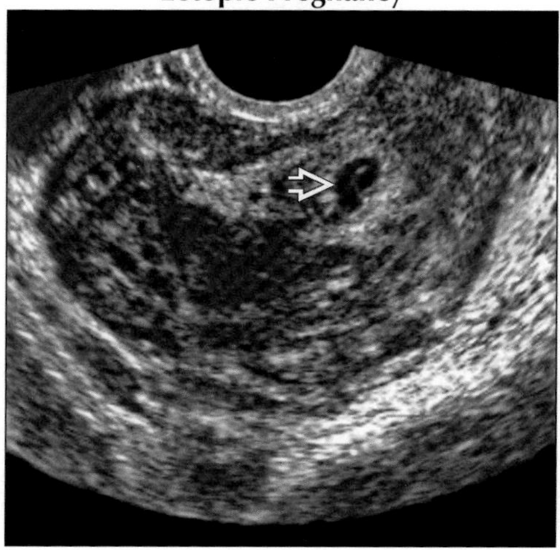

Ectopic Pregnancy

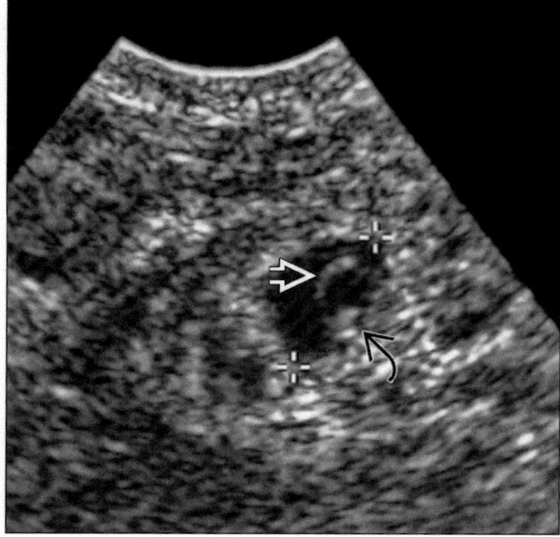

*(**Left**) Transvaginal ultrasound shows an enlarged and heterogeneous right adnexa containing a small cyst ➔ (GEST SAC) in this teenager with vaginal bleeding, pelvic pain, and a fainting episode. (**Right**) Transvaginal ultrasound at higher magnification shows the gestational sac (calipers). A tiny fetal pole ➔ and yolk sac ➔ are visible within the gestational sac in this case of right adnexal ectopic pregnancy.*

OVARIAN MASS

(***Left***) *AP radiograph shows mass effect in the pelvis displacing the bowel superiorly in this 12 year old with periumbilical pain and a palpable mass.* (***Right***) *Axial CECT shows a very large mass with some cystic areas* ↷ *and patchy contrast enhancement* ➭ *rising out of the pelvis. Only 1 ovary could be identified on CT and US scans, which helped to determine the organ of origin of this large ovarian tumor.*

Dysgerminoma

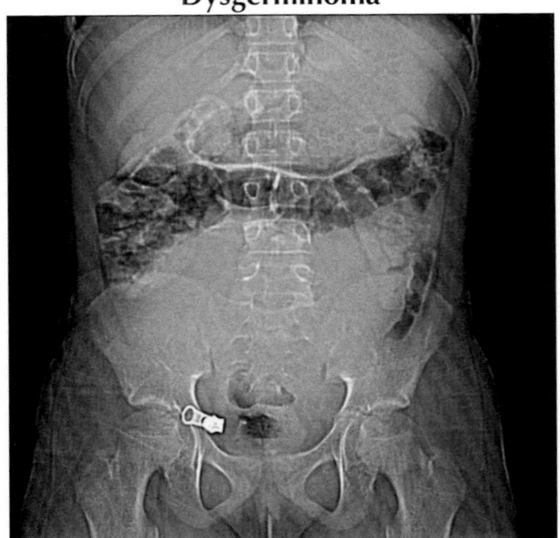

Dysgerminoma

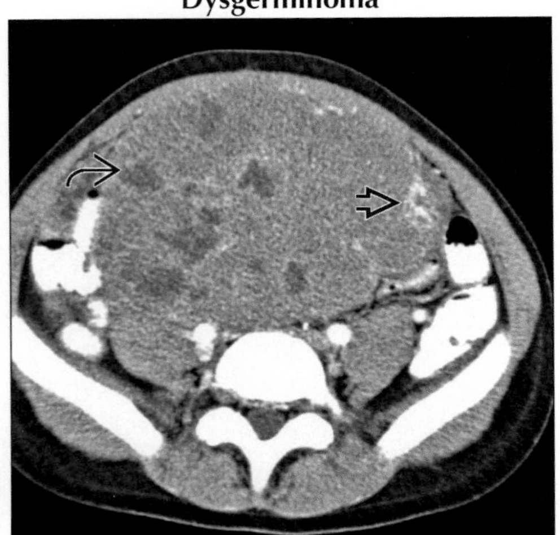

(***Left***) *Spatial compounding ultrasound with extended field of view was needed to show the extent of another large mass arising in the pelvis in a 14-year-old girl. The mass practically fills the abdomen, extending from bladder to liver margin.* (***Right***) *Color Doppler ultrasound in the same patient shows the heterogeneous, partially cystic* ➭ *tumor. Ovary/tumor, fallopian tube, and omentum were resected in this stage II malignant germ cell tumor.*

Yolk Sac Tumor

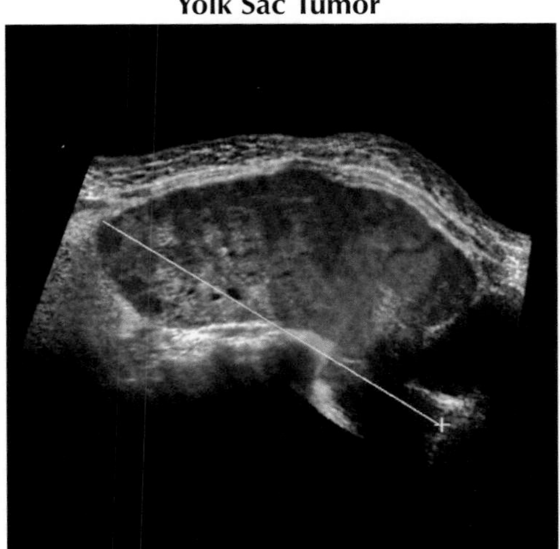

Yolk Sac Tumor

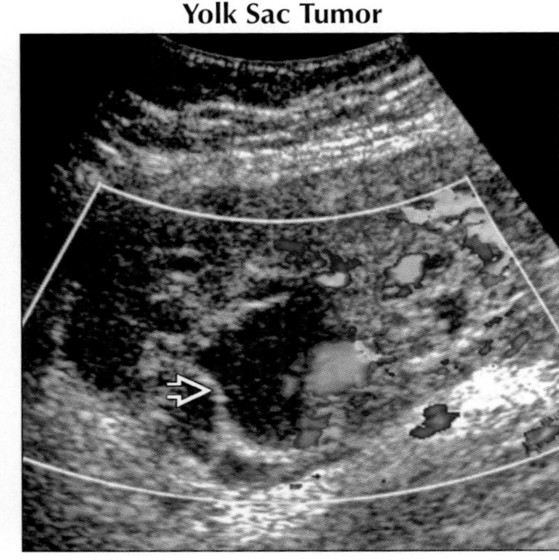

(***Left***) *Longitudinal harmonic ultrasound shows another, very large, heterogeneous mass* ➭ *extending up from the pelvis in front of the right kidney in this 9 year old with vomiting and a palpable mass.* (***Right***) *Coronal reformat CECT in the same patient shows linear areas of enhancement* → *in the large mass and a relatively well-defined capsule. This patient had a right salpingo-oophorectomy and received chemotherapy with good response.*

Sertoli-Leydig Cell Tumor

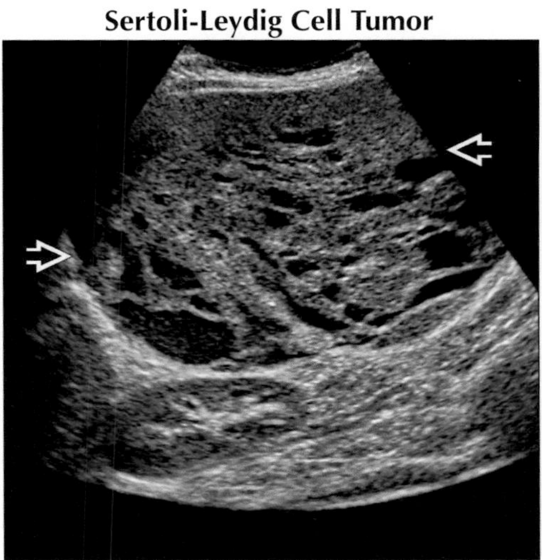

Sertoli-Leydig Cell Tumor

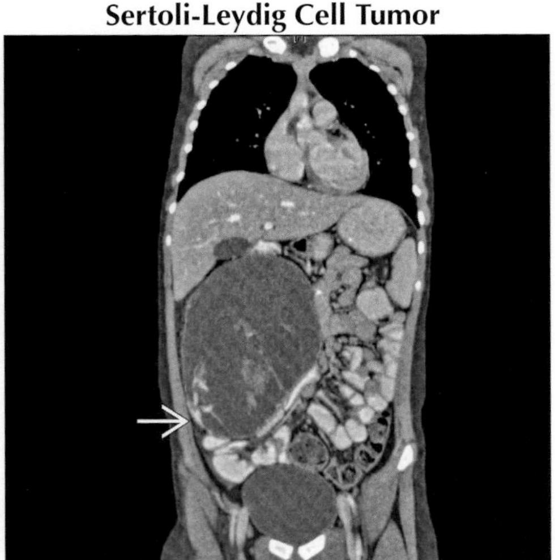

Sertoli-Leydig Cell Tumor

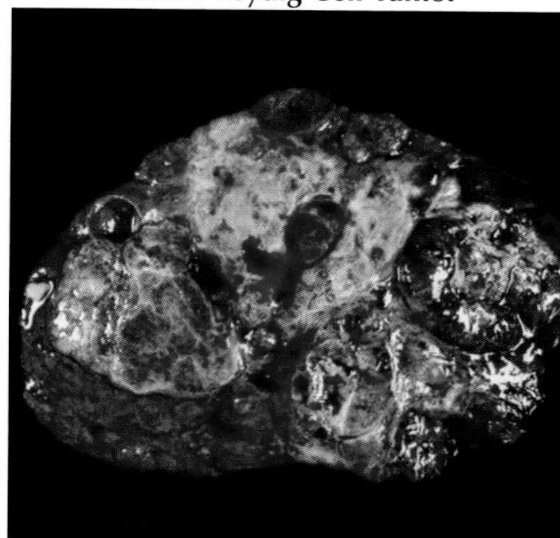

Ovarian Fibroma

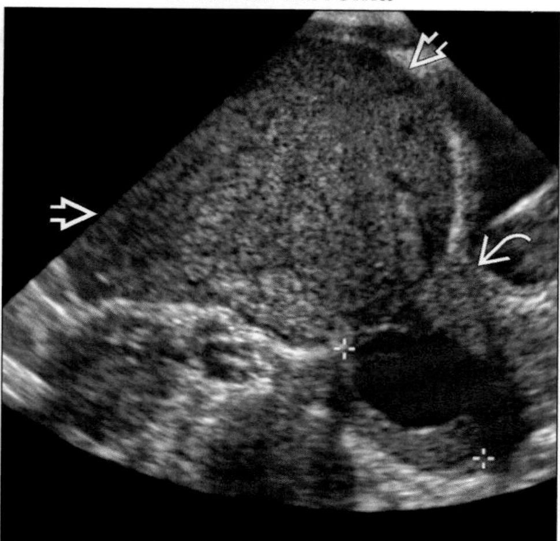

*(**Left**) Gross pathology, section from the same patient shows the resected, large, heterogeneous tumor. There is no recognizable ovarian tissue remaining on the gross examination. (**Right**) Longitudinal transabdominal ultrasound shows the left ovary (calipers), which is located deep to a solid, soft tissue, palpable mass ➡ just above the bladder. The uterus ➡ is partially seen between the bladder and left ovary.*

Ovarian Fibroma

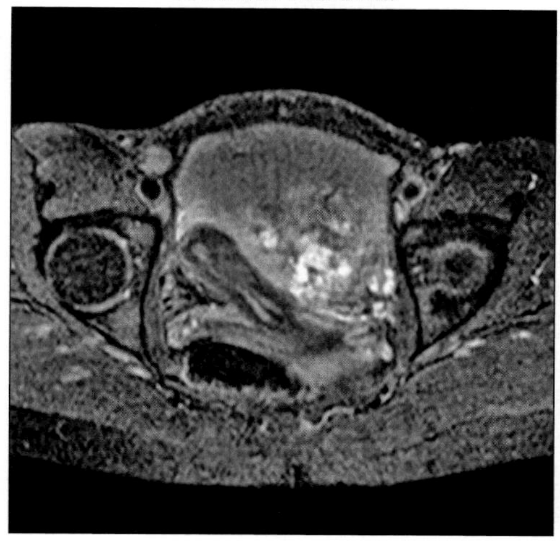

Granulosa Cell Tumor, Juvenile

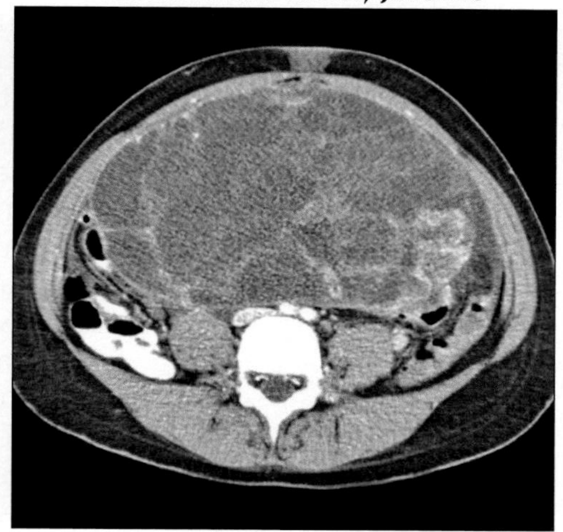

*(**Left**) Axial T2WI FS MR shows mixed, high signal intensity in the mass, which abuts the uterus but does not appear to invade the myometrium. Only 1 ovary was identified on imaging, helping to confirm the ovarian origin of the mass. (**Right**) Axial CECT shows a large mass at the level of the umbilicus and extending out of the pelvis in this 12-year-old girl. The mass enhances heterogeneously and has some cystic areas.*

Granulosa Cell Tumor, Juvenile

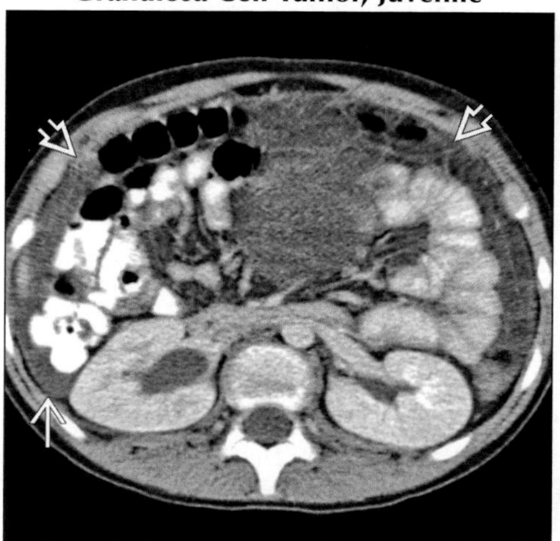

Granulosa Cell Tumor, Juvenile

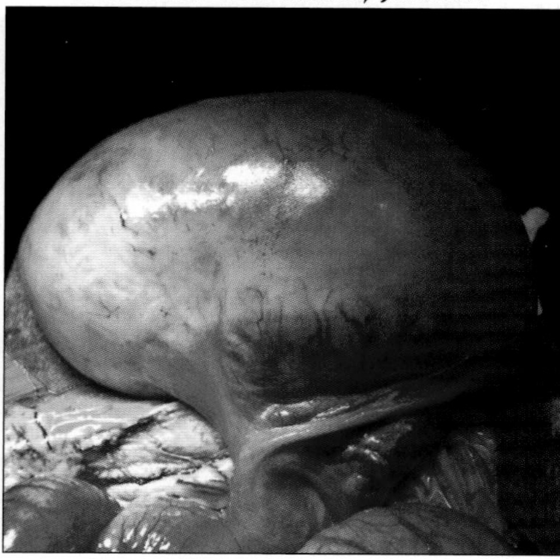

*(**Left**) Axial CECT shows a small amount of ascites in the paracolic gutters ➡, nodular thickening of the omentum ➡, and mild right side pelviectasis due to mass effect. (**Right**) Intra-operative photograph shows the massive tumor, weighing 1200 grams, that was surgically incised. The tumor was adherent to the omentum, but histology showed no extraovarian spread. The patient was treated with chemotherapy and was disease free 5 years later.*

SCROTAL MASS

DIFFERENTIAL DIAGNOSIS

Common
- Inguinal-Scrotal Hernia
- Epididymoorchitis
- Hydrocele
- Varicocele
- Testicular Torsion
- Torsion of Testicular Appendage
- Testicular Rupture/Hematoma

Less Common
- Spermatocele/Epididymal Cyst
- Pyocele
- Tubular Ectasia
- Testicular Tumors

Rare but Important
- Meconium Peritonitis
- Scrotal Pneumatosis
- Henoch-Schönlein Purpura

ESSENTIAL INFORMATION

Key Differential Diagnosis Issues
- Begin by determining structural origin of scrotal mass
  - Testicle
  - Epididymis
  - Tunica, surrounding testicle
  - Spermatic cord
  - Fat and connective tissues
- Next, determine if mass is
  - Soft tissue
  - Cystic or fluid
  - Vascular
  - Peristalsing
  - Or mixture of these
- Finally, confirm normal blood flow in testicle
  - Testicular ischemia can be complication of many scrotal masses

Helpful Clues for Common Diagnoses
- **Inguinal-Scrotal Hernia**
  - Typically heterogeneous, mixed soft tissue mass
  - Look for hernia neck pointing to inguinal canal or frank communication with peritoneal cavity
  - Peristalsis may be diminished/absent when incarcerated
  - Testicle is usually displaced to bottom of scrotal sac
- **Epididymoorchitis**
  - Enlarged, hypoechoic epididymis
  - May show increased echoes if there is hemorrhage
  - Marked hyperemia on Doppler
  - Associated hydrocele common
- **Hydrocele**
  - Fluid within tunica
  - Surrounds testicle
  - Should not displace or compress testicle
  - Debris present with infection or trauma
  - Very common in baby boys
- **Varicocele**
  - Dilated veins of pampiniform plexus
  - Left side > > right
  - Idiopathic type: Due to incompetent valves in internal spermatic vein
  - Secondary type: Due to increased pressure on draining veins
  - Most common correctable cause of male infertility
  - Varicoceles increase in size during Valsalva
- **Testicular Torsion**
  - Twisting of testis and spermatic cord in scrotum
  - Spontaneous or traumatic
  - Results in ischemia/venous congestion
  - Surgical emergency
  - Testicular salvage rate drops with symptom duration
  - Doppler hypoperfusion is key to diagnosis
  - Always compare to asymptomatic side
  - Spontaneous detorsion, may appear hyperemic
- **Torsion of Testicular Appendage**
  - Twisting of testicular or epididymal remnant
  - Hypoechoic mass adjacent to testis OR
  - Hyperechoic mass between testis and epididymis
  - Absent Doppler flow in mass with surrounding hyperemia
  - Associated hydrocele common
  - Typically less painful than testicular torsion
- **Testicular Rupture/Hematoma**
  - Variable appearance depending on severity and acuity

- Hematoma initially appears as echogenic avascular mass
- Subsequently liquifies and contracts
- Search testicular capsule for any breaks
- Confirm testicular perfusion
- Ruptured testicle is surgical emergency
  - Salvage rate drops with symptom duration
- Extratesticular hematoma treated nonsurgically

Helpful Clues for Less Common Diagnoses

- **Spermatocele/Epididymal Cyst**
  - Both result from dilated epididymal tubule
  - Spermatoceles
    - Contain spermatozoa and sediment
    - Most often in epididymal head
  - Epididymal cysts
    - Contain clear serous fluid
    - Found anywhere in epididymis
- **Pyocele**
  - Infected collection
    - May be complication of prior trauma, surgery, bacteremia
  - Loculations and debris characteristic
- **Tubular Ectasia**
  - Dilation of rete testis
  - Variably sized cysts or tubules
  - Radiate from mediastinum testis
  - No flow on Doppler
- **Testicular Tumors**
  - Only 1-2% of all pediatric tumors
  - Bimodal age peaks
    - < 2 years old and young adults
  - Germ cell variety (60-77%)
    - Teratomas: Benign in pediatric patients (malignant in adults)
    - Yolk sac tumors: Elevated α-fetoprotein
    - Mixed: Variable behavior
  - Seminomas: Rare in children
  - Sertoli cell and Leydig cell tumors
    - Hormonally active: Gynecomastia, precocious puberty
  - Juvenile granulosa cell tumors
    - 27% of all neonatal testicular tumors, benign
  - Gonadoblastoma: Intersex disorders
  - Leukemia/lymphoma secondary involvement, bilateral
  - Cystic dysplasia: Benign, associated ipsilateral renal agenesis/dysplasia
  - Extratesticular rhabdomyosarcoma
    - Highly aggressive malignancy
    - 70% retroperitoneal nodal spread at diagnosis

Helpful Clues for Rare Diagnoses

- **Meconium Peritonitis**
  - Extension into scrotum from peritoneum
  - Calcification common
- **Scrotal Pneumatosis**
  - Extension from peritoneum or perineum
  - Benign or infectious varieties
- **Henoch-Schönlein Purpura**
  - Marked swelling and hyperemia of peritesticular soft tissues
  - Usually bilateral
  - Testicles are normal

Inguinal-Scrotal Hernia

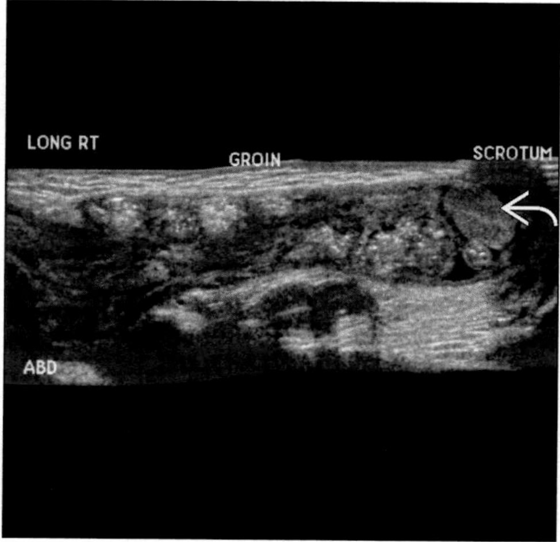

Longitudinal ultrasound with extended field of view shows bowel and fat extending through the inguinal canal into the scrotum in this child with scrotal fullness. The testicle ➡ is displaced inferiorly.

Inguinal-Scrotal Hernia

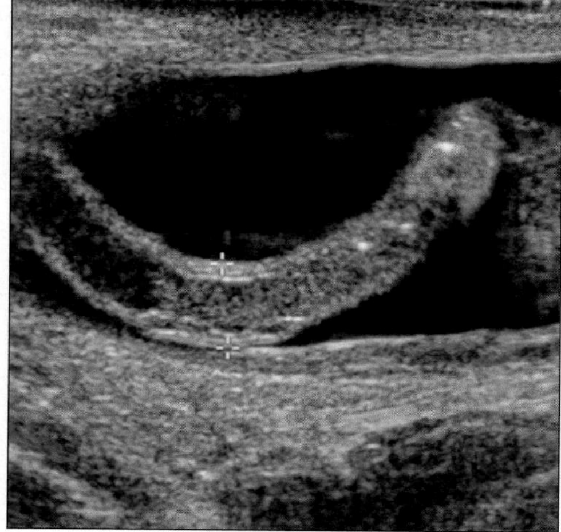

Transverse ultrasound shows the tubular appendix (calipers) extending into the right scrotal sac surrounded by fluid in this 2-month-old boy with scrotal swelling and pain.

SCROTAL MASS

Epididymoorchitis

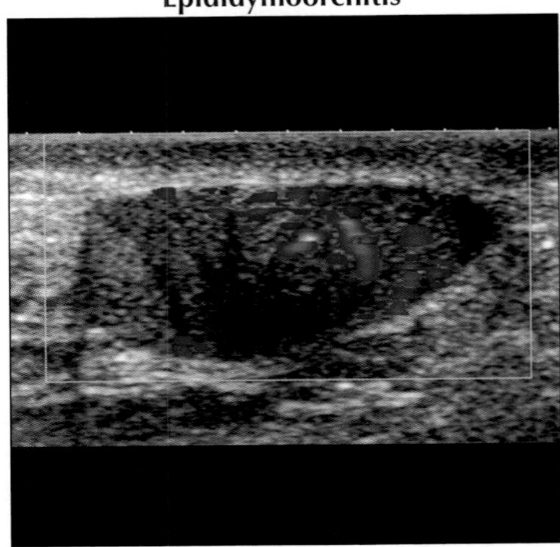

Epididymoorchitis

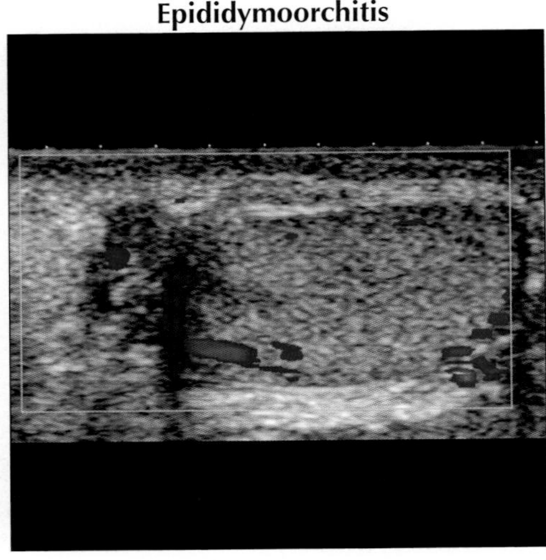

(Left) *Longitudinal color Doppler ultrasound shows hyperemia in an inflamed, relatively hypoechoic epididymis, consistent with epididymitis. The testicles (not shown) were normal bilaterally.* ***(Right)*** *Longitudinal color Doppler ultrasound shows normal echotexture and blood flow in the asymptomatic contralateral testicle.*

Hydrocele

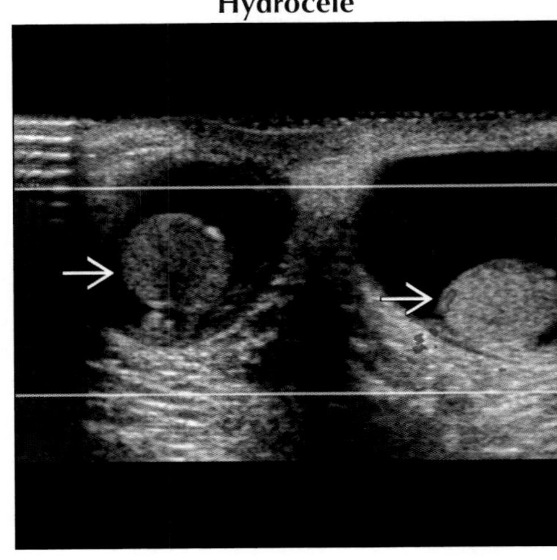

Varicocele

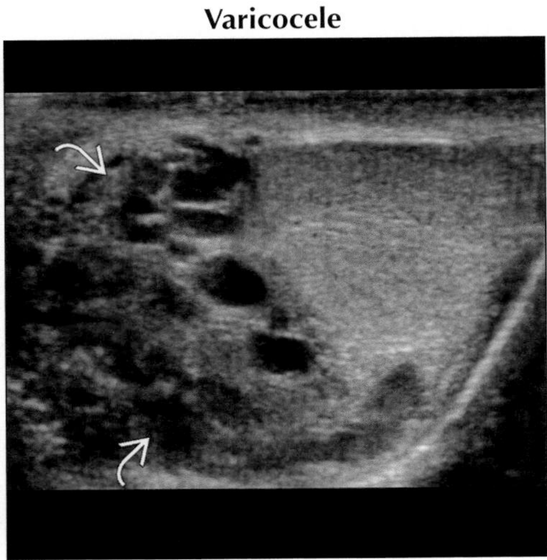

(Left) *Transverse color Doppler ultrasound shows normal perfusion of both testes ➔, which are surrounded by anechoic fluid, more on the left side than the right. This baby had large, bilateral hydroceles causing scrotal enlargement.* ***(Right)*** *Transverse harmonic ultrasound shows a normal testicle adjacent to the serpiginous anechoic tubes ➔, consistent with a varicocele. Varicoceles enlarge during Valsalva and show flow on color Doppler.*

Testicular Torsion

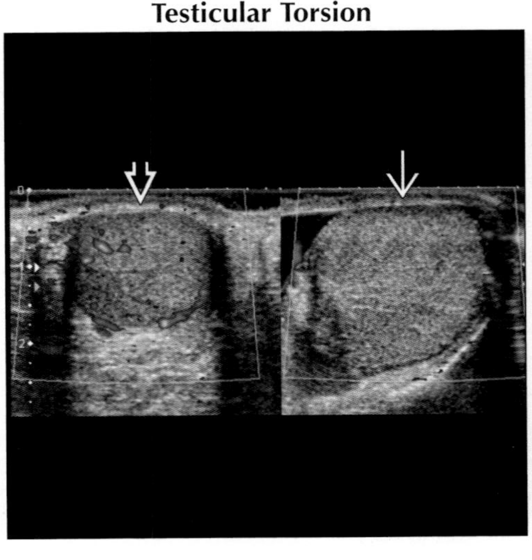

Testicular Torsion

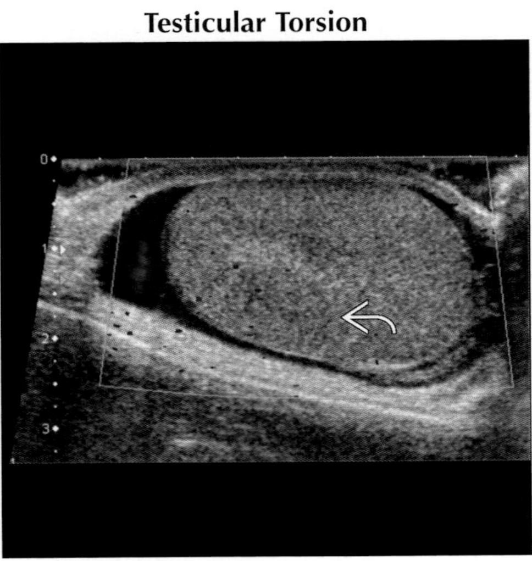

(Left) *Transverse power Doppler ultrasound shows a side-by-side split screen view of both testicles during power Doppler examination. The right testicle ➔ is well perfused, while the large left testicle ➔ is not.* ***(Right)*** *Longitudinal color Doppler ultrasound shows a small hydrocele surrounding the symptomatic left testicle and mild prominence of the rete testis ➔ radiating out from the mediastinum testis, reflecting swelling/edema.*

Torsion of Testicular Appendage

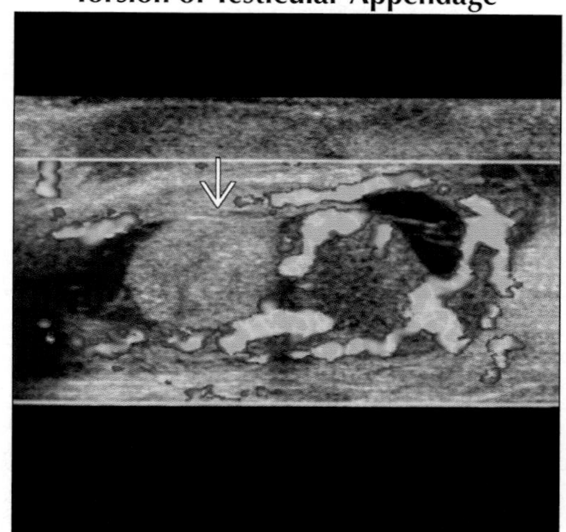

Testicular Rupture/Hematoma

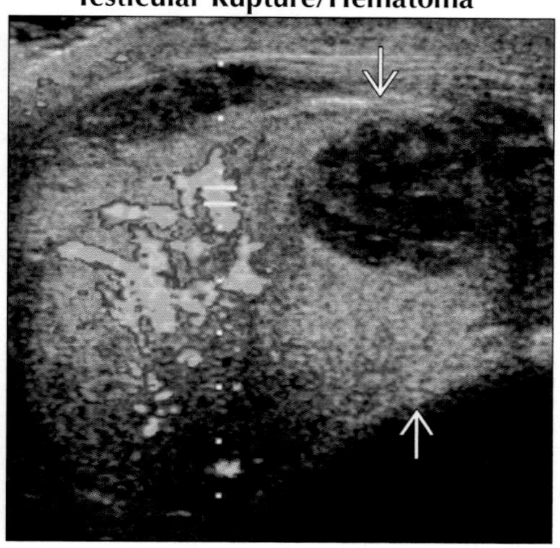

(Left) *Transverse color Doppler ultrasound shows absent flow in a round, hyperechoic nodule ➡ adjacent to the normally perfused epididymis. This teenager had focal pain in the upper scrotum for several days.* ***(Right)*** *Longitudinal color Doppler ultrasound shows perfusion of only 1/2 of the testicle after a direct blow to the scrotum during a lacrosse game. The area of absent perfusion ➡ was irregular in contour, due to disruption of the capsule (seen in the OR).*

Spermatocele/Epididymal Cyst

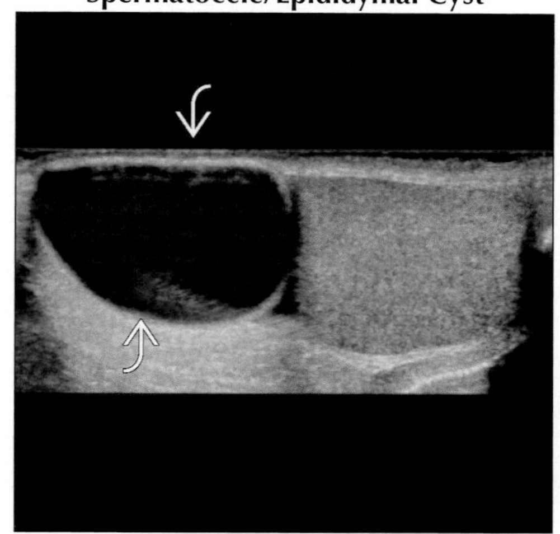

Pyocele

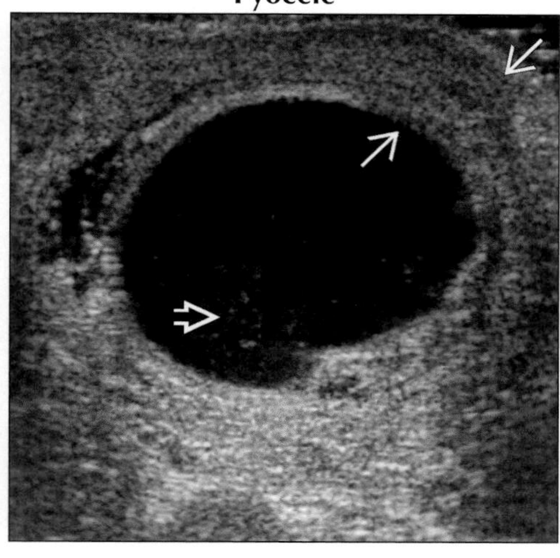

(Left) *Longitudinal ultrasound shows a large cyst ➡ in the upper aspect of the left scrotum, abutting the epididymis. This palpable cyst may represent a spermatocele, epididymal cyst, or cyst of the spermatic cord.* ***(Right)*** *Transverse harmonic ultrasound shows faintly echogenic debris ➡ within the hydrocele fluid in a young boy who recently had ureteral reimplant surgery. Note the scrotal wall thickening ➡.*

Tubular Ectasia

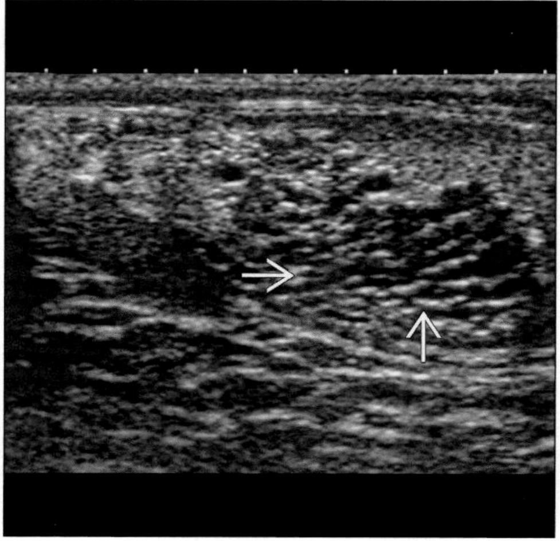

Tubular Ectasia

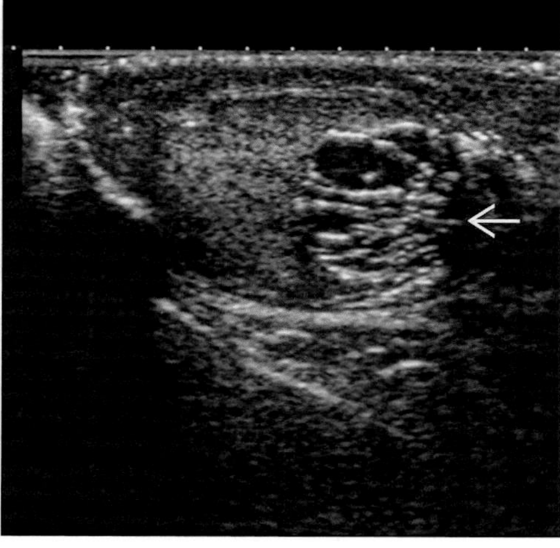

(Left) *Longitudinal harmonic ultrasound shows dilated anechoic tubes ➡ in a portion of the right testicle in this asymptomatic patient. The epididymis (EPI) is normal.* ***(Right)*** *Transverse harmonic ultrasound shows the characteristic dilated rete testis ➡ radiating from the mediastinum testis in this 7 year old. Tubular ectasia is often bilateral and asymmetric.*

SCROTAL MASS

*(**Left**) Transverse color Doppler ultrasound shows a heterogeneous mass in the testicle of this teenager who was subsequently diagnosed with a testicular embryonal cell tumor. (**Right**) Longitudinal US with extended field of view shows complete replacement of the left testicle with a heterogeneous soft tissue mass. There is a large, complex hydrocele with septations and debris in this 17 yo who reported the left scrotum had been enlarged for many months.*

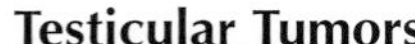

Testicular Tumors

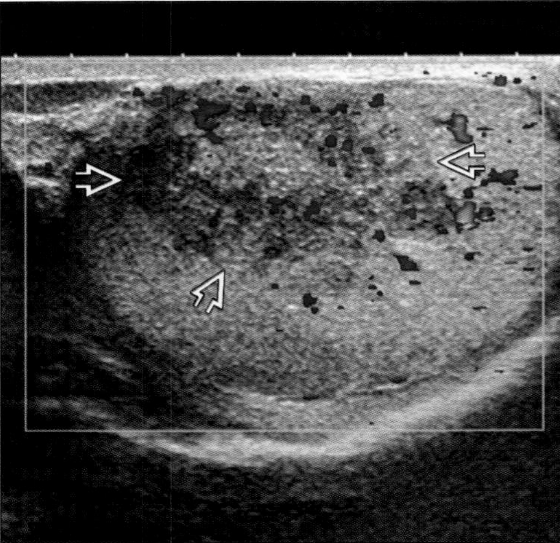

Testicular Tumors

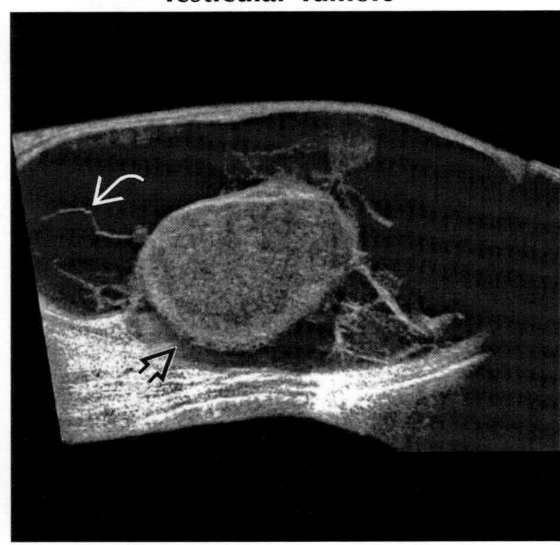

*(**Left**) Axial CECT in the same patient shows bulky periaortic adenopathy, some ascites, and a delayed left nephrogram from hydronephrosis. The findings are most consistent with a metastatic testicular tumor, though lymphoma and infection were also considered. (**Right**) Axial CECT shows numerous lung metastases in the same teenage boy, consistent with a metastatic testicular tumor. The cell type was later shown to be a germ cell tumor.*

Testicular Tumors

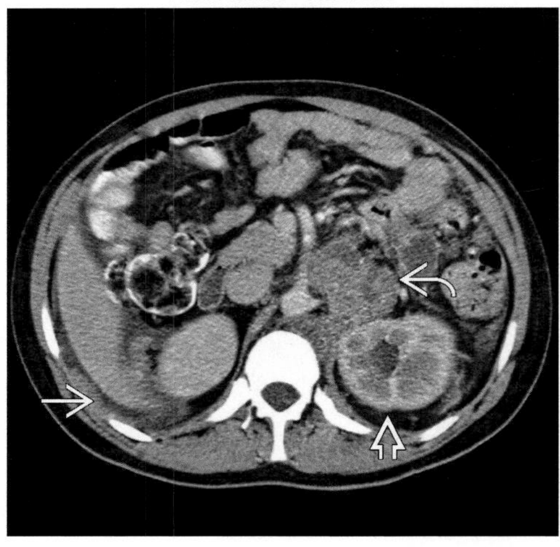

Testicular Tumors

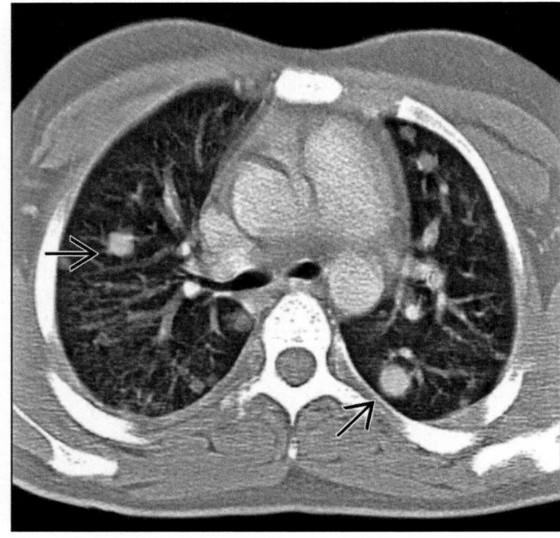

*(**Left**) Transverse harmonic ultrasound shows a heterogeneous mass in the right testicle with an echogenic shadowing focus suggesting calcification. (**Right**) Longitudinal harmonic ultrasound shows the same mass in a perpendicular plane. The mass appears heterogeneous but relatively well circumscribed. It was subsequently removed and found to be a testicular teratoma.*

Testicular Tumors

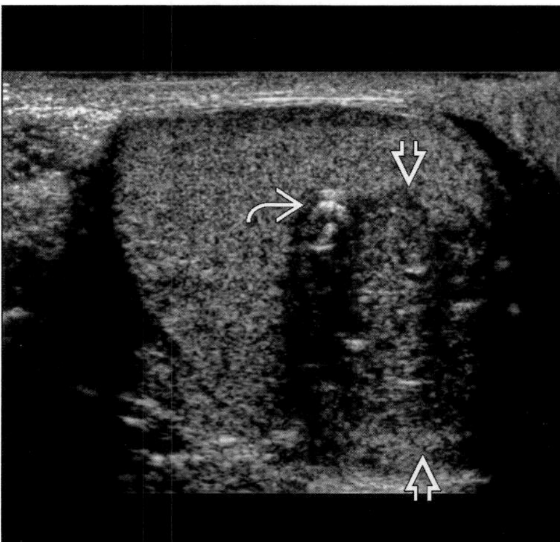

Testicular Tumors

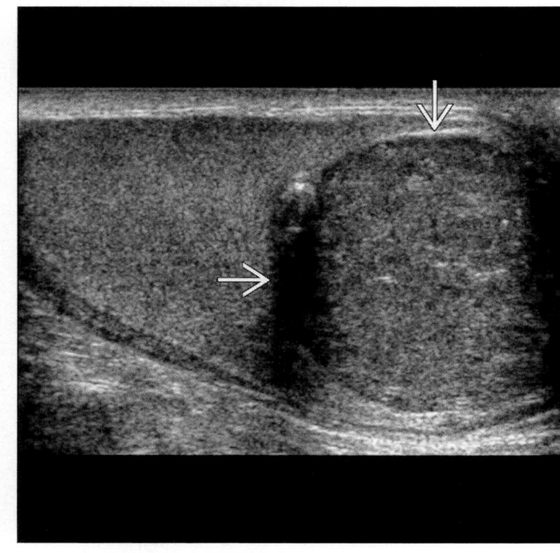

Testicular Tumors

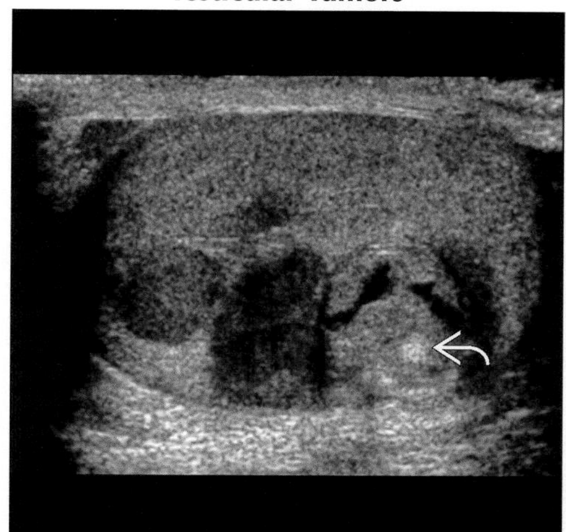

Testicular Tumors

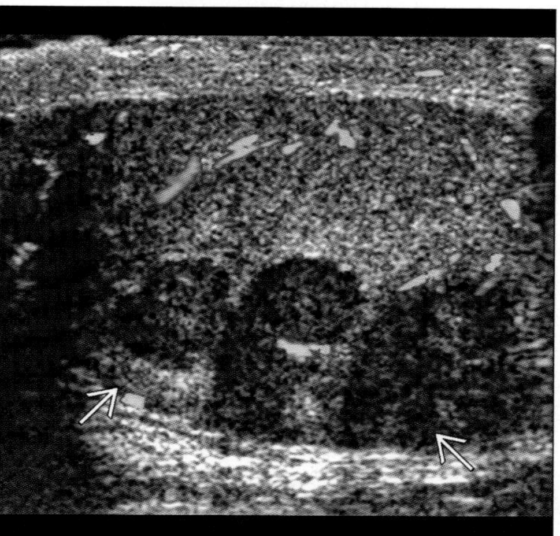

(Left) *Longitudinal harmonic ultrasound shows another heterogeneous mass in a testicle but with a more lobulated outer contour. No defined capsule is seen. The hyperechoic focus ⮫ does not shadow but may still represent calcification.* ***(Right)*** *Longitudinal color Doppler US shows relatively decreased blood flow in the tumor ➡ compared with the normal portion of the testicle in the near field. The mass was resected and found to be a malignant mixed germ cell tumor.*

Meconium Peritonitis

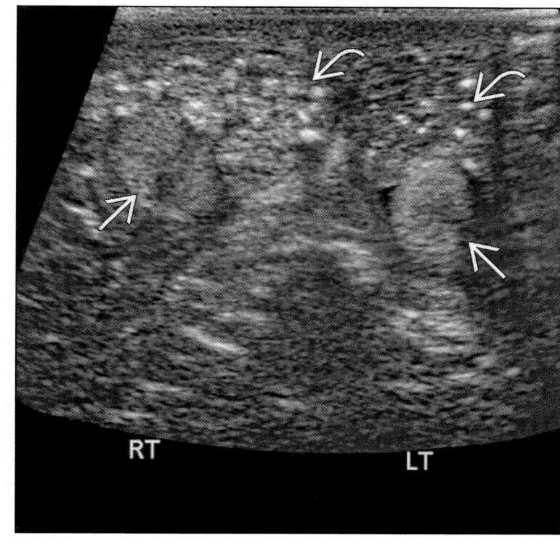

Scrotal Pneumatosis

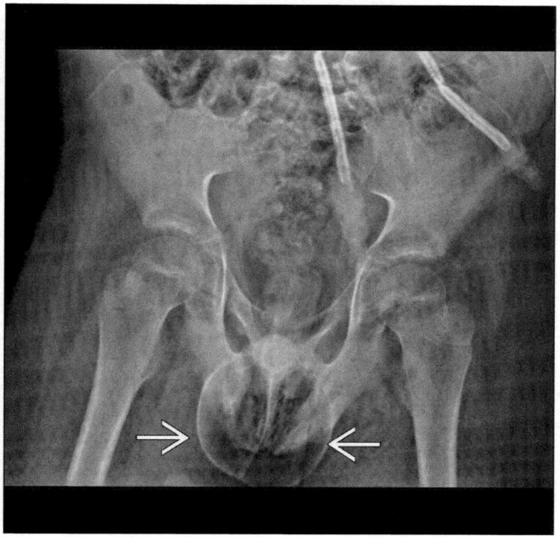

(Left) *Transverse harmonic ultrasound shows marked scrotal wall edema and tiny echogenic foci ⮫ in the soft tissue surrounding both normal testicles ➡ in this newborn. The baby had in utero bowel perforation and meconium peritonitis, which extended into the scrotal sac.* ***(Right)*** *AP radiograph shows air ➡ tracking into the scrotal sac in this child with pneumatosis intestinalis and bowel perforation.*

Henoch-Schönlein Purpura

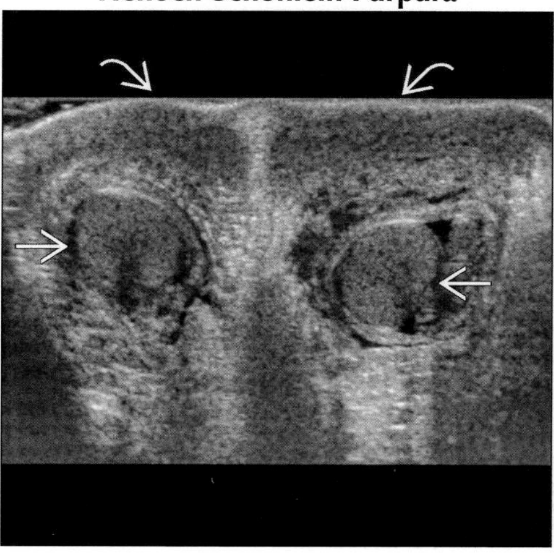

Henoch-Schönlein Purpura

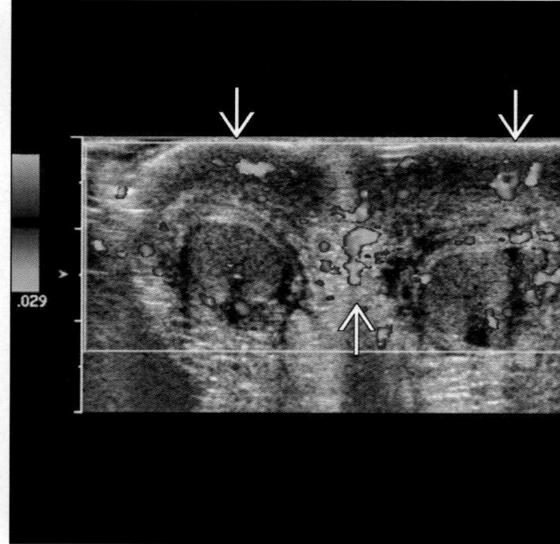

(Left) *Transverse harmonic ultrasound shows marked scrotal wall edema and thickening ⮫. Tiny hydroceles are present bilaterally, and the testicles ➡ are normal in this patient with Henoch-Schönlein purpura.* ***(Right)*** *Transverse color Doppler ultrasound shows hyperemia in the scrotal wall ➡ and normal perfusion of the testicles, which appear relatively diminished.*

SCROTAL PAIN

DIFFERENTIAL DIAGNOSIS

Common
- Epididymoorchitis
- Testicular Torsion
- Inguinal Hernia
- Torsion of Testicular/Epididymal Appendage
- Varicocele
- Hydrocele, Primary or Secondary

Less Common
- Primary Neoplasm: Germ Cell Tumors, Stromal Cell Tumors
- Metastases: Lymphoma, Leukemia, Neuroblastoma

ESSENTIAL INFORMATION

Key Differential Diagnosis Issues
- Specific duration/timing of pain
- Known prior medical history

Helpful Clues for Common Diagnoses
- **Epididymoorchitis**
  - Epididymis/testis often enlarged, hypoechoic/heterogeneous, hypervascular
  - Reactive hydrocele often present
  - If recurrent, consider congenital anomaly
- **Testicular Torsion**
  - Appearance depends on duration
    - Acute: Enlarged, hypoechoic, absent flow
    - Subacute/chronic: Heterogeneous, hydrocele, or peritesticular hyperemia
- **Inguinal Hernia**
  - Loops of bowel in scrotum usually peristalse, though not always
  - Hernia contents can be mesentery only
- **Torsion of Testicular/Epididymal Appendage**
  - May involve appendix testis, appendix epididymis, paradidymis
  - US appearance
    - Small, echogenic or hypoechoic knot
    - Hyperemia/hydrocele may mimic epididymitis
- **Varicocele**
  - Tubular anechoic structures with blood flow on color Doppler with Valsalva
  - Usually left sided, occasionally bilateral
    - If unilateral on right, search for underlying venous obstruction
- **Hydrocele, Primary or Secondary**
  - May be simple fluid or complex with septations, debris

Helpful Clues for Less Common Diagnoses
- **Primary Neoplasms: Germ Cell Tumors, Stromal Cell Tumors**
  - US characteristics nonspecific
    - Focal or diffuse abnormality
    - Hydrocele or hyperemia may be present
    - Hematoma after minor trauma: Follow to resolution to exclude underlying lesion
- **Metastases: Leukemia, Lymphoma, Neuroblastoma**
  - US characteristics nonspecific
    - Focal or diffuse abnormality
    - May be unilateral or bilateral

Epididymoorchitis

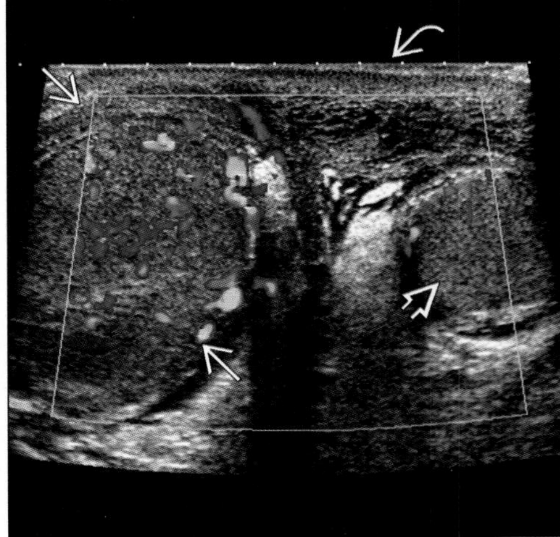

Transverse color Doppler ultrasound shows an enlarged, painful right testis ➡ with diffuse scrotal wall thickening ➡ and exuberant blood flow. The left testis is normal ➡.

Testicular Torsion

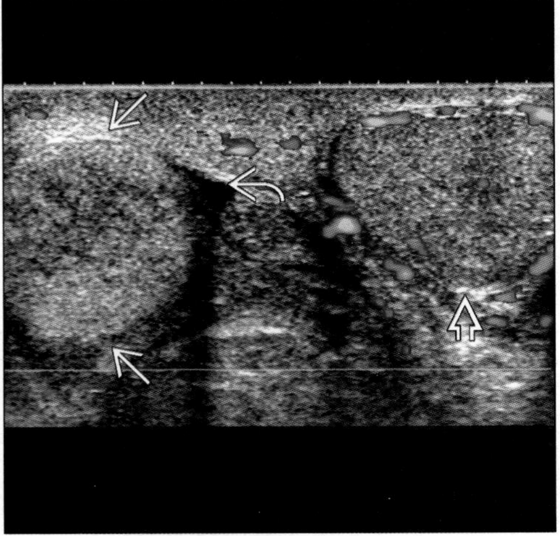

Transverse power Doppler ultrasound shows no blood flow in an acutely torsed right testis ➡, which is mildly heterogeneous in echotexture compared with the normal left testis ➡. Note the small hydrocele ➡.

SCROTAL PAIN

Inguinal Hernia

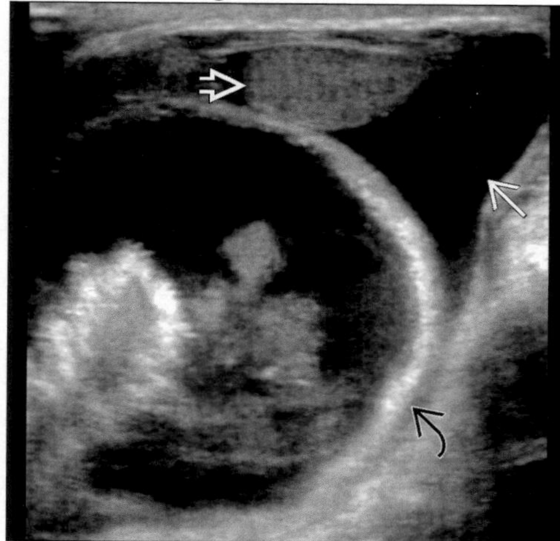

Torsion of Testicular/Epididymal Appendage

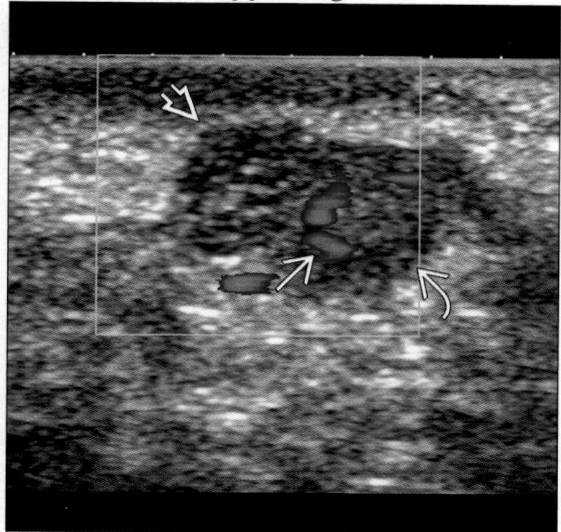

*(**Left**) Transverse ultrasound shows a fluid- and debris-filled loop of bowel wall within the scrotal sac. There is a simple hydrocele, which is also consistent with a patent processus vaginalis. The testis is normal. (**Right**) Longitudinal power Doppler echocardiogram shows a small, round, hypoechoic structure with surrounding hyperemia but no internal blood flow. The otherwise normal epididymis is adjacent.*

Varicocele

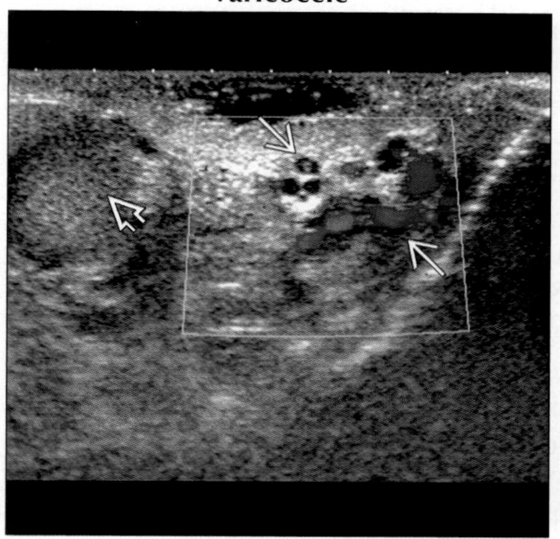

Hydrocele, Primary or Secondary

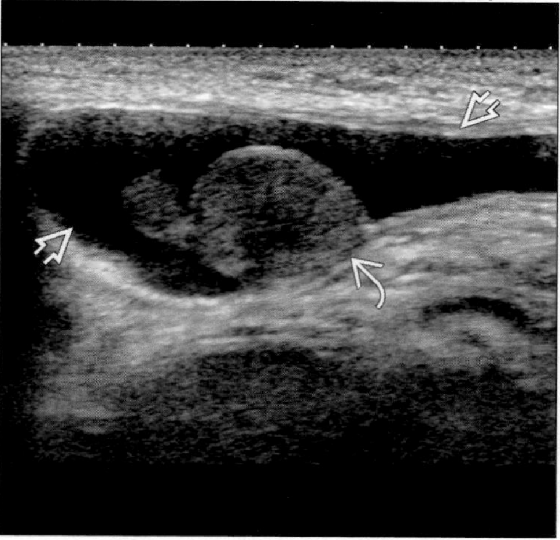

*(**Left**) Transverse color Doppler ultrasound shows the anechoic tubular and round structures adjacent to the left testis; many promptly fill in with color flow when the patient performs a mild Valsalva maneuver. (**Right**) Longitudinal US shows the source of scrotal pain in this 4 year old: A large hydrocele comprised of simple anechoic fluid surrounding the left testis and extending into the inguinal canal. The left testis and epididymis are normal.*

Primary Neoplasm: Germ Cell Tumors, Stromal Cell Tumors

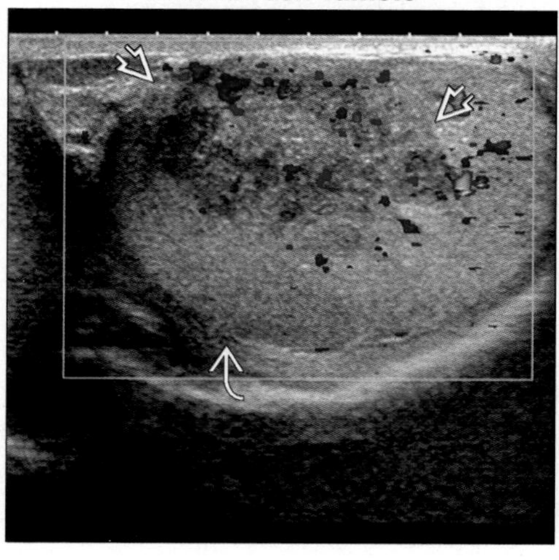

Metastases: Lymphoma, Leukemia, Neuroblastoma

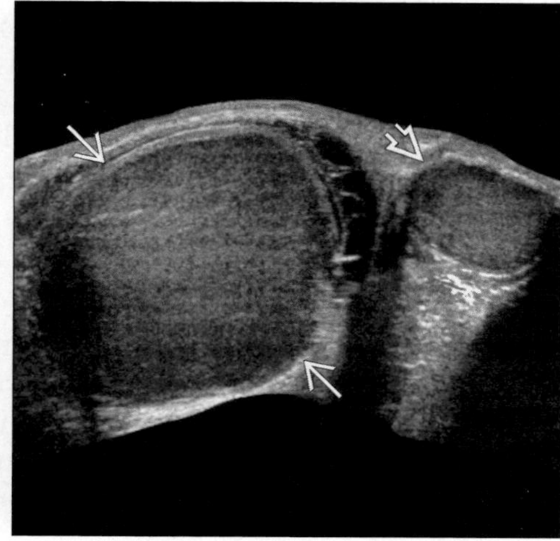

*(**Left**) Longitudinal ultrasound shows a vascular, heterogeneous lesion within the left testis discovered to be an embryonal carcinoma. These primary neoplasms often do not present with pain unless there has been infarction, hemorrhage, or development of a hydrocele. (**Right**) Transverse ultrasound shows massive enlargement and subtle heterogeneity of the right testis in a child with relapsed acute lymphocytic leukemia. The left testis is normal.*

ANOMALIES OF THE URETHRA

DIFFERENTIAL DIAGNOSIS

Common
- Normal Urethra (Male)
- Normal Urethra (Female)
- Posterior Urethral Valve (PUV)
- Prostatic Utricle
- Bladder Sphincter Dyssynergia

Less Common
- Cowper Duct Syringocele
- Anterior Urethral Valve
- Ejaculatory Duct Reflux
- Prostatic Reflux
- Reflux into Ectopic Ureter
- Urethral Stricture
- Urethral Trauma

Rare but Important
- Megalourethra
- Urethral Polyp
- Lacuna Magna
- Urethral Duplication

ESSENTIAL INFORMATION

Key Differential Diagnosis Issues
- Location of urethral anomaly on VCUG
- Symptoms: Infection, hematuria, dysuria, obstructive
- Associated bony anomaly, i.e., pubic symphysis diastasis

Helpful Clues for Common Diagnoses
- **Posterior Urethral Valve (PUV)**
  - Important treatable cause of urethral obstruction in males
  - Prenatal diagnosis in many cases
  - Suspect in males born with thick bladder and bilateral hydroureteronephrosis (HUN)
  - Type 1: Abnormal migration of mesonephric ducts resulting in abnormal insertion of valvulae colliculi
  - Type 2: Considered by most to not represent PUV
  - Type 3: Incomplete dissolution of urogenital membrane (near membranous urethra)
  - Ultrasound
    - Bladder wall thickening, HUN, ± renal dysplasia, ascites
  - Voiding cystourethrogram
    - Dilated posterior urethra to level of valvulae colliculi
    - ± periureteral diverticula
    - Thick bladder wall
    - ± vesicoureteral reflux, intrarenal reflux
  - Fetal imaging
    - Bladder may be thick
    - Bladder distended with keyhole configuration at outlet
    - ± HUN, renal dysplasia, cortical thinning, ascites, oligohydramnios
- **Prostatic Utricle**
  - Also called utriculus masculinus
  - Blind-ending pouch/diverticulum
  - From posterior urethra at verumontanum
  - Mesodermal remnant of müllerian tubercle
  - Associated with hypospadias in males
    - Larger size correlated with more severe hypospadias
  - On VCUG, posterior urethral diverticulum
    - Optimally imaged during voiding in steep obliquity
  - Incidentally on US, CT, or MR performed for other indication
  - In males after repair of imperforate anus
    - Posterior urethral diverticulum vs. residual of rectourethral fistula
- **Bladder Sphincter Dyssynergia**
  - Dyscoordination of bladder and urethral sphincter
  - Disruption of central nervous system regulation of micturition
  - During bladder detrusor contraction, urethral sphincter fails to relax
  - On VCUG, results in dilation of posterior urethra to urethral sphincter
  - "Spinning top" appearance in females
  - Usually due to underlying neurologic condition
    - Spinal cord injury
    - Myelomeningocele

Helpful Clues for Less Common Diagnoses
- **Cowper Duct Syringocele**
  - Cystic dilation at end of Cowper duct
  - Frequently asymptomatic
  - Can present as urinary infection, hematuria, dysuria, obstructive symptoms
  - Possible findings on VCUG
    - Lucent defect with mass effect on bulbous urethra at orifice of duct

- Larger defect → contrast filling of distal Cowper duct
- **Anterior Urethral Valve**
  - Most caused by anterior urethral diverticulum
  - Diverticulum expands into urethral lumen during voiding, occluding urethral flow
  - Variable obstruction, mild to severe
- **Ejaculatory Duct Reflux**
  - Reflux into ejaculatory duct during voiding
  - Associated with neurogenic bladder
    - Bladder-sphincter dyssynergia, anorectal malformation
    - Associated with variable degree of urethral obstruction
  - Multiple episodes of epididymitis
- **Prostatic Reflux**
  - Associated with variable degree of urethral obstruction
  - "Cloudy" increased density in distribution surrounding prostatic urethra
- **Reflux into Ectopic Ureter**
  - Single system, predominantly in males
  - Upper pole of duplex kidneys, usually in females
- **Urethral Stricture**
  - Post-traumatic, straddle injuries
  - Infectious
  - Post-repair hypospadias, epispadias
- **Urethral Trauma**
  - Type 1, 2, 3, 4, 5A, 5
  - Type 3 (tear at urogenital diaphragm) most common

Helpful Clues for Rare Diagnoses

- **Megalourethra**
  - Nonobstructive urethral dilation
  - Abnormal development of corpus spongiosum, sometimes cavernosa
    - Scaphoid type: Focally abnormal segment spongiosum; association with prune belly
    - Fusiform: Abnormal spongiosum and cavernosa
  - Focally or diffusely dilated, no obstruction
- **Urethral Polyp**
  - Symptoms of obstruction or hematuria
  - Usually solitary, pedunculated, urothelial-lined benign mass from verumontanum
  - Mobile filling defect in prostatic urethra
- **Lacuna Magna**
  - Dorsal diverticulum roof of fossa navicularis
  - Dysuria, end-void gross hematuria, or hematospermia
- **Urethral Duplication**
  - Dorsal (epispadiac), ventral (hypospadiac), and "Y" types
  - Complete (2 orifices) vs. incomplete
  - Epispadiac: Abnormal orifice above glanular meatus
  - Hypospadiac: Abnormal orifice below meatus
  - Often incidentally discovered
    - Catheterize largest orifice

Normal Urethra (Male)

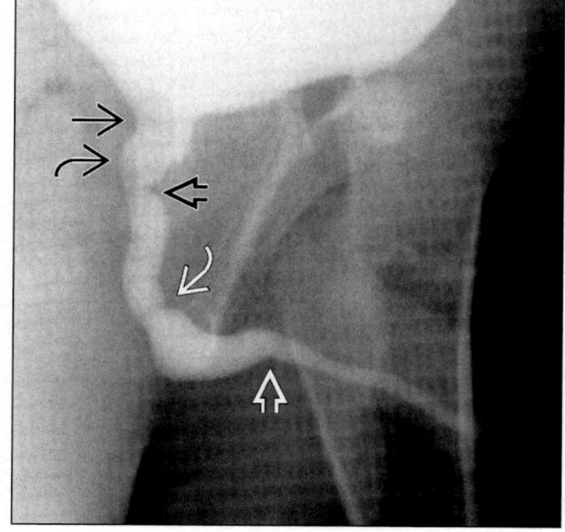

Oblique voiding cystourethrogram demonstrates bladder neck ➔, intermuscular incisura ➔, verumontanum ➔, urethral sphincter (membranous urethra) ➔, and suspensory ligament of penis ➔.

Normal Urethra (Female)

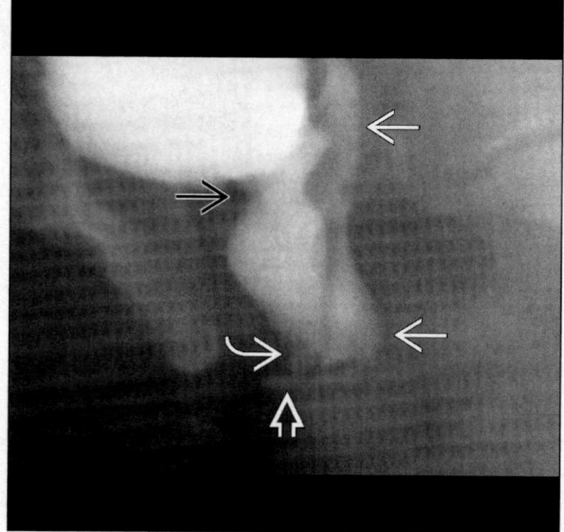

Oblique voiding cystourethrogram shows the bladder neck ➔, urethral sphincter ➔, external urethral meatus ➔, and incidental vaginal reflux ➔.

ANOMALIES OF THE URETHRA

(**Left**) *Oblique voiding cystourethrogram shows a dilated posterior urethra ➔ to the level of the obstructing valvulae colliculi ➔. The rest of the urethra emanates from the posterior aspect of the dilated proximal urethra, a characteristic appearance for type 1 PUV. Note the thick-walled bladder ➔, right Hutch diverticulum ➔, and reflux ➔.* (**Right**) *Oblique voiding cystourethrogram in another patient shows concentric narrowing of a type 3 PUV ➔.*

Posterior Urethral Valve (PUV)

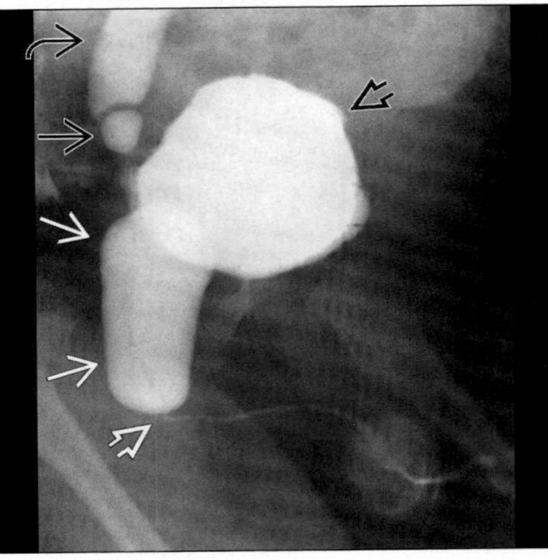

Posterior Urethral Valve (PUV)

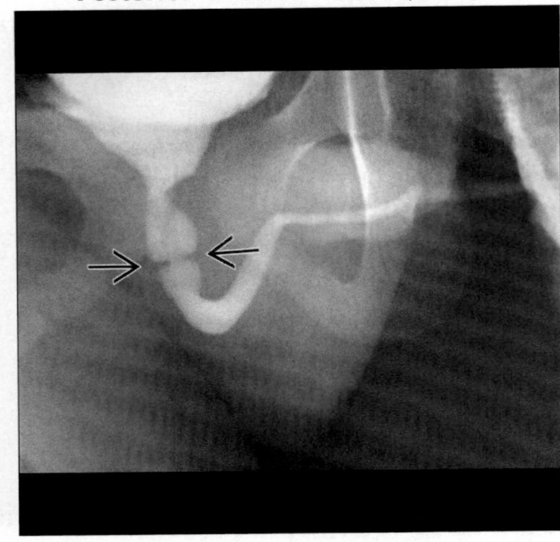

(**Left**) *Oblique voiding cystourethrogram shows minor PUV ➔ and incidental lacuna magna ➔.* (**Right**) *Longitudinal ultrasound of the same patient is oriented similar to the VCUG and shows the anechoic fluid-filled posterior urethra ➔ just below the bladder neck ➔.*

Posterior Urethral Valve (PUV)

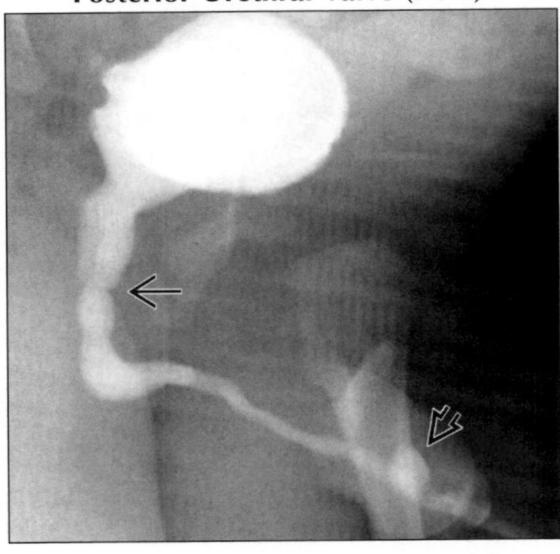

Posterior Urethral Valve (PUV)

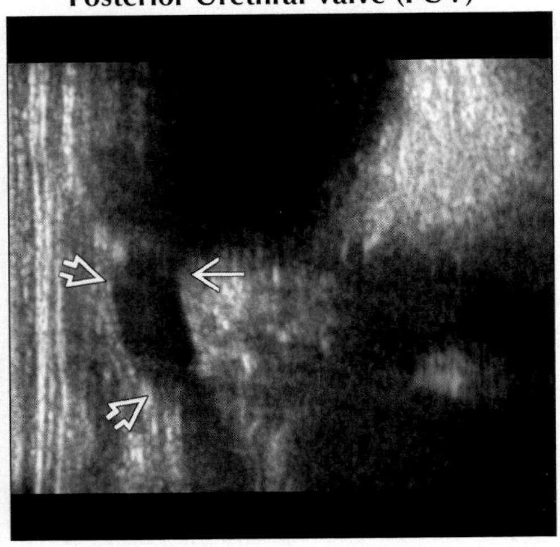

(**Left**) *Oblique voiding cystourethrogram in a 1-week-old male shows prominent plicae colliculae ➔, which can mimic subtle PUV. Secondary signs of bladder outlet obstruction, such as bladder thickening, hypertrophy of interureteric ridge, VUR, and HUN, were not present.* (**Right**) *Oblique voiding cystourethrogram shows a dilated posterior urethra ➔, prominent interureteric ridge ➔, valvulae ➔, and a subtle syringocele ➔.*

Posterior Urethral Valve (PUV)

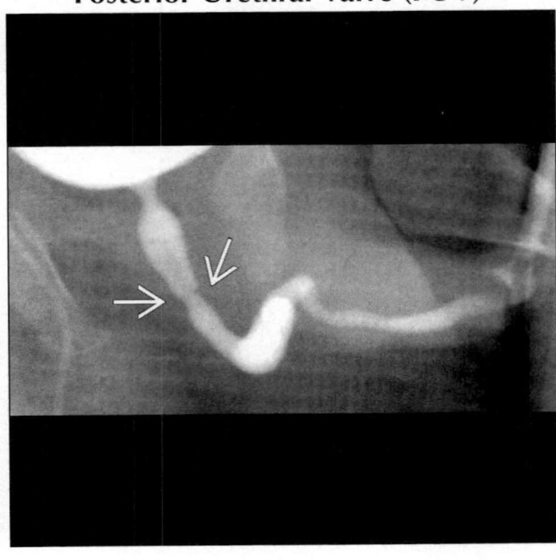

Posterior Urethral Valve (PUV)

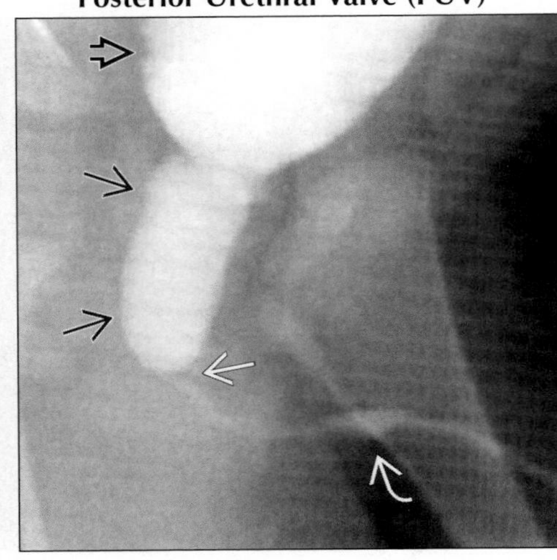

ANOMALIES OF THE URETHRA

Prostatic Utricle

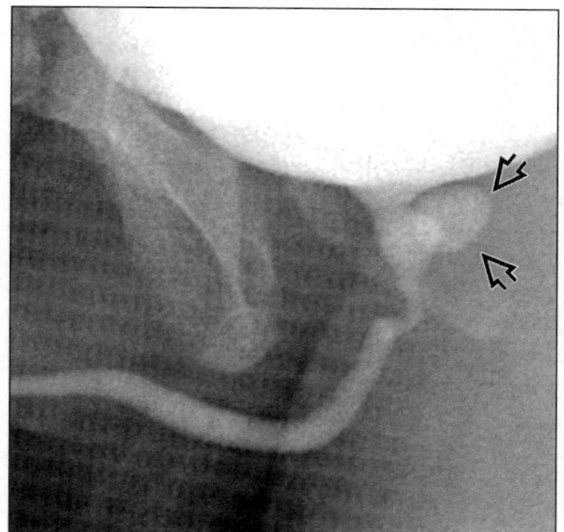

Bladder Sphincter Dyssynergia

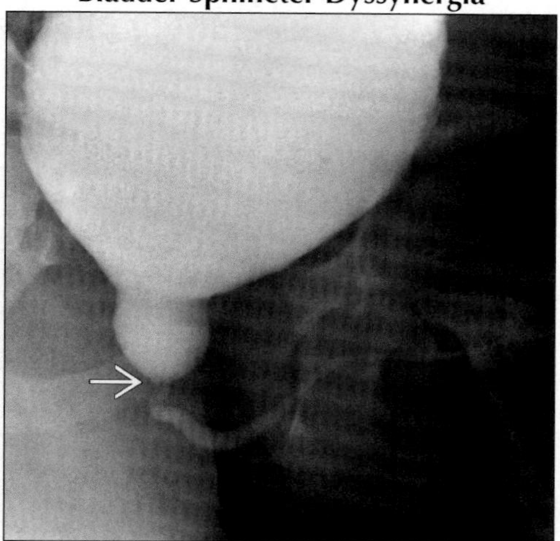

(Left) *Oblique voiding cystourethrogram in a 2-year-old male shows a contrast-filled diverticulum ➩ from the prostatic urethra, consistent with a utricle in this patient who also had hypospadias.* ***(Right)*** *Oblique voiding cystourethrogram in a male with mild myelomeningocele shows intermittent dilation of the posterior urethra to the level of the urethral sphincter ➡ and bladder thickening.*

Bladder Sphincter Dyssynergia

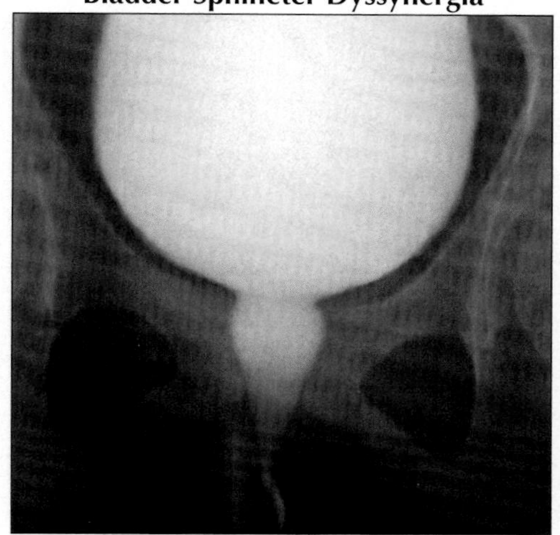

Cowper Duct Syringocele

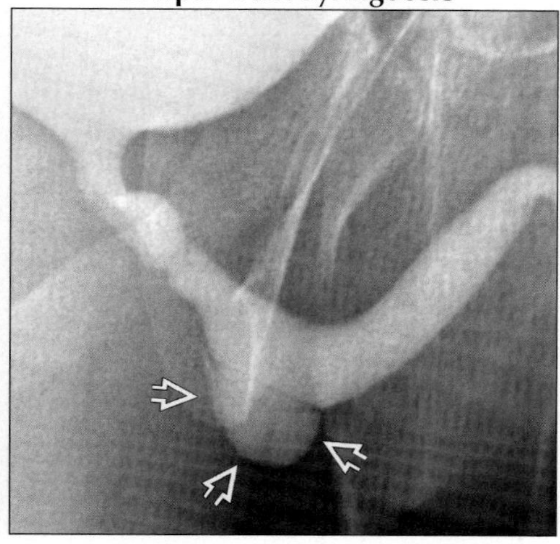

(Left) *AP voiding cystourethrogram in a young girl with day and night wetting and tethered spinal cord shows a "spinning top" appearance of the urethra during intermittent start-stop voiding, which can be seen in bladder sphincter dyssynergia.* ***(Right)*** *Oblique voiding cystourethrogram shows outpouching of contrast toward the undersurface of the bulbous urethra ➩, characteristic of a syringocele.*

Anterior Urethral Valve

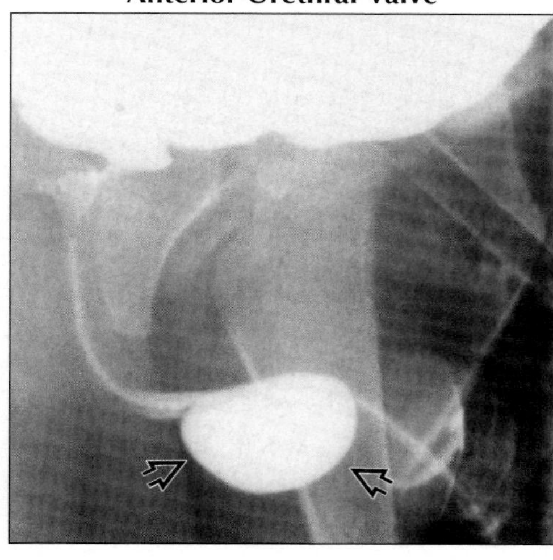

Ejaculatory Duct Reflux

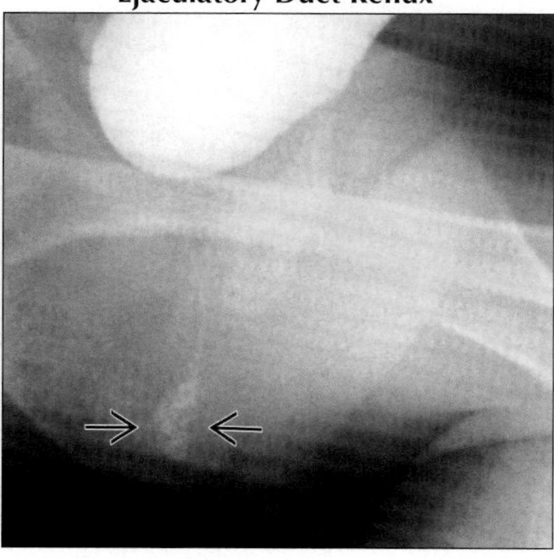

(Left) *Oblique voiding cystourethrogram in a 2 day old shows contrast filling an anterior urethral diverticulum ➩, which made catheterization difficult by causing obstruction. This differs from syringocele, which is usually located more proximally and not usually associated with obstruction.* ***(Right)*** *Lateral voiding cystourethrogram in a patient with anorectal malformation shows contrast extending along the ejaculatory duct to the epididymis ➔.*

ANOMALIES OF THE URETHRA

(**Left**) *Oblique voiding cystourethrogram in a patient with neurogenic bladder and bladder sphincter dyssynergia shows prominence of the posterior urethra to the urethral sphincter and significant prostatic reflux as a cloud of density surrounding the prostate* ➡. (**Right**) *Oblique voiding cystourethrogram in a male patient shows ectopic insertion of the left ureter into the prostatic urethra* ⇨. *In males it is more commonly a single system ectopic ureter.*

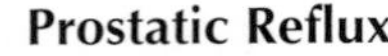

Prostatic Reflux

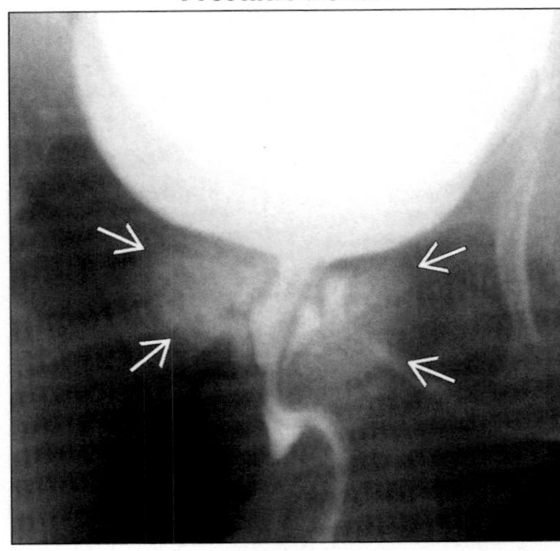

Reflux into Ectopic Ureter

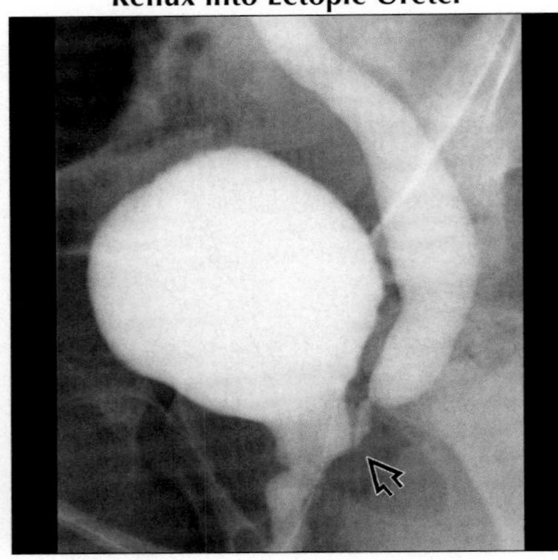

(**Left**) *Oblique voiding cystourethrogram shows fairly long segment narrowing of the bulbous urethra* ➡ *in this adolescent male who had a urethral swab positive for gonorrhea.* (**Right**) *Oblique retrograde urethrogram shows an anterior urethral stricture* ➡ *in this patient treated for hypospadias as an infant. VCUG could not be performed because the catheter could not pass through the stricture.*

Urethral Stricture

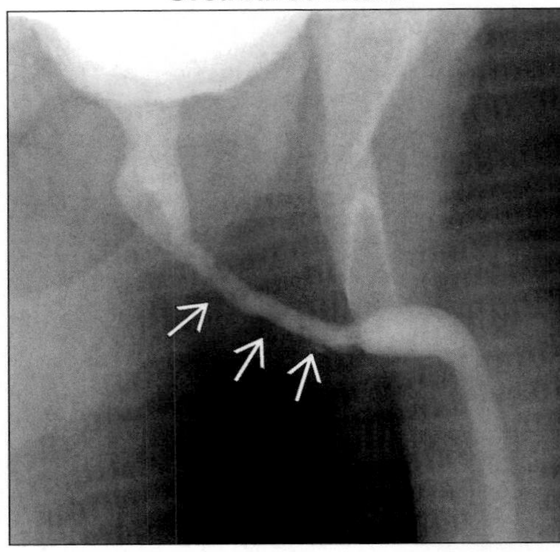

Urethral Stricture

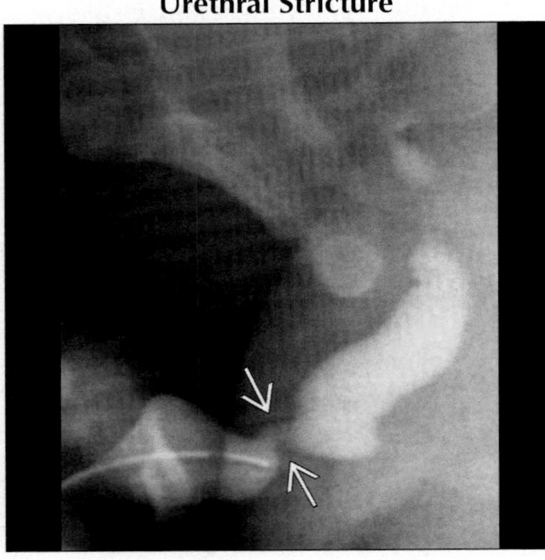

(**Left**) *Oblique retrograde urethrogram shows contrast extravasation at the level of the urogenital diaphragm* → *and extending toward the perineum* ⇨ *and scrotum* ↗. (**Right**) *Oblique retrograde urethrogram of the same patient several weeks post-trauma shows the urethral catheter in place, as well as persistent but smaller urethral contrast extravasation* → *after conservative treatment. Risk of future stricture at this site is high.*

Urethral Trauma

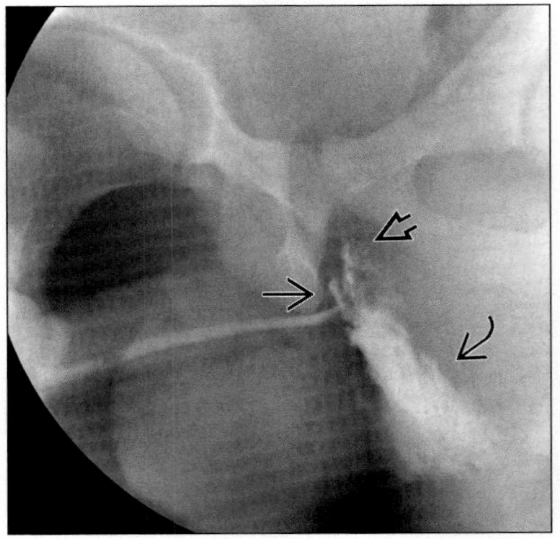

Urethral Trauma

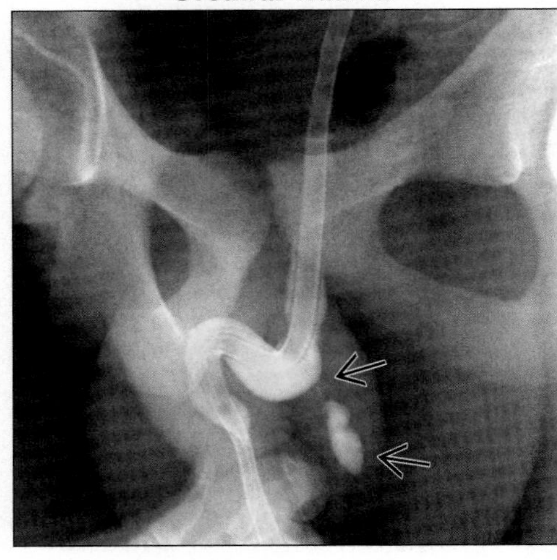

- **Chondrodysplasia Punctata**
  - Stippled epiphyses
  - Nonrhizomelic type: Conradi Hunermann; nonlethal & autosomal dominant
  - Rhizomelic type: Lethal autosomal recessive; multiple other abnormalities
- **Trevor Fairbank (Dysplasia Epiphysealis Hemimelica)**
  - Cartilaginous proliferation at epiphysis
    - Considered analogous to epiphyseal osteochondroma
  - Irregular lobulations superimposed on epiphyses
  - Lower limb (knee, ankle, hip) most frequently affected
  - May be polyarticular
  - Monomelic
- **Spondyloepiphyseal Dysplasia**
  - Group of disorders resulting in short trunk dwarfism
  - Congenita and tarda forms, with spectrum of abnormalities
  - Platyspondyly
  - Generalized delay in epiphyseal ossification
  - Once epiphysis forms, it is flattened and irregular
  - May have metaphyseal flaring
  - Develops coxa vara, genu valgum
  - Early osteoarthritis
- **Nail Patella Disease (Fong)**
  - a.k.a. Fong disease, osteo-onychodysplasia
  - Absent or small patellae
  - Posterior iliac "horns"
  - Nail dysplasia
  - Radial head hypoplasia, subluxation
  - Irregularity and flattening of epiphyses; less constant finding than nail and patella abnormalities

Helpful Clues for Rare Diagnoses

- **Thermal Injury, Frostbite**
  - Epiphyses at risk for vascular injury with vasoconstriction from cold temperature
  - May become dense, fragmented
  - Early fusion results in short phalanges
  - Thumb generally not involved (folded into palm in cold temperatures)
- **Multiple Epiphyseal Dysplasia**
  - Hereditary disease, usually autosomal dominant
  - Delayed and irregular mineralization of epiphyses
  - Results in coxa vara and genu vara or valgum
  - Early osteoarthritis
  - Vertebral involvement variable and generally mild
- **Pseudoachondroplasia**
  - Heterogeneous inherited skeletal dysplasia with dwarfism
  - Malformations not apparent until early childhood
  - Shortening of tubular bones
    - Flaring of metaphyses
    - Variable irregularity of epiphyses

Normal Variant in Child (Mimic)

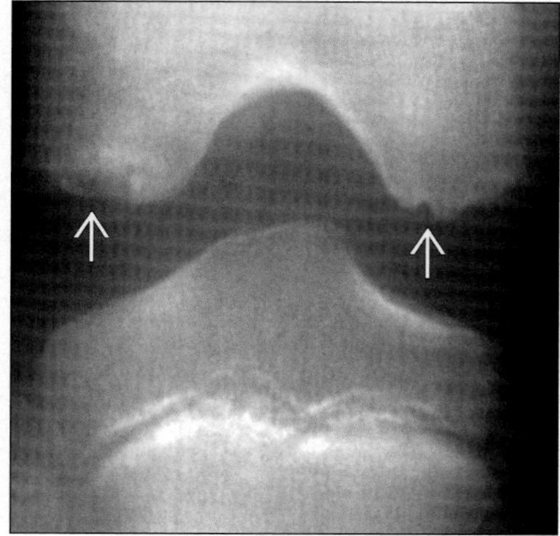

AP notch view shows irregularity of the medial and lateral femoral condyles ➔ in a child. The notch view profiles the posterior portions of the femoral condyles, the expected location of this normal variant.

Normal Variant in Child (Mimic)

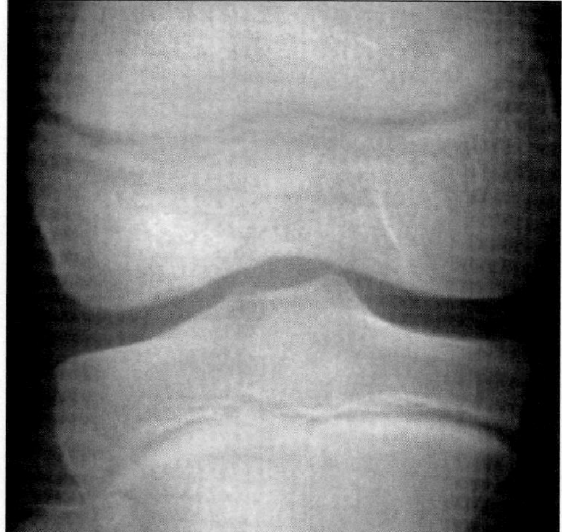

AP radiograph of the same knee shows smooth, normal femoral condyles. This, in combination with the notch view, localizes the epiphyseal irregularities to the posterior condyles.

LONG BONE, EPIPHYSEAL, IRREGULAR OR STIPPLED

*(**Left**) Anteroposterior radiograph shows fragmentation of the humeral head ➡. This is in the weight-bearing portion and is typical of both the location and appearance of osteonecrosis. (**Right**) Anteroposterior radiograph shows irregularity, flattening, and increased density in the femoral capital epiphysis ➡. This child has typical Legg-Calvé-Perthes. (†MSK Req).*

Osteonecrosis

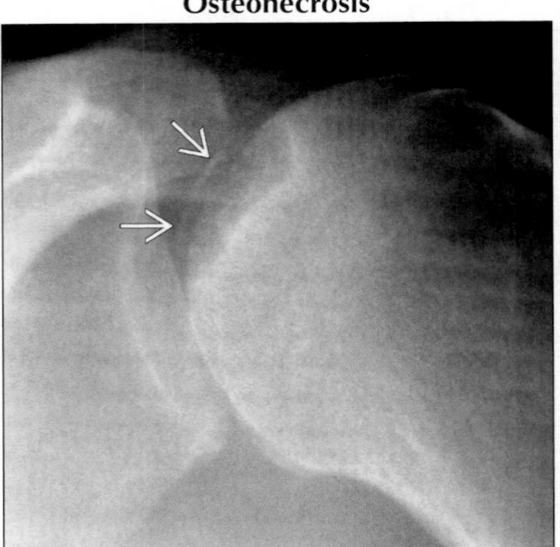

Legg-Calvé-Perthes (LCP)

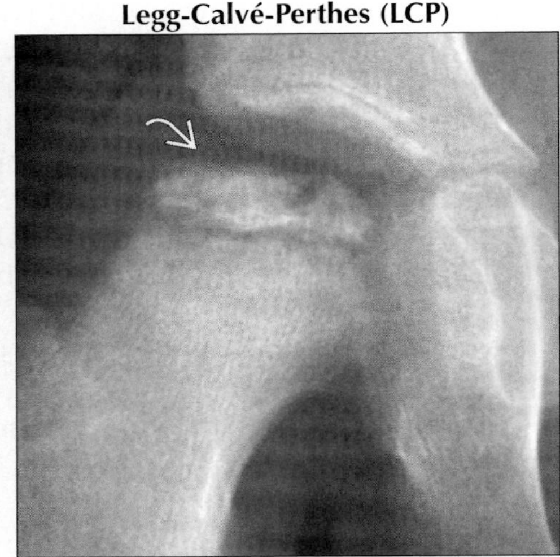

*(**Left**) Lateral radiograph shows irregularity involving the entire surface of the femoral condyles ➡ in this patient with JIA. Such "crenulation" may be seen involving carpal bones as well. (**Right**) AP radiograph shows irregularity of the femoral capital epiphysis ➡, along with fraying of the metaphysis ➡, a widened zone of provisional calcification, and a slipped epiphysis. These are typical changes of rickets in a patient with renal osteodystrophy.*

Juvenile Idiopathic Arthritis (JIA)

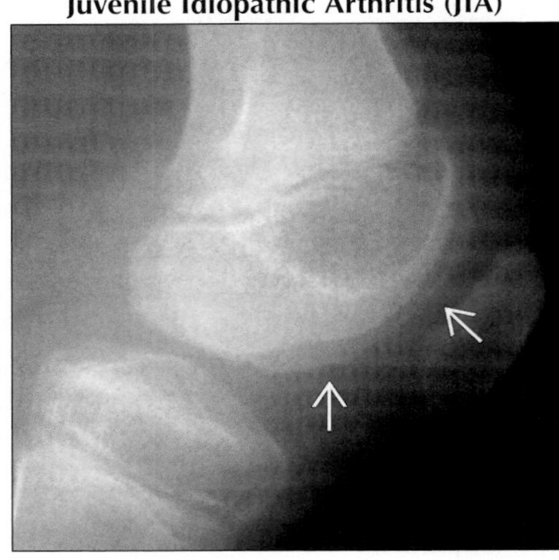

Rickets

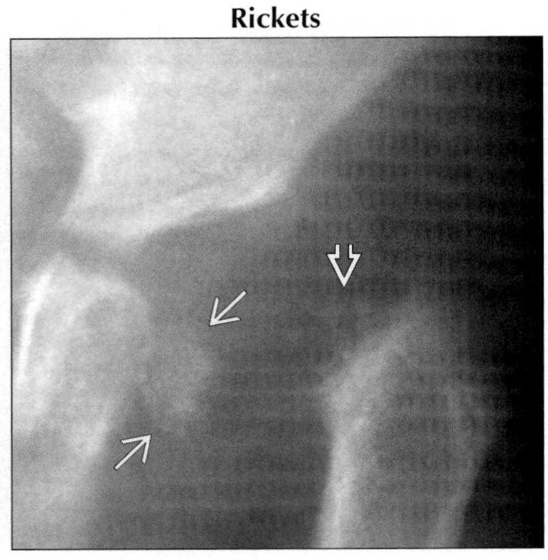

*(**Left**) Anteroposterior radiograph shows fragmentation of the femoral capital epiphysis ➡. This patient also had severely delayed skeletal maturation. This appearance suggests LCP, but it is also seen in hypothyroidism. (**Right**) Anteroposterior radiograph in an infant shows stippled epiphyses ➡ at the femoral head/greater trochanter. Hypothyroidism is 1 of several entities that may present with stippled epiphyses.*

Hypothyroidism

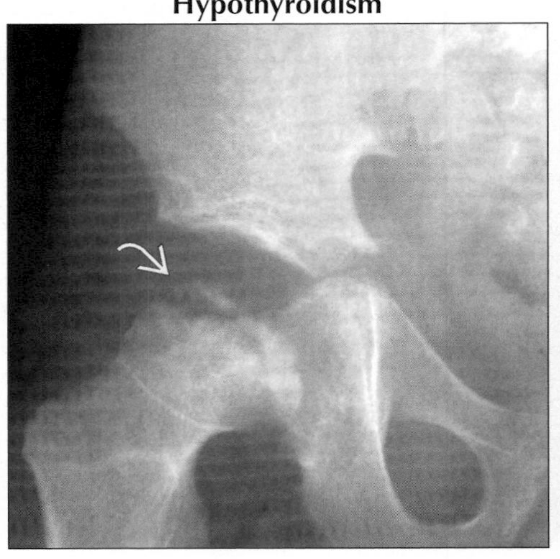

Hypothyroidism

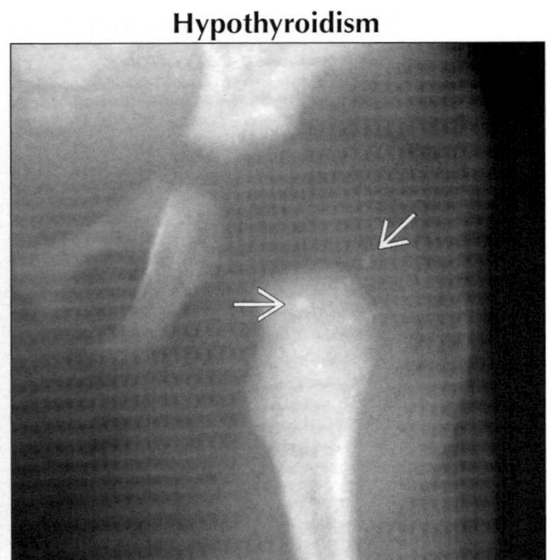

Osteomyelitis

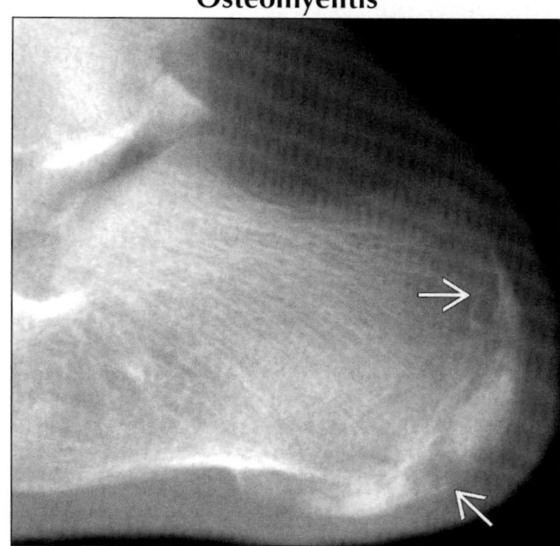

Complications of Warfarin (Coumadin)

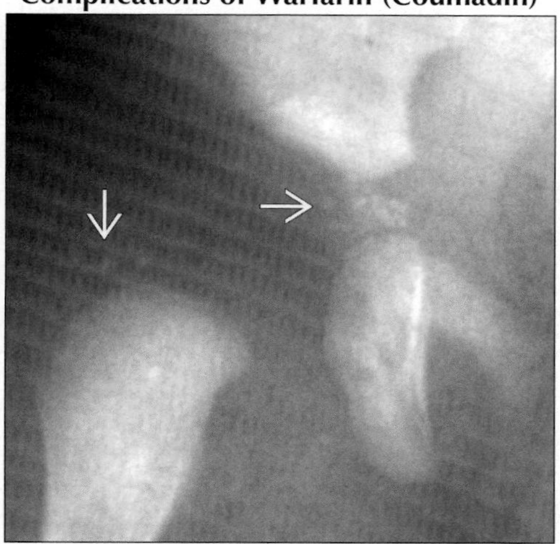

*(**Left**) Lateral radiograph shows irregularity and fragmentation of the calcaneal apophysis ➔. This patient has osteomyelitis, with associated destruction. (**Right**) AP radiographs show stippling of the epiphyses and apophyses ➔ of the acetabulum and femoral head. This infant's mother had been given warfarin during pregnancy; stippled epiphyses are 1 manifestation of warfarin embryopathy.*

Chondrodysplasia Punctata

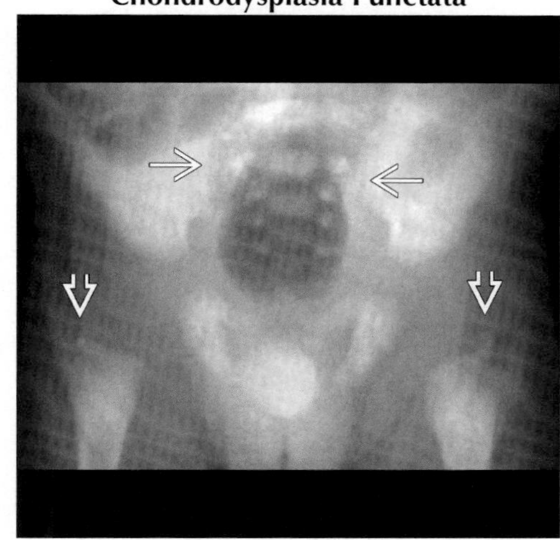

Trevor Fairbank (Dysplasia Epiphysealis Hemimelica)

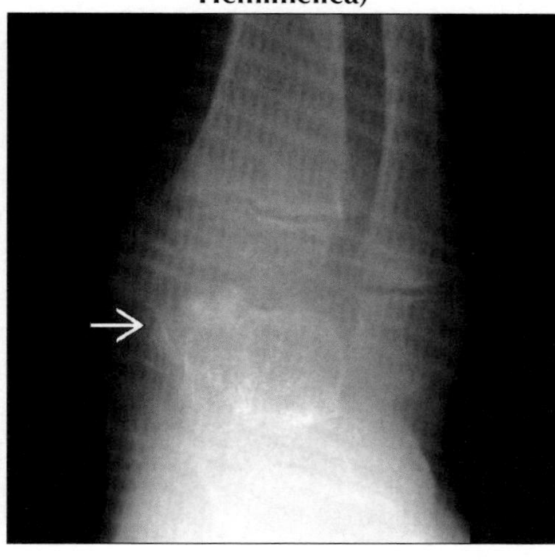

*(**Left**) Anteroposterior radiograph shows stippled epiphyses at the sacrum ➔ and femoral heads ➔. This finding is nonspecific, but this patient had other manifestations of chondrodysplasia punctata. (**Right**) Anteroposterior radiograph shows irregularity of the epiphyses of the tibiotalar joint ➔. This is actually an epiphyseal osteochondroma, termed Trevor Fairbank dysplasia. The irregular bone results in joint damage.*

Spondyloepiphyseal Dysplasia

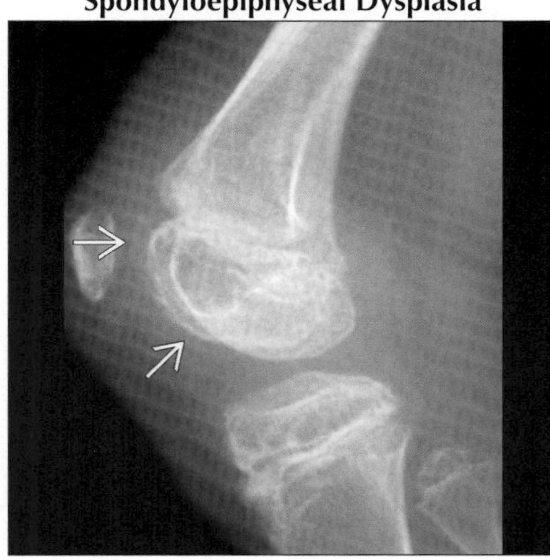

Nail Patella Disease (Fong)

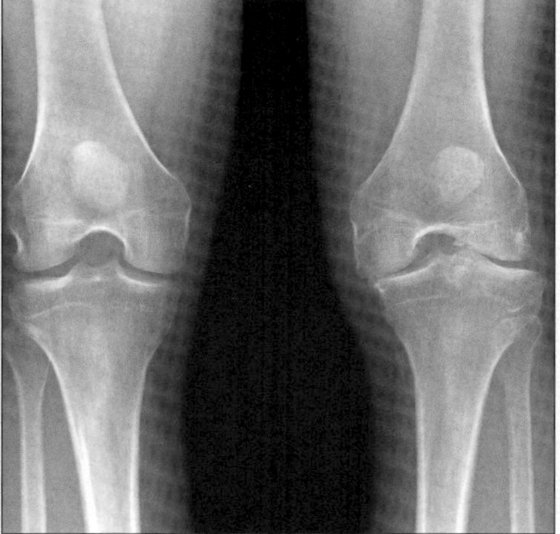

*(**Left**) Lateral radiograph shows irregularity of the femoral condyles ➔. This is the appearance of a relatively mild form of spondyloepiphyseal dysplasia. (**Right**) Anteroposterior radiograph shows irregularity and flattening of the femoral condyles of the left knee. There is also hypoplasia of the patellae. Both findings are seen in nail patella (Fong) disease.*

LONG BONE, EPIPHYSEAL, OVERGROWTH/BALLOONING

DIFFERENTIAL DIAGNOSIS

Common
- Juvenile Idiopathic Arthritis (JIA)
- Hemophilia: MSK Complications

Less Common
- Septic Joint
- Epiphyseal Fracture, Pediatric
- Epiphyseal Dysplasia
- Hyperemia, Other Causes
- Turner Syndrome (Mimic)
- Blount Disease (Mimic)

Rare but Important
- Meningococcemia (Mimic)

ESSENTIAL INFORMATION

Key Differential Diagnosis Issues
- Hyperemia is fundamental cause of overgrowth in several cases
  - In skeletally immature patient
    - Prolonged hyperemia adjacent to joint → overgrowth (ballooning) of epiphysis
    - In addition to enlarged epiphysis, hyperemia → early physeal fusion → short limb
  - Etiologies of overgrowth secondary to hyperemia include
    - Hemophilia
    - Juvenile idiopathic arthritis
    - Septic joint, particularly tuberculosis or fungal etiology
    - Epiphyseal or metaphyseal fracture

Helpful Clues for Common Diagnoses
- **Juvenile Idiopathic Arthritis (JIA)**
  - Hemophilia: Similar to JIA
  - Chronic hyperemia from synovitis (JIA) or recurrent intraarticular bleed (hemophilia)
  - Knee > elbow > ankle
  - Erosion of intercondylar or trochlear notch
  - Erosions, cartilage loss in both
    - JIA may be distinguished by carpal fusion
    - Hemophilia may be distinguished by dense effusion (hemosiderin deposition)

Helpful Clues for Less Common Diagnoses
- **Septic Joint**
  - Effusion, cartilage loss, erosions
  - Tuberculosis or fungal etiologies more likely to result in overgrowth than bacterial
    - Slower joint destruction, so occurs over longer period of time, allowing chronic hyperemia
    - Less likely to have reactive osseous change than bacterial etiology
- **Epiphyseal Fracture, Pediatric**
  - Hyperemia with fracture healing results in overgrowth
  - Watch for malunion
- **Epiphyseal Dysplasia**
  - May be fragmented in severe cases or overgrown if less severe
- **Turner and Blount Disease (Mimics)**
  - Underdevelopment or collapse of medial tibial condyle results in relative overgrowth of medial femoral condyle

Juvenile Idiopathic Arthritis (JIA)

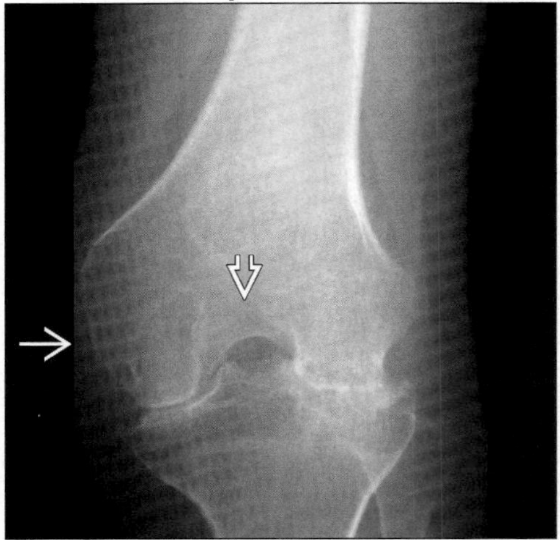

AP radiograph shows significant enlargement (overgrowth) of the femoral epiphyses ➡ relative to the diaphyses. There are severe erosions and widening of the intercondylar notch ➡ in this patient with JIA.

Hemophilia: MSK Complications

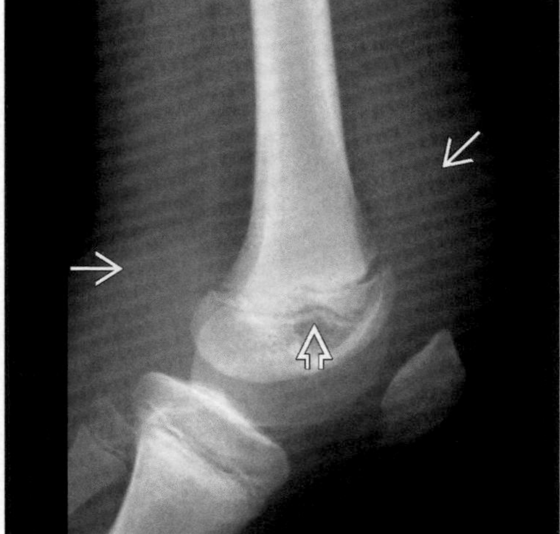

Lateral radiograph shows no erosions but a huge effusion ➡ in a hemophilic. There is a widened notch (displacement of Blumensaat line ➡). The epiphyses & patella are overgrown relative to the diaphyses.

Septic Joint

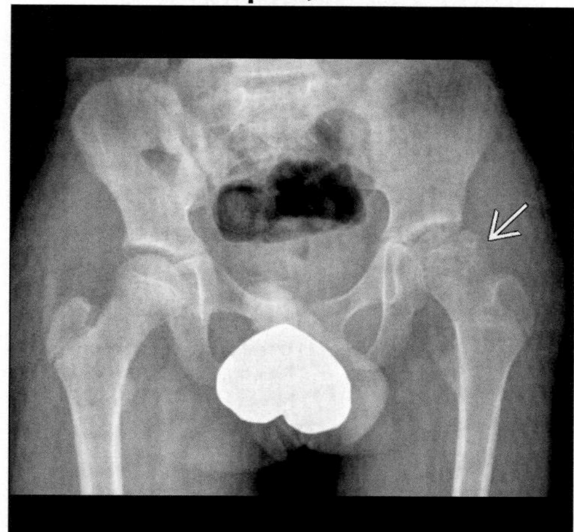

Epiphyseal Fracture, Pediatric

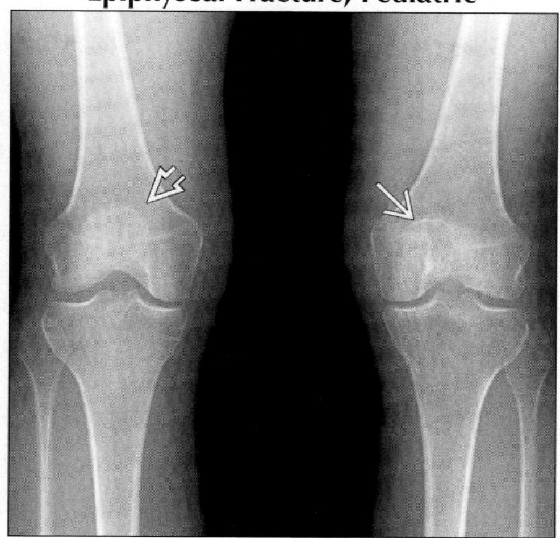

*(**Left**) AP radiograph shows an enlarged left femoral head and neck ➔. This 12 year old had a septic joint treated 9 months earlier. The hyperemia from the process resulted in overgrowth in this child. (**Right**) AP radiograph demonstrates relative overgrowth of the left patella and epiphyses ➔ (compare to normal right side ➔). The patient had a patellar fracture as a child, resulting in hyperemia, enough to result in overgrowth of the patella and adjacent femoral epiphyses.*

Epiphyseal Dysplasia

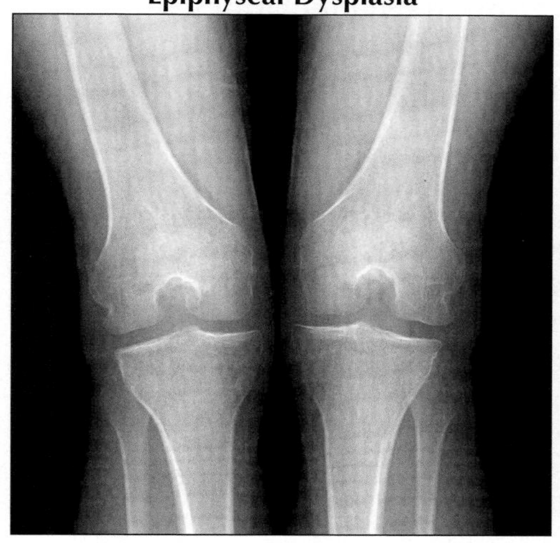

Turner Syndrome (Mimic)

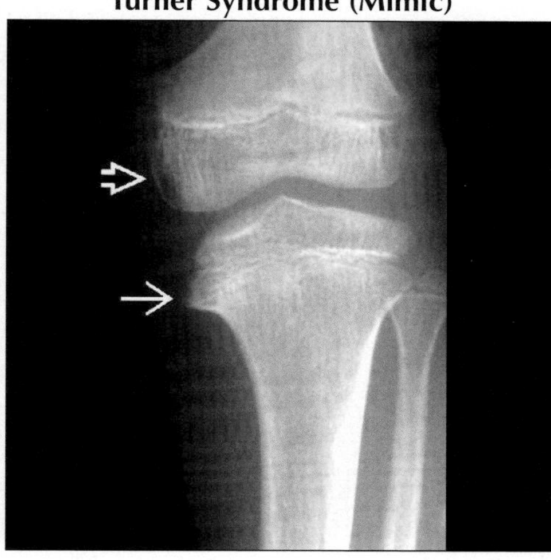

*(**Left**) AP radiograph shows symmetric enlarged femoral epiphyses, giving a "ballooned" appearance. Note also the morphologic flattening of the tibial plateaus. The patient is short; the diagnosis is spondyloepiphyseal dysplasia. (**Right**) AP radiograph shows relative flattening/underdevelopment of the medial tibial condyle ➔, which results in an overgrowth of the medial femoral condyle ➔. This appears as focal ballooning of the femoral epiphysis.*

Blount Disease (Mimic)

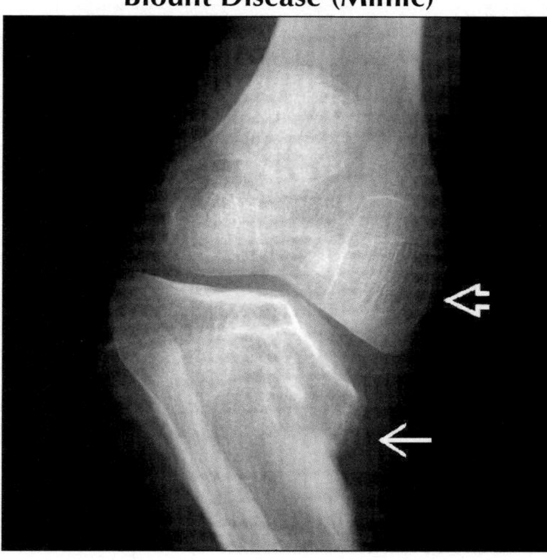

Meningococcemia (Mimic)

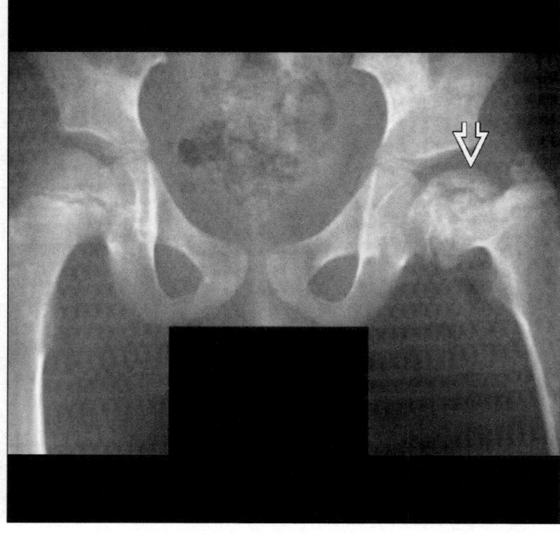

*(**Left**) AP radiograph shows collapse of the medial tibial metaphysis ➔ in Blount disease. There may be compensatory overgrowth of the medial femoral condyle ➔ but rarely enough to prevent a significant varus deformity. (**Right**) AP radiograph shows fragmentation and dysmorphic changes in the femoral capital epiphysis ➔ typical of meningococcemia. This mimics a ballooned epiphysis but is due to ischemia from thrombotic episodes.*

LONG BONE, EPIPHYSIS, SCLEROSIS/IVORY

DIFFERENTIAL DIAGNOSIS

Common
- Osteonecrosis (AVN)
- Renal Osteodystrophy

Less Common
- Cement & Bone Fillers, Normal
- Neoplasm
  - Chondroblastoma
  - Ewing Sarcoma
  - Osteosarcoma, Conventional
- Legg-Calvé-Perthes (LCP)
- Osteopoikilosis
- Osteopetrosis
- Pycnodysostosis

Rare but Important
- Down Syndrome (Trisomy 21)
- Hypopituitarism
- Hypothyroidism
- Turner Syndrome
- Morquio Syndrome
- Thiemann Disease
- Deprivation Dwarfism
- Multiple Epiphyseal Dysplasia
- Trichorhinophalangeal Dysplasia
- Seckel Syndrome
- Lesch-Nyhan
- Idiopathic Hypercalcemia
- Homocystinuria
- Complications of Fluoride

ESSENTIAL INFORMATION

Key Differential Diagnosis Issues
- Differentiate between extent of sclerosis
  - Focal, isolated to epiphysis
    - Osteonecrosis
    - Chondroblastoma
    - Legg-Calvé-Perthes
  - Epiphyseal/metaphyseal
    - Ewing sarcoma
    - Chondrosarcoma
    - Osteopoikilosis
  - Diffuse
    - Renal osteodystrophy
    - Osteopetrosis
    - Pycnodysostosis
    - All diagnoses listed as "rare but important"

Helpful Clues for Common Diagnoses
- **Osteonecrosis (AVN)**
  - Sclerosis is secondary to surrounding osteopenia (relative sclerosis)
    - Classic appearance is central sclerosis in femoral head
  - Later, sclerosis is secondary to osseous impaction from collapse
  - Even later, sclerosis is due to reparative bone formation
- **Renal Osteodystrophy**
  - Diffuse sclerosis, including epiphyses
    - May be part of primary disease, due to activation of osteoblasts
    - More prominent, as neostosis, when undergoing effective treatment
  - Indistinct trabeculae
  - Other signs of renal osteodystrophy
    - Rickets: Widened zone of provisional calcification, frayed metaphyses
    - Hyperparathyroidism: Resorption patterns (subperiosteal, endosteal, subchondral, subligamentous)
    - Soft tissue calcification

Helpful Clues for Less Common Diagnoses
- **Cement & Bone Fillers, Normal**
  - Commonly used to fill lesion sites following curettage
    - Most common lesion in epiphyseal region treated this way is giant cell tumor
  - Cement: Homogeneous, more dense than cortical bone
  - Nonstructural bone graft: Round or square pieces, same density as cortical bone
    - As it incorporates, approaches normal bone density
  - Rare use of coral as structure with haversian canal-like morphology to allow substitution by normal bone
- **Neoplasm**
  - **Chondroblastoma**
    - Most common epiphyseal neoplasm
    - Generally arise in skeletally immature (teenage, young adult) patients
    - Margin generally sclerotic
    - May contain chondroid matrix, resulting in greater sclerosis
    - Often elicits dense periosteal reaction
  - **Ewing Sarcoma**

- Generally metadiaphyseal lesion, but may cross into epiphysis (physis is only a relative barrier)
- Age range: 5-30 years
- Lesion generally is highly aggressive, with permeative destruction, cortical breakthrough, and soft tissue mass
- Rarely may be more indolent, remaining contained for variable amount of time
- Elicits significant osseous reaction, in form of new bone formation; this is source of sclerosis

- **Osteosarcoma, Conventional**
  - Generally metaphyseal in location but may cross into epiphysis
  - Highly aggressive lesion, with permeative bone destruction, cortical breakthrough, soft tissue mass
  - Tumor osteoid results in amorphous sclerosis, both in bone and in soft tissue mass

- **Legg-Calvé-Perthes (LCP)**
  - Osteonecrosis of femoral head in child
    - Age 4-8 most common
  - Early sign: Sclerosis of femoral head
  - Later signs
    - Fragmentation of femoral head
    - Flattening of femoral head
  - Late appearance
    - Coxa magna deformity (short, broad femoral head and neck)
    - Early development of osteoarthritis
- **Osteopoikilosis**
  - Round, regular, generally subcentimeter sclerotic lesions
    - Bone islands (hamartoma)
  - Epiphyseal and metaphyseal
  - Generally bilaterally symmetric
  - 1 of sclerosing dysplasias
  - Incidental finding
- **Osteopetrosis**
  - Severe sclerosing dysplasia, involving entire skeleton (axial and appendicular)
  - Homogeneously dense bones
  - Undertubulation of long bones
    - Due to poor function of osteoclasts; inhibits remodeling
    - May also be manifest as "bone-in-bone" appearance
- **Pycnodysostosis**
  - Severe sclerosing dysplasia, involving entire skeleton (axial & appendicular)
  - Homogeneously dense bones
  - Undertubulation of long bones
  - Similar in appearance to osteopetrosis
  - Morphologic differentiating factors
    - Wormian bones
    - Acroosteolysis
    - Small angle of jaw

Helpful Clues for Rare Diagnoses

- Those listed under "rare but important" are extraordinarily uncommon
  - Disease process itself is rare
  - Manifestation of sclerotic epiphyses in these diagnoses is even more rare

Osteonecrosis (AVN)

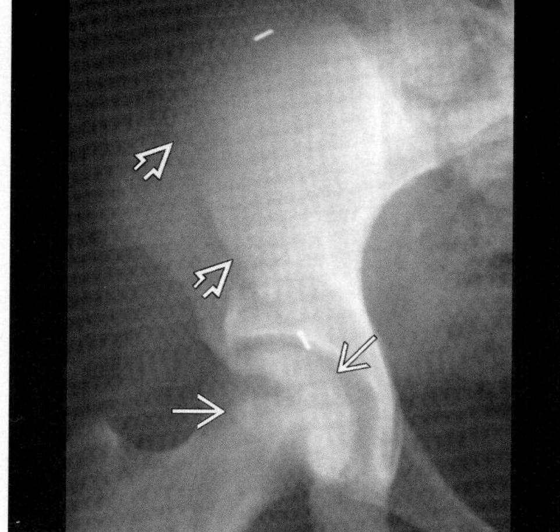

AP radiograph shows sclerosis in the femoral head ➡, an early indication of osteonecrosis. An outline of a renal transplant is seen in the iliac fossa ➡, indicating steroids as the etiology of the osteonecrosis.

Osteonecrosis (AVN)

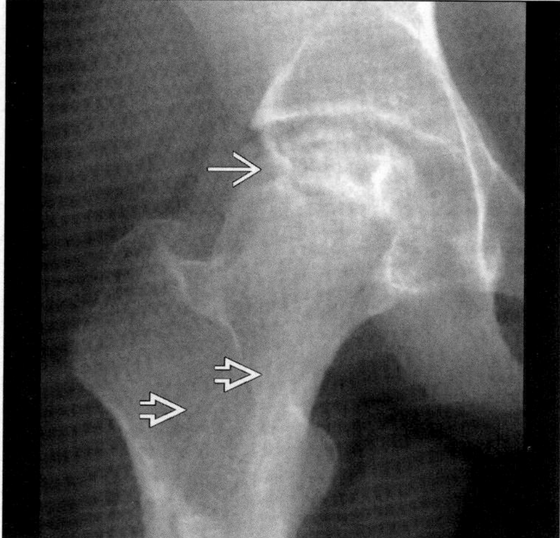

Anteroposterior radiograph shows sclerosis, flattening, and irregularity of the femoral head ➡ in a young adult. There are linear densities in the neck ➡, indicating pin tracks; the patient had SCFE, complicated by AVN.

LONG BONE, EPIPHYSIS, SCLEROSIS/IVORY

(Left) Anteroposterior radiograph shows diffuse increased density, including the humeral epiphysis. There is also subperiosteal resorption ➔ and a brown tumor ➔; the patient has renal osteodystrophy. *(Right)* Posteroanterior radiograph shows sclerosis in the radial epiphysis ➔, but there is also generalized increased density as well as indistinctness of the trabeculae. Endosteal resorptive pattern adds to the findings of renal osteodystrophy.

Renal Osteodystrophy

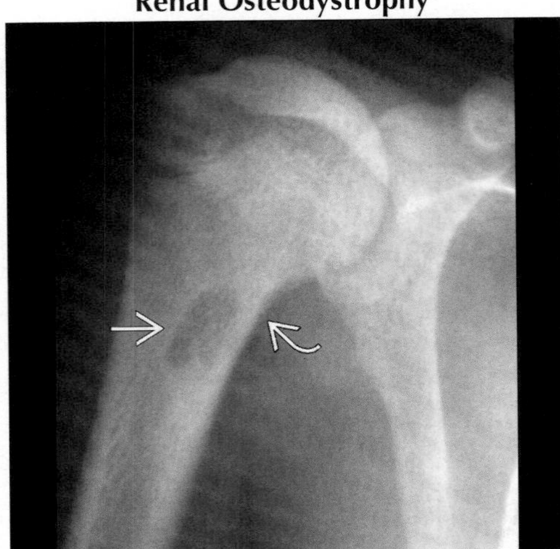

Renal Osteodystrophy

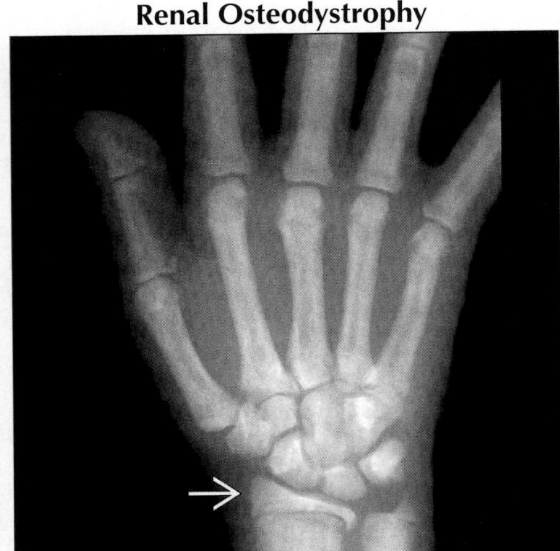

(Left) Lateral radiograph shows sclerosis of the ring apophyses and endplates ➔ in a patient with renal osteodystrophy, termed "rugger jersey" sign. *(Right)* Posteroanterior radiograph shows an expanded lytic lesion of the distal radius, which has been treated by curettage and bone grafting ➔. Nonstructural bone graft may have rounded or square pieces and should be differentiated from chondroid or osteoid matrix.

Renal Osteodystrophy

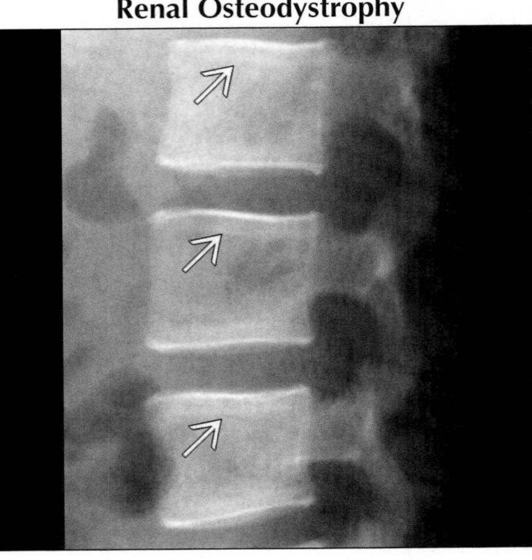

Cement & Bone Fillers, Normal

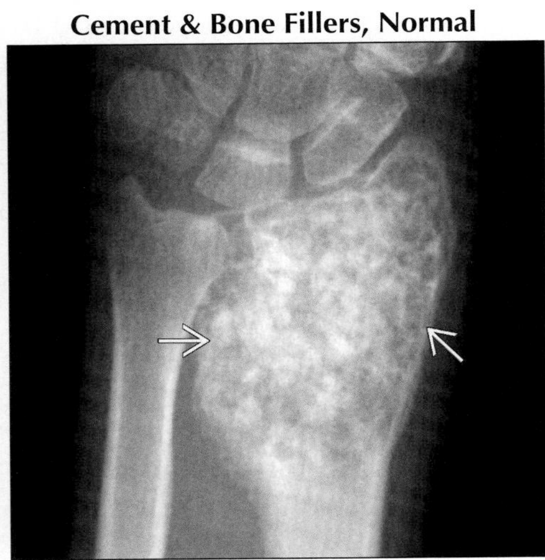

(Left) Anteroposterior radiograph shows dense material placed at the MTP joint ➔ following resection of a failed arthroplasty ➔. The material has canals the width of Haversian canals; it is a coral graft. *(Right)* Frog lateral radiograph shows an epiphyseal lesion with a dense sclerotic margin ➔, containing a small amount of chondroid matrix. The appearance is typical of a chondroblastoma.

Cement & Bone Fillers, Normal

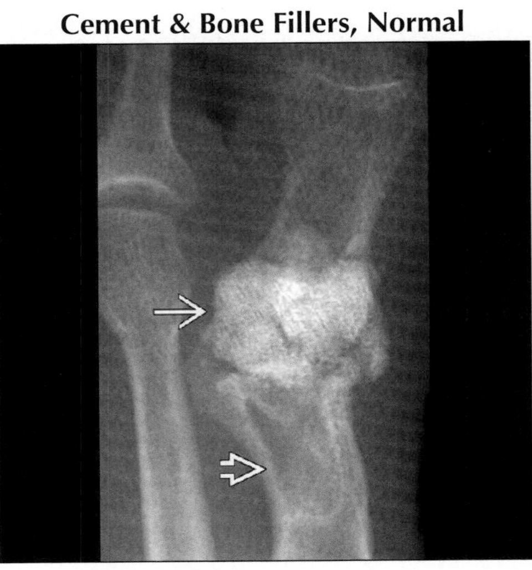

Chondroblastoma

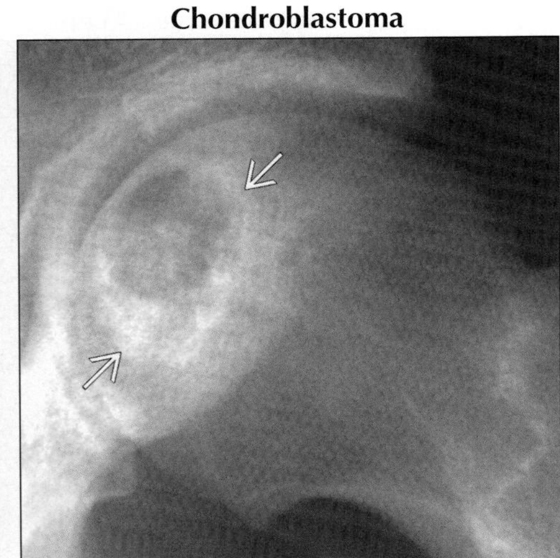

LONG BONE, EPIPHYSIS, SCLEROSIS/IVORY

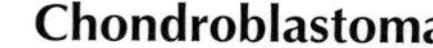

Chondroblastoma

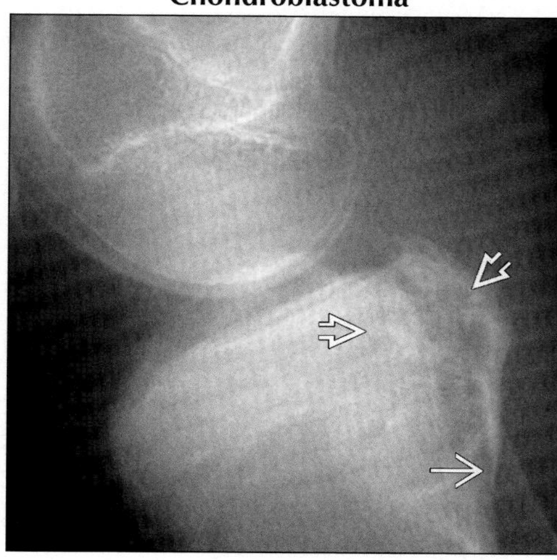

Ewing Sarcoma

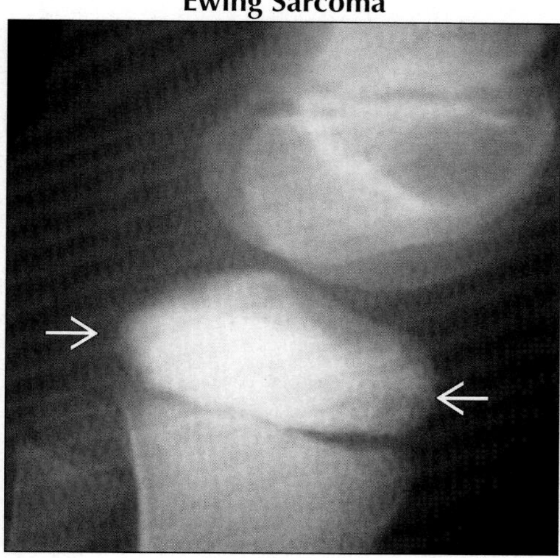

(Left) *Lateral radiograph shows a lytic lesion with surrounding dense sclerosis ⇨. There is thick, dense periosteal reaction →. The lesion is typical of a chondroblastoma.* ***(Right)*** *Lateral radiograph shows uniform sclerosis of the epiphysis → without destructive changes. This patient had Ewing sarcoma that originated in the metaphysis and extended to involve the epiphysis; the density is due to reactive change.*

Osteosarcoma, Conventional

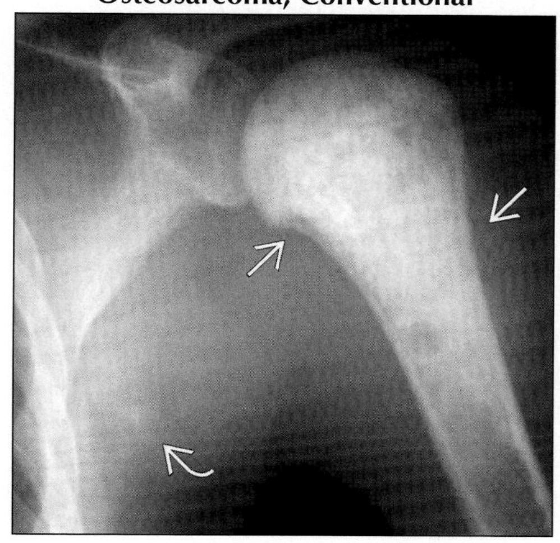

Legg-Calvé-Perthes (LCP)

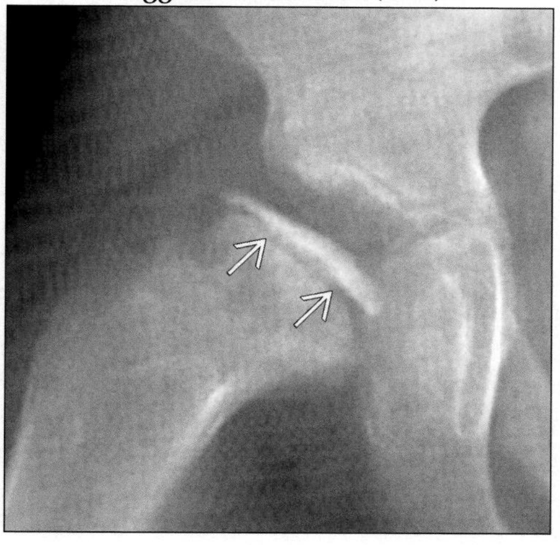

(Left) *Anteroposterior radiograph shows a densely sclerotic metaphysis, extending to the epiphysis, with periosteal reaction and a soft tissue mass →, all typical of osteosarcoma. There is an ossified lymph node metastasis ↪.* ***(Right)*** *Anteroposterior radiograph shows a flattened and sclerotic femoral capital epiphysis →. This is typical of advanced Legg-Calvé-Perthes disease and will develop into a coxa magna deformity.*

Osteopoikilosis

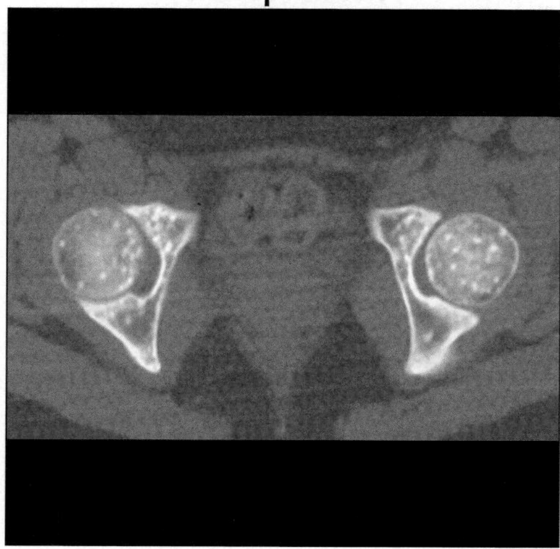

Osteopetrosis

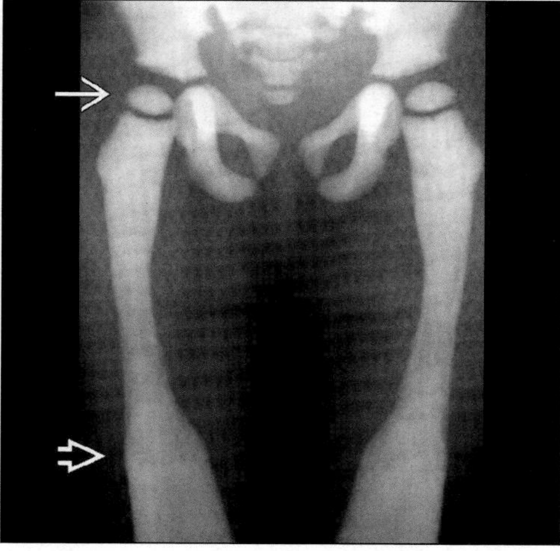

(Left) *Axial NECT shows multiple small, round, sclerotic densities in both femoral epiphyses and both acetabulae. The appearance is typical of osteopoikilosis, a sclerosing dysplasia.* ***(Right)*** *Anteroposterior radiograph shows uniform density of the epiphyses → as well as the remainder of the bones in this child. Note also the undertubulation of the femora ⇨, indicating poor remodeling with growth. This is typical osteopetrosis.*

LONG BONE, METAPHYSEAL BANDS AND LINES

DIFFERENTIAL DIAGNOSIS

Common
- Growth Arrest Lines
- Chronic Illness
- Trauma
- Normal Variant
- Disuse Osteoporosis
- Chemotherapy
- Malnutrition or Prolonged Hyperalimentation
- Hyperemia
- Heavy Metal or Chemical Ingestion
- Rickets
- Radiation

Less Common
- Leukemia
- Juvenile Idiopathic Arthritis (JIA)
- Ankylosing Spondylitis
- Complications of High Dose Drug Therapy (Non-Chemotherapeutic)
- Metastases
- Osteoporosis

Rare but Important
- Complications of Vitamin D
- Osteopetrosis
- Hypothyroidism, Treated
- Complications of Fluoride
- Hypoparathyroidism
- Pseudohypoparathyroidism
- Idiopathic Hypercalcemia
- Scurvy
- Congenital Infection
- Aminopterin Fetopathy
- Hypophosphatasia
- Erythroblastosis Fetalis
- Osteopathia Striata
- Primary Oxalosis

ESSENTIAL INFORMATION

Key Differential Diagnosis Issues
- Manifestations include: Dense horizontal bands (DB), lucent bands (LB), alternating dense and lucent bands (AB), vertical dense bands (VB)
  - AB indicate multiple insults separated in time
- Most are systemic, involve multiple physes
  - Especially at knee, wrist (sites of greatest growth)
- Isolated physeal involvement: Trauma, radiation, metastatic disease, disuse osteoporosis, hyperemia

Helpful Clues for Common Diagnoses
- **Growth Arrest Lines**
  - DB, VB: Sharply defined, thin dense lines
  - Variable distance from metaphysis depending on age of insult
  - Underlying insult may not be identifiable
- **Chronic Illness**
  - LB, VB: Any illness, including sickle cell anemia, rickets, osteogenesis imperfecta, neoplasm
  - LB: Nonspecific manifestation of illness
  - May develop DB during healing
- **Trauma**
  - LB: Acute injury, early healing
  - DB, VB: Healing Salter fractures, chronic injury, stress fracture
    - ± metaphyseal cupping/fraying
- **Normal Variant**
  - DB, LB: Otherwise normal skeleton
  - Normal fibula helps differentiate from other conditions, such as lead poisoning
- **Disuse Osteoporosis**
  - LB: Regional distribution
- **Chemotherapy**
  - LB, VB
- **Malnutrition or Prolonged Hyperalimentation**
  - LB
- **Hyperemia**
  - LB: Bone resorption leads to osteoporosis
  - Arthritis, infection
- **Heavy Metal or Chemical Ingestion**
  - DB, AB: Lead most common; lines are late manifestation
- **Rickets**
  - LB, VB (healing): Manifestation of bone resorption of hyperparathyroidism
- **Radiation**
  - VB, LB, DB; ± physeal widening, fraying
  - DB, AB during healing

Helpful Clues for Less Common Diagnoses
- **Leukemia**
  - LB: May also see osteolytic lesions, periostitis
  - DB, during healing
  - 2-5 years old
- **Juvenile Idiopathic Arthritis (JIA)**
  - LB due to hyperemia and chronic illness

- Monoarticular to symmetric polyarticular
- Uniform joint space narrowing, marginal erosions, periostitis

- **Ankylosing Spondylitis**
  - LB due to osteoporosis, hyperemia
  - Anterior and posterior spinal fusion
  - Symmetric sacroiliitis
  - Hip, shoulder arthritis; enthesopathy
- **Complications of High Dose Drug Therapy (Non-Chemotherapeutic)**
  - DB
- **Metastases**
  - LB, DB (during healing), especially neuroblastoma, lymphoma
    - Osteolytic lesions and periostitis from direct tumor invasion
- **Osteoporosis**
  - LB: Juvenile idiopathic, Cushing disease

Helpful Clues for Rare Diagnoses

- **Complications of Vitamin D**
  - DB, AB: Variable manifestations; osteoporosis, osteosclerosis, cortical thickening, soft tissue calcification
- **Osteopetrosis**
  - DB, LB, AB: Generalized osteosclerosis
  - Metaphyseal expansion
- **Hypothyroidism, Treated**
  - DB: Abnormal epiphyses
- **Complications of Fluoride**
  - DB: ↑ bone density, osteophytes, ligament calcification
  - Axial changes dominate
- **Hypoparathyroidism**
  - DB: Ligament and tendon ossification, axial and appendicular
  - Osteosclerosis, abnormal dentition, subcutaneous calcification
- **Pseudohypoparathyroidism**
  - DB: Same as hypoparathyroidism
  - Differentiating features
    - Short stature, developmental delay
    - Short metacarpals, especially 4 and 5
    - Subcutaneous calcification, ossification
- **Idiopathic Hypercalcemia**
  - DB: Diffuse bone sclerosis
- **Scurvy**
  - DB, LB: Orientation of growth plate to lucent line (scurvy line) to dense line
  - Metaphyseal beaks, periostitis
- **Congenital Infection**
  - DB, VB, "celery stalk"
  - Includes rubella, CMV, syphilis, herpes simplex, toxoplasmosis
- **Aminopterin Fetopathy**
  - DB
- **Hypophosphatasia**
  - LB, VB: Physis mimics rickets
- **Erythroblastosis Fetalis**
  - LB: Diffuse soft tissue edema
- **Osteopathia Striata**
  - VB: Mild metaphyseal expansion
  - Asymptomatic
- **Primary Oxalosis**
  - DB, AB ± renal osteodystrophy
  - "Drumstick" metacarpals
  - Renal calculi, parenchymal calcification
  - Vascular calcification

Growth Arrest Lines

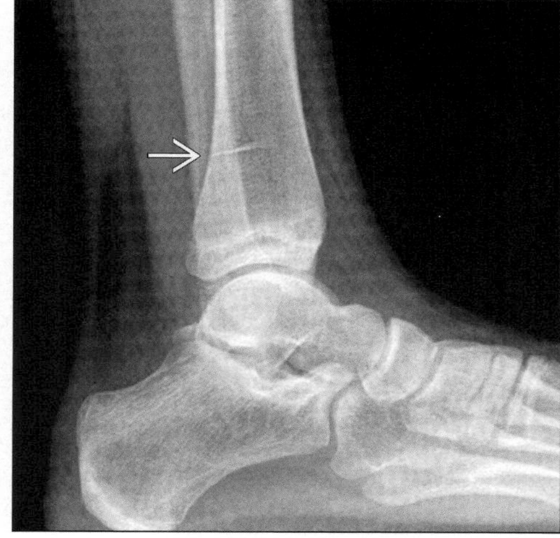

Lateral radiograph shows a single growth recovery line in the distal tibia ➔. In many cases, an underlying contributing cause is not known.

Growth Arrest Lines

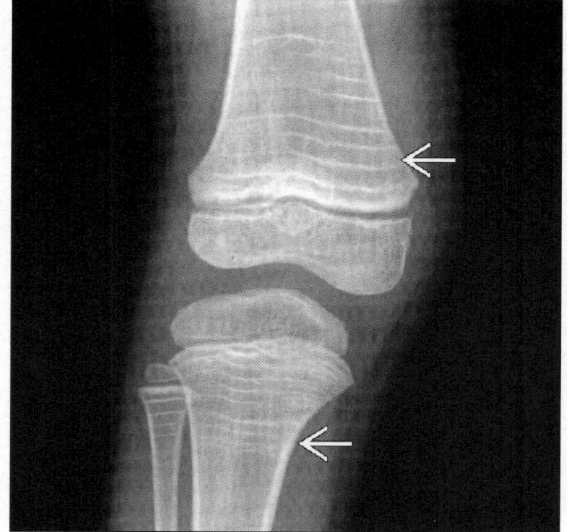

Anteroposterior radiograph shows diffuse osteopenia from osteogenesis imperfecta. Multiple metaphyseal lines ➔ are present,. corresponding to growth lines associated with bisphosphonate therapy.

LONG BONE, METAPHYSEAL BANDS AND LINES

*(**Left**) Anteroposterior radiograph shows irregularity of the physis with sclerosis along the metaphyseal margin ➔ in this Little League pitcher with a chronic repetitive injury. (**Right**) Anteroposterior radiograph shows a typical stress fracture with an ill-defined sclerotic line ➔ and adjacent periosteal new bone formation ➔.*

Trauma

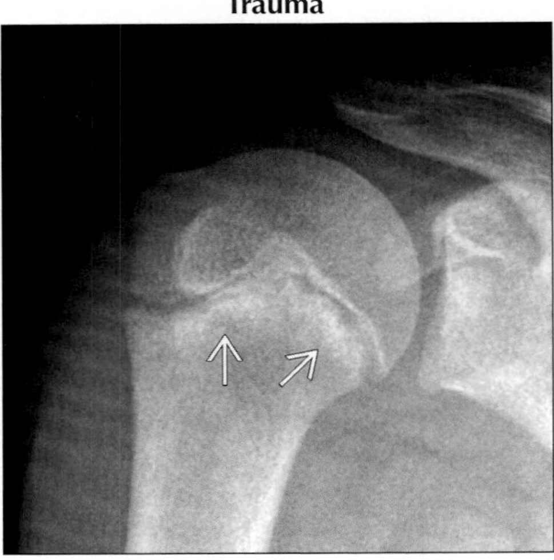

Trauma

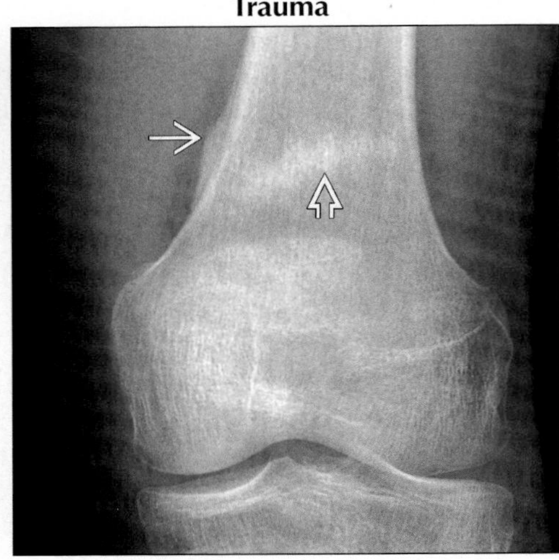

*(**Left**) Anteroposterior radiograph shows the appearance of normal physes ➔, mimicking dense metaphyseal bands. Differentiation from other entities, such as lead poisoning, can be difficult. (**Right**) Anteroposterior radiograph shows lucent metaphyseal band ➔, caused by disuse osteoporosis following immobilization after open reduction and internal fixation (ORIF) of a tibial diaphyseal fracture.*

Normal Variant

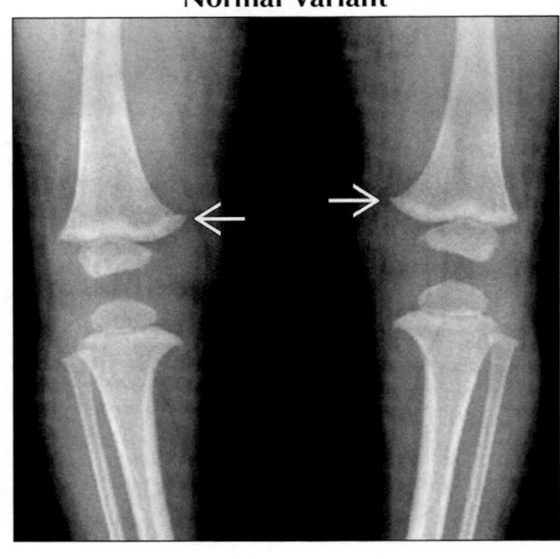

Disuse Osteoporosis

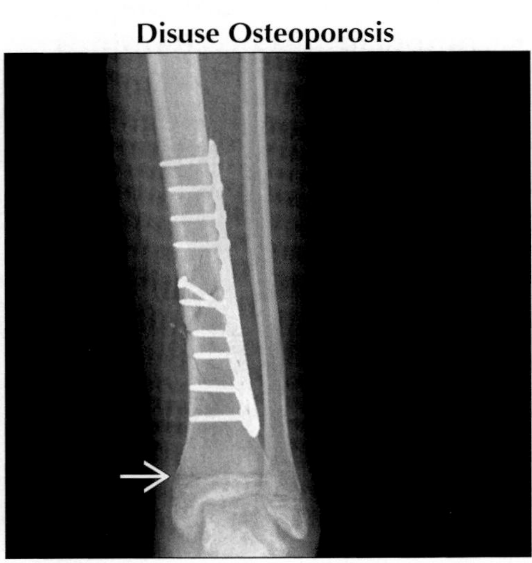

*(**Left**) Anteroposterior radiograph shows the classic dense metaphyseal lines ➔ seen with lead poisoning. Involvement of the fibula helps distinguish this appearance from a normal variant. (**Right**) Anteroposterior radiograph shows markedly abnormal physis in this patient with renal rickets. The physes are cupped and frayed with lucent and sclerotic metaphyseal bands ➔.*

Heavy Metal or Chemical Ingestion

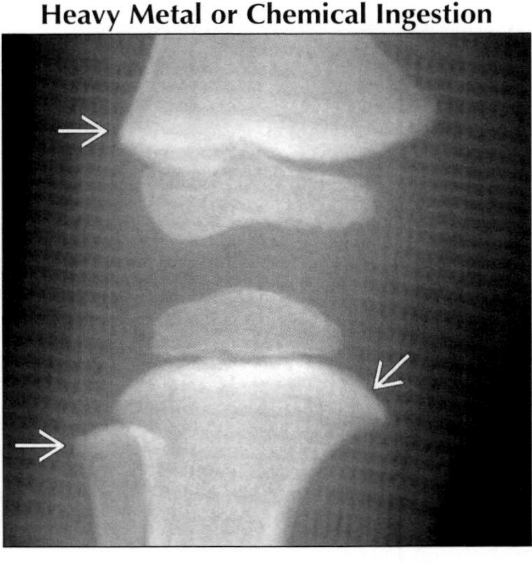

Rickets

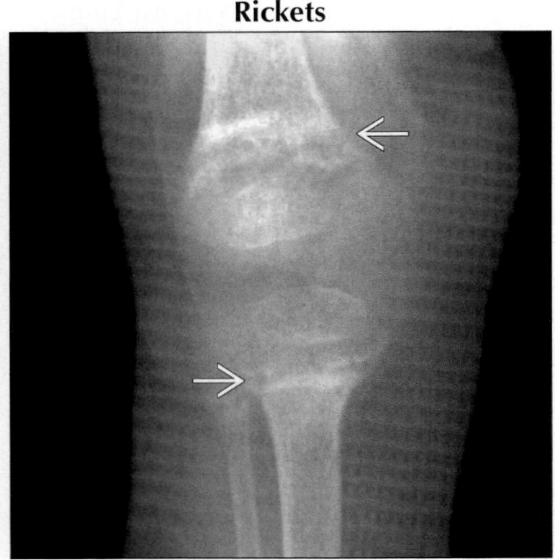

LONG BONE, METAPHYSEAL BANDS AND LINES

Leukemia

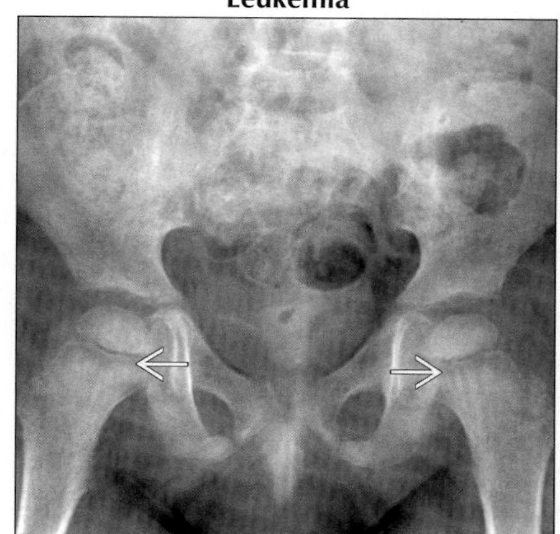

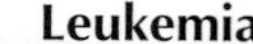

Leukemia

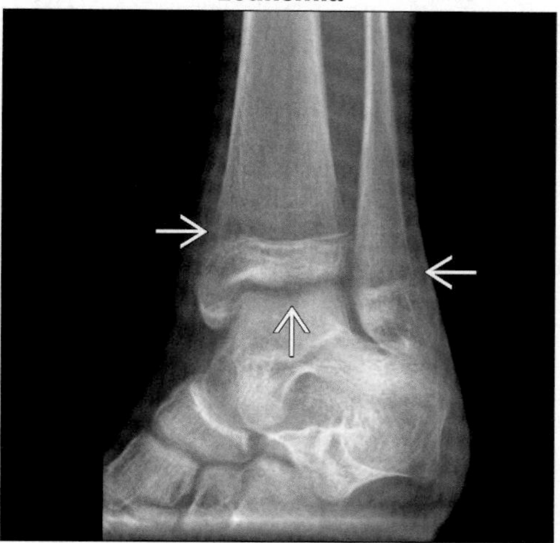

(Left) *Anteroposterior radiograph shows diffuse osteopenia and subtle lucent metaphyseal bands ➡ in this patient with leukemia.* ***(Right)*** *Oblique radiograph shows the typical appearance of leukemic metaphyseal lucent lines ➡ at the ankle.*

Ankylosing Spondylitis

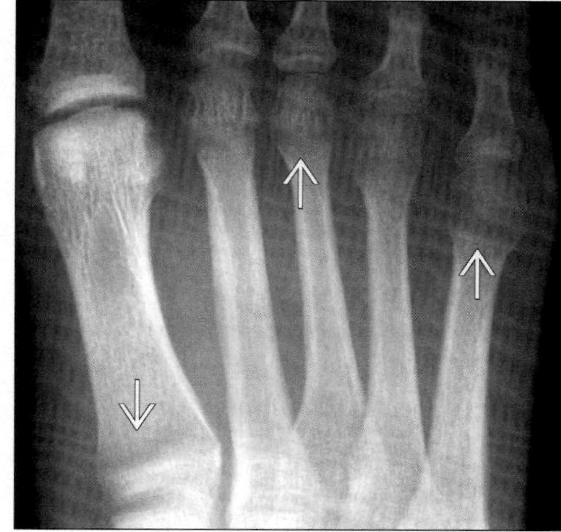

Scurvy

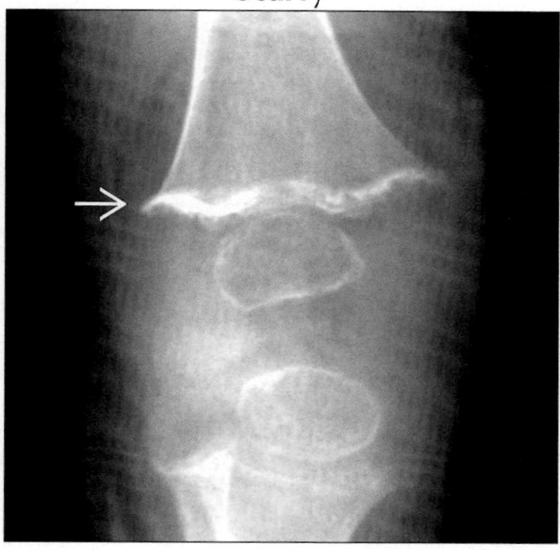

(Left) *Anteroposterior radiograph shows lucent bands at the metaphyses ➡ as an early manifestation of osteoporosis in a patient with hyperemia from ankylosing spondylosis.* ***(Right)*** *Anteroposterior radiograph shows classic signs of scurvy, including diffuse osteopenia and dense lines at the metaphyses and epiphyses. The dense metaphyseal line ➡ is known as the white line of Frankel.*

Congenital Infection

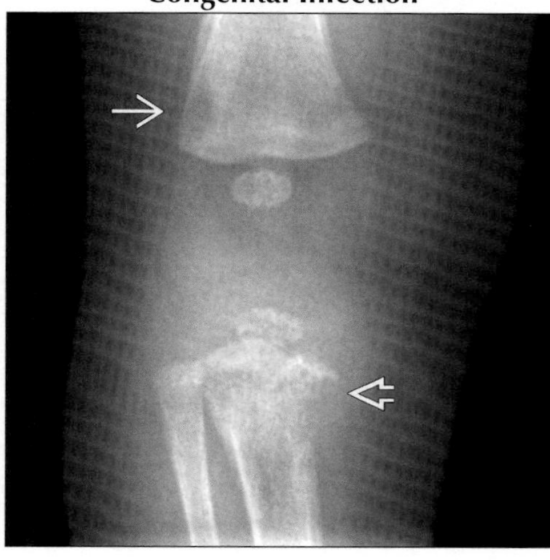

Congenital Infection

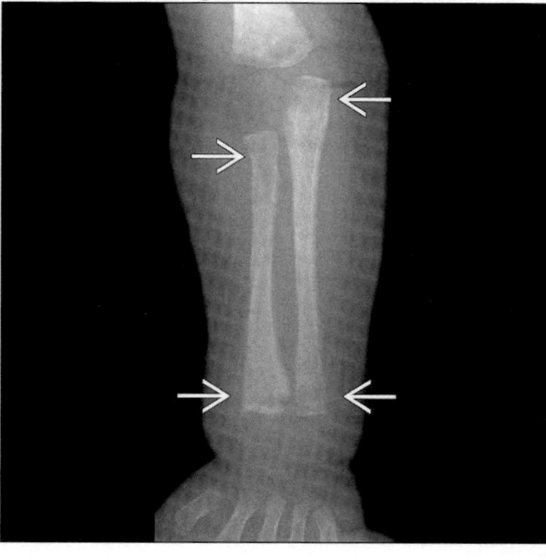

(Left) *Anteroposterior radiograph shows typical appearance of syphilis on radiographs. The tibias show Wimberger signs ➡ and generalized metaphyseal osteitis, which appears as lucent bands ➡.* ***(Right)*** *Anteroposterior radiograph shows a typical appearance of congenital syphilis with generalized metaphyseal osteitis manifesting as metaphyseal lucencies ➡.*

LONG BONE, METAPHYSEAL CUPPING

DIFFERENTIAL DIAGNOSIS

Common
- Normal Variant
- Child Abuse, Metaphyseal Fx (Mimic)

Less Common
- Renal Osteodystrophy
- Rickets
- Pediatric Fracture
- Prolonged Immobilization
- Sickle Cell Anemia

Rare but Important
- Post Infection
- Radiation Induced
- Scurvy
- Hypophosphatasia
- Achondroplasia
- Metaphyseal Dysplasias
- Polio (Prolonged Immobilization)
- Hypervitaminosis A

ESSENTIAL INFORMATION

Key Differential Diagnosis Issues
- Rickets, renal osteodystrophy, and hypophosphatasia: Overgrowth of disorganized chondrocytes
  - **Hint**: Involves sites of rapid growth: Distal radius/ulna, distal femur, proximal tibia, costochondral articulations
- Other entities: Oligemia, thrombosis create central metaphyseal depression; causative insult need not be at growth plate
  - May be isolated or involve random sites

Helpful Clues for Common Diagnoses
- **Child Abuse, Metaphyseal Fx (Mimic)**
  - Horizontal shear through growth plate; periostitis during healing

Helpful Clues for Less Common Diagnoses
- **Renal Osteodystrophy**
  - Combination of rickets & hyperparathyroidism
- **Pediatric Fracture**
  - Delayed complication
- **Prolonged Immobilization**
  - Associated disuse osteoporosis
- **Sickle Cell Anemia**
  - Metacarpals, metatarsals; AVN, infarcts, coarse trabecula, dactylitis, osteomyelitis

Helpful Clues for Rare Diagnoses
- **Radiation Induced**
  - Regional mixed ↑ & ↓ bone density
- **Scurvy**
  - Subperiosteal hemorrhage, osteopenia
- **Hypophosphatasia**
  - Coarse trabecula, osteopenia
- **Achondroplasia**
  - Short femora and humeri; spine and pelvic anomalies
- **Metaphyseal Dysplasias**
  - Short stature, bowing of long bones
- **Polio (Prolonged Immobilization)**
  - Especially knees, metatarsals; muscle wasting, thin gracile osteoporotic bones
- **Hypervitaminosis A**
  - Hyperostosis, premature physeal fusion

Child Abuse, Metaphyseal Fx (Mimic)

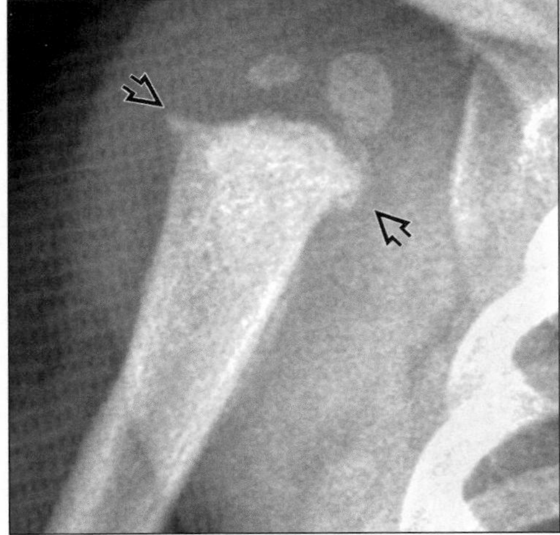

Anteroposterior radiograph shows 2 metaphyseal corner fractures ⇨ of the upper humerus in this victim of child abuse. The fractures mimic the appearance of a widened and cupped metaphysis.

Renal Osteodystrophy

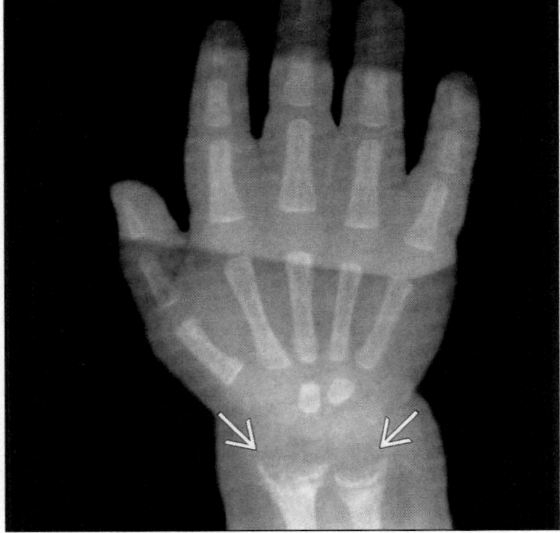

Posteroanterior radiograph shows a widened zone of provisional calcification and cupping/fraying of the metaphyses of the radius and ulna ➔ in this child with chronic renal disease.

LONG BONE, METAPHYSEAL CUPPING

Rickets

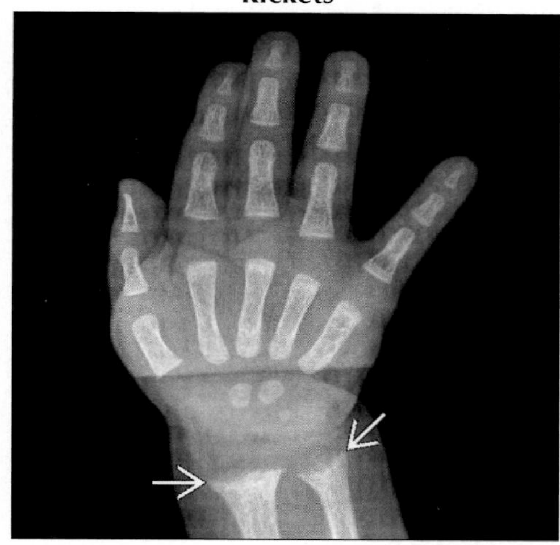

Rickets

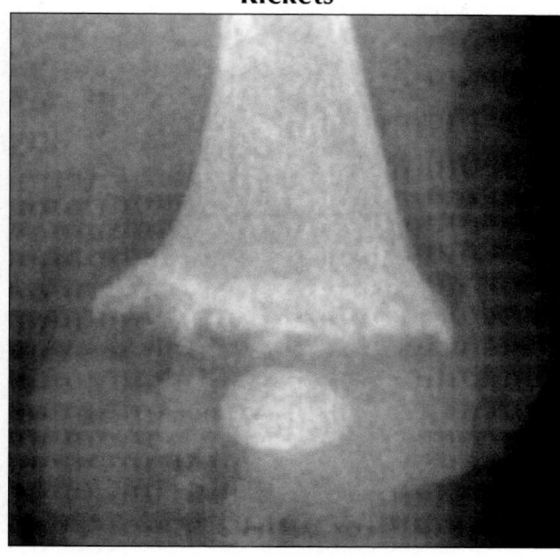

*(**Left**) Anteroposterior radiograph shows changes of nutritional deficiency rickets, including metaphyseal cupping and fraying of the distal radius and ulna ➡. (**Right**) Anteroposterior radiograph shows changes of rickets. The growth plate changes are due to an increase in the number of chondrocytes with loss of the normal columnar organization, leading to widening and cupping of the growth plate.*

Scurvy

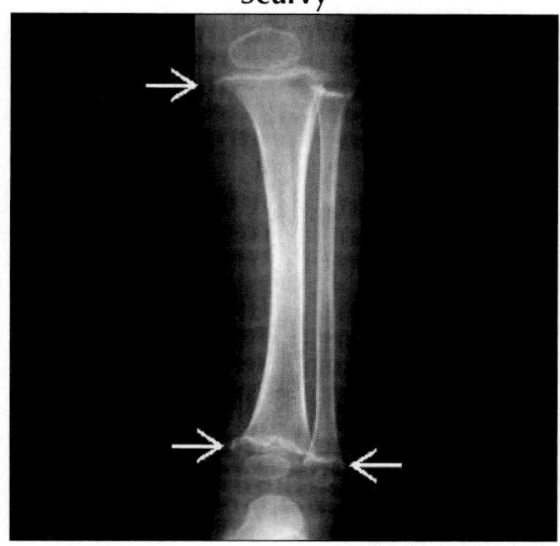

Hypophosphatasia

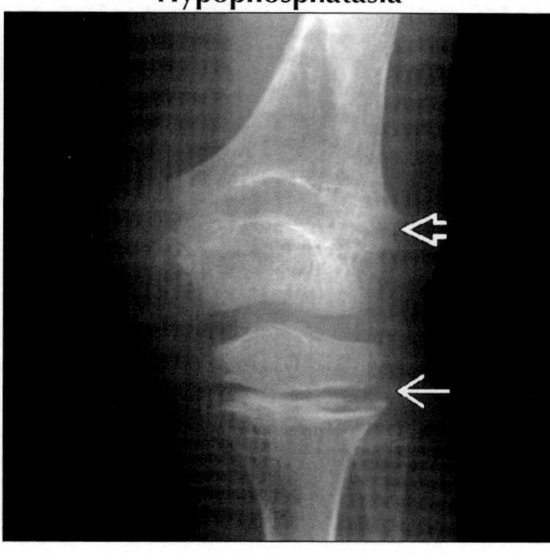

*(**Left**) Anteroposterior radiograph shows classic signs of scurvy, including osteopenia and dense lines at the metaphyses and epiphyses. Mild cupping is present at the proximal and distal metaphyses of both tibia and fibula ➡. (**Right**) Anteroposterior radiograph of a patient with hypophosphatasia shows osteopenia and a widened zone of provisional ossification of the growth plates ➡ with mild cupping of the distal femur ➡.*

Achondroplasia

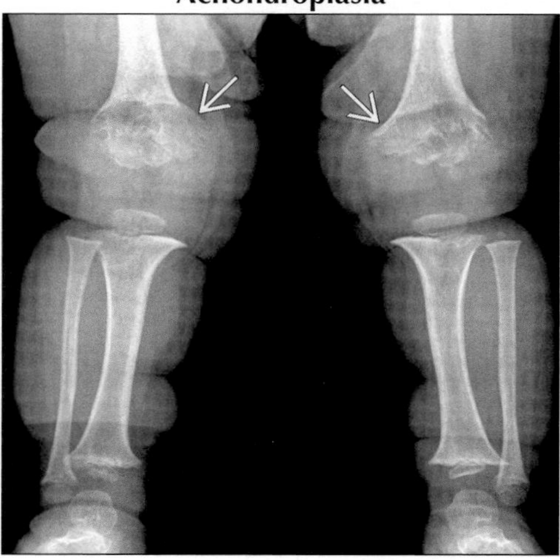

Metaphyseal Dysplasias

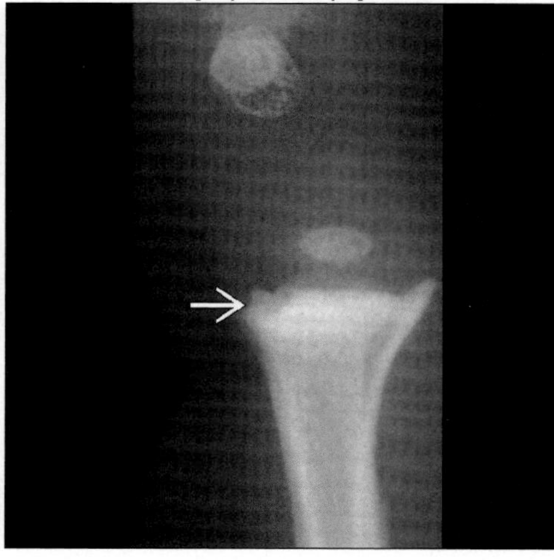

*(**Left**) Anteroposterior radiograph shows flaring (cupping) of the metaphyses of the distal femora ➡ in this patient with achondroplasia. (**Right**) Lateral radiograph shows widening of the distal radial metaphysis ➡ with mild irregularity of the growth plate in this patient with metaphyseal dysplasia.*

LONG BONE, METAPHYSEAL FRAYING

DIFFERENTIAL DIAGNOSIS

Common
- Chronic Repetitive Trauma
- Osteomyelitis, Pediatric
- Physeal Fractures, Pediatric
- Child Abuse, Metaphyseal Fracture

Less Common
- Rickets
- Thermal Injury
- Neuropathic Disease

Rare but Important
- Radiation
- Hypophosphatasia
- Copper Deficiency, Infantile
- Metaphyseal Chondrodysplasias

ESSENTIAL INFORMATION

Key Differential Diagnosis Issues
- **Hint**: Differentiate isolated/multisite from systemic involvement
  - Systemic: Sites of rapid growth = proximal and distal tibia/fibula, distal radius/ulna
  - Isolated/multisite: Chronic repetitive trauma, osteomyelitis, fracture, thermal injury, neuropathic disease, radiation
- Metaphyseal sclerosis common
- Periosteal new bone with fractures, trauma, osteomyelitis, neuropathic disease

Helpful Clues for Common Diagnoses
- **Chronic Repetitive Trauma**
  - Sport/situation and site specific
- **Osteomyelitis, Pediatric**
  - Focal metaphyseal osteopenia and destruction
- **Physeal Fractures, Pediatric**
  - Any healing fracture or avulsion
- **Child Abuse, Metaphyseal Fracture**
  - Corner fractures, cupping late

Helpful Clues for Less Common Diagnoses
- **Rickets**
  - Metaphyseal osteolysis & cupping, coarse ill-defined trabecula, rachitic rosary, enlarged knees, ankles, & wrists
  - Generalized osteopenia, delayed skeletal maturation, bowing
- **Thermal Injury**
  - Soft tissues changes, including calcification
- **Neuropathic Disease**
  - Exaggerated changes, including extensive fragmentation

Helpful Clues for Rare Diagnoses
- **Radiation**
  - Regional osteopenia
- **Hypophosphatasia**
  - **Hint**: Distinct finger-like lucent extension into metaphysis from growth plate
  - Osteopenia, cranial synostosis, bowing, fractures, metaphyseal spurs
- **Copper Deficiency, Infantile**
  - Metaphyseal cupping and spurs, hypotonia, seizures, mental retardation
- **Metaphyseal Chondrodysplasia**
  - Metaphyseal cupping, short stature, bowing

Chronic Repetitive Trauma

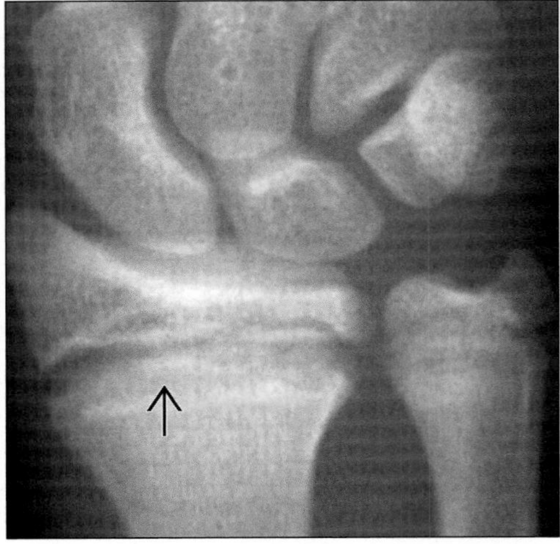

Anteroposterior radiograph shows osteolysis of the distal radius ⇒ in a skeletally immature patient. This is a form of chronic Salter 1 injury that is seen particularly in young gymnasts.

Chronic Repetitive Trauma

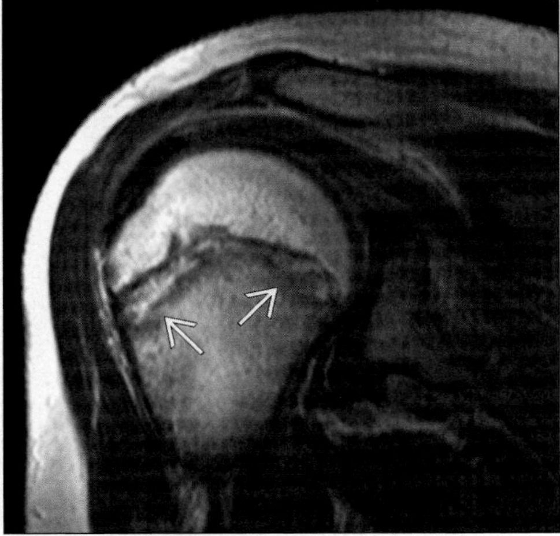

Coronal oblique T1WI MR shows widening and irregularity of the physis ➡ in this Little League pitcher with chronic injury from throwing curve balls.

Osteomyelitis, Pediatric

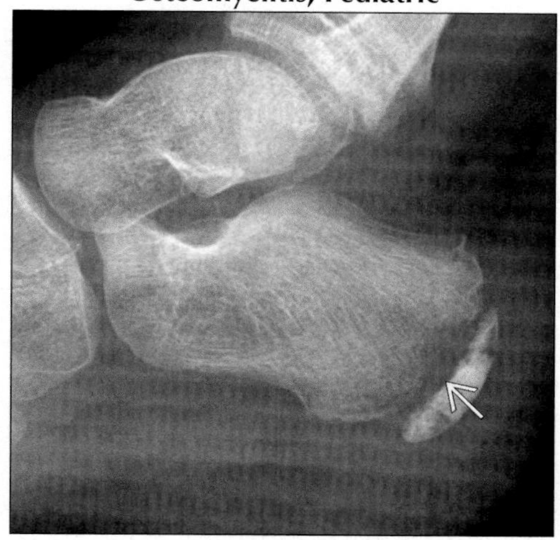

Physeal Fractures, Pediatric

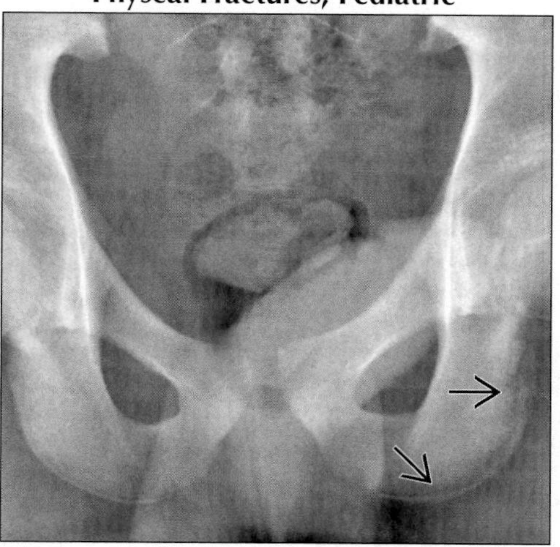

*(**Left**) Lateral radiograph shows demineralization of the posterior calcaneus with irregularity of the central portion of the metaphyseal side of the growth plate ➡ in this patient with biopsy and culture-proven osteomyelitis. (**Right**) Anteroposterior radiograph shows changes of a healing ischial tuberosity avulsion. The growth plate is widened and irregular ➡ when compared to the opposite normal physis.*

Child Abuse, Metaphyseal Fracture

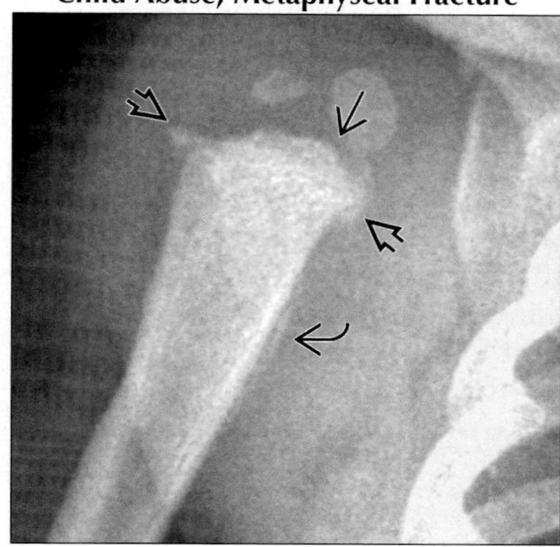

Rickets

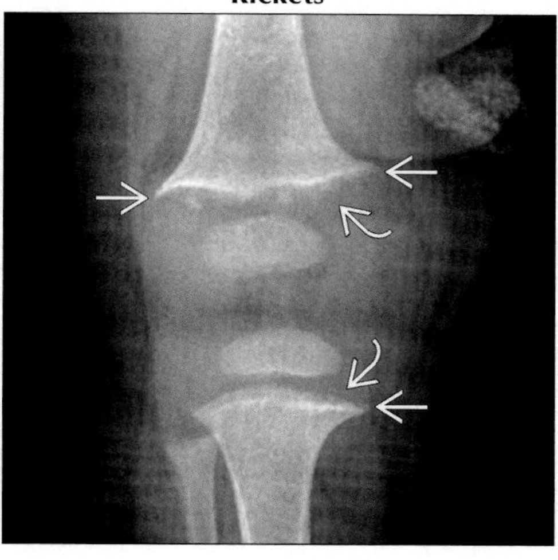

*(**Left**) Anteroposterior radiograph shows 2 metaphyseal corner fractures ➡ of the upper humerus. Periosteal reaction is occurring along the shaft ➡. The metaphyseal margin of the growth plate has lost its normal sharp margin ➡, indicating injury throughout the physis. (**Right**) Anteroposterior radiograph shows typical bone changes in nutritional rickets. The metaphyses are widened (cupping) ➡, and the margins of the growth plate are irregular (fraying) ➡.*

Rickets

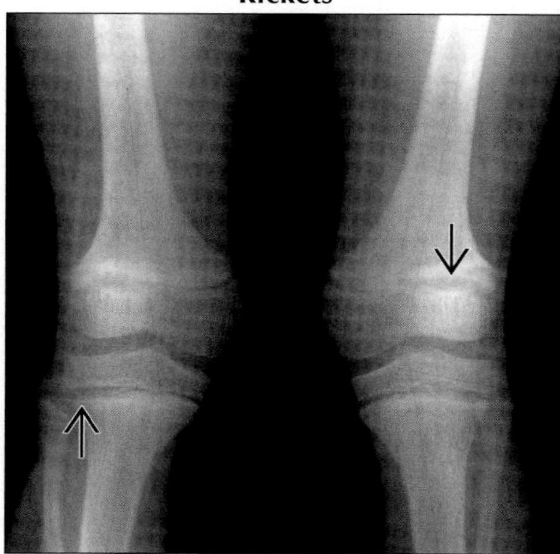

Hypophosphatasia

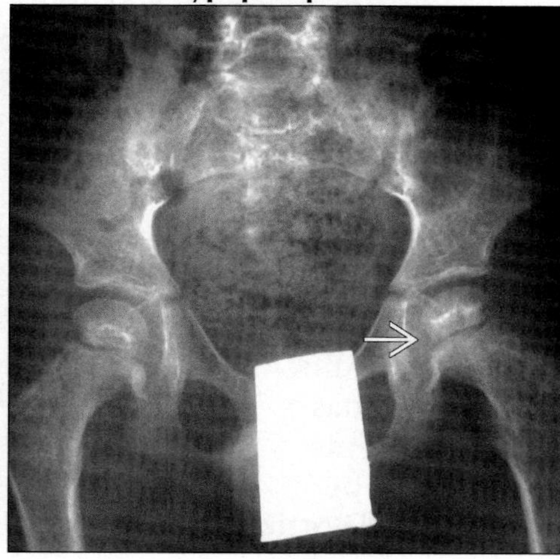

*(**Left**) Anteroposterior radiograph shows a widened zone of provisional calcification at all the physes of the knee ➡ in this patient with nutritional rickets. The weakened physes have caused a valgus deformity to develop. (**Right**) Anteroposterior radiograph shows a widened zone of provisional ossification at the physes ➡ as well as diffuse osteopenia. Serological studies proved hypophosphatasia.*

LONG BONE, DIAPHYSEAL LESION, AGGRESSIVE

DIFFERENTIAL DIAGNOSIS

Common
- Osteomyelitis, Pediatric
- Ewing Sarcoma
- Langerhans Cell Histiocytosis (LCH)
- Leukemia
- Osteosarcoma
- Metastases, Bone Marrow
- Lymphoma

Less Common
- Sickle Cell Anemia
- Malignant Fibrous Histiocytoma, Bone
- Chondrosarcoma, Conventional
- Adamantinoma
- Radiation-Induced Sarcoma

Rare but Important
- Hemophilia
- Congenital Syphilis

ESSENTIAL INFORMATION

Key Differential Diagnosis Issues
- **Hint**: Most common of these lesions fall into small, round, blue cell category
  - All have appearance that may be indistinguishable from one another
  - Must consider each of these diagnoses with this aggressive appearance
    - Osteomyelitis
    - Ewing sarcoma
    - Langerhans cell histiocytosis
    - Leukemia
    - Metastases
    - Lymphoma
  - **Hint**: Note that in each of these cases, lesion may be polyostotic
- **Hint**: Ewing sarcoma and osteosarcoma usually have distinct appearance from one another
  - Occasionally they can be indistinguishable, if
    - Osteosarcoma is diaphyseal and lytic
    - Ewing sarcoma is metadiaphyseal and has sclerotic reactive bone formation
    - **Hint**: In these cases, watch for tumor osteoid formation in soft tissue mass; this can only occur in osteosarcoma
- **Hint**: Rarely, 4 of these lesions may be aggressive, yet induce endosteal and cortical thickening
  - Osteomyelitis
  - Ewing sarcoma
  - Lymphoma
  - Chondrosarcoma

Helpful Clues for Common Diagnoses
- **Osteomyelitis, Pediatric**
  - Usually metaphyseal in children but diaphyseal with direct trauma
  - Highly aggressive and permeative, often with reactive sclerosis and periosteal reaction
- **Ewing Sarcoma**
  - Common in long bones in children
  - Highly aggressive permeative lesion, cortical breakthrough, and soft tissue mass
  - Elicits reactive bone formation
    - May have appearance of tumor osteoid & mimic osteosarcoma
    - Reactive bone NOT in soft tissue mass in Ewing but present in osteosarcoma
  - May appear polyostotic since it may present with osseous metastases
- **Langerhans Cell Histiocytosis (LCH)**
  - Ranges in appearance between geographic nonaggressive and highly aggressive
    - When aggressive, is permeative and may have soft tissue mass
    - May be indistinguishable from malignant lesions in differential
  - Often polyostotic
  - Beveled edge of skull lesion may help distinguish
- **Leukemia**
  - Usually polyostotic
  - May be so highly infiltrative that it is not visible on radiograph; MR makes diagnosis
- **Osteosarcoma**
  - Common lesion but usually is metaphyseal
  - Less frequently is diaphyseal; if it is lytic in this location, may not be distinguished from other lesions in differential
  - Usually some tumor osteoid is visible
- **Metastases, Bone Marrow**
  - Usually polyostotic in children
  - Metaphyseal is more frequent but may be diaphyseal
  - Neuroblastoma is most frequent in children
- **Lymphoma**
  - 50% of childhood lymphomas are polyostotic at presentation

- Highly aggressive; metaphyseal more frequent than diaphyseal

Helpful Clues for Less Common Diagnoses

- **Sickle Cell Anemia**
  - Early bone infarcts (particularly dactylitis) present with periosteal reaction
  - With evolution of infarct, will see mixed lytic and sclerotic pattern
    - Often longitudinal, involving entire diaphysis
    - Remember that bone infarct need not be serpiginous and subchondral, especially in sickle cell patients
- **Malignant Fibrous Histiocytoma, Bone**
  - Unusual lesion in children; may be seen in teenagers
  - Aggressive; may be metaphyseal or diaphyseal
  - No other distinguishing characteristics
- **Chondrosarcoma, Conventional**
  - Uncommon in children
  - Should be considered if subtle matrix is seen in diaphyseal lesion of teenager
  - May induce endosteal thickening rather than showing cortical breakthrough
- **Adamantinoma**
  - Almost invariably tibial metadiaphysis; cortically based
  - Generally only moderately aggressive initially
    - May become aggressive and malignant
- **Radiation-Induced Sarcoma**
  - Generally at least 7 years post-radiation (RT), so typically seen in teenagers
  - Highly aggressive lesion in bone that shows underlying radiation-related abnormality
    - Usually osteosarcoma, tumor osteoid
  - Consider locations likely to be radiated in childhood
    - Long bones (Ewing sarcoma, lymphoma)
    - Spine (Wilms tumor, leukemia)
  - Watch for underlying signs of radiation osteonecrosis
    - Mixed lytic and sclerotic, disordered bone
  - Watch for growth deformities associated with radiation
    - Long bone may be short if subjected to whole bone radiation (physes at risk for vascular injury in RT)
    - Spine may develop scoliosis if not completely included in radiation field
  - Watch for port-like distribution of osseous abnormalities, indicating RT

Helpful Clues for Rare Diagnoses

- **Hemophilia**
  - Pseudotumor appears aggressive: Soft tissue, intraosseous, and subperiosteal bleeds
  - Femur most commonly involved long bone
- **Congenital Syphilis**
  - Periosteal reaction, infiltrative appearance

Osteomyelitis, Pediatric

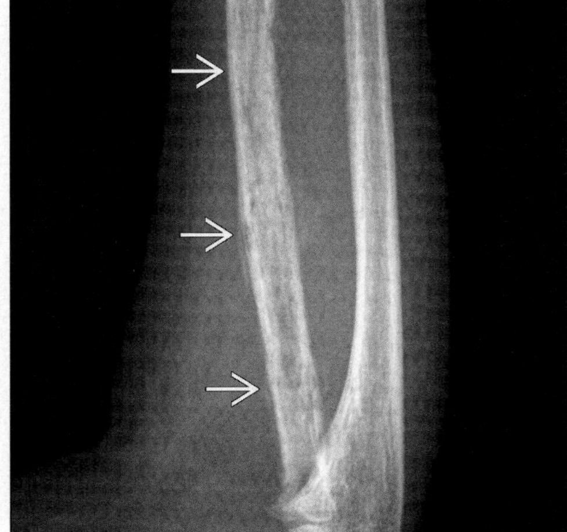

AP radiograph shows a highly aggressive lesion in the radial diaphysis ➔ in a 7 year old. There is prominent periosteal reaction and cortical breakthrough. The fat planes are obliterated, indicating osteomyelitis.

Osteomyelitis, Pediatric

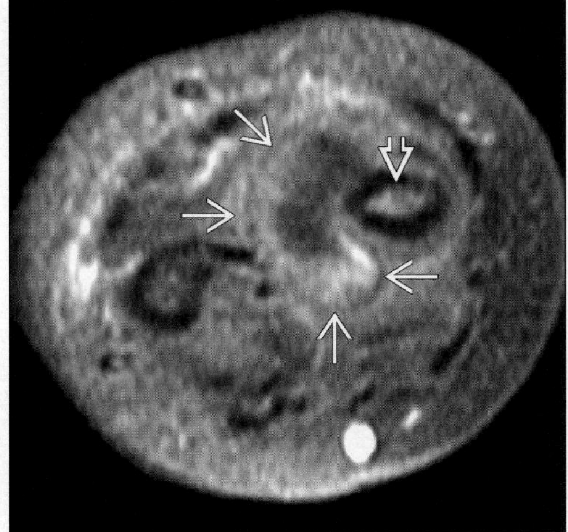

Axial T1 C+ MR in the same patient shows infiltration of the marrow of the radius ➔ and a large soft tissue abscess ➔, confirming the diagnosis of osteomyelitis. This child had direct trauma to the forearm.

LONG BONE, DIAPHYSEAL LESION, AGGRESSIVE

Ewing Sarcoma

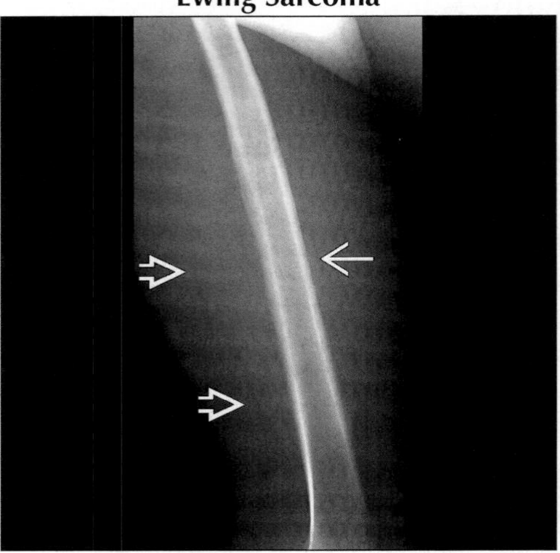

Langerhans Cell Histiocytosis (LCH)

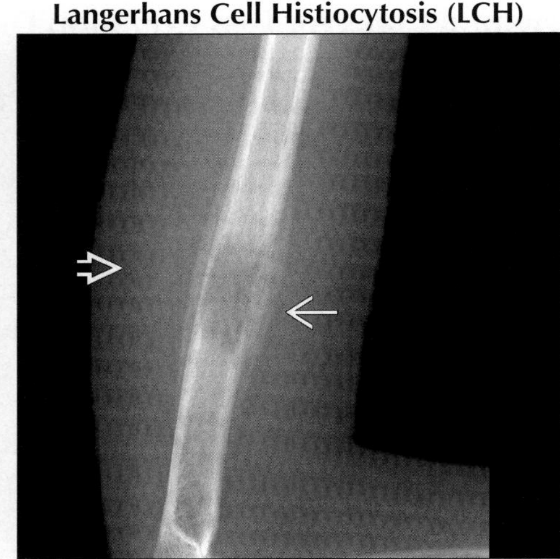

(Left) Lateral radiograph shows a permeative mid-diaphyseal lesion in a 10 year old. There is periosteal reaction ➡ and a large soft tissue mass ⇨; this is the classic age and appearance for Ewing sarcoma. (Right) Lateral radiograph shows a highly permeative diaphyseal lesion with prominent periosteal reaction ➡, cortical breakthrough, and a soft tissue mass ⇨ in an 8 year old. This case appears as aggressive as the previous case of Ewing sarcoma but proved to be LCH.

Leukemia

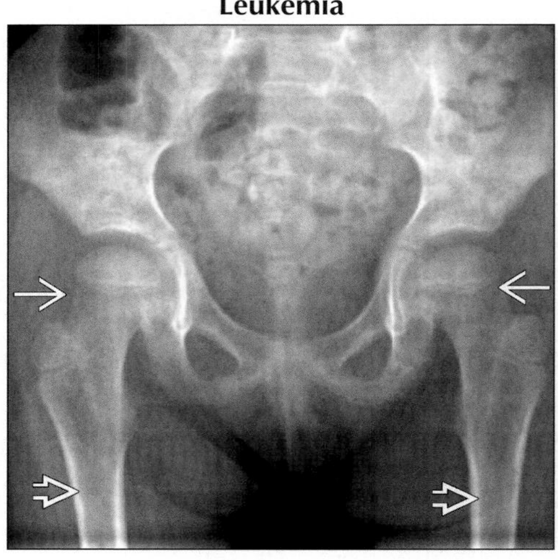

Osteosarcoma

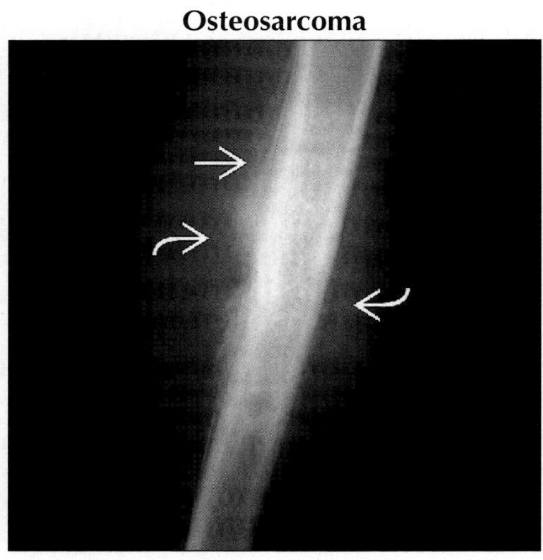

(Left) AP radiograph shows diffuse osteopenia in both femoral diaphyses ⇨ along the lucent metaphyseal lines ➡ in a 5 year old. Though no periosteal reaction is seen, this must be interpreted as aggressive; leukemia was proven. (Right) Lateral radiograph shows a highly aggressive mid-diaphyseal humeral lesion with a Codman triangle ➡, an aggressive periosteal reaction. There is tumor osteoid forming in the soft tissue mass ↪, diagnostic of osteosarcoma.

Metastases, Bone Marrow

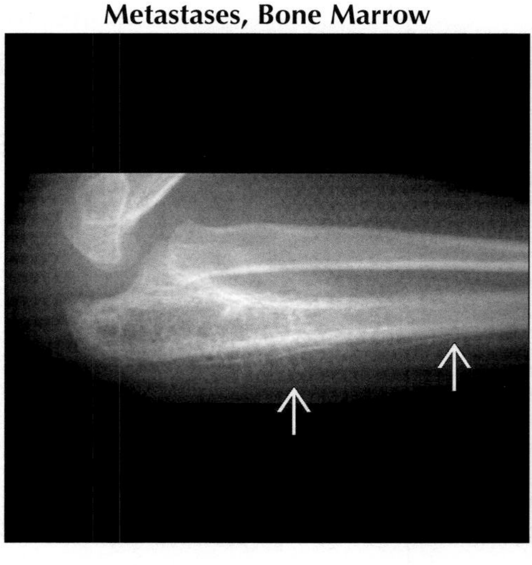

Lymphoma

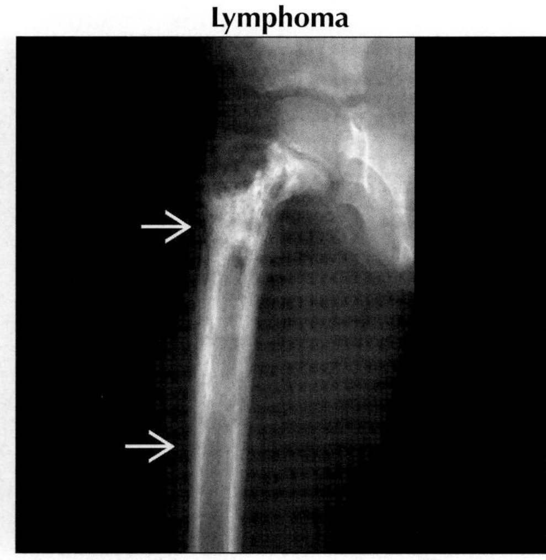

(Left) Lateral radiograph shows a permeative lesion occupying the entire length of the ulna, with extensive periosteal reaction ➡. This 6-month-old patient has medulloblastoma metastases. (Right) AP radiograph shows a lytic lesion with reactive sclerosis occupying the entire diaphysis and metaphysis of the femur in a 7-year-old African-American child ➡. There is periosteal reaction and a soft tissue mass. The lesion is polyostotic and proved to be lymphoma.

Sickle Cell Anemia

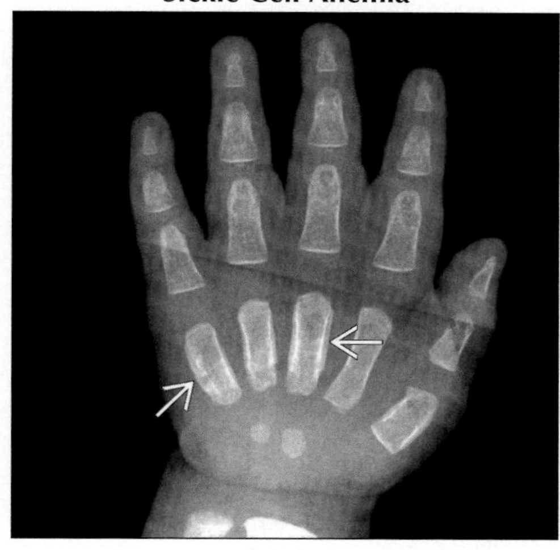

Malignant Fibrous Histiocytoma, Bone

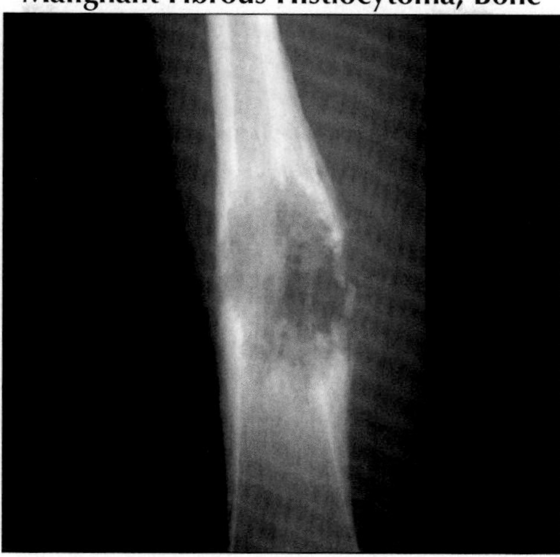

*(**Left**) AP radiograph shows periosteal reaction ➡ and a permeative appearance in most of the metacarpals and phalanges in the hand of this 1-year-old African-American child. This is sickle cell dactylitis. (**Right**) AP radiograph shows a lytic permeative lesion occupying the mid-diaphysis in a 13 year old. The lesion is aggressive, with cortical breakthrough, a soft tissue mass, and prominent periosteal reaction. MFH is rare in children but certainly does occur.*

Chondrosarcoma, Conventional

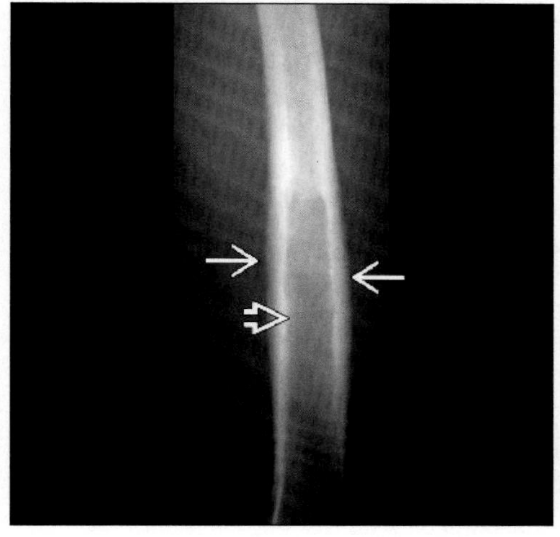

Chondrosarcoma, Conventional

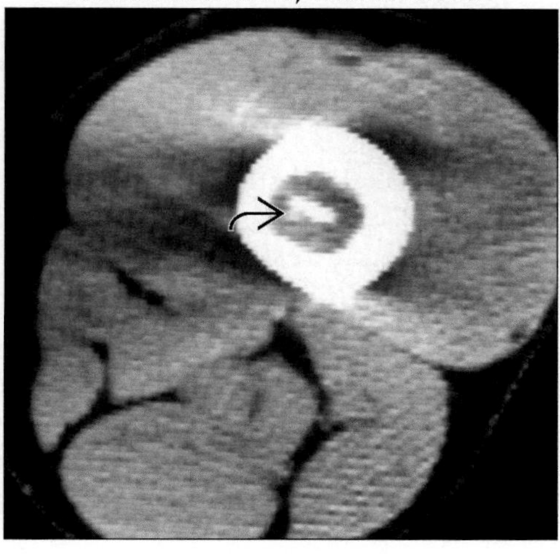

*(**Left**) Lateral radiograph shows mild expansion of the diaphysis ➡ with endosteal thickening ➡ in a 17 year old. This is suggestive of osteomyelitis or Ewing sarcoma, but chondrosarcoma must also be considered. (**Right**) Axial NECT in the same patient shows endosteal thickening, with a central chondroid matrix ➡. This matrix makes the diagnosis of chondrosarcoma. It is an unusual diagnosis in teenagers but must be considered.*

Adamantinoma

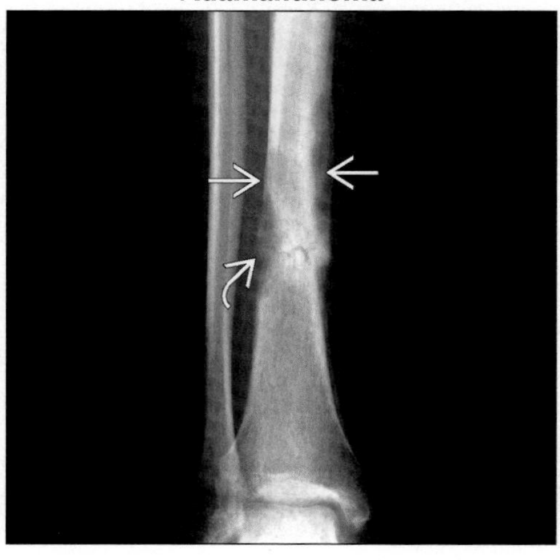

Adamantinoma

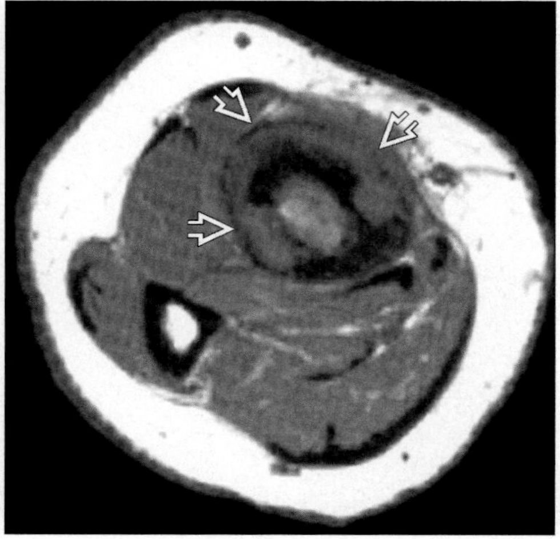

*(**Left**) AP radiograph shows a lytic lesion in the diaphysis of the tibia of a 17 year old. The lesion proved to be entirely restricted to the cortex ➡, which is typical of adamantinoma. Note the pathologic fracture ➡. (**Right**) Axial T1WI MR in the same patient shows that the tibial lesion is indeed based entirely in the cortex ➡. The marrow is not entirely normal, suggesting involvement, which contributes to the aggressive appearance and behavior of this lesion. (†MSK Req).*

GROWTH PLATE, PREMATURE PHYSEAL CLOSURE

DIFFERENTIAL DIAGNOSIS

Common
- Fracture

Less Common
- Osteomyelitis
- Septic Joint
- Iatrogenic (Surgical)
- Juvenile Idiopathic Arthritis (JIA)
- Ollier/Maffucci Syndrome (Mimic)
- Radiation-Induced Growth Deformities
- Thermal Injury

Rare but Important
- Complications of Vitamin A
- Hemophilia: MSK Complications
- Meningococcemia

ESSENTIAL INFORMATION

Key Differential Diagnosis Issues
- Number/distribution of physes is diagnostic

Helpful Clues for Common Diagnoses
- **Fracture**
  - Hyperemia in metadiaphyseal fracture may result in early fusion of physis
  - Salter injury (usually 3, 4, or 5) may result in focal early bony bridging

Helpful Clues for Less Common Diagnoses
- **Osteomyelitis**
  - Usually located in metaphysis in child
    - Occasionally, process will cross physis to involve epiphysis → early fusion
  - Hyperemia from chronic infection may result in early fusion of entire physis
- **Septic Joint**
  - Early fusion: Chronic hyperemia or direct extension to physis if intracapsular (hip)
- **Iatrogenic (Surgical)**
  - Epiphysiodesis performed for angular deformity or short contralateral limb
- **Juvenile Idiopathic Arthritis (JIA)**
  - Chronic hyperemia at involved joints has 2 growth-related consequences
    - Epiphyseal/metaphyseal overgrowth
    - Early fusion of physis → short limb
  - Knee > elbow > ankle, not symmetric
- **Ollier/Maffucci Syndrome (Mimic)**
  - Short, broad, abnormally tubulated metaphyses; often chondroid matrix
- **Radiation-Induced Growth Deformities**
  - Vasculitis from radiation puts physis at risk
  - Nonviable physis → fusion and hypoplasia
  - Watch for port-like distribution
- **Thermal Injury**
  - Vessels supplying physes at risk, particularly in hands or feet
    - → short, stubby fingers in adults
  - Burn: Contractures and calcification
  - Frostbite: Abnormality spares thumb

Helpful Clues for Rare Diagnoses
- **Complications of Vitamin A**
  - Focal bony bridging across physis
  - Diffuse periostitis, coned epiphyses
- **Hemophilia: MSK Complications**
  - Same as JIA, with dense effusions

Fracture

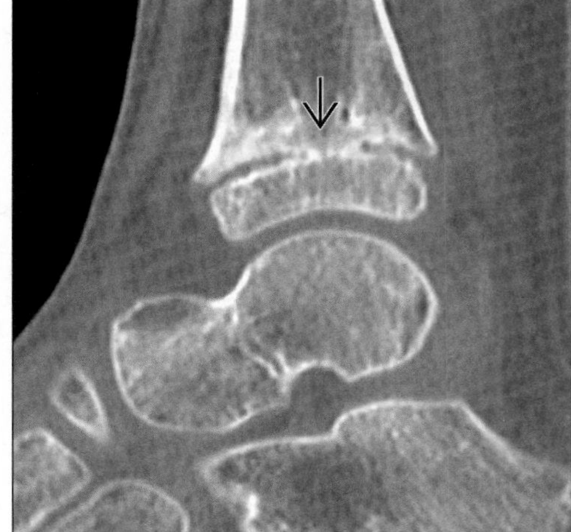

Sagittal bone CT shows a premature bony bridge (physeal bar) formed at site of physeal fracture ⇨. This partial early fusion will result in relative overgrowth anteriorly and posteriorly, deforming the distal tibia.

Osteomyelitis

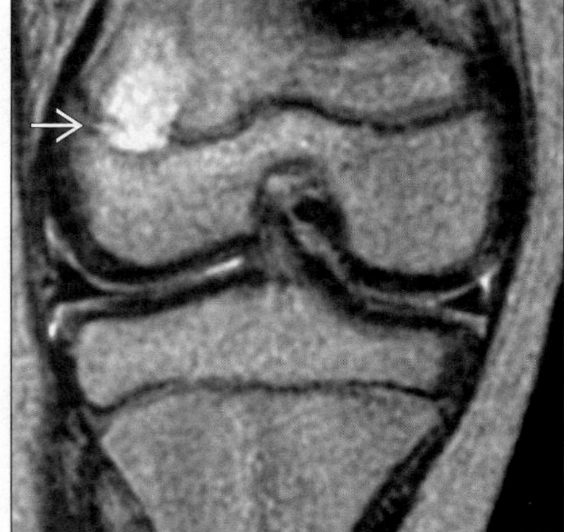

Coronal T2WI MR shows a metaphyseal focus of osteomyelitis crossing the physis ➡ and involving the epiphysis in an 8 yo. This involvement of the physis may result in early focal bridging of the physis. (†MSK Req).

Iatrogenic (Surgical)

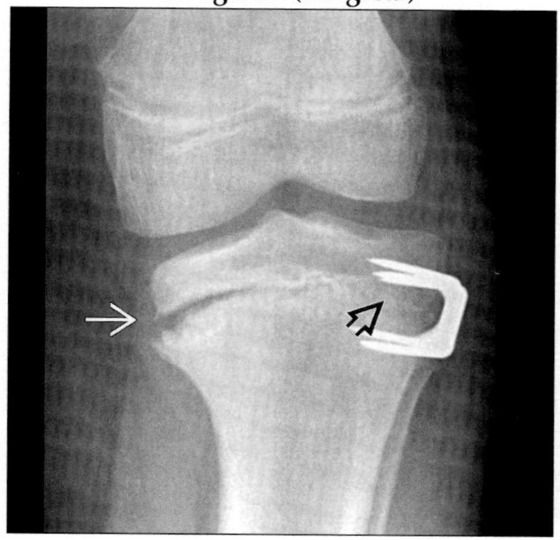

Juvenile Idiopathic Arthritis (JIA)

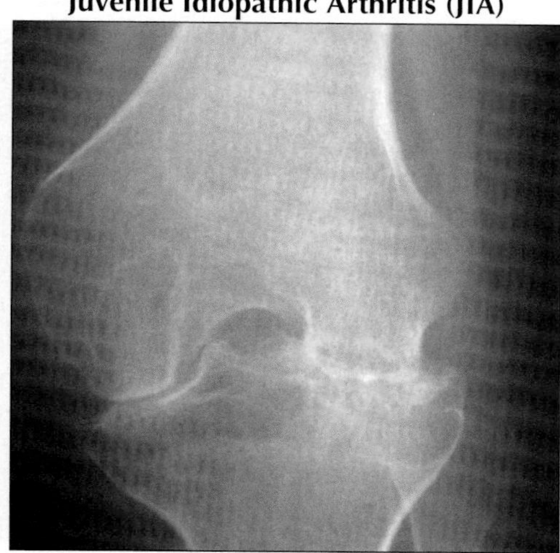

(Left) *Anteroposterior radiograph shows typical Blount disease ➡ involving the medial tibia. Since this results in tibia vara, prophylactic epiphysiodesis is performed laterally ⇨, now showing closure of this portion of the physis.* ***(Right)*** *Anteroposterior radiograph shows early physeal closure in this 16 year old with JIA. This joint shows severe involvement with overgrowth of the epiphyses, joint destruction, and widening of the intercondylar notch.*

Ollier/Maffucci Syndrome (Mimic)

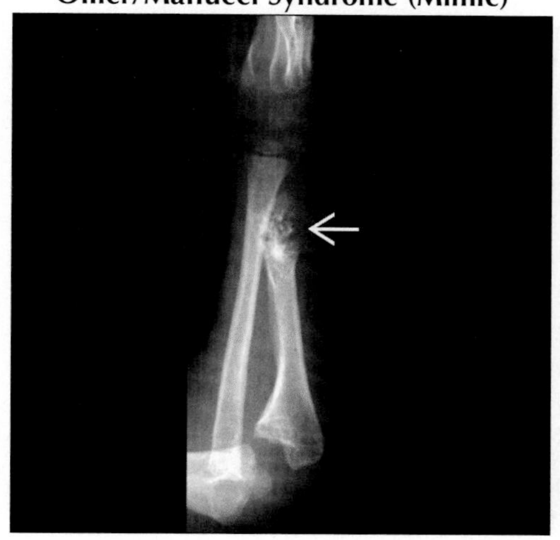

Radiation-Induced Growth Deformities

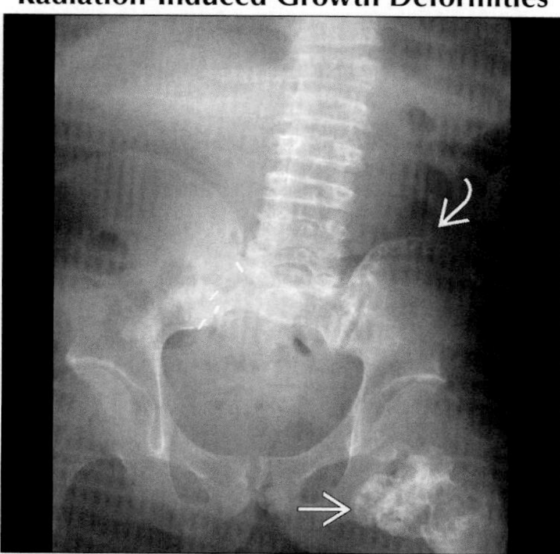

(Left) *Lateral radiograph shows a short ulna in a patient with Ollier disease ➡, mimicking early physeal closure. Short bones result from metaphyseal dysplasia rather than true early fusion.* ***(Right)*** *AP radiograph shows a hypoplastic left iliac wing ➡ in a 20 year old who had radiation therapy to the left hemipelvis as a child. Vascular damage results in early fusion of epiphyses and apophyses, with cessation of growth. Exostosis ➡ is also a complication of radiation.*

Thermal Injury

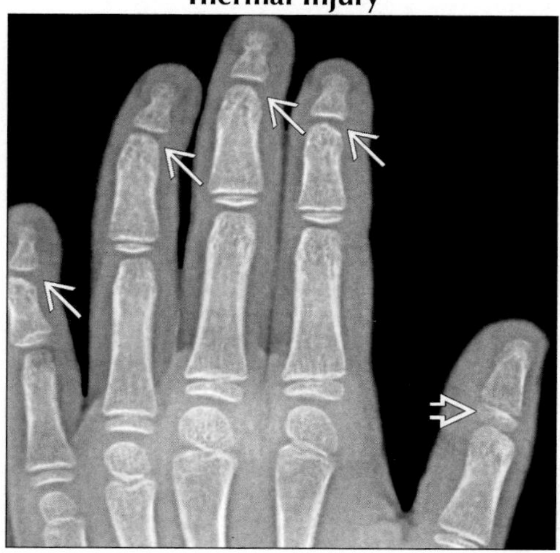

Meningococcemia

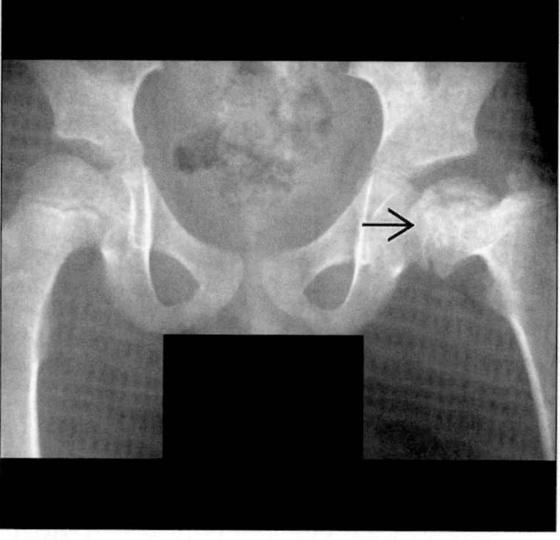

(Left) *Posteroanterior radiograph shows premature closure of the physes of the distal phalanges of digits 2-5 ➡, resulting in short, stubby digits. This is due to vascular damage from frostbite. Note the normal physis and distal phalanx of the thumb ⇨, typical of frostbite.* ***(Right)*** *Anteroposterior radiograph shows early bony bridging of a portion of the physis of the left hip ➡ in a patient with meningococcemia. Short limbs are often a consequence of this process.*

GROWTH PLATE, WIDENED PHYSIS

DIFFERENTIAL DIAGNOSIS

Common
- Physeal Fracture
- Chronic Repetitive Trauma
- Slipped Capital Femoral Epiphysis (SCFE)
- Renal Osteodystrophy (Renal OD)
- Rickets

Less Common
- Osteomyelitis
- Legg-Calvé-Perthes (LCP)
- Blount Disease
- Total Parenteral Nutrition
- Gigantism
- Mucopolysaccharidoses
- Osteogenesis Imperfecta (OI)
- Hypophosphatasia

Rare but Important
- Hypothyroidism
- Scurvy
- Copper Deficiency (Menkes Kinky-Hair Syndrome)
- Metaphyseal Dysplasias

ESSENTIAL INFORMATION

Key Differential Diagnosis Issues
- Involvement of all physes rather than a single or few sites seen in several processes
  - Rickets and renal OD
  - Total parenteral nutrition
  - Gigantism
  - Mucopolysaccharidoses
  - Osteogenesis imperfecta
  - Hypophosphatasia
  - Hypothyroidism
  - Copper deficiency
  - Metaphyseal dysplasias

Helpful Clues for Common Diagnoses
- **Physeal Fracture**
  - Salter 1: Fracture through physis; difficult to visualize unless displaced
  - Salter 2: Fracture through physis, extending through metaphysis
    - Metaphyseal portion may be subtle; easier to visualize if displaced
  - Salter 3: Fracture through physis, extending through epiphysis
  - Salter 4: Fracture through epiphysis, physis, & metaphysis; generally does not result in physeal widening
  - Salter 5: Crush fracture of physis; does not result in widening
- **Chronic Repetitive Trauma**
  - In child, repeated microtrauma to a physis results in resorption and appearance of widening
  - Analogous to Salter 1 injury
  - Associated with competitive athletes
    - Distal radius/ulna: Gymnasts
    - Distal tibia/fibula: Runners
    - Proximal humerus: Baseball pitchers
- **Slipped Capital Femoral Epiphysis (SCFE)**
  - Slip direction generally posterior and medial
  - Results in appearance of widened physis and "short" capital epiphysis
  - Bilateral in 20-25% but need not be synchronous
  - Optimal age range: 8-14
- **Renal Osteodystrophy (Renal OD)**
  - Combined findings of rickets and hyperparathyroidism (HPTH)
  - Rickets results in widening of physis
  - Watch for HPTH as well
    - Subperiosteal resorption
    - Subchondral resorption with collapse (particularly sacroiliac joints)
- **Rickets**
  - Similar appearance, whether renal or nutritional etiology
  - Results from lack of mineralization of osteoid laid down at metaphyseal zone of provisional calcification
  - Widened physis, often with fraying of metaphyses
  - Decreased bone density, smudgy trabeculae

Helpful Clues for Less Common Diagnoses
- **Osteomyelitis**
  - If metaphyseal osteomyelitis crosses physis, may result in slip of physis and appearance of widening
  - Watch for osseous destruction, periosteal reaction
- **Legg-Calvé-Perthes (LCP)**
  - Osteonecrosis of femoral capital epiphysis
  - Increased density, flattening, fragmentation of epiphysis

- Associated appearance of widened physis
- Optimal age range: 4-8

- **Blount Disease**
  - Fragmentation and abnormal ossification of medial tibial metaphysis
  - Focal "widening" of physis medially
  - Usually bilateral; results in tibia vara
- **Total Parenteral Nutrition**
  - Premature infant dependent on total parenteral nutrition for long period of time
  - Diffuse widening of physes, thought to be due to nutritional deficiency of copper
  - Indistinguishable from rickets, though true rickets does not appear prior to 6 months of age
- **Gigantism**
  - With overgrowth of gigantism, physes may appear mildly widened diffusely
- **Mucopolysaccharidoses**
  - Delay in epiphyseal ossification may give appearance of relatively widened physis
  - Other manifestations: Fan-shaped carpus, oar-shaped ribs, narrow inferior ilium with steep acetabular roof
- **Osteogenesis Imperfecta (OI)**
  - OI tarda may show physeal widening and mild slip of epiphyses
  - Other manifestations: Osteoporosis and more fractures than normally expected in a child
- **Hypophosphatasia**
  - Nearly indistinguishable from rickets
  - Diffuse widening of physes
  - Osteopenia
  - Ranges from mild tarda form to severe destructive form
  - Bowing of long bones with excrescences may help differentiate from rickets
  - May have "button sequestra" in skull

Helpful Clues for Rare Diagnoses

- **Hypothyroidism**
  - Severe retardation of skeletal maturation
  - Widened physes, short broad phalanges
  - Hip may show fragmentation of femoral capital epiphysis
    - Appearance may be similar to Legg-Calvé-Perthes; watch for abnormal bone age to differentiate
  - Infant shows stippled epiphyses
- **Scurvy**
  - Osteopenia, with sclerotic metaphyseal line (white line of Frankel) and sclerotic rim of epiphysis (Wimberger sign)
  - Corner metaphyseal fracture may cause a slip and mild physeal widening
    - Wide periosteal "reaction" due to subperiosteal hemorrhage
- **Copper Deficiency (Menkes Kinky-Hair Syndrome)**
  - Rare disorder resulting in physeal widening
  - Myeloneuropathy
- **Metaphyseal Dysplasias**
  - Metaphyses flared and irregular with apparent physeal widening

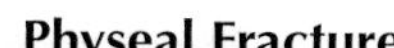

Physeal Fracture

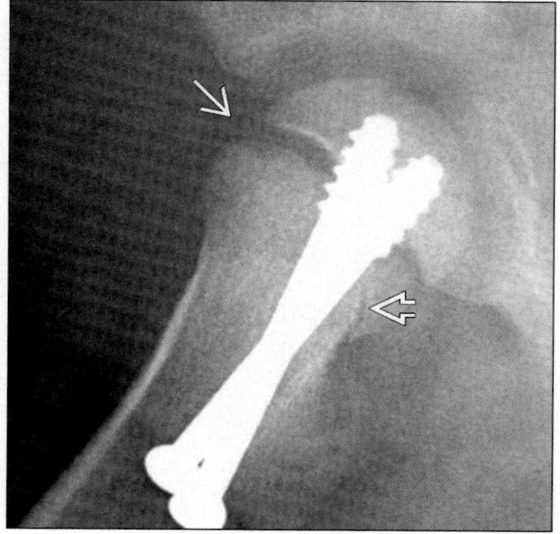

Frog lateral radiograph shows widening of the physis →, due to a Salter 2 fracture. The fracture line extends on through the metaphysis ➔. Salter 2 fractures are rarely subtle; Salter 1 is more difficult to recognize.

Chronic Repetitive Trauma

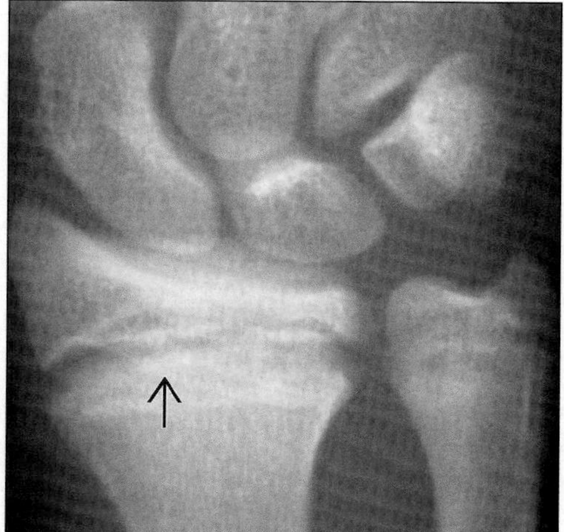

Anteroposterior radiograph shows osteolysis at the distal radial epiphyseal plate →, a type of Salter 1 injury occurring in gymnasts due to chronic repetitive trauma. Note the similar abnormality involving the ulna.

GROWTH PLATE, WIDENED PHYSIS

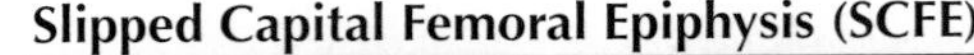

Slipped Capital Femoral Epiphysis (SCFE)

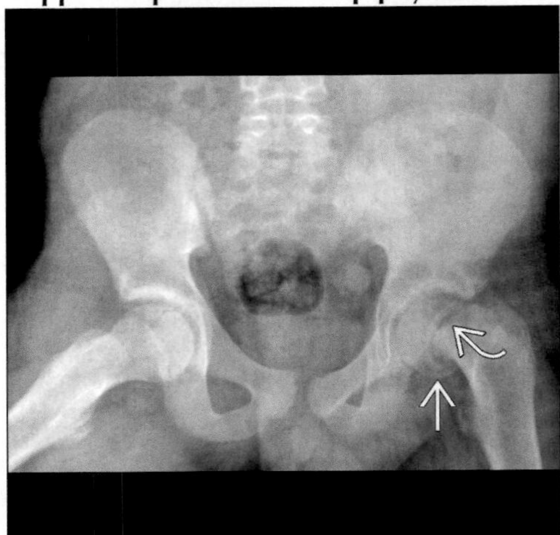

Renal Osteodystrophy (Renal OD)

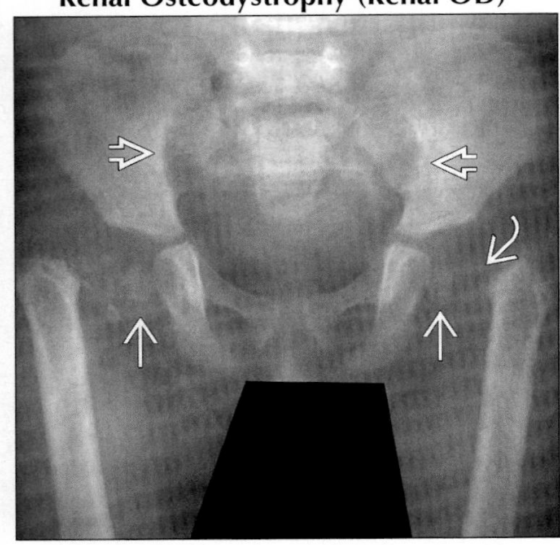

(Left) *Frog lateral radiograph shows a left SCFE (compare with normal right side). With the posteromedial slip of the head, the physis appears to widen.* ***(Right)*** *AP radiograph shows severe renal OD, manifest in the hips as rickets, with widening of the zone of provisional calcification and slip of the capital epiphyses. There is also typical hyperparathyroidism, with widened sacroiliac joints due to subchondral resorption and collapse on the iliac side.*

Rickets

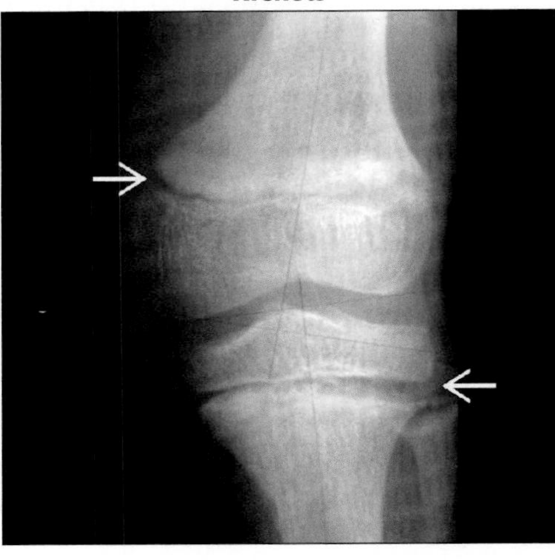

Osteomyelitis

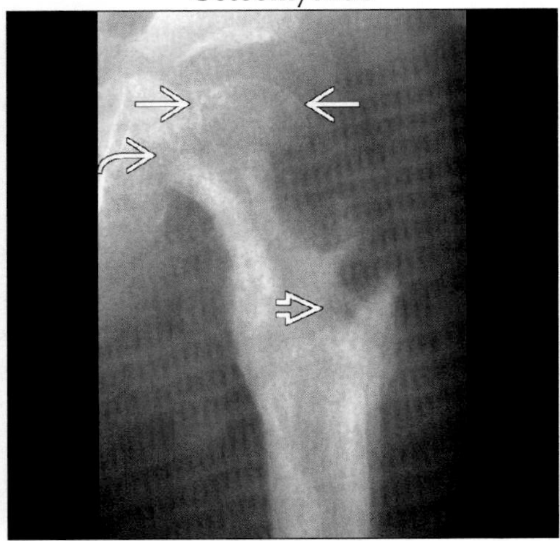

(Left) *Anteroposterior radiograph shows a widened physis at both the tibia and femur due to nutritional rickets. The abnormality is secondary to the formation of osteoid, which is not mineralized; the appearance is identical in rickets due to renal OD.* ***(Right)*** *Anteroposterior radiograph shows metaphyseal destruction and periosteal reaction secondary to osteomyelitis. Infection has crossed the physis, resulting in widening and slip of the epiphysis.*

Legg-Calvé-Perthes (LCP)

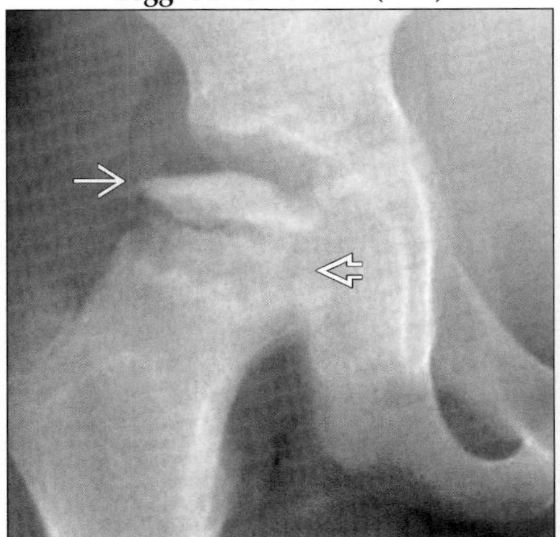

Blount Disease

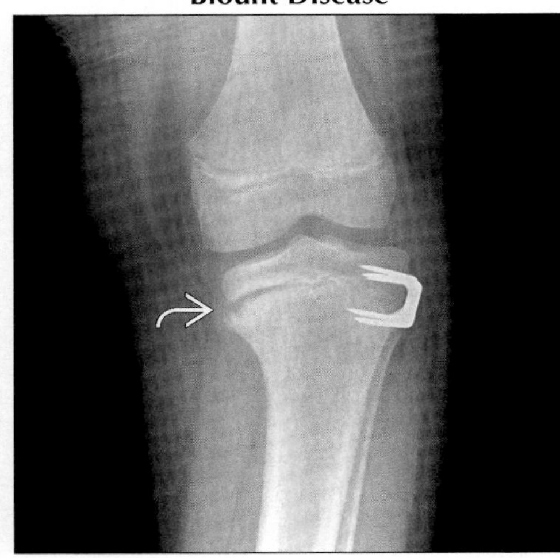

(Left) *AP radiograph shows a dense, flattened femoral capital epiphysis in a young child; this is LCP or osteonecrosis. The abnormality may result in widening and fraying of the metaphysis, as in this case.* ***(Right)*** *Anteroposterior radiograph shows beaking and underdevelopment of the medial metaphysis of the left tibia. This results in an appearance of physeal widening. The patient has undergone epiphysiodesis laterally to address the growth inequity.*

Total Parenteral Nutrition

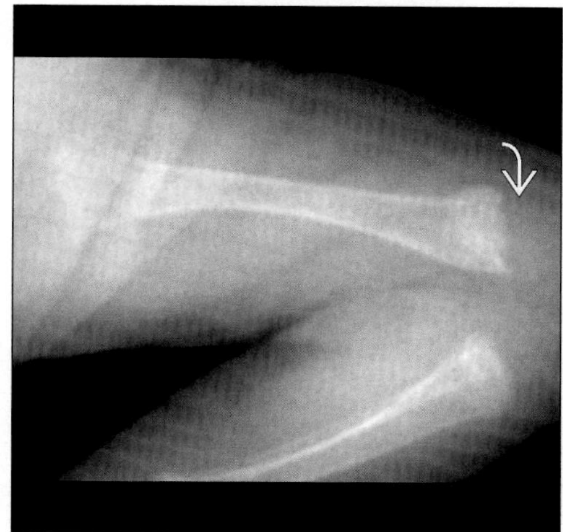

Mucopolysaccharidoses

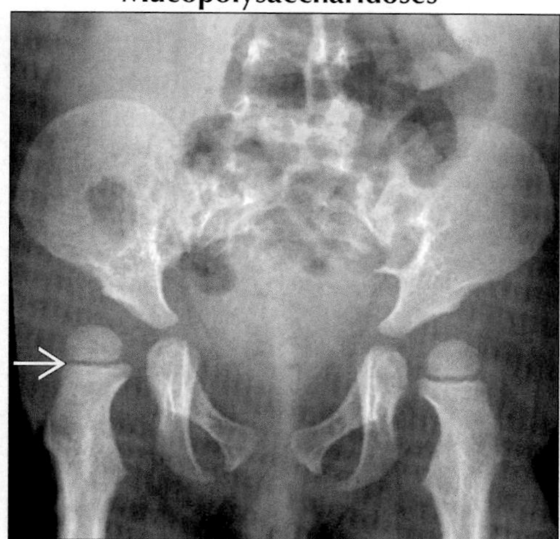

(Left) *Lateral radiograph shows widening of the physis and fraying of the metaphyses ➲ in a case of neonatal rickets; the patient was a 26-week premature infant, now 3 months old. Infants nourished for long periods with total parenteral nutrition may develop the appearance of rickets.* ***(Right)*** *AP radiograph shows typical skeletal findings of dysostosis multiplex, with inferior tapering of ilia, steep acetabular roofs, and coxa valga. The physes may appear widened ➔.*

Osteogenesis Imperfecta (OI)

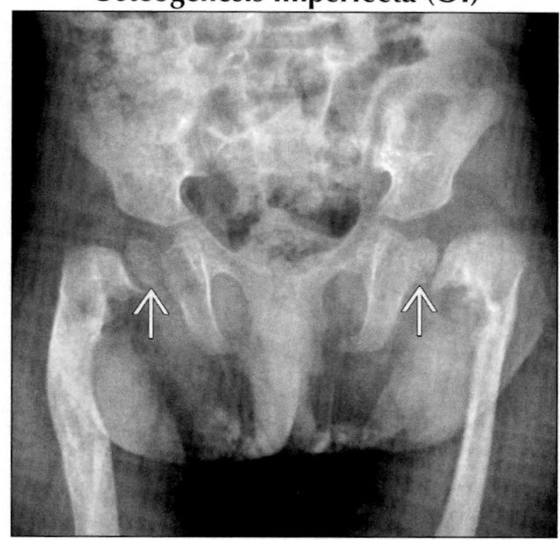

Hypophosphatasia

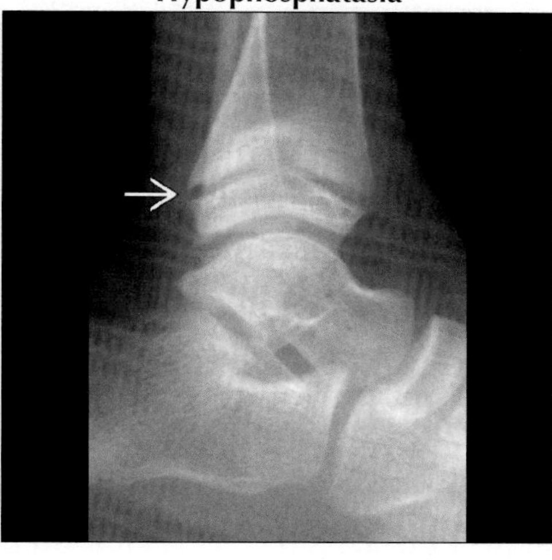

(Left) *Anteroposterior radiograph shows osteopenia and multiple healed fractures typical of OI tarda. The physes are mildly widened and slipped ➔.* ***(Right)*** *Lateral radiograph shows widening of the physis ➔ that is reminiscent of rickets. This is a mild case of hypophosphatasia. In severe cases, the bone density is significantly reduced and the physes show more significant widening, with fraying of the metaphyses.*

Hypothyroidism

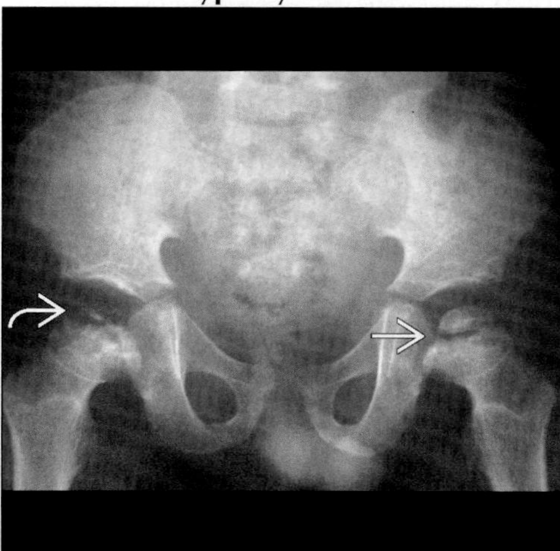

Scurvy

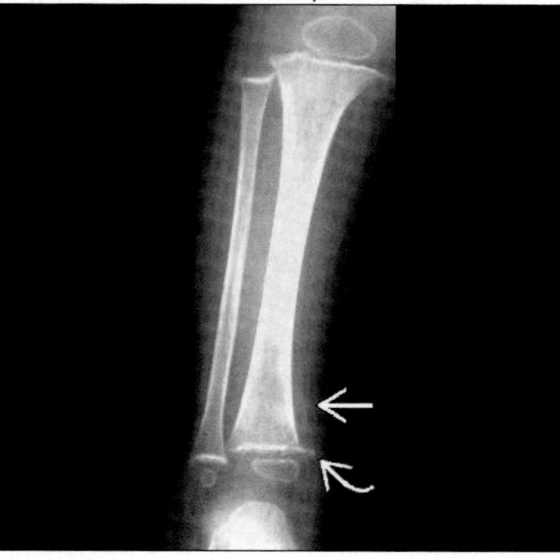

(Left) *AP radiograph shows widening of the physes ➔ & severe growth retardation in this 4 year old with hypothyroidism. There is also fragmentation of the right femoral capital epiphysis ➲, which has been termed the "cretinoid" hip.* ***(Right)*** *AP radiograph shows typical findings of scurvy, with a metaphyseal corner ➲ fracture. With such a fracture, the physis may be displaced & appear widened. Note the wide periosteal reaction ➔ related to subperiosteal hemorrhage.*

BOWING BONES

DIFFERENTIAL DIAGNOSIS

Common
- Physiologic Bowing
- Blount Disease

Less Common
- Rickets
- Fibrous Dysplasia
- Neurofibromatosis
- Osteogenesis Imperfecta

Rare but Important
- Congenital Tibial Dysplasia
- Congenital Bowing
- Achondroplasia
- Camptomelic Dysplasia

ESSENTIAL INFORMATION

Key Differential Diagnosis Issues
- Must determine which causes of lower extremity bowing are physiologic vs. pathologic
- Isolated or generalized bowing
- Cortical thickening along convex side and thinning along concave side of curve
- Neonates and infants have normal varus angulation of lower extremities
    - Correction of bowing by 6 months after beginning to walk or aged 1.5-2 years old
    - **Hint**: Considered abnormal if varus angulation of knee in child > 2 years old
- Changes to valgus angulation by 1.5-3 years old (11° in 3 year old)
- 5-6° of valgus angulation by 13 years old

Helpful Clues for Common Diagnoses
- **Physiologic Bowing**
    - a.k.a. developmental bowing
    - Exaggerated varus angulation when younger than 2 years old
        - If exaggerated during 2nd year of life, probably normal but follow to exclude development of Blount disease
    - More common in early walkers, heavier children, and African-American children
    - Tibial metaphysis appears prominent, depressed with small beaks of distal medial and posterior tibia and femur
        - Not fragmented, thickened medial tibial cortex
        - Tilted distal tibial growth plate laterally
    - Usually resolves without treatment
- **Blount Disease**
    - Infantile type: 1-3 years old, bilateral in 60-80%
        - Must differentiate from physiologic bowing
    - Adolescent type: 8-14 years old, more commonly unilateral
    - Thought to result from abnormal stress on proximal medial tibial physis
        - May reflect normal physiologic bowing that progresses and fails to predictably correct
    - Diagnosed by progressive clinical bowing on clinical examination in combination with characteristic radiographic changes
    - Predisposed: Early walkers, obese children, and African-Americans
    - Medial tibial metaphysis depression and fragmentation, constriction ± bone bridging of proximal medial tibial physis, genu varum
    - Enlarged epiphyseal cartilage and medial meniscus on MR
    - Metaphyseal-diaphyseal angle
        - Angle between line drawn parallel to proximal tibial metaphysis and another line drawn perpendicular to long axis of tibial diaphysis
        - Abnormal if > 11° on standing radiographs
        - Indeterminate angle (8-11°), should follow clinically ± radiographically

Helpful Clues for Less Common Diagnoses
- **Rickets**
    - Generalized bowing, changes at sites of rapid growth
    - Deficiency in mineralization of normal osteoid, widening zone of provisional calcification
    - Metaphyseal flaring and fraying
- **Fibrous Dysplasia**
    - Hamartomatous lesion, replacement of portions of medullary cavity with fibroosseous tissue
    - Long bone medullary space widening, endosteal scalloping, coarse or obliterated trabeculation
        - Lytic, ground-glass, or sclerotic
    - 70% monostotic
    - 90% of polyostotic lesions are unilateral

- Sarcomatous degeneration: 0.5%
- **Neurofibromatosis**
  - Anterolateral bowing of tibia, ± hypoplastic fibula, often narrowing or intramedullary sclerosis or cystic change at apex of angulation
    - Hamartomatous fibrous tissue
  - Bowing typically at junction of middle and distal 1/3 of tibia
  - May develop pathologic fracture, pseudoarthrosis of tibia ± fibula, tapering or penciling ends of bones at fracture site
- **Osteogenesis Imperfecta**
  - History of osteogenesis imperfecta
  - Bowing results from soft bones
  - Generalized bowing of long bones, osteoporosis, and multiple fractures

Helpful Clues for Rare Diagnoses

- **Congenital Tibial Dysplasia**
  - a.k.a. congenital pseudoarthrosis
  - Rare
  - 70% will eventually be diagnosed with neurofibromatosis (NF)
  - 1-2% of neurofibromatosis patients
  - Anterolateral tibia bowing or fracture
  - If fibular bowing is absent, tends to resolve spontaneously
- **Congenital Bowing**
  - Abnormal intrauterine or fetal positioning
  - Convex posteromedially, rarely laterally
    - Calcaneovalgus deformity of ipsilateral foot
    - ± diaphyseal broadening
  - Tends to resolve
  - ± protective bracing
- **Achondroplasia**
  - Generalized bowing
  - Most common form of short-limb dwarfism
  - Autosomal dominant or spontaneous mutation
  - Small thorax with short ribs
  - Short and thick long bones with metaphyseal cupping and flaring, short broad phalanges
  - Short rectangular iliac bones (elephant ear-shaped), narrow sacrosciatic notches, flat acetabular roof
  - Bullet-shaped vertebral bodies with posterior scalloping, narrowed interpedicular distances in lumbar spine
- **Camptomelic Dysplasia**
  - a.k.a. campomelic dysplasia
  - Autosomal dominant
  - Often fatal in infancy
  - Anterolateral bowing of lower extremities > upper extremities
    - Bowed femur with short-bowed tibia
  - Pretibial skin dimples
  - Large skull with small face, hypoplastic scapula, narrow pelvis, dislocated hips, bell-shaped chest

Physiologic Bowing

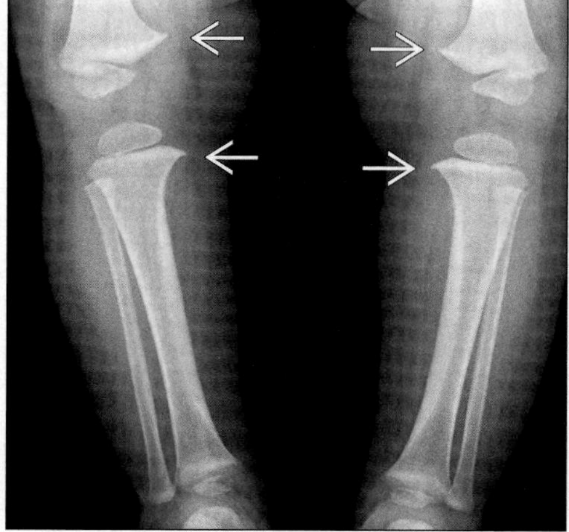

Anteroposterior radiograph shows the typical medial beaking of the bilateral tibia and femur ➡ and cortical thickening along the convex margin of the tibia.

Physiologic Bowing

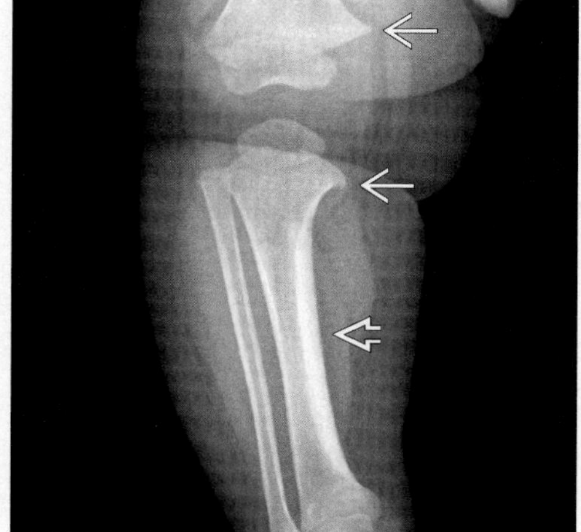

Anteroposterior radiograph shows the typical metaphyseal beaks ➡ of physiologic bowing of the right lower leg. Note the thickened medial cortex ⇨ along the convexity of the curve.

BOWING BONES

*(**Left**) AP radiograph of the left lower leg in the same patient shows beaking ➡ of the medial tibia without fragmentation. Notice the thickened medial cortex ➡ of the tibia and tilting of the distal tibial growth plate laterally ➡. (**Right**) AP radiograph shows the more vertically oriented medial growth plate, fragmentation, and spurring ➡. Notice the medial joint space widening. Adolescent Blount disease may be the result of segmental arrest of the medial tibial physis.*

Physiologic Bowing

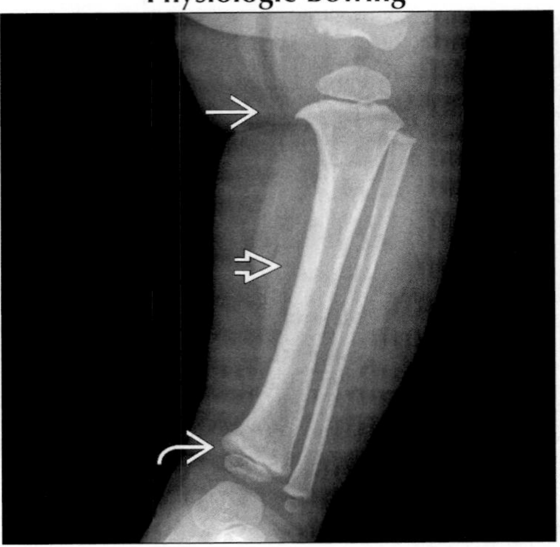

Blount Disease

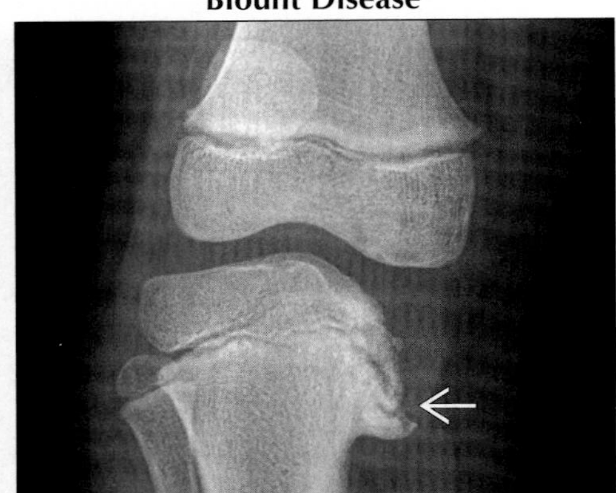

*(**Left**) Coronal T2WI FS MR shows fragmentation and widening of the proximal tibial growth plate. Notice that the more vertically oriented growth plate causes beaking of the proximal tibial metaphysis ➡. (**Right**) Anteroposterior radiograph shows medial depression and fragmentation of the left medial tibial metaphysis ➡ and widening of the medial joint space and genu varum. The adolescent form of Blount disease tends to be unilateral.*

Blount Disease

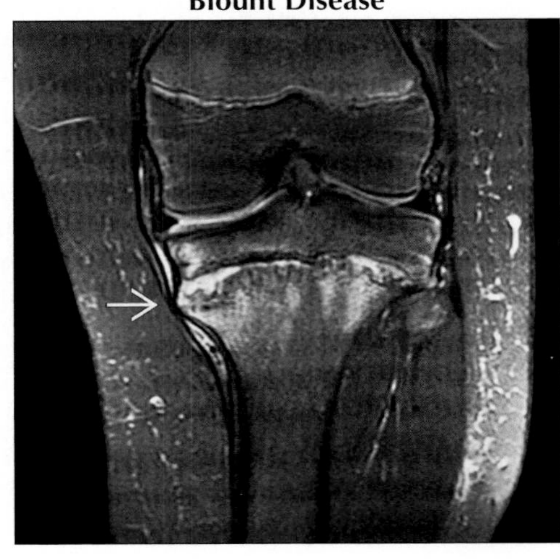

Blount Disease

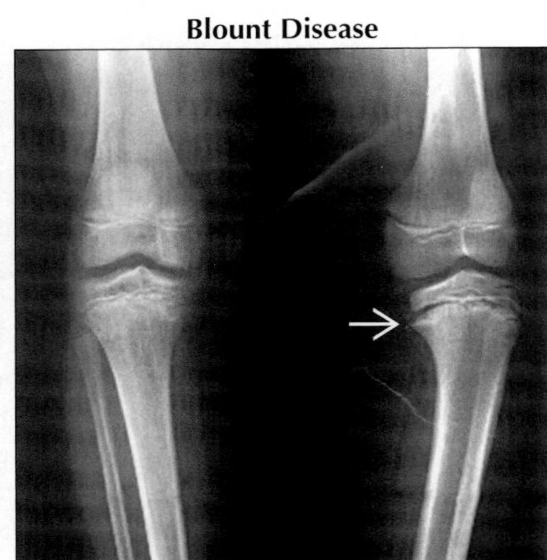

*(**Left**) Anteroposterior radiograph shows fragmentation, fraying, and growth plate widening ➡. Rickets is a cause of generalized bowing of the bones. (**Right**) Anteroposterior radiograph shows osteopenia, metaphyseal fragmentation, flaring, and growth plate widening of the distal femur ➡. There was more severe involvement of the femur, rather than the tibia, in this patient.*

Rickets

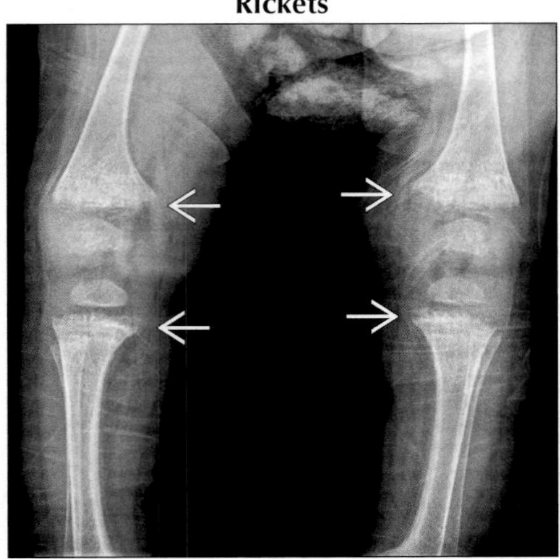

Rickets

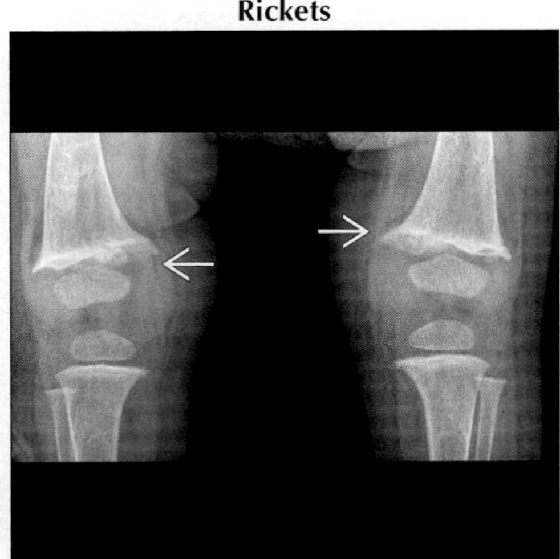

BOWING BONES

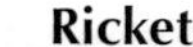

Rickets

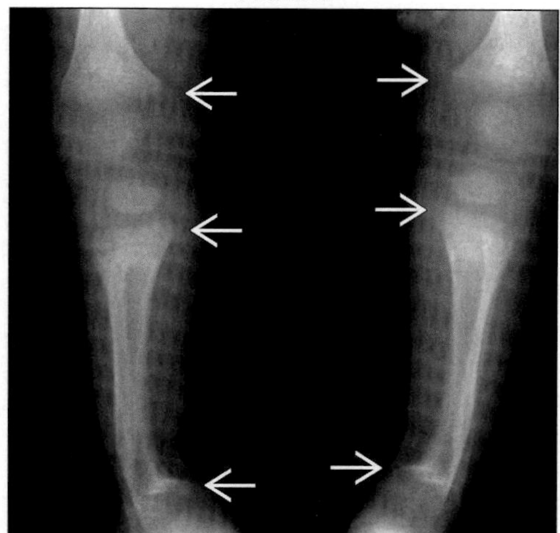

Rickets

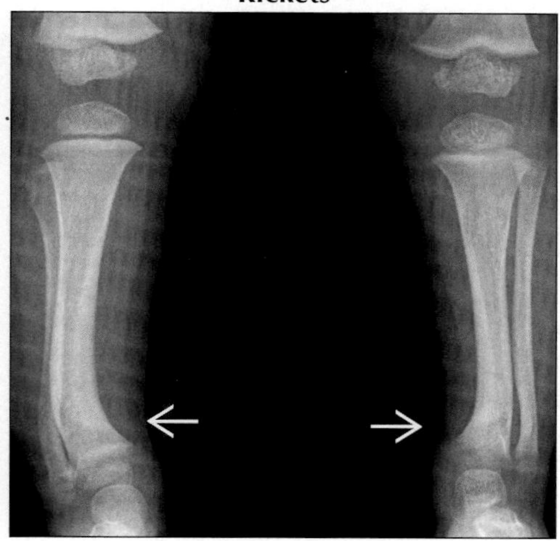

*(**Left**) Anteroposterior radiograph shows the typical findings of rickets with metaphyseal flaring, cupping, fragmentation, and growth plate widening →. Notice the more prominent focal bowing at the ankles. (**Right**) Anteroposterior radiograph in the same patient a few years later shows residual bowing of the distal tibia and fibula → with marked thickening of the distal medial tibial cortex. The previous radiographic changes of rickets have resolved.*

Fibrous Dysplasia

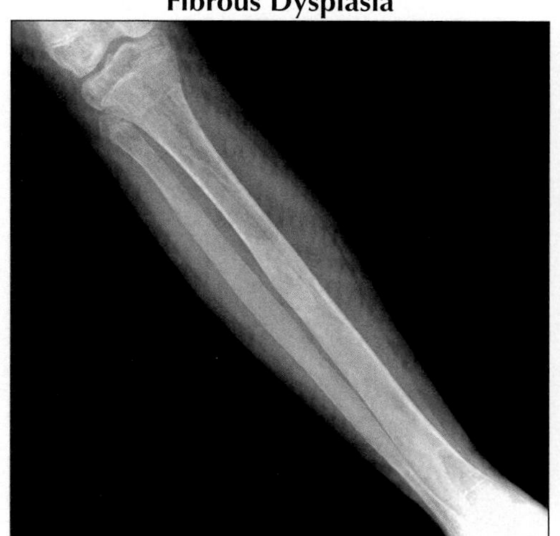

Fibrous Dysplasia

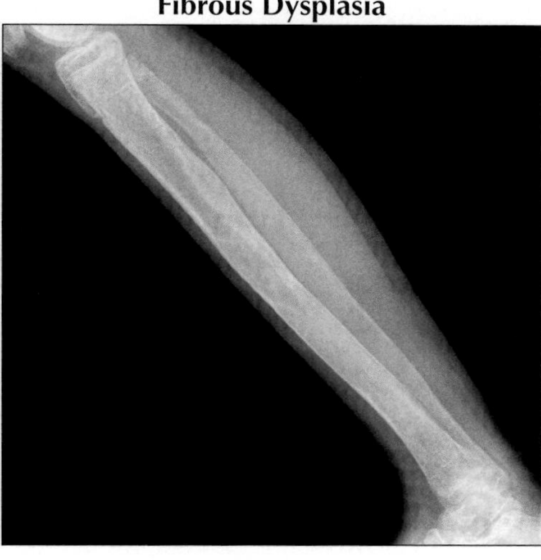

*(**Left**) Anteroposterior radiograph shows intramedullary ground-glass and mildly sclerotic lesions throughout the tibia and fibula, with endosteal scalloping and mild expansion. The ground-glass lesions are typical for fibrous dysplasia. (**Right**) Lateral radiograph in the same patient shows central and eccentric ground-glass and mildly sclerotic lesions within both the tibia and fibula. No pathologic fracture was seen in this patient.*

Neurofibromatosis

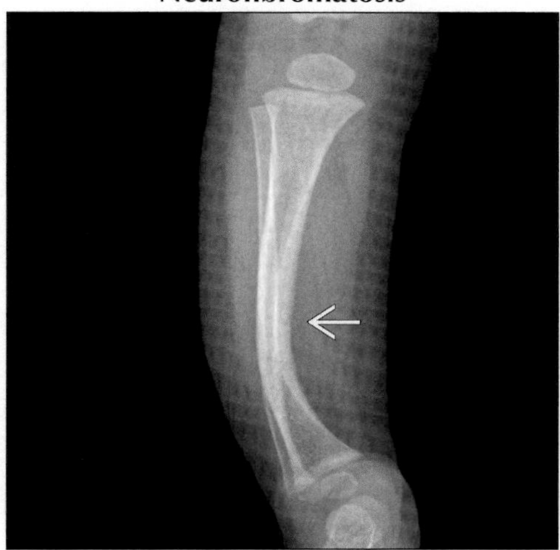

Neurofibromatosis

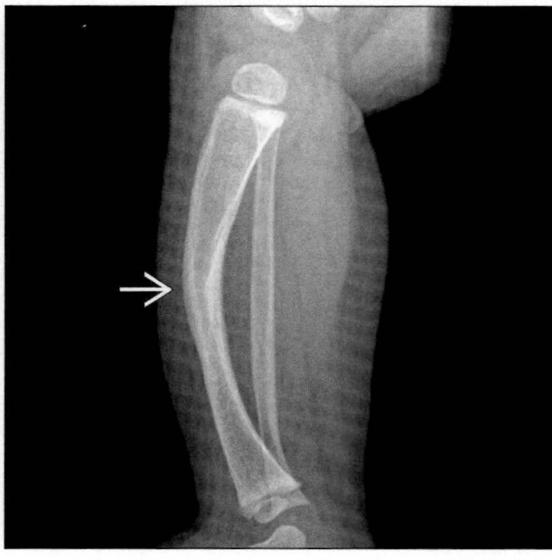

*(**Left**) Anteroposterior radiograph shows lateral bowing of the tibia → and, to a lesser degree, the fibula. Bowing in neurofibromatosis usually involves the middle or distal 1/3 of the tibial diaphysis. Pseudoarthrosis can develop as a complication. (**Right**) Anteroposterior radiograph shows anterior bowing of the mid-tibia → with mild constriction of the medullary space. The fibula may be hypoplastic in patients with neurofibromatosis, though it is not in this case.*

BOWING BONES

*(**Left**) Anteroposterior radiograph shows moderate lateral bowing of the tibia. Notice a pathologic fracture along the medial cortex of the tibia ➔. Pseudoarthrosis is a complication of tibial bowing with fractures in patients with neurofibromatosis. (**Right**) Lateral radiograph in the same patient shows anterior bowing of the tibial diaphysis. Notice the diaphyseal narrowing and intramedullary sclerosis at the apex of the curve ➔.*

Neurofibromatosis

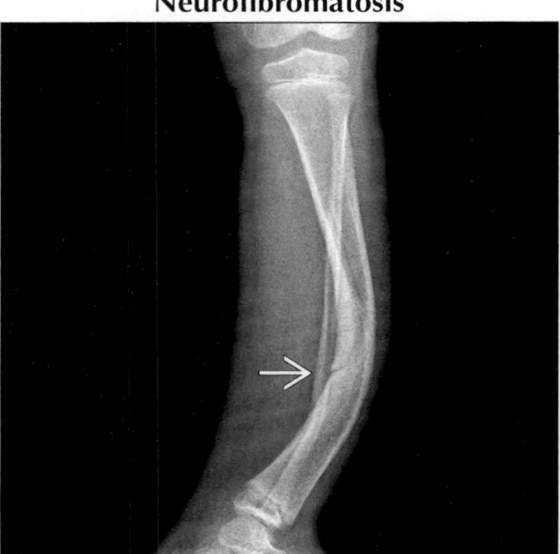

Neurofibromatosis

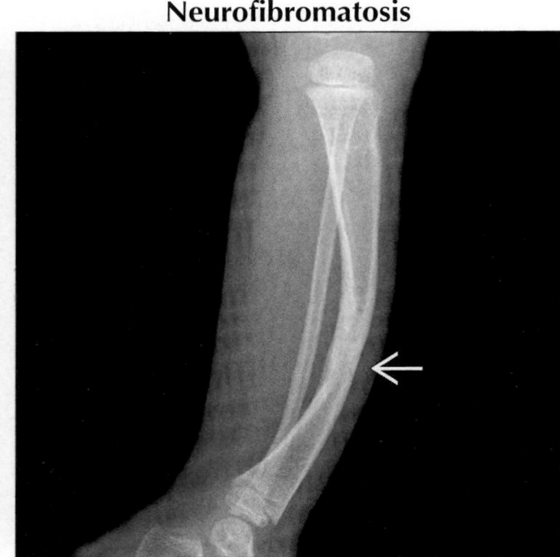

*(**Left**) Anteroposterior radiograph shows a pseudoarthrosis of both the tibia ➔ and fibula ➔. Notice the penciling of the margins of the fibular pseudoarthrosis. (**Right**) Anteroposterior radiograph shows mild medial bowing of the tibia and osteoporosis. Notice the growth arrest or recovery lines within the proximal tibia and fibula. Periosteal reaction ➔ is present along the distal tibial fracture ➔.*

Neurofibromatosis

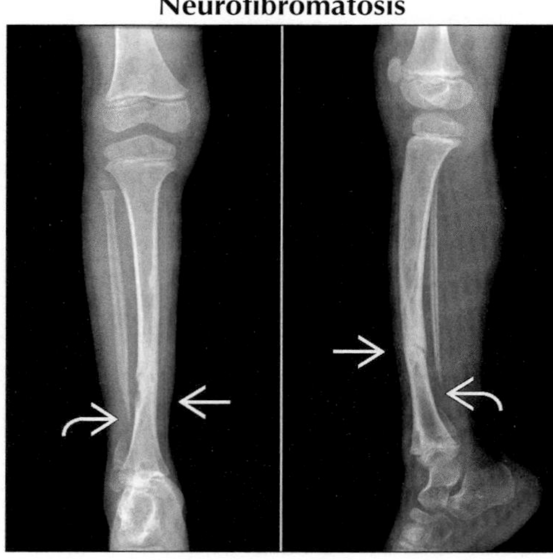

Osteogenesis Imperfecta

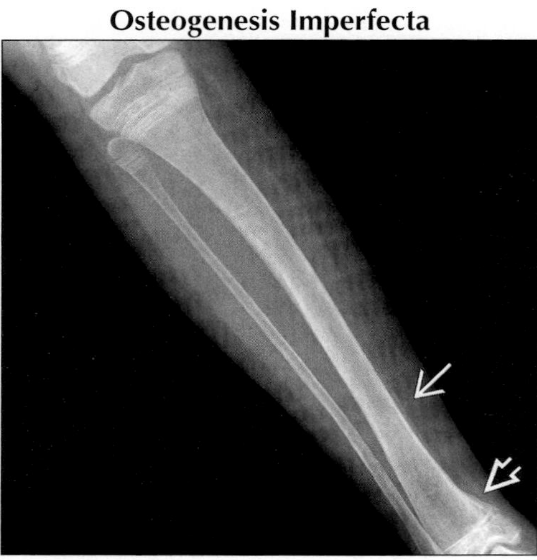

*(**Left**) Anteroposterior radiograph shows multiple fractures of both the tibia and femur. Considerable anterior bowing of the tibia is also present. (**Right**) Lateral radiograph shows moderate osteoporosis with marked anterior bowing of the tibia and, to a lesser degree, the fibula. There is a mid-tibia diaphyseal fracture ➔. Notice the multiple growth recovery lines within the femur and tibia.*

Osteogenesis Imperfecta

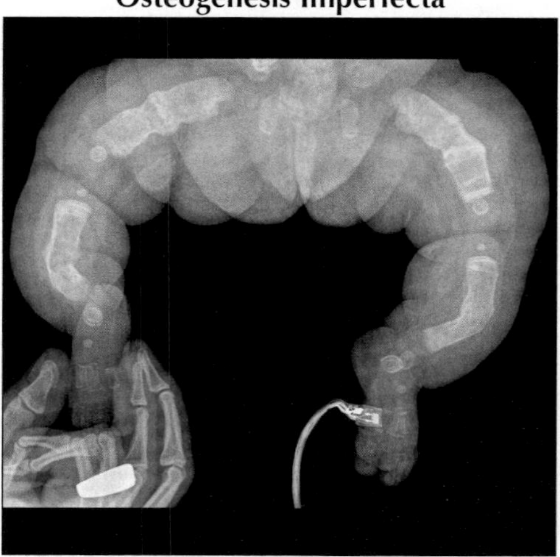

Osteogenesis Imperfecta

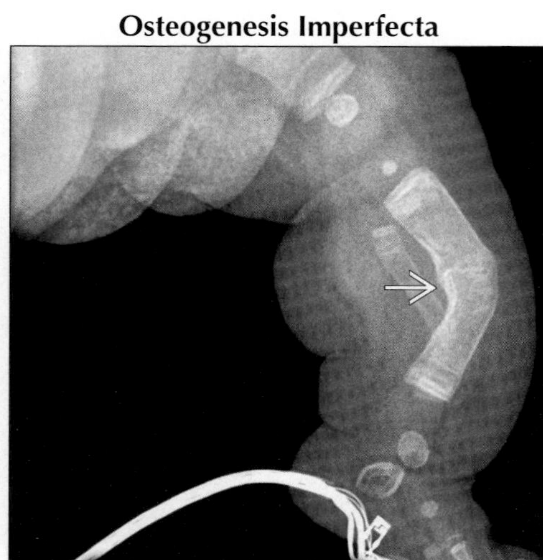

Congenital Tibial Dysplasia

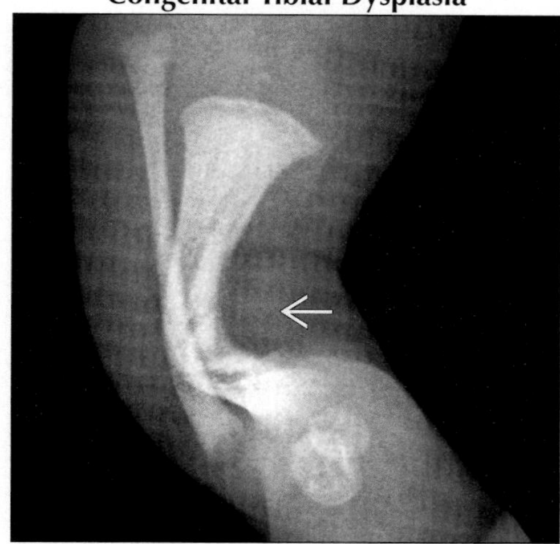

Congenital Tibial Dysplasia

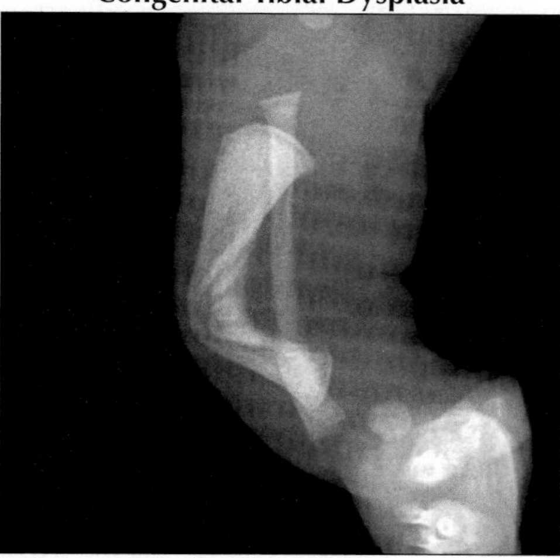

(Left) *Anteroposterior radiograph in a 6 day old shows marked lateral bowing of the tibia ➡. There is moderate thickening of the medial cortex of the tibia.* *(Right)* *Lateral radiograph in the same patient shows anterior bowing of the tibia. 70% of congenital tibial dysplasia patients are eventually diagnosed with neurofibromatosis, though this diagnosis has not yet been made in this patient, now 3 years old.*

Congenital Bowing

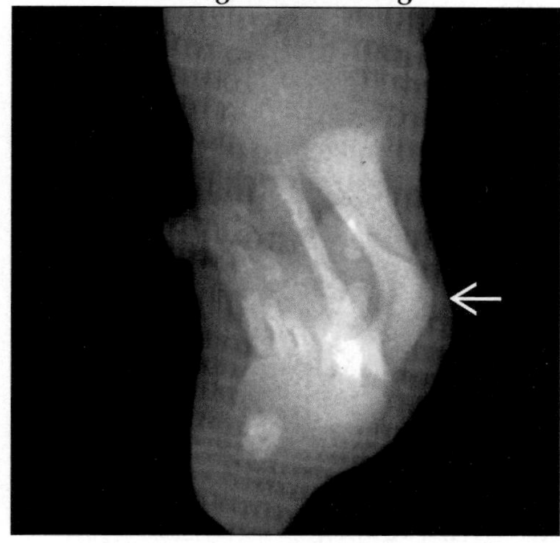

Congenital Bowing

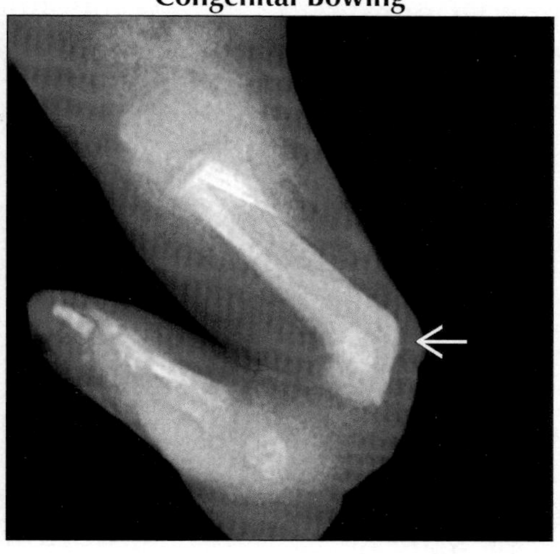

(Left) *Anteroposterior radiograph in a newborn shows convex medial tibial bowing ➡. Notice the complex foot deformity with the toes obscuring the distal tibia and fibula.* *(Right)* *Lateral radiograph in the same newborn shows the typical posterior tibial bowing ➡ seen in congenital tibial bowing.*

Achondroplasia

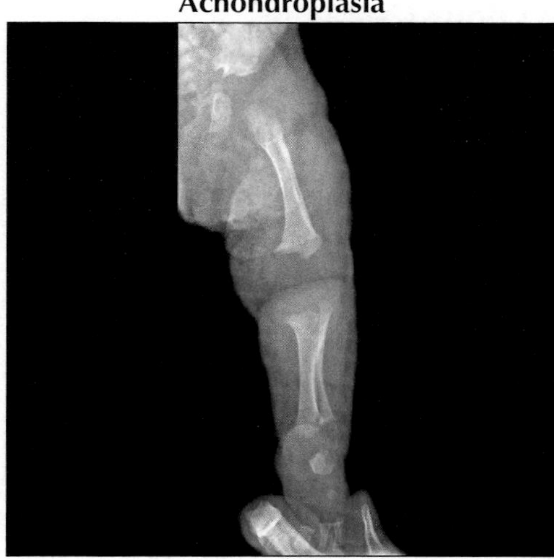

Camptomelic Dysplasia

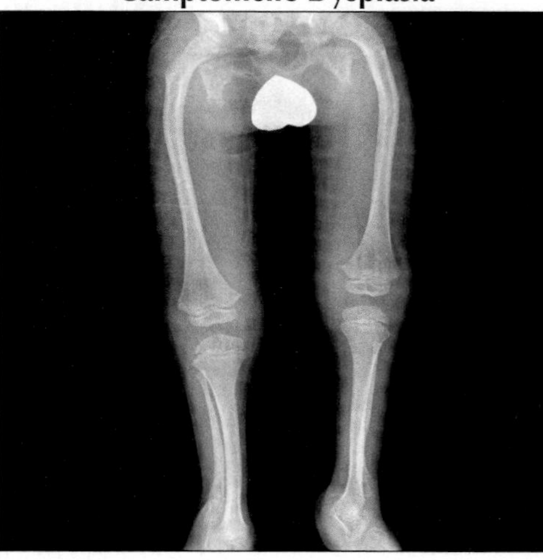

(Left) *Anteroposterior radiograph shows a horizontal acetabular roof, small sacrosciatic notch, and flaring of the proximal femoral metaphysis with shortening of the femur and tibia/fibula.* *(Right)* *Anteroposterior radiograph shows lateral bowing of the proximal femur. Notice the mild medial bowing of the right tibia and short bilateral fibula.*

BUBBLY BONE LESION

DIFFERENTIAL DIAGNOSIS

Common
- Nonossifying Fibroma (NOF)

Less Common
- Aneurysmal Bone Cyst (ABC)
- Unicameral Bone Cyst (UBC)
- Fibrous Dysplasia (FD)
- Langerhans Cell Histiocytosis (LCH)
- Enchondroma
- Primary Sarcoma or Metastatic Disease

Rare but Important
- Osteoblastoma
- Giant Cell Tumor (GCT)
- Chondroblastoma
- Chondromyxoid Fibroma (CMF)

ESSENTIAL INFORMATION

Helpful Clues for Common Diagnoses
- **Nonossifying Fibroma (NOF)**
  - a.k.a. fibroxanthoma, fibrous cortical defect (FCD)
  - Developmental defect, usually discovered as incidental finding on radiograph or MR of knee
  - Age: 2-20 years
  - M:F = 2:1; 30-40% of all children
  - Diametaphyseal of long bones
    - Femur (38%), tibia (43%), knee (55%), fibula (8%), humerus (5%)
  - Eccentric, multiloculated, subcortical; no mineralized matrix; cortex may appear absent; scalloped sclerotic margin
    - Size differentiates FCD and NOF
    - FCD: < 2 cm, within cortex
    - NOF: > 2 cm, extends into medullary cavity
  - T1WI: Hypointense with hypointense rim (sclerotic margin)
  - T2WI: Low to intermediate intensity with hypointense rim (sclerotic margin)
  - T1 C+: Enhances
  - Jaffe-Campanacci syndrome
    - Café-au-lait lesions, mental retardation, hypogonadism, ocular and cardiovascular abnormalities
  - Usually asymptomatic and requires no treatment
  - Most spontaneously regress with time, progressive ossification
  - Curettage and bone grafting if lesion is > 50% diameter of weight bearing bone; increased risk of pathologic fracture

Helpful Clues for Less Common Diagnoses
- **Aneurysmal Bone Cyst (ABC)**
  - Not true neoplasm: Intraosseous AVM
  - Thin-walled, blood-filled cystic cavities
  - Age: 10-30 years; rare in ≤ 5 years old; slight female predominance
  - Primary (1°) or secondary (2°) in preexisting lesion in 1/3 of cases
    - 1°: No recognized preexisting lesion
    - 2°: GCT, chondroblastoma, fibrous dysplasia, osteoblastoma, chondromyxoid fibroma, NOF
    - 2°: Osteosarcoma (e.g., telangiectatic variant), chondrosarcoma, malignant fibrous histiocytoma
  - Typically metaphyseal, most commonly around knee
  - Tubular long bones (70-80%), lower leg (29%), pelvis (5-10%), clavicle and ribs (5%), spinal posterior elements (16%)
  - Geographic eccentric expansile lucent lesion ± multiloculated, markedly thinned cortex (may need CT to see) ± periosteal reaction (if fractured)
  - MR: Characteristic fluid-fluid level (blood products) containing cavities of differing signal intensity; hypointense rim surrounds ABC
    - Enhancement of cyst walls and septations without enhancing cyst contents, "honeycomb"
  - Treatment: Curettage and bone grafting with 20% recurrence rate
- **Unicameral Bone Cyst (UBC)**
  - a.k.a. simple or solitary bone cyst
  - Age: 10-20 years; ~ 2/3 present with pathologic fracture
  - Proximal humerus and femur in up to 80-90%
  - Central metaphyseal, well defined, lucent, lacks periosteal reaction unless fractured
  - **Hint**: Pathognomonic, fallen fragment sign
    - Pathologic fracture with cortical bone fragment floating dependently with UBC
  - MR: May contain fluid-fluid level if traumatized; no solid enhancing component

- **Fibrous Dysplasia (FD)**
  - Age: 5-20 years, peak 10-20 years
  - Monostotic (70-80%) or polyostotic
  - Expansile, ground-glass, lucent, sclerotic (skull base lesions), no periosteal reaction, bowing
  - Associations
    - McCune-Albright: Female predominance, polyostotic, unilateral FD, precocious puberty, hyperthyroidism, café-au-lait spots
    - Mazabraud syndrome: Polyostotic FD with intramuscular myxoma, rare
- **Langerhans Cell Histiocytosis (LCH)**
  - Age: 50% < 10 years
  - Lytic, sharply demarcated lesion without sclerotic margin unless healing
  - Skull (50%), axial skeleton (25%), proximal long bones (15%)
- **Enchondroma**
  - Age: 10-30 years
  - Lucent, scalloped endosteum; ring and arc calcified matrix
  - Small bones of hand and wrist; metadiaphysis of long bones
- **Primary Sarcoma or Metastatic Disease**
  - Telangiectatic osteosarcoma: Radiographically, lytic lesion could look like ABC

Helpful Clues for Rare Diagnoses

- **Osteoblastoma**
  - Age: 80% < 30 years old
  - 1-10 cm in size, > 1.5 cm osteoblastoma, < 1.5 cm considered osteoid osteoma
  - Lytic, expansile, sclerotic margin, variable central calcification, radiolucent nidus
  - Spine (40%), long bones (30%), hands and feet (15%), skull and face (15%)
  - May present with painful scoliosis
  - Extensive inflammatory change can mimic malignancy or infection
- **Giant Cell Tumor (GCT)**
  - Occurs after growth plate closure
  - Metaepiphyseal, eccentric, lytic, nonsclerotic margin, extends subarticular bone ± periosteal reaction
  - Long bones (75-90%), around knee (50%)
  - Pathologic fracture (30%)
- **Chondroblastoma**
  - Eccentric, epiphyseal, expansile; periosteal reaction in 50%
  - Immature skeleton
  - Most commonly around knee and proximal humerus
    - Long bones (80%), hands and feet (10%)
  - Thin sclerotic margin with chondroid calcification in 1/3
  - MR: Solid with no fluid-fluid levels
    - T1WI: Low to intermediate
    - T2WI: Intermediate to low with surrounding edema
- **Chondromyxoid Fibroma (CMF)**
  - Eccentric, lucent with sclerotic margin
  - Male predominance; CMFs present with pain
  - Treatment: Curettage, recurrence in 25%

Nonossifying Fibroma (NOF)

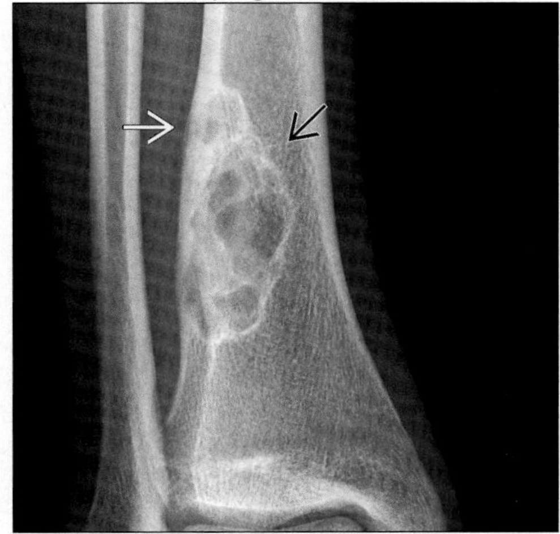

Anteroposterior radiograph shows a bubbly eccentric lesion ⇒ with a scalloped sclerotic margin within the distal tibial diaphysis. Notice the thinned cortical margin ➡ of the NOF.

Nonossifying Fibroma (NOF)

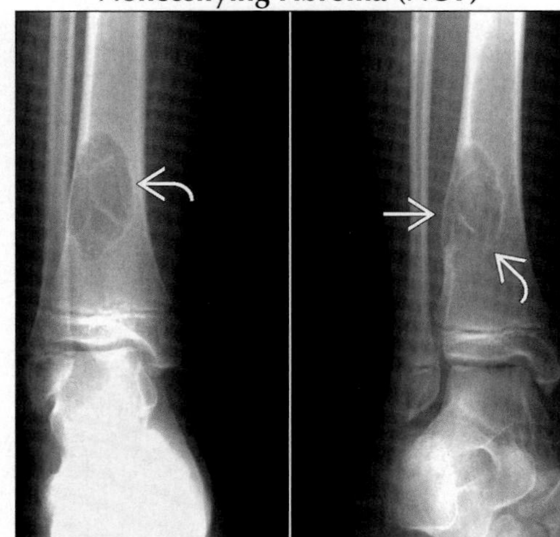

Anteroposterior and oblique radiographs show an eccentric, multiloculated, lucent lesion ➡ with a thin sclerotic margin within the distal tibia. Notice the thinned lateral cortical margin ➡.

*(**Left**) Anteroposterior radiograph shows an eccentric lucent lesion ➔ with a thin sclerotic scalloped margin within the proximal lateral aspect of the tibia. NOFs are most commonly seen about the knee. (**Right**) Lateral radiograph in the same child shows the NOF ⇨, which was discovered incidentally in this patient presenting with knee pain. Notice the Osgood-Schlatter changes ➔ with fragmented anterior tibial apophysis & thickening of the patellar tendon.*

Nonossifying Fibroma (NOF)

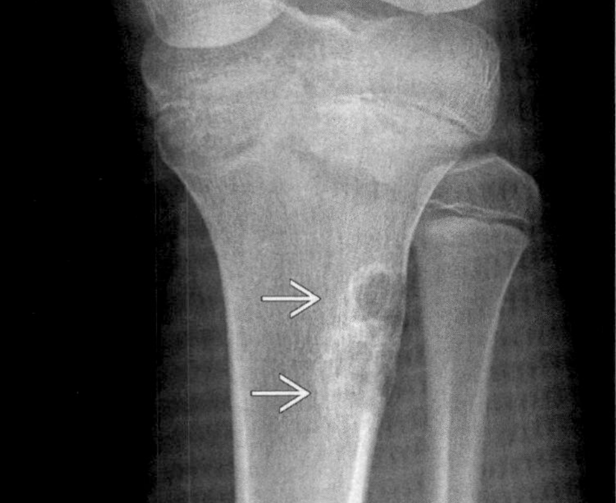

Nonossifying Fibroma (NOF)

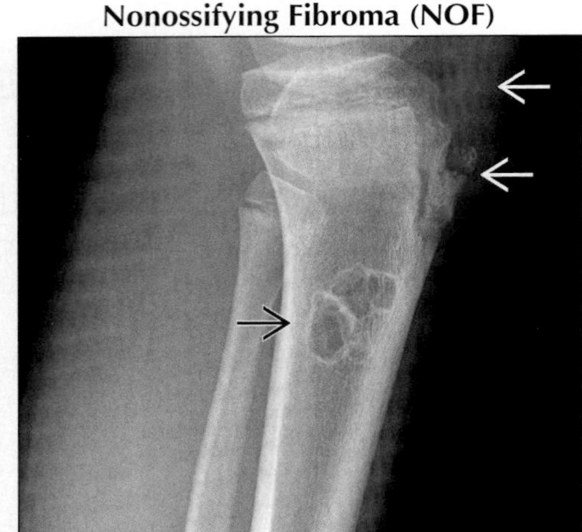

*(**Left**) Lateral radiograph shows a pathologic fracture ➔ through the distal tibial NOF ➔. This patient was prone to fracturing the NOF due to the large size of the lesion, which was greater than 50% of the diameter of the tibia. (**Right**) Anteroposterior radiograph shows a lucent lesion ⇨ within the distal humerus. There was slight expansion on the lateral view (not shown).*

Nonossifying Fibroma (NOF)

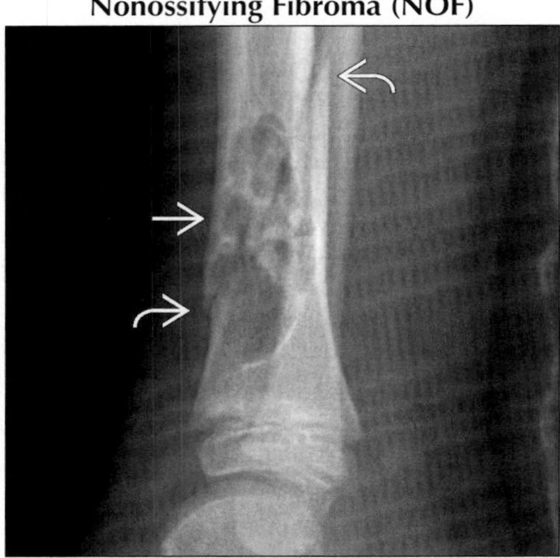

Aneurysmal Bone Cyst (ABC)

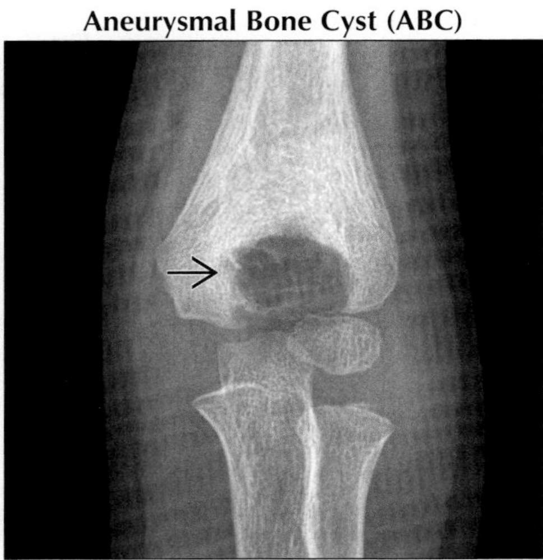

*(**Left**) Anteroposterior radiograph shows a bubbly multiloculated lesion ➔ expanding the proximal tibial metadiaphysis. There is an approximately 20% recurrence rate of ABC following curettage. (**Right**) Axial T2WI FS MR in the same child shows multiple fluid-fluid levels ➔ contained within the cystic cavities. Note the lack of soft tissue mass, which may help differentiate ABCs from telangiectatic osteosarcoma, a look-alike.*

Aneurysmal Bone Cyst (ABC)

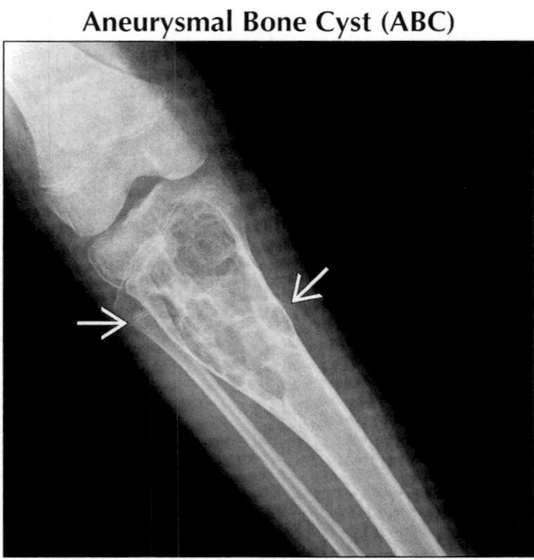

Aneurysmal Bone Cyst (ABC)

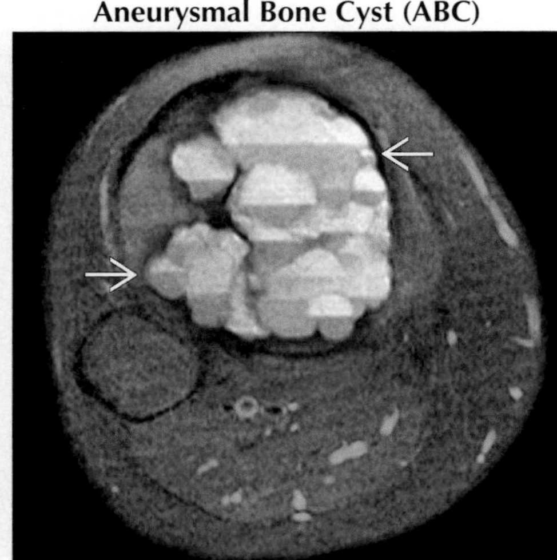

BUBBLY BONE LESION

Unicameral Bone Cyst (UBC)

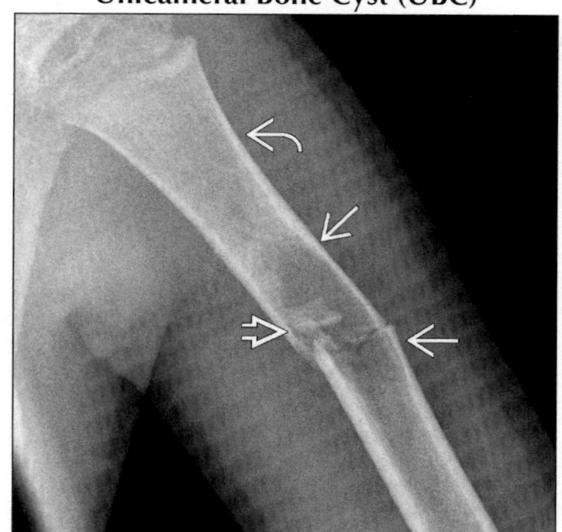

Unicameral Bone Cyst (UBC)

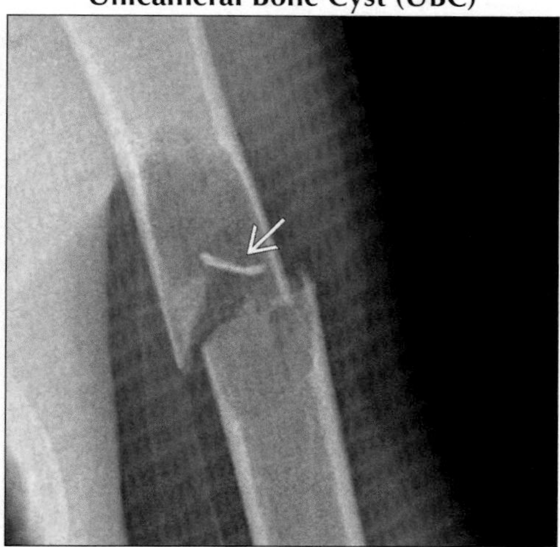

(Left) *Oblique radiograph shows a pathologic fracture through a UBC ➔, which contains a fragment of bone ➔ in a pathognomic fallen fragment sign. An additional, more proximal lucent lesion ➔ is also shown, believed to be a NOF.* ***(Right)*** *Anteroposterior radiograph in the same patient shows a bone fragment ➔. The majority of UBCs are seen within either the proximal humerus or the femur.*

Unicameral Bone Cyst (UBC)

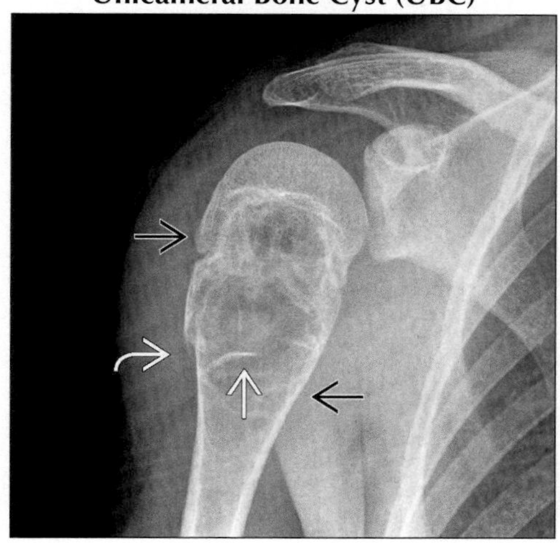

Unicameral Bone Cyst (UBC)

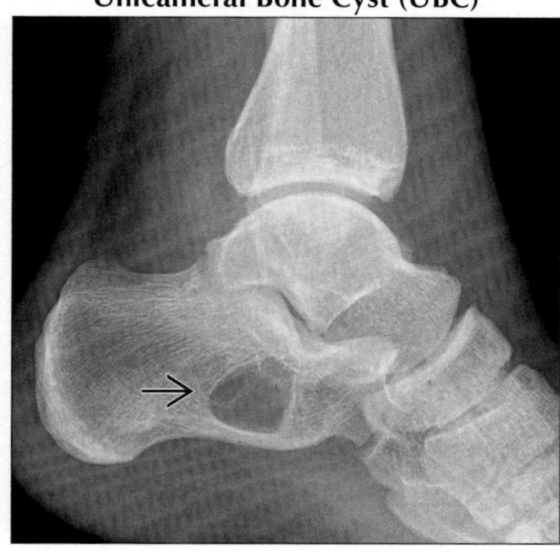

(Left) *Oblique radiograph shows a pathologic fracture ➔ through an expansile bubbly lesion → within the proximal right humerus. This lesion may contain a fragment of bone ➔.* ***(Right)*** *Lateral radiograph shows a lucent → calcaneal lesion. This was confirmed on a MR to be a unicameral bone cyst. UBCs should be differentiated from a normal region of lucency in the anterior calcaneus (seen as a triangular lucent area between the major trabecular groups).*

Fibrous Dysplasia (FD)

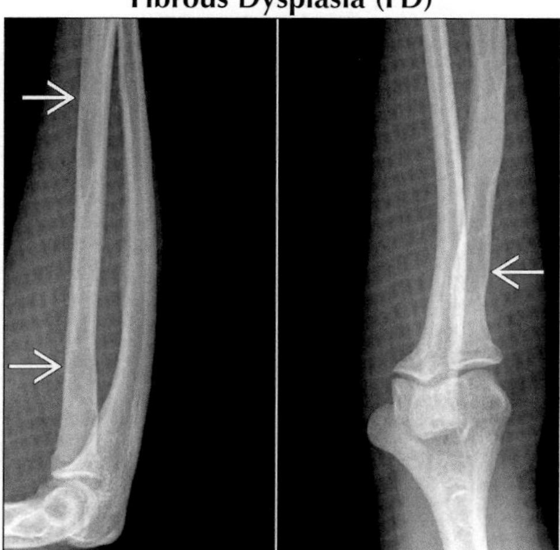

Fibrous Dysplasia (FD)

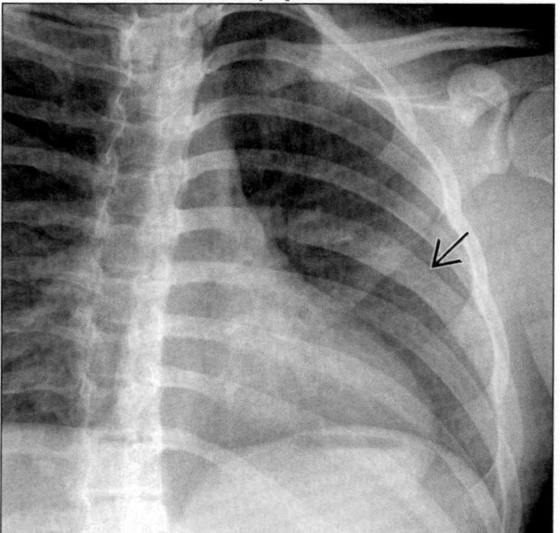

(Left) *AP and lateral views of the forearm show ground-glass and lucent lesions ➔ throughout the radius in this patient with known multifocal fibrous dysplasia.* ***(Right)*** *Anteroposterior radiograph in the same patient shows expansion of the left posterior 6th rib →. Fibrous dysplasia is the most common benign tumor of the ribs.*

BUBBLY BONE LESION

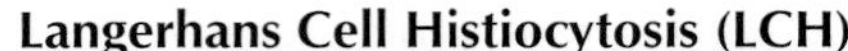

Langerhans Cell Histiocytosis (LCH)

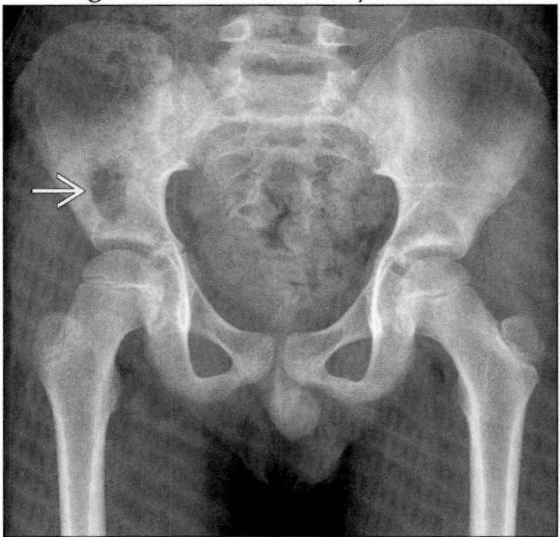

Langerhans Cell Histiocytosis (LCH)

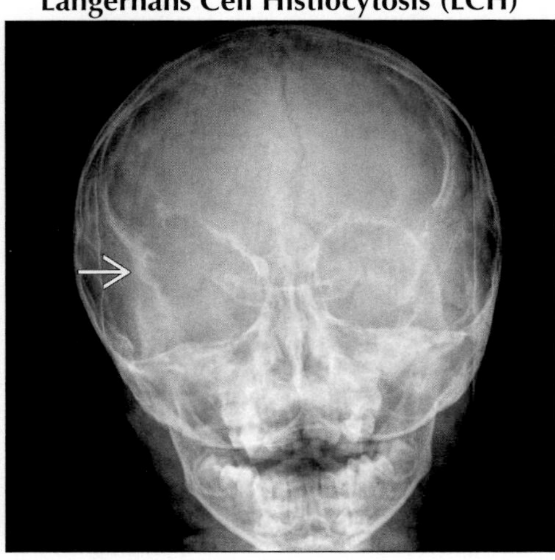

(Left) *Anteroposterior radiograph shows a geographic, well-defined, lucent lesion ➔ without a sclerotic margin within the right iliac wing. This patient has a known history of LCH.* ***(Right)*** *Anteroposterior radiograph in the same patient shows destruction of the right lateral orbital wall ➔. Solitary lesions tend to be more common than multiple lesions. When multiple, the new osseous lesions are usually seen within 1-2 years. Any bone can be involved.*

Enchondroma

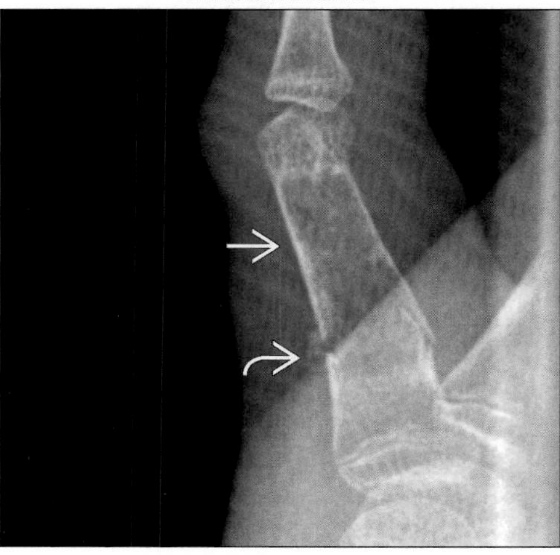

Primary Sarcoma or Metastatic Disease

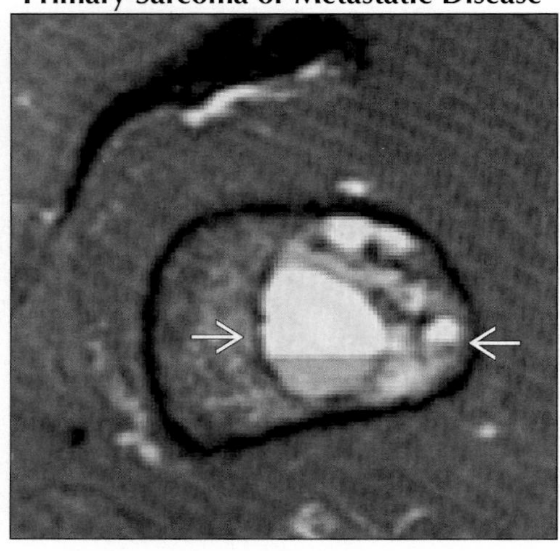

(Left) *Anteroposterior radiograph shows a lucent lesion ➔ with a pathologic fracture ➔ within the 5th digit. Approximately 1/2 of solitary enchondromas are found in the hands. When lesions are painful or grow rapidly, malignant transformation should be excluded. Enchondromas and chondrosarcomas may be indistinguishable by imaging.* ***(Right)*** *Axial T2WI FS MR shows multiple fluid-fluid levels ➔ in a femoral osteosarcoma.*

Osteoblastoma

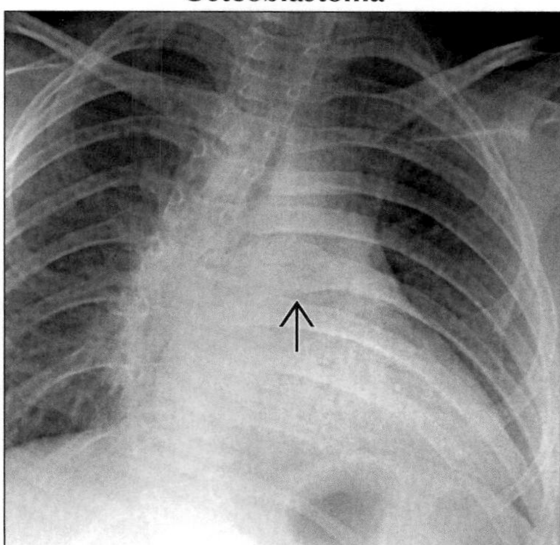

Osteoblastoma

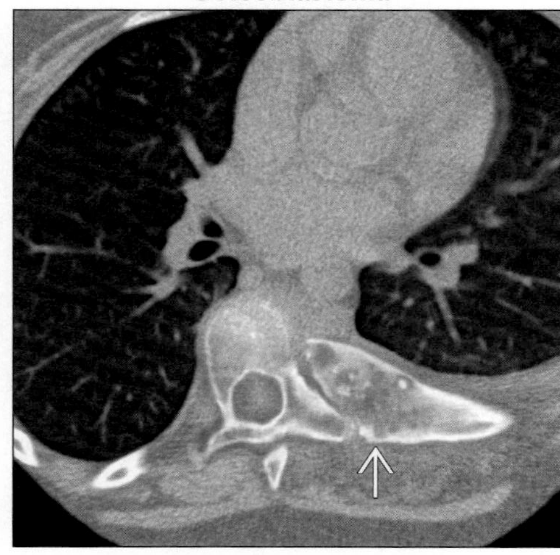

(Left) *Anteroposterior radiograph shows an expansile posterior left rib lesion ➔. This patient presented with a painful scoliosis.* ***(Right)*** *Axial NECT in the same patient shows the expansile posterior rib lesion ➔ with an osteoid matrix. Typically osteoblastomas lack soft tissue extension/mass. A more aggressive form of osteoblastoma may rapidly resorb bone and extend into surrounding soft tissues. Osteoblastomas account for 1% of primary bone tumors.*

BUBBLY BONE LESION

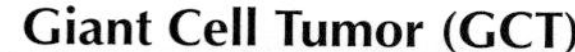

Giant Cell Tumor (GCT)

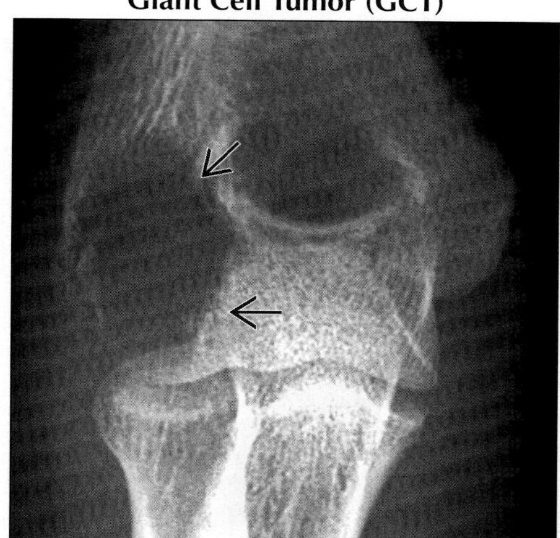

Chondroblastoma

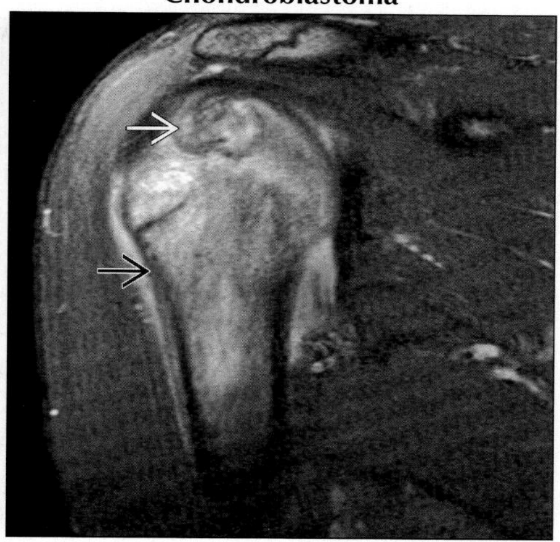

(Left) *Anteroposterior radiograph shows a lytic lesion → within the distal lateral humerus. Notice the closed physis and extension to the articular surface. Although benign, GCTs have a tendency for bone destruction, local recurrence, and occasional metastasis. GCTs account for 5% of all primary bone tumors and may mimic osteomyelitis.* ***(Right)*** *Coronal T2WI FS MR shows an epiphyseal lesion → with a hypointense margin and significant marrow edema →.*

Chondroblastoma

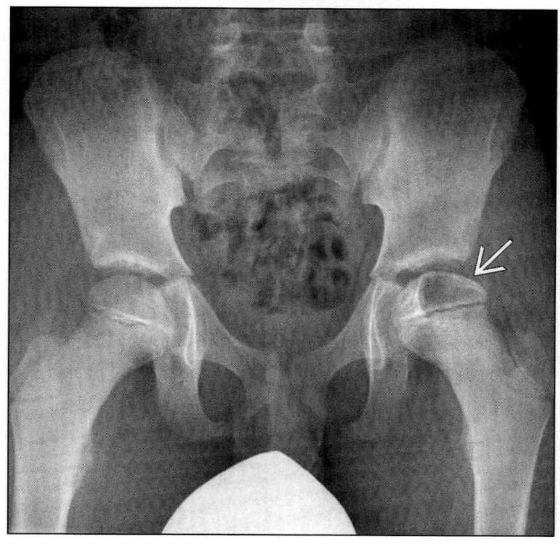

Chondroblastoma

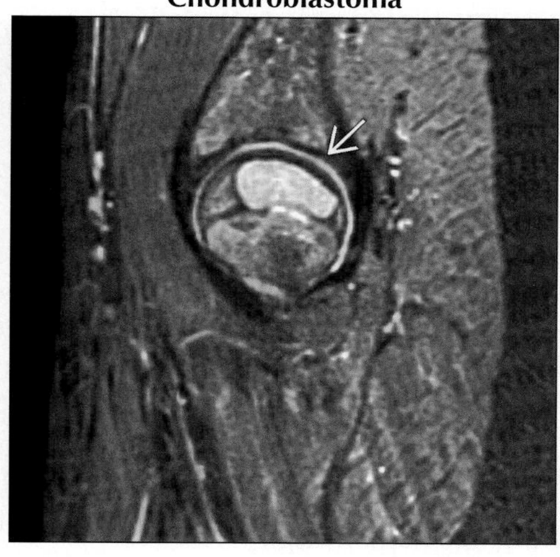

(Left) *AP radiograph shows a lucent epiphyseal lesion → within the left femoral head with mild flattening of the superior lateral femoral head. Chondroblastomas account for ~ 1% of all bone tumors, and more than 90% of patients presenting with chondroblastoma are younger than 30 years old.* ***(Right)*** *Sagittal inversion recovery FSE MR shows a hyperintense oval lesion → within the left femoral head. Most patients are diagnosed during the 2nd decade of life.*

Chondromyxoid Fibroma (CMF)

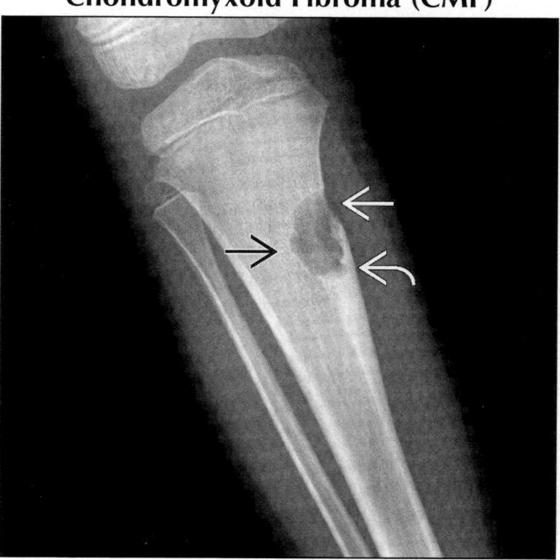

Chondromyxoid Fibroma (CMF)

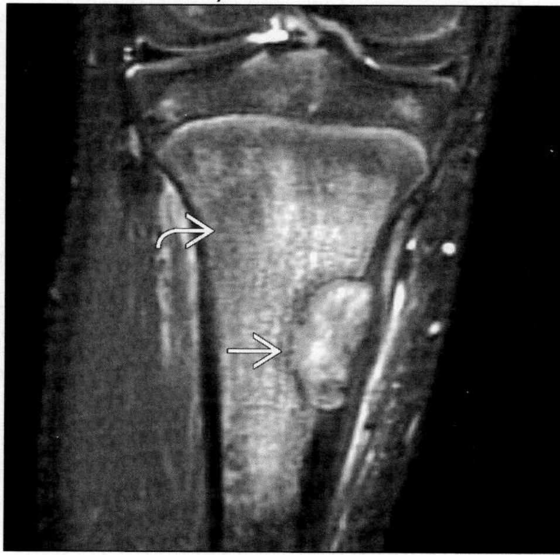

(Left) *Anteroposterior radiograph shows a lucent, slightly expansile, proximal tibial lesion → with a thin sclerotic margin, focal cortical defect →, and cortical buttressing ↪. 75% of CMFs occur in the lower extremity, particularly around the knee joint.* ***(Right)*** *Coronal inversion recovery FSE MR in the same patient shows a hyperintense eccentric lesion → within the proximal tibia. Note the diffuse marrow edema ↪.*

PERIOSTEUM: PERIOSTITIS MULTIPLE BONES

DIFFERENTIAL DIAGNOSIS

Common
- Physiologic Periostitis
- Child Abuse
- Multifocal Osteomyelitis
- Juvenile Idiopathic Arthritis (JIA)
- Hypervitaminosis A
- Polyostotic Aggressive Bone Tumor

Less Common
- Prostaglandin Periostitis
- Sickle Cell Dactylitis

Rare but Important
- Caffey Disease
- Renal Osteodystrophy (Mimic)
- Leukemia
- Scurvy
- Complications of Chemotherapeutic Drugs, Methotrexate
- Hypertrophic Osteoarthropathy, Cystic Fibrosis
- Complications of Retinoids

ESSENTIAL INFORMATION

Key Differential Diagnosis Issues
- Periosteal reaction is common in a single bone, with a multitude of etiologies
- Polyostotic periostitis is much less common; the polyostotic nature and patient age helps to limit the diagnosis
- **Hint**: Some etiologies are limited by patient age
  - 1st appearance BEFORE 6 months of age
    - Physiologic (should disappear by age 6 months)
    - Congenital osteomyelitis
    - Caffey disease
    - Prostaglandin periostitis
  - 1st appearance AFTER 6 months of age
    - Juvenile idiopathic arthritis
    - Hypervitaminosis A
    - Sickle cell dactylitis
    - Renal osteodystrophy
    - Scurvy
- **Hint**: Always consider the possibility of child abuse/nonaccidental trauma

Helpful Clues for Common Diagnoses
- **Physiologic Periostitis**
  - Normal growth may be so rapid during first 6 months that new periosteal bone is produced
    - Symmetric, regular
    - Resolves by 6 months of age
- **Child Abuse**
  - Always consider this diagnosis when periosteal reaction is seen in a child!
  - Often not symmetric
  - Often 2° to metaphyseal corner fracture
    - Fracture causes subperiosteal bleeding and lifting of periosteum
  - May occur without fracture 2° to normally loose periosteum and a twisting injury
- **Multifocal Osteomyelitis**
  - Congenital infections
    - TORCH infections
    - Congenital syphilis (may have "celery stalking" at metaphyses as well)
  - Infections from newborn ICU: Generally *Streptococcus*
  - Multifocal osteomyelitis later in childhood
    - Hematogenous spread (metaphyseal)
    - Consider underlying disease: HIV/AIDS or sickle cell anemia
  - Tuberculosis (TB) involvement in hands: Dactylitis is termed spina ventosa
- **Juvenile Idiopathic Arthritis (JIA)**
  - 1st osseous manifestation may be periostitis of hand or foot phalanges
  - Later, joints will be involved
  - Differential is sickle cell and TB dactylitis
- **Hypervitaminosis A**
  - Excessive intake of vitamin A results initially in periosteal reaction
    - Subtle at first but may become quite dense and thick
    - Painful
  - Continued use of excessive vitamin A may lead to coned epiphyses
- **Polyostotic Aggressive Bone Tumor**
  - Bone metastases
    - Ewing sarcoma presents with osseous metastases as frequently as lung mets
    - Others to consider: Medulloblastoma, neuroblastoma, osteosarcoma
  - Leukemia: Common but usually presents with lucent metaphyseal bands or diffuse osteoporosis
    - Periostitis is a rare manifestation

- Langerhans cell histiocytosis: Often polyostotic; may be aggressive enough to elicit periosteal reaction

Helpful Clues for Less Common Diagnoses

- **Prostaglandin Periostitis**
  - Prostaglandins used for congenital heart disease in infancy to keep ductus open
  - Dense, nonspecific periosteal reaction on long bones
- **Sickle Cell Dactylitis**
  - Generally young children (< 7 years of age)
  - Cold temperature → vasoconstriction of terminal vessels in phalanges → sludging of sickled red blood cells → bone infarct
  - Bone infarct may initially elicit periostitis; eventually has mixed lytic and sclerotic appearance

Helpful Clues for Rare Diagnoses

- **Caffey Disease**
  - Rare disease manifests at birth
  - Painful periostitis of long bones
  - Involvement of clavicle and mandible is suggestive of diagnosis since not usually seen with other diagnoses
  - Self-limited; spontaneously resolves over 1st 2 years of life
- **Renal Osteodystrophy (Mimic)**
  - Severe subperiosteal resorption, especially at proximal humeral, tibial, or femoral metaphysis or at radial aspect of middle phalanx, may mimic fluffy periostitis
    - Watch for underlying abnormal bone density, signs of rickets (widening at zone of provisional calcification)
  - Severe renal osteodystrophy may result in bone accretion when effective treatment is initiated; mimics periosteal reaction
- **Scurvy**
  - Rare metabolic disease affecting collagen
  - Osseous manifestations
    - Osteopenia
    - Sclerotic ring around epiphyses (Wimberger sign)
    - Sclerotic metaphyseal line (white line of Frankel)
    - Corner fractures at metaphyses
    - Subperiosteal bleed (especially with corner fracture) → elevates periosteum → reparative bone formation, which mimics periosteal reaction
- **Complications of Chemotherapeutic Drugs, Methotrexate**
  - Rare periosteal reaction, nonspecific
- **Hypertrophic Osteoarthropathy, Cystic Fibrosis**
  - Lung disease may elicit hypertrophic osteoarthropathy, just as in adults
  - Periosteal reaction that is painful, referred to joints
- **Complications of Retinoids**
  - May induce productive bone changes
    - Most frequently, large syndesmophytes at anterior vertebral bodies
    - Rarely, periostitis

Physiologic Periostitis

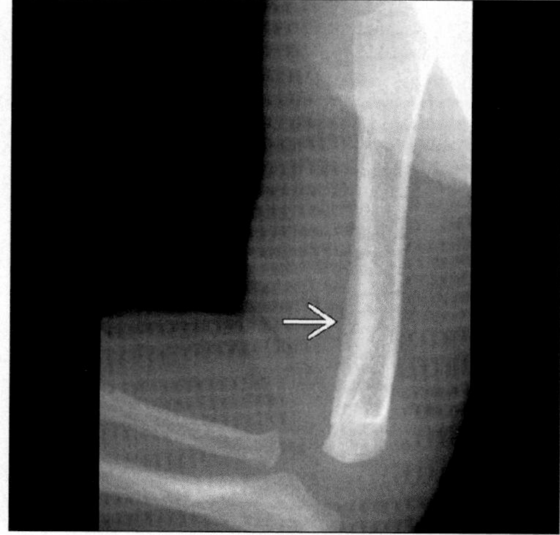

Lateral radiograph shows dense, regular periosteal reaction ➔ that was symmetric in this 6 week old. There were no other abnormalities. Under the age of 6 months, rapid growth results in this normal appearance.

Child Abuse

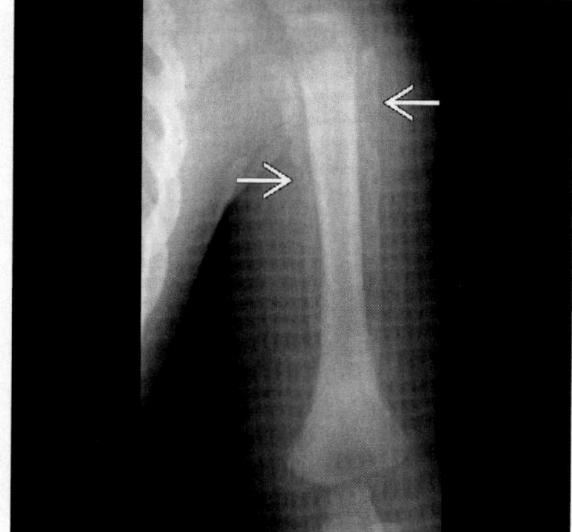

AP radiograph shows dense periosteal reaction ➔ representing healing following a subperiosteal bleed from a proximal metaphyseal corner fracture. The child had other sites of periosteal reaction and fractures.

PERIOSTEUM: PERIOSTITIS MULTIPLE BONES

(Left) *Anteroposterior radiograph shows periosteal reaction ➡ related to a metaphyseal corner fracture seen only on the lateral view; fracture occurred 19 days earlier. Periosteal reaction should alert radiologist to seek other signs of nonaccidental trauma.* ***(Right)*** *Anteroposterior radiograph shows periosteal reaction along the tibia ➡ of an infant. Other bones were similarly involved. Finding is nonspecific but can be seen with congenital infections such as syphilis in this case.*

Child Abuse

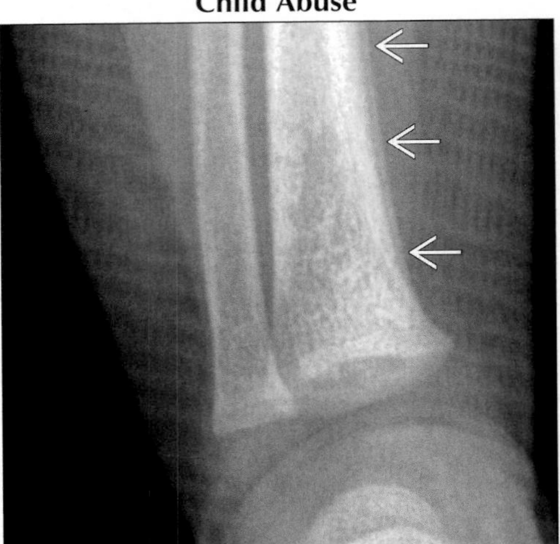

Multifocal Osteomyelitis

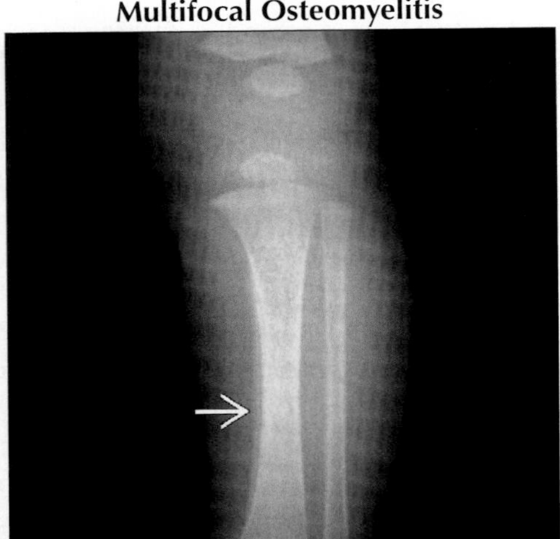

(Left) *Lateral radiograph shows thin regular periosteal reaction along many of the phalanges ➡ in this child, along with soft tissue swelling.* ***(Right)*** *Posteroanterior radiograph in the same patient also demonstrates the periosteal reaction ➡. The findings are not specific but in this case were the 1st manifestation of JIA. Sickle cell dactylitis would be considered if the child was African-American.*

Juvenile Idiopathic Arthritis (JIA)

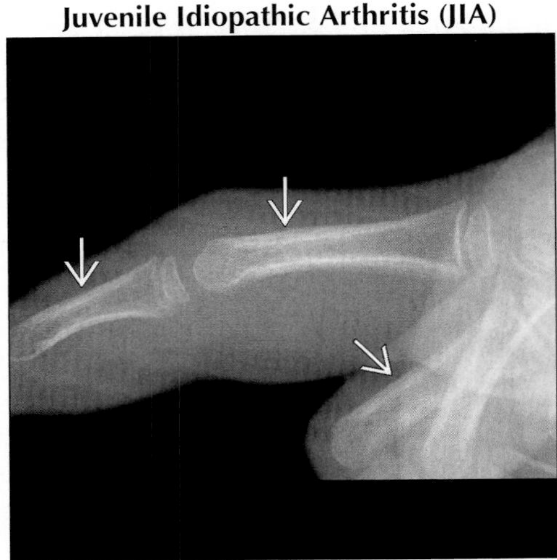

Juvenile Idiopathic Arthritis (JIA)

(Left) *Posteroanterior radiograph shows dense periosteal accretion along the ulnar diaphysis ➡. This was seen on other bones, including both legs. This 1 year old was being given large doses of vitamin A.* ***(Right)*** *Lateral radiograph shows thick and prominent periosteal reaction along the ulna ➡. Other bones showed lytic lesions and others showed simply periosteal reaction in this child with metastatic medulloblastoma.*

Hypervitaminosis A

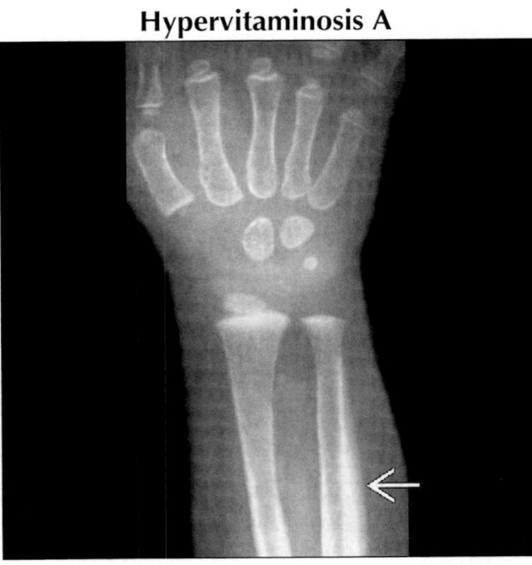

Polyostotic Aggressive Bone Tumor

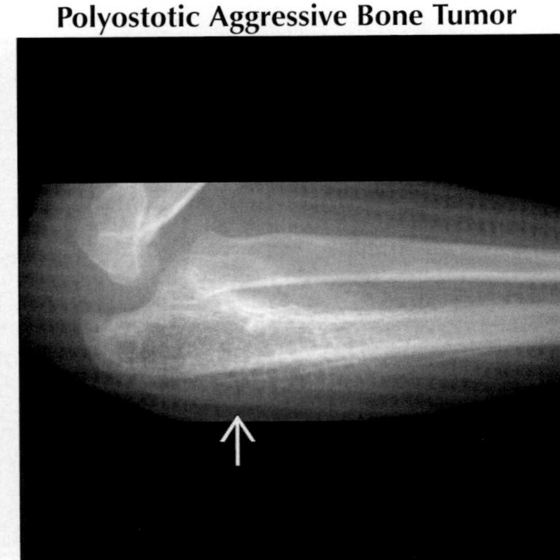

Prostaglandin Periostitis

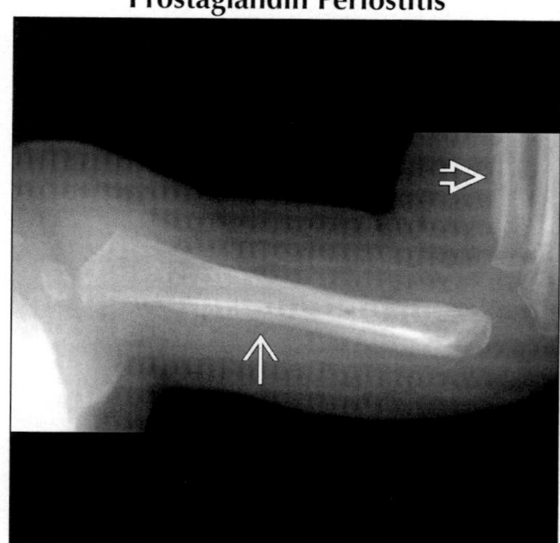

Sickle Cell Dactylitis

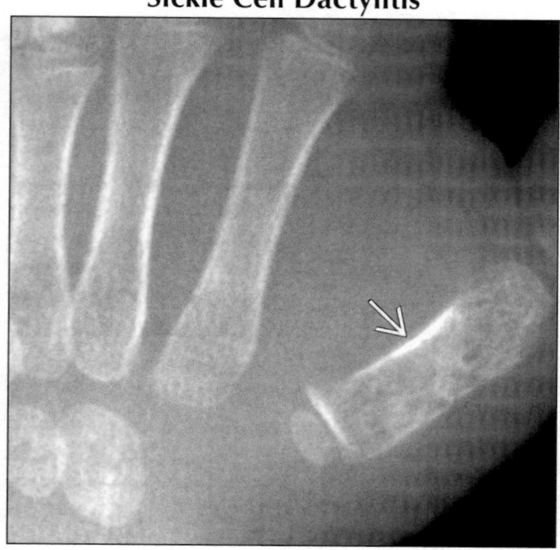

(Left) *Lateral radiograph shows thick, dense periosteal reaction in the humerus ➡ as well as the bones of the forearm ➡. This infant had been treated with prostaglandins for a cardiac defect.* ***(Right)*** *Anteroposterior radiograph shows subtle periosteal reaction ➡ and underlying bone abnormality in this African-American child who developed hand pain on the 1st cold day of winter. This represents a bone infarct in sickle cell disease.*

Caffey Disease

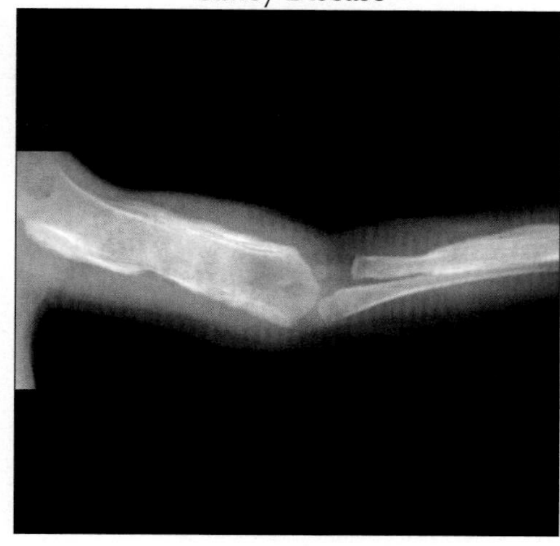

Caffey Disease

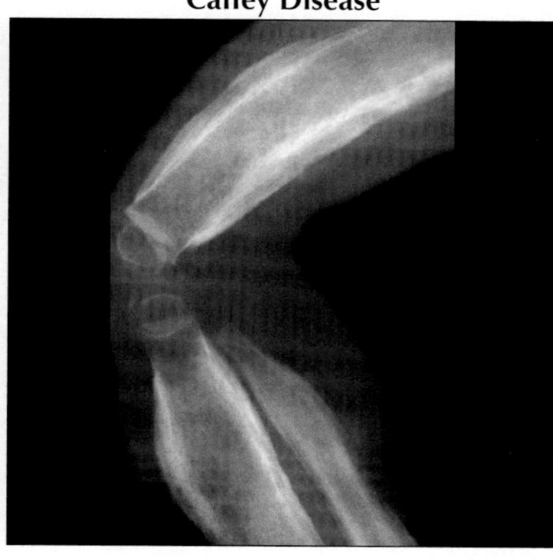

(Left) *Lateral radiograph shows dense periosteal new bone formation along the humerus as well as the radius in this child. The child also had mandibular periosteal bone change, which is considered highly suggestive of Caffey disease.* ***(Right)*** *Lateral radiograph shows thick, dense periosteal new bone formation along all long bones in a severe case of Caffey disease. The process is painful but self-limited; this patient returned to normal by 3 years of age.*

Renal Osteodystrophy (Mimic)

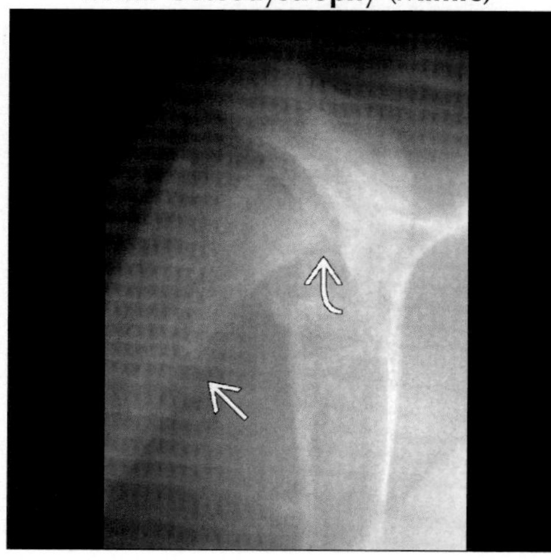

Scurvy

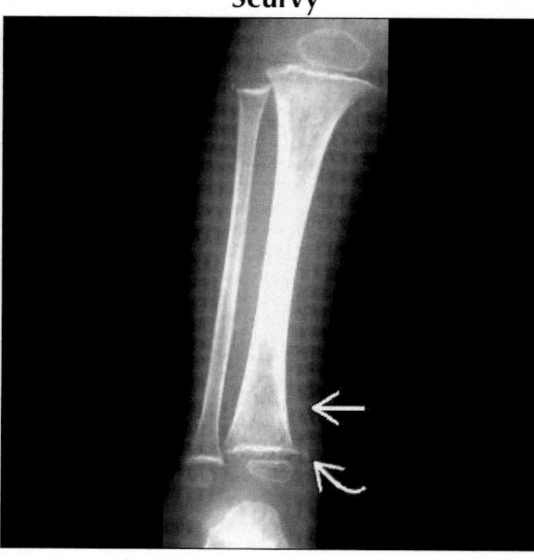

(Left) *AP radiograph shows what might be mistaken for fluffy periostitis ➡ along the proximal humerus. This is aggressive subperiosteal resorption in a patient with renal disease. Note the rickets and slipped humeral epiphysis ➡.* ***(Right)*** *AP radiograph shows dense metaphyseal lines of Frankel as well as a metaphyseal corner fracture ➡ in this patient with scurvy. There was a subperiosteal bleed, and periosteal bone formation is developing ➡ along the tibia.*

PSEUDOARTHROSIS

DIFFERENTIAL DIAGNOSIS

Common
- Fracture, Nonunion
- Failed Graft

Rare but Important
- Neurofibromatosis (NF)
- Congenital Pseudoarthrosis
- Osteogenesis Imperfecta (OI)
- Fibrous Dysplasia
- Ankylosing Spondylitis, Post-Trauma

ESSENTIAL INFORMATION

Helpful Clues for Common Diagnoses
- **Postoperative (Nonunion & Failed Graft)**
  - **Hint**: Motion, especially in spine
  - **Hint**: Look for hardware failure
  - Tibia common due to poor blood supply
  - Radiographic findings
    - Nonbridging callus, may be hypertrophic
    - Smooth sclerotic margins

Helpful Clues for Rare Diagnoses
- **Neurofibromatosis (NF)**
  - Tibia, clavicle, radius, ulna
  - Congenital pseudoarthrosis similar
    - a.k.a. congenital tibial dysplasia
    - 70% eventually develop NF
    - 1-2% of NF patients
- **Osteogenesis Imperfecta (OI)**
  - Defect in type 1 collagen
  - Radiographic findings (severity) depends on type of OI
    - Generalized osteoporosis
    - Thinning of skull, multiple wormian bones, platybasia
    - Scoliosis, kyphosis, wedging vertebral bodies
    - Thin gracile bones, bowing bones, pseudoarthrosis, epiphyseal and physeal broadening and irregularity, "popcorn bones"
    - Multiple fractures of varying ages
    - Narrow pelvis, protrusio acetabuli
- **Fibrous Dysplasia**
  - Radiographic findings
    - Mildly expansile, ground-glass matrix
    - Well-defined ± sclerotic margins
  - Monostotic or polyostotic
- **Ankylosing Spondylitis, Post-Trauma**
  - 2-3x more common in males
  - Approximately 90% HLA-B27 positive
  - Affects all age groups
    - Most common in 2nd and 3rd decades of life
  - Following disruption of fused spine
  - Radiographic findings
    - Syndesmophytes
    - Facet joint ankylosis
    - Interspinous, supraspinous ligament ossification
    - Sacroiliac joint fusion
    - Enthesopathy, hip & shoulder arthritis

Fracture, Nonunion

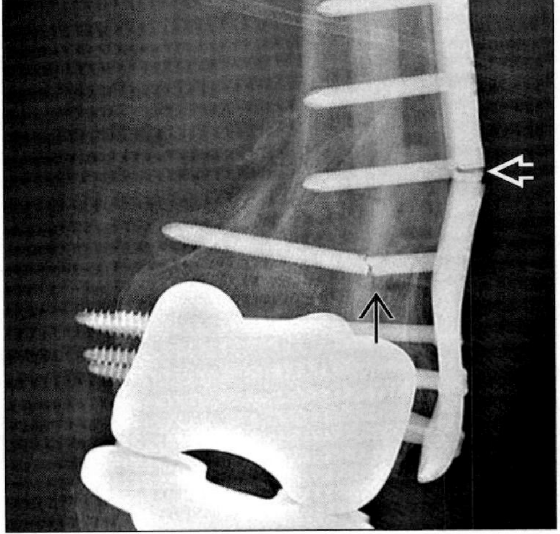

AP radiograph shows screw ➔ & plate ➔ fractures in a patient who has developed pseudarthrosis. The original construct was too rigid to permit the micromotion required to promote osteoblastic activity.

Failed Graft

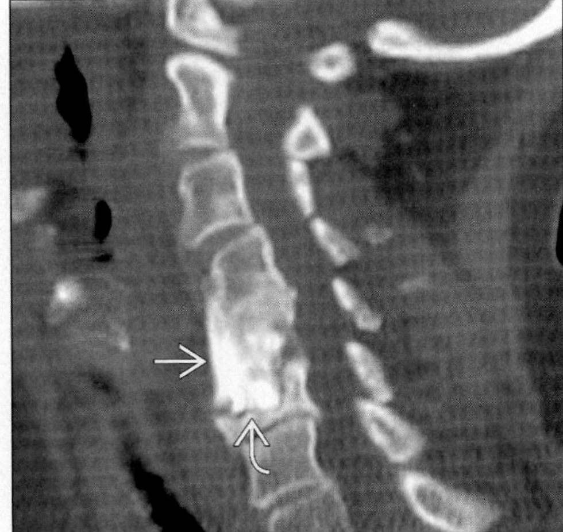

Sagittal NECT reveals a C5 corpectomy and a strut graft from C4 to C6 ➔. The margins of the graft-C6 interface are smooth and sclerotic ➔, consistent with pseudoarthrosis.

Neurofibromatosis (NF)

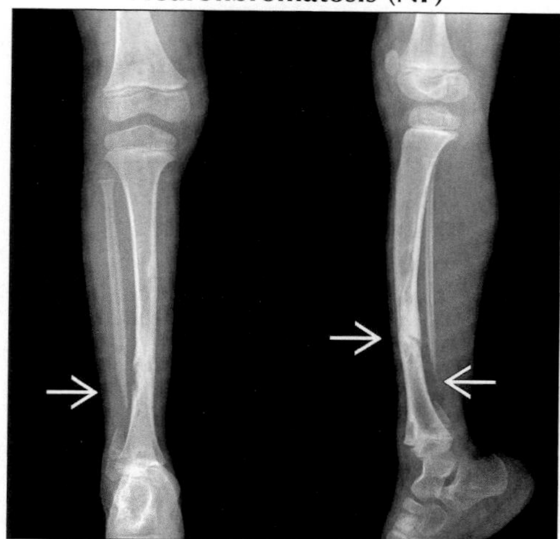

Neurofibromatosis (NF)

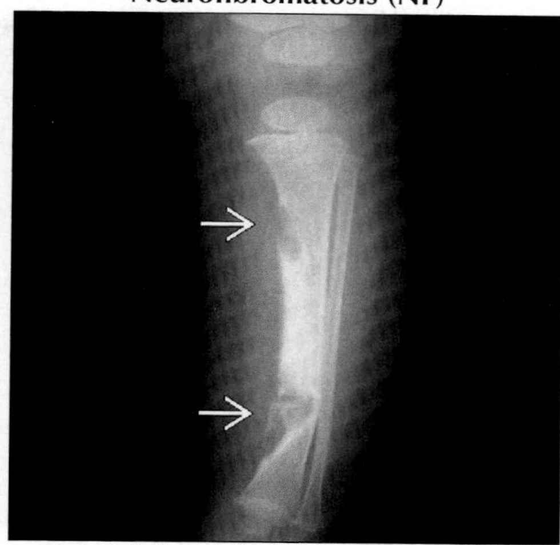

(Left) *AP and lateral radiographs show pseudoarthrosis ➡ of both the tibia and fibula. Tibial bowing in neurofibromatosis usually is at the junction of the middle and distal 1/3 of the tibial diaphysis.* ***(Right)*** *Anteroposterior radiograph shows 2 sites of osseous dysplasia ➡ in a child with the cystic type of pseudoarthrosis associated with neurofibromatosis.*

Congenital Pseudoarthrosis

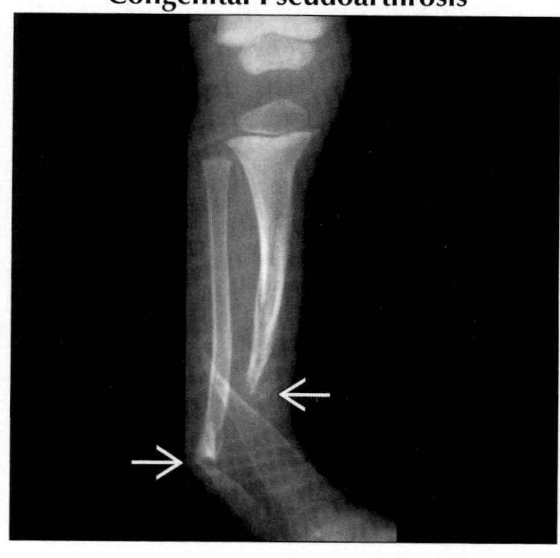

Osteogenesis Imperfecta (OI)

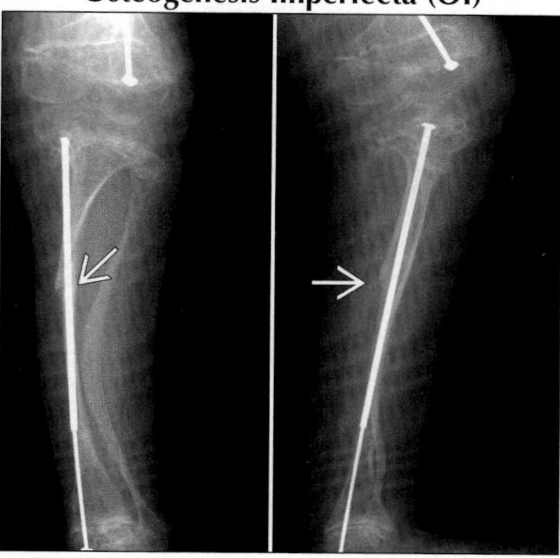

(Left) *Anteroposterior radiograph shows complete fracture through the tibia and fibula with smoothly tapered fracture margins ➡. The appearance is classic for congenital pseudoarthrosis.* ***(Right)*** *AP and lateral radiographs show an intramedullary rod transfixing a tibial pseudoarthrosis ➡. Notice the osteopenia and gracile bones with both tibial and fibular bowing in this patient with osteogenesis imperfecta.*

Osteogenesis Imperfecta (OI)

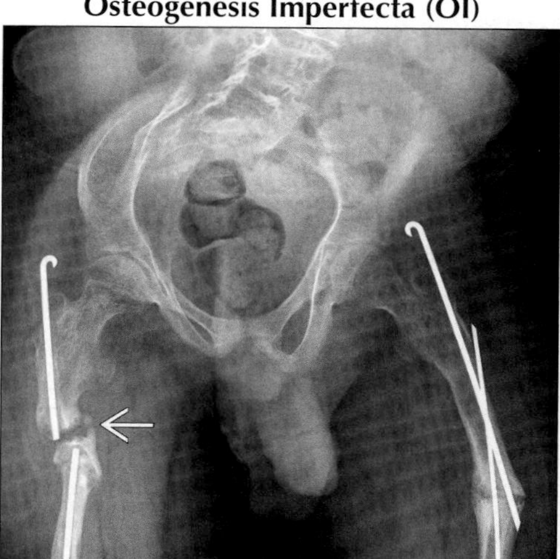

Ankylosing Spondylitis, Post-Trauma

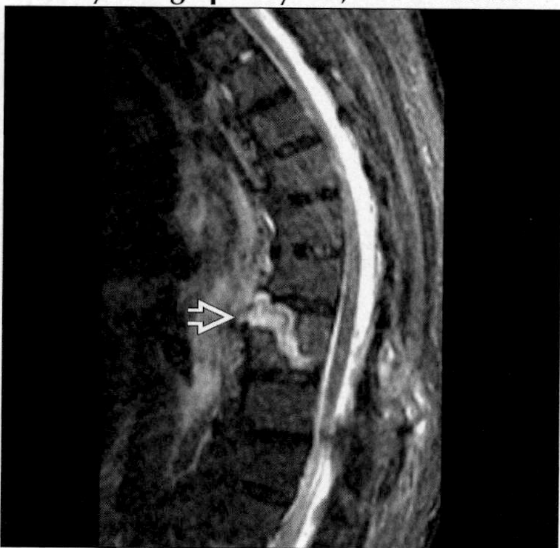

(Left) *Anteroposterior radiograph shows a intramedullary rodding of both femora. The right femoral rod is fractured with pseudoarthrosis of the mid-femoral diaphysis ➡ in this patient with osteogenesis imperfecta.* ***(Right)*** *Sagittal STIR MR shows a pronounced oblique fracture involving the lower thoracic spine with a fluid-filled pseudoarthrosis ⇨ in this patient with ankylosing spondylitis.*

GENERALIZED INCREASED BONE DENSITY

DIFFERENTIAL DIAGNOSIS

Common
- Physiologic Periosteal Reaction of Newborn (Mimic)
- Renal Osteodystrophy (Healing)
- Child Abuse (Mimic)

Less Common
- Sickle Cell Anemia: MSK Complications
- Complications of Prostaglandins (Mimic)
- Congenital Cyanotic Heart Disease
- Complications of Vitamin A
- Complications of Vitamin D
- Scurvy (Mimic)
- Neuroblastoma (Mimic)
- Leukemia (Mimic)
- Osteomyelitis

Rare but Important
- Caffey Disease (Infantile Cortical Hyperostosis) (Mimic)
- Idiopathic Hypercalcemia of Infancy
- Erythroblastosis Fetalis
- Osteopetrosis
- Pycnodysostosis
- Polyostotic Fibrous Dysplasia
- Hypoparathyroidism
- Complications of Fluoride
- Engelmann-Camurati Disease
- Osteosclerotic Dysplasias
- Hyperphosphatasia (Juvenile Paget)
- Melorheostosis
- Tuberous Sclerosis
- Van Buchem Disease
- Ribbing Disease

ESSENTIAL INFORMATION

Key Differential Diagnosis Issues
- Generalized density due to intrinsic alteration of bone vs. dense circumferential overlay of periosteal new bone
- **Hint**: Consider age at presentation
- **Hint**: May involve diaphysis, metaphysis, &/or epiphysis

Helpful Clues for Common Diagnoses
- **Physiologic Periosteal Reaction of Newborn (Mimic)**
  - Seen in 35% of infants age 1-4 months
  - Thin, uniform symmetric periosteal new bone; in humerus, femur, tibia
- **Renal Osteodystrophy (Healing)**
  - Patchy sclerosis as unmineralized osteoid (osteomalacia) calcifies and bone resorption (hyperparathyroidism) heals
  - Coarsened trabeculae, periosteal new bone, widened metaphyses
- **Child Abuse (Mimic)**
  - Average age: 1-4 years
  - Fractures of varying ages, metaphyseal corner fractures, periosteal new bone

Helpful Clues for Less Common Diagnoses
- **Sickle Cell Anemia: MSK Complications**
  - Bone pain begins after age 2-3
  - Multiple bone infarctions may create "bone within bone" appearance
  - Long bone periostitis and generalized patchy increased density
- **Complications of Prostaglandins (Mimic)**
  - IV prostaglandins used in ductus-dependent congenital heart disease
  - Soft tissue swelling, periosteal elevation, and extensive periosteal new bone
- **Congenital Cyanotic Heart Disease**
  - Represents 2° hypertrophic osteoarthropathy
  - Thick, widespread periostitis in diaphysis, metaphysis, and epiphysis
- **Complications of Vitamin A**
  - Excessive intake; occurs after age 1
  - Cortical thickening, soft tissue nodules
  - Involves ulna, metatarsal, clavicle, tibia, other tubular bones, ribs
- **Complications of Vitamin D**
  - Excessive intake; given for rickets
  - Dense metaphyseal bands; variable cortical thickening and thinning
- **Scurvy (Mimic)**
  - Occurs later than 8 months of age
  - Typically osteopenic but coarsened trabeculae, subperiosteal hemorrhage, and periosteal new bone may dominate
- **Neuroblastoma (Mimic)**
  - Typically aggressive osteolytic process but may have periostitis & periosteal new bone
- **Leukemia (Mimic)**
  - Similar to neuroblastoma, particularly metadiaphyseal
- **Osteomyelitis**
  - Congenital syphilis-transplacental

- Symmetric diaphyseal periosteal reaction; widened, serrated metaphysis; epiphyses spared
- Rubella: 1st trimester maternal infection
  - Irregular, alternating sclerotic and lytic areas create "celery stick" pattern

Helpful Clues for Rare Diagnoses

- **Caffey Disease (Mimic)**
  - Seen in 1st 5 months
  - Involves mandible, clavicles, scapulae, ribs, tubular bones; ± asymmetric
  - Spindle-shaped bones due to diaphyseal involvement; lamellated periosteal reaction when healing
- **Idiopathic Hypercalcemia of Infancy**
  - Seen after 1st 5 months; looks similar to hypervitaminosis D
- **Erythroblastosis Fetalis**
  - Diffuse diaphyseal sclerosis and transverse metaphyseal bands
- **Osteopetrosis**
  - Osteosclerosis with mottled metaphyses; "bone-within-bone" appearance
- **Pycnodysostosis**
  - Like osteopetrosis but with short stature, short broad hands, acroosteolysis
- **Polyostotic Fibrous Dysplasia**
  - Triad: Polyostotic fibrous dysplasia, cutaneous pigmentation, precocious puberty; female > male
  - Mildly expanded, ground-glass matrix; generally not diffuse dense sclerosis
- **Hypoparathyroidism**
  - Axial skeleton osteosclerosis with sclerotic metaphyseal bands
- **Complications of Fluoride**
  - Excessive intake; axial skeletal changes predominate
  - Coarsened trabeculae, ± diffuse periosteal new bone, extensive ligament calcification
- **Engelmann-Camurati Disease**
  - Presents within 4-12 years with waddling gait, muscle weakness
  - Spindle-shaped with diaphyseal cortical thickening; metaepiphyses spared
- **Osteosclerotic Dysplasias**
  - Frontometaphyseal: Prominent cranial involvement, flared iliac wings
  - Craniometaphyseal: Prominent cranial involvement, normal pelvis
  - Pyle: Minimal cranial involvement, marked metaphyseal flaring
- **Hyperphosphatasia (Juvenile Paget)**
  - Sclerosis with narrowed medullary space
  - Short, large skull; bowed long bone
- **Melorheostosis**
  - Cortical &/or endosteal hyperostosis; usually limited to 1 extremity
- **Tuberous Sclerosis**
  - Sclerotic bone blends with normal bone; involves hands, feet, long bones, & spines
- **Van Buchem Disease**
  - a.k.a. hyperostosis corticalis generalisata
  - Normal stature, diffuse osteosclerosis, enlarged mandible, ribs, clavicles
- **Ribbing Disease**
  - Hyperostosis, predilection for femur/tibia

Physiologic Periosteal Reaction of Newborn (Mimic)

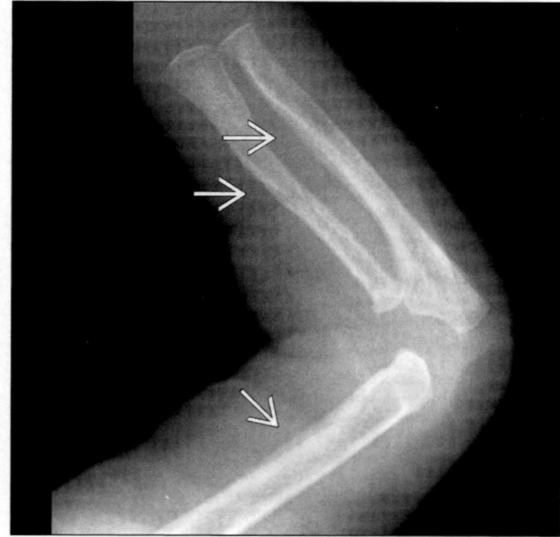

Anteroposterior radiograph shows subtle diffuse increased density of the upper extremity long bones which is bilaterally symmetric and results from subtle diaphyseal periostitis ➔.

Renal Osteodystrophy (Healing)

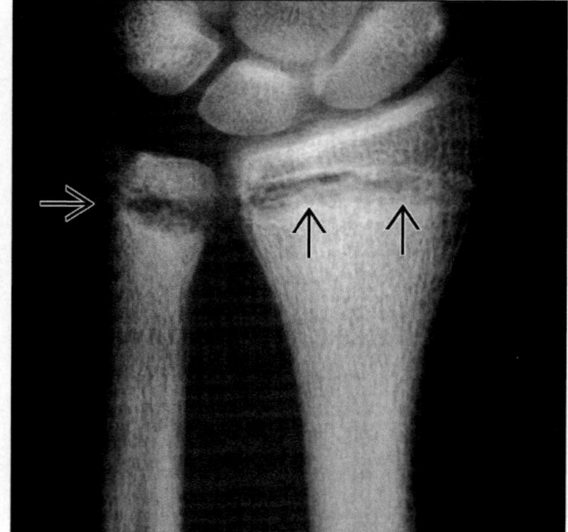

Posteroanterior radiograph shows growth plate widening ➔ as a result of unmineralized osteoid of osteomalacia. The trabeculae are coarsened, and there is generalized increased density.

GENERALIZED INCREASED BONE DENSITY

(**Left**) Lateral radiograph shows new bone formation ➩ resulting from subperiosteal hemorrhage in this child with nonaccidental trauma. Note the metaphyseal corner fracture ➔, typical of this trauma. (**Right**) Anteroposterior radiograph shows sclerosis in the proximal tibial metaphysis due to infarction and dystrophic calcification ➚. Multiple long bone infarctions in sickle cell anemia can result in apparent diffuse increased bone density.

Child Abuse (Mimic)

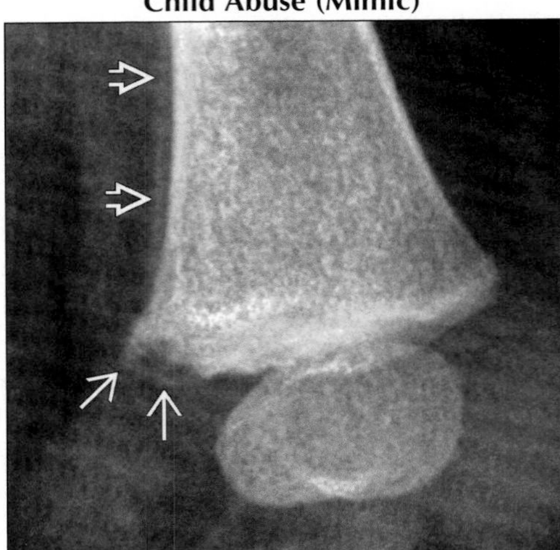

Sickle Cell Anemia: MSK Complications

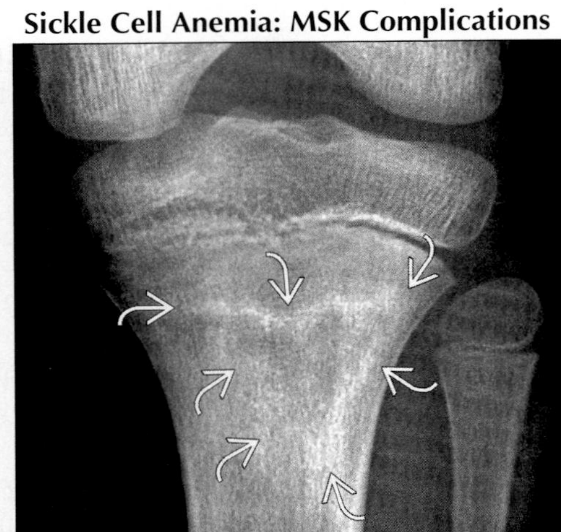

(**Left**) Anteroposterior radiograph shows uniform, thick, periosteal new bone formation in the humerus ➔ in this patient who received prostaglandins for several days to maintain a patent ductus arteriosus. (**Right**) Anteroposterior radiograph shows cortical hyperostosis of the ulna ➔, which does not involve the metaphysis or epiphysis. If the hypervitaminosis continues, it may result in deformity of the metaphyses and epiphyses.

Complications of Prostaglandins (Mimic)

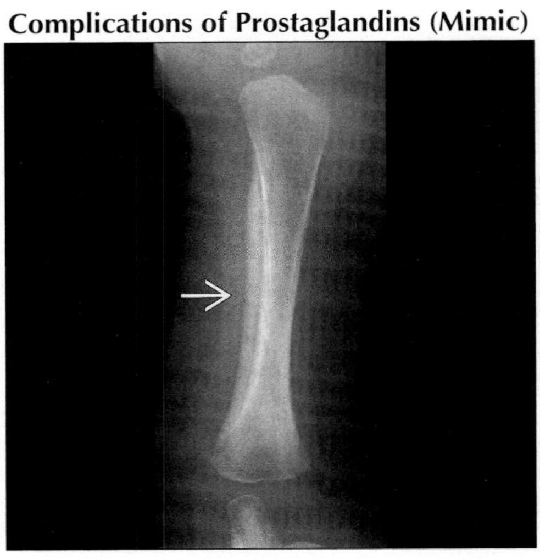

Complications of Vitamin A

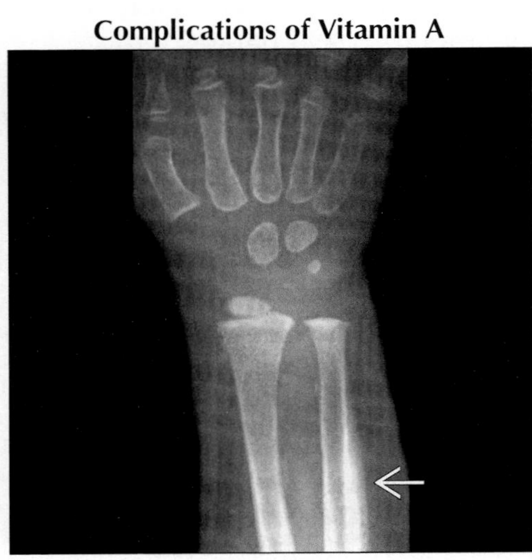

(**Left**) Anteroposterior radiograph shows diffuse increased density of diaphyses ➔ due to subperiosteal hemorrhage and periosteal new bone. Note the dense metaphyseal bands (white line of Frankel) ➩ and metaphyseal (Pelken) fracture ➚. (**Right**) Lateral radiograph shows diffuse soft tissue swelling and a moth-eaten-appearing humerus with extensive cloaking periostitis resulting in increased density. Findings represent metastatic neuroblastoma.

Scurvy (Mimic)

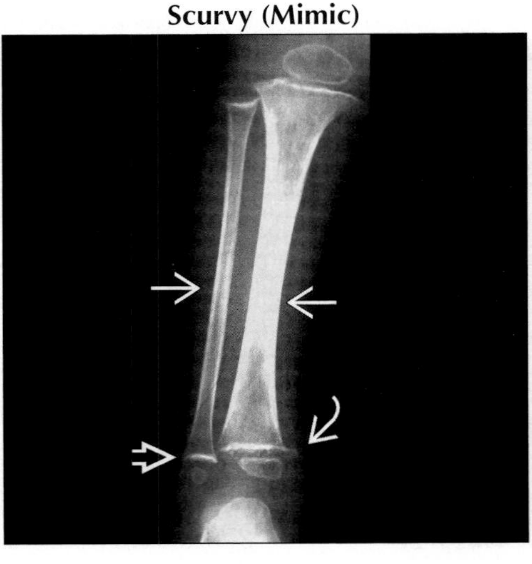

Neuroblastoma (Mimic)

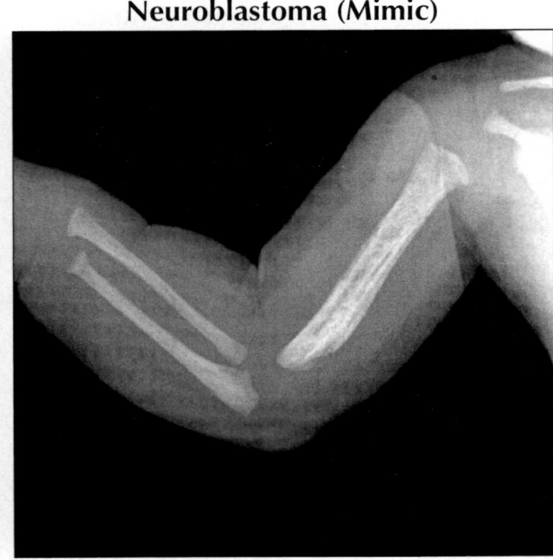

Osteomyelitis

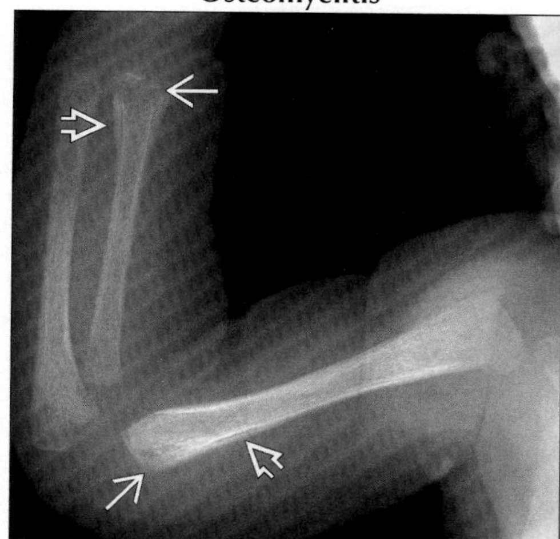

Caffey Disease (Infantile Cortical Hyperostosis) (Mimic)

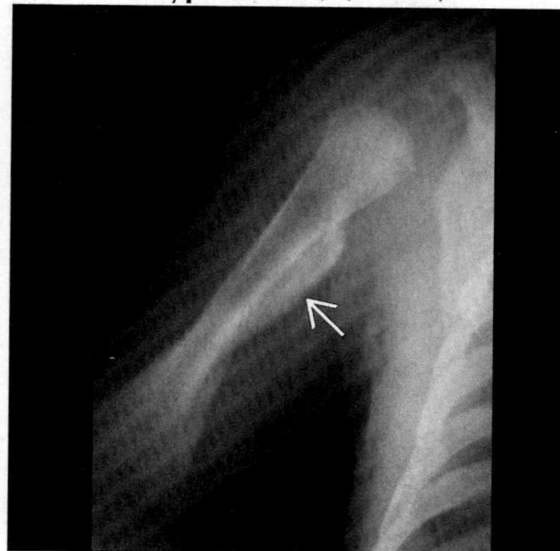

(Left) *Anteroposterior radiograph shows a widened provisional calcification zone of syphilitic osteochondritis. There are lucent metaphyseal bands ➡ with subtle diaphyseal periostitis ⇨ along the long bones, typical of congenital syphilis.* ***(Right)*** *Anteroposterior radiograph shows Caffey disease at age 1 month with the typical marked, thick, wavy periosteal new bone ➡, typical of cortical hyperostosis. This patient's mandible was also involved (not shown).*

Osteopetrosis

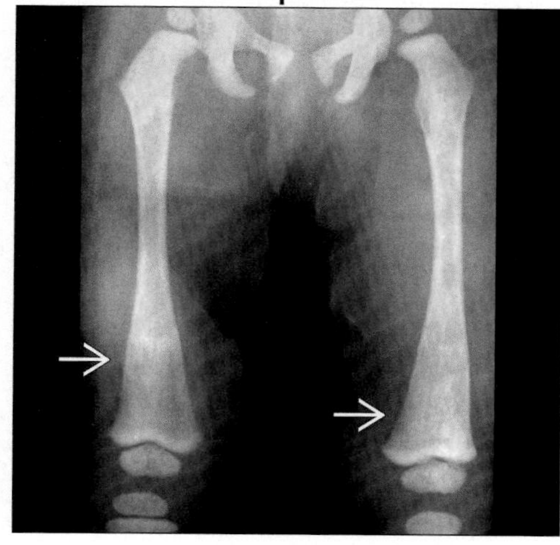

Pycnodysostosis

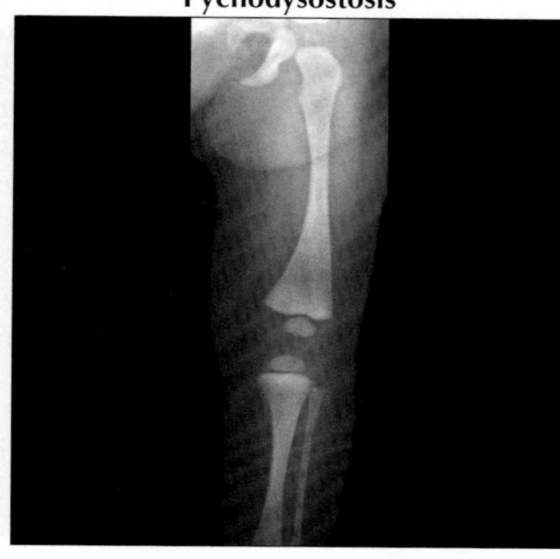

(Left) *Anteroposterior radiograph shows uniform increased density in this patient with osteopetrosis. There is mild undertubulation ➡, with relative widening of the distal femoral metadiaphyses.* ***(Right)*** *Anteroposterior radiograph in a child with pycnodysostosis also shows uniformly dense bone, similar to osteopetrosis. This short-limbed dwarf has micrognathia and shortened fingers (not shown), typical of pycnodysostosis.*

Polyostotic Fibrous Dysplasia

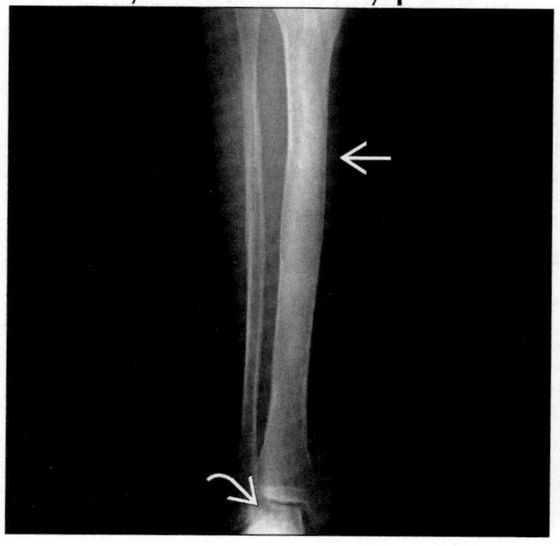

Engelmann-Camurati Disease

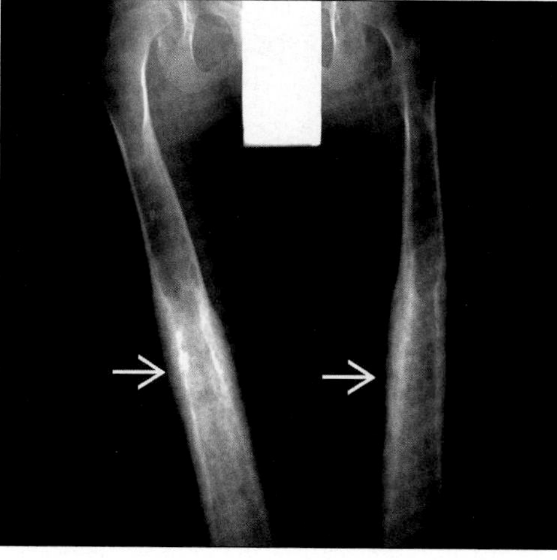

(Left) *Anteroposterior radiograph shows a long, mildly expansile tibial diaphyseal lesion ➡ with ground-glass matrix, typical of fibrous dysplasia. Additional lesions are present in the distal tibia and talus ➡ in this female with precocious puberty.* ***(Right)*** *Anteroposterior radiograph shows bilateral diaphyseal cortical thickening ➡ with normal metaphyses and epiphyses. Process becomes smoother and thicker, involving entire diaphysis, as patient matures.*

POLYOSTOTIC LESIONS

DIFFERENTIAL DIAGNOSIS

Common
- Fibroxanthoma (Nonossifying Fibroma)
- Fibrous Dysplasia, Polyostotic
- Langerhans Cell Histiocytosis (LCH)
- Osteomyelitis
- Osteochondroma, Multiple Hereditary Exostosis
- Leukemia
- Ewing Sarcoma, Metastatic
- Metastases, Bone Marrow

Less Common
- Lymphoma, Multifocal
- Osteosarcoma, Metastatic
- Hyperparathyroidism/Renal Osteodystrophy, Brown Tumor
- Melorheostosis

Rare but Important
- Ollier Disease
- Maffucci Syndrome
- Chronic Recurrent Multifocal Osteomyelitis
- Sarcoidosis
- Trevor Fairbank

ESSENTIAL INFORMATION

Key Differential Diagnosis Issues
- Polyostotic nature of lesion can narrow differential substantially and is highly valuable characteristic
  - Information regarding multiple sites can be gained by bone scan, PET/CT, or clinical exam
- Lesions listed above range from benign ("leave me alone") lesions → "Aunt Minnie" lesions → highly aggressive lesions
  - Most use this alternative approach to sort these out

Helpful Clues for Common Diagnoses
- **Fibroxanthoma (Nonossifying Fibroma)**
  - Benign fibrous cortical defects (same histologically as NOF but smaller) are often multiple in children
  - Nonossifying fibroma (NOF) not commonly multiple, except in patients with neurofibromatosis
  - Both have same natural history of healing
  - Both are cortically based and metadiaphyseal
- **Fibrous Dysplasia, Polyostotic**
  - Lesion may have different appearance in different locations
    - Skull: Sclerotic
    - Pelvis: Bubbly, lytic
    - Long bones: Generally central, metadiaphyseal, mildly expanded, with variable homogeneous ground-glass density
- **Langerhans Cell Histiocytosis (LCH)**
  - Lesions may be lytic, geographic, and nonaggressive
  - Lesions may also be extremely aggressive in appearance: Permeative, cortical breakthrough, soft tissue mass, periosteal reaction, with rapid growth
  - **Hint**: Skull lesions may have beveled edge appearance due to differential involvement of inner and outer tables
- **Osteomyelitis**
  - Hematogenous spread usually results in metaphyseal sites
  - Osteomyelitis can appear extremely aggressive, with permeative change and cortical breakthrough with soft tissue mass; may not be distinguishable from aggressive tumor
  - Sickle cell patients at risk for multifocal osseous infection; higher predilection for *Salmonella*
- **Osteochondroma, Multiple Hereditary Exostosis**
  - Not difficult diagnosis if exophytic (cauliflower) lesions are present
  - May have only sessile exostoses at metaphyses, which can give appearance of dysplasia; diagnosis often missed
- **Leukemia**
  - Diffuse marrow infiltration may result in appearance of osteopenia, easily overlooked
  - Metaphyseal lucent bands may highlight degree of osteopenia
  - MR shows extent of abnormalities
- **Ewing Sarcoma, Metastatic**
  - Primary lesion usually highly aggressive; lytic, permeative, cortical breakthrough, large soft tissue mass

- May have extensive reactive bone formation, giving appearance of osteoid, with potential confusion with osteosarcoma
  - Reactive bone formation restricted to bone, does not extend into soft tissue mass (as it does in osteosarcoma)
- Most common sarcoma to have osseous metastases; lung and osseous metastases present with equal frequency

Helpful Clues for Less Common Diagnoses

- **Lymphoma, Multifocal**
  - 50% of childhood bone lymphoma is polyostotic (much less frequent in adults)
  - Lesions highly aggressive: Permeative, cortical breakthrough with soft tissue mass
  - Generally lytic but may have reactive sclerosis within osseous lesion
  - In same differential as Ewing sarcoma with metastases, multifocal osteomyelitis, LCH, and metastases

Alternative Differential Approaches

- "Aunt Minnie" lesions can generally be identified immediately
  - Fibroxanthoma (nonossifying fibroma)/benign fibrous cortical defect
  - Osteochondroma (multiple hereditary exostoses); remember they can be sessile and resemble a metaphyseal dysplasia
  - Melorheostosis
  - Sarcoidosis (when lacy appearance is obvious)
  - Trevor Fairbank
- Polyostotic lesions, which are usually monomelic
  - Fibrous dysplasia (generally unilateral)
  - Melorheostosis
  - Ollier disease
  - Trevor Fairbank
  - Maffucci syndrome
- Polyostotic lesions with an intermediately aggressive appearance
  - Fibrous dysplasia: Generally central, poorly marginated, but geographic
  - Langerhans cell histiocytosis: Appearance ranges from nonaggressive geographic to extremely aggressive permeative
  - Hyperparathyroidism/renal osteodystrophy, brown tumor: Generally lesion is geographic, but surrounding bone abnormal in density & trabecular pattern
- Polyostotic lesions with aggressive appearance: These can be indistinguishable from one another by imaging
  - Langerhans cell histiocytosis: Range in appearance from nonaggressive to highly aggressive
  - Osteomyelitis
  - Leukemia
  - Ewing sarcoma, metastatic
  - Metastases, bone marrow
  - Lymphoma, multifocal
  - Osteosarcoma, metastatic
  - Chronic recurrent multifocal osteomyelitis

Fibroxanthoma (Nonossifying Fibroma)

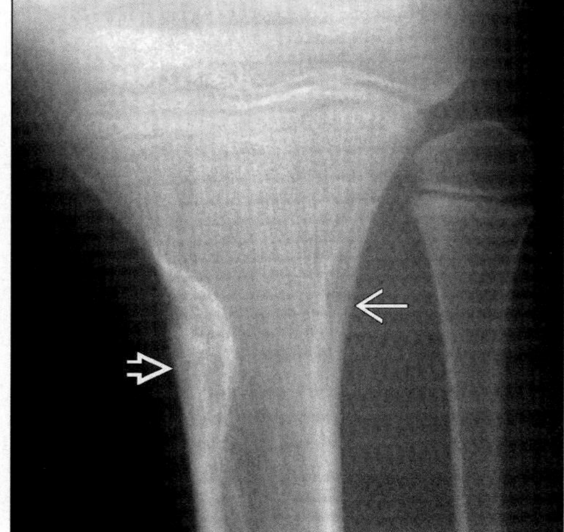

Anteroposterior radiograph shows a small lytic cortical lesion ➔ (benign fibrous cortical defect) and a sclerotic healing nonossifying fibroma ⇨. The 2 lesions have the same histology, and the natural history is to heal.

Fibroxanthoma (Nonossifying Fibroma)

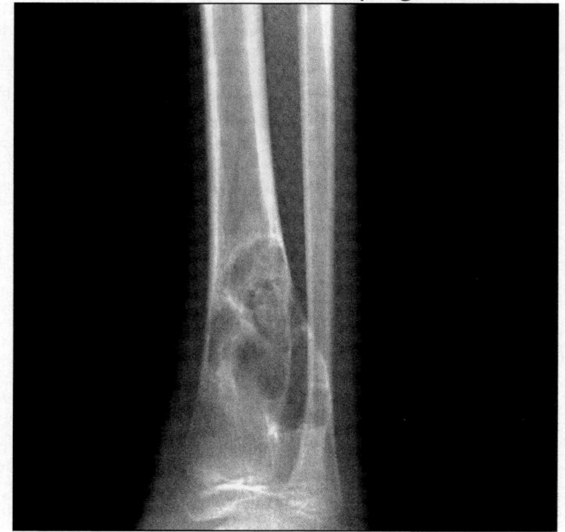

Oblique radiograph in the same patient shows a lytic cortically based lesion; this is another NOF, but 1 which is still active in this child. These images show the 3 different appearances for this lesion.

POLYOSTOTIC LESIONS

(Left) Anteroposterior radiograph shows mixed lytic and sclerotic lesion involving the metadiaphysis of the femur, tibia, and fibula. The lesions are central and nonaggressive, typical of fibrous dysplasia. ***(Right)*** Anteroposterior radiograph shows the mildly expanded and sclerotic, otherwise featureless "ground-glass" appearance of fibrous dysplasia in the tibial diaphysis ➡, with a lytic talar lesion ➡ in this teenager with polyostotic fibrous dysplasia.

Fibrous Dysplasia, Polyostotic

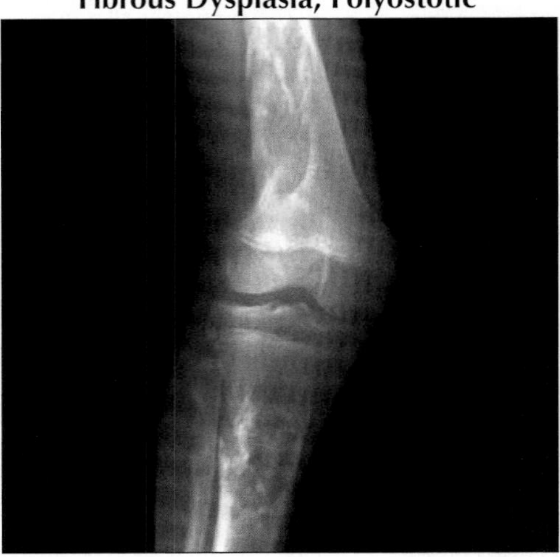

Fibrous Dysplasia, Polyostotic

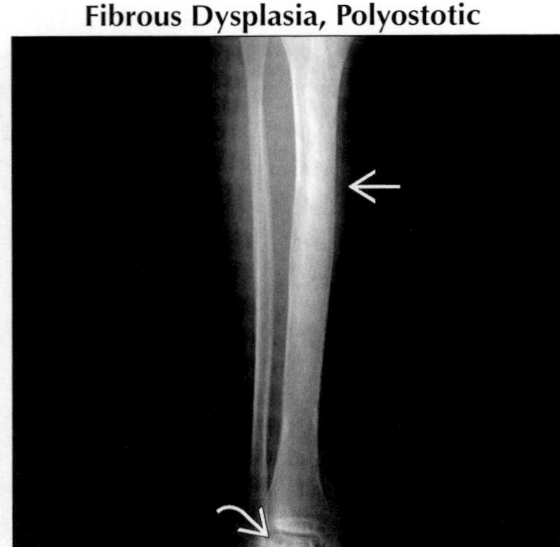

(Left) Anteroposterior radiograph shows a geographic lytic lesion of the femoral neck ➡. This is compatible with a diagnosis of Langerhans cell histiocytosis (LCH). ***(Right)*** Lateral radiograph in the same child shows multiple skull lesions. These lesions have a more aggressive appearance, and in fact, grew quite rapidly. The polyostotic and relatively geographic appearance overall makes the diagnosis of LCH highly probable, proven in this case.

Langerhans Cell Histiocytosis (LCH)

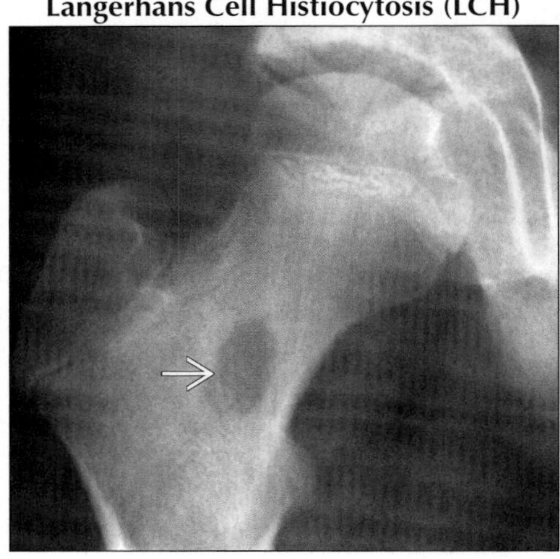

Langerhans Cell Histiocytosis (LCH)

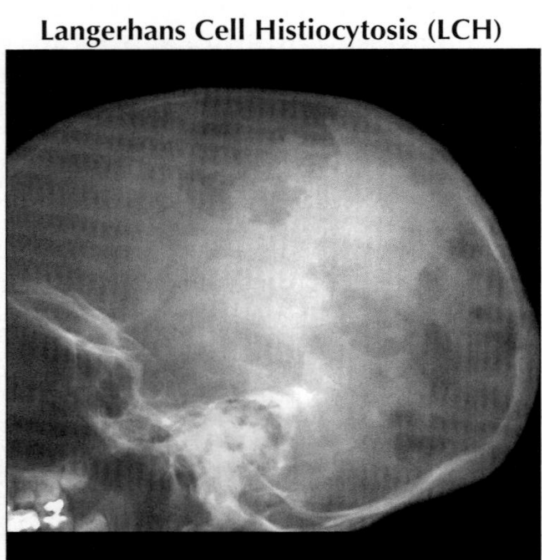

(Left) Anteroposterior radiograph shows lytic lesions within the metaphysis ➡, which have an aggressive appearance. ***(Right)*** Lateral radiograph of the contralateral heel in the same patient as previous image, at the same setting shows lytic lesions within both the metaphysis and apophysis ➡. The metaphyseal location makes hematogenous spread of osteomyelitis the most likely diagnosis, proven here.

Osteomyelitis

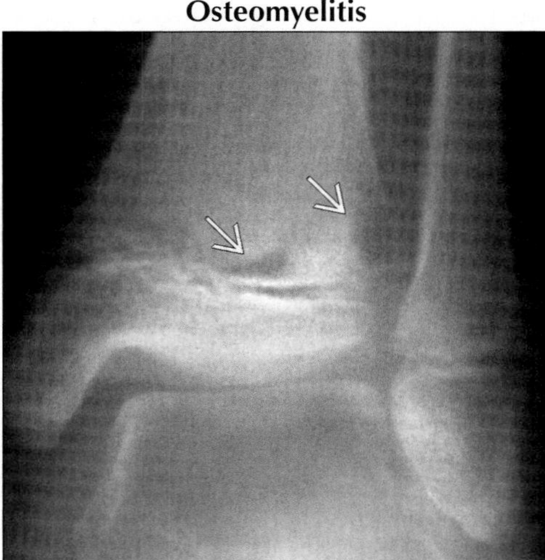

Osteomyelitis

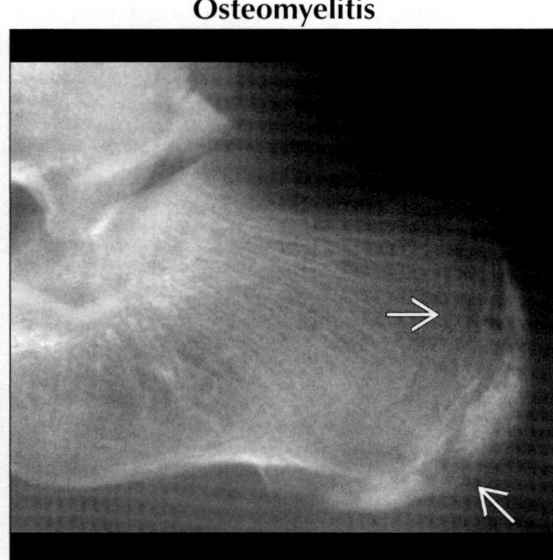

POLYOSTOTIC LESIONS

Osteochondroma, Multiple Hereditary Exostosis

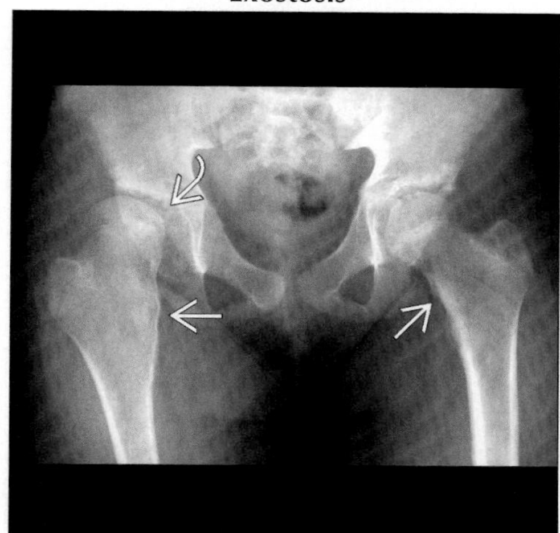

Leukemia

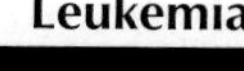

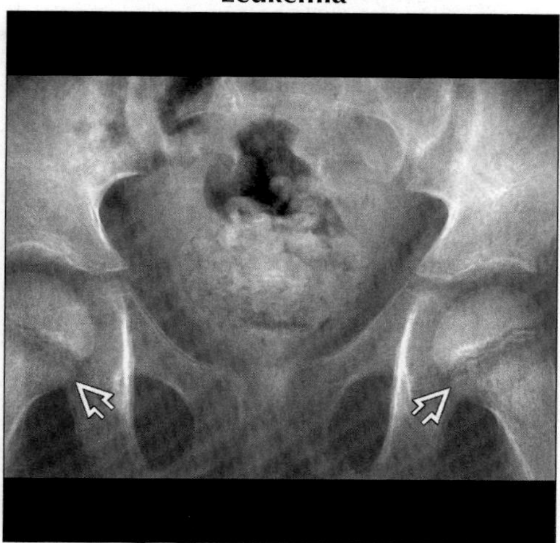

(Left) *Anteroposterior radiograph shows sessile osteochondromas along the medial femoral metaphyses → in this teenager. Note the subluxation of the right femoral head →; this was proven to be an intraarticular exostosis.* ***(Right)*** *AP radiograph shows diffuse osteopenia and metaphyseal lucent lines → in this child. He also had mild compression fractures in the spine. Leukemia may present as diffuse osteopenia rather than focal lesions, as in this case.*

Ewing Sarcoma, Metastatic

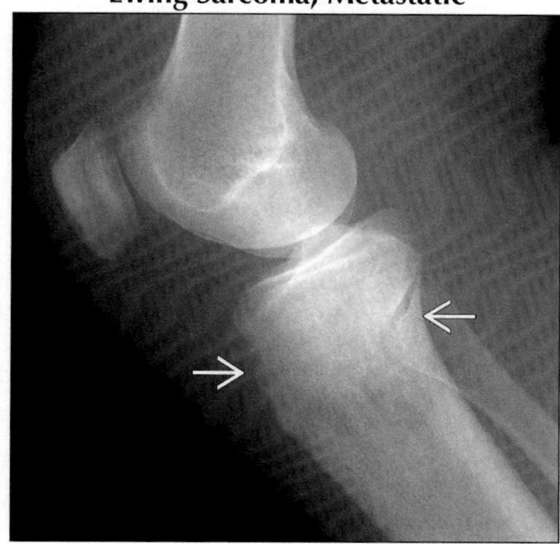

Ewing Sarcoma, Metastatic

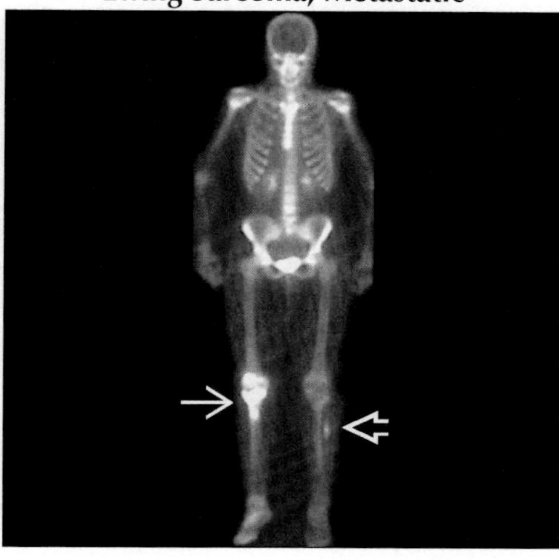

(Left) *Lateral radiograph shows faint permeative change and sclerosis within the proximal tibia → in a teenager. The lesion is so subtle as to be easily missed; this makes it aggressive. With the reactive sclerosis, Ewing sarcoma is highly probable.* ***(Right)*** *Anteroposterior bone scan in the same patient, shows the tibial lesion, with extended uptake →. However, there is also a lesion within the contralateral fibula →; the diagnosis is Ewing sarcoma with osseous metastasis.*

Metastases, Bone Marrow

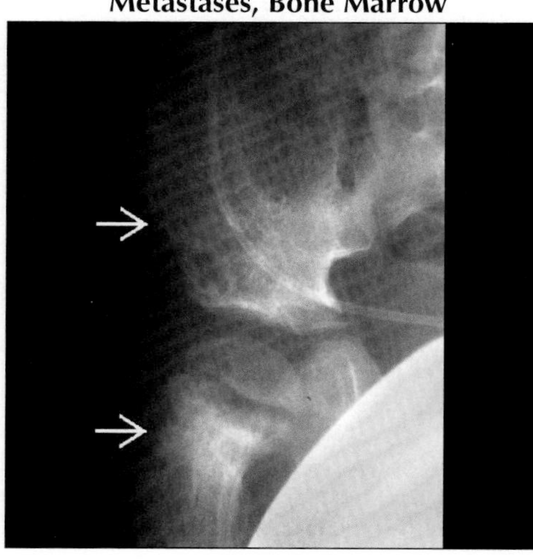

Lymphoma, Multifocal

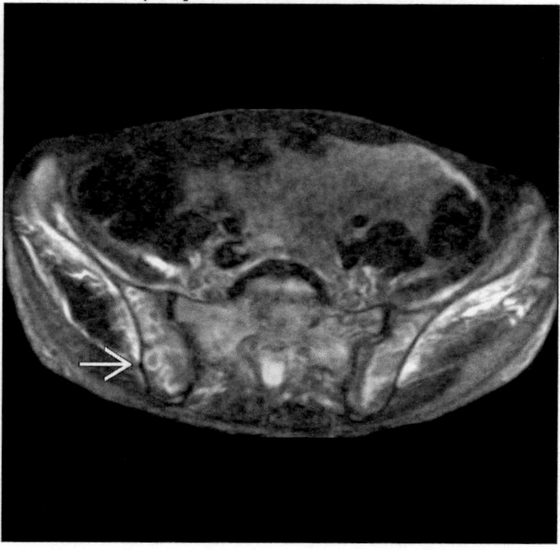

(Left) *AP radiograph shows multiple lesions in a child →. These are metaphyseal, suggesting hematogenous spread. The major differential is multifocal osteomyelitis and metastases; the primary was medulloblastoma (note the VP shunt).* ***(Right)*** *Axial STIR MR shows polyostotic lesions involving the iliac wings and sacrum in this child. A typical serpiginous pattern is seen →. 50% of children developing lymphoma of bone present with polyostotic lesions.*

POLYOSTOTIC LESIONS

*(**Left**) Anteroposterior radiograph shows multiple osseous sites of amorphous bone formation ➔ within the spine and pelvis in a teenager whose left hip was disarticulated 1 year earlier for osteosarcoma (note the recurrence in the acetabulum ➔). (**Right**) Posteroanterior radiograph shows severe renal osteodystrophy in a teenager with end-stage renal disease. Besides the subperiosteal and tuft resorption, there are multiple lytic lesions, and brown tumors ➔.*

Osteosarcoma, Metastatic

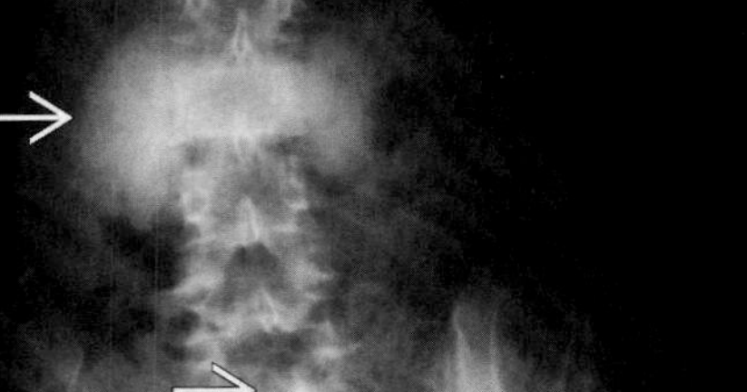

Hyperparathyroidism/Renal Osteodystrophy, Brown Tumor

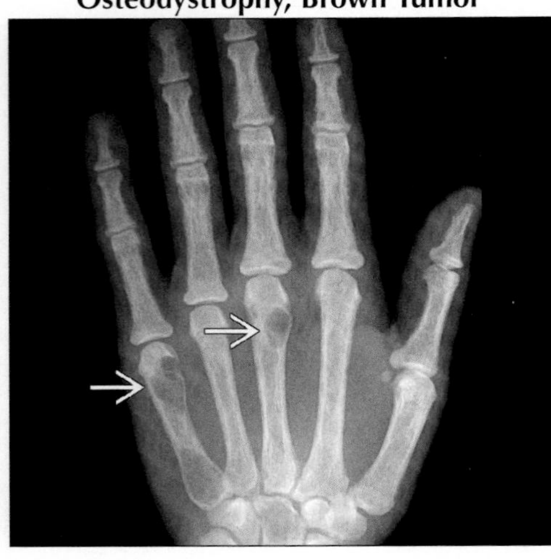

*(**Left**) Anteroposterior radiograph shows dense sclerotic endosteal bone extending down the femur ➔ with what has been termed a "dripping candle wax" appearance. This is typical melorheostosis, a sclerosing dysplasia. (**Right**) Oblique radiograph in the same patient shows linear as well as punctate regions of sclerosis ➔ in a sclerotomal pattern. The lesions are restricted to 1 extremity (monomelic).*

Melorheostosis

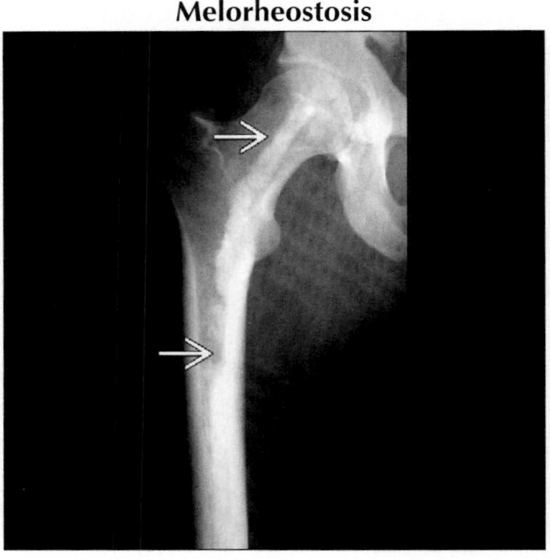

Melorheostosis

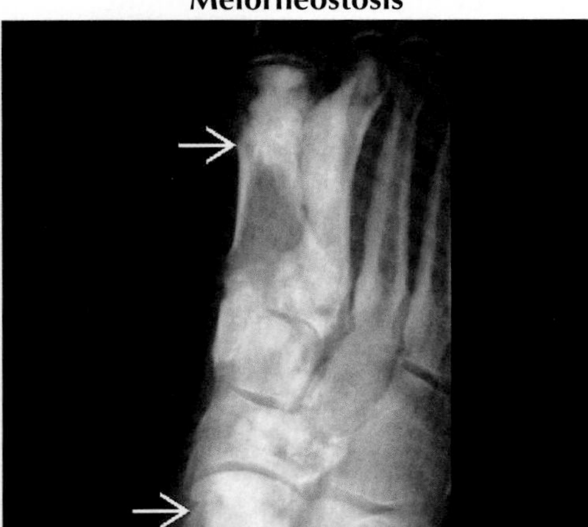

*(**Left**) Oblique radiograph shows multiple lytic lesions in the hand ➔, some with prominent expansion. These do not have distinct cartilage matrix, but nonetheless are typical for multiple enchondromatosis. (**Right**) AP radiograph shows a lytic lesion occupying the metaphysis, with faintly seen linear striations ➔. No distinct matrix is seen. Remember that the lesions in Ollier disease often do not have the same appearance as solitary enchondromas.*

Ollier Disease

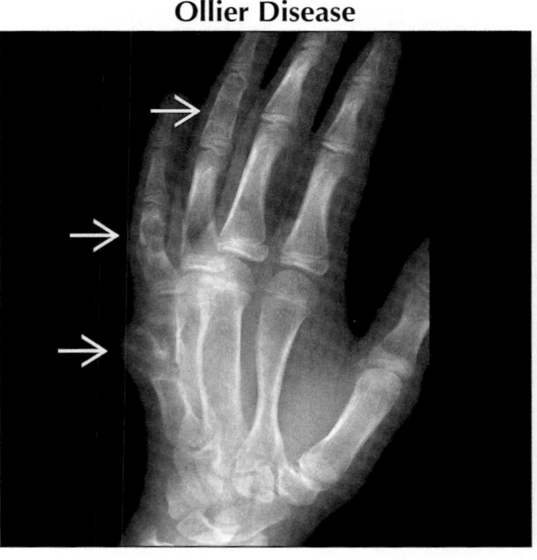

Ollier Disease

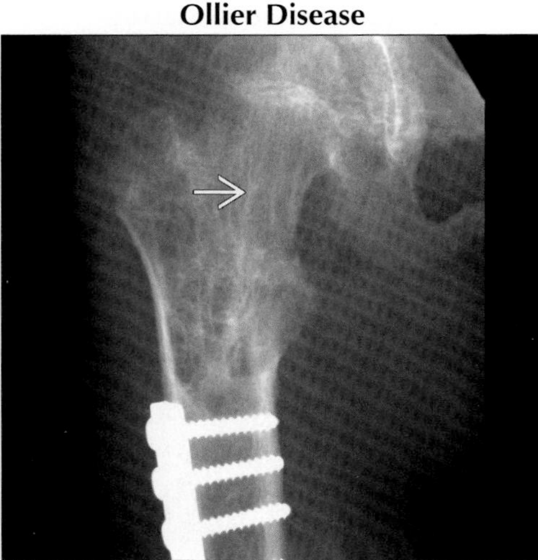

Maffucci Syndrome

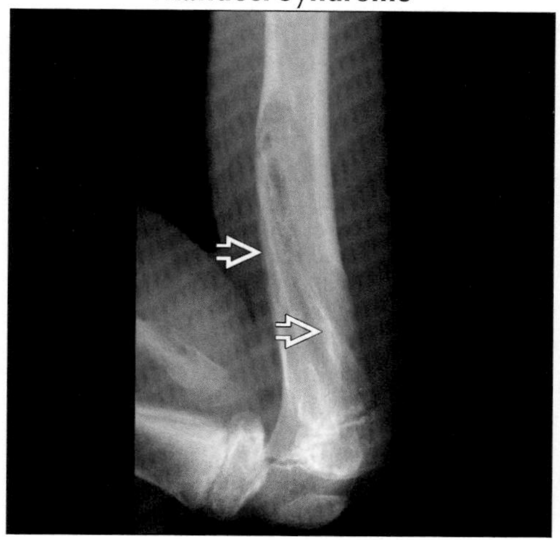

Maffucci Syndrome

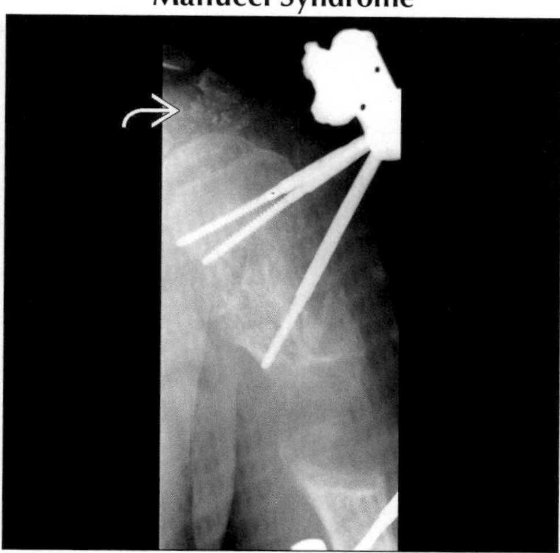

(Left) *Lateral radiograph shows the linear striations within a lytic metaphyseal lesion ➨; note the proximal fibula is abnormal as well. The findings are typical of multiple enchondromatosis.* ***(Right)*** *Anteroposterior radiograph in the same patient shows a lytic lesion in the proximal humerus, as well as phleboliths in the adjacent soft tissues ➨; these change the diagnosis to Maffucci syndrome. The patient is undergoing limb lengthening. (†MSK Req).*

Chronic Recurrent Multifocal Osteomyelitis

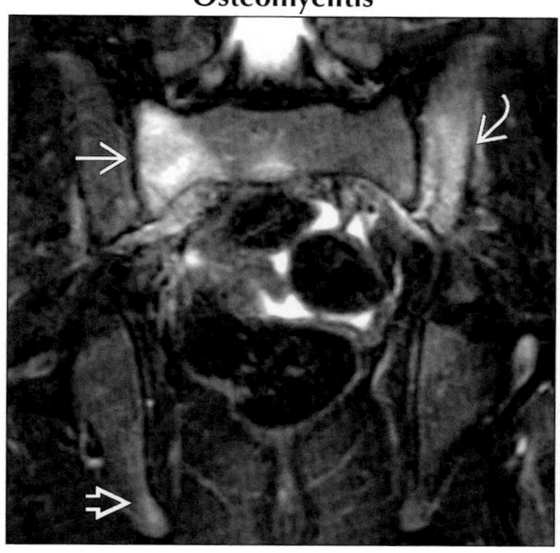

Sarcoidosis

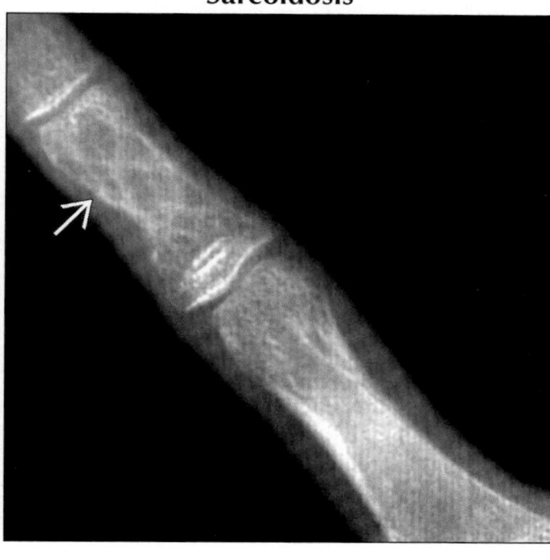

(Left) *Coronal T2WI FS MR shows signal abnormalities in the sacrum ➡, iliac wing ➨, and ischium ➨. There is no soft tissue mass. The patient had chronic pain for 1 year but normal radiograph and no constitutional symptoms.* ***(Right)*** *Posteroanterior radiograph shows the lacy lytic lesion ➡ typical of sarcoidosis of the hands and feet. This teenage patient had lesions in her foot as well and massive pulmonary fibrosis.*

Trevor Fairbank

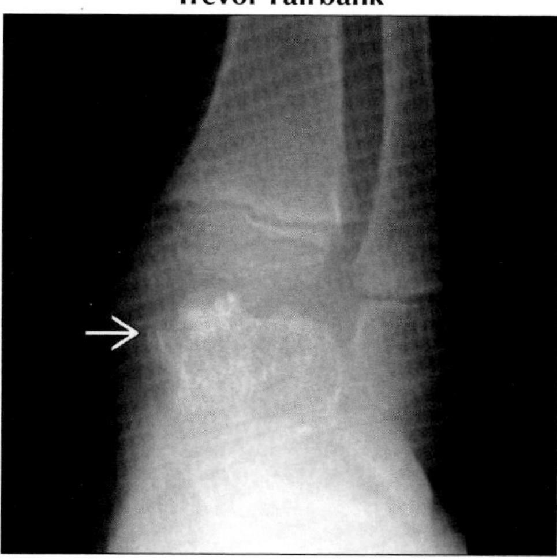

Trevor Fairbank

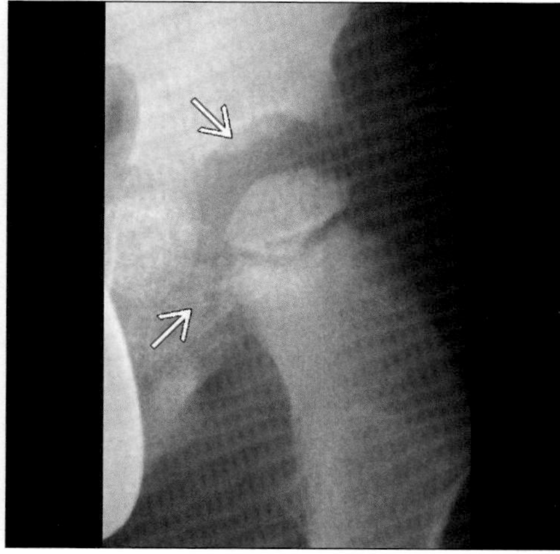

(Left) *Anteroposterior radiograph shows abnormal bone formation in the ankle ➡. Other radiographs demonstrate this to be intraarticular and attached to the talus. This represents an intraarticular exostosis, or Trevor disease.* ***(Right)*** *Anteroposterior radiograph of the hip in the same patient, shows abnormal ossification arising from the acetabulum ➡. It is not uncommon for Trevor disease to be polyarticular; it is monomelic.*

SKELETAL METASTASES

DIFFERENTIAL DIAGNOSIS

Common
- Neuroblastoma
- Leukemia

Less Common
- Rhabdomyosarcoma
- Ewing Sarcoma
- Osteosarcoma
- Retinoblastoma
- Lymphoma
- Medulloblastoma

Rare but Important
- Clear Cell Sarcoma

ESSENTIAL INFORMATION

Key Differential Diagnosis Issues
- Neuroblastoma, sometimes leukemia, rarely lymphoma, may present with multiple skeletal metastases (mets)
- Langerhans cell histiocytosis and multifocal osteomyelitis may mimic skeletal mets
- Metastatic bone disease looks alike; can be lytic, sclerotic, or mixed

Helpful Clues for Common Diagnoses
- **Neuroblastoma**
  - Most common metastatic bone tumor in pediatrics
    - Bone mets: Lucent, sclerotic, or mixed
    - Liver mets also common
- **Leukemia**
  - 1/4 of children with leukemia have bone mets
  - Children: Long bones
    - Femur > humerus > pelvis > spine > tibia
    - Spectrum of radiographic findings: Normal, diffuse osteopenia, "leukemic lines," periostitis, bone destruction, sclerosis, pathologic fracture, chloroma

Helpful Clues for Less Common Diagnoses
- **Rhabdomyosarcoma**
  - Lung mets most common
  - Bone mets has poorer prognosis
- **Ewing Sarcoma**
  - More commonly metastasizes to lung, 15-30% at presentation
  - Mets to bone less frequent
- **Osteosarcoma**
  - More commonly metastasizes to lungs (calcifying nodules)
  - Bone mets may be blastic
- **Retinoblastoma**
  - May have blastic bone mets
- **Lymphoma**
  - Focal or patchy marrow involvement
- **Medulloblastoma**
  - Often blastic mets

Helpful Clues for Rare Diagnoses
- **Clear Cell Sarcoma**
  - a.k.a. bone metastasizing renal tumor of childhood
  - Looks like Wilms in kidney but with bone mets
  - Also commonly mets to lung and liver

Neuroblastoma

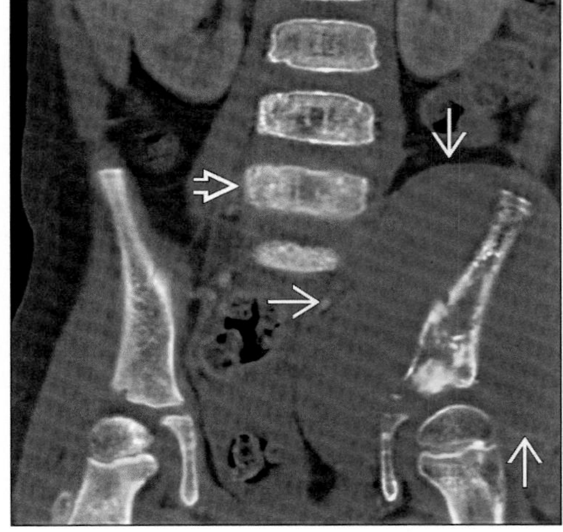

Coronal CECT shows the lytic destructive left iliac wing metastasis with a large soft tissue mass ➡. Notice the L5 met ➡. This is a nearly 6 year old with known relapsed neuroblastoma.

Leukemia

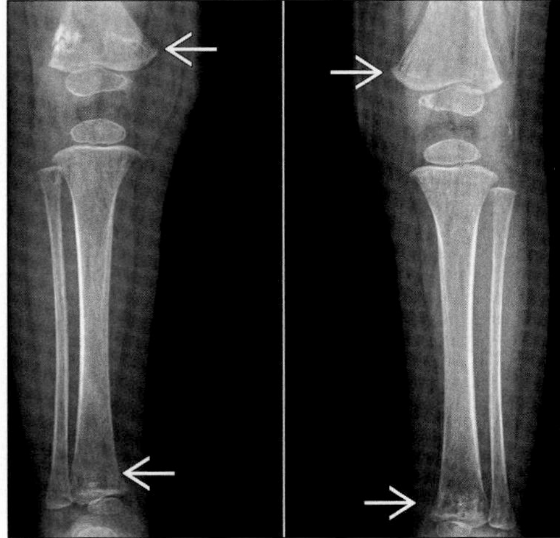

Anteroposterior radiograph shows destructive lesions ➡ within the bilateral distal femoral, distal tibial, and distal fibular metaphyses with a pathologic fracture within the distal right femur.

Rhabdomyosarcoma

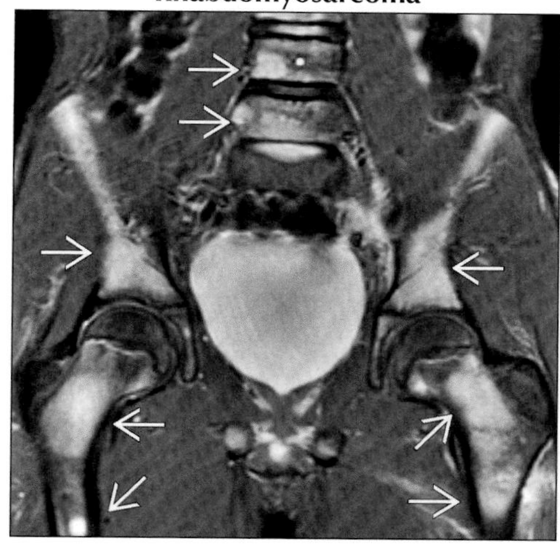

Ewing Sarcoma

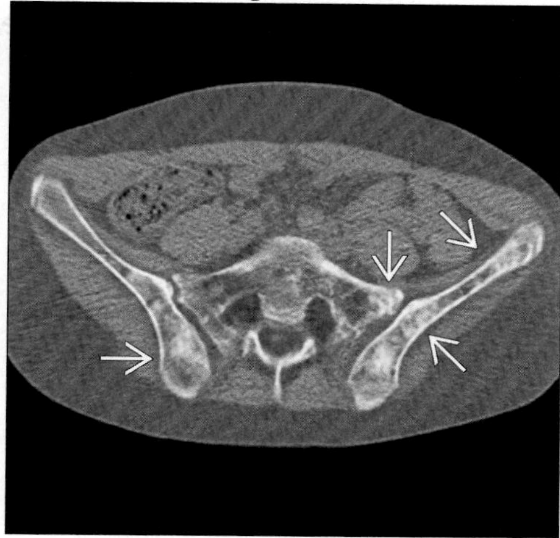

*(**Left**) Coronal STIR MR shows numerous hyperintense mets ➡ throughout the pelvis, lower lumbar spine, and proximal femurs. Extremity and alveolar rhabdomyosarcoma (RMS) tend to have a worse prognosis compared to embryonal RMS. (**Right**) Axial NECT shows diffuse mixed lytic and sclerotic mets ➡ of Ewing sarcoma within both iliac wings and S1 vertebral body. Metastatic disease is more common to the lungs, 15-30% at presentation.*

Osteosarcoma

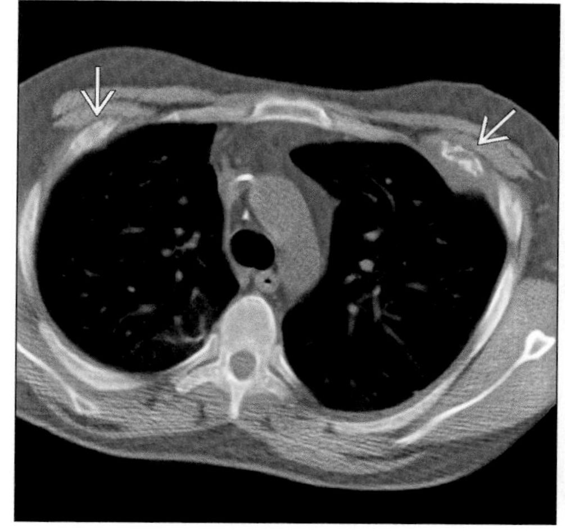

Retinoblastoma

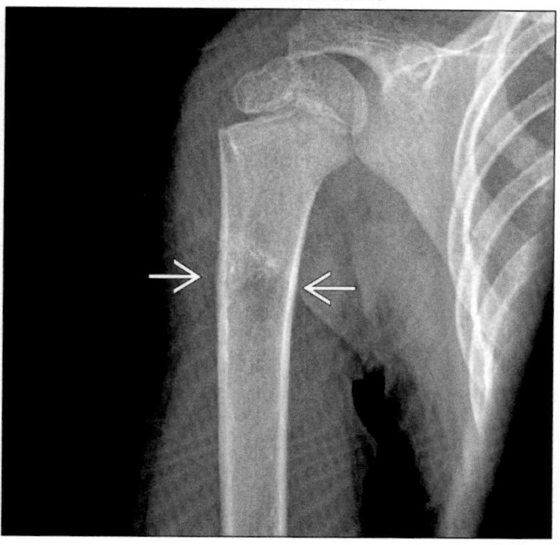

*(**Left**) Axial CECT shows destruction of bilateral anterior ribs ➡ from mets disease in this patient with mandibular osteosarcoma. Pulmonary mets may calcify. Other mets from osteosarcoma would include lymph nodes, liver, and brain. Bone mets are uncommon. (**Right**) Anteroposterior radiograph shows a subtle lytic met ➡ within the proximal humeral diaphysis. There is mild adjacent periostitis along the lateral cortical margin of the humerus.*

Lymphoma

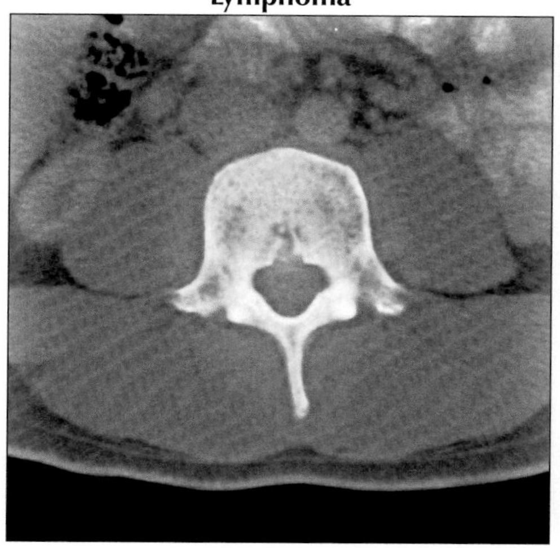

Medulloblastoma

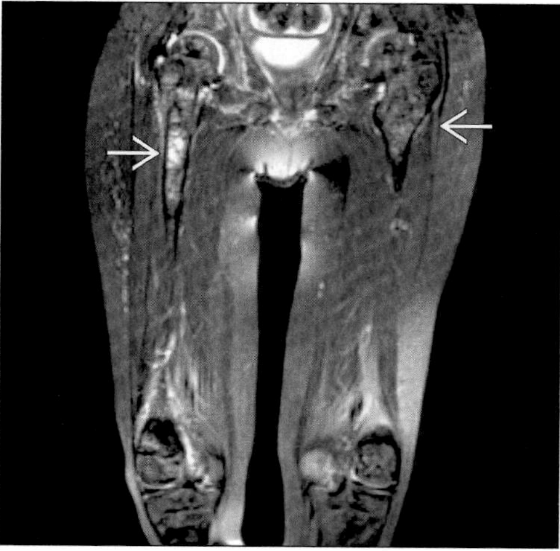

*(**Left**) Axial NECT shows diffuse sclerosis of a lumbar vertebral body. This was a known metastasis in this child with lymphoma. (**Right**) Coronal T2WI FS MR shows diffuse marrow replacement by met disease ➡ in this patient with known metastatic medulloblastoma. The patient was diagnosed with medulloblastoma 6 years ago and has had diffuse met disease for several years.*

DESTROYED FEMORAL HEADS

DIFFERENTIAL DIAGNOSIS

Less Common
- Legg-Calvé-Perthes (LCP) Disease
- Avascular Necrosis
- Septic Arthritis
- Juvenile Idiopathic Arthritis (JIA)
- Slipped Capital Femoral Epiphysis (SCFE)

Rare but Important
- Meyer Dysplasia
- Idiopathic Chondrolysis
- Epiphyseal Bone Tumors
- Epiphyseal Dysplasias

ESSENTIAL INFORMATION

Key Differential Diagnosis Issues
- Age and clinical presentation
- Need to exclude infection in child with hip pain and femoral head destruction

Helpful Clues for Less Common Diagnoses
- **Legg-Calvé-Perthes (LCP) Disease**
  - Avascular necrosis of femoral head of unknown etiology
  - Age: 3-12 years old, peak 6-8 years old
  - Bilateral (10-20%)
  - Radiographs
    - Normal
    - Flattening, sclerosis, fragmentation of femoral head ± subchondral fracture (best seen on frog leg lateral view)
  - Bone scintigraphy: Earlier diagnosis than radiographs with decreased or absent perfusion
  - MR: Earlier diagnosis than radiographs with decreased perfusion; loss of fatty marrow signal T1WI within femoral head
  - 3 stages (initial ⇒ fragmentation ⇒ reparative)
    - Initial: Necrosis, vascular invasion, cartilage hypertrophy, overgrowth
    - Fragmentation: Necrotic/dead bone is resorbed, ± metaphyseal cysts (cartilage) and cartilage hypertrophy
    - Reparative: Healing and replacement of necrotic/dead bone
  - Key: Prognosis heavily depends on containment of femoral head
    - Femoral head grows laterally (extrusion of femoral head) with widening of medial joint space
    - Incongruency between femoral head and acetabulum
    - Point of maximum weight bearing shifts laterally and leads to labral degeneration ⇒ osteoarthritis 3rd or 4th decade of life
- **Avascular Necrosis**
  - Most commonly located: Anterolateral weight bearing portion of femoral head but can occur anywhere within femoral head
  - Important to detect and treat prior to subchondral fracture ⇒ subchondral collapse
  - T2WI: "Double line" sign
  - Many causes, including sickle cell disease, trauma, steroids, vasculitis, Gaucher disease, hemophilia
  - Children with acute lymphoblastic leukemia (ALL) and those treated with steroids particularly at risk
- **Septic Arthritis**
  - *Staphylococcus aureus* most common
  - May extend into joint from femoral epiphysis, metaphysis, joint capsule, or acetabulum
  - Key: Early diagnosis and treatment
    - Ultrasound: Detect joint effusion (cannot distinguish infected vs. aseptic fluid)
    - Complications: Cartilage destruction (joint space narrowing), erosions, periosteal reaction, osteonecrosis, and soft tissue abscesses
- **Juvenile Idiopathic Arthritis (JIA)**
  - a.k.a. juvenile rheumatoid arthritis (JRA)
  - < 16 years old and symptoms > 6 weeks in duration
  - Joint space narrowing is a late finding
- **Slipped Capital Femoral Epiphysis (SCFE)**
  - Femoral head or joint destruction as complication in treatment
  - Acute or chronic presentations
  - Salter-Harris 1 femoral physeal fracture
  - More common in boys
  - Bilateral in up to 36%
    - When bilateral, contralateral SCFE usually occurs within 18 months
  - Age
    - Girls: 8-15 years old
    - Boys: 10-17 years old
  - Predisposition
    - Obesity (most significant)

- Growth spurt, endocrine deficiencies, Down syndrome, and renal rickets
  - Complications
    - Chondrolysis (10%)
    - Avascular necrosis (1%), increase in open reduction with fixation or pins across superolateral quadrant of femoral head ossification center
    - Pin penetration

Helpful Clues for Rare Diagnoses

- **Meyer Dysplasia**
  - Age: 2-4 years old
  - Mostly boys
  - Bilateral (60%)
  - Asymptomatic
  - When clinical sign or symptoms present, consider early LCP disease
- **Idiopathic Chondrolysis**
  - Destruction of articular cartilage of femoral head and acetabulum
  - Stiffness, limp, and pain around hip
  - Radiographs: Concentrically joint space narrowing, < 3 mm with osteopenia, pelvic tilt
  - MR: Rectangular hypointense T1 and hyperintense T2 signal abnormality of center 1/3 of femoral head, ± ill defined within acetabulum
- **Epiphyseal Bone Tumors**
  - Chondroblastoma
    - 1% of primary bone tumors
    - 2nd decade of life, > 90% are seen in patients < 30 years old
    - M:F = 2:1
    - Well-defined, eccentric, lucent, sclerotic borders
    - Calcified matrix (50%)
  - Giant cell tumor
    - 4-5% of primary bone tumors
    - Considered benign, but malignant in up to 10% (can metastasize to lungs)
    - Slight female predominance
    - After growth plate closure
- **Epiphyseal Dysplasias**
  - Diastrophic dysplasia
    - Characteristic: "Hitchhiker thumb"
    - Cervical platyspondyly and kyphosis, clubfoot
  - Multiple epiphyseal dysplasia
    - Ribbing (milder form) or Fairbank forms
    - Should differentiate from LCP
    - Bilateral and symmetric changes, short limbs
  - Spondyloepiphyseal dysplasia
    - Congenita: Evident at birth; short trunk, mildly short limbs, pear-shaped vertebral body, atlantoaxial instability
    - Tarda: Presents at age 5-10; short trunks, disc spaces widened anteriorly and narrowed posteriorly, flattening vertebral bodies, dysplastic epiphyses

Legg-Calvé-Perthes (LCP) Disease

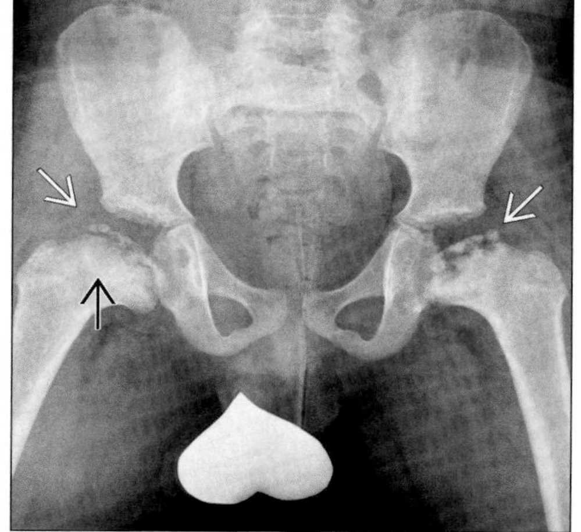

Anteroposterior radiograph shows fragmented, flattened, femoral head ossification centers ➔. Notice the metaphyseal cysts (cartilage) ➔ and femoral neck widening.

Legg-Calvé-Perthes (LCP) Disease

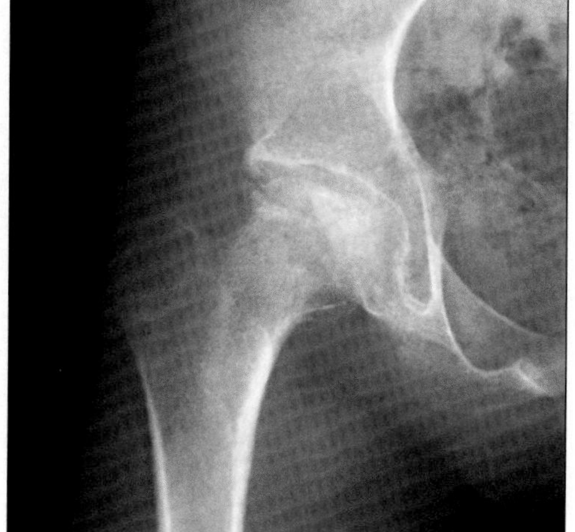

Anteroposterior radiograph shows partial collapse and mixed lucency and sclerosis within the femoral head. The ossified lateral femoral head appears well contained within the hip joint.

DESTROYED FEMORAL HEADS

Legg-Calvé-Perthes (LCP) Disease

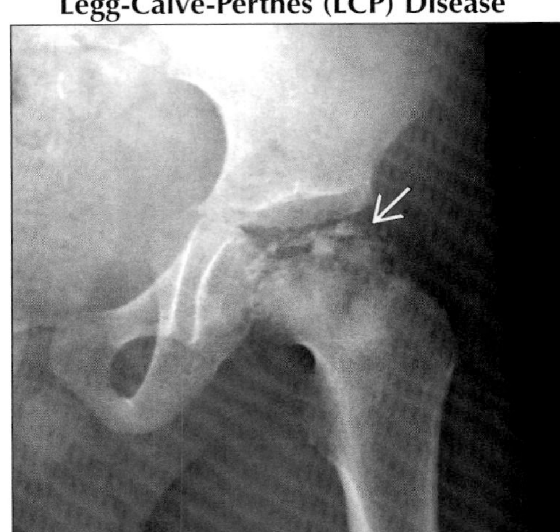

Legg-Calvé-Perthes (LCP) Disease

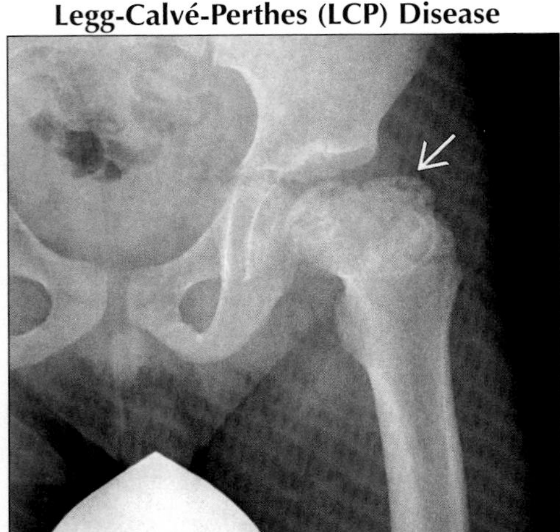

(Left) *Anteroposterior radiograph shows a fragmented and flattened femoral head ➡ with widening of the femoral neck.* ***(Right)*** *Anteroposterior radiograph in the same child 2 years later shows extrusion of the femoral head ➡ laterally and widening of the medial joint space. Notice the increasing ossification of the femoral head.*

Legg-Calvé-Perthes (LCP) Disease

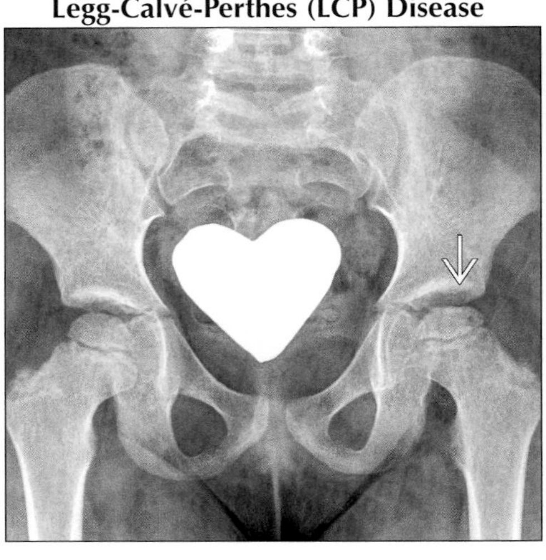

Legg-Calvé-Perthes (LCP) Disease

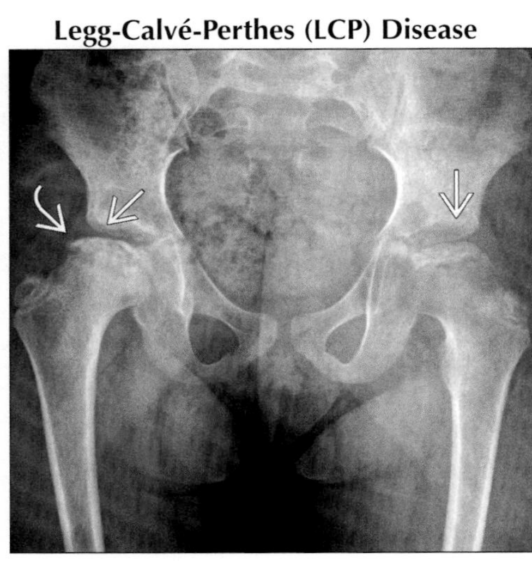

(Left) *Anteroposterior radiograph in this 5-year-old child with left hip pain shows subtle flattening and irregularity of the left femoral head ➡.* ***(Right)*** *Anteroposterior radiograph follow-up study in the same child shows bilateral femoral head ➡ flattening and sclerosis. The right femoral head was initially normal on radiograph. Now there are bilateral LCP changes, worse on the right, with lateral extrusion of the right femoral head ➡.*

Legg-Calvé-Perthes (LCP) Disease

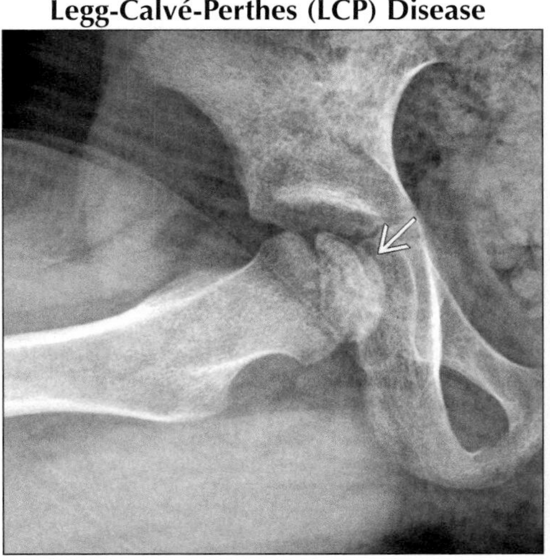

Legg-Calvé-Perthes (LCP) Disease

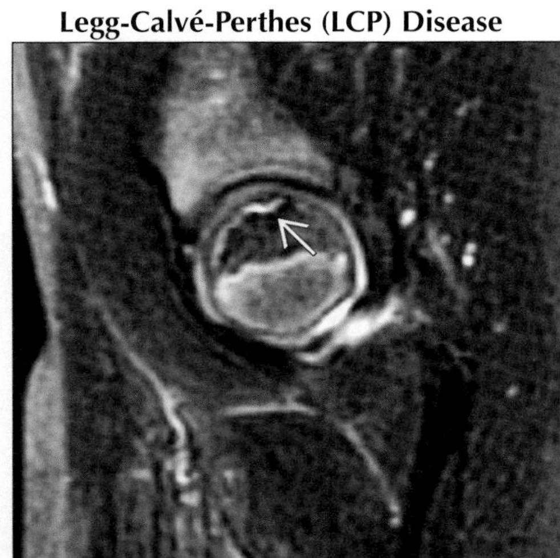

(Left) *Frog leg lateral radiograph shows a subchondral fracture ➡, fragmentation, and sclerosis of the femoral head in this child with LCP disease. Subchondral fractures are best detected on frog leg lateral images.* ***(Right)*** *Sagittal T2WI FS MR shows a subchondral hyperintense signal band ➡ and fracture in this patient with LCP disease. The femoral head on follow-up studies (not shown) demonstrated progressive fragmentation, sclerosis, and collapse.*

DESTROYED FEMORAL HEADS

Avascular Necrosis

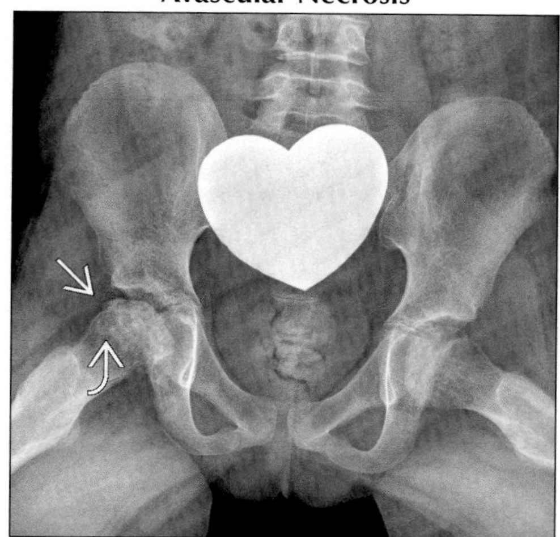

Avascular Necrosis

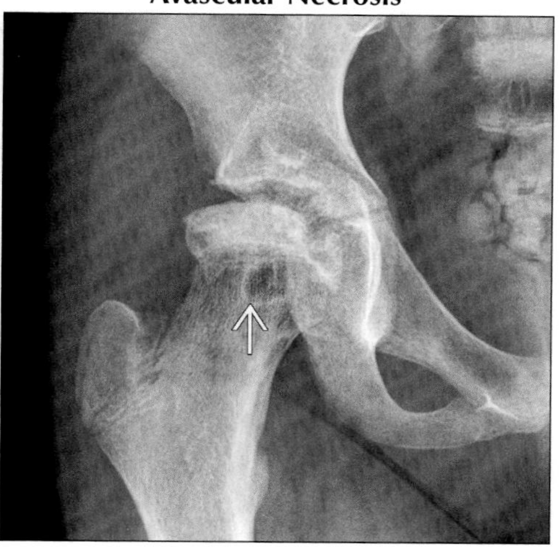

*(**Left**) Frog leg lateral radiograph shows irregularity, flattening, and sclerosis of the right femoral head ➡. Notice the metaphyseal lucencies ➡ and femoral neck widening. This child had a predisposing avascular necrosis history of ALL and steroid therapy. (**Right**) Anteroposterior radiograph in the same child shows sclerosis and flattening of the right femoral head. Notice the large metaphyseal cyst ➡ and medial femoral neck thickening.*

Avascular Necrosis

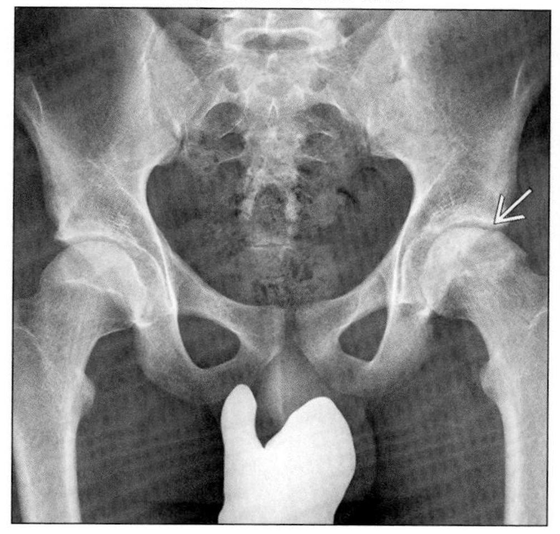

Avascular Necrosis

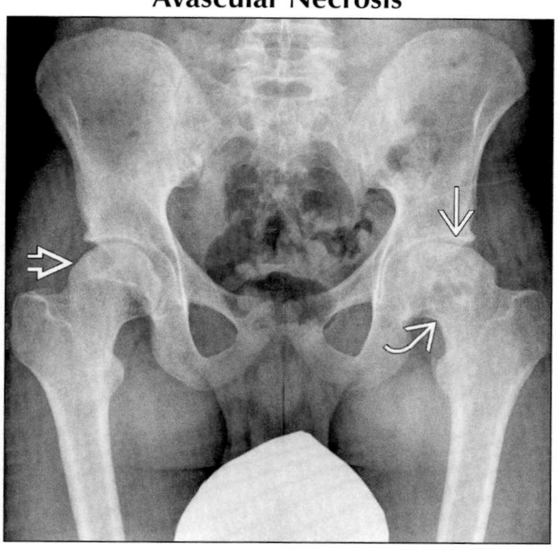

*(**Left**) Anteroposterior radiograph shows a left femoral head irregularity ➡. There is slight increased sclerosis of both femoral heads in this child with a history of dermatomyositis and steroid therapy. (**Right**) Anteroposterior radiograph in the same child 1 year later shows increasing deformity of the left ➡ with similar sclerosis of the right ➡ femoral head. Note the interval core decompression with multiple lucencies within the femoral neck ➡.*

Avascular Necrosis

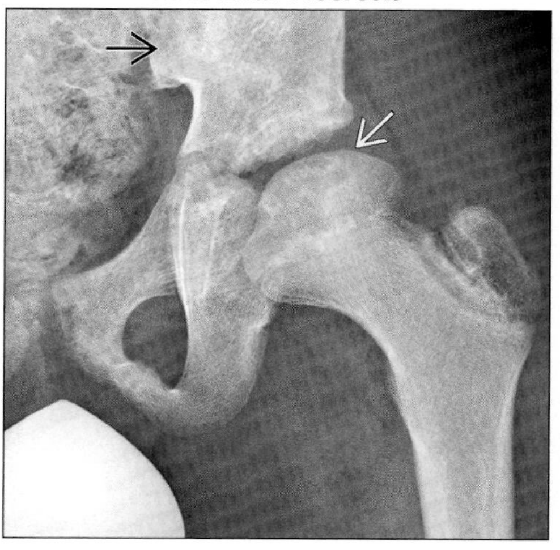

Avascular Necrosis

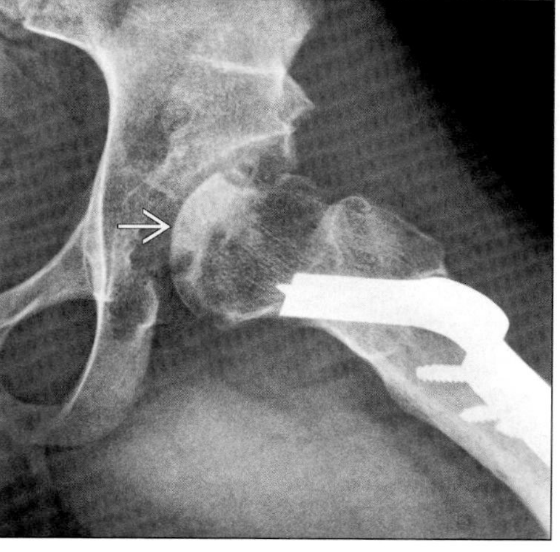

*(**Left**) Anteroposterior radiograph in a child with sickle cell disease shows enlargement of the left femoral head with subchondral lucencies ➡ and iliac wing infarct →, findings consistent with AVN and bone infarcts. (**Right**) Frog leg lateral radiograph shows subchondral lucency and sclerosis ➡ within the left femoral head. Note the surgical plate from a varus rotation osteotomy for hip dislocation. AVN was a complication of the surgical procedure.*

DESTROYED FEMORAL HEADS

(Left) *Coronal T1 C+ FS MR shows periarticular and intraarticular nonenhancing fluid collections →. There is diffuse myositis. Notice the subluxation the left femoral head laterally.* ***(Right)*** *Anteroposterior radiograph shows progressive destruction of the right femoral head → and adjacent acetabulum. This teenager had a history of paraplegia from a motor vehicle crash and deep decubitus ulcers and septic hips.*

Septic Arthritis

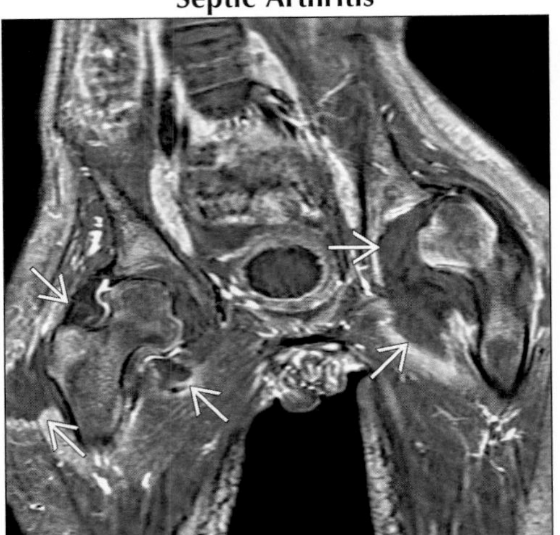

Septic Arthritis

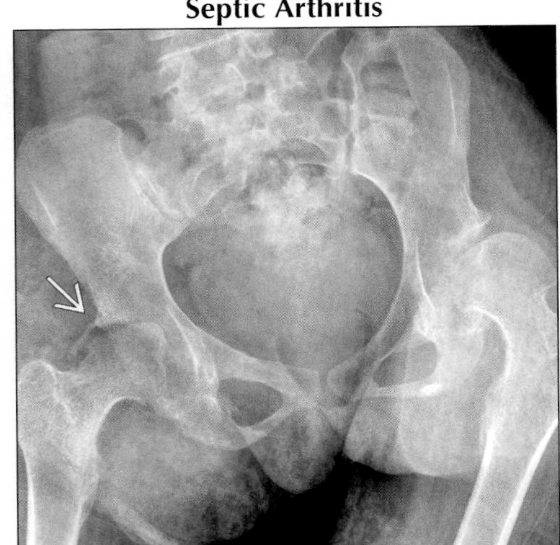

(Left) *Anteroposterior radiograph shows lateral dislocation of the right hip with destruction of the femoral head →. An adjacent fragment of the femoral head is detected ↷.* ***(Right)*** *Coronal T2WI FS MR in the same patient shows a completely destroyed femoral head with extensive hyperintense material → within the hip joint and surrounding soft tissues.*

Septic Arthritis

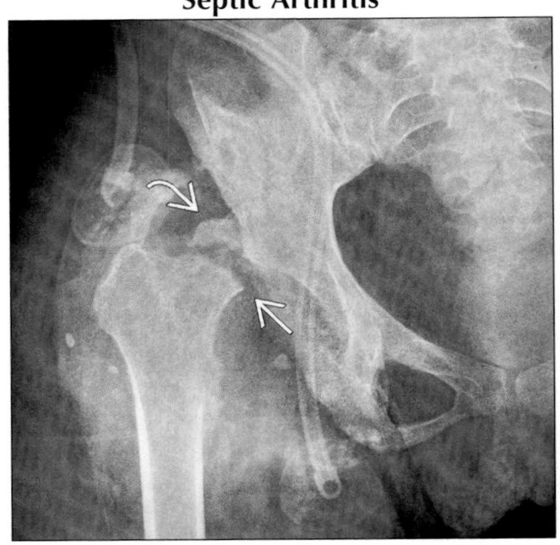

Septic Arthritis

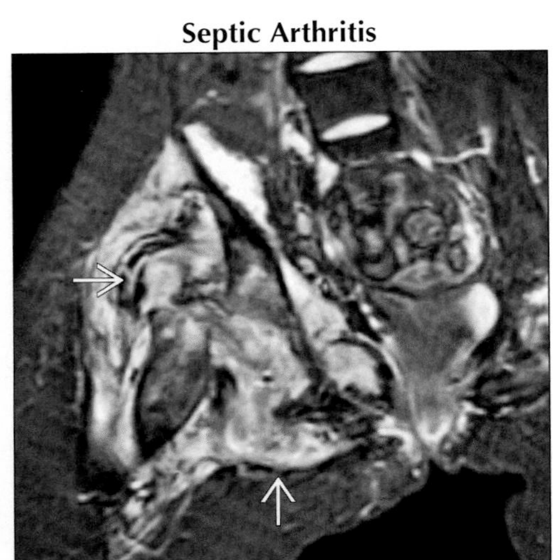

(Left) *Coronal T2WI FS MR shows joint space narrowing with loss of articular cartilage along both sides of the bilateral hip joints. Note the full thickness defects within the acetabular cartilage → and mild synovitis.* ***(Right)*** *Frog leg lateral radiograph in a patient with chronic SCFE shows slippage of the femoral head posteromedially →. There are also changes of AVN of the femoral head with increased sclerosis and lucency, a complication of SCFE.*

Juvenile Idiopathic Arthritis (JIA)

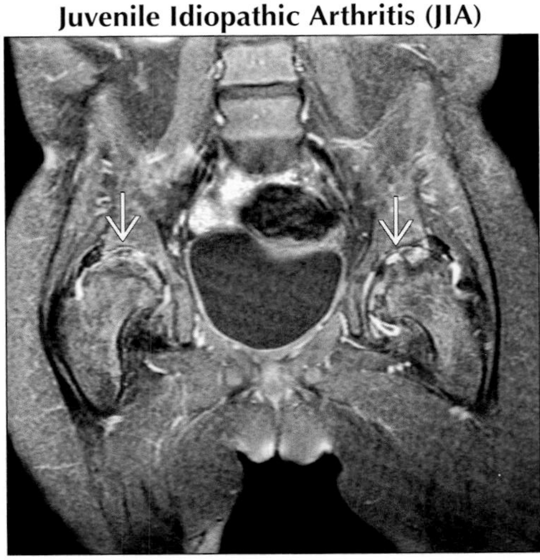

Slipped Capital Femoral Epiphysis (SCFE)

Meyer Dysplasia

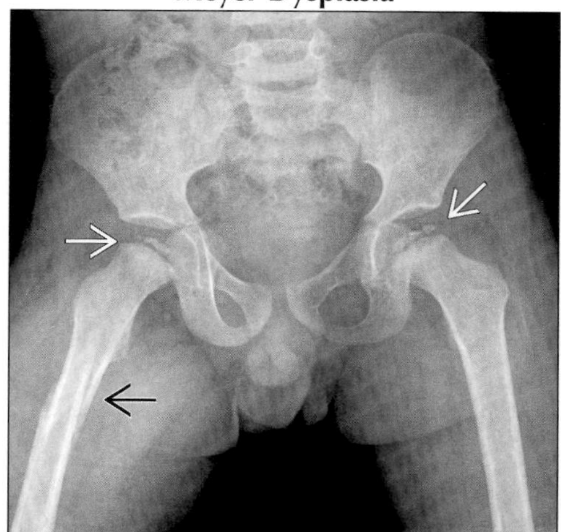

Idiopathic Chondrolysis

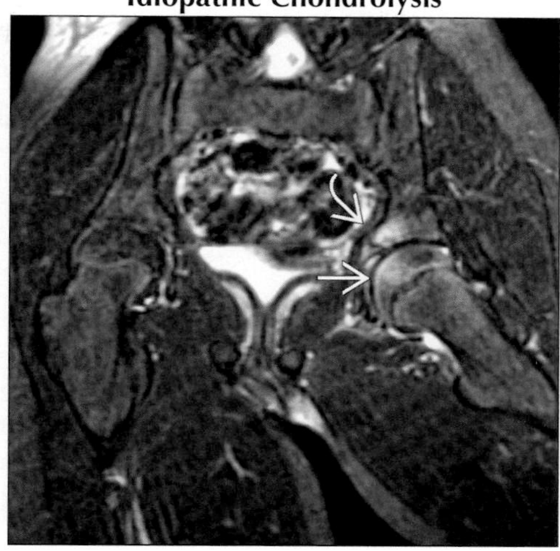

(Left) *Anteroposterior radiograph shows small, fragmented, femoral head ossification centers ➡. This 2 year old presented with trauma and a right femur fracture ➡. Some children initially diagnosed with Meyer dysplasia eventually develop LCP disease.* ***(Right)*** *Coronal T2WI FSE MR shows rectangular-shaped hyperintense signal within the medial left femoral head ➡. Note also that mild hyperintense signal is present within the adjacent acetabulum ➡.*

Idiopathic Chondrolysis

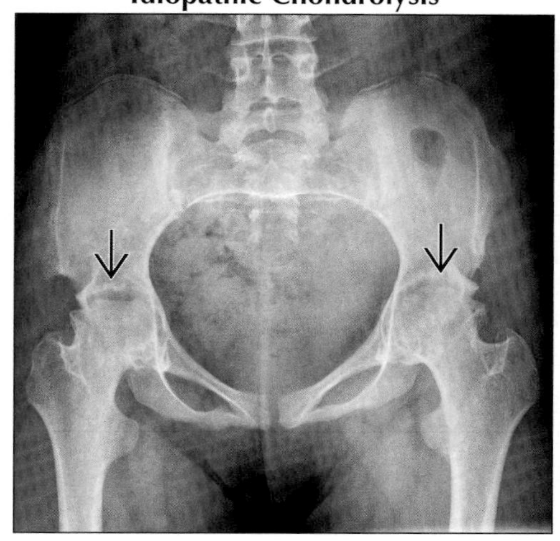

Epiphyseal Bone Tumors

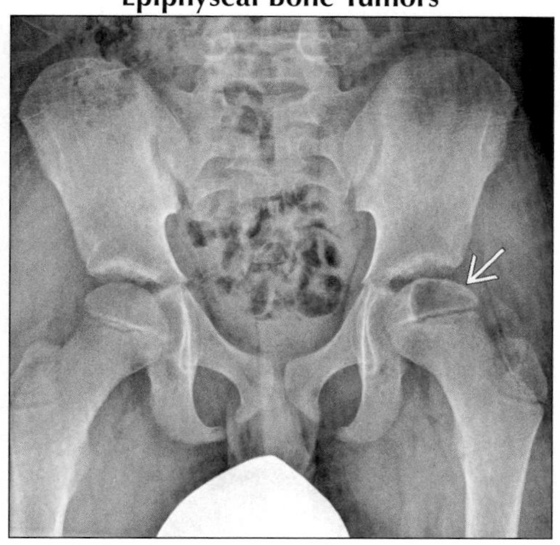

(Left) *Anteroposterior radiograph in the same patient 4 years later shows destruction of both femoral heads ➡, joint space narrowing, and joint margin spurring. This patient developed chondrolysis on the right hip in the interval.* ***(Right)*** *Anteroposterior radiograph shows a well-defined lytic lesion with a medial sclerotic margin within the left femoral head ➡. There is mild femoral head flattening. This was pathologically proven to be chondroblastoma.*

Epiphyseal Dysplasias

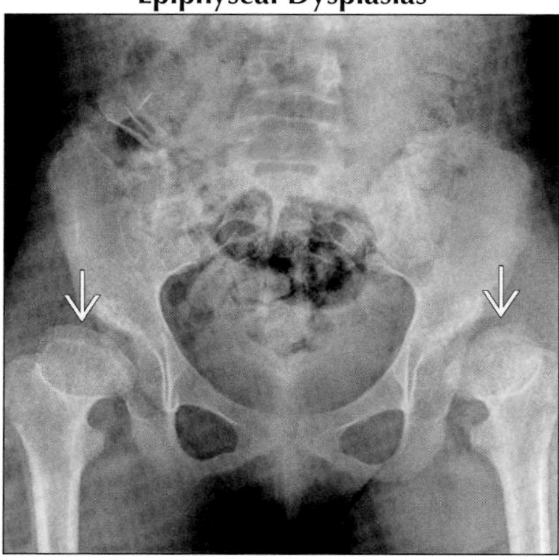

Epiphyseal Dysplasias

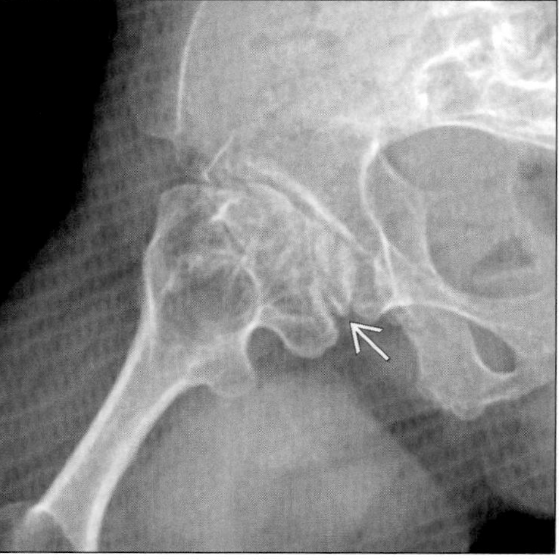

(Left) *Anteroposterior radiograph shows mild bilateral femoral head flattening, with enlargement and lateral subluxation ➡. The acetabuli are shallow in this patient with spondyloepiphyseal dysplasia.* ***(Right)*** *Frog leg lateral radiograph shows enlargement, deformity, and fragmentation of the femoral head ➡. This patient was diagnosed with diastrophic dysplasia.*

COXA MAGNA DEFORMITY

DIFFERENTIAL DIAGNOSIS

Common
- Developmental Dysplasia Hip (DDH)

Less Common
- Slipped Capital Femoral Epiphysis (SCFE)
- Legg-Calvé-Perthes (LCP)

Rare but Important
- Septic Hip
- Hip/Femur Trauma

ESSENTIAL INFORMATION

Key Differential Diagnosis Issues
- Coxa magna: Short, broad femoral head sitting on short, broad femoral neck
  - Results in limb length discrepancy
  - Relatively proximal displacement of greater and lesser trochanters
- Coxa magna is secondary to insult to femoral head or epiphysis

Helpful Clues for Common Diagnoses
- **Developmental Dysplasia Hip (DDH)**
  - Lack of coverage of femoral head during development due to deficient acetabulum
  - Without coverage, head cannot develop spherical shape
    - Head becomes short, broad
    - With head and neck shortening, limb becomes short, with proximal displacement of both trochanters
  - Congenital abnormality
    - Severe DDH develops coxa magna
    - Subtle DDH does not show coxa magna but seen as ↓ center-edge angle of Wiberg
  - **Hint**: Shallow acetabulum distinguishes coxa magna of DDH from other etiologies of coxa magna

Helpful Clues for Less Common Diagnoses
- **Slipped Capital Femoral Epiphysis (SCFE)**
  - Femoral capital epiphysis slips medially and posteriorly
    - As head slips, appears short and broad, on short and broad neck
  - Most frequently occurs 8-14 years of age
  - **Hint**: Position of femoral head on neck and a normal acetabulum distinguish coxa magna of SCFE from other etiologies
- **Legg-Calvé-Perthes (LCP)**
  - Avascular necrosis of femoral head in child, generally 4-8 years of age
  - Flattening of head leads to coxa magna deformity
  - **Hint**: Head remains centered on femoral neck and acetabulum is normal, distinguishing this etiology of coxa magna from others

Helpful Clues for Rare Diagnoses
- **Septic Hip**
  - Chronic hip infection during childhood
    - Hyperemia results in overgrowth of femoral head and neck
- **Hip/Femur Trauma**
  - Resorption/impaction of neck or malalignment mimics coxa magna
  - Salter fracture with early fusion

Developmental Dysplasia Hip (DDH)

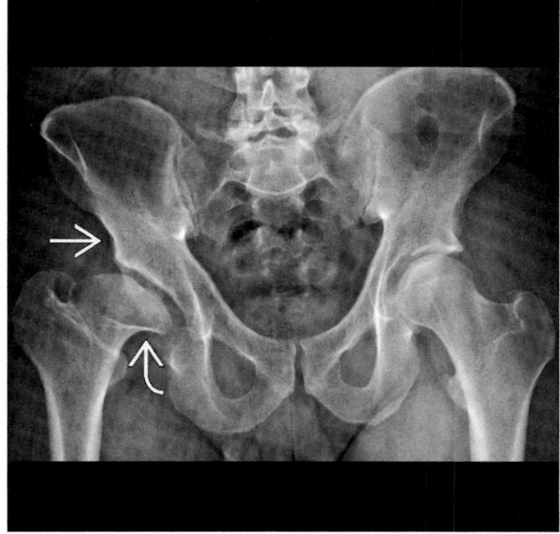

AP radiograph shows right DDH. Note the short, broad head ➔ and neck, compared with normal left side. Coxa magna is due to DDH, with shallow acetabulum ➔, resulting in decrease in femoral head coverage.

Slipped Capital Femoral Epiphysis (SCFE)

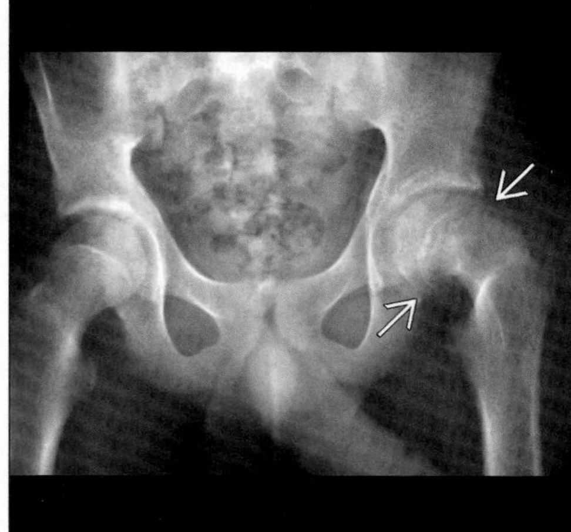

AP radiograph shows SCFE with medial and posterior femoral head slip ➔. This results in the appearance of a short, broad femoral head; the neck also appears broad. Note the lateral femoral neck is not covered by head.

Legg-Calvé-Perthes (LCP)

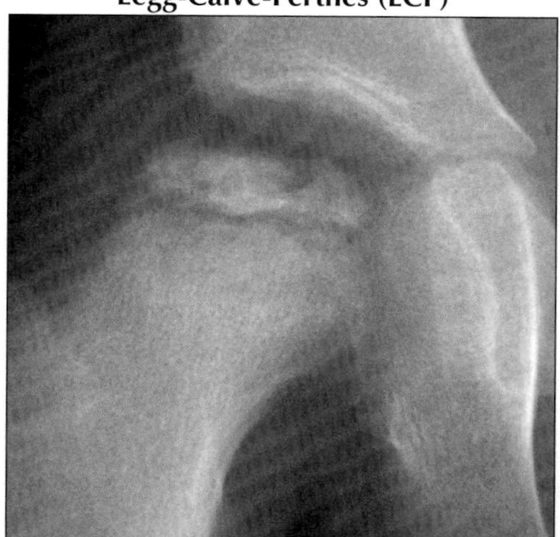

Legg-Calvé-Perthes (LCP)

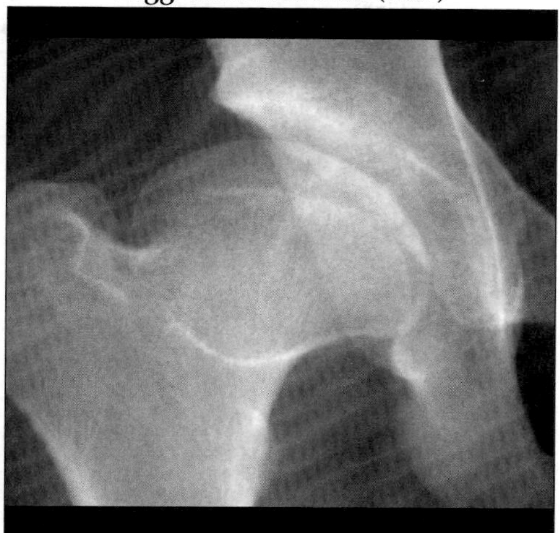

(Left) *AP radiograph shows flattened & dense femoral capital epiphysis typical of LCP. This is already chronic disease, & morphologic change of short, broad head & neck is seen in its early form. (†MSK Req).* ***(Right)*** *AP radiograph in the same patient 12 years later shows typical coxa magna deformity. Head is not medially displaced to suggest SCFE, & acetabulum is normal, ruling out DDH. Even without prior X-ray, this should be diagnosed as coxa magna due to LCP.*

Legg-Calvé-Perthes (LCP)

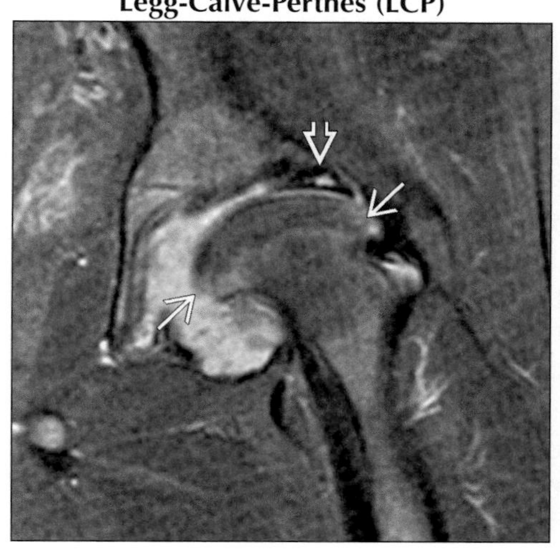

Septic Hip

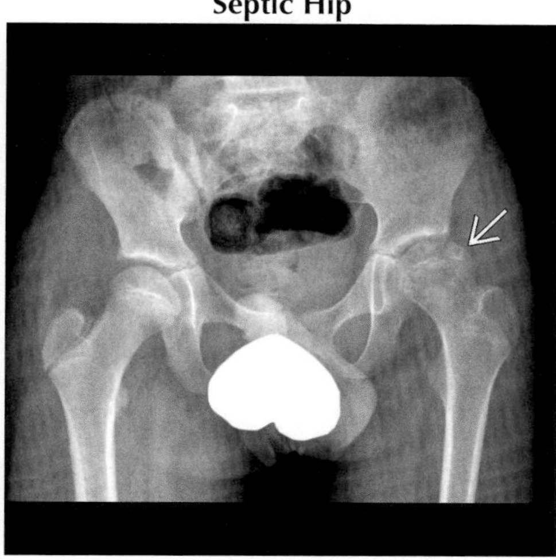

(Left) *Coronal T2WI FS MR shows old LCP, with the short, broad femoral head ➡ on a shortened femoral neck, resulting in a coxa magna deformity. This has resulted in a significant labral tear ⇨ and early arthritic change.* ***(Right)*** *AP radiograph shows an enlarged, short femoral capital femoral epiphysis ➡, with broadening and slight shortening of the femoral neck. This 12 year old had a septic hip treated 9 months earlier. The growth deformity results from hyperemia.*

Hip/Femur Trauma

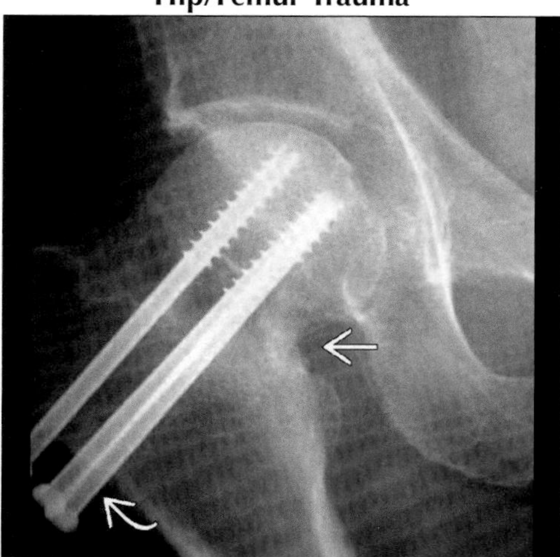

Hip/Femur Trauma

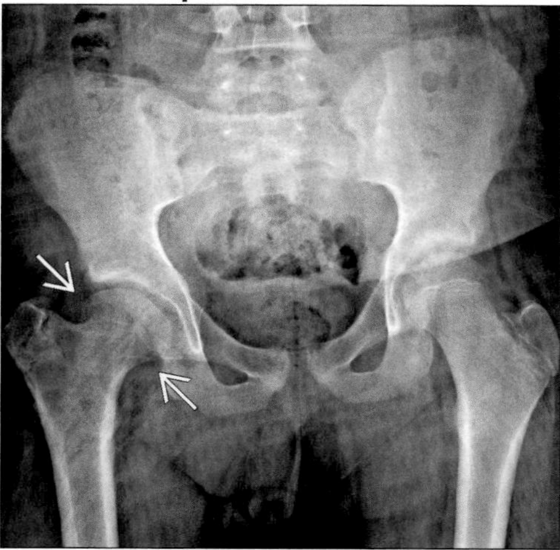

(Left) *AP radiograph shows an old subcapital fracture treated with pins. The fracture has impacted, with resorption of much of the neck ➡ and backing out of the pins ↪. This results in the appearance of a short femoral head on a short broad neck, similar to a coxa magna deformity.* ***(Right)*** *AP radiograph shows an enlarged femoral head with early fusion ➡ and subsequent limb shortening in a teenager. This coxa magna deformity resulted from Salter 2 fracture.*

PAINFUL HIP

DIFFERENTIAL DIAGNOSIS

Common
- Transient Synovitis
- Septic Arthritis
- Osteomyelitis
- Slipped Capital Femoral Epiphysis (SCFE)
- Legg-Calvé-Perthes (LCP)
- Juvenile Idiopathic Arthritis (JIA)
- Trauma

Less Common
- Idiopathic Chondrolysis
- Osteoid Osteoma
- Osteonecrosis
- Malignancy

ESSENTIAL INFORMATION

Key Differential Diagnosis Issues
- Age and history are helpful in narrowing differential diagnosis

Helpful Clues for Common Diagnoses
- **Transient Synovitis**
  - a.k.a. irritable hip, toxic synovitis
  - Age: 18 months to 10 years; most common from age 4-7
  - Typically follows recent upper respiratory infection
  - Radiographs
    - Normal
    - Widening of medial joint space, lateral displacement of femoral head
  - 70% hip effusion on ultrasound
  - Hip held in flexion, external rotation, and abduction, restricted abduction and internal rotation
  - ± fever (often < 38° C)
  - May have mildly elevated erythrocyte sedimentation rate and white blood cell
  - Symptoms improve (usually within 48 hours) in 1-5 weeks
    - If symptoms persists beyond 1 week, consider another diagnosis
    - Recur in up to 17%
    - Legg-Calvé-Perthes develops in 1-3%
- **Septic Arthritis**
  - Important to diagnose early to avoid destruction of joint
    - Delay in treatment ≥ 4 days results in suboptimal recovery
  - Age: < 4 years old
  - *Staphylococcus aureus* most common cause
    - Umbilical catheter, sepsis, and prior venous puncture have been implicated
  - Hip held in flexion
  - Infants can present with low-grade fever and feeding intolerance
  - Radiographs
    - Normal
    - Periostitis of proximal femur in neonates within days after start of symptoms
  - Treatment: Surgical drainage, IV antibiotics, traction
- **Osteomyelitis**
  - *Staphylococcus aureus* most common
  - *Streptococcus pneumonia* (hypogammaglobinemia, sickle cell disease, asplenia)
  - Referred pain from spine or sacroiliac joints
    - Importance of scrutinizing spine and sacroiliac joints when imaging hips
  - May take up to 10-14 days before radiographs depict changes or osteomyelitis
  - Treatment: Abscess drainage, debridement, IV antibiotics
- **Slipped Capital Femoral Epiphysis (SCFE)**
  - Salter-Harris type 1 femoral epiphyseal fracture
  - Age: 10-15 years old
  - M:F = 2:1; occurs earlier in girls
  - Predisposed: Obesity and endocrine disorders
  - Bilateral (18-36%)
    - Opposite side occurs within 18-24 months of 1st occurrence
  - Presentations: Acute, chronic, and acute on chronic
  - Radiographs
    - Widened femoral physis, medial and posterior displacement of femoral head (best seen frog leg lateral view)
    - Capital femoral epiphysis displacement without intersection of Klein line
    - Klein line: Line along lateral femoral neck and continuing toward acetabulum; ordinarily crosses small portion of femoral ossification center
- **Legg-Calvé-Perthes (LCP)**
  - Osteonecrosis of femoral head of unknown etiology

- Age: 3-12 years old; peak: 6-8 years old
- Bilateral (10-20%)
- Radiographs
  - Normal
  - Flattening, fragmentation, and sclerosis of femoral head
- **Key**: Prognosis heavily depends on containment of femoral head

- **Juvenile Idiopathic Arthritis (JIA)**
  - a.k.a. juvenile rheumatoid arthritis (JRA)
  - Age: < 16 years old
  - Symptoms with > 6 week duration
  - Other causes of arthritis are excluded
  - Stiff, swollen, painful, warm, and decreased motion in joint involved
  - MR: Synovitis, ± erosions, ± rice bodies
  - Joint space narrowing and ankylosis are late findings
- **Trauma**
  - Acute (fracture) or repetitive (stress fracture) trauma

Helpful Clues for Less Common Diagnoses

- **Idiopathic Chondrolysis**
  - Destruction of articular cartilage of femoral head and acetabulum
  - Stiffness, limpness, and pain around hip
  - Radiographs
    - Concentrically joint space narrowing, < 3 mm with osteopenia and pelvic tilt
  - MR: Rectangular hypointense T1 and hyperintense T2WI signal abnormality of center 1/3 of femoral head, ± ill defined within acetabulum
- **Osteoid Osteoma**
  - Benign composed of osteoid and woven bone
  - 3 types: Cortical (most common), cancellous, or subperiosteal
  - < 2 cm nidus surrounded by dense sclerotic bone
  - Most common location is femur
  - Age: 10-30 years old, uncommon before age 5
  - Classic history: Pain at night relieved by nonsteroidal anti-inflammatory agents
  - NECT: Depicts nidus better than MR
  - Bone scan: Increased flow, "double density" pattern
    - Intense uptake by nidus surrounded by less intense activity of reactive bone
- **Osteonecrosis**
  - Most commonly located in anterolateral weightbearing portion of femoral head
  - T2WI: "Double line" sign
  - Many causes, including sickle cell disease, trauma, steroid therapy, vasculitis, Gaucher disease, hemophilia
- **Malignancy**
  - Primary such as chondroblastoma
  - Metastatic disease: Most commonly neuroblastoma
  - ± pathologic fracture

Transient Synovitis

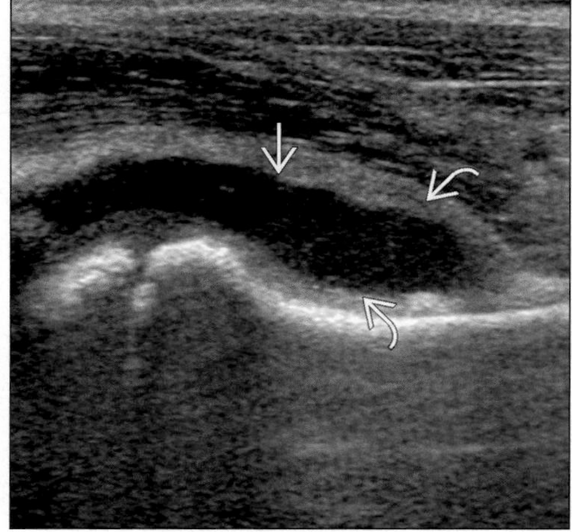

Longitudinal ultrasound shows a widened anechoic joint space ➔ with a convex outer margin, consistent with a hip effusion. Note the synovial thickening ➔ along the femoral neck and joint lining.

Transient Synovitis

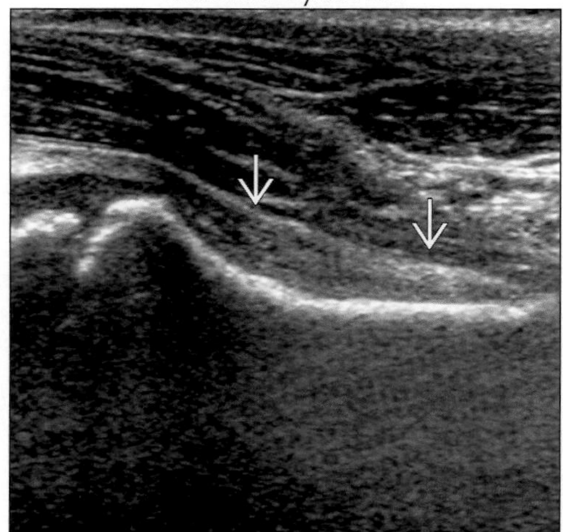

Longitudinal ultrasound shows a normal hip for comparison with no significant joint fluid, evidenced by a normal joint space with a concave anterior margin ➔ along the anterior femoral neck.

PAINFUL HIP

Septic Arthritis

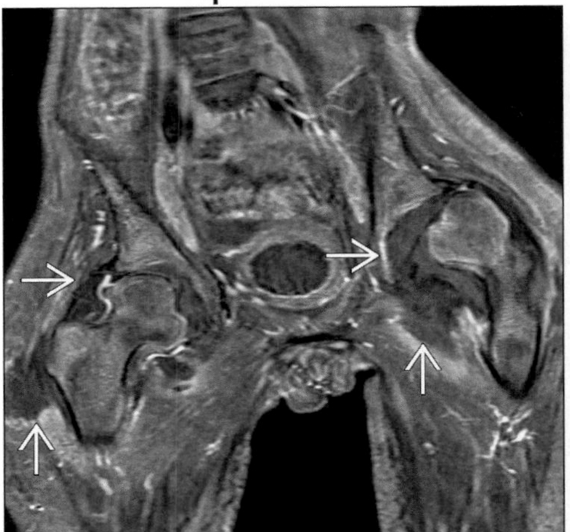

Septic Arthritis

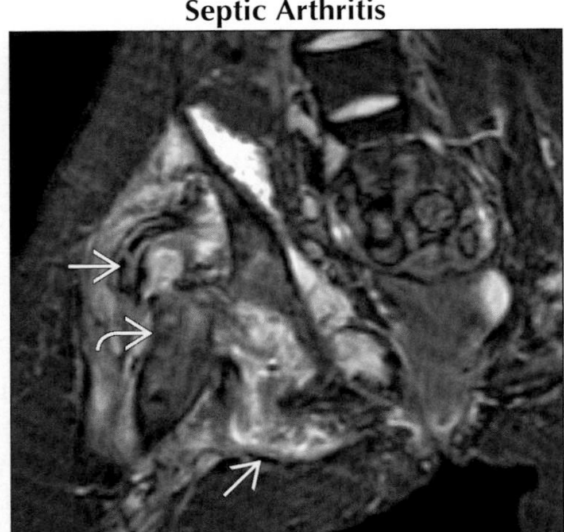

(Left) *Coronal T1WI C+ FS MR shows nonenhancing intra- and periarticular fluid collections ➔. The left femoral head is subluxed laterally.* ***(Right)*** *Coronal T2WI FS MR in the same patient 8 months later shows a completely destroyed femoral head with hyperintense material ➔ within the hip joint and periarticular soft tissues. The proximal femur is displaced superolaterally ↪. Early detection and treatment are very important to avoid joint destruction.*

Septic Arthritis

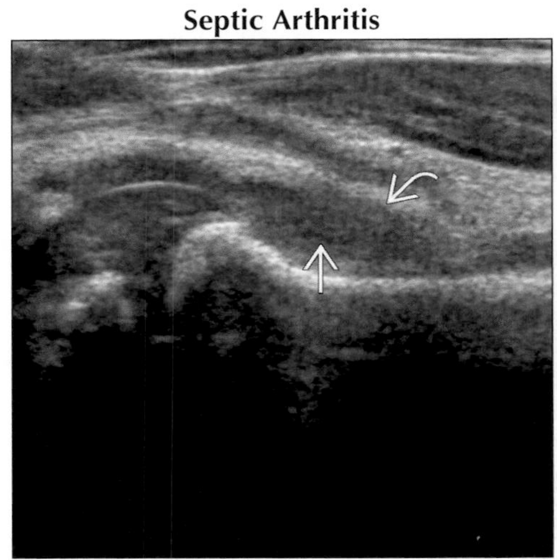

Osteomyelitis

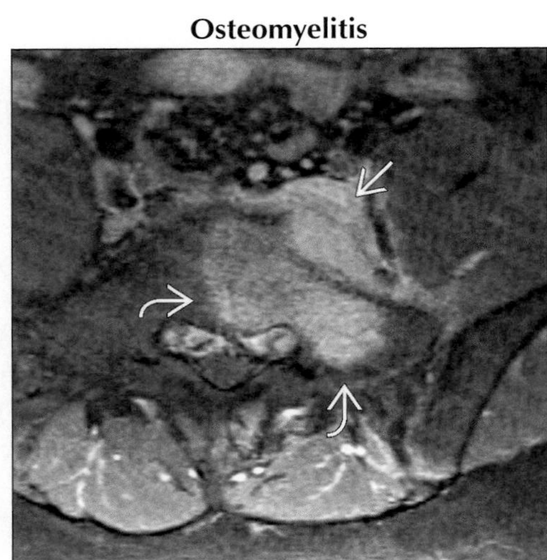

(Left) *Longitudinal ultrasound shows complex fluid (infected fluid) ➔ with convex anterior bowing ↪ of the hip joint. One cannot predict on ultrasound alone if the fluid is infected or not.* ***(Right)*** *Axial T1WI C+ MR shows enhancing, left, presacral soft tissue ➔ (phlegmon). Note the S1 marrow enhancement ↪ in this child with L5-S1 discitis and osteomyelitis.*

Osteomyelitis

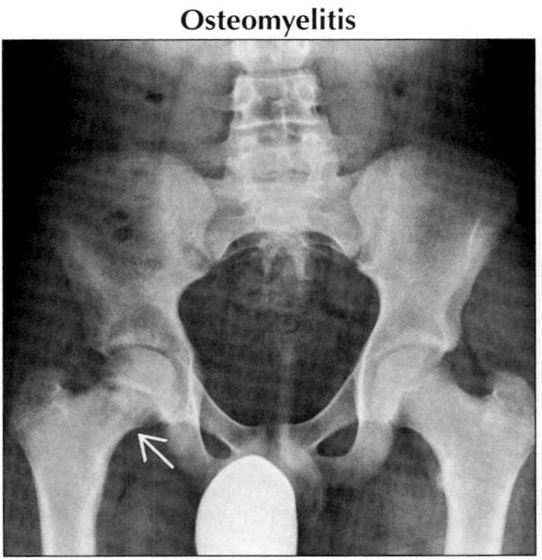

Osteomyelitis

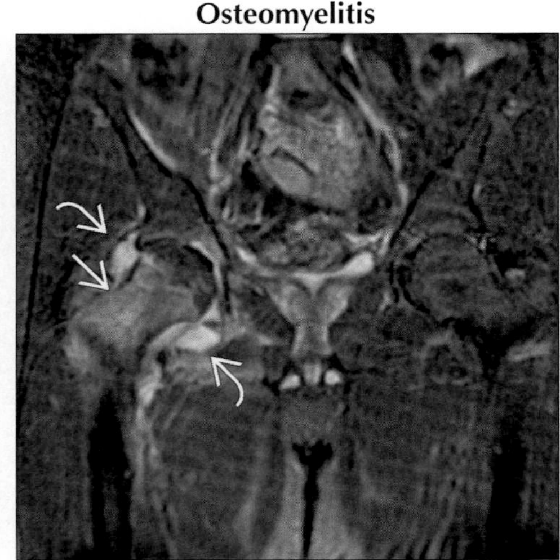

(Left) *AP radiograph shows focal rarefaction of the femoral neck ➔. This child was diagnosed and treated for a septic hip 1 month before imaging, and the hip pain recurred 2 weeks later. A hip aspiration and biopsy of the femoral neck were performed. The hip fluid was sterile, while the femoral neck specimen grew S. aureus.* ***(Right)*** *Coronal T2WI FS MR in the same patient shows hyperintense signal within the femoral neck ➔ and a hip effusion ↪.*

Osteomyelitis

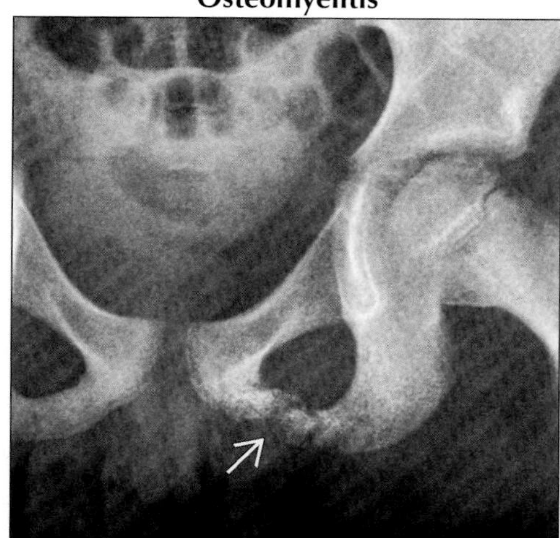

Osteomyelitis

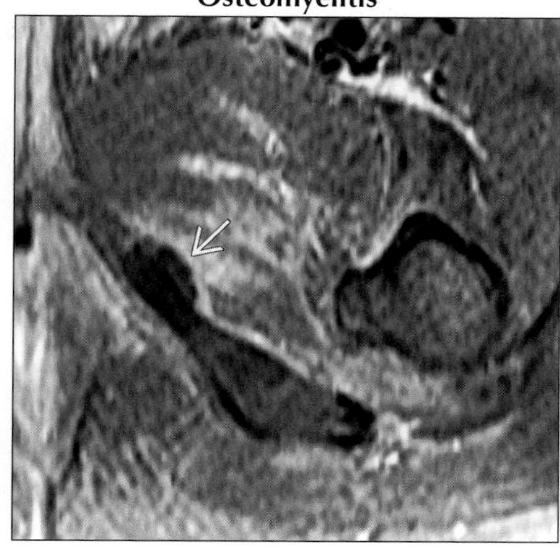

(Left) *Anteroposterior radiograph shows fragmentation of the left ischiopubic synchondrosis ➡ in an 8-year-old boy who presented with left hip pain, swelling, and a fever.* ***(Right)*** *Axial T1WI C+ FS MR in the same child shows decreased intramedullary enhancement with a small fluid collection and subperiosteal abscess ➡ within the left ischiopubic bone. Staphylococcal aureus is the most common cause for osteomyelitis in children.*

Slipped Capital Femoral Epiphysis (SCFE)

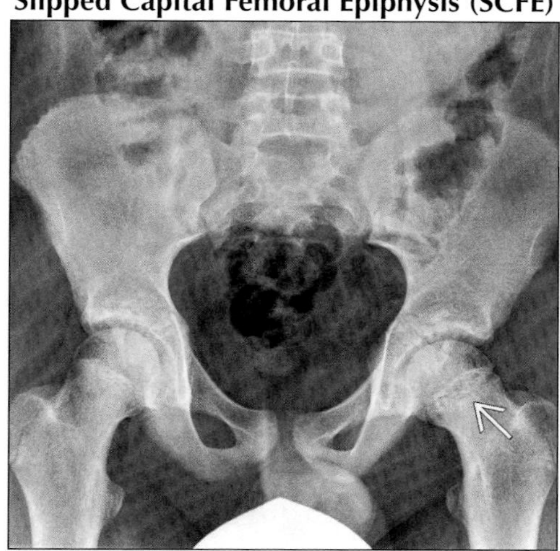

Slipped Capital Femoral Epiphysis (SCFE)

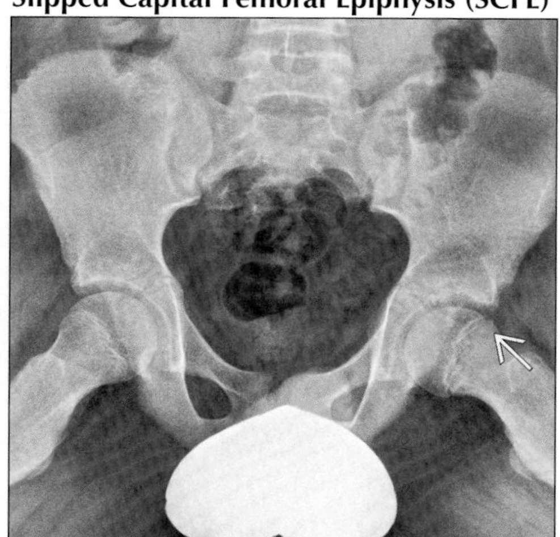

(Left) *Anteroposterior radiograph shows widening and irregularity ➡ of the left femoral physis.* ***(Right)*** *Frog leg lateral radiograph in the same patient shows subtle posteromedial slippage of the left capital femoral epiphysis ➡. SCFE is more commonly seen with obesity and during growth spurts. Most cases are idiopathic, but there may be increased incidence in hypothyroidism, other endocrine deficiencies, and renal osteodystrophy.*

Slipped Capital Femoral Epiphysis (SCFE)

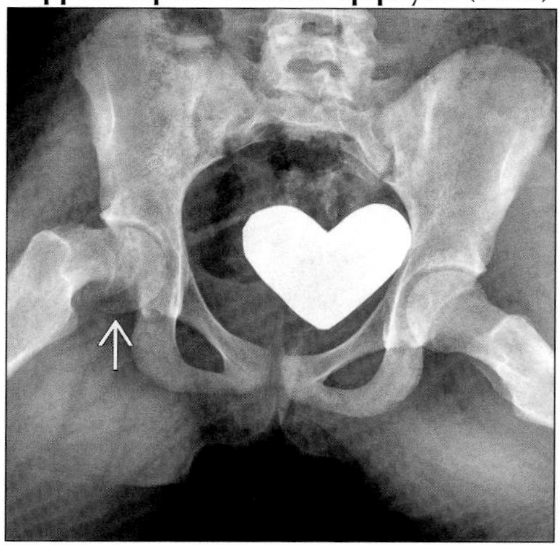

Legg-Calvé-Perthes (LCP)

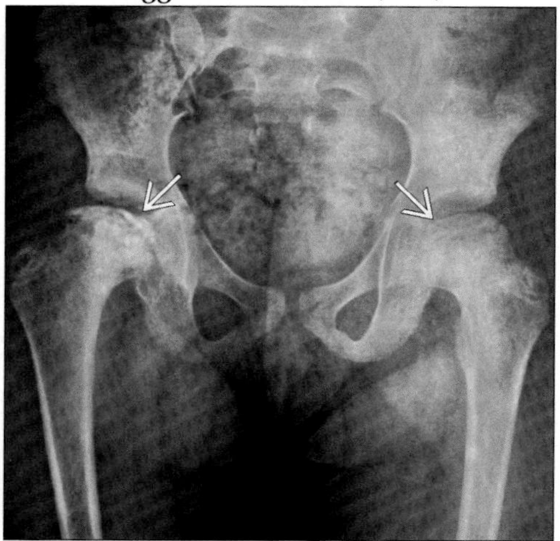

(Left) *Frog leg lateral radiograph shows posteromedial slippage of the right femoral head ➡. Osteonecrosis and chondrolysis are potential complications of SCFE.* ***(Right)*** *Coronal radiograph shows bilateral femoral head flattening (coxa plana) and sclerosis ➡, as well as widening of the femoral necks. Bilateral hip involvement is seen in 10-20% of patients with LCP.*

*(**Left**) Coronal T2WI FSE MR shows a mild right hip joint effusion ➔. (**Right**) Coronal T1WI C+ FS MR in the same child shows diffuse synovial enhancement ➔ (synovitis). Mild, diffuse joint space narrowing, especially superolaterally, had progressed when compared to prior studies (not shown).*

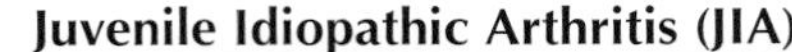

Juvenile Idiopathic Arthritis (JIA)

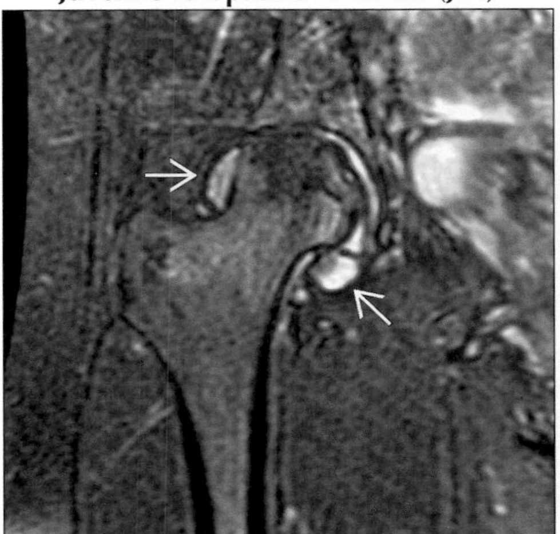

Juvenile Idiopathic Arthritis (JIA)

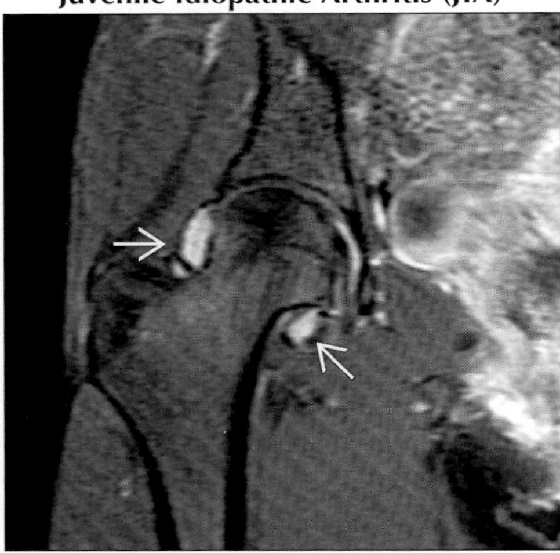

*(**Left**) Anteroposterior radiograph shows an ill-defined band of sclerosis ➔ along the femoral neck. This was shown to be a stress fracture along the tensile and compression portions of the femoral neck. This was transfixed by 2 Synthes screws. This child was a gymnast presenting with 3-4 months of hip pain. (**Right**) Coronal T2WI FS MR shows a linear dark band ➔ along the medial femoral neck with surrounding edema. This is consistent with a stress fracture.*

Trauma

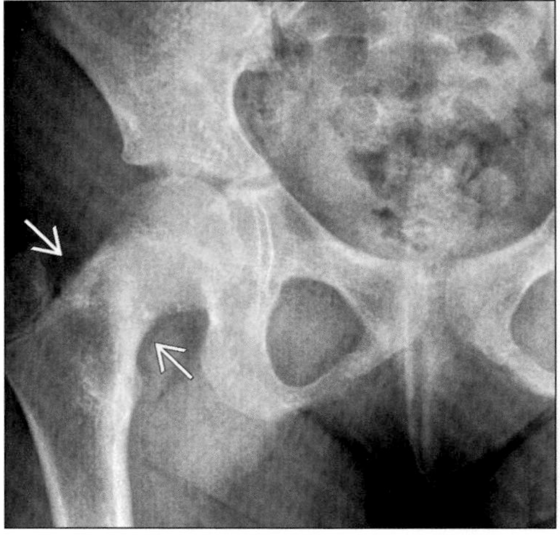

Trauma

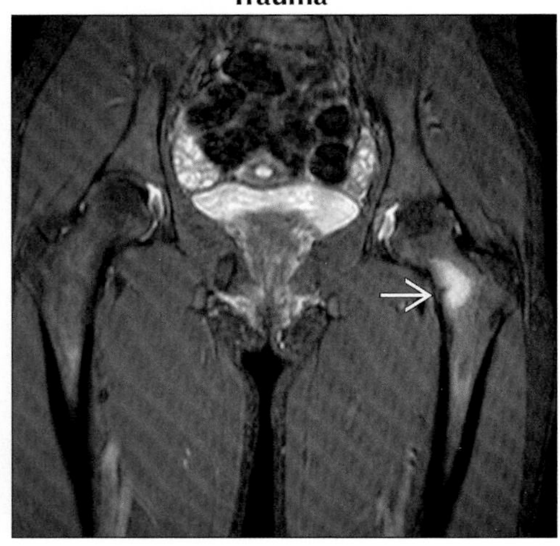

*(**Left**) Coronal T2WI FS MR shows a rectangular-shaped hyperintense signal within the medial left femoral head ➔. Notice the mild hyperintense signal within the adjacent acetabulum ➔. (**Right**) Axial NECT shows a sclerotic focus nidus ➔ contained within a radiolucent nidus in the medial wall of the left acetabulum. This was subsequently drilled and removed by interventional radiology.*

Idiopathic Chondrolysis

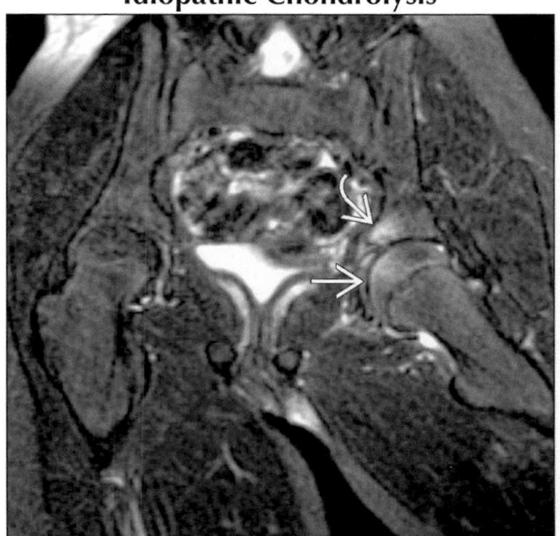

Osteoid Osteoma

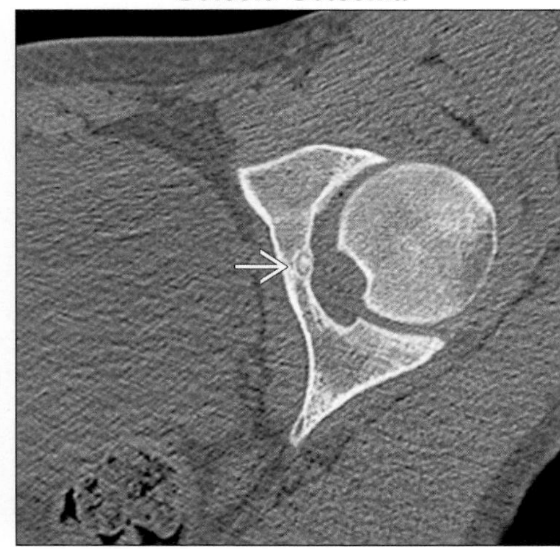

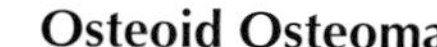

Osteoid Osteoma

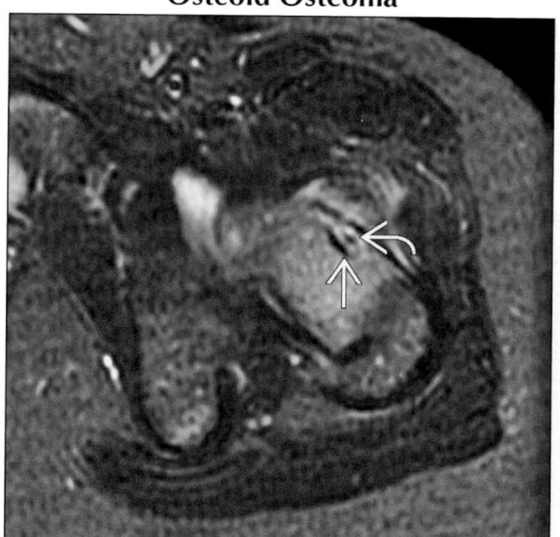

Osteoid Osteoma

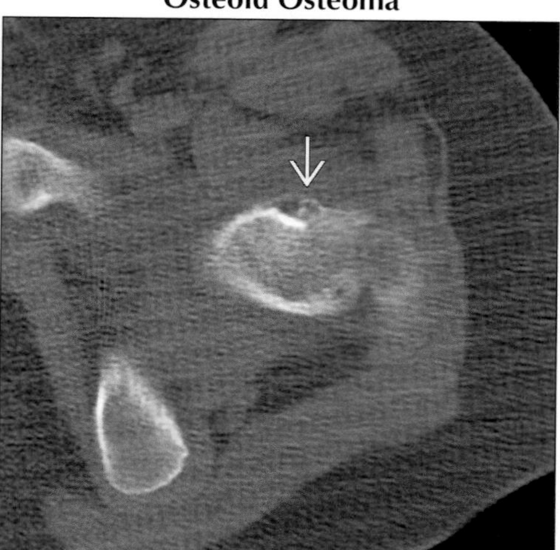

(Left) *Axial T2WI FS MR shows a cortically based lesion ➡ within the anterior femoral neck. There is a central hypointense focus ↪ with surrounding muscle and marrow edema.* ***(Right)*** *Axial NECT in the same patient shows a tiny sclerotic focus within a radiolucent nidus ➡ (characteristic of an osteoid osteoma) along the anterior left femoral neck.*

Osteonecrosis

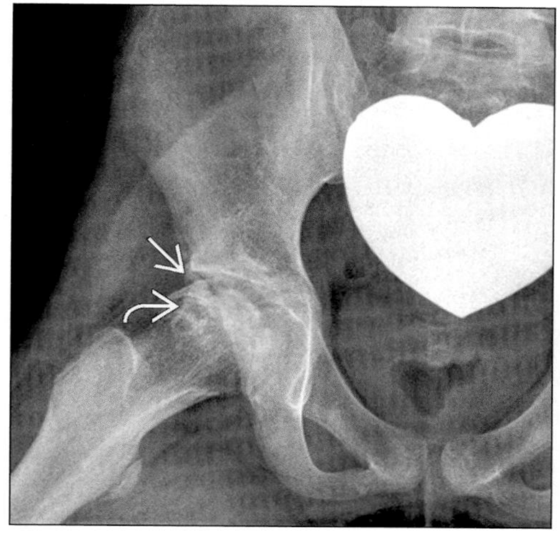

Osteonecrosis

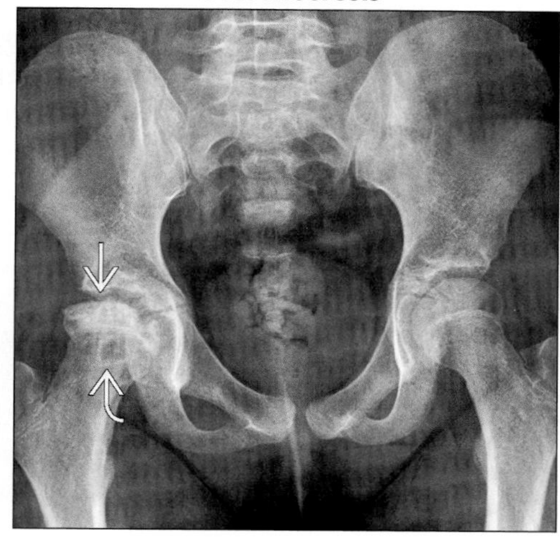

(Left) *Frog leg lateral radiograph shows irregularity, flattening, and sclerosis of the right femoral head ➡. Notice the metaphyseal lucencies ↪ and femoral neck widening. This child had a predisposing history of acute lymphoblastic leukemia and steroid therapy.* ***(Right)*** *Anteroposterior radiograph in the same child shows sclerosis and flattening of the right femoral head ➡. Note the large metaphyseal cyst ↪.*

Osteonecrosis

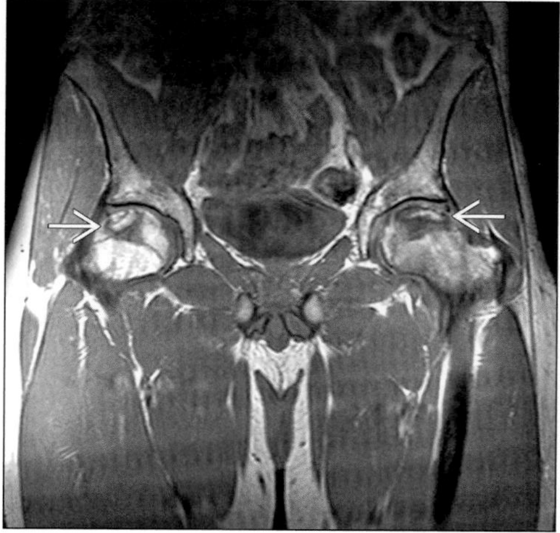

Malignancy

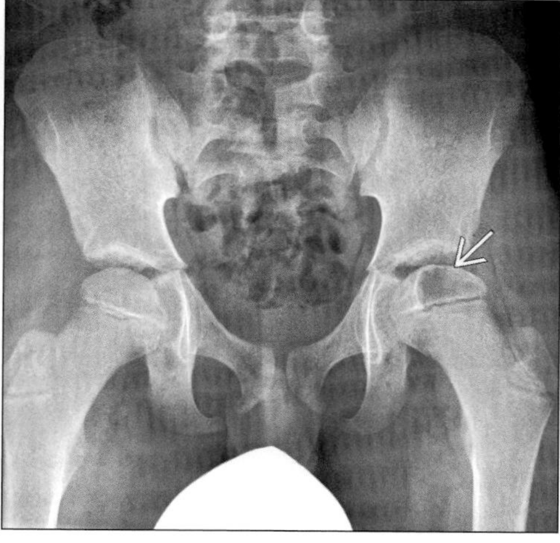

(Left) *Coronal T1WI MR shows an area of osteonecrosis within both femoral heads, in which serpentine hypointense bands ➡ surround hyperintense signal (similar to fat).* ***(Right)*** *Anteroposterior radiograph shows a lucent left epiphyseal lesion ➡ and subtle flattening of the superolateral femoral head. The lesion was biopsied and pathologically proven to be a chondroblastoma.*

ELBOW EFFUSION

DIFFERENTIAL DIAGNOSIS

Common
- Supracondylar Fracture
- Lateral Condylar Fracture
- Medial Epicondyle Avulsion
- Trauma without Fracture
- Radial Neck Fracture
- Other Less Common Fractures

Less Common
- Osteochondritis Dissecans
- Juvenile Idiopathic Arthritis (JIA)
- Septic Arthritis
- Panner Disease

Rare but Important
- Tumor
- Hemophilia

ESSENTIAL INFORMATION

Key Differential Diagnosis Issues
- Anatomy
  - Elbow ossification center appearance (**CRITOE**)
    - **C**apitellum, **r**adial head, medial (**i**nternal) epicondyle, **t**rochlea, **o**lecranon, lateral (**e**xternal) epicondyle
- Trauma
  - Anterior humeral line
    - Lateral view: Line should pass through middle 1/3 of capitellum
    - When anterior humeral line is abnormal, may indicate minimally displaced supracondylar fracture (fx)
  - Coronoid line
    - Line along volar border of coronoid process should barely contact volar portion of lateral condyle on lateral view
  - Radiocapitellar line
    - Line drawn from center of radial shaft that normally extends through capitellar ossification center
    - Not necessarily passing through middle 1/3 of capitellum
    - When abnormal, radial head dislocation is likely
  - Teardrop
    - On lateral view, dense anterior line reflects posterior margin of coronoid fossa
    - Posterior dense line reflects anterior margin of olecranon fossa
  - Fat pad signs
    - Anterior fat pad: Nondisplaced and visualized in normal elbows
    - If elevated ("sail" sign), consider joint effusion; if trauma history, must exclude occult fx
    - Supinator fat pad: Anterior aspect of supinator muscle along proximal radius; if displaced, consider radial neck fx
    - Posterior fat pad sign more sensitive to underlying occult elbow fx
    - Joint capsule must be intact to detect fat pad displacement

Helpful Clues for Common Diagnoses
- **Supracondylar Fracture**
  - ~ 50-70% of elbow fxs in children
  - Most commonly extension type injury
  - Age: 3-10 years old
  - Cubitus varus (calculated by Baumann angle) most common complication
  - Vascular injury: Most serious complication
  - Displaced fx: 10-15% injury rate for anterior interosseous branch of median nerve injury
- **Lateral Condylar Fracture**
  - ~ 20% of elbow fxs in children
  - Age: typically 4-10 years old
  - Fx line parallels metaphyseal margin of lateral physis
  - Oblique views are often helpful in detection and assessing amount of displacement
  - ≥ 2 mm of displacement may require open surgical reduction and pinning
  - Nondisplaced fxs: Posterior splint and lateral gutter
- **Medial Epicondyle Avulsion**
  - Displacement > 5 mm, surgical reduction
  - Valgus stress with avulsion from flexor-pronator muscle group
  - 50% associated with elbow dislocations
  - Should see medial epicondyle on AP radiograph if trochlea is identified
  - May become displaced and trapped into elbow joint; simulates trochlear ossification center
  - Unreliable fat pad sign; tends to be extracapsular in location in children > 2 years old

ELBOW EFFUSION

- **Trauma without Fracture**
  - If elbow effusion initially found without detection of fx, > 80% likelihood of seeing fx on follow-up radiographs
- **Radial Neck Fracture**
  - Most cases are Salter-Harris type 2 fxs (90%); average age of 10 years
- **Other Less Common Fractures**
  - Transphyseal fracture
    - < 2 years old, > 50% result of nonaccidental trauma
    - May be mistaken for elbow dislocation; in true dislocation, radiocapitellar (RC) line is disrupted
    - Capitellum still aligns with radial head
  - Olecranon (normal ossification center can be mistaken for fx), intercondylar, medial condylar, radial head dislocation

Helpful Clues for Less Common Diagnoses

- **Osteochondritis Dissecans**
  - a.k.a. osteochondral lesion
  - Medial femoral condyle is most common site
  - Elbow: Most commonly anterolateral aspect of capitellum
  - Typically adolescent boys (> 13 years old)
  - Related to repetitive valgus stress and impaction with radial head
- **Juvenile Idiopathic Arthritis (JIA)**
  - Begins < 16 years old, symptoms > 6 weeks
  - Systemic, pauciarticular, polyarticular
  - Pannus, synovial proliferation, joint effusion, erosions
- **Septic Arthritis**
  - Infection via bloodstream but may become infected due to injection, surgery, or injury
  - *Staphylococcus aureus* most common pathogen
  - Most common symptoms: Fever, arthralgia, and joint swelling
  - < 1/2 have arthritis and osteomyelitis
- **Panner Disease**
  - Osteochondrosis of capitellum
  - Capitellar ossification center irregular mineralization, similar changes to Legg-Calvé-Perthes disease
  - Most commonly: Boys 5-12 years old, dominant arm
    - Distinguish from osteochondritis dissecans (patients > 13 years old)
  - ± effusion

Helpful Clues for Rare Diagnoses

- **Tumor**
  - Chondroblastoma, giant cell tumor, Langerhans cell histiocytosis, etc.
- **Hemophilia**
  - Bleeding disorder; knee, elbow, ankle, hip, and shoulder most commonly involved joints
  - Diagnosis usually known prior to imaging
  - Joint effusion may appear radiodense on conventional radiographs
  - MR: Subchondral erosion, synovial proliferation, joint effusion, hemosiderin deposition

Supracondylar Fracture

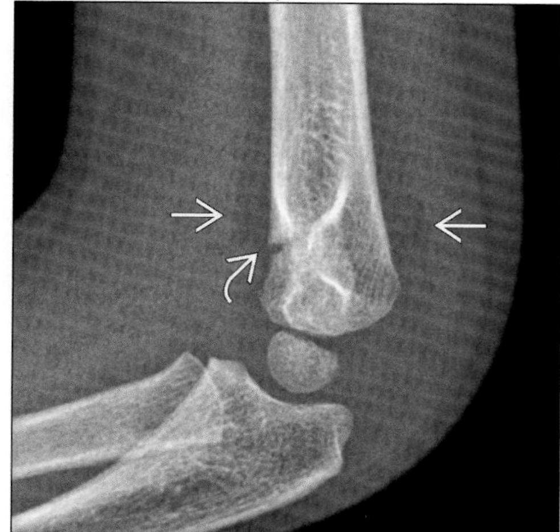

Lateral radiograph shows displacement of the anterior ("sail" sign) and posterior fat pads ➔ due to hemarthrosis. Note the fracture line ➔ through the volar cortex of the distal humerus.

Supracondylar Fracture

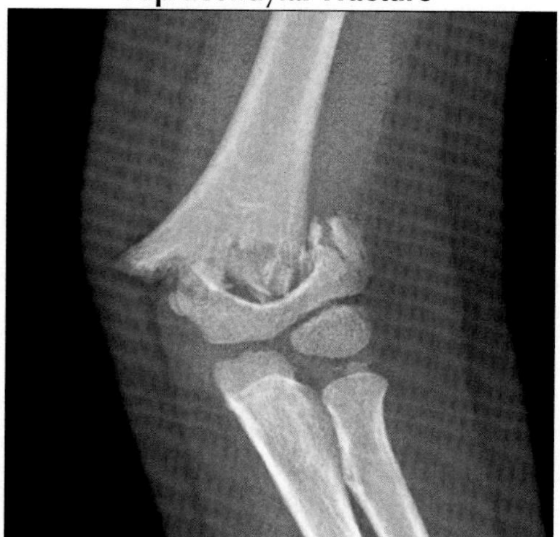

Anteroposterior radiograph shows a comminuted supracondylar fx. The distal humeral fracture fragments are displaced laterally. The peak incidence of supracondylar fxs is seen in children ages 5-8 years.

ELBOW EFFUSION

*(**Left**) Lateral radiograph shows elevation of the anterior ("sail" sign) ➡ and posterior fat pads ⮫, indicating a hemarthrosis. In this case a lateral condylar fx was detected on follow-up imaging. (**Right**) Anteroposterior radiograph shows a lateral condylar fx ➡. Oblique views may be helpful in determining the extent of displacement of the fx fragment. Inadequate reduction may result in significant loss of range of motion.*

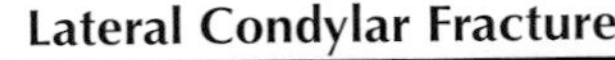

Lateral Condylar Fracture

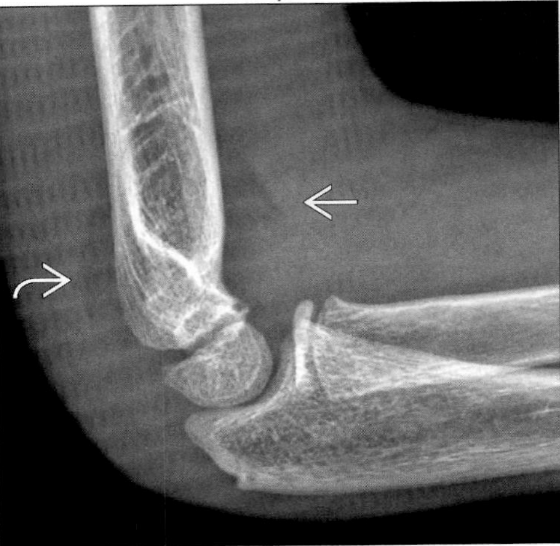

Lateral Condylar Fracture

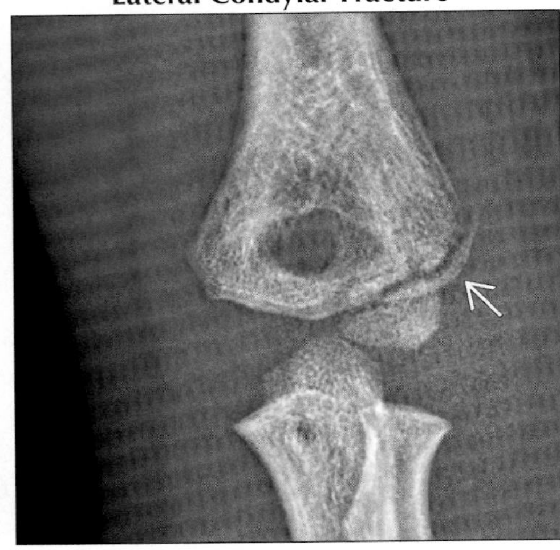

*(**Left**) Anteroposterior radiograph shows a subtle example of a nondisplaced lateral condylar fx ➡. Lateral condylar fxs are most commonly seen in children age 4-10 years. (**Right**) Anteroposterior radiograph shows a displaced medial epicondyle avulsion fx ➡. The ME fx fragment may become incarcerated in the elbow joint. This injury may be the result of acute valgus stress, elbow dislocation, or repetitive traction from throwing ("Little Leaguer's elbow").*

Lateral Condylar Fracture

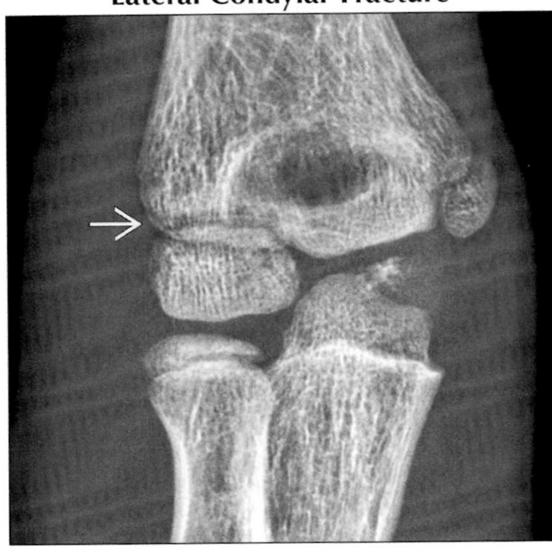

Medial Epicondyle Avulsion

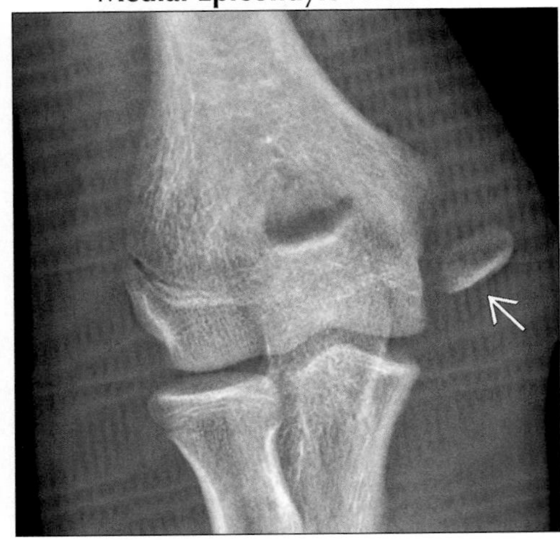

*(**Left**) Lateral radiograph shows elevation of both the anterior ➡ and posterior ⮫ fat pads in this 14 year old with elbow trauma. Follow-up radiographs at 6 days and 3 weeks did not reveal a healing fracture. (**Right**) Anteroposterior radiograph shows a healing radial neck fracture. Notice the cortical step-off ➡ and subtle sclerosis ⮫. Proximal radial fractures in children primarily involve the radial neck; radial head fxs occur primarily in adults.*

Trauma without Fracture

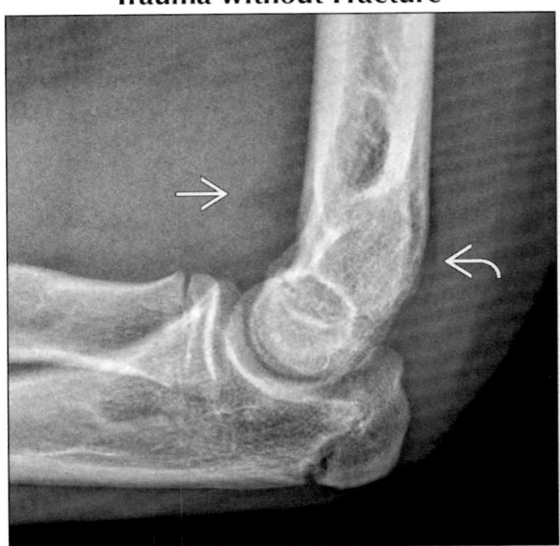

Radial Neck Fracture

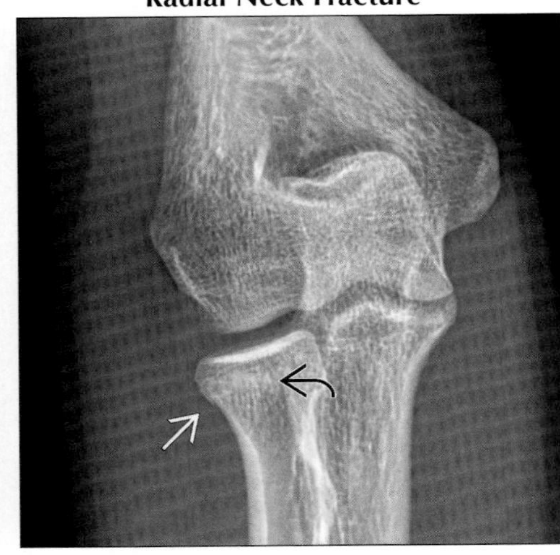

Other Less Common Fractures

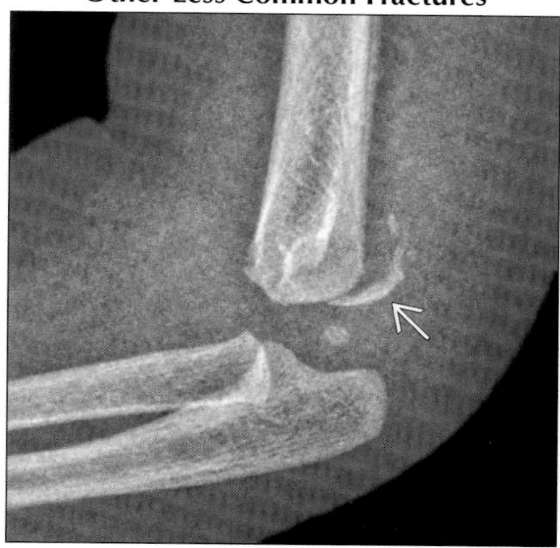

Other Less Common Fractures

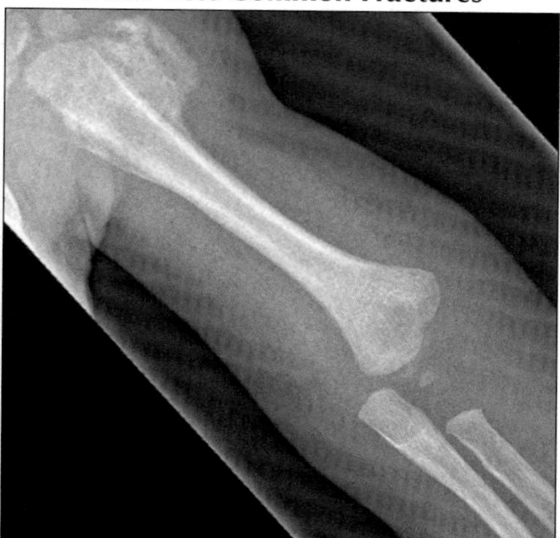

(Left) *Lateral radiograph shows a transphyseal fx ➡.* ***(Right)*** *Anteroposterior radiograph in the same child shows the typical medial displacement of the radius and ulna in relation to the distal humerus. Note a healing proximal humeral fx related to abuse. As the RC alignment is maintained on both views, the elbow is not dislocated. In true elbow dislocations, the radius and ulna are dislocated either laterally and posteriorly or primarily posteriorly.*

Other Less Common Fractures

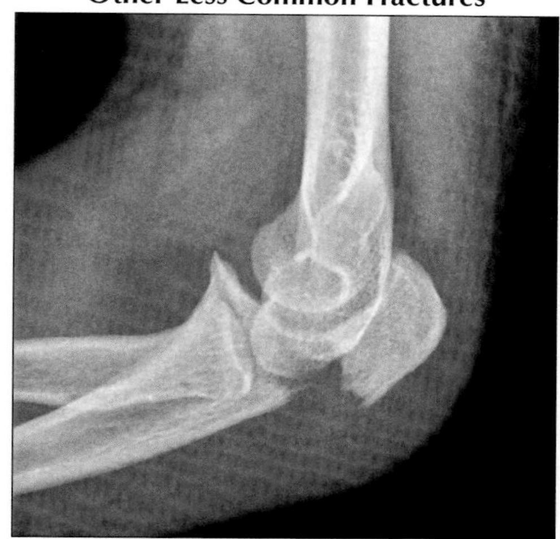

Other Less Common Fractures

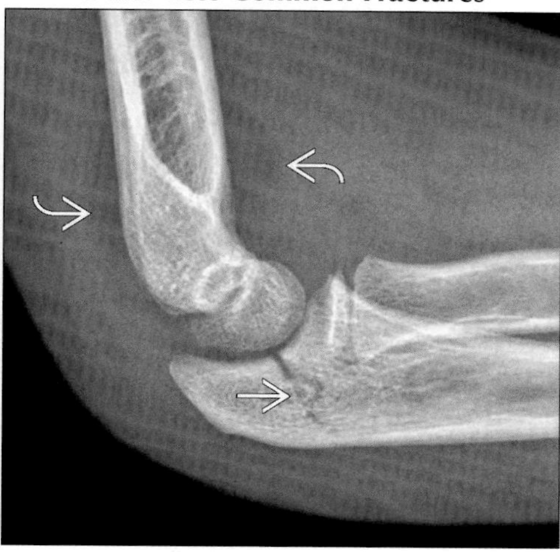

(Left) *Lateral radiograph shows a proximal olecranon process fracture of the ulna with distraction. This fracture in this child required open reduction and screw fixation.* ***(Right)*** *Lateral radiograph shows an intraarticular olecranon fracture ➡ with elevation of both the anterior and posterior fat pads ➡. Olecranon fractures account for 4-7% of all childhood elbow fractures.*

Other Less Common Fractures

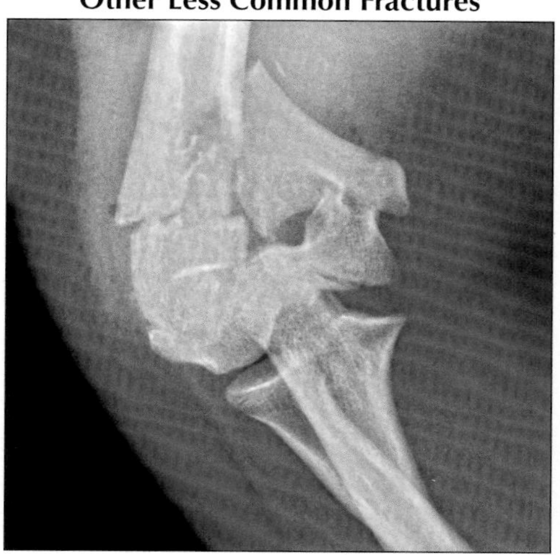

Osteochondritis Dissecans

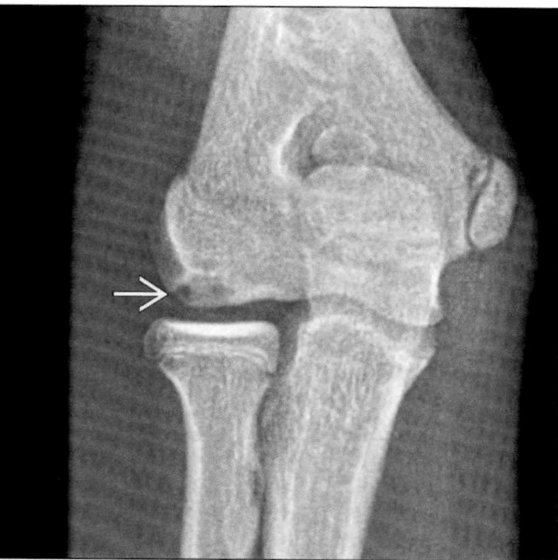

(Left) *Anteroposterior radiograph shows a comminuted displaced intercondylar fracture of the elbow. This 10-year-old girl sustained this open (clinically noted) fracture while playing kickball; she fell directly onto her flexed elbow.* ***(Right)*** *Anteroposterior radiograph shows a well-defined lucent lesion ➡ within the capitellum. The osteochondritis dissecans was found incidentally in this 13-year-old male who presented with acute trauma.*

ELBOW EFFUSION

*(**Left**) Lateral radiograph shows bulging of both the anterior and posterior fat pads →. This indicates either a joint effusion &/or pannus in this child with a history of JIA. (**Right**) Lateral radiograph shows spurring of the radial head → and diffuse joint space narrowing from longstanding JIA. No significant joint effusion was detected on this image.*

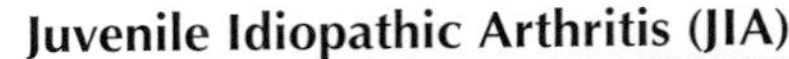

Juvenile Idiopathic Arthritis (JIA)

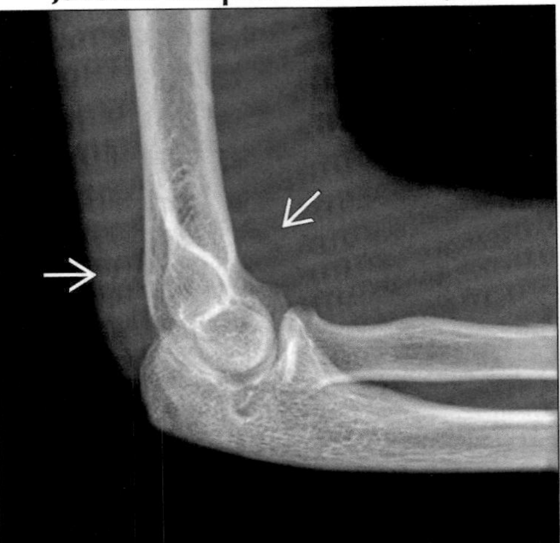

Juvenile Idiopathic Arthritis (JIA)

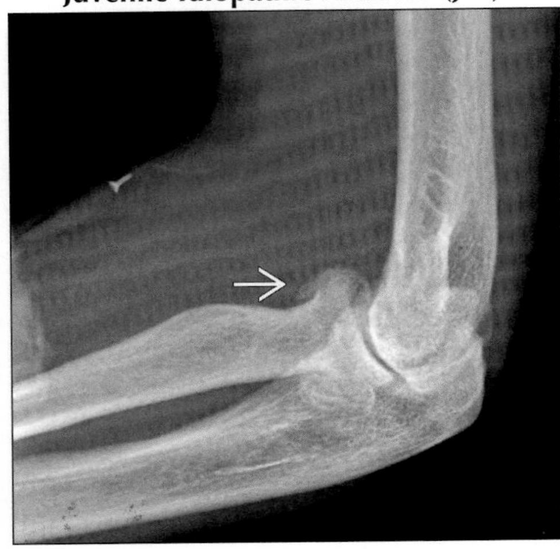

*(**Left**) Lateral radiograph shows elevation of both the anterior and posterior fat pads →, indicating an elbow effusion. This 1-year-old child presented with a history of refusing to use the arm. MR (not shown) revealed osteomyelitis, joint effusion, and synovitis. (**Right**) Anteroposterior radiograph shows a lateral condylar fracture →. Notice the irregular ossification of the capitellum ↪ in this 5-year-old boy. This could reflect Panner disease.*

Septic Arthritis

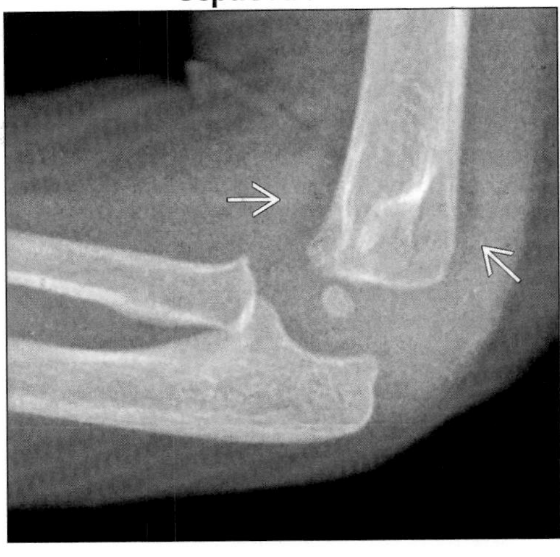

Panner Disease

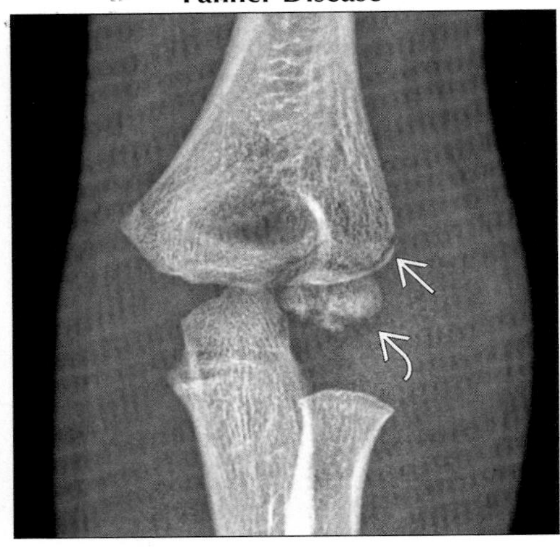

*(**Left**) Lateral radiograph shows elevation of the anterior and posterior fat pads →, indicating an elbow joint effusion. MR demonstrated that the effusion was moderate in size (not shown). (**Right**) Anteroposterior radiograph in the same teenager shows an eccentric lucent expansile lesion →, extending to the subchondral plate in this skeletally mature female. This lesion was pathologically proven to be a giant cell tumor.*

Tumor

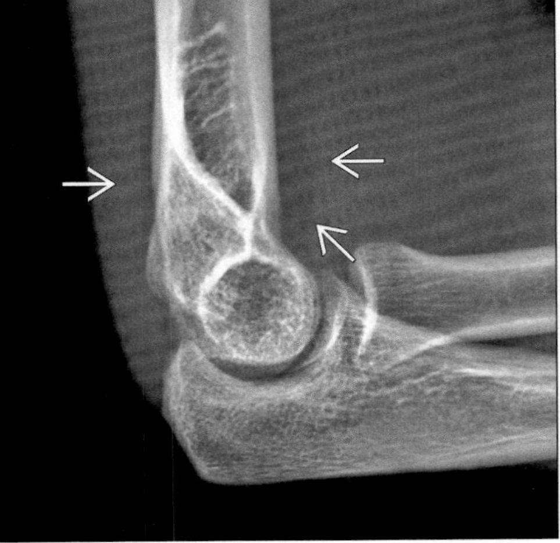

Tumor

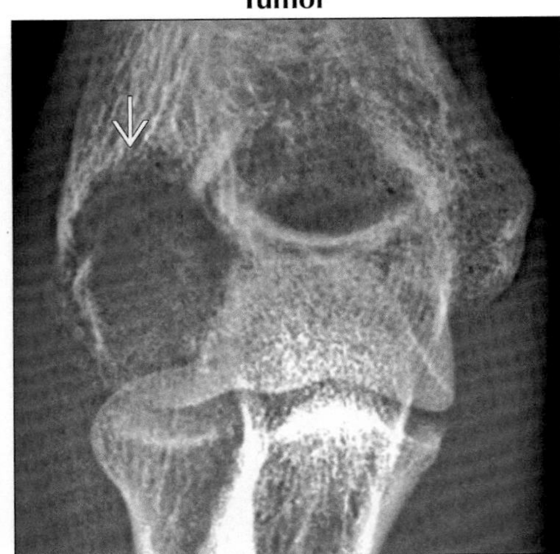

Tumor

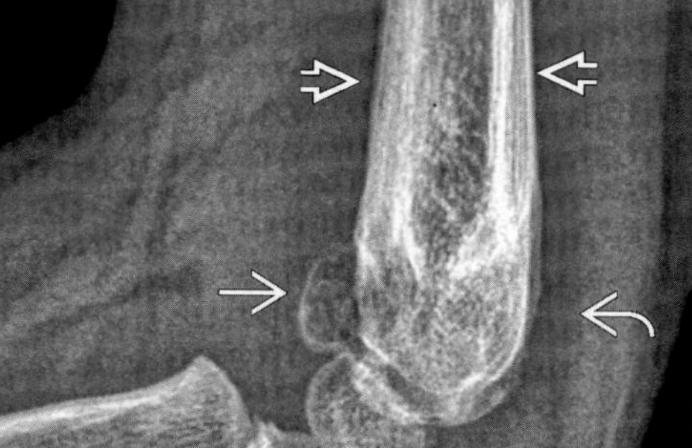

Tumor

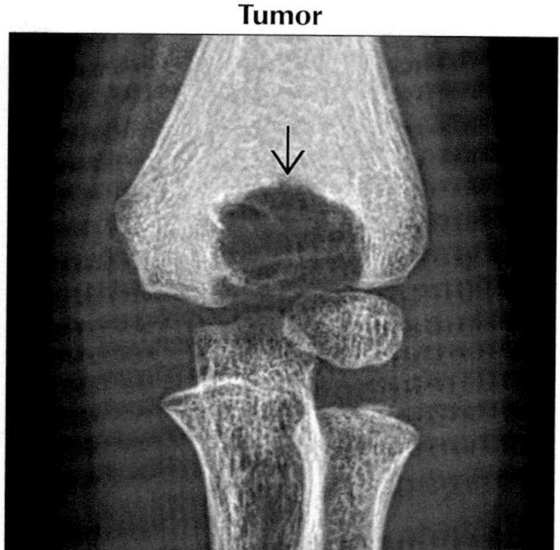

(Left) *Lateral radiograph shows a lucent expansile lesion → within the distal humerus of this 6 year old presenting with elbow pain. Note the elevation of the posterior fat pad → indicating a joint effusion (present on MR, not shown) and diffuse periosteal thickening →.* ***(Right)*** *Anteroposterior radiograph in the same child shows a distal humeral lucent lesion →. The lesion was pathologically proven to be an aneurysmal bone cyst.*

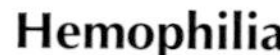

Hemophilia

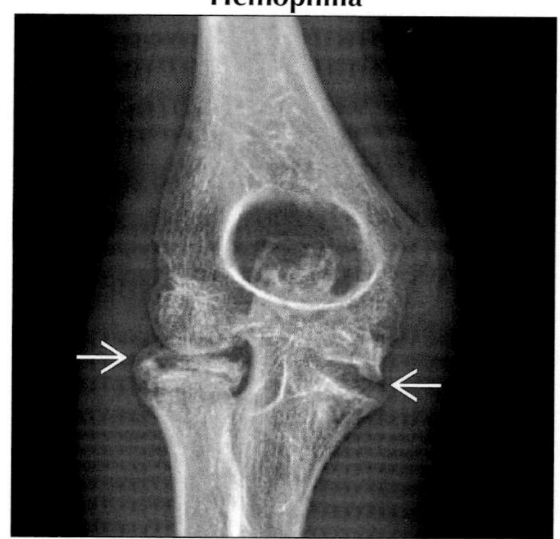

Hemophilia

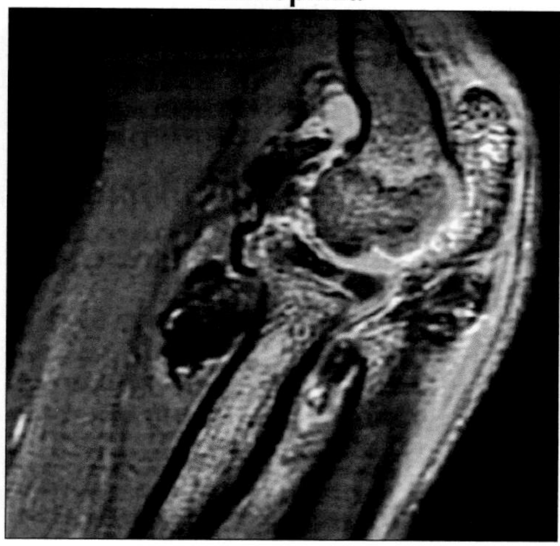

(Left) *Anteroposterior radiograph shows joint space narrowing →, spurring, radial head overgrowth, and subchondral lucencies. This study was obtained in 13-year-old male with a history of hemophilia and progressively worsening elbow pain.* ***(Right)*** *Sagittal PDWI FS MR in the same teenager shows hypointense hemosiderin deposits filling the elbow joint.*

Hemophilia

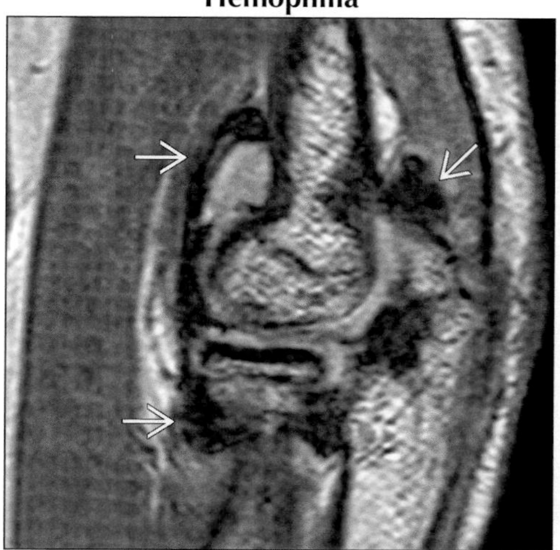

Hemophilia

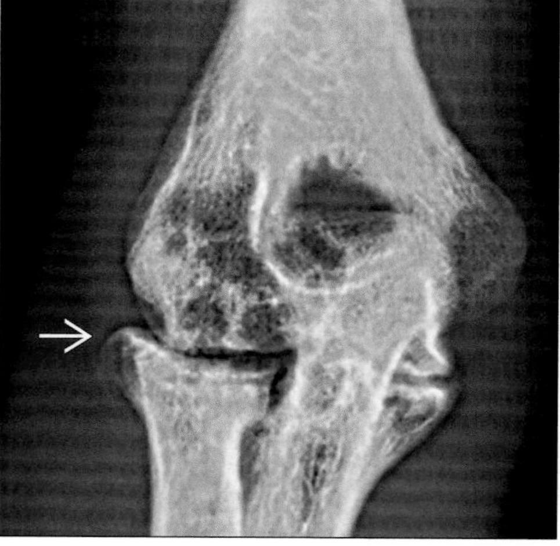

(Left) *Sagittal 3D SPGR shows hypointense, hemosiderin-laden synovium → outlining the capsule of the elbow joint. Hemosiderin deposition is related to prior hemarthrosis. The most common type, hemophilia A (80-85%), is due to factor VIII deficiency. Hemophilia B, a.k.a. Christmas disease, is due to factor IX deficiency.* ***(Right)*** *Anteroposterior radiograph shows degenerative radiocapitellar joint space narrowing and marginal spurring →.*

RADIAL DYSPLASIA/APLASIA

DIFFERENTIAL DIAGNOSIS

Common
- Fanconi Anemia
- Holt-Oram Syndrome
- Thrombocytopenia-Absent Radius (TAR) Syndrome

Less Common
- Klippel Feil
- VATER Association
- Trisomy 18
- Trisomy 13-15
- Radioulnar Synostosis
- Dyschondrosteosis

Rare but Important
- Pseudothalidomide Syndrome
- Thalidomide Embryopathy
- Fetal Varicella Syndrome
- Fetal Valproic Acid Exposure
- Cornelia de Lange Syndrome
- Radial Clubhand
- Ulnar Clubhand
- Mesomelic Dysplasias
- Oculo-Auriculo-Vertebral Spectrum
- Nail Patella Disease (Fong)

ESSENTIAL INFORMATION

Key Differential Diagnosis Issues
- Radial hypoplasia, dysplasia, and aplasia are associated with many congenital syndromes and skeletal dysplasias
  - Forearm radiographs are often nonspecific

Helpful Clues for Diagnoses
- **Fanconi Anemia**
  - Thumb aplasia or short metacarpal
  - Absent or malformed navicular
  - Brachydactyly, clinodactyly
- **Holt-Oram Syndrome**
  - Brachydactyly, camptodactyly, and clinodactyly
  - Thumb aplasia or malformation ± triphalangeal thumb
  - Abnormal navicular ± fusion
  - Os centrale
- **Trisomy 18**
  - Thumb aplasia or short metacarpal
  - Ulnar deviation of MCP joints
  - Clinodactyly, syndactyly
- **Trisomy 13-15**
  - Polydactyly, clinodactyly
  - Triphalangeal thumb
  - Broad thumb distal phalanx
- **Dyschondrosteosis**
  - Decreased carpal angle
  - Carpal fusion
  - Cone-shaped epiphyses
- **Cornelia de Lange Syndrome**
  - Short, wide thumb metacarpal
  - Clinodactyly, brachydactyly
  - Volar-radial curvature of 5th digit distal phalanx (Kirner deformity)
- **Ulnar Clubhand**
  - Aplasia or hypoplasia of ulna with radius deformity
  - Thumb present, absent 4th and 5th digits

Fanconi Anemia

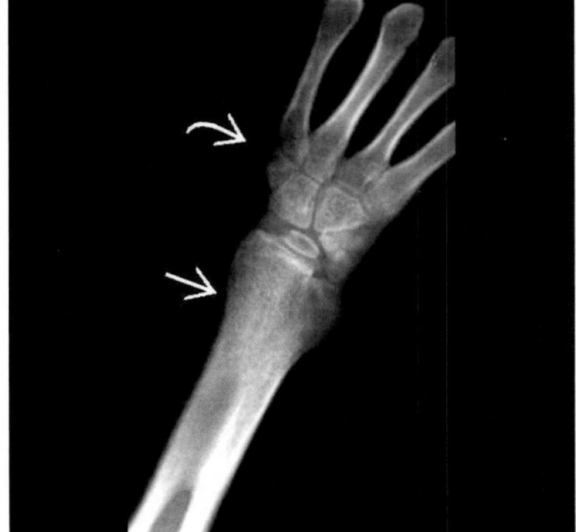

Anteroposterior radiograph shows a dysplastic radius ➔ that is fused to the ulna. The thumb is absent ➔, as are the trapezium and scaphoid bones. The distal carpal row is dysplastic.

Fanconi Anemia

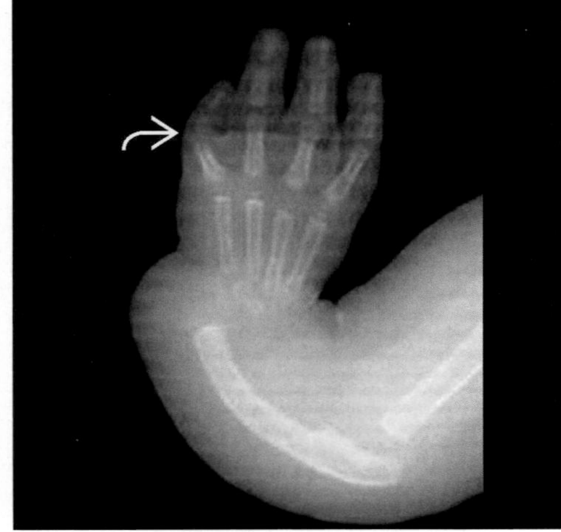

Posteroanterior radiograph shows an absence of the radius and thumb. There is clinodactyly of the fifth digit ➔. Skeletal changes in this entity range from nonexistent to major congenital malformations.

RADIAL DYSPLASIA/APLASIA

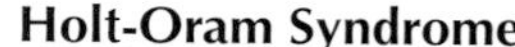

Holt-Oram Syndrome

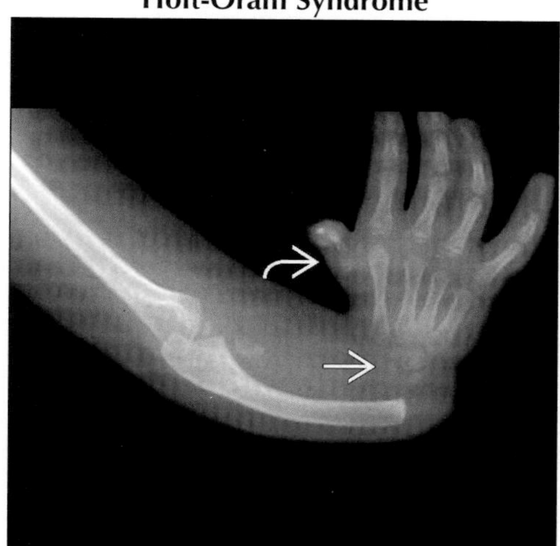

VATER Association

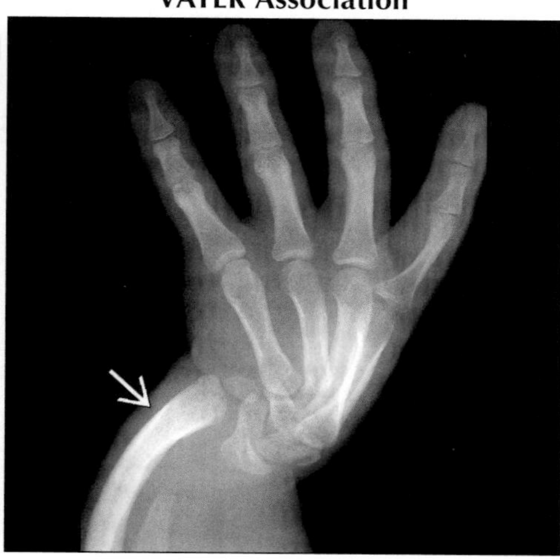

*(**Left**) AP radiograph shows an absence of the radius, trapezium, and scaphoid. The thumb is severely dysplastic →. A small triangular bone proximal and radial to the capitate likely represents an os centrale → anatomic variant. (**Right**) PA radiograph shows phocomelia with near complete aplasia of the radius, a short curved ulna →, and absent scaphoid and thumb. The findings were bilateral, and the patient also had renal abnormalities.*

Trisomy 18

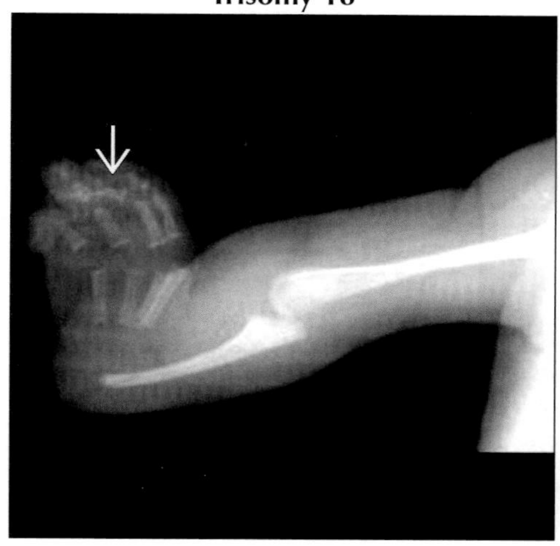

Radioulnar Synostosis

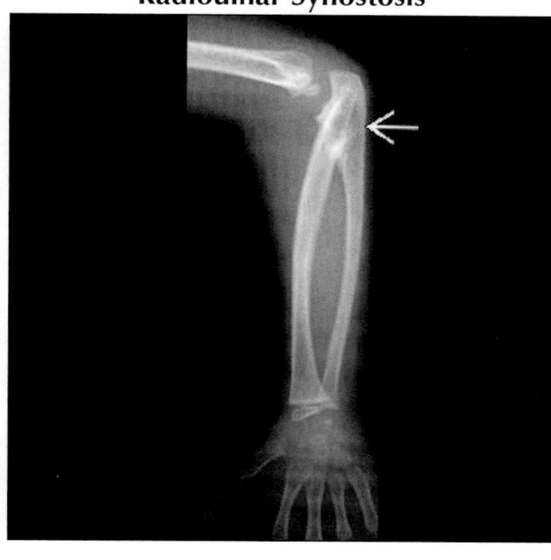

*(**Left**) AP radiograph shows aplasia of the radius and hypoplastic thumb. Overlapping fingers → and ulnar deviation of the metacarpophalangeal joints are common findings. (**Right**) Lateral radiograph shows fusion of the proximal radius to the ulna →. The degree of fusion and location in the forearm is variable. This bony fusion can be congenital, due to lack of segmentation, or post-traumatic, due to fracture or heterotopic ossification most commonly.*

Ulnar Clubhand

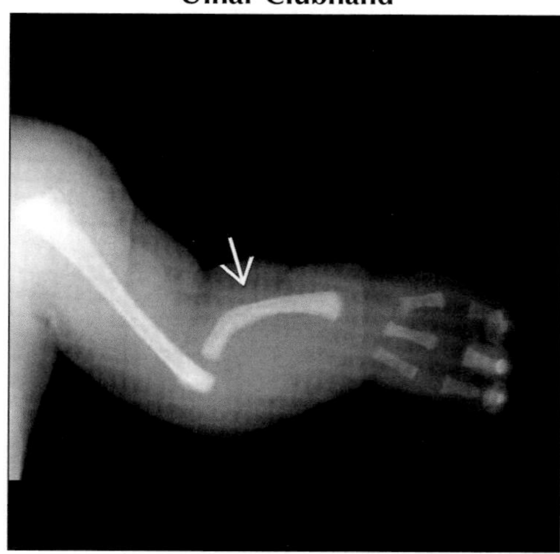

Nail Patella Disease (Fong)

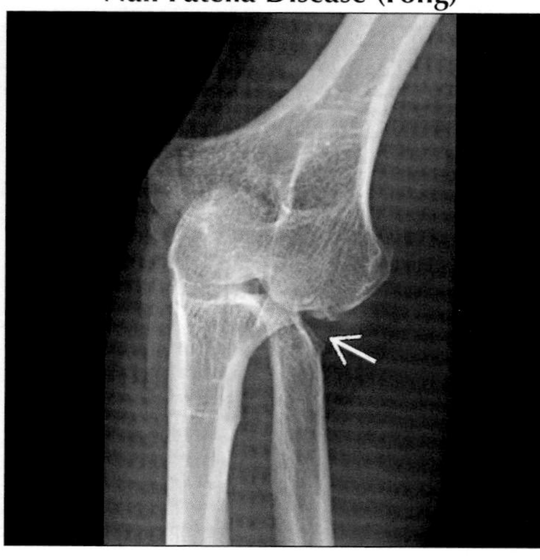

*(**Left**) Anteroposterior radiograph shows absence of the ulna. The radius → is dysplastic and bowed. The thumb and index finger are absent, which is unusual. This infant is too young to definitively assess for carpal abnormalities. (**Right**) Oblique radiograph shows a hypoplastic radial head →, which results in osteoarthritis of the elbow and an increased carrying angle. This also causes relative elongation of the ulna, with subluxation of the distal radioulnar joint.*

FOCAL GIGANTISM/MACRODACTYLY

DIFFERENTIAL DIAGNOSIS

Common
- Juvenile Idiopathic Arthritis (Epiphyses)
- Venous Malformation
- Arteriovenous Malformation
- Lymphatic Malformation
- Neurofibromatosis

Less Common
- Macrodystrophia Lipomatosa
- Klippel-Trenaunay-Weber Syndrome (KTW)
- Ollier Disease (Phalanges)
- Maffucci Syndrome (Phalanges)
- Hemophilia (Epiphyses)
- Hyperemia, Any Cause
  - Chronic Osteomyelitis
  - Fracture During Childhood
  - Tuberculosis

Rare but Important
- Epidermal Nevus Syndrome
- Proteus Syndrome

ESSENTIAL INFORMATION

Key Differential Diagnosis Issues
- Key features to aid in differentiation
  - Overgrowth: Osseous, soft tissue, or both
  - Cutaneous manifestations
- **Hint**: Macrodystrophia lipomatosa, neurofibromatosis, KTW, and Maffucci have similar appearance
  - Soft tissue and osseous involvement
- **Hint**: Hyperemia underlying cause with osseous overgrowth only
  - Juvenile idiopathic arthritis
  - Hemophilia
  - Chronic osteomyelitis
  - Tuberculosis
  - See hyperemia, any cause below
- **Hint**: Juvenile idiopathic arthritis and hemophilia have similar appearance
  - Osseous overgrowth only
    - Ballooned epiphyses
    - Widened intercondylar notch
    - Knee (femoral condyles), elbow (capitellum) overgrowth common

Helpful Clues for Common Diagnoses
- **Juvenile Idiopathic Arthritis (Epiphyses)**
  - Overgrowth mainly knee, elbow
  - No cutaneous changes
  - Other disease manifestations
    - Monoarticular to polyarticular disease
    - Small joints, hands, feet; also wrist, elbow, knee, shoulder, ankle
    - Periarticular osteoporosis
    - Marginal erosions
    - Periosteal new bone formation
    - Uniform joint space narrowing
- **Venous Malformation**
  - Soft tissue mass
    - Phleboliths
    - Variable amount of fatty stroma
  - Osseous changes variable
    - Overgrowth secondary to hyperemia
    - Periosteal new bone
    - Cortical thickening
    - Pressure erosions
  - Cutaneous changes
    - Skin discoloration
    - Prominent veins
- **Arteriovenous Malformation**
  - Soft tissue lesion
    - No phleboliths
    - Tangled dilated vessels, no discrete mass
  - Intra-osseous extension may be seen
  - Cutaneous changes absent
    - Dilated vessels may be visible beneath skin
- **Lymphatic Malformation**
  - Soft tissue mass with multiple cystic spaces
  - No osseous overgrowth
  - No cutaneous changes
- **Neurofibromatosis**
  - Gigantism may be bilateral
  - Involved digits may not be contiguous
  - Most severe involvement at any site along digit
  - Secondary plexiform neurofibroma (soft tissue) and mesodermal dysplasia (osseous)
  - Cutaneous changes: Café-au-lait spots
  - Other disease manifestations
    - Neurofibromas
    - Mesodermal dysplasia: Bowing, pseudoarthrosis, abnormal healing, periosteal abnormalities
    - Optic glioma, Lisch nodule (iris nevi)

Helpful Clues for Less Common Diagnoses
- **Macrodystrophia Lipomatosa**
  - Unilateral; 1 or more contiguous digits
  - Most severe involvement along distal digit

- Volar surface more affected than dorsal surface creating dorsal bowing deformity
- 2nd and 3rd digits most common
- Overgrowth soft tissue and bone
  - Prominent adipose overgrowth
- Neural enlargement
  - Median nerve > plantar nerve
- No cutaneous changes

- **Klippel-Trenaunay-Weber Syndrome (KTW)**
  - Unilateral soft tissue and osseous overgrowth
    - Gigantism ranges from macrodactyly to hemihypertrophy
  - Lower extremity more common than upper extremity
  - Syndrome: Capillary hemangiomas (port wine), varicose veins, local gigantism
    - ± Arteriovenous malformations
- **Ollier Disease (Phalanges)**
  - a.k.a. enchondromatosis
  - Gigantism of hands/feet only
  - Osseous involvement only: Multiple enchondromas of phalanges
    - Expansile lytic ± ground-glass matrix
    - Bilateral asymmetric distribution
- **Maffucci Syndrome (Phalanges)**
  - Ollier disease plus soft tissue venous malformations
  - Venous malformations
    - Phleboliths
    - Any site throughout body
    - Hands, feet especially involved
- **Hemophilia (Epiphyses)**
  - Typically 1 joint suffers repeated hemorrhage, which leads to hyperemia then osseous overgrowth
    - Commonly affects knee (femoral condyles), elbow (radial head)
  - Associated arthritic changes
    - Periarticular osteoporosis
    - Uniform joint space narrowing
    - Dense effusion
    - Subchondral cysts
    - Secondary osteoarthritis
- **Hyperemia, Any Cause**
  - Osseous overgrowth
  - Random sites of involvement
    - Typically 1 site or multiple sites in 1 extremity
  - Hyperemia prior to skeletal maturation, often from fracture healing

Helpful Clues for Rare Diagnoses

- **Epidermal Nevus Syndrome**
  - Soft tissue and osseous overgrowth
  - No typical site of involvement
  - Cutaneous changes: Multiple nevi
  - Variable other manifestations, including cerebral atrophy
- **Proteus Syndrome**
  - Syndrome has protean manifestations
    - Focal gigantism and lymphangiomatous hamartomas are consistent features
  - Soft tissue and osseous overgrowth
  - No cutaneous changes
  - Osteochondroma-like osseous lesions
  - Skull, face, spine abnormalities common

Juvenile Idiopathic Arthritis (Epiphyses)

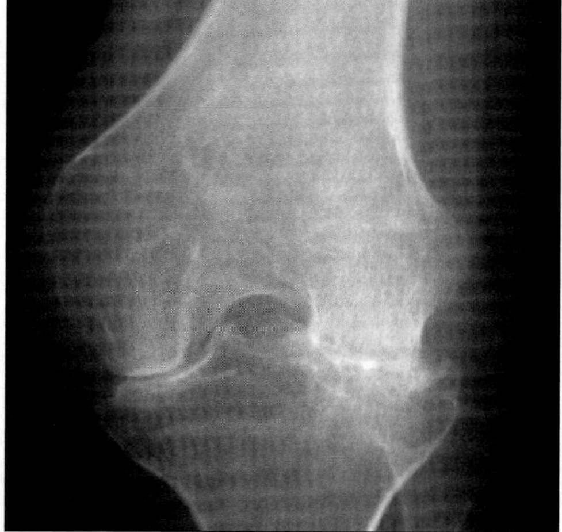

Anteroposterior radiograph shows a classic example of severe juvenile idiopathic arthritis with overgrowth of the femoral condyles especially medially and widening of the intercondylar notch.

Juvenile Idiopathic Arthritis (Epiphyses)

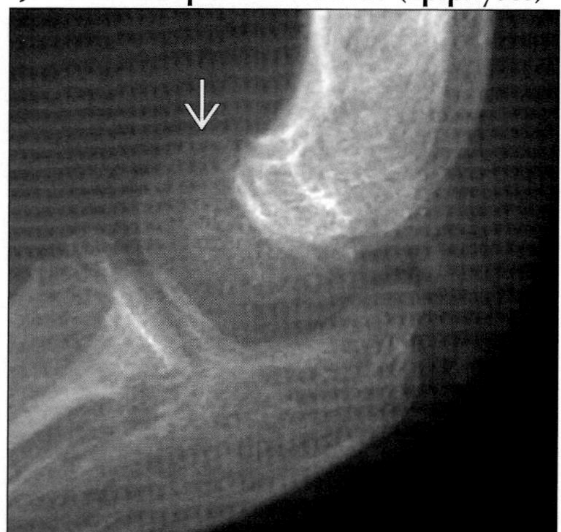

Lateral radiograph of this patient with juvenile idiopathic arthritis reveals overgrowth of the capitellum ➔ secondary to hyperemia. (†MSK Req).

FOCAL GIGANTISM/MACRODACTYLY

(Left) Lateral radiograph shows bulky soft tissues of the forearm and hand ➡ secondary to soft tissue vascular malformation. Associated overgrowth of the 1st and 2nd digits was present but is not seen on this image. *(Right)* Anteroposterior radiograph shows focal overgrowth of the 2nd digit of the left foot ➡. The overgrowth was due to hyperemia from a vascular malformation.

Venous Malformation

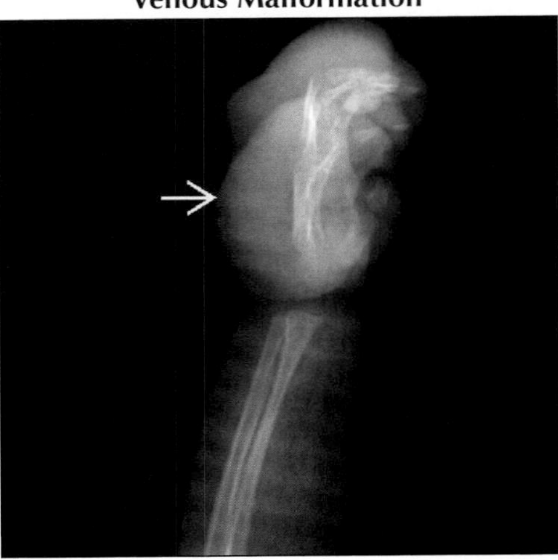

Arteriovenous Malformation

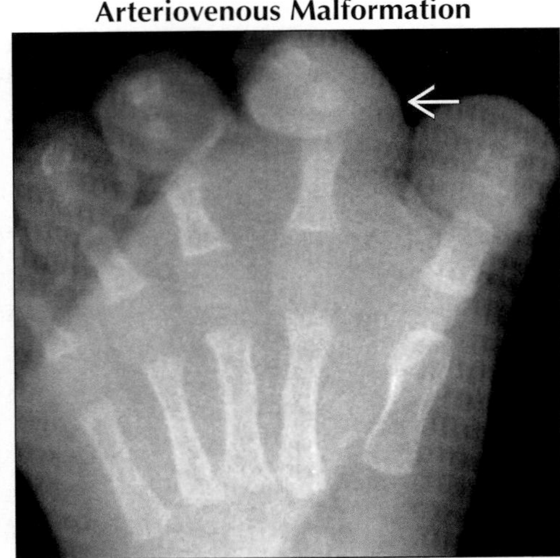

(Left) Axial T2* GRE MR shows multiple flow void from the enlarged vessels in this arteriovenous malformation ➡; the adjacent osseous structures showed overgrowth. *(Right)* Posteroanterior radiograph shows focal giantism secondary to macrodystrophia lipomatosa, involving a single ray of the hand ➡. The osseous and soft tissues are both involved.

Arteriovenous Malformation

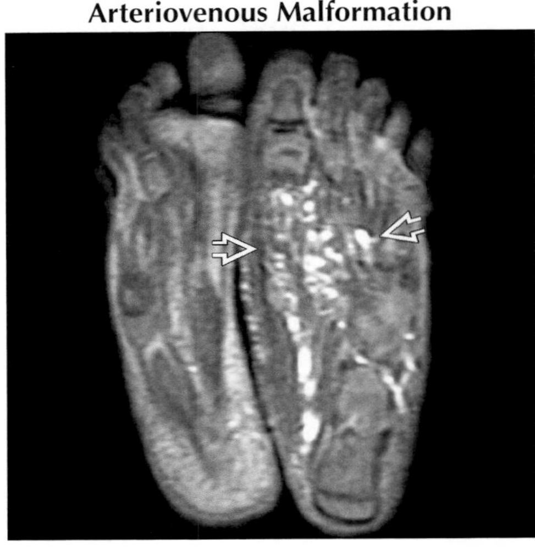

Macrodystrophia Lipomatosa

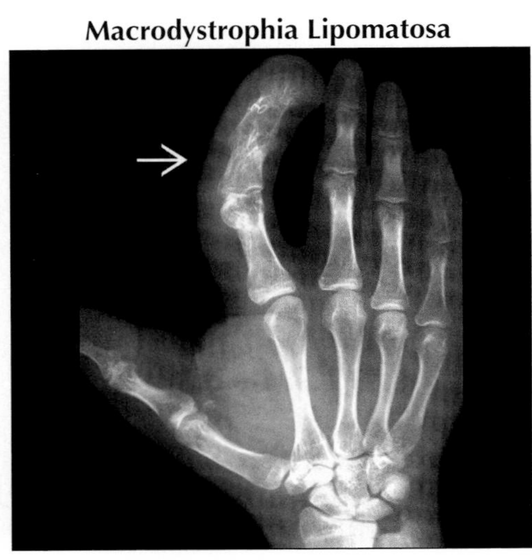

(Left) Lateral radiograph shows a normal hindfoot and midfoot with giantism of both the soft tissues and osseous structures of the forefoot in this patient with macrodystrophia lipomatosa. *(Right)* Posteroanterior radiograph of the hand of a patient with Ollier disease demonstrates multiple enchondromas ➡.

Macrodystrophia Lipomatosa

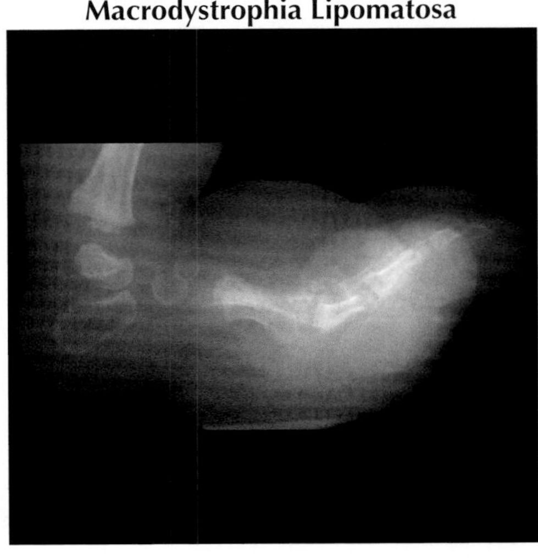

Ollier Disease (Phalanges)

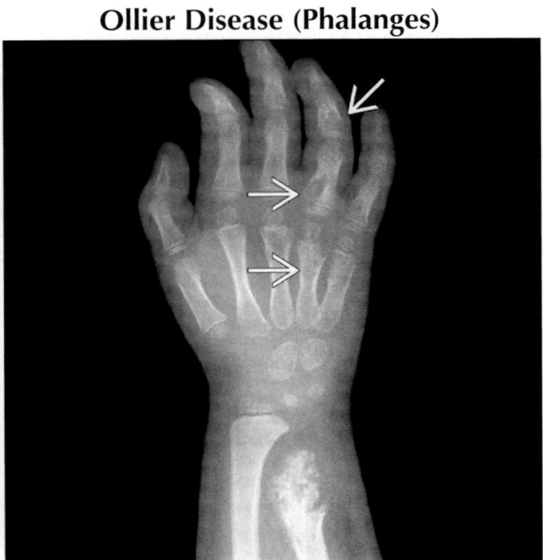

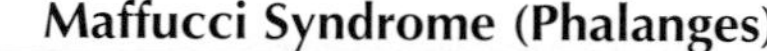

Ollier Disease (Phalanges)

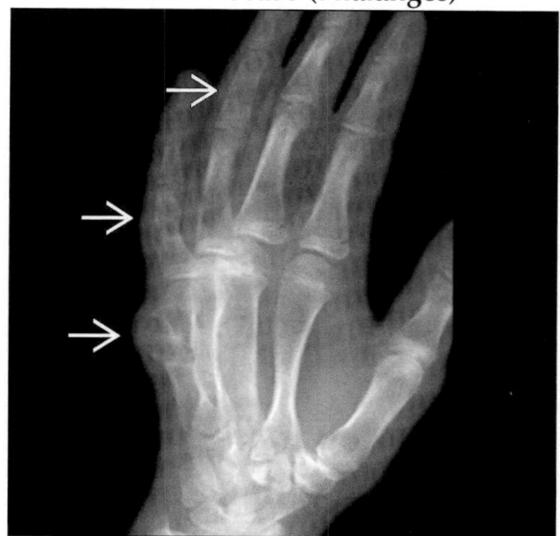

Maffucci Syndrome (Phalanges)

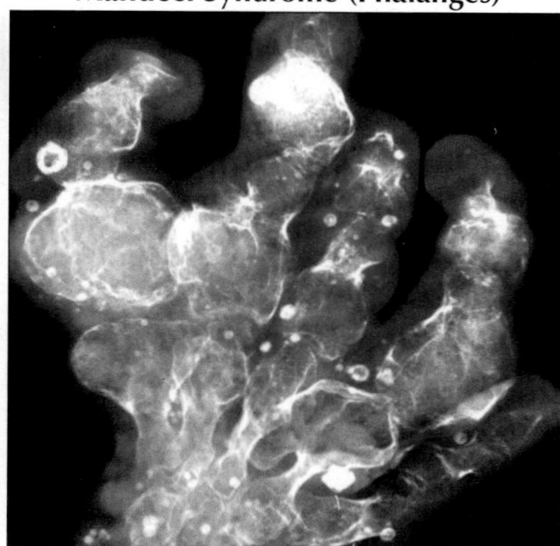

*(**Left**) Oblique radiograph shows a skeletally immature child with multiple enchondromas ➡ consistent with Ollier disease. The lesions are expansile especially in the 5th metacarpal. (**Right**) PA radiograph shows bizarre expansion of all the bones of the hand, associated with multiple phleboliths. The diagnosis is Mafucci syndrome, but clinically it manifests as focal gigantism of the hand.*

Maffucci Syndrome (Phalanges)

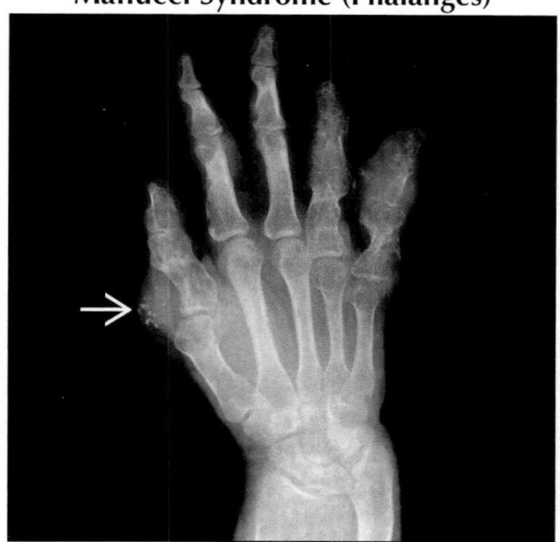

Hemophilia (Epiphyses)

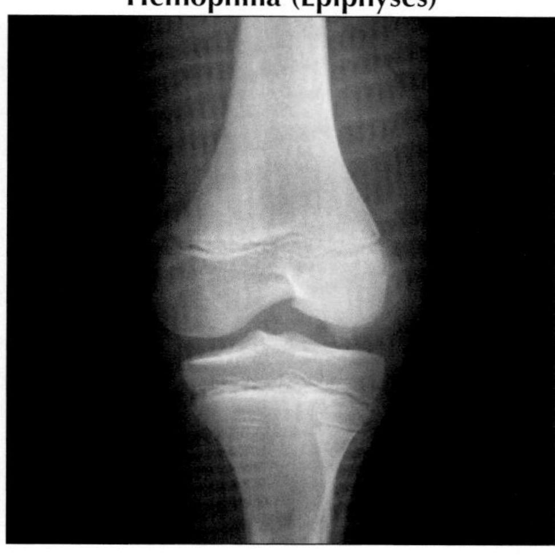

*(**Left**) Posteroanterior radiograph shows a classic case of Maffucci syndrome with multiple enchondromas in the phalanges and multiple soft tissue venous malformations with phleboliths ➡. (†MSK Req). (**Right**) Anteroposterior radiograph shows enlargement of the femoral condyles and widening of the intercondylar notch in this patient with hemophilia.*

Hemophilia (Epiphyses)

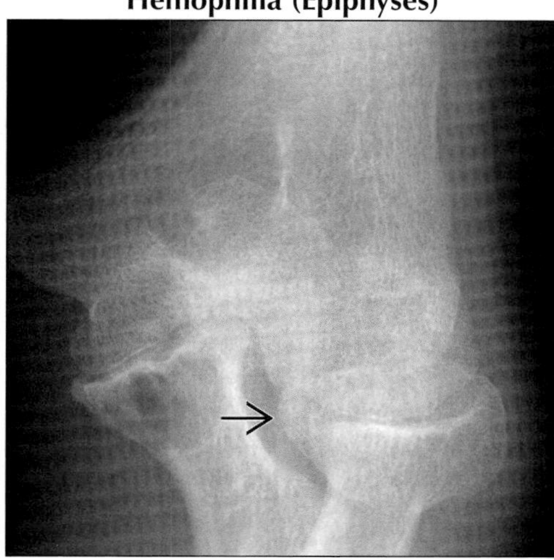

Hyperemia, Any Cause

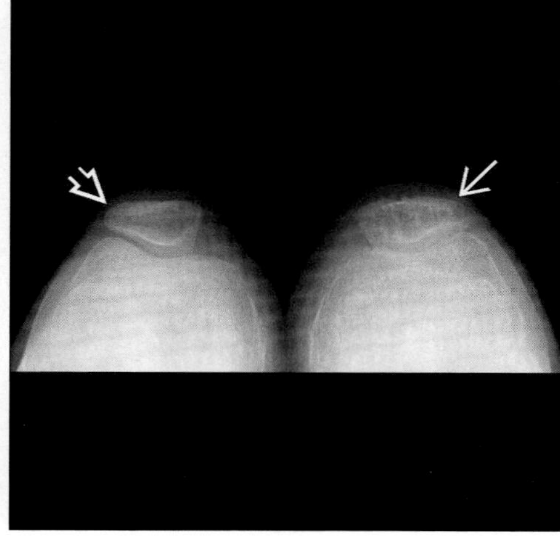

*(**Left**) Anteroposterior radiograph shows capitellar overgrowth ➡ in this patient with hemophilia. Associated changes include subchondral cyst formation and joint space narrowing. (**Right**) Axial radiograph shows relative overgrowth of the left patella ➡ compared to the right ➡, resulting from a patellar fracture that occurred prior to skeletal maturation.*

DWARFISM WITH SHORT EXTREMITIES

DIFFERENTIAL DIAGNOSIS

Common
- Achondroplasia
- Pseudoachondroplasia
- Achondrogenesis
- Chondrodysplasia Punctata
- Dyschondrosteosis
- Mesomelic Dysplasia
- Multiple Epiphyseal Dysplasia

Less Common
- Hypochondroplasia
- Chondroectodermal Dysplasia (Ellis-van Creveld)
- Camptomelic Dysplasia

Rare but Important
- Thanatophoric Dwarf
- Asphyxiating Thoracic Dystrophy of Jeune
- Kniest Dysplasia

ESSENTIAL INFORMATION

Helpful Clues for Diagnoses
- **Achondroplasia**
  - Short, thick tubular bones with flared metaphyses
  - Hemispheric femoral head
  - Overgrown fibulae
- **Pseudoachondroplasia**
  - Splayed, fragmented, irregular metaphyses
- **Achondrogenesis**
  - Short tubular bones and long bones
  - Nonossified sacrum and pubis
- **Chondrodysplasia Punctata**
  - Punctate calcifications in cartilage and periarticular regions
- **Dyschondrosteosis**
  - Madelung deformity of forearms
  - Beaking of medial tibial metaphysis
- **Mesomelic Dysplasia**
  - Hypoplastic fibula
- **Multiple Epiphyseal Dysplasia**
  - Marked epiphyseal ossification delay
  - Small, fragmented epiphyses
  - Femoral head avascular necrosis
- **Hypochondroplasia**
  - Shortened long bones with wide diaphyses
  - Brachydactyly
- **Chondroectodermal Dysplasia (Ellis-van Creveld)**
  - Short, heavy tubular bones
  - Spur at medial distal humeral metaphysis
  - Cone-shaped epiphyses of middle phalanges and polydactyly
- **Camptomelic Dysplasia**
  - 5th digit clinodactyly
- **Thanatophoric Dwarf**
  - Short, bowed limbs, "French telephone receiver femurs"
  - Flared metaphyses
- **Asphyxiating Thoracic Dystrophy of Jeune**
  - Hands with cone-shaped epiphyses
  - Handlebar clavicles
- **Kniest Dysplasia**
  - "Swiss cheese" cartilage dysplasia
  - Short, dumbbell-shaped long bones

Achondroplasia

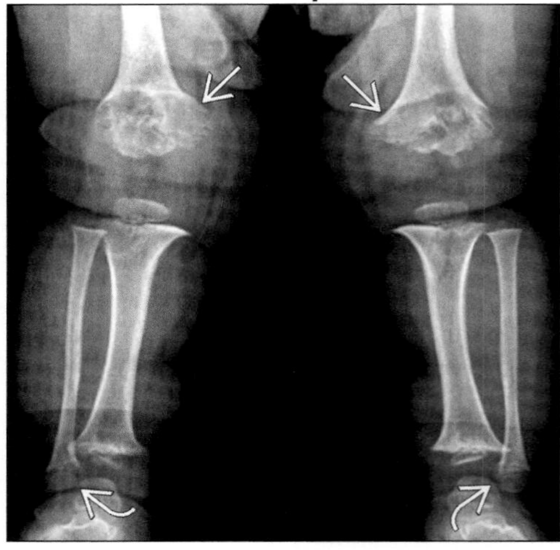

Anteroposterior radiograph of the lower legs shows flaring of the lower femoral metaphyses ➔. The fibulae ➔ are longer than the tibiae, a reversal of the normal relationship.

Pseudoachondroplasia

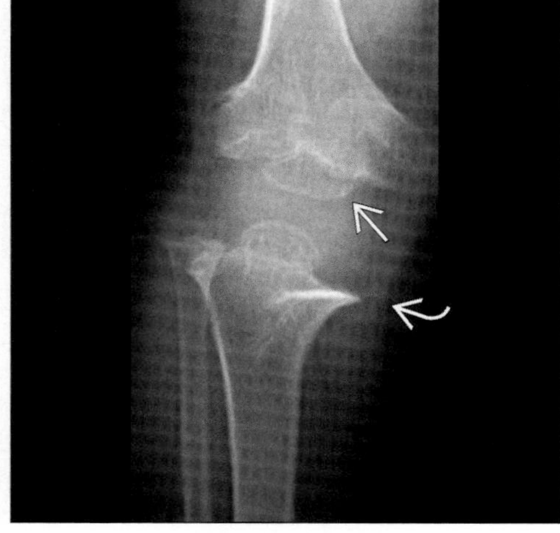

Anteroposterior radiograph shows delayed skeletal maturation, with abnormal epiphyses ➔, resulting in short, stubby long bones. Note the excrescences arising from the metaphyses ➔.

DWARFISM WITH SHORT EXTREMITIES

Chondrodysplasia Punctata

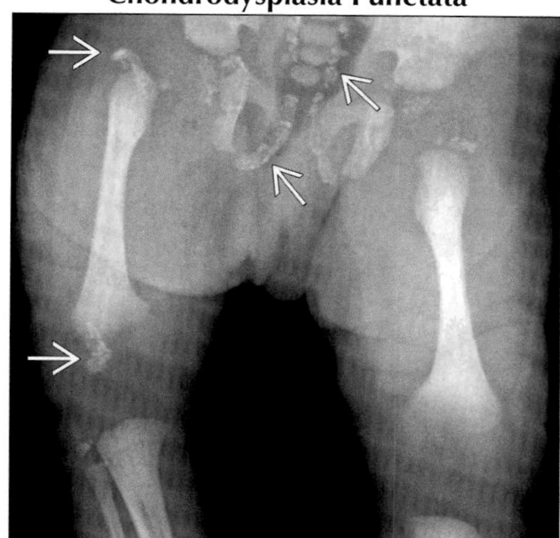

Chondroectodermal Dysplasia (Ellis-van Creveld)

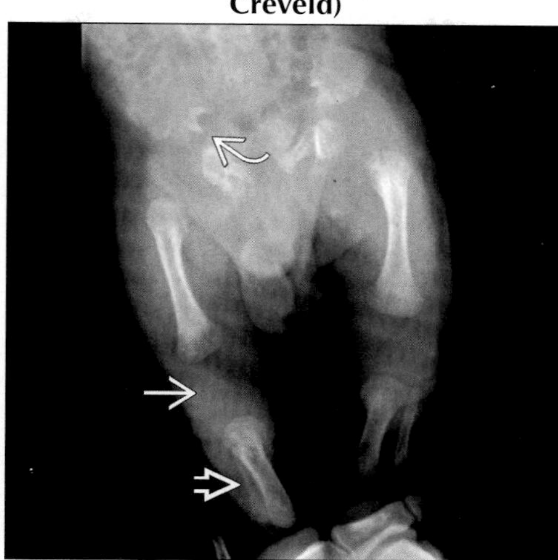

(Left) *Anteroposterior radiograph shows diffuse stippling ➔ in the pelvis and epiphyses of the lower extremities. These patients also have long fibulae with respect to the shortened tibiae.* ***(Right)*** *Anteroposterior radiograph shows flared iliac wings with a trident deformity of the acetabulum ➔. The knees lack epiphyseal ossification centers ➔. Each fibula is very short relative to the tibia ➔.*

Thanatophoric Dwarf

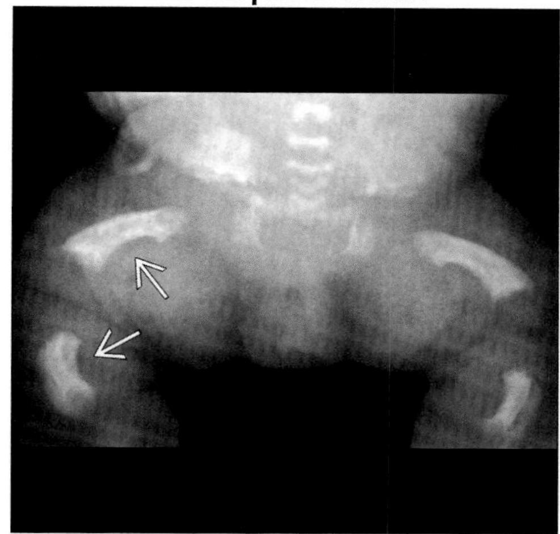

Thanatophoric Dwarf

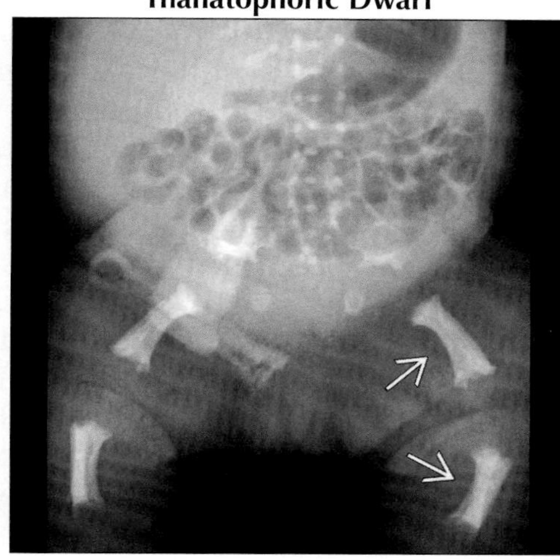

(Left) *Anteroposterior radiograph of the pelvis and legs shows the short, bowed tubular bones ➔. These have been likened to "telephone receivers" (the old fashioned, pre-cell phone types).* ***(Right)*** *Anteroposterior radiograph shows short, bowed tubular bones ➔. Flaring of the metaphyseal regions is a typical finding. This infant died shortly after birth. On prenatal ultrasound, the femurs may appear short or curved.*

Asphyxiating Thoracic Dystrophy of Jeune

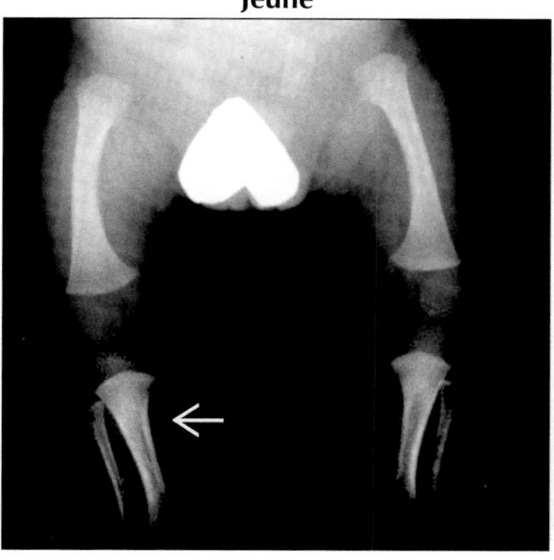

Kniest Dysplasia

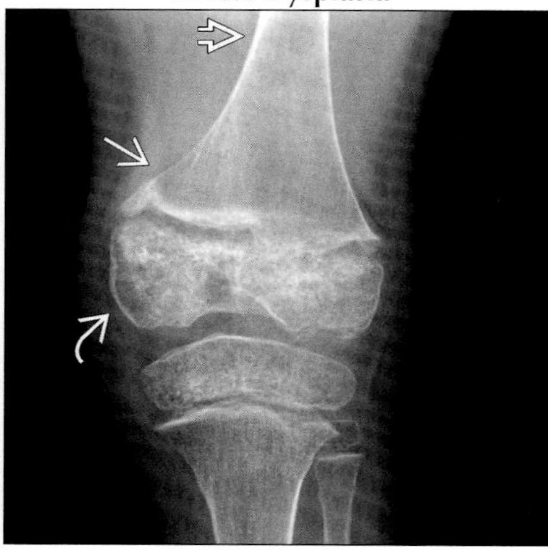

(Left) *Anteroposterior radiograph of the lower extremities shows shortened long bones that have normal tubulation. The lower legs ➔ are shorter than the upper legs (mesomelic shortening). Premature femoral head ossification is commonly present.* ***(Right)*** *Anteroposterior radiograph shows markedly splayed metaphyses ➔ and epiphyses compared with the diaphyseal diameter ➔. The epiphyseal regions ➔ are squared and have irregular ossification.*

DWARFISM WITH SHORT RIBS

DIFFERENTIAL DIAGNOSIS

Common
- Achondroplasia

Less Common
- Cleidocranial Dysplasia
- Chondroectodermal Dysplasia (Ellis-van Creveld)

Rare but Important
- Mucopolysaccharidoses
- Thanatophoric Dwarf
- Asphyxiating Thoracic Dystrophy of Jeune
- Camptomelic Dysplasia
- Achondrogenesis
- Mucolipidosis 2 and 3
- Otopalatodigital Syndrome
- Short-Rib Polydactyly Syndrome

ESSENTIAL INFORMATION

Helpful Clues for Diagnoses
- **Achondroplasia**
  - Short trunk with short, wide ribs that do not extend around chest
- **Cleidocranial Dysplasia**
  - Cone-shaped chest with short ribs due to long cartilaginous segments
  - Hypoplastic clavicles
  - Small scapulae
- **Chondroectodermal Dysplasia (Ellis-van Creveld)**
  - Short, heavy tubular bones (including ribs)
  - Handlebar clavicles
- **Mucopolysaccharidoses**
  - Oar-shaped, short ribs
  - Short clavicles
  - Morquio syndrome = thin posterior portion of rib
- **Thanatophoric Dwarf**
  - Short ribs with cupped costochondral junctions
  - Long trunk with small chest
- **Asphyxiating Thoracic Dystrophy of Jeune**
  - Horizontal, short ribs with bulbous ends
  - Bell-shaped thoracic cage
  - Handlebar clavicles
- **Camptomelic Dysplasia**
  - Bell-shaped thorax
  - 11 pairs of shortened ribs
  - Hypoplastic cervical vertebrae
- **Achondrogenesis**
  - Short tubular bones & long bones
  - Minimal mineralization of vertebral bodies
- **Mucolipidosis 2 and 3**
  - Short, wide ribs similar to mucopolysaccharidoses
- **Otopalatodigital Syndrome**
  - Ribs are short, wavy and angled
  - Long scapular bodies
  - Precocious fusion of sternum
  - Sloped clavicles
- **Short-Rib Polydactyly Syndrome**
  - Very short, horizontal ribs
  - Deformed, elevated clavicles
  - Small scapulae
  - Polydactyly

Achondroplasia

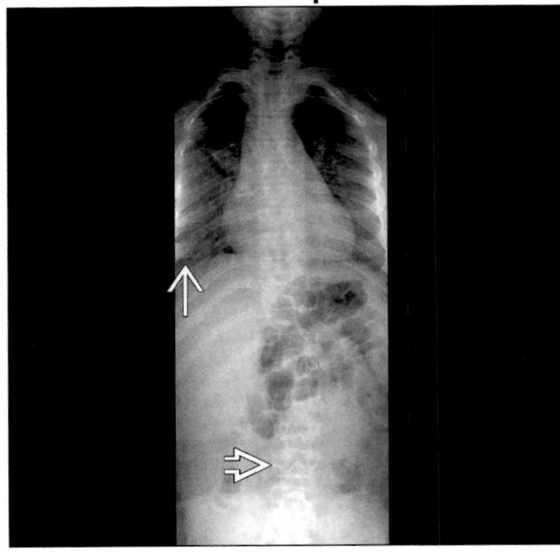

Anteroposterior radiograph shows a short trunk with wide, short ribs ➡. Additional findings include scoliosis and a narrow mediolateral dimension of the spinal canal in the lumbar region ➡.

Cleidocranial Dysplasia

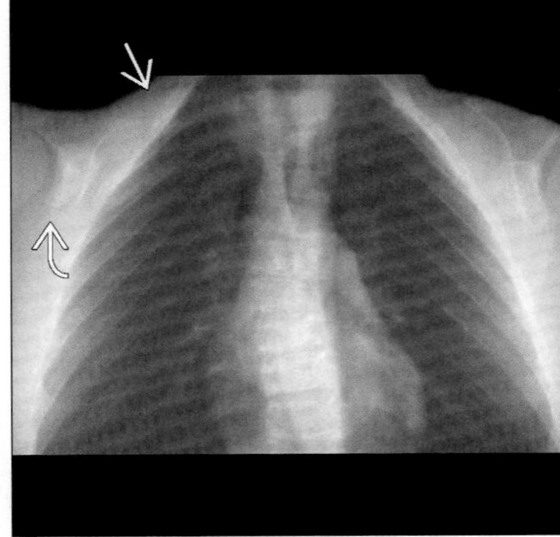

Anteroposterior radiograph shows short ribs, absence of both clavicles ➡, as well as hypoplastic glenoid fossae ➡. A midline defect was also present at the pubic symphysis.

Mucopolysaccharidoses

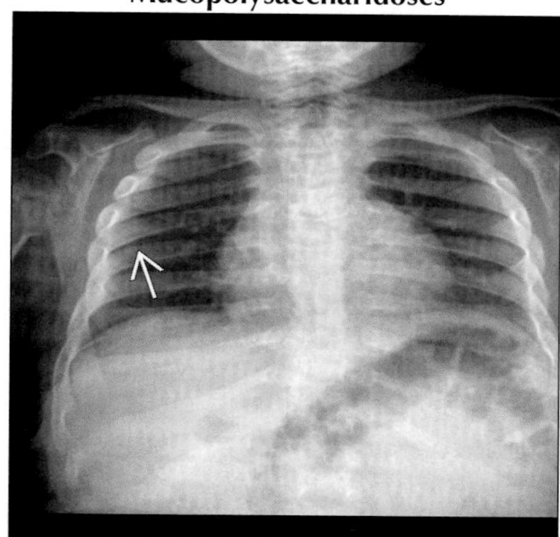

Mucopolysaccharidoses

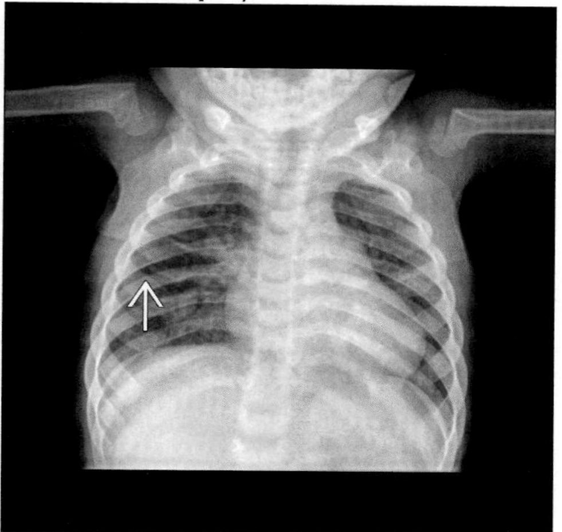

(Left) *Anteroposterior radiograph shows wide, short, paddle-shaped ribs* ➡ *with relatively small intercostal spaces in this patient with Morquio syndrome.* ***(Right)*** *Anteroposterior radiograph shows wide ribs* ➡ *with narrow intercostal spaces. Additional findings include humeral neck varus and short thick clavicles, which are typical skeletal findings of Hurler syndrome.*

Thanatophoric Dwarf

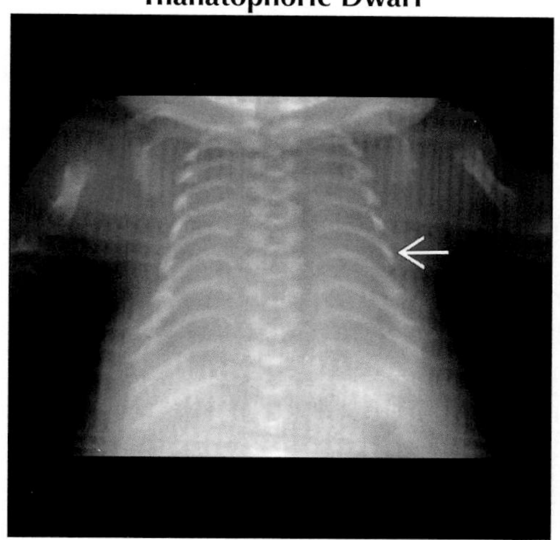

Thanatophoric Dwarf

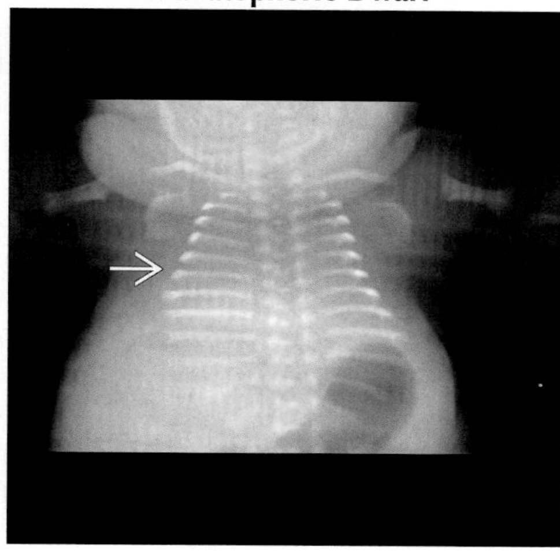

(Left) *Anteroposterior radiograph shows very short ribs* ➡ *with cupped costochondral junctions. The vertebral bodies are flat with the widened intervertebral disk spaces maintaining the normal truncal length.* ***(Right)*** *Anteroposterior radiograph shows platyspondyly but maintenance of normal trunk length by means of widened intervertebral disk spaces. Note the very short ribs* ➡ *that do not encircle the chest.*

Asphyxiating Thoracic Dystrophy of Jeune

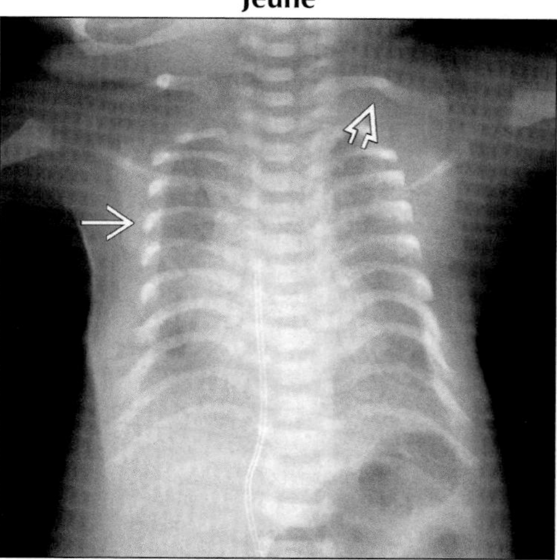

Asphyxiating Thoracic Dystrophy of Jeune

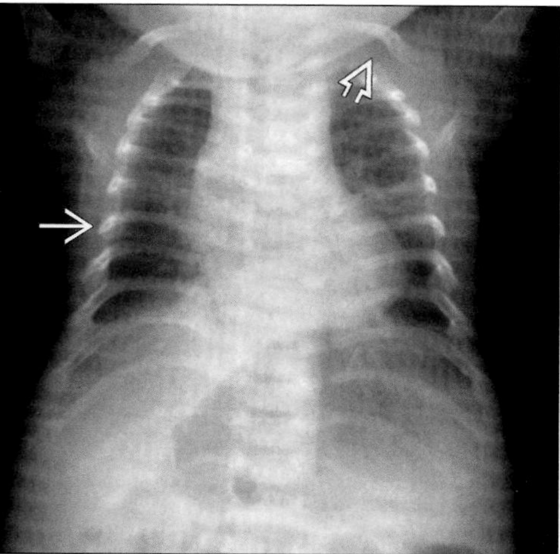

(Left) *Anteroposterior radiograph shows short ribs* ➡ *with bulbous ends. The chest has a mild "bell" shape, and the clavicles show "handlebar" deformities* ➡*.* ***(Right)*** *Anterior radiograph shows a narrow chest with short ribs* ➡*. Handlebar clavicles* ➡ *are also evident. Other commonly seen associated skeletal anomalies include a small pelvis with a trident acetabular margin, a femoral head ossification center present at birth, and mesomelic limb shortening.*

DWARFISM WITH HORIZONTAL ACETABULAR ROOF

DIFFERENTIAL DIAGNOSIS

Common
- Achondroplasia

Less Common
- Achondrogenesis
- Chondrodysplasia Punctata

Rare but Important
- Thanatophoric Dwarf
- Asphyxiating Thoracic Dystrophy of Jeune
- Chondroectodermal Dysplasia (Ellis-van Creveld)
- Caudal Regression
- Hypochondroplasia
- Down Syndrome (Mimic)
- Nail Patella Syndrome (Fong) (Mimic)

ESSENTIAL INFORMATION

Helpful Clues for Diagnoses
- **Achondroplasia**
  - Short, thick tubular bones
  - Short trunk with short ribs
  - Large skull with narrow foramen magnum
  - Short, flat vertebral bodies lacking normal widened interpediculate distance caudally
  - Posterior vertebral body scalloping
  - Square iliac wing with horizontal acetabular roof
  - Hemispheric femoral head
  - Overgrown fibulae
- **Achondrogenesis**
  - Short tubular bones and long bones
  - Short ribs
  - Minimal mineralization of vertebral bodies
  - Short iliac wing
  - Nonossified sacrum and pubis
- **Chondrodysplasia Punctata**
  - Short long bones
  - Punctate calcifications in cartilage and periarticular regions
  - Coronal clefts of vertebral bodies
  - Delayed brain myelination, cortical atrophy
- **Thanatophoric Dwarf**
  - Large "cloverleaf" skull with small face and frontal bossing
  - Long trunk with small chest
  - Short ribs with cupped costochondral junctions
  - Short, bowed limbs, "French telephone receiver femurs"
  - Flared metaphyses
  - Platyspondyly with rounded anterior vertebral bodies
  - Short, small iliac bones with horizontal acetabular roof
  - Lethal shortly after birth
- **Asphyxiating Thoracic Dystrophy of Jeune**
  - Bell-shaped thoracic cage
  - Handlebar clavicles
  - Horizontal, short ribs with bulbous ends
  - Short iliac bones with spur of sciatic notch
  - Horizontal acetabular roof and trident acetabular margin
  - Hands with cone-shaped epiphyses

Achondroplasia

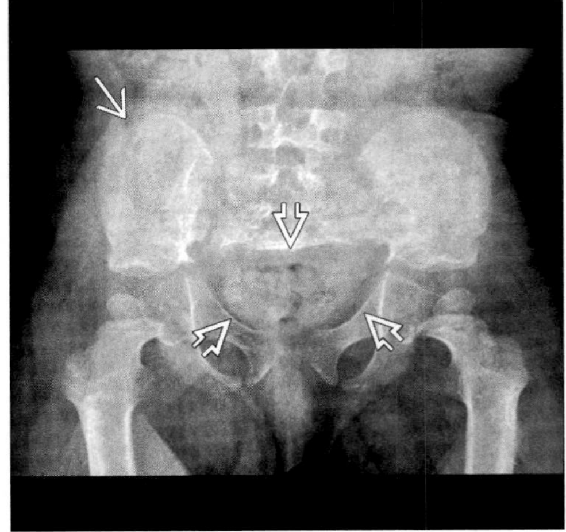

Anteroposterior radiograph shows short, wide iliac wings → and horizontal acetabular roofs with the inner margin of the pelvis ⇨ resembling a champagne glass. There is coxa valga with short femoral necks.

Chondrodysplasia Punctata

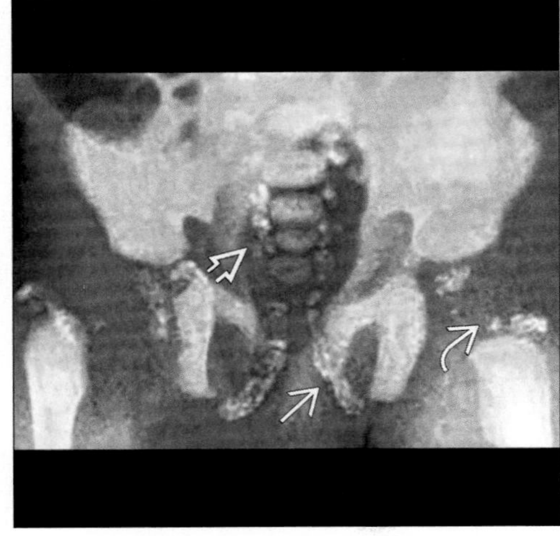

Anteroposterior radiograph shows stippled calcification in the pubic →, hip ↪, and sacral ⇨ regions that is typical for chondrodysplasia punctata. Each acetabular roof has a horizontal orientation.

DWARFISM WITH HORIZONTAL ACETABULAR ROOF

Thanatophoric Dwarf

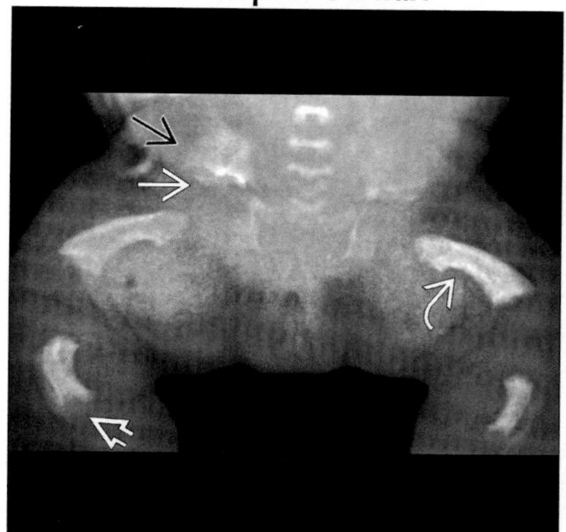

Asphyxiating Thoracic Dystrophy of Jeune

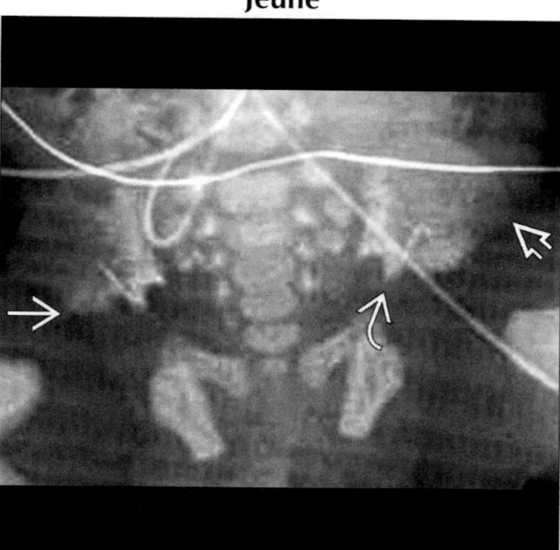

*(**Left**) Anteroposterior radiograph shows short, small iliac bones ➔, horizontal acetabular roofs ➔, "French telephone receiver"-shaped femora ➔, and bowed long bones with irregular flared metaphyses ➔. (**Right**) Anteroposterior radiograph shows short, flared iliac wings ➔ and horizontal acetabular roofs ➔ with a trident margin due to an inferolateral spur along the sciatic notch ➔.*

Chondroectodermal Dysplasia (Ellis-van Creveld)

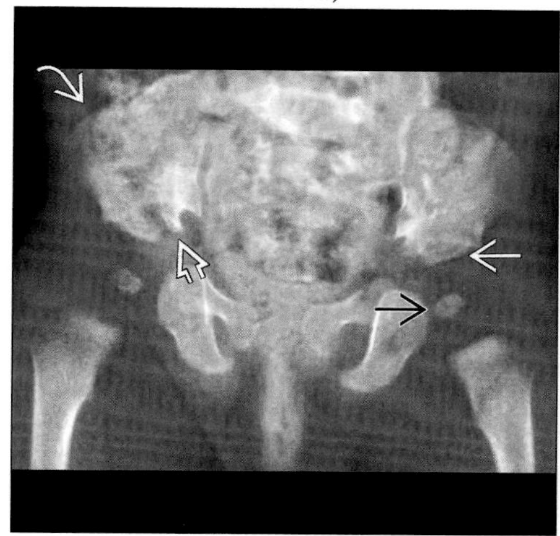

Caudal Regression

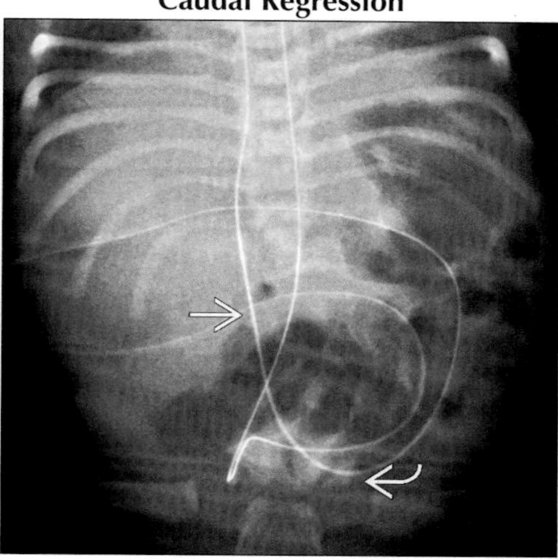

*(**Left**) Anteroposterior radiograph shows iliac wings that are flared and hypoplastic ➔. Acetabular roofs are somewhat horizontal ➔ and have a trident configuration ➔. The femoral heads are prematurely ossified ➔. (**Right**) Anteroposterior radiograph shows agenesis of the lumbar vertebrae ➔ and dysplastic, fused iliac bones with horizontal acetabular roofs ➔. Hip dislocation is a common finding.*

Down Syndrome (Mimic)

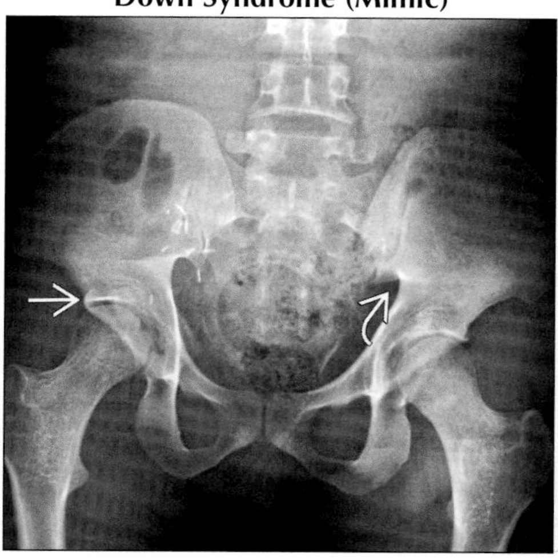

Nail Patella Syndrome (Fong) (Mimic)

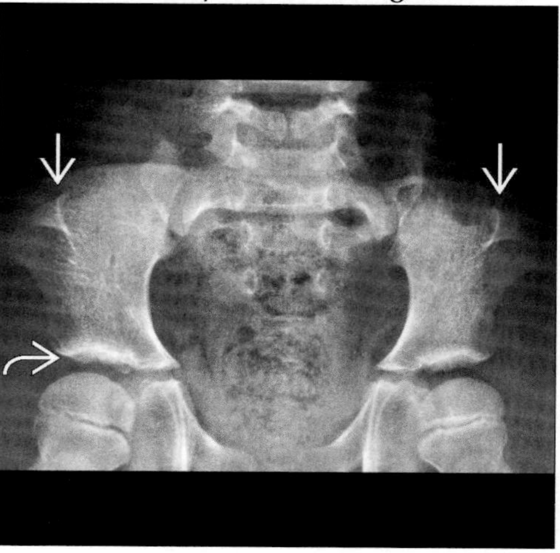

*(**Left**) Anteroposterior radiograph shows broad iliac wings, narrow sacrosciatic notch ➔, and horizontal acetabular roof ➔ seen in a patient with Down syndrome. Although Down patients are not dwarfs, this appearance of the pelvis, along with delayed skeletal maturation, may mimic dwarfism. (**Right**) Anteroposterior radiograph shows horizontal acetabular roofs ➔. The classic finding is the presence of symmetric, bilateral, central-posterior, iliac horns ➔.*

DWARFISM WITH MAJOR SPINE INVOLVEMENT

DIFFERENTIAL DIAGNOSIS

Common

- Achondroplasia
- Thanatophoric Dwarf
- Spondyloepiphyseal Dysplasia

Less Common

- Hypothyroidism, Child (Mimic)
- Noonan Syndrome
- Morquio Syndrome
- Hurler Syndrome
- Hunter Syndrome

Rare but Important

- Progeria
- Hypochondroplasia
- Metatropic Dwarfism
- Diastrophic Dwarfism
- Kniest Dysplasia
- Camptomelic Dysplasia
- Osteoglophonic Dysplasia
- Dyssegmental Dysplasia

ESSENTIAL INFORMATION

Helpful Clues for Diagnoses

- **Achondroplasia**
  - Short, flat vertebral bodies; decreasing interpediculate distance L1 → L5
  - Posterior vertebral body scalloping
  - Hypoplastic upper lumbar vertebral bodies
- **Thanatophoric Dwarf**
  - Platyspondyly with rounded anterior vertebral bodies
- **Spondyloepiphyseal Dysplasia**
  - Ovoid or pear-shaped vertebrae in infancy
  - Central, anterior vertebral body beak
  - Odontoid hypoplasia
- **Hypothyroidism, Child (Mimic)**
  - Congenital vertebral anomalies: Hemivertebrae, abnormal rib-vertebral articulations, platyspondyly
    - "Sail" vertebrae = upper lumbar vertebra with wedge or hook shape
- **Noonan Syndrome**
  - Klippel-Feil anomaly
  - Scoliosis & kyphosis
- **Morquio Syndrome**
  - Extensive vertebra plana
  - Central, anterior vertebral body beak
  - Diminutive or disappearing dens of axis
- **Hurler Syndrome**
  - Anterior inferior vertebral body beak
  - Oval to biconvex vertebral bodies
  - Absent dens → atlantoaxial subluxation
- **Hunter Syndrome**
  - Inferior beak similar to Hurler syndrome
  - Posterior vertebral body scalloping
- **Progeria**
  - Infantile central notching retained
- **Hypochondroplasia**
  - Decreased interpediculate distance L1 → L5
- **Kniest Dysplasia**
  - Platyspondyly with narrow interpediculate distance
  - Coronal vertebral body clefts, infants
- **Camptomelic Dysplasia**
  - Hypoplastic cervical vertebrae

Achondroplasia

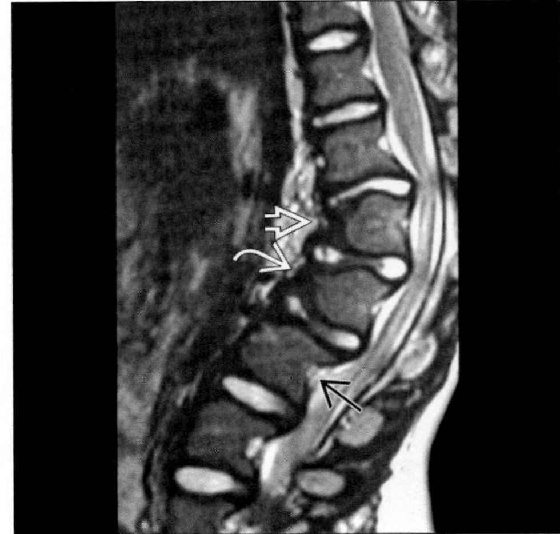

Sagittal T2WI MR shows posterior vertebral scalloping ➡, anterior beaking ➡, as well as hypoplasia of L1 and L2. This results in a focal kyphosis ➡.

Achondroplasia

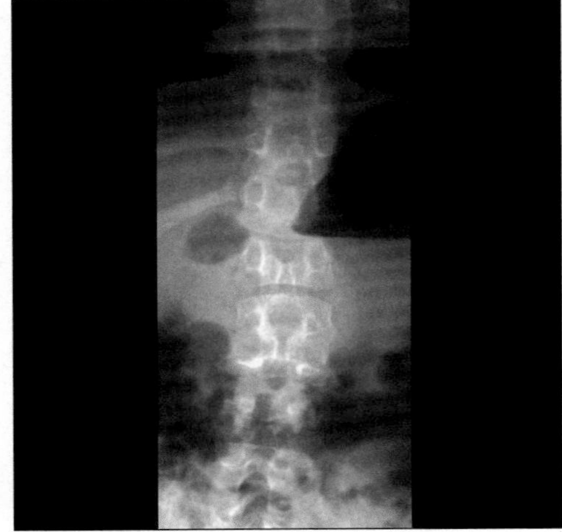

Anteroposterior radiograph shows progressive narrowing of the interpediculate distance in the lower lumbar spine, typical of achondroplasia.

Thanatophoric Dwarf

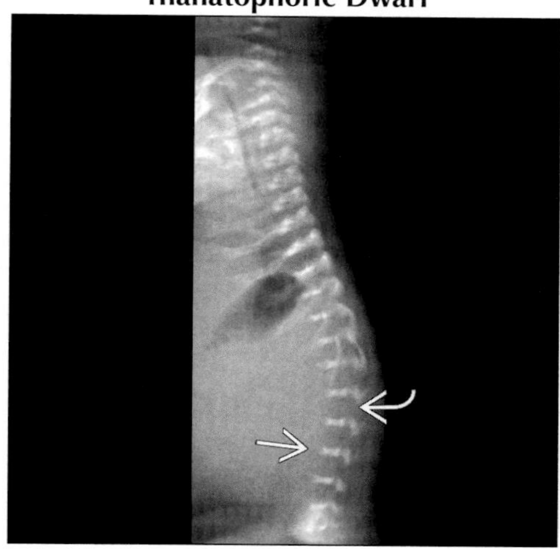

Spondyloepiphyseal Dysplasia

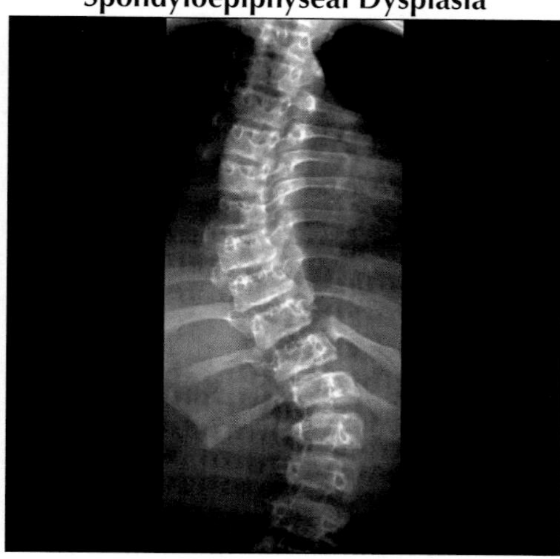

*(**Left**) Lateral radiograph shows the classic platyspondyly ➔, with widened intervertebral disk spaces ➔. Thus, the normal truncal length is maintained despite the flat vertebral bodies. This is a lethal form of dwarfism. (**Right**) Anteroposterior radiograph shows universal platyspondyly and scoliosis. Images of the extremities (not shown) demonstrated severely deformed epiphyses. The combination of findings helps make the diagnosis.*

Noonan Syndrome

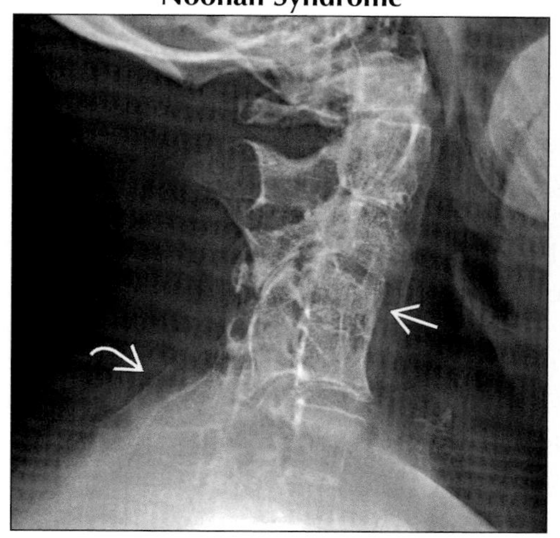

Morquio Syndrome

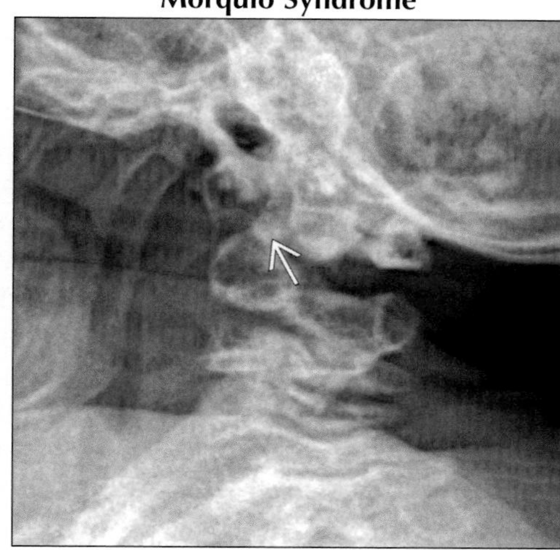

*(**Left**) Lateral radiograph shows a Klippel-Feil anomaly that is typical in Noonan syndrome but is also seen incidentally, as in this patient. The cervical vertebral bodies are small and fused ➔, and there is an adjacent omovertebral bone ➔. (**Right**) Lateral radiograph shows hypoplasia of the odontoid ➔. This anomaly can contribute to atlantoaxial subluxation in these patients.*

Morquio Syndrome

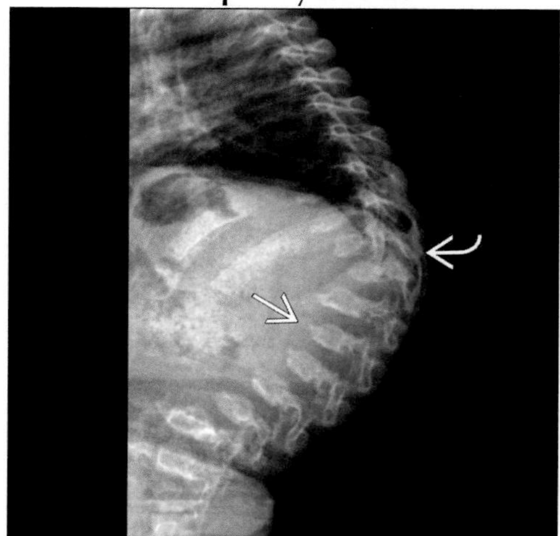

Hurler Syndrome

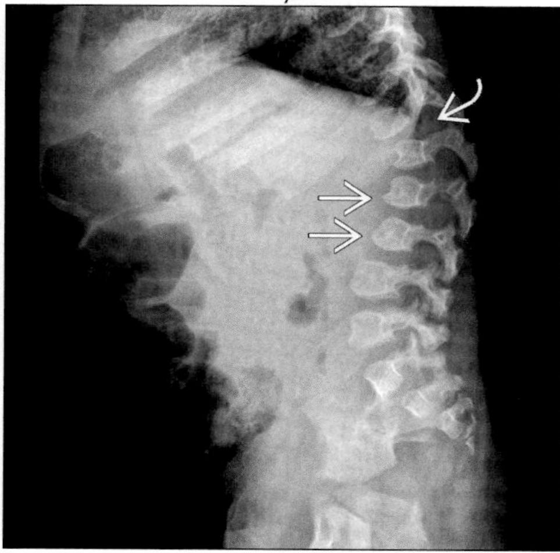

*(**Left**) Lateral radiograph shows dorsolumbar kyphosis ➔, flattened vertebral bodies, and central, anterior beaking of the vertebral bodies ➔. (**Right**) Lateral radiograph shows a focal dorsolumbar kyphosis ➔, oval vertebral bodies, and typical anterior inferior beaks ➔. The mucopolysaccharidoses, including Morquio, Hunter, and Hurler syndrome all have variably short, rounded vertebral bodies with anterior beaks.*

SOFT TISSUE MASS

DIFFERENTIAL DIAGNOSIS

Common
- Ganglion Cyst
- Lipoma
- Hematoma
- Vascular Malformation
- Hemangioma
- Fat Necrosis

Less Common
- Rhabdomyosarcoma (RMS)
- Myositis Ossificans
- Neurofibroma (NF)
- Synovial Sarcoma

Rare but Important
- Extraosseous Ewing Sarcoma (EOES)
- Fibromatosis
- Fibrosarcoma (FS)
- Malignant Peripheral Nerve Sheath Tumor
- Lipoblastoma
- Liposarcoma
- Other Sarcomas
- Congenital or Infantile

ESSENTIAL INFORMATION

Key Differential Diagnosis Issues
- Some soft tissue masses can be diagnosed by clinical exam
  - Lipoma: Superficial & doughy by palpation
  - Ganglion cyst: Transilluminates and near joint
  - Others need further evaluation by radiographs and then MR
- MR will help differentiate determinate from indeterminate lesions
  - Determinant lesions: Neurofibroma, vascular malformations, hematoma, lipoma
    - Excision biopsy or monitoring
  - Indeterminate: Underlying pathology is uncertain
    - Needle biopsy to determine management

Helpful Clues for Common Diagnoses
- **Ganglion Cyst**
  - MR: Homogeneous hyperintense T2 signal cystic mass, peripheral enhancement
  - Communicates with joint space or tendon sheath
- **Lipoma**
  - May represent up to 1/3 of all soft tissue masses
  - May appear lucent on radiographs
  - MR: Follows subcutaneous fat signal on all pulse sequences
    - **Hint**: Use fat-suppression sequences
    - May have thin septations
    - Intramuscular lipomas may appear more complex with infiltration and poor definition
- **Hematoma**
  - MR: Hemorrhagic products
    - Hyperintense T1 and hypo- to hyperintense on T2 with "blooming" on gradient echo sequences
  - Must use caution; may be difficult to differentiate from soft tissue sarcoma with hemorrhage
- **Vascular Malformation**
  - Present at birth
  - Venous: Low-flow lesion on gradient echo MR images with thrombi, phleboliths, and diffuse contrast enhancement
    - May see calcified phleboliths on radiographs
  - Lymphatic: Low-flow lesion on gradient echo MR images with septal enhancement and often fluid-fluid levels
  - Arteriovenous: High-flow lesion on gradient echo MR images; tangle of vessels without enhancing soft tissue mass
- **Hemangioma**
  - True neoplasm
  - Small or absent at birth, rapid growth over 1st several months, involutes over months to years
  - MR: Hyperintense on T2, vascular flow voids (high flow on GE images), intense post-contrast enhancement
    - May have fatty component when involuting
  - Ultrasound: High vessel density (> 5 vessels/cm^2)
  - Strawberry skin discoloration if superficial or bluish in deeper hemangiomas
- **Fat Necrosis**
  - Most commonly follows trauma (may not recall) and over bony protuberances
  - Small, stellate, spiculated, linear with lack of soft tissue mass

  - May possess peripheral or irregular marginal contrast enhancement

Helpful Clues for Less Common Diagnoses

- **Rhabdomyosarcoma (RMS)**
  - Most common soft tissue sarcoma in children
  - Embryonal RMS: 60-70% of childhood RMS
    - Typically < 15 years old; more common in GU and head and neck
  - Alveolar RMS: Adolescents; most common in extremity, trunk, perianal/perirectal
  - Alveolar and extremity RMS tend to have worse prognosis
- **Myositis Ossificans**
  - Ring-like peripheral calcifications
- **Neurofibroma (NF)**
  - Frequently multiple and seen in neurofibromatosis type 1
  - May be sporadic and solitary
  - "Target" sign or "bag of worms"
- **Synovial Sarcoma**
  - 2nd most common sarcoma in childhood, 15-35 years old
  - Calcifications in 1/3 can appear nonaggressive on MR, near joint; when extensive, improved prognosis

Helpful Clues for Rare Diagnoses

- **Extraosseous Ewing Sarcoma (EOES)**
  - May erode adjacent bone
- **Fibromatosis**
  - MR: Typically hypointense to skeletal muscle on T1 and hyperintense with areas of hypointensity on T2, may enhance
- **Fibrosarcoma (FS)**
  - Infantile FS < 5 years old; more common in lower extremities, heterogeneous enhancement, local recurrence
  - Rarely metastasizes, better prognosis than adult FS
- **Malignant Peripheral Nerve Sheath Tumor**
  - Most commonly associated with NF1 (50%); more common in lower extremities
  - Must consider malignant degeneration of neurofibroma if erodes bone, painful, rapid growth, and loss of "target" sign
- **Lipoblastoma**
  - Primarily < 3 years old, superficial arms and legs (deeper in lipoblastomatosis)
  - MR: Composed of fat and myxoid tissue, hyperintense on T1, heterogeneous on T2
- **Liposarcoma**
  - Myxoid subtype more common, bright on T2 with heterogeneous enhancement
  - Well-differentiated subtype; looks like lipoblastoma (but > 3 years old)
- **Other Sarcomas**
  - PPNET, epithelioid sarcoma, MFH, ASPS
- **Congenital or Infantile**
  - Infantile myofibromatosis, fibrous hamartoma of infancy, congenital-infantile fibrosarcoma, etc.

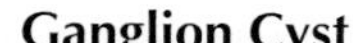

Ganglion Cyst

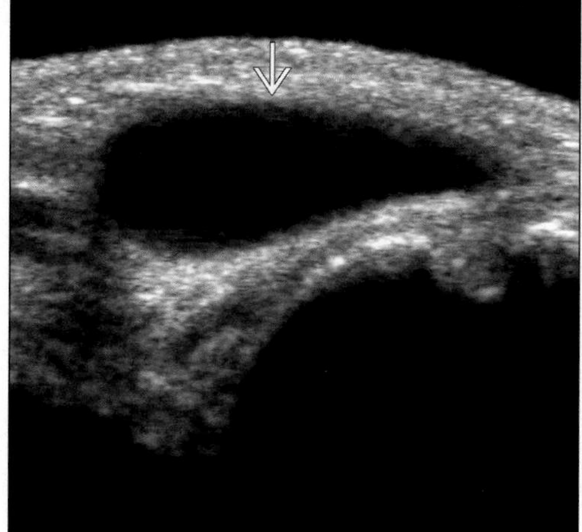

Longitudinal ultrasound shows a well-defined anechoic fluid collection ➡ in the volar aspect of the wrist. Connection to the joint or tendon sheath was not seen, but this is still likely a ganglion cyst.

Ganglion Cyst

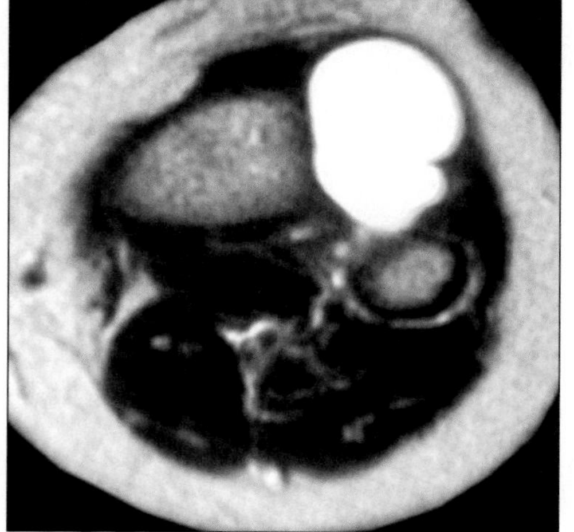

Axial T2WI MR shows a bright hyperintense signal mass extending from the proximal tibia-fibia joint. The mass demonstrated peripheral enhancement (not shown), typical of a ganglion cyst.

SOFT TISSUE MASS

Lipoma

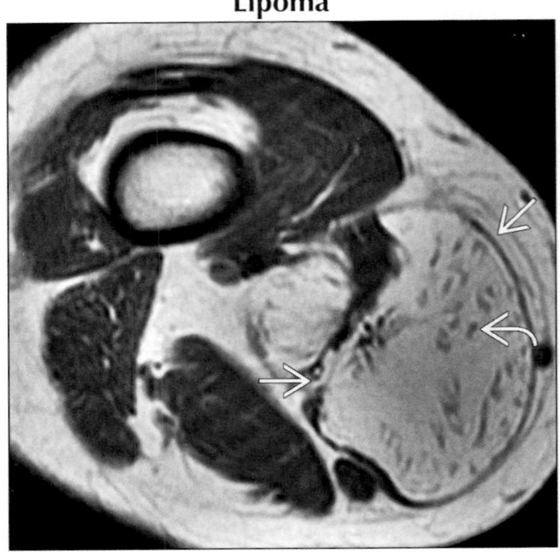

Lipoma

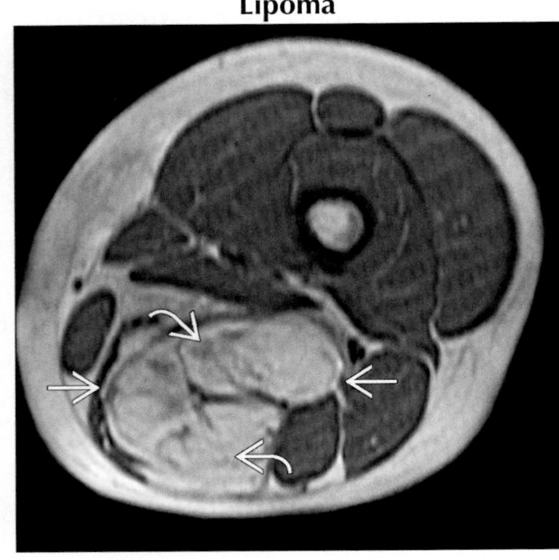

__(Left)__ Axial T1WI MR shows a mass → with signal equal to subcutaneous fat replacing the sartorius muscle in the left thigh. Note the linear hypointense intermingled muscle fibers ↪ within this intramuscular lipoma. __(Right)__ Axial T1WI MR shows a lobulated posterior thigh mass →. The mass followed subcutaneous fat signal on all the other imaging sequences (not shown) without contrast enhancement. Notice the hypointense intermingled muscle fibers ↪.

Hematoma

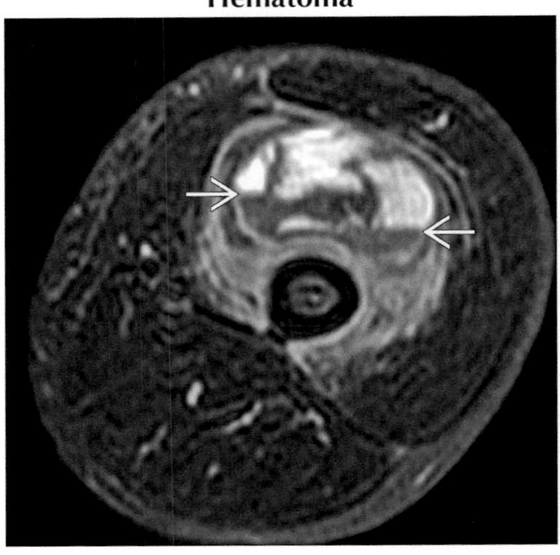

Hematoma

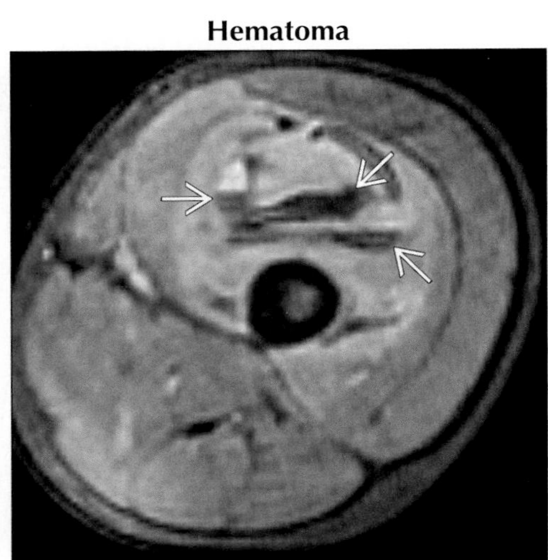

__(Left)__ Axial T2WI FS MR shows fluid-fluid levels → in a complex anterior thigh mass. __(Right)__ Axial MPGR image shows "blooming" →, indicating hemorrhagic components in this anterior thigh hematoma. This 9 year old had a history of direct trauma and pain. The mass decreased in size and resolved over time.

Vascular Malformation

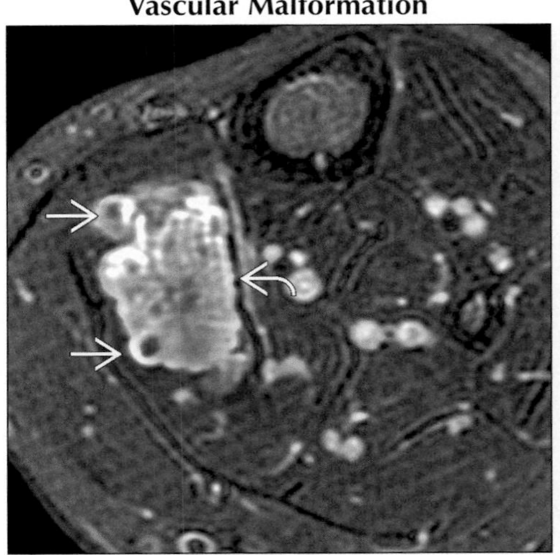

Vascular Malformation

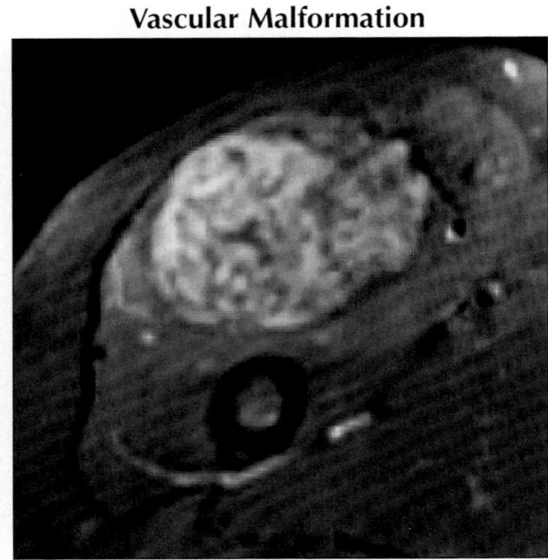

__(Left)__ Axial T2WI FS MR shows a hyperintense mass ↪ in the lower extremity. Notice the hypointense signal thrombus → or phlebolith in this venous malformation. Venous malformations are typically low-flow vascular malformations with diffuse enhancement. __(Right)__ Axial T1WI FS MR C+ shows diffuse enhancement in this anterior thigh venous malformation.

Vascular Malformation

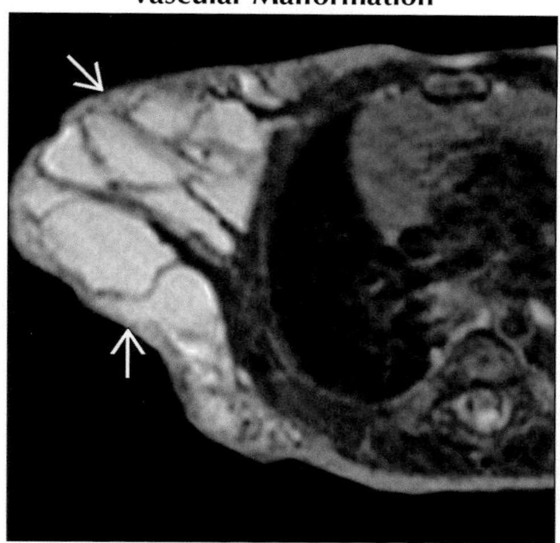

Hemangioma

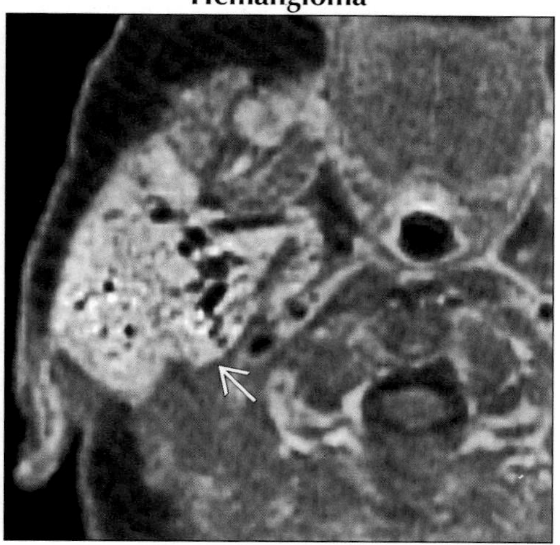

*(**Left**) Axial T2WI FSE MR shows a septated hyperintense signal mass ➡ (lymphatic malformation) within the right axilla. Lymphatic malformations are low-flow lesions with septal enhancement (not shown). (**Right**) Axial T2WI FS MR shows a hyperintense right parotid mass ➡. Notice the numerous flow voids in this highly vascular lesion.*

Fat Necrosis

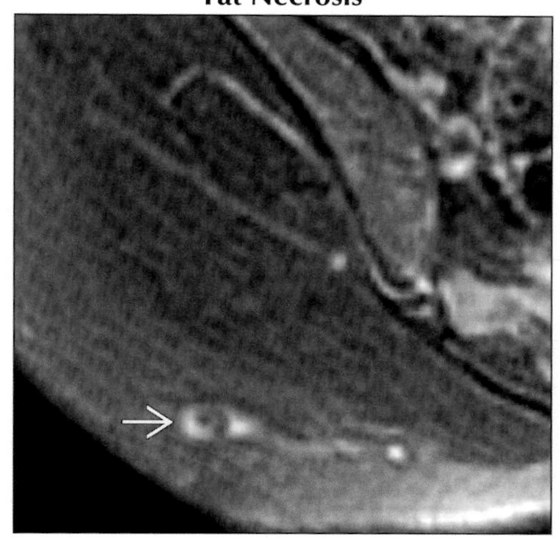

Fat Necrosis

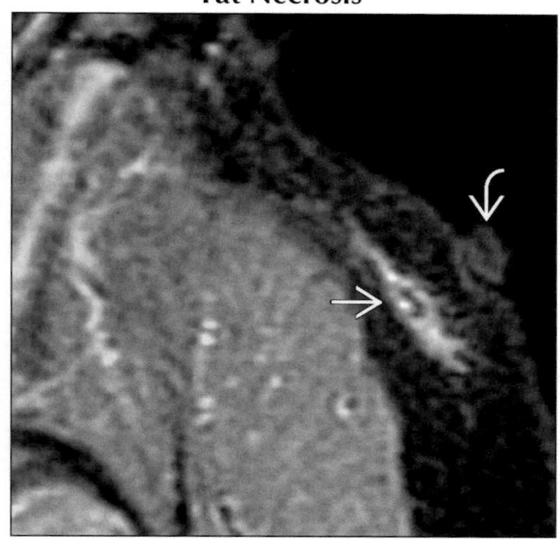

*(**Left**) Axial T2WI FS MR shows an irregular region of hyperintense signal ➡ abnormality in the posterior gluteal subcutaneous fat. (**Right**) Coronal STIR MR in the same child shows a stellate spiculated lesion ➡ within the subcutaneous fat with a hypointense central component (signal similar to fat). Notice the overlying vitamin E capsule ➡ marking the clinical soft tissue mass.*

Rhabdomyosarcoma (RMS)

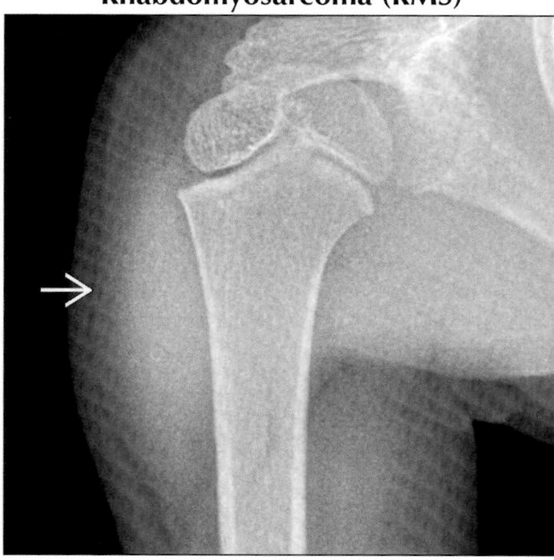

Rhabdomyosarcoma (RMS)

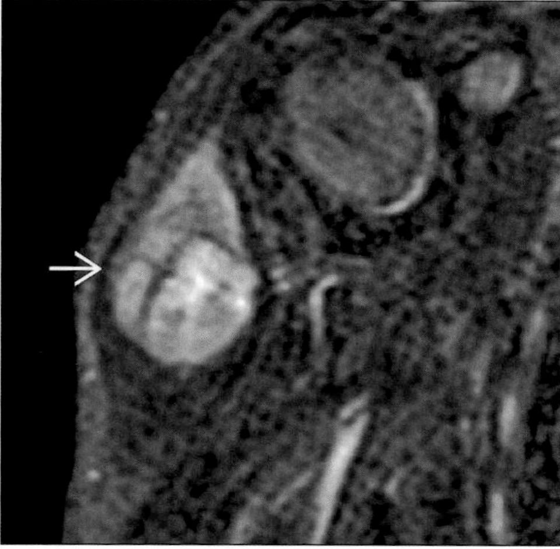

*(**Left**) Anteroposterior radiograph shows a soft tissue mass ➡ within the lateral aspect of the right shoulder. Neither calcifications nor underlying bone destruction was detected. (**Right**) Coronal T2WI FS MR shows a heterogeneous hyperintense soft tissue mass ➡ within the lateral deltoid muscle. This mass was indeterminate by imaging but biopsy proven to be RMS, the most common soft tissue sarcoma in children.*

SOFT TISSUE MASS

(Left) Axial MPGR image shows a left iliopsoas mass with a hypointense dark signal band ➡. The mass was heterogeneous in signal on other imaging sequences in this football player with 3 weeks of pain. When there is dark signal band on the GE sequences, consider myositis ossificans. ***(Right)*** *Axial NECT in the same patient 2 weeks later shows a peripherally calcified ➡ anterior thigh mass. The findings are characteristic of myositis ossificans.*

Myositis Ossificans

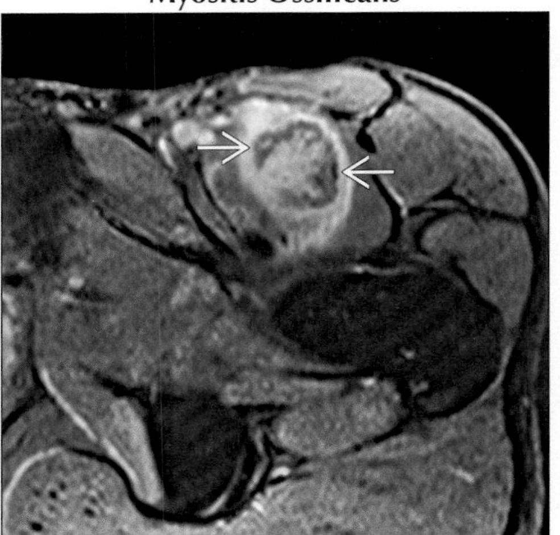

Myositis Ossificans

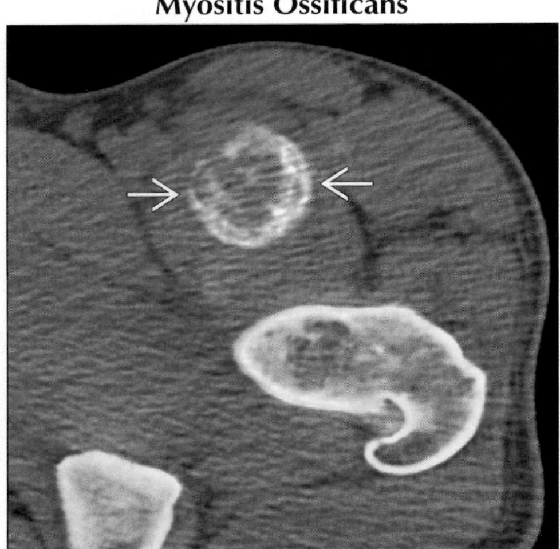

(Left) Axial T2WI FS MR shows tubular worm-like masses ➡ (hyperintense signal margin with relatively hypointense center) within the posterior paraspinal muscles of the neck. The masses ➡ extend between and displace the carotid arteries and internal jugular veins bilaterally. This is a determinant soft tissue lesion. ***(Right)*** *Axial T2WI FS MR shows the classic "target" sign ➡ of extensive intrapelvic neurofibromas ➡.*

Neurofibroma (NF)

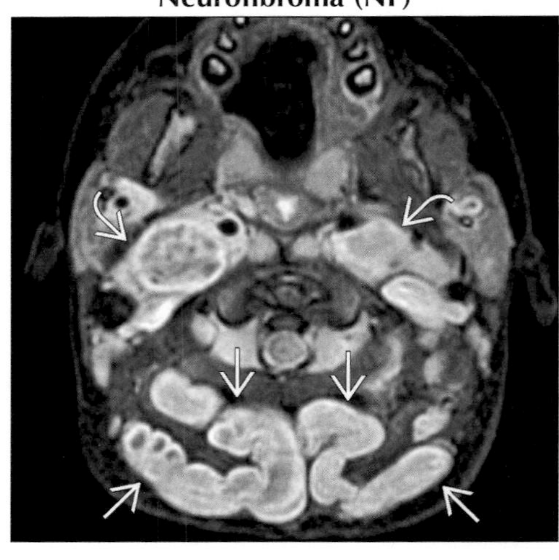

Neurofibroma (NF)

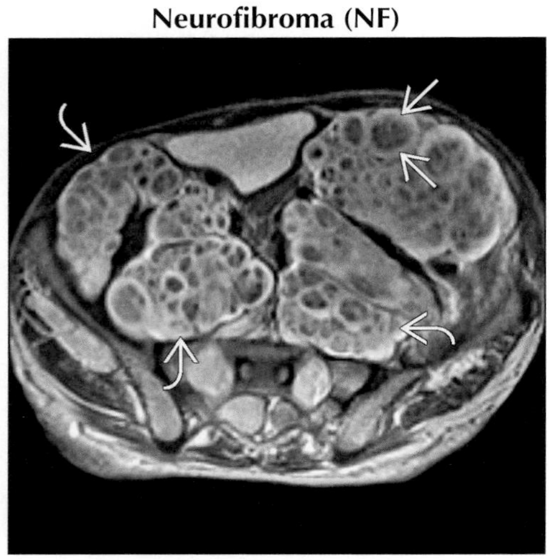

(Left) Anteroposterior radiograph shows irregular calcifications ➡ within the medial soft tissue of the lower leg. Calcifications are seen radiographically in approximately 1/3 of synovial sarcoma tumors. ***(Right)*** *Coronal T2WI FS MR shows a heterogeneous hyperintense mass ➡. Notice the proximal and distal hyperintense edema ➡ or "tail" extending along the fascial planes.*

Synovial Sarcoma

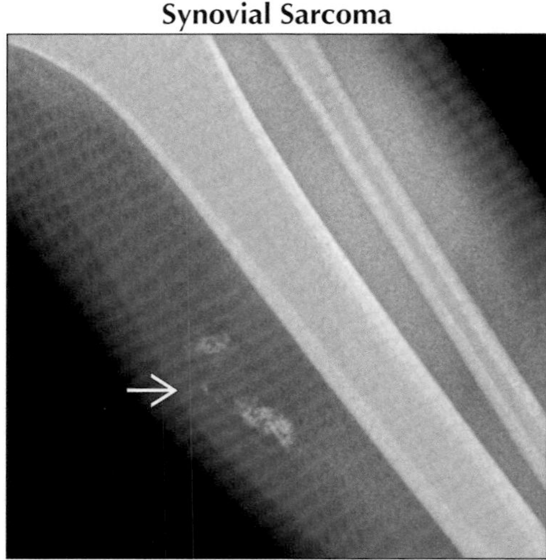

Synovial Sarcoma

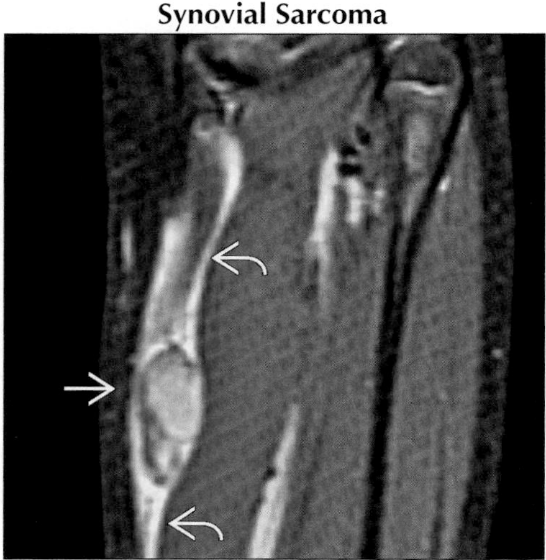

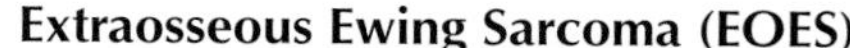

Extraosseous Ewing Sarcoma (EOES)

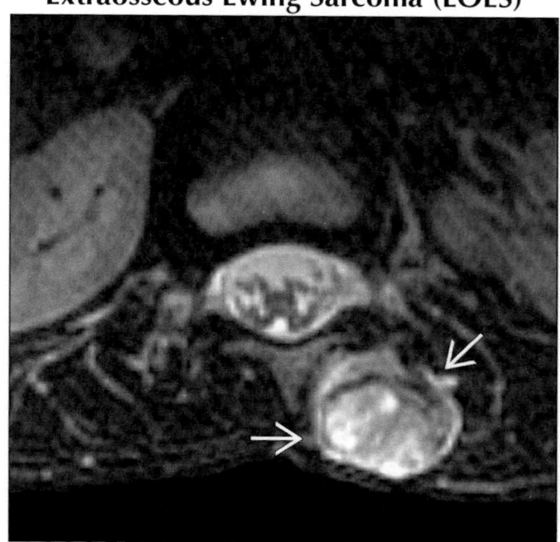

Fibromatosis

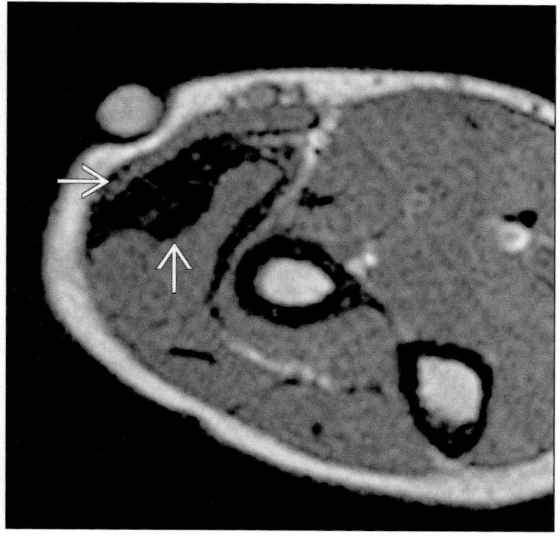

(Left) Axial T2WI FS MR shows a heterogeneous hyperintense signal mass ➔ within the left posterior paraspinal muscles. *(Right)* Axial T1WI MR shows a dark signal mass ➔ within the right forearm. This lesion was more infiltrative distally within the forearm, insinuating along the fascial planes.

Fibrosarcoma (FS)

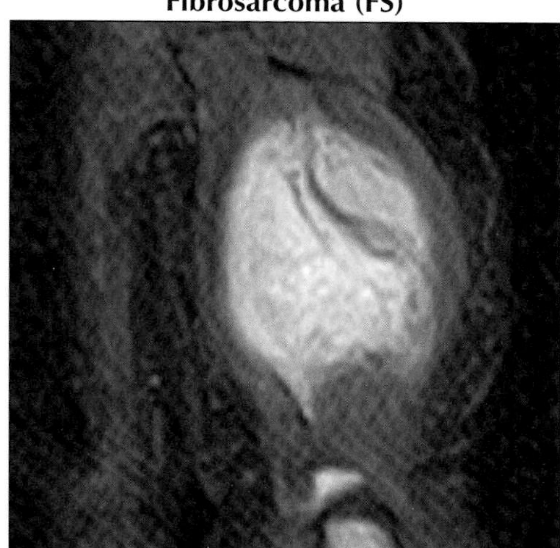

Malignant Peripheral Nerve Sheath Tumor

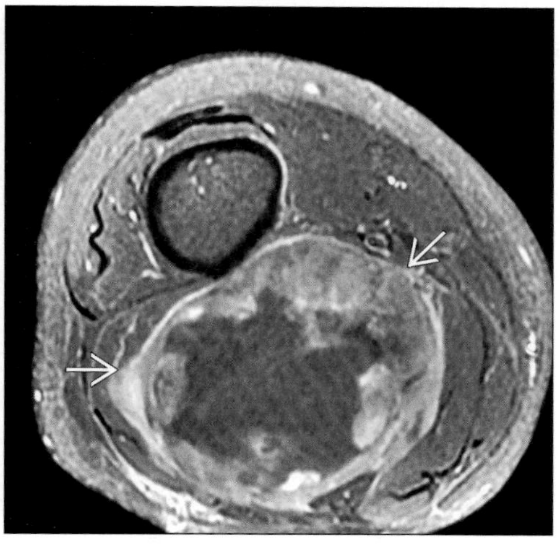

(Left) Coronal T2WI FS MR shows a heterogeneous hyperintense soft tissue mass within the posterior left upper arm. This is a pathologically proven infantile fibrosarcoma in this 2 month old. The mass was detected shortly after birth and imaged due to its increased growth. *(Right)* Axial T1WI MR C+ shows a heterogeneous necrotic mass ➔ with peripheral enhancement.

Lipoblastoma

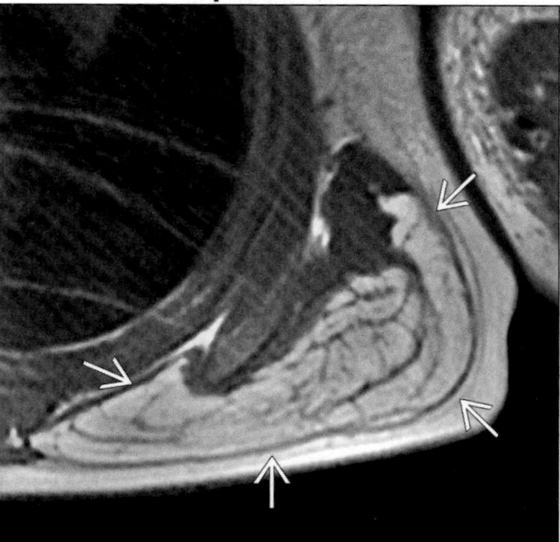

Lipoblastoma

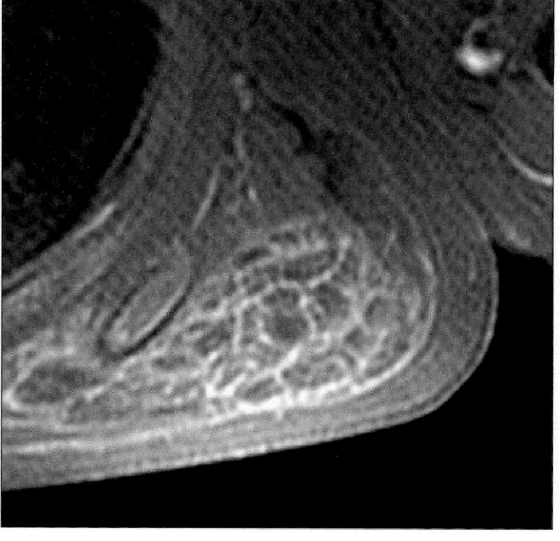

(Left) Axial T1WI MR shows a septated mass ➔ with internal signal equal to the fat posterior to the left scapula. *(Right)* Axial T1WI FS MR C+ shows diffuse enhancement of the septae. No nodular or soft tissue enhancement was found. Notice the internal signal (fat) suppressing on this fat-suppressed image. 80-90% of lipoblastomas are seen in patients younger than 3 years. Lipoma should also be considered for this imaging appearance.

SOFT TISSUE CALCIFICATIONS

DIFFERENTIAL DIAGNOSIS

Common
- Venous Malformation
- Heterotopic Ossification (HO)
  - Myositis Ossificans Circumscripta (MO)
- Dermatomyositis (DM)

Less Common
- Other Collagen Vascular Diseases
- Neoplastic

Rare but Important
- Metabolic/Hypercalcemia
- Ehlers-Danlos
- Parasitic
- Tumoral Calcinosis
- Myositis Ossificans Progressiva

ESSENTIAL INFORMATION

Helpful Clues for Common Diagnoses
- **Venous Malformation**
  - Present at birth and grows proportional to child
  - MR
    - Lack of high-flow vessel on GE imaging
    - Phleboliths or thrombi
    - Diffuse contrast enhancement
- **Heterotopic Ossification (HO)**
  - HO and MO in literature are commonly used interchangeably
    - But MO is subtype of HO
  - HO: Lamellar bone inside soft tissue (ST) structures where bone does not exist
    - MO: When HO occurs within muscles or ST
  - Ectopic calcification differs from MO: Mineralization of ST as result of chemical or physical trauma
    - Calcification deposits rather than bone formation
  - MO: Most commonly in arms or in quadriceps of thighs
  - HO: Adjacent to large joints
    - 1-4 months (up to 18 months) following injury
  - HO
    - Trauma: Spinal fusion, total hip arthroplasty, intraoperative fixation of acetabular fracture, burns, etc.
    - Neurogenic: Spinal cord injury, CNS tumors, CNS infections, MS, etc.
    - Myositis ossificans progressiva: Rare
  - MO
    - Radiographically calcifications are seen at 4-6 weeks following injury
    - Bone scan (BS) used for earliest detection
    - BS: Positive 2-6 weeks earlier than ossification is visible on radiographs
    - BS: Early in course, only blood pool images may be positive whereas abnormal uptake during soft tissue phase is seen later
    - NECT: Used for osseous architecture
    - Mature phase; well-defined calcified mass with internal fat marrow
  - Alkaline phosphatase is commonly elevated up to 3.5x normal with peak at ~ 12 weeks following injury
- **Dermatomyositis (DM)**
  - Collagen vascular disease
  - Gottron papules and heliotrope rash are pathognomic
  - Bimodal age distribution (seen at any age)
    - Peak: 40-50 years old
    - Children: 5-14 years old
  - Calcifications in 1/4 to 1/2; typically seen 6 months to 3 years after onset of disease
    - Typically elbows, knees, digits, and extremities
  - 5 major criteria for diagnosis of DM
    - Symmetric muscle weakness
    - Characteristic changes on muscle biopsy
    - Increased muscle enzymes in serum
    - EMG abnormality of myopathy and denervation
    - Characteristic skin rash

Helpful Clues for Less Common Diagnoses
- **Other Collagen Vascular Diseases**
  - Scleroderma
    - Anywhere can be affected
    - Most commonly fingers and extremities; usually extensor side of forearms and prepatellar ST
  - Polymyositis, SLE, CREST syndrome
- **Neoplastic**
  - Synovial sarcoma
    - Calcifications in 1/3
    - Age: 15-35 years old
    - Typically adjacent to joints and tendon sheaths
  - Lipoma, infantile myofibromatosis, etc.

Helpful Clues for Rare Diagnoses

- **Metabolic/Hypercalcemia**
  - Metastatic calcification
    - Any process that causes elevated calcium-phosphate product; may lead to precipitation of calcium phosphate in ST
    - Secondary hyperparathyroidism, hypervitaminosis D, sarcoidosis, milk-alkali syndrome
    - Fat necrosis: May lead to widespread subcutaneous calcifications in young infants
    - May also see vascular calcifications in chronic renal failure
- **Ehlers-Danlos**
  - Autosomal dominant disorder, abnormal or deficient collagen
  - Characterized by hyperextensibility of "cigarette paper" skin, joint hypermobility and dislocation, bone and ST fragility, and ST calcification
- **Parasitic**
  - Cysticercosis: "Rice grain" calcifications
    - Caused by pork tapeworm (Taenia solium) found worldwide
  - Dracunculiasis: Crescentic calcifications
    - a.k.a. guinea worm disease
    - Most commonly seen in Africa
- **Tumoral Calcinosis**
  - Rare familial disease
  - Massive periarticular calcifications along extensor surfaces (hip, elbow, shoulder, foot, wrist)
  - Seen primarily in 1st 2 decades of life
  - Similar radiographic appearance to other ST calcifications but more similar to ST calcifications seen in chronic renal failure
- **Myositis Ossificans Progressiva**
  - Mean age at onset: 5 years old
  - Progressive ossifications in trunk and shoulders
  - Short great toe with synostosis

Alternative Differential Approaches

- Congenital
  - Venous malformation
  - Myositis ossificans progressiva
- Traumatic
  - Myositis ossificans circumscripta, heterotopic ossification
  - Frostbite, burn, post-injection, fat necrosis, hematoma
- Inflammatory
  - Dermatomyositis, systemic lupus erythematosus (SLE), scleroderma, Ehlers-Danlos
  - Parasitic: Cysticercosis, guinea worm, loiasis, hydatid disease, trichinosis
- Metabolic/hypercalcemia
  - Renal osteodystrophy
  - Hypervitaminosis D, sarcoid, milk-alkali syndrome, fat necrosis
- Idiopathic
  - Tumoral calcinosis
- Neoplastic
  - Synovial sarcoma, lipoma, etc.

Venous Malformation

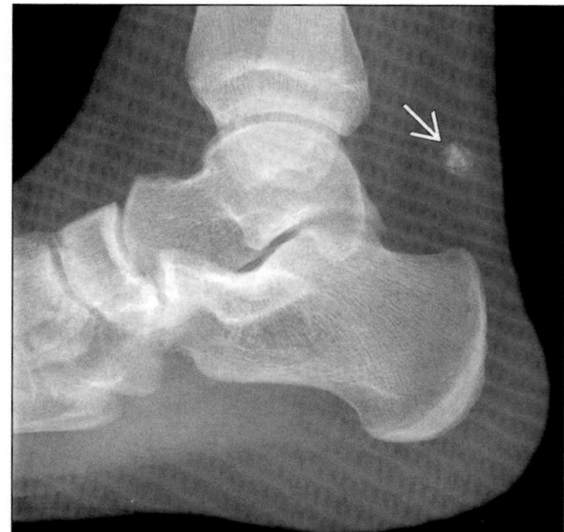

Lateral radiograph shows a "rock," well-defined calcification ➔ within the posterior ST of the ankle. Venous malformations are low-flow vascular malformations containing thrombi or phleboliths.

Venous Malformation

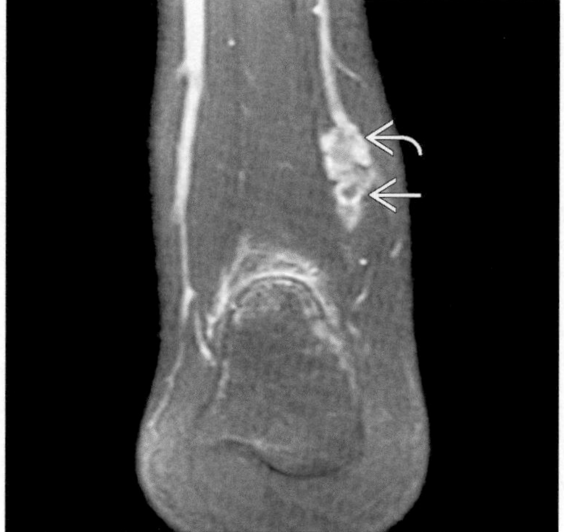

Coronal T1WI FS MR C+ in the same child shows diffuse enhancement ➔ in the venous malformation. Notice the hypointense phlebolith ➔, which represents the calcification on the previous image.

SOFT TISSUE CALCIFICATIONS

(Left) Axial T2WI FS MR shows a hyperintense mass ➔ in the medial calf. Note the hypointense signal thrombus ➔ or phlebolith in this venous malformation. Venous malformations are typically low-flow vascular malformations with diffuse enhancement. (Right) Anteroposterior radiograph shows faint ST calcification or ossification ➔ along the diaphysis of the left femur. Note the surgical plate and decompression screw transfixing the femoral fracture.

Venous Malformation

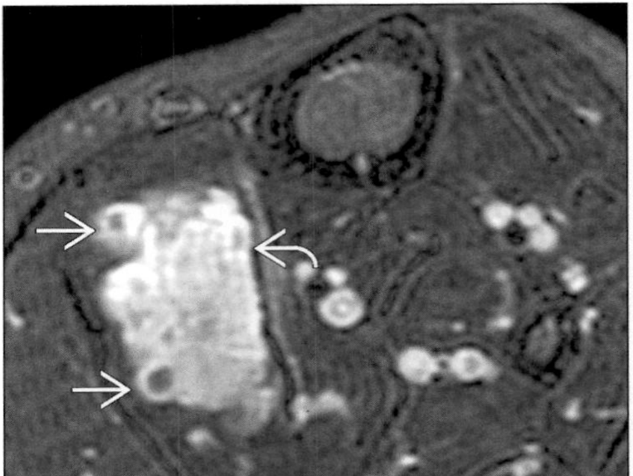

Heterotopic Ossification (HO)

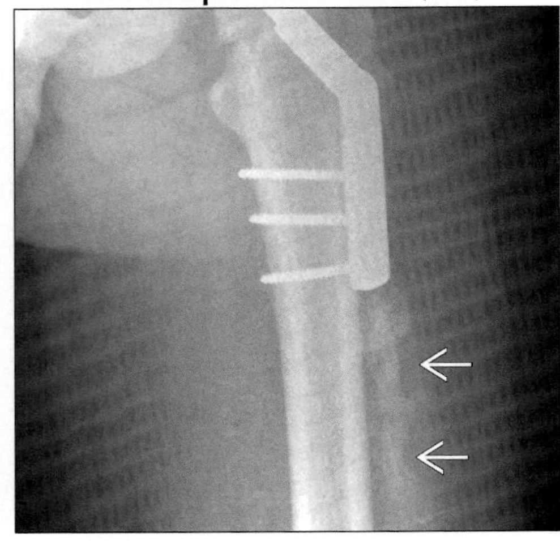

(Left) Axial NECT in the same teenager 2 weeks later shows a peripherally ring-like calcified ➔ iliopsoas mass. The findings are characteristic of MO. In the mature phase of MO, there is a peripherally calcified mass containing internal fatty marrow. (Right) Oblique radiograph in the same teenager weeks later shows a well-defined, peripherally calcified mass with decreased density centrally (marrow fat).

Myositis Ossificans Circumscripta (MO)

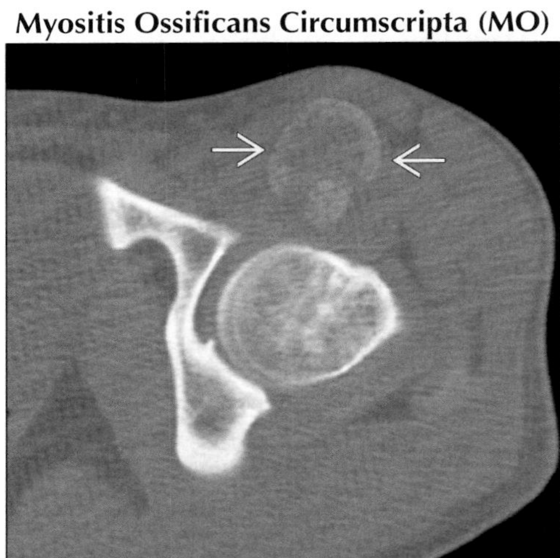

Myositis Ossificans Circumscripta (MO)

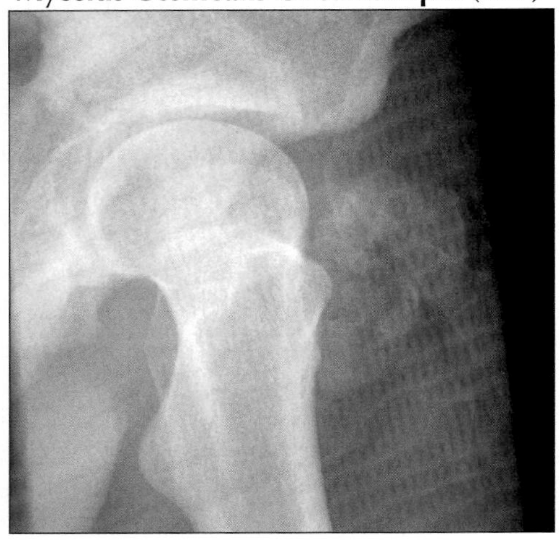

(Left) Anteroposterior radiograph shows extensive periarticular calcifications ➔ around the knee in this child with dermatomyositis. Soft tissue calcifications develop in 25-50% of patients with DM. (Right) Lateral radiograph shows periarticular and subcutaneous calcifications ➔ around the elbow in this child several years after the onset of dermatomyositis.

Dermatomyositis (DM)

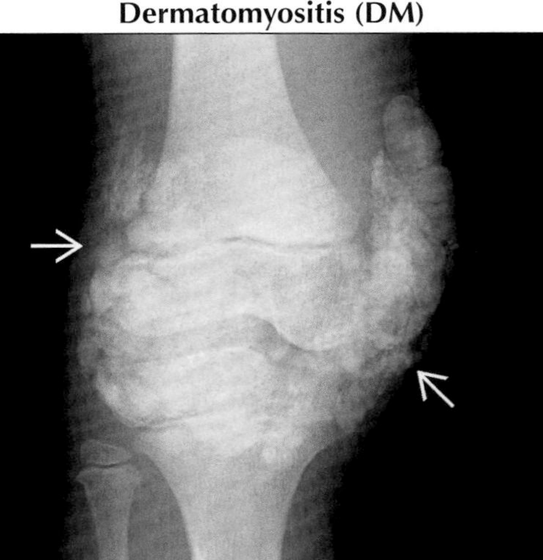

Dermatomyositis (DM)

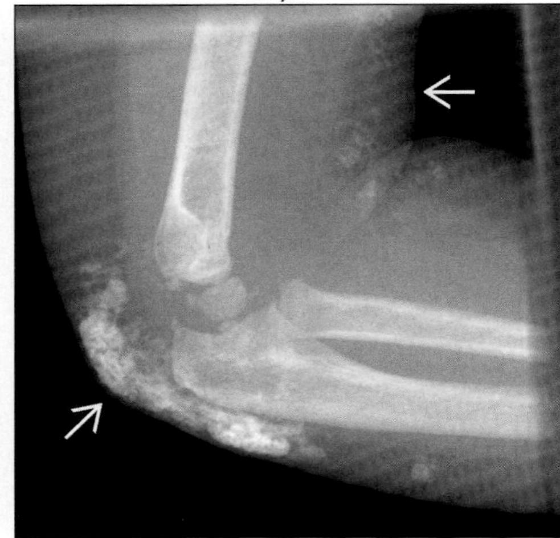

Other Collagen Vascular Diseases

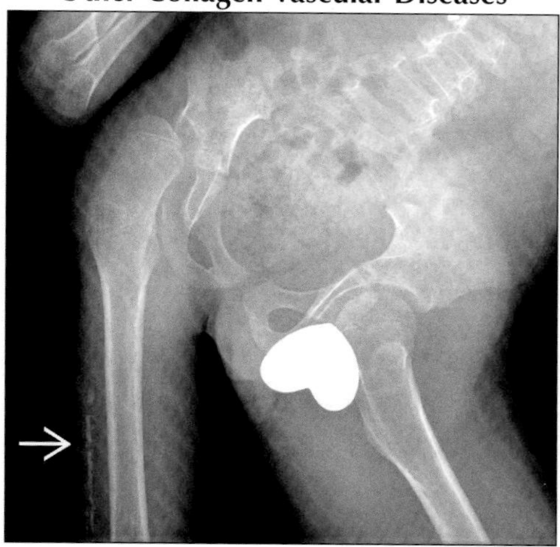

Neoplastic

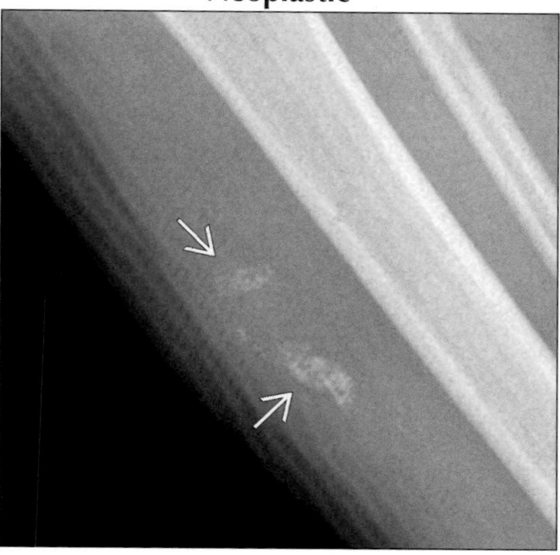

(Left) *Anteroposterior radiograph shows sheet-like calcifications ➡ within the lateral soft tissues of the right lateral thigh in this child with scleroderma. Soft tissue calcifications are seen in up to 1/4 of patients with scleroderma.* ***(Right)*** *Anteroposterior radiograph shows irregular calcifications ➡ within an soft tissue mass of the lower leg. Calcifications are seen in approximately 1/3 of synovial sarcoma tumors and are typically more irregular than venous malformations.*

Neoplastic

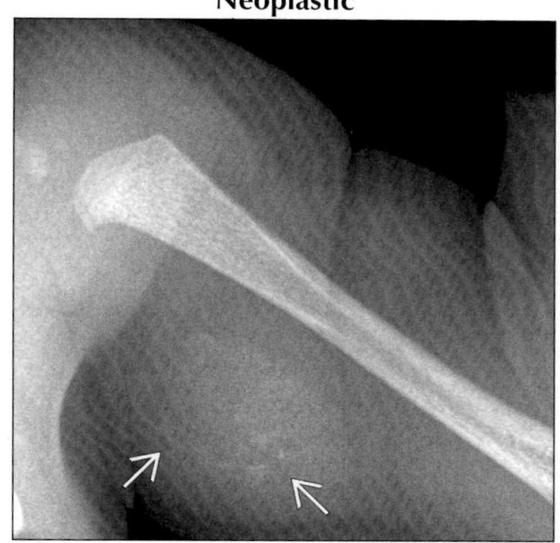

Metabolic/Hypercalcemia

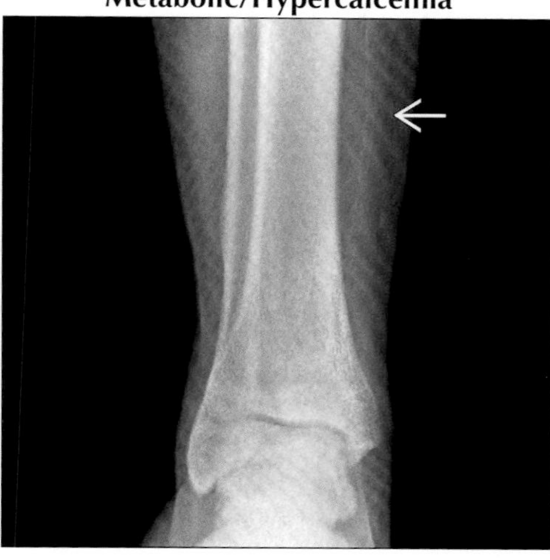

(Left) *Anteroposterior radiograph shows stippled calcifications ➡ in this upper extremity soft tissue mass. In this infant only 27 days old, the mass was pathologically proven to be infantile myofibromatosis.* ***(Right)*** *Anteroposterior radiograph shows diffuse vascular calcifications ➡. This patient had a history of chronic renal failure and was currently on hemodialysis. The left lower quadrant renal transplant (not shown) was no longer functioning.*

Metabolic/Hypercalcemia

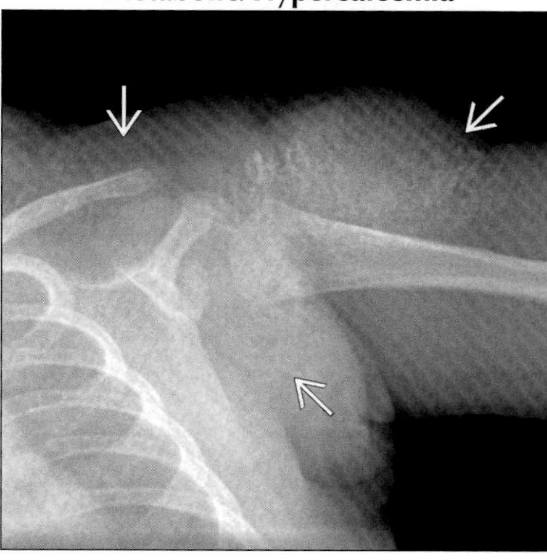

Parasitic

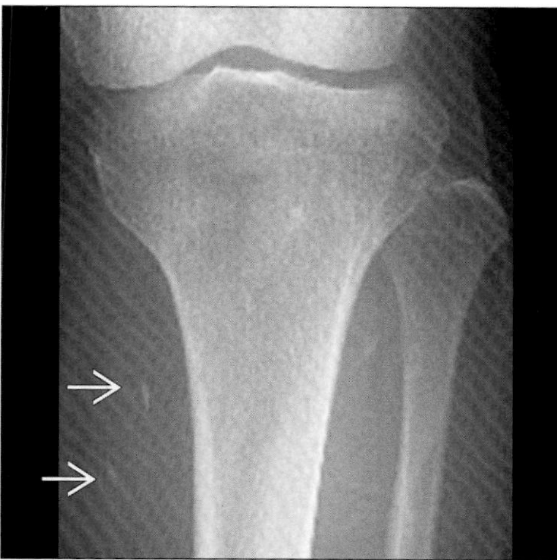

(Left) *Radiograph of the left shoulder shows diffuse soft tissue calcifications ➡. Diffuse calcifications of all extremities (not shown) were detected in this 7 week old with a large region of fat necrosis on the back.* ***(Right)*** *Anteroposterior radiograph shows multiple rice-shaped, calcified bodies in the soft tissues ➡. The size and shape of these bodies is typical for the parasitic infection of cysticercosis.*

CONGENITAL FOOT DEFORMITY

DIFFERENTIAL DIAGNOSIS

Common
- Metatarsus Adductus
- Pes Planovalgus (Flexible Flatfoot)
- Club Foot (Talipes Equinovarus)
- Tarsal Coalition

Less Common
- Congenital Vertical Talus (Rocker Bottom Foot)
- Pes Cavus (Mimic)
- Polio (Mimic)
- Cerebral Palsy (Mimic)

Rare but Important
- Metaphyseal Bar

ESSENTIAL INFORMATION

Key Differential Diagnosis Issues
- **Hint**: Do not attempt to diagnosis foot deformities without weight-bearing films
- **Hint**: Most congenital foot deformities can be diagnosed by evaluation of 3 relationships
  - Hindfoot equinus or calcaneus
    - On lateral radiograph, normal angle between lines bisecting calcaneus and tibia ranges between 60° and 90°
    - Hindfoot equinus: Tibiocalcaneal angle > 90° (excessive plantarflexion of calcaneus)
    - Hindfoot calcaneus: Tibiocalcaneal angle < 60° (excessive dorsiflexion of calcaneus); also termed "cavus"
  - Hindfoot varus or valgus
    - On lateral radiograph, normal angle between lines bisecting talus and calcaneus ranges between 25° and 55° (termed Kite angle or lateral talocalcaneal angle)
    - On AP radiograph, normal angle between lines bisecting talus and calcaneus ranges between 15° and 40°
    - Varus hindfoot: ↓ talocalcaneal angle (bones approach parallel), < 25° on lateral and < 15° on AP
    - Valgus hindfoot: ↑ talocalcaneal angle (bones diverge): > 55° on lateral and > 40° on AP
  - Forefoot varus or valgus
    - On lateral radiograph, metatarsals normally are moderately superimposed, with 5th in plantar-most position; angle of inclination of metatarsals gradually ↑ from 5° for 5th to 20° for 1st
    - On AP radiograph, metatarsals normally show moderate convergence of bases
    - Varus forefoot: Inversion and supination; on lateral, ↓ superimposition of metatarsals (ladder-like) with 5th MT in plantar-most position; on AP, ↑ overlap of MT bases
    - Valgus forefoot: Eversion and pronation; on lateral, ↑ superimposition of metatarsals with 1st MT in plantar-most position; on AP, ↓ convergence of MT bases
- **Hint**: Most congenital foot deformities match type of hindfoot and forefoot deformities
  - Varus hindfoot with varus forefoot
  - Valgus hindfoot with valgus forefoot
- **Hint**: If hindfoot and forefoot deformities are unmatched (i.e., varus hindfoot and valgus forefoot or valgus hindfoot and varus forefoot), usually due to spastic foot

Helpful Clues for Common Diagnoses
- **Metatarsus Adductus**
  - Most common structural foot abnormality of infants
  - Adduction of metatarsals; normal hindfoot
  - Rarely imaged, since it is flexible deformity and self-correcting
- **Pes Planovalgus (Flexible Flatfoot)**
  - Common (4% of population)
  - Note: It is **flexible**; non-weight-bearing radiographs are normal
  - Abnormalities on weight-bearing radiographs
    - Hindfoot valgus, forefoot valgus, **no** equinus
- **Club Foot (Talipes Equinovarus)**
  - Incidence 1:1,000 births
  - M > F = 2-3:1
  - Constant structural abnormalities
    - Hindfoot equinus, hindfoot varus, forefoot varus
- **Tarsal Coalition**
  - Painful flatfoot: Persistent or intermittent spasm of peroneal muscles

- Usually secondary to congenital lack of segmentation of bones of hindfoot
- Symptoms begin in late 1st or 2nd decade
- Secondary signs
  - Talar beak: Due to excessive motion at talonavicular joint because of rigid subtalar joint
  - "Ball and socket" tibiotalar joint: Conversion of this hinge joint to rounded articulation; generally due to unusually extensive subtalar coalition
- Calcaneonavicular coalition
  - Anterior process of calcaneus extends and broadens at union with navicular
  - Directly visualized on oblique radiograph
- Talonavicular coalition
  - Generally mid subtalar joint (sustentaculum tali) and not directly visualized
  - Diagnosed by CT or MR where this portion of subtalar joint is directly visualized on radiographs
  - Rarely will involve posterior &/or anterior subtalar facets
- 25% bilaterality

Helpful Clues for Less Common Diagnoses

- **Congenital Vertical Talus (Rocker Bottom Foot)**
  - Rigid flatfoot
  - Isolated, or part of several syndromes (frequently associated with meningomyelocele)
  - Constant structural abnormalities
    - Hindfoot equinus
    - Hindfoot valgus
    - Plantarflexed talus, dislocated from navicular
    - Forefoot valgus
- **Pes Cavus (Mimic)**
  - Multiple etiologies; none are strictly congenital, hence "mimic" designation
    - Upper motor neuron lesions (Friedrich ataxia)
    - Lower motor neuron lesions (poliomyelitis)
    - Vascular ischemia, Charcot-Marie-Tooth, Chinese bound foot
- **Polio (Mimic) and Cerebral Palsy (Mimic)**
  - Spastic abnormalities, often with mismatch of hindfoot and forefoot abnormalities (varus-valgus)
  - Soft tissues show muscle atrophy

Helpful Clues for Rare Diagnoses

- **Metaphyseal Bar**
  - a.k.a. longitudinally bracketed epiphysis or δ phalanx
  - Rare congenital link between proximal and distal epiphyses of 1st metatarsal
  - Link is on medial side, resulting in curved 1st MT, concave medially
  - Clinical appearance is of metatarsus adductus, but deformity is rigid

Pes Planovalgus (Flexible Flatfoot)

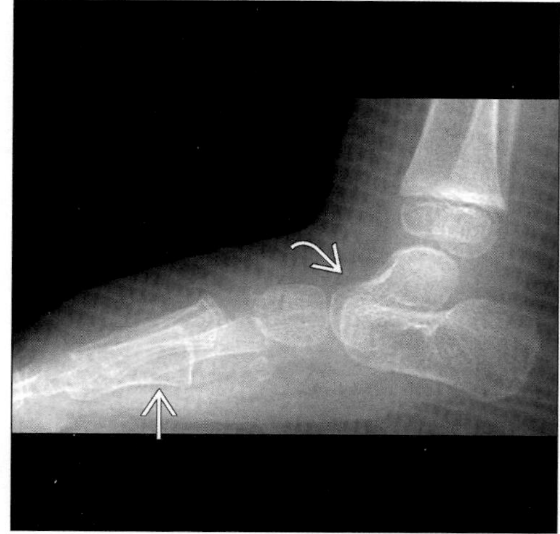

Lateral radiograph shows increased plantar flexion of the talus ➡, forming hindfoot valgus. There is also pronation of the forefoot, with superimposition of the metatarsals & decreased inclination angle of MT 1-3 ➡.

Pes Planovalgus (Flexible Flatfoot)

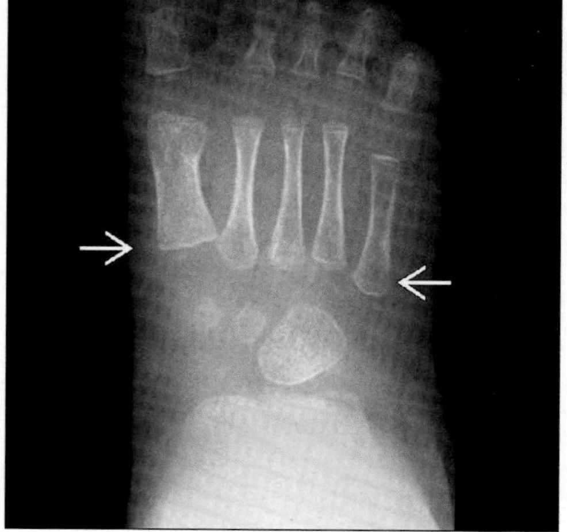

AP radiograph in the same patient shows a wide T-C angle (hindfoot valgus), with lack of convergence at the metatarsal bases ➡ (forefoot pronation/valgus). The abnormalities reduce on non-weight-bearing.

CONGENITAL FOOT DEFORMITY

(Left) AP radiograph shows near superimposition of talus ➔ and calcaneus ➔ (decreased talocalcaneal angle, hindfoot varus). There is increased convergence at the bases of the metatarsals ➔, typical of forefoot supination/varus. ***(Right)*** *Lateral radiograph in the same patient shows equinus of the calcaneus ➔. The calcaneus & talus are nearly parallel, confirming hindfoot varus. The forefoot shows severe supination, with the metatarsals ➔ appearing stacked, typical of clubfoot.*

Club Foot (Talipes Equinovarus)

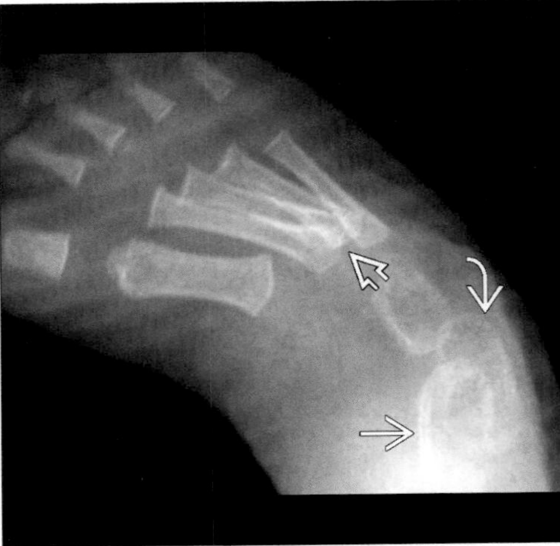

Club Foot (Talipes Equinovarus)

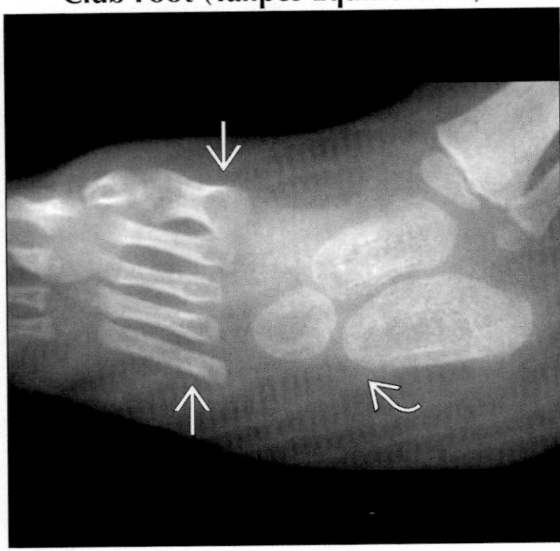

(Left) *Lateral radiograph shows the "anteater" sign of an elongated anterior process of the calcaneus ➔. This long process extends to the navicular and is highly suggestive of calcaneonavicular coalition. In this case, there is no talar beak.* ***(Right)*** *Oblique radiograph confirms the calcaneonavicular coalition ➔. This type of coalition can usually be diagnosed with oblique radiograph. If there is further question, CT is confirmatory.*

Tarsal Coalition

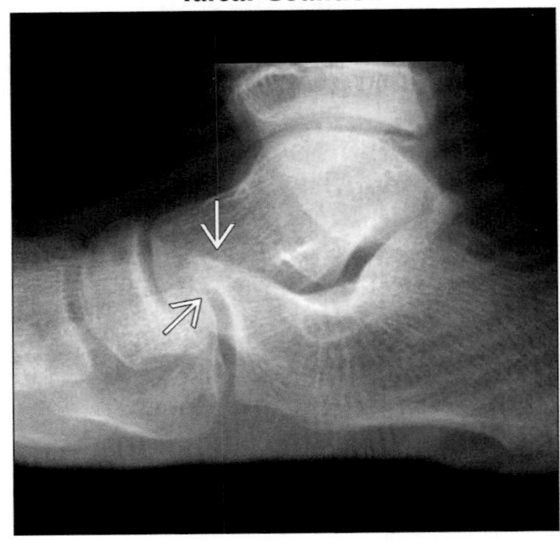

Tarsal Coalition

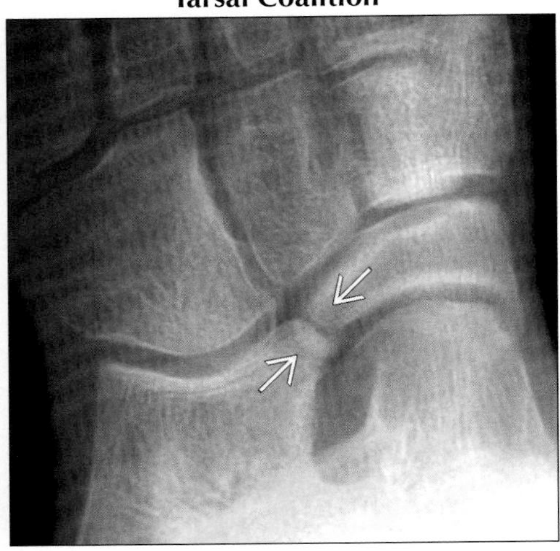

(Left) *Lateral radiograph shows a large talar beak ➔, a secondary sign of tarsal coalition. The coalition itself is not seen, but there is a sclerotic "C" sign in the region of the subtalar joint ➔, which is highly suggestive.* ***(Right)*** *Angled axial bone CT shows the broad and sclerotic talocalcaneal coalition at the middle facet ➔, compared with the normal left side ➔. Talocalcaneal coalitions most frequently involve this portion of the subtalar joint.*

Tarsal Coalition

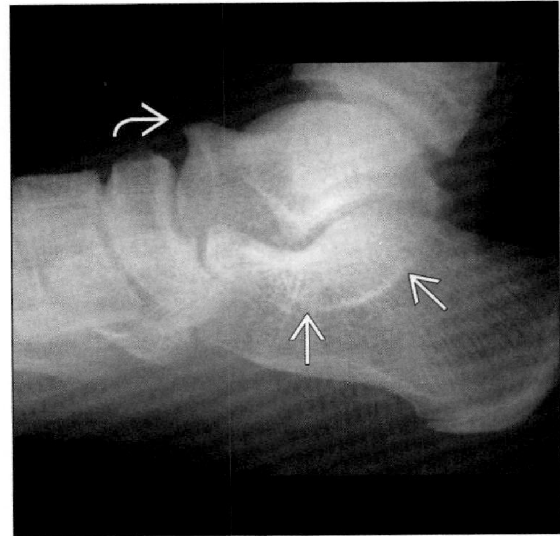

Tarsal Coalition

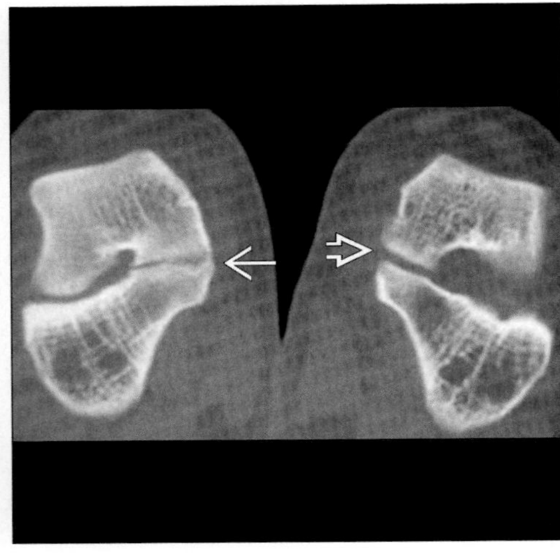

Congenital Vertical Talus (Rocker Bottom Foot)

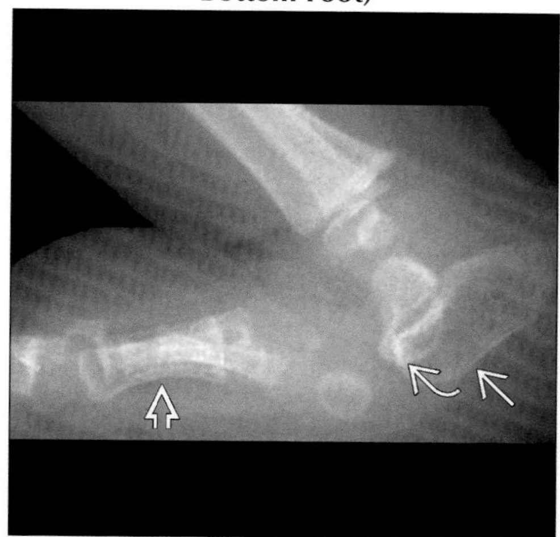

Congenital Vertical Talus (Rocker Bottom Foot)

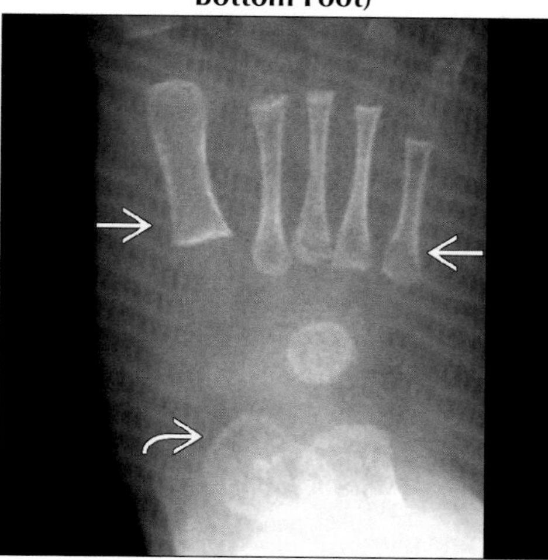

*(**Left**) Lateral radiograph shows all the elements of congenital vertical talus, including calcaneal equinus ➡ & hindfoot valgus. Note the severe plantar flexion of the talus ➡, contributing to the valgus. The forefoot is severely pronated ➡. (**Right**) AP radiograph in the same patient shows ↑ talocalcaneal angle with severe medial angulation of the talus ➡. There is pronation/valgus of the forefoot with lack of convergence at the MT bases ➡.*

Pes Cavus (Mimic)

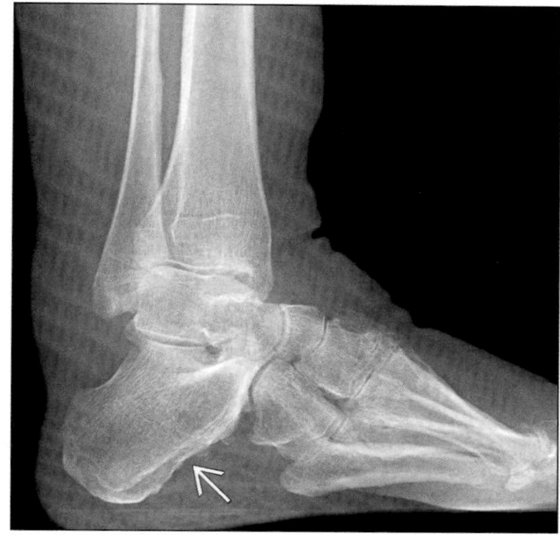

Polio (Mimic)

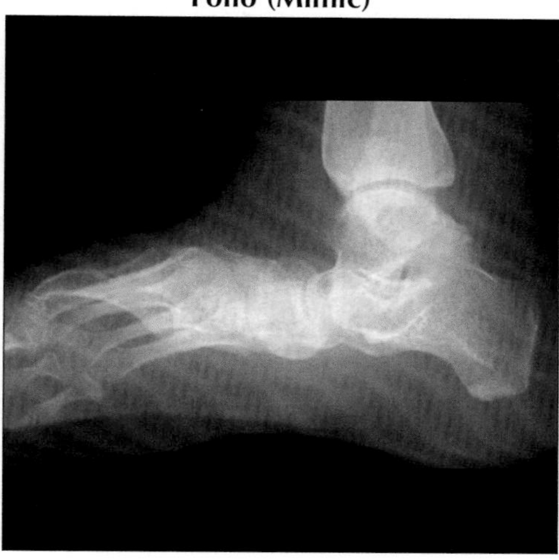

*(**Left**) Lateral radiograph shows abnormal dorsiflexion of the calcaneus ➡ and varus deformity of the forefoot. This cavovarus pattern is typically seen in Charcot-Marie-Tooth, as in this case, but may be seen with other spastic conditions as well. (**Right**) Lateral radiograph shows a mixed pattern of hindfoot valgus (increased talocalcaneal angle) and forefoot varus/supination. This unusual combination is seen in spastic conditions, including polio.*

Cerebral Palsy (Mimic)

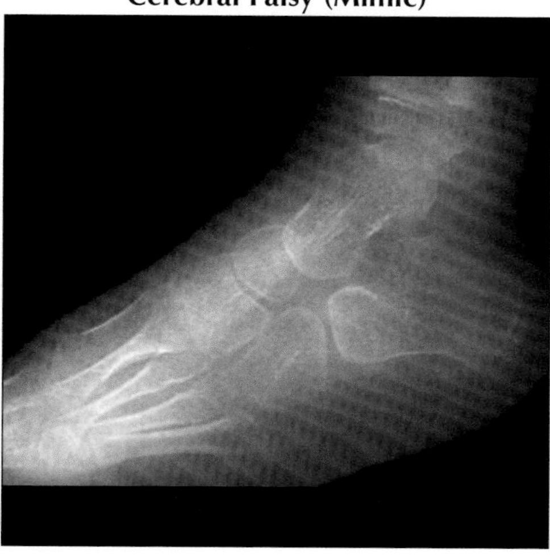

Metaphyseal Bar

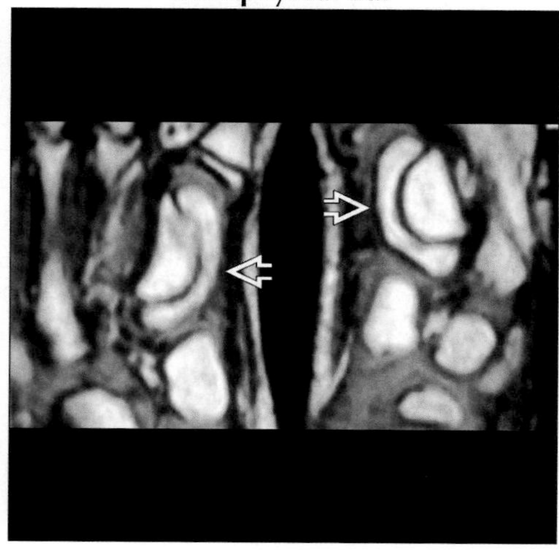

*(**Left**) Lateral radiograph shows equinus of the calcaneus, valgus hindfoot, and supinated forefoot. This is another pattern of a spastic foot, this time in a patient with cerebral palsy. (**Right**) Axial T1WI MR shows bridging bone extending from the proximal to distal epiphysis, across the diaphysis of the 1st metatarsal ➡. It is bilaterally symmetric and causes bowing and shortening of the bone. It results in overall fixed metatarsus adductus.*

ARTHRITIS IN A TEENAGER

DIFFERENTIAL DIAGNOSIS

Common

- Juvenile Idiopathic Arthritis (JIA)
- Ankylosing Spondylitis (AS)
- Psoriatic Arthritis
- Septic Joint
- Pigmented Villonodular Synovitis (PVNS)
- Femoral Acetabular Impingement (FAI)
- Developmental Dysplasia of Hip

Less Common

- Hemophilia: MSK Complications
- Synovial Osteochondromatosis
- Legg-Calvé-Perthes, Secondary Changes
- Chronic Reactive Arthritis
- Inflammatory Bowel Disease Arthritis
- Osteoid Osteoma of Hip, 2° Changes

Rare but Important

- Congenital Insensitivity/Indifference to Pain

ESSENTIAL INFORMATION

Key Differential Diagnosis Issues

- Surprising number of arthridities originate during childhood or teenage years
- Early and accurate diagnosis is important to initiate treatment and avoid later debilitating joint disease

Helpful Clues for Common Diagnoses

- **Juvenile Idiopathic Arthritis (JIA)**
  - May have 1 of several manifestations
    - 5% appear indistinguishable from adult rheumatoid arthritis (RA); most become seropositive
    - 40% are pauciarticular, affecting knee, elbow, and ankle most frequently; seronegative; 25% develop iridocyclitis
    - 20% have Still disease: Acute systemic disease with fever, anemia, hepatosplenomegaly; 25% of these have polyarticular destructive arthritis, affecting small and large joints alike
    - 25% have seronegative polyarticular disease, symmetric & widespread in adult distribution; no systemic complaints & seronegative
  - Specific features generally distinguishing JIA from other teenage arthridities
    - Enlarged metaphyses and epiphyses ("balloon joints") due to overgrowth, secondary to hyperemia from inflammatory process
    - Cartilage narrowing & widened notches related to pannus formation & erosion
    - Often asymmetric
  - Other distinguishing features
    - Periostitis may be 1st manifestation in young child
    - Fusion frequently occurs in carpals
    - Interbody fusion in cervical spine limits growth of vertebral bodies, giving "waisted" appearance
- **Ankylosing Spondylitis (AS)**
  - Earliest manifestations (clinical and radiographic) occur during teenage years
  - Spinal manifestations initiate radiographic disease process
    - Osteitis at anterior corners of vertebral bodies
    - SI joint widening and erosions; may be asymmetric initially
    - Teenagers normally have wide SI joints with indistinct cortices; do not overcall!
  - Appendicular disease most frequently is in large proximal joints, particularly hips; may be erosive or productive
- **Psoriatic Arthritis**
  - 30-50% of psoriatic patients develop spondyloarthropathy
    - Bilateral asymmetric erosive disease; may eventually fuse
  - 20% of psoriatic patients develop arthropathy prior to skin and nail changes
  - Distinguishing features
    - May have "sausage" digit with periostitis
    - DIP disease predominates; hands > feet
    - Aggressive erosive disease ("pencil-in-cup") and eventual fusion
- **Septic Joint**
  - Monostotic; cartilage damage and osseous deformity eventually leads to secondary osteoarthritis
  - If longstanding & slow process in child (especially tuberculous or fungal septic joint), hyperemia leads to overgrowth of epiphyses & metaphyses: "Balloon" joint
- **Pigmented Villonodular Synovitis (PVNS)**
  - Monoarticular; nodular mass or nodules lining synovium

- Causes erosion if longstanding
- Large effusion; iron deposition results in foci of low signal, which bloom on GRE

- **Femoral Acetabular Impingement (FAI)**
  - Often bilateral abnormalities, though complaints usually begin unilaterally
  - Morphologic abnormalities of femoral head, neck, or acetabulum → impingement
    - Lateral femoral neck "bump," limiting normal head/neck cutback: Cam type
    - Acetabular rim overgrowth or retroversion: Pincer type
    - Multiple etiologies: Trauma, DDH, SCFE
    - → labral tear and cartilage damage → early osteoarthritis
    - Onset of complaints 2nd or 3rd decade
- **Developmental Dysplasia of Hip**
  - Multiple types of dysplasia
    - Shallow acetabulum
    - Femoral varus or valgus
    - Acetabular or femoral retroversion
  - Develop labral hypertrophy; with shear stress, labrum tears; eventual cartilage damage and early osteoarthritis

Helpful Clues for Less Common Diagnoses

- **Hemophilia: MSK Complications**
  - Similar appearance to JIA, with "balloon" overgrowth of epiphyses/metaphyses due to hyperemia
  - Pauciarticular; knee > elbow > ankle
  - Hemosiderin deposits lead to low signal on MR, "blooming" on GRE sequence
- **Chronic Reactive Arthritis**
  - Rare compared with psoriatic arthritis; appendicular manifestations usually foot/ankle
- **Inflammatory Bowel Disease Arthritis**
  - Less frequent, but manifestations are similar to AS
- **Osteoid Osteoma of Hip, 2° Changes**
  - Intraarticular OO elicits synovitis → subluxation of joint → altered weight bearing & development of osteophytes

Alternative Differential Approaches

- Consider number of joints involved (some diagnoses belong in more than 1)
  - Monoarticular
    - Septic joint
    - Pigmented villonodular synovitis (PVNS)
    - Synovial osteochondromatosis
    - Osteoid osteoma of hip, 2° changes
  - Pauciarticular
    - Juvenile idiopathic arthritis (JIA)
    - Ankylosing spondylitis
    - Psoriatic arthritis
    - Femoral acetabular impingement (FAI)
    - Developmental dysplasia of hip
    - Hemophilia: MSK complications
    - Legg-Calvé-Perthes, secondary changes
    - Chronic reactive arthritis
    - Inflammatory bowel disease arthritis
    - Congenital insensitivity/indifference to pain
  - Polyarticular
    - Juvenile idiopathic arthritis (JIA)
    - Psoriatic arthritis

Juvenile Idiopathic Arthritis (JIA)

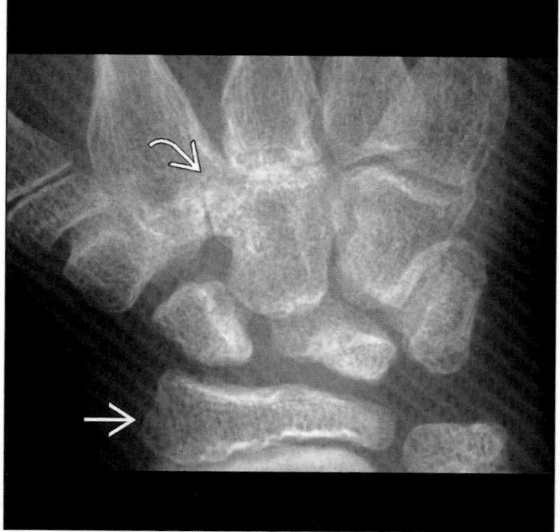

AP radiograph shows a combination of overgrowth of the radial epiphysis ➡ and erosions with fusion at the carpometacarpal joint ➡. This combination indicates hyperemia plus an inflammatory arthritis, typical of JIA.

Ankylosing Spondylitis (AS)

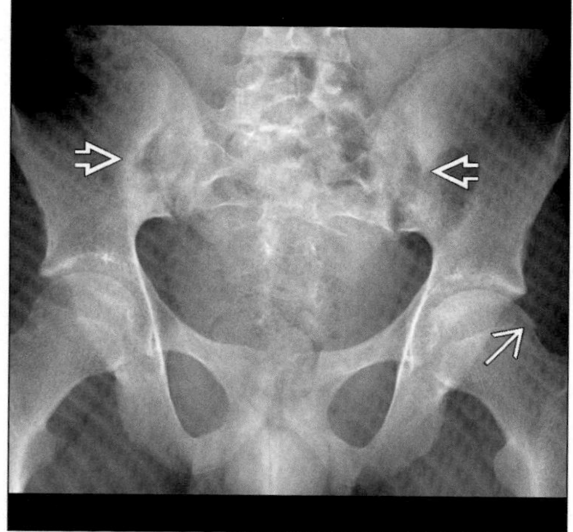

AP radiograph shows bilateral widening and erosion of the sacroiliac joints ➡, as well as a small osteophyte on the femoral neck ➡. This 18-year-old male has had back pain for 3 years; findings are typical of AS.

ARTHRITIS IN A TEENAGER

(Left) AP x-ray shows near complete loss of cartilage in this 17 yo female's hip ➡, with mild erosive change. There were hand and foot erosions, but also 1 site of periostitis and unilateral sacroiliitis (not shown). The patient developed psoriatic skin changes within a year. *(Right) AP radiograph shows a chronic septic hip ➡ in a teenager with L2 paraplegia and chronic decubitus ulcer leading to the hip joint. There is complete cartilage destruction, with associated osseous deformity.*

Psoriatic Arthritis

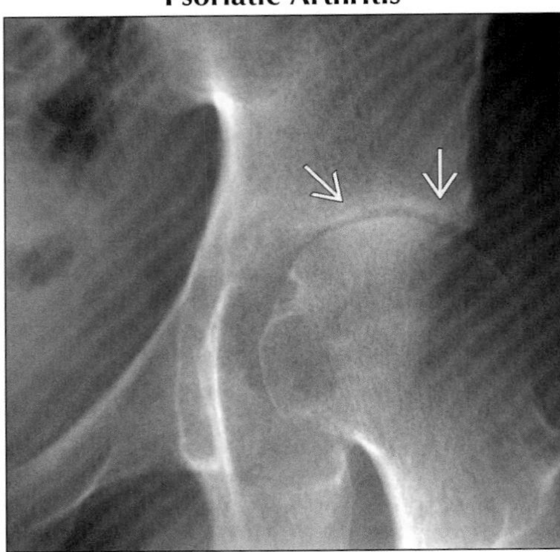

Septic Joint

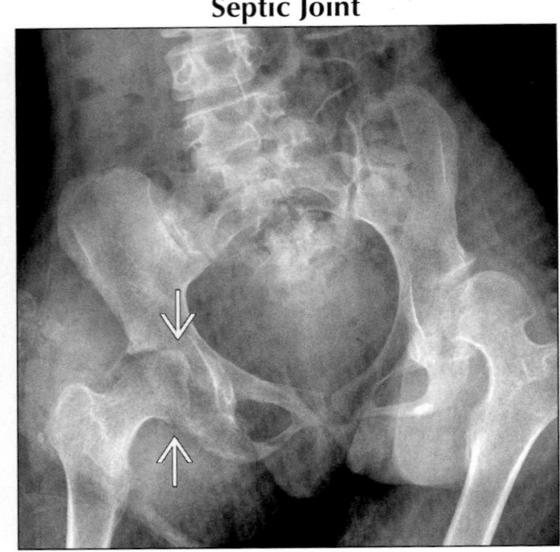

(Left) Coronal T2WI MR shows a huge glenoid erosion ➡ in a 15 yo. Note nodular synovial masses scattered throughout joint ⇨. Appearance is typical for PVNS, proven at biopsy. *(Right) AP radiograph shows a bump at the lateral femoral junction of the head and neck ➡, eliminating the normal cutback at this site. This configuration puts the patient at risk for cam-type FAI; this 20 yo already had a labral tear and cartilage damage, despite minimally abnormal appearance.*

Pigmented Villonodular Synovitis (PVNS)

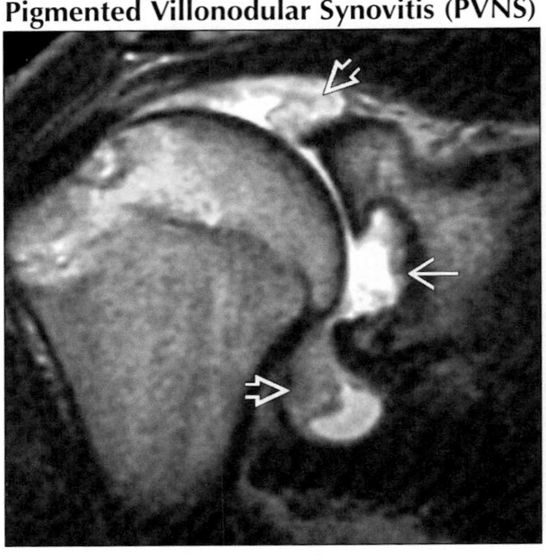

Femoral Acetabular Impingement (FAI)

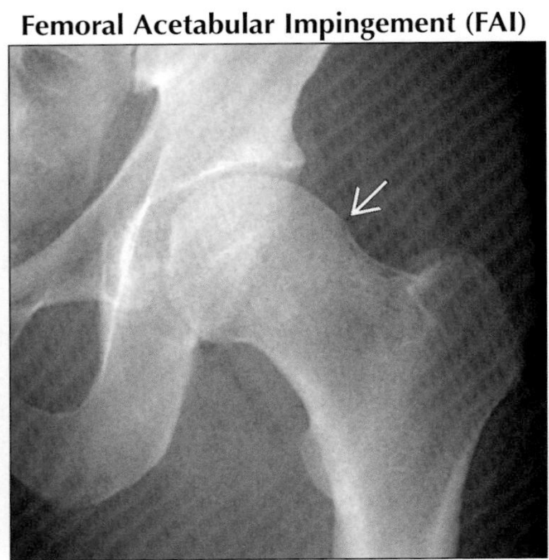

(Left) AP radiograph in a 15 yo shows severe DDH, with a shallow acetabulum, superolateral subluxation of the femoral head, and coxa magna deformity. Patient is developing a painful arthritis. *(Right) Lateral radiograph shows a large dense effusion ➡. There is erosive change throughout the joint. Note the overgrowth of the epiphyses, particularly the femoral condyles and patella. This overgrowth is due to chronic hyperemia from multiple hemophilic bleeds.*

Developmental Dysplasia of Hip

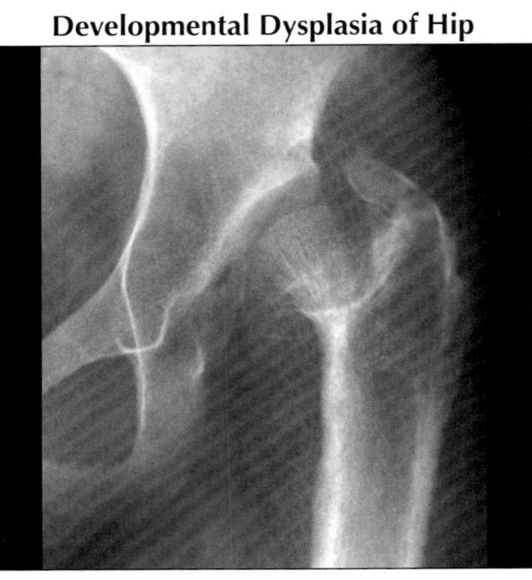

Hemophilia: MSK Complications

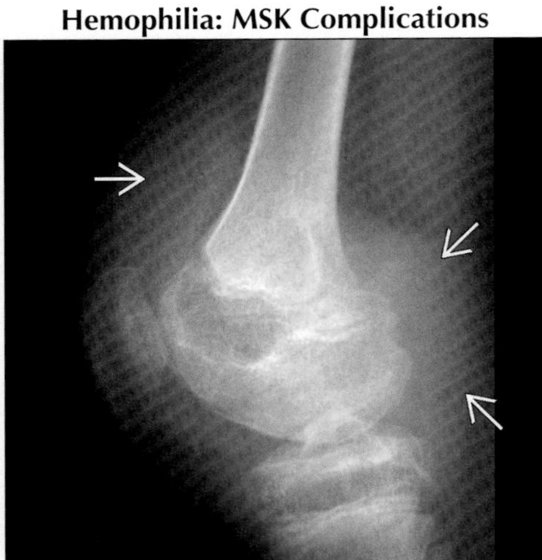

ARTHRITIS IN A TEENAGER

Synovial Osteochondromatosis

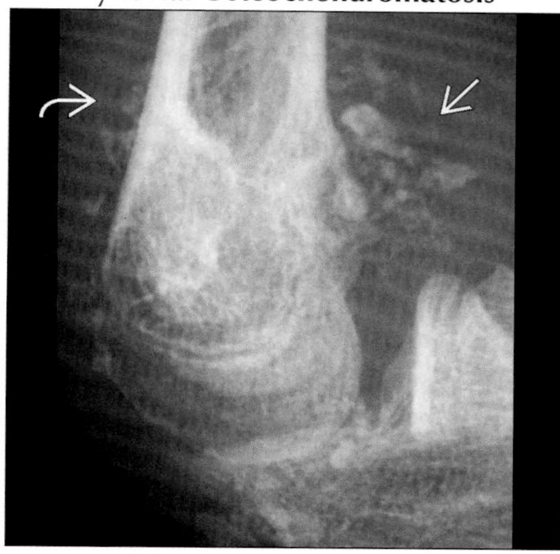

Legg-Calvé-Perthes, Secondary Changes

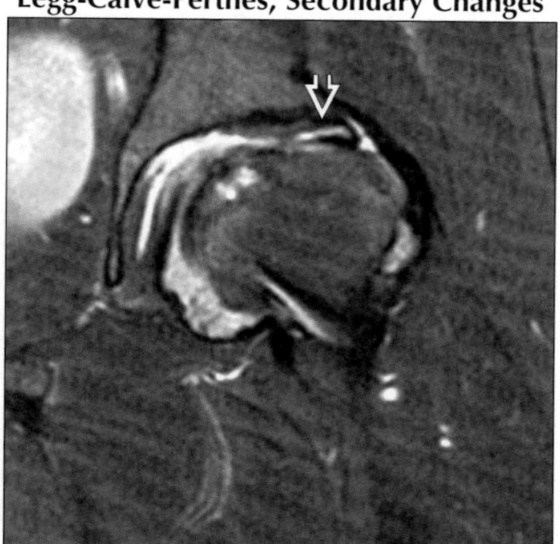

*(**Left**) Lateral radiograph shows multiple loose bodies within a distended elbow joint of a 12 yo. Note the bodies distending the anterior → as well as posterior → fat pads. Synovial osteochondromatosis is unusual in children but not rare. (**Right**) Coronal T2WI FS MR in this 15 yo with LCP shows findings of secondary arthritis, with a large labral tear →, subchondral cysts, and diffuse cartilage loss. This is a severely damaged hip.*

Chronic Reactive Arthritis

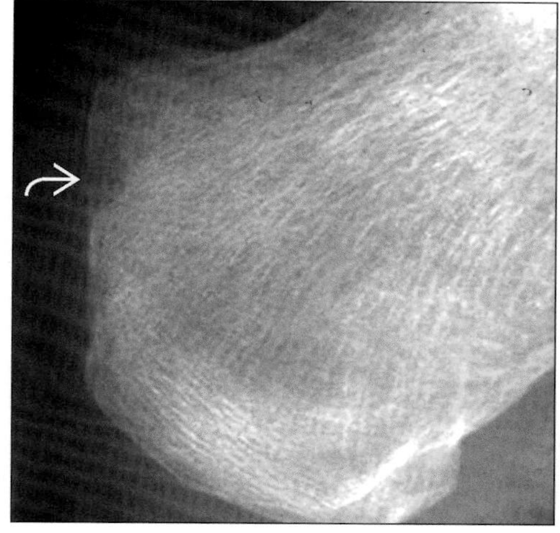

Inflammatory Bowel Disease Arthritis

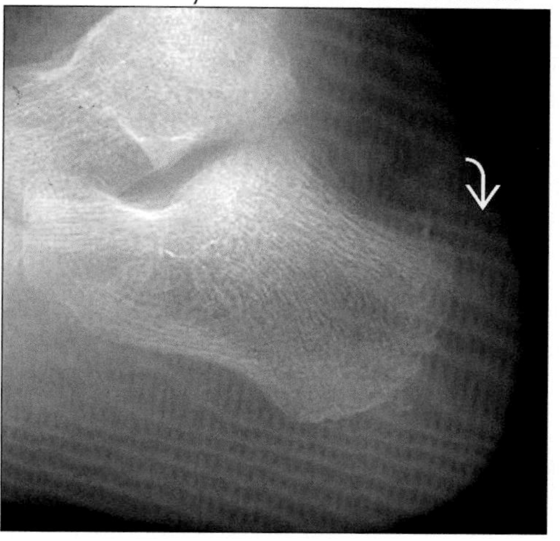

*(**Left**) Lateral radiograph shows early erosion of the posterior calcaneus →. There is also soft tissue inflammatory change, which obliterates the pre-Achilles fat pad. These are early heel changes in a 19 yo with chronic reactive arthritis. (**Right**) Lateral radiography shows soft tissue swelling and inflammatory change at the posterior calcaneus → in a 10 yo who had diarrhea for 3 months. The heel is so painful that he cannot walk. This is inflammatory bowel disease arthropathy.*

Osteoid Osteoma of Hip, 2° Changes

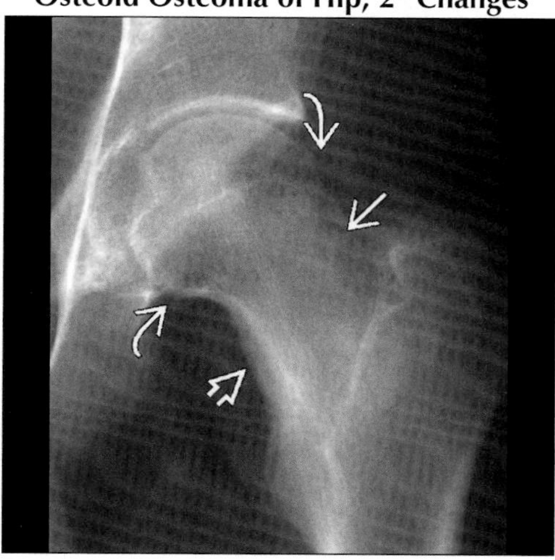

Congenital Insensitivity/Indifference to Pain

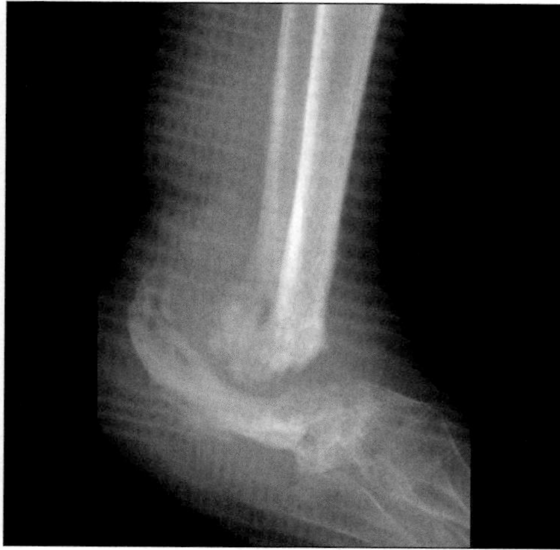

*(**Left**) AP radiograph in a 17 yo shows surprising findings of femoral neck osteophytes → & calcar buttressing →. These relate to the chronic synovitis developed in conjunction with an intraarticular osteoid osteoma, faintly seen in the neck →. (†MSK Req). (**Right**) Lateral radiograph in a 16 yo shows severe destruction of the foot and ankle. He had congenital indifference to pain (felt pain with ambulation but continued to walk on it, destroying the joints).*

BONE AGE, DELAYED

DIFFERENTIAL DIAGNOSIS

Common

- Constitutional Delay of Puberty (Normal Variant)
- Chronic Disease
  - Chronic Liver Disease
  - Renal Osteodystrophy
  - Congenital Heart Disease
  - Rickets
  - Juvenile Idiopathic Arthritis
  - Thalassemia
  - Cerebral Palsy
- Excessive Exercise
- Malnutrition
  - Anorexia
  - Malabsorption Conditions
- Complications of Steroids
- Fetal Alcohol Syndrome

Less Common

- Lead Poisoning
- Down Syndrome (Trisomy 21)
- Cushing Disease
- Hypopituitarism
- Pseudohypoparathyroidism
- Craniopharyngioma

Rare but Important

- HIV-AIDS: MSK Complications
- Growth Hormone Deficiency
- Hypogonadism
- Hypothyroidism
- Warfarin Embryopathy

ESSENTIAL INFORMATION

Key Differential Diagnosis Issues

- Skeletal maturation more than 2 standard deviations below mean
  - Formally evaluated with serial PA radiographs of left hand
  - Standards of Greulich and Pyle classically used for comparison

Helpful Clues for Common Diagnoses

- Majority of common diagnoses cause delayed bone age due to delay of puberty
  - Identifiable by clinical history

Helpful Clues for Less Common Diagnoses

- **Lead Poisoning**
  - Widened metaphyses, dense metaphyseal lines
- **Down Syndrome (Trisomy 21)**
  - Additional findings: Flared iliac wing, flat acetabular roof, clinodactyly, microcephaly, atlantoaxial instability

Helpful Clues for Rare Diagnoses

- **Hypogonadism**
  - Results in long limbs with disproportionally short trunk

Alternative Differential Approaches

- Stippled epiphyses: Hypothyroidism, warfarin embryopathy, chondrodysplasia punctata, multiple epiphyseal dysplasia, trisomy 21, trisomy 18, prenatal infection, Morquio syndrome

Chronic Disease

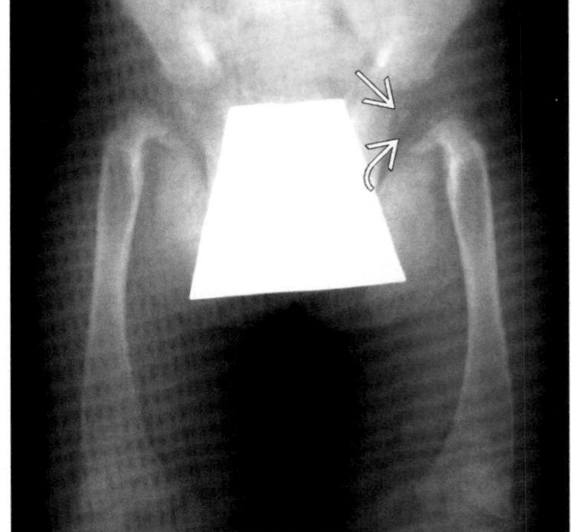

AP radiograph shows delayed skeletal maturation in this 5 year old. Note the tiny femoral head ossification centers ➔. The widened metaphyses ➔ indicate rickets in this patient with long-term renal disease.

Renal Osteodystrophy

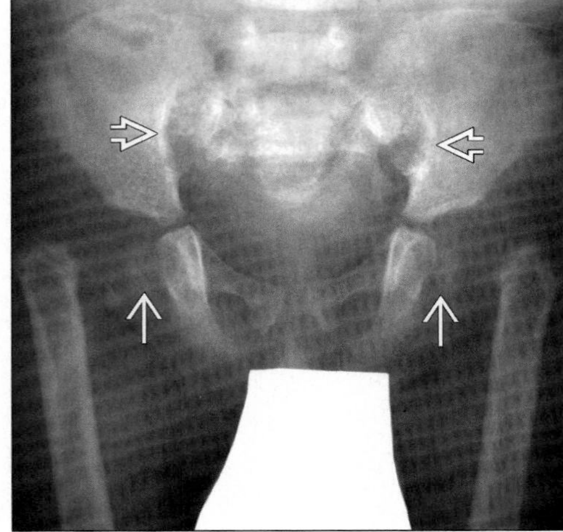

AP radiograph shows subchondral resorption at the SIJ ➔ and slipped capital femoral epiphyses from rickets ➔ in this 10 year old with renal osteodystrophy. The skeletal maturation is severely delayed.

BONE AGE, DELAYED

Rickets

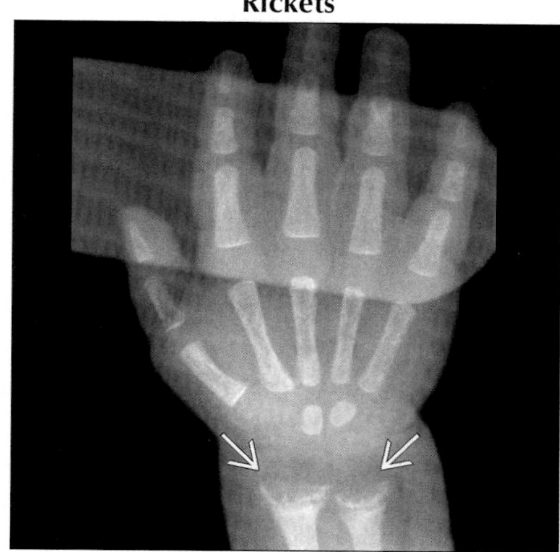

Juvenile Idiopathic Arthritis

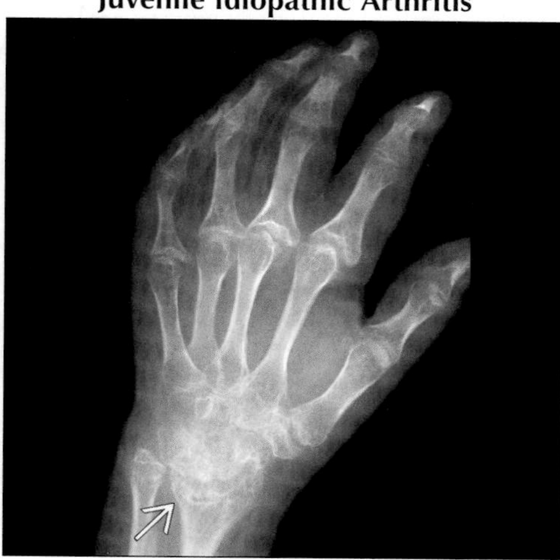

*(**Left**) Posteroanterior radiograph shows the widened zone of provisional calcification with frayed, cupped metaphysis at the distal radius and ulna ➡, typical of rickets. Note that despite the chronologic age of 1 year, the skeletal maturation is severely delayed. (**Right**) Posteroanterior radiograph shows an open physis ➡ in a 22-year-old patient with JIA, indicating delayed bone age. Note the fused carpals and significant metacarpal erosive disease.*

Excessive Exercise

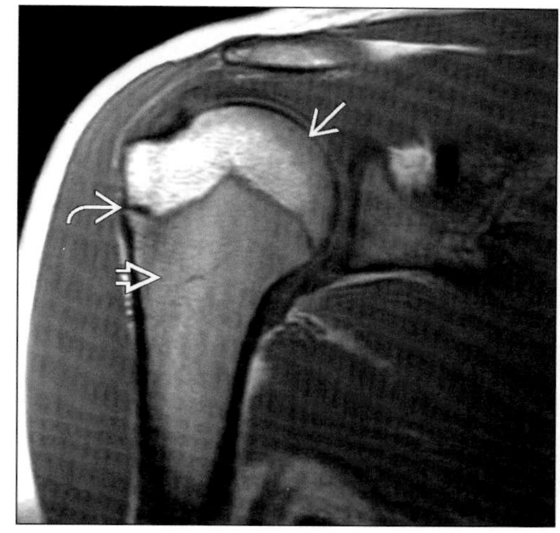

Excessive Exercise

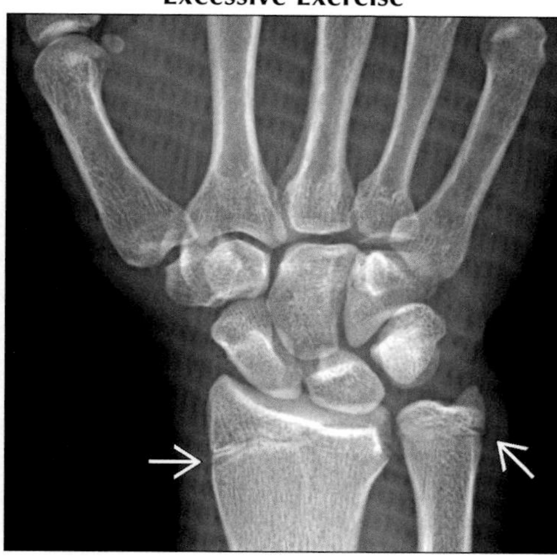

*(**Left**) Coronal T1WI MR shows open physis ➡, as well as immature bone marrow distribution with a crescent of red marrow in the epiphysis ➡ and solid red marrow in the metadiaphysis ➡. The patient is a 19-year-old competitive gymnast who practices 5 hours daily. (**Right**) PA radiograph of the wrist in the same patient, shows open physes at the distal radius and ulna ➡. This patient is at least 2 standard deviations younger than her chronologic age.*

Thalassemia

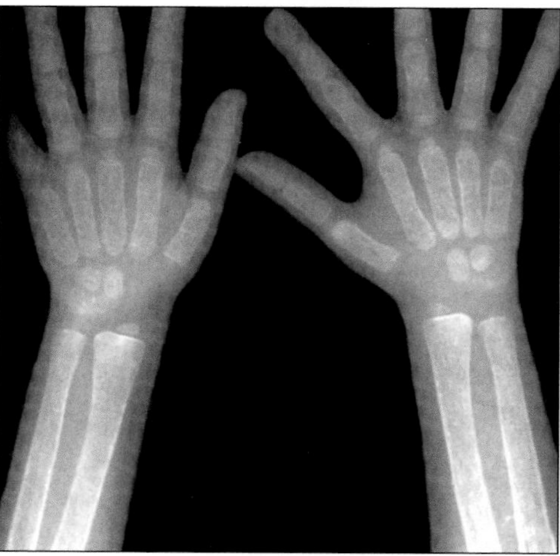

Lead Poisoning

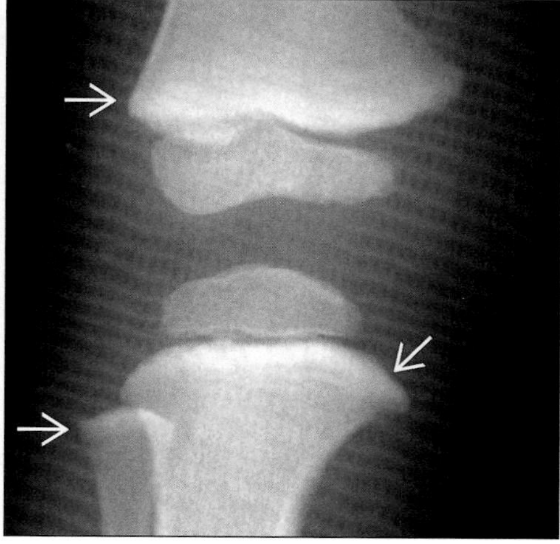

*(**Left**) Anteroposterior radiograph shows the squared bones, indicating severe marrow packing in a patient with thalassemia. This 5 year old also shows delayed bone age, related to the chronicity of the disease. (**Right**) Anteroposterior radiograph shows the dense metaphyseal lines ➡ resulting from deposition of lead during growth. Chronic lead poisoning can lead to a delay in skeletal maturation.*

BONE AGE, ADVANCED

DIFFERENTIAL DIAGNOSIS

Common
- Familial Tall Stature
- Idiopathic Precocious Puberty
- Excessive Sex Hormone
- Juvenile Idiopathic Arthritis (JIA)
- Hemophilia
- Physeal Fractures
- Radiation-Induced Growth Deformities

Less Common
- Hyperthyroidism
- Hypothalamic Mass
- Pituitary Gigantism
- Adrenocortical Tumor
- Adrenal Hyperplasia
- Exogenous Obesity
- Ectopic Gonadotropin Tumor
- Polyostotic Fibrous Dysplasia, McCune-Albright

Rare but Important
- Chronic Septic Arthritis, Nonbacterial
- Encephalitis
- Primary Hyperaldosteronism
- Beckwith-Wiedemann Syndrome

ESSENTIAL INFORMATION

Key Differential Diagnosis Issues
- Skeletal maturation more than 2 standard deviations above mean
- Determining etiology highly dependent on lab findings and clinical presentation
- Marked advancement in bone age is more likely to indicate elevated sex hormones

Helpful Clues for Common Diagnoses
- **Excessive Sex Hormone**
  - Induces early growth plate maturation
- **Juvenile Idiopathic Arthritis (JIA)**
  - Chronic hyperemia causes growth centers to ossify early, enlarge, & fuse prematurely
- **Hemophilia**
  - Similar JIA, + dense effusion
- **Radiation-Induced Growth Deformities**
  - Vascular obliteration → premature fusion
  - Associated with bone hypoplasia, slipped capital femoral epiphysis, scoliosis
  - Watch for port-like distribution
  - Associated radiation-induced sarcoma

Helpful Clues for Less Common Diagnoses
- **Hypothalamic Mass**
  - Early onset of normal maturation process
  - Hypothalamic hamartoma or mass effect from suprasellar tumors
- **Adrenocortical Tumor or Hyperplasia**
  - Hypersecretion of androgens and cortisol
- **Ectopic Gonadotropin Tumor**
  - Hepatoblastoma/teratoma/chorioepithelioma
- **Polyostotic Fibrous Dysplasia, McCune-Albright**
  - "Ground-glass" bone lesions + café-au-lait spots + precocious puberty

Other Essential Information
- MR brain to exclude hypothalamic lesion
- Pelvic ultrasound (females) for evidence of gonadotropin/estrogen stimulation

Juvenile Idiopathic Arthritis (JIA)

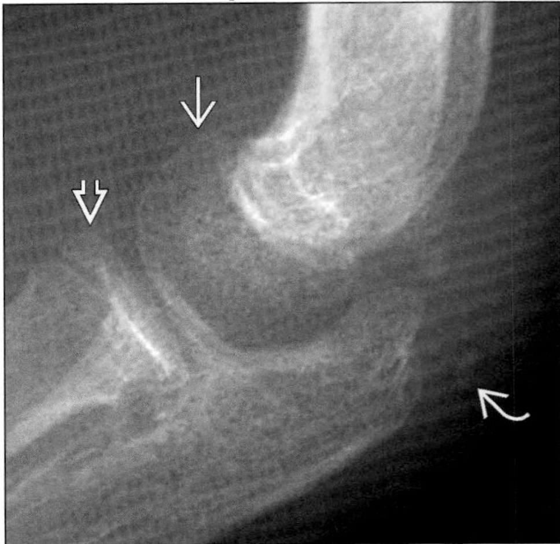

Lateral radiograph of the affected left elbow shows advanced skeletal maturation in the capitellum ➡, radial head ➡, & olecranon ➡. This early skeletal maturation is due to chronic hyperemia. (†MSK Req).

Juvenile Idiopathic Arthritis (JIA)

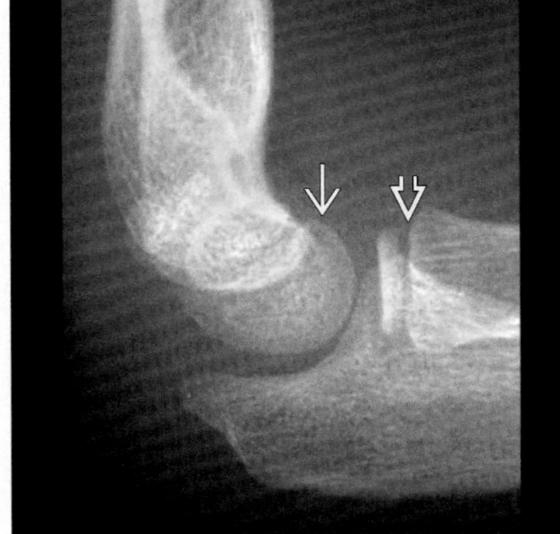

Lateral radiograph shows the unaffected right elbow in the same patient, for comparison. The capitellum ➡ and radial head ➡ are normal. (†MSK Req).

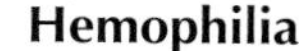

Hemophilia

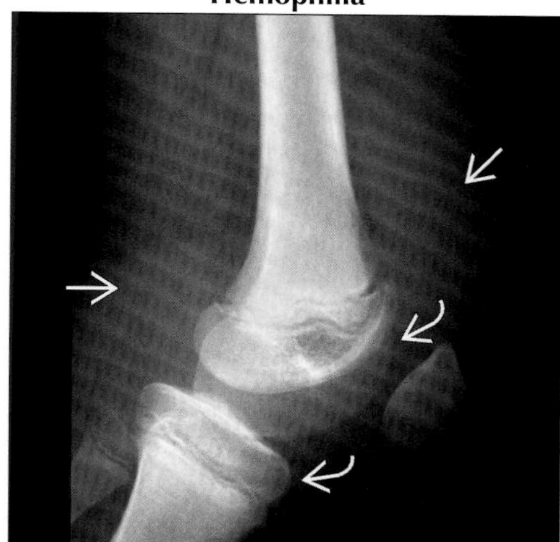

Hemophilia

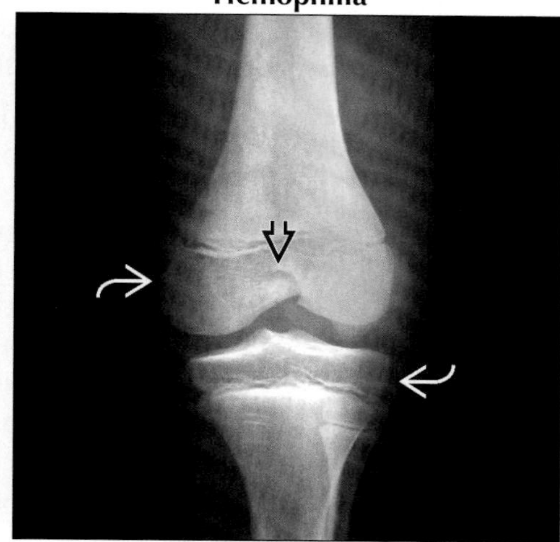

(Left) *Lateral radiograph of a knee of a teenager shows a huge effusion → and overgrowth of the epiphyses →, with the femoral condyles particularly enlarged, in a male patient with hemophilia.* ***(Right)*** *Anteroposterior radiograph of the same knee as previous image, shows epiphyseal overgrowth → and intercondylar notch widening ⇨, which can be seen with hemophilia or juvenile idiopathic arthritis. The bone age was advanced.*

Physeal Fractures

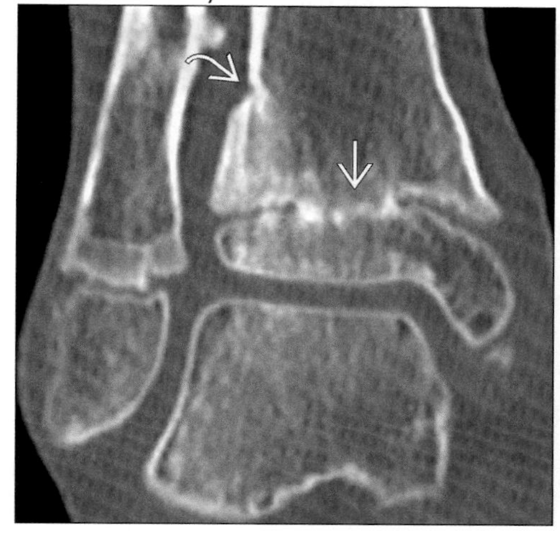

Radiation-Induced Growth Deformities

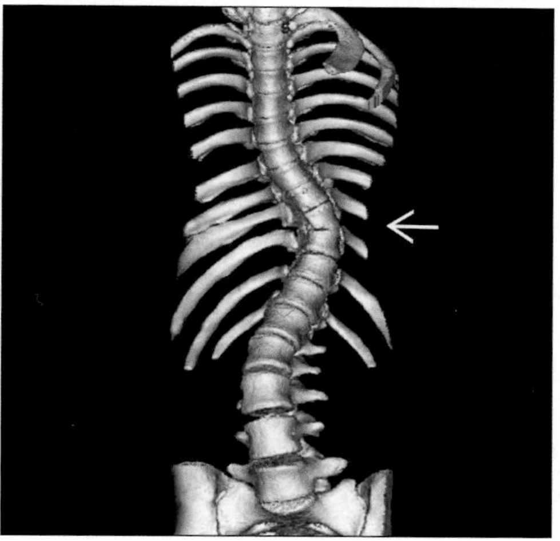

(Left) *Coronal bone CT shows a remote fracture of the distal tibia → and the development of bone bridging across the physeal plate →. This will result in a short limb from premature growth plate closure.* ***(Right)*** *3D bone CT shows focal convex left scoliosis → in a patient treated with radiation therapy for neuroblastoma. The affected thoracolumbar vertebrae are short on the right from early physeal fusion, yielding a flattened curvature without congenital segmentation anomalies.*

Radiation-Induced Growth Deformities

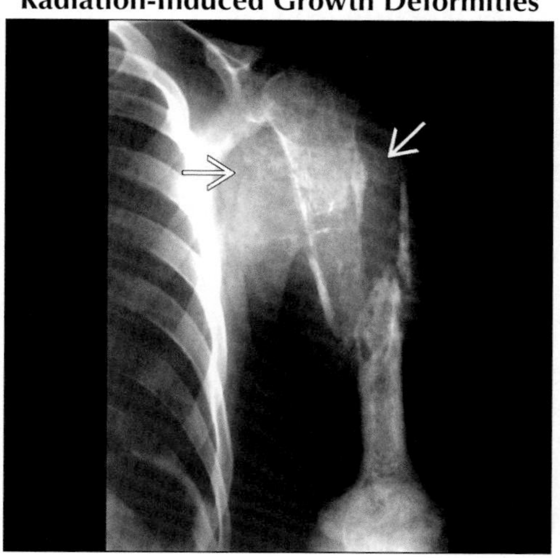

Polyostotic Fibrous Dysplasia, McCune-Albright

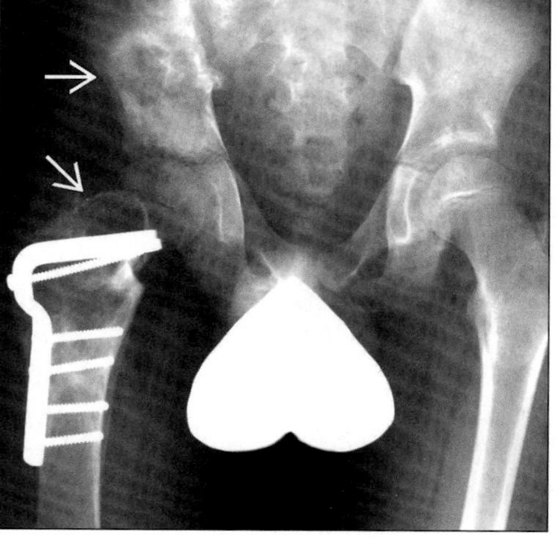

(Left) *Anteroposterior radiograph shows a short humerus (relative to thorax) in a patient radiated at a young age for Ewing sarcoma. Note the aggressive osteoid-producing tumor →, an associated radiation-induced osteosarcoma.* ***(Right)*** *AP radiograph shows numerous lesions → of mixed density with a narrow zone of transition. The right femoral lesion extends to the epiphyseal plate, resulting in a "shepherd's crook" deformity.*

CHILD ABUSE

DIFFERENTIAL DIAGNOSIS

Common
- Long Bone Fractures
- Posterior, Lateral, Anterior Rib Fractures
- Skull Fractures
- Classic Metaphyseal Lesion
- Solid Organ Lacerations
- Inflicted Head Injury
- Mimics of Child Abuse
  - Physiologic Periosteal Reaction (Mimic)
  - Nutritional Deficiency (Mimic)
  - Leukemic Lines (Mimic)
  - Birth Injuries (Mimic)
  - Infection (Mimic)
  - Osteogenesis Imperfecta (Mimic)
  - Menkes Syndrome (Mimic)

Less Common
- Small Bone Fractures
- Spinous Process Fractures
- Scapular Fractures
- Sternal Fractures
- Vertebral Compression Fractures
- Bowel Injury

ESSENTIAL INFORMATION

Key Differential Diagnosis Issues
- Age of child
  - Posterior rib fractures and intracranial injures more common in children < 1 year
  - Solid organ injury/blunt trauma more common at toddler age and older
- Clinical presentation
  - Ranges from fussy/failure to thrive to frankly obtunded
  - Clinicians may detect inconsistent or implausible stories explaining injuries
  - Suspicious bruising patterns or soft tissue injuries
- American College of Radiology Guidelines for Skeletal Survey
  - Dedicated AP views each of humeri, forearms, femurs, tibia/fibula, hands, feet
  - AP chest, AP abdomen
  - Lateral views of cervical, thoracic, lumbar spine
  - AP and lateral views of skull
  - Additional orthogonal views should be obtained of any suspected abnormality
  - Consider bilateral oblique rib views
  - "Babygram" images are inadequate
  - Follow-up skeletal survey performed 10-12 days after initial study is useful to detect fractures not initially seen, confirm equivocal findings

Helpful Clues for Common Diagnoses
- **Long Bone Fractures**
  - Femur, humerus most common
    - Common but nonspecific injury
    - May be innocent fractures once children are mobile/toddling
  - Metatarsal/metacarpal fractures
    - Often buckled appearance, can be subtle
- **Posterior, Lateral, Anterior Rib Fractures**
  - More common on left
  - May be subtle if minimally displaced, or acute without callus formation
    - Oblique views may increase detection
- **Skull Fractures**
  - Common but nonspecific injury
  - Features that raise suspicion
    - Complex, displaced fractures
    - Crossing suture lines
- **Classic Metaphyseal Lesion**
  - Accepted mechanism is shear injury through primary spongiosa of distal metaphysis due to grabbing, twisting
  - Common locations
    - Tibia, femur, humerus
- **Solid Organ Lacerations**
  - Liver lacerations/contusions
    - Linear or branching, low-attenuation, intraparenchymal foci on CT
    - CT bone windows may reveal additional rib fractures overlying organ injury
  - Splenic lacerations/contusions
    - Linear or branching, low-attenuation, intraparenchymal foci on CT
  - Adrenal laceration/hematoma
    - Usually globular abnormality
    - High attenuation on CT if acute; low attenuation if subacute/chronic
- **Inflicted Head Injury**
  - Subdural hematoma
    - Fluid collection overlying brain convexity, layering along tentorium and interhemispheric falx
    - Swirling low attenuation within high attenuation fluid may indicate active bleeding or dural injury with CSF leak

- Interhemispheric hematoma increases suspicion for inflicted trauma
- Subarachnoid hemorrhage
  - Wispy/linear high density following sulci
- Anoxic injury
  - Early: Ill-defined, low-attenuation areas
  - Late: Progressively low-attenuating parenchyma, loss of gray-white matter differentiation, sulcal effacement

- **Mimics of Child Abuse**
  - **Physiologic Periosteal Reaction (Mimic)**
    - Typically seen ages 1-6 months
    - Often symmetric but not exclusively
    - Appearance: Thin, smooth, diaphyseal
  - **Nutritional Deficiency (Mimic)**
    - Children with liver failure, TPN dependency, short gut syndrome
    - Rib and extremity fractures may be seen from normal patient handling
  - **Leukemic Lines (Mimic)**
    - Usually in older age group; neonatal leukemia very rare, associated with hepatosplenomegaly and chromosomal abnormalities
    - Expect symmetric manifestation
  - **Birth Injuries (Mimic)**
    - Most common: Clavicle, humerus fractures; subdural hematomas
    - Timing/manner of delivery important
  - **Infection (Mimic)**
    - Osteomyelitis, TORCH infections, especially syphilis
  - **Osteogenesis Imperfecta (Mimic)**
    - Appearance of bones ranges from near normal to osteopenic and dysmorphic
  - **Menkes Syndrome (Mimic)**
    - Intracranial parenchymal volume loss, hemorrhages, and metaphyseal lesions can be mistaken for abuse
    - X-linked disorder

Helpful Clues for Less Common Diagnoses

- **Small Bone Fractures**
  - Buckle fractures of metatarsals, metacarpals
- **Spinous Process Fractures**
  - Avulsion fractures of spinous process tips uncommon but highly specific for abuse
- **Scapular Fractures**
  - Fractures of acromion, scapular body uncommon but highly specific for abuse
- **Sternal Fractures**
  - Associated with blunt trauma
  - Consider vascular/cardiac injury
- **Vertebral Compression Fractures**
  - Thoracolumbar compression fractures occur with axial loading force
- **Bowel Injury**
  - Duodenum
    - Hematoma protruding as intraluminal mass or intramural lesion
    - Perforation: Look for retroperitoneal air
  - Jejunum
    - Perforation somewhat more likely than hematoma

Long Bone Fractures

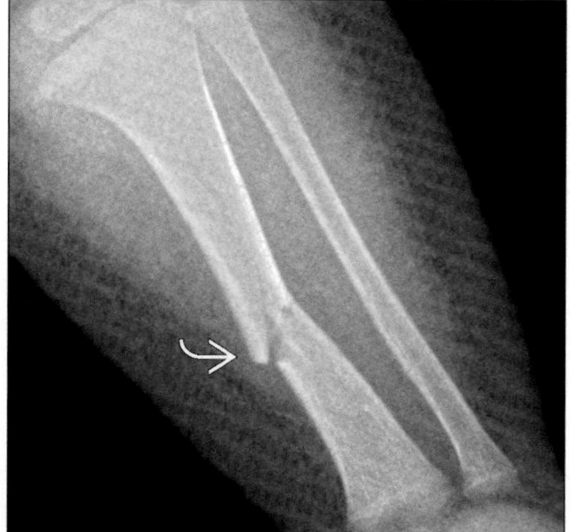

Frontal radiograph obtained as part of a postmortem skeletal survey shows a midshaft left tibial fracture ➔ in this 3 month old with numerous fractures and devastating intracranial injury.

Long Bone Fractures

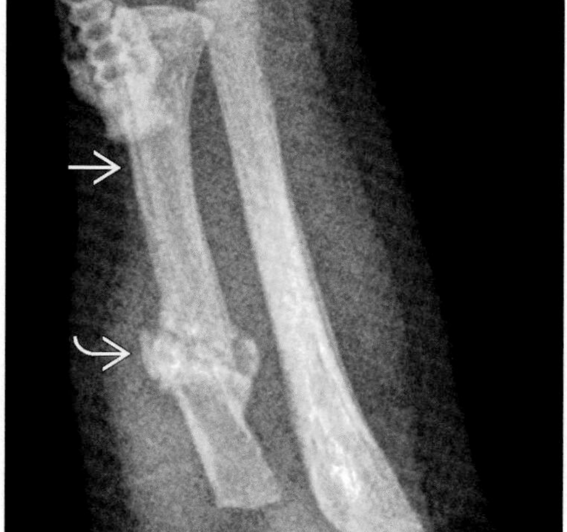

AP radiograph shows callus ➔ and periosteal reaction ➔ around a radial fracture in a 2 month old with multiple fractures of varying ages and intracranial hemorrhage.

CHILD ABUSE

*(**Left**) AP radiograph shows multiple healing posterior and lateral rib fractures in this infant who presented with rectal prolapse. (**Right**) Frontal radiograph shows bulbous callus around multiple bilateral posterior rib fractures, bilateral clavicle fractures, and a proximal left humeral fracture in this 2-month-old infant. A prior radiograph (from the 1st week of life) had demonstrated no fractures.*

Posterior, Lateral, Anterior Rib Fractures

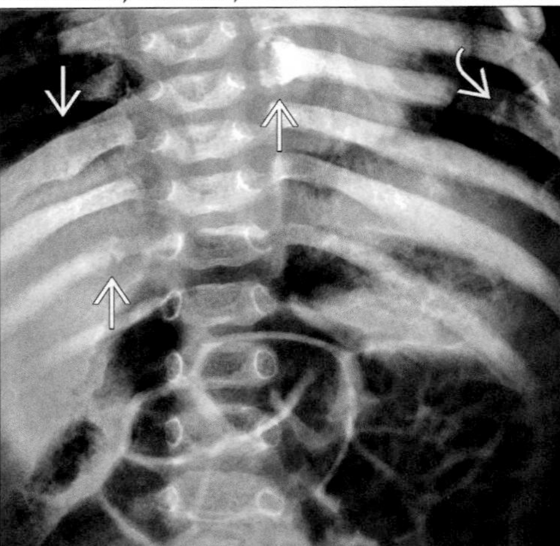

Posterior, Lateral, Anterior Rib Fractures

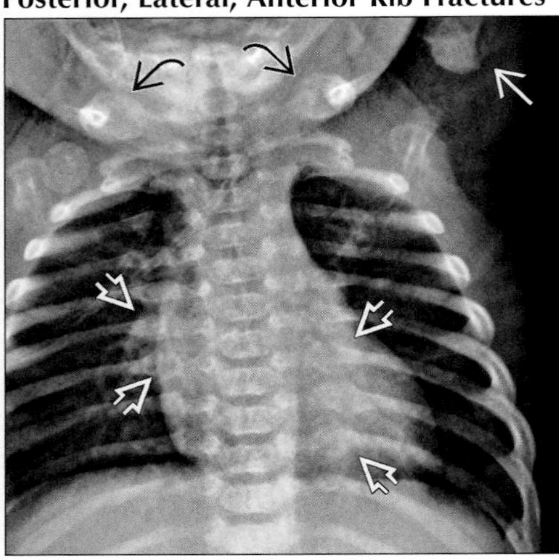

*(**Left**) Frontal radiograph shows multiple bilateral posterior rib fractures with healing bony callus in a 6-week-old infant referred to oncology for bruising. All laboratory values were normal. The father confessed to abusing the infant. (**Right**) Coronal CECT shows the same fractures as depicted on bone windows. Again note the preponderance of fractures on the left.*

Posterior, Lateral, Anterior Rib Fractures

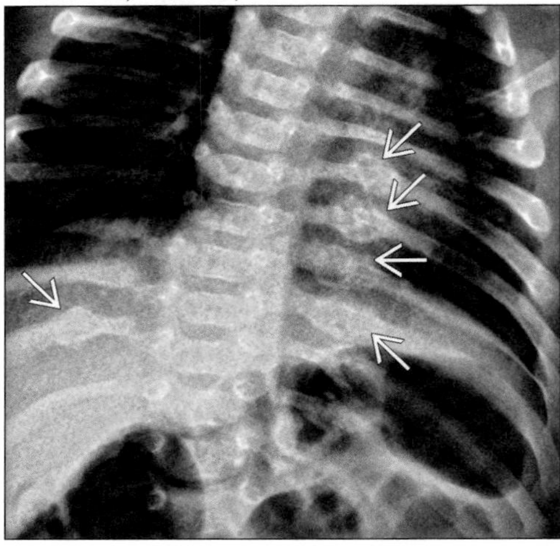

Posterior, Lateral, Anterior Rib Fractures

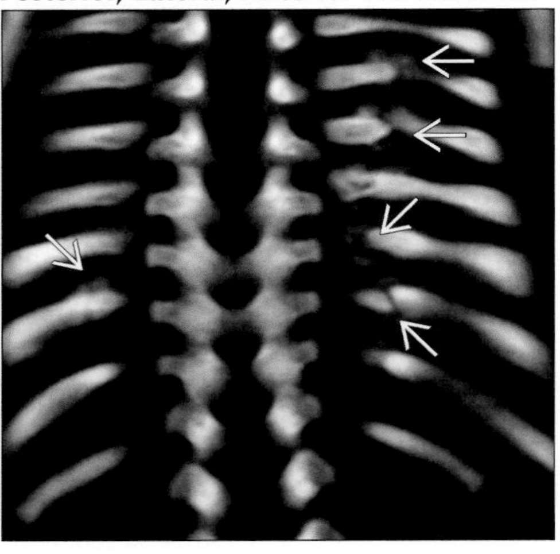

*(**Left**) Lateral radiograph shows a long, markedly diastatic parietal skull fracture and a large overlying soft tissue hematoma in this 1 month old with numerous rib and metaphyseal lesions. (**Right**) Axial NECT shows the same skull fracture and an overlying hematoma. Skull fractures that occur in the plane of imaging may be missed on CT; it is helpful to scrutinize the scout view and obtain coronal reformatted images.*

Skull Fractures

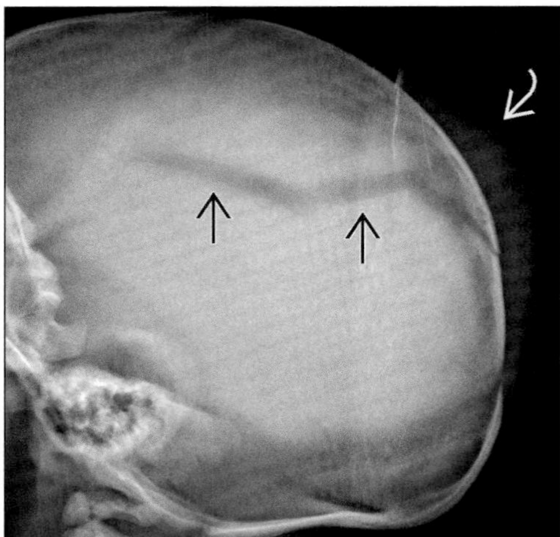

Skull Fractures

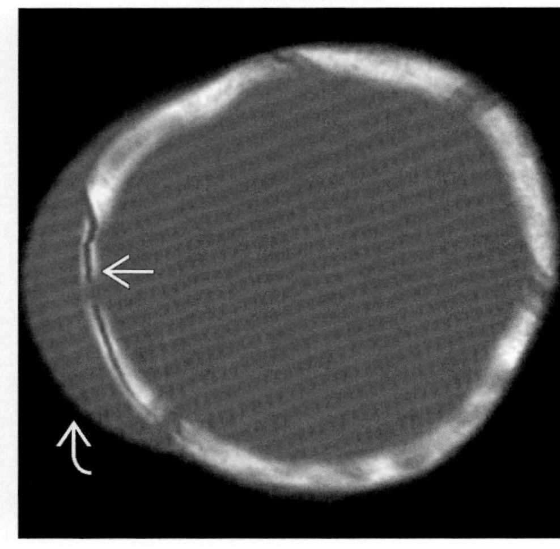

Classic Metaphyseal Lesion

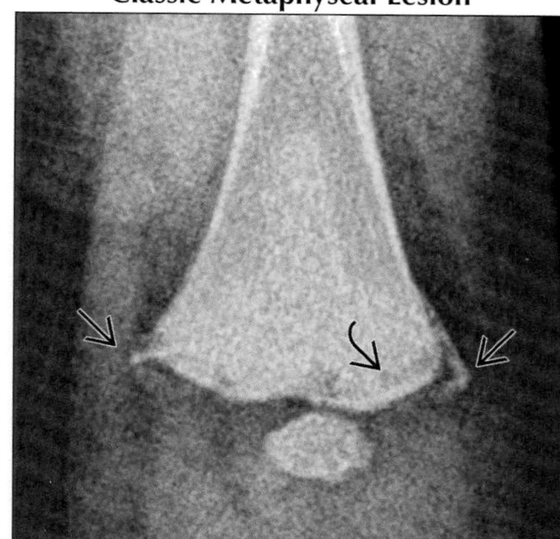

Classic Metaphyseal Lesion

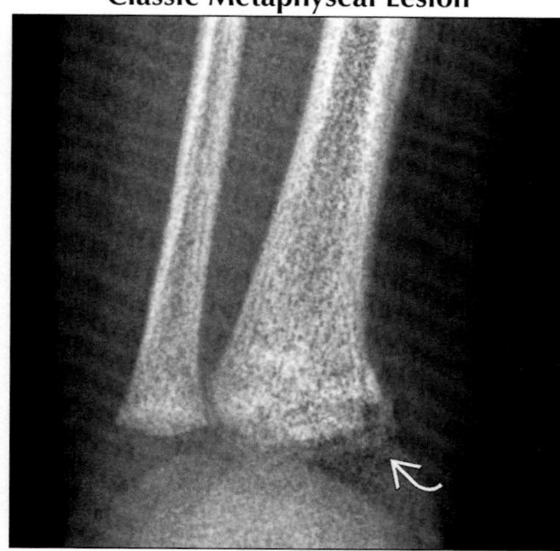

*(**Left**) Frontal radiograph shows uplifted periosteum ➙ and lucency of the primary spongiosum ➙ in the distal left femur. This is the typical appearance of a classic metaphyseal lesion, also called a "bucket handle" fracture or a "corner" fracture. (**Right**) AP radiograph shows a classic "bucket handle" appearance of a distal tibial metaphyseal fracture ➙ in this 2 month old with multiple injuries.*

Classic Metaphyseal Lesion

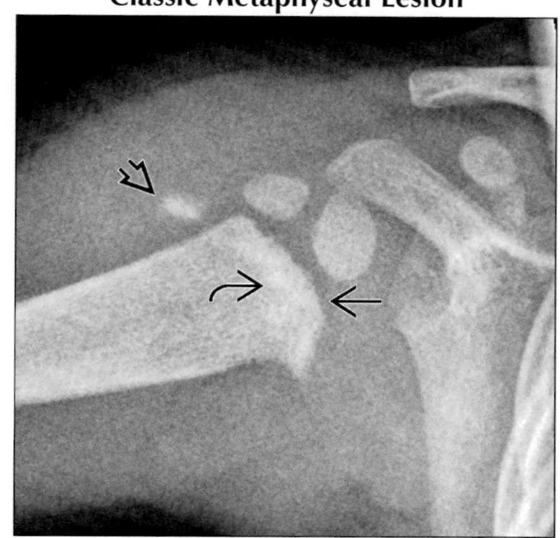

Classic Metaphyseal Lesion

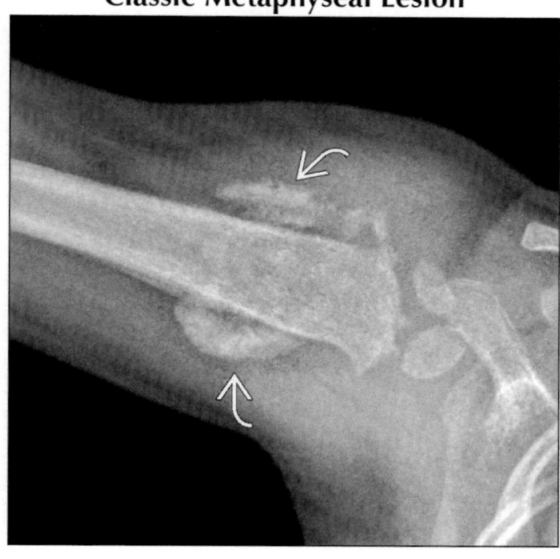

*(**Left**) Frontal radiograph shows irregular shaggy margins ➙, sclerosis ➙, and an ossific fragment ➙ adjacent to the proximal right humerus in this 10-month-old child with multiple bilateral long bone fractures. Such fractures of the proximal humeri are frequently overlooked. (**Right**) Frontal radiograph shows exuberant callus around the fracture ➙ 11 days later. Disproportionate callus formation may be seen with nonimmobilized fractures.*

Solid Organ Lacerations

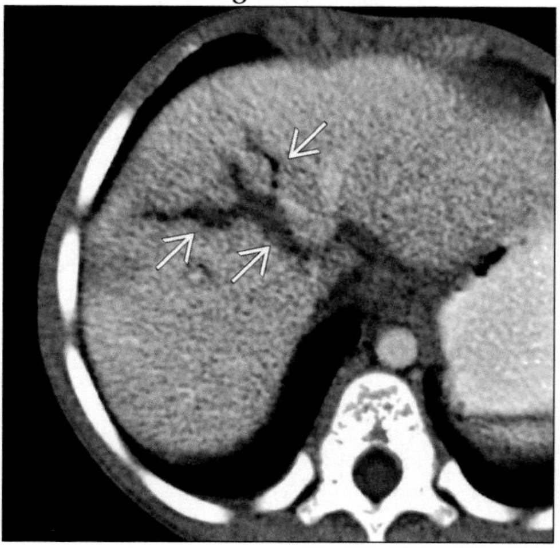

Solid Organ Lacerations

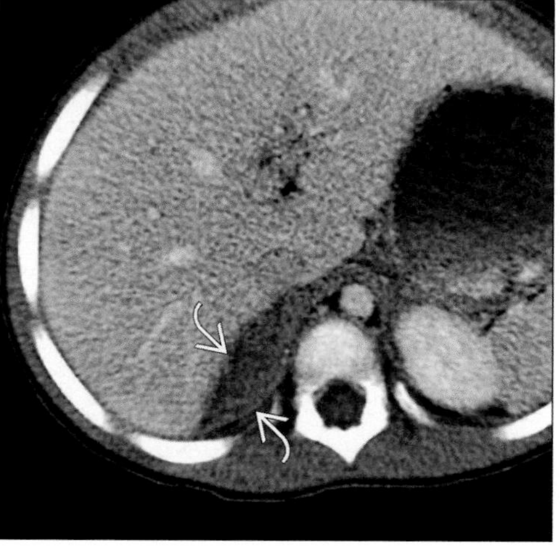

*(**Left**) Axial CECT shows a branching, low attenuation area ➙ in the hepatic parenchyma, consistent with a hepatic laceration. This 4-year-old child presented with elevated liver enzymes and failure to thrive. (**Right**) Oblique CECT shows globular low-attenuation in the region of the right adrenal gland ➙, consistent with hematoma, in this 3-year-old child with extensive skin bruising, liver laceration (not shown), and healing pubic ramus fracture.*

CHILD ABUSE

*(**Left**) Axial NECT shows hyperattenuating collections of acute blood overlying the occipital cortex and within the interhemispheric fissure in this 2 month old with more than 15 skeletal fractures of varying ages. Five months later, the child's brain was nearly normal by MR imaging. (**Right**) Axial NECT shows a linear high-density focus ➔ following the sulcal groove. There is also a scalp hematoma ➔ and a skull fracture (not shown).*

Inflicted Head Injury

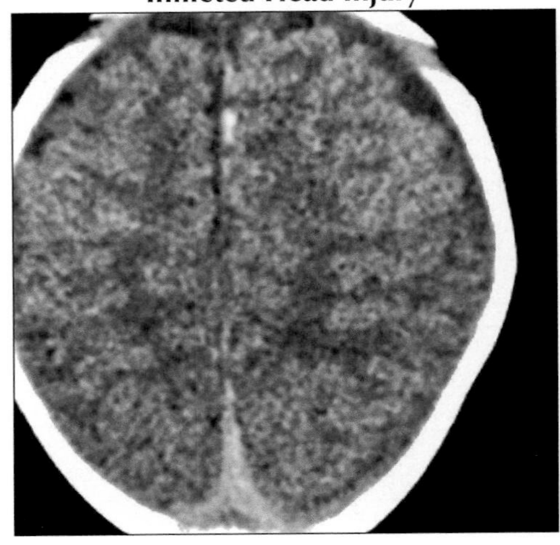

Inflicted Head Injury

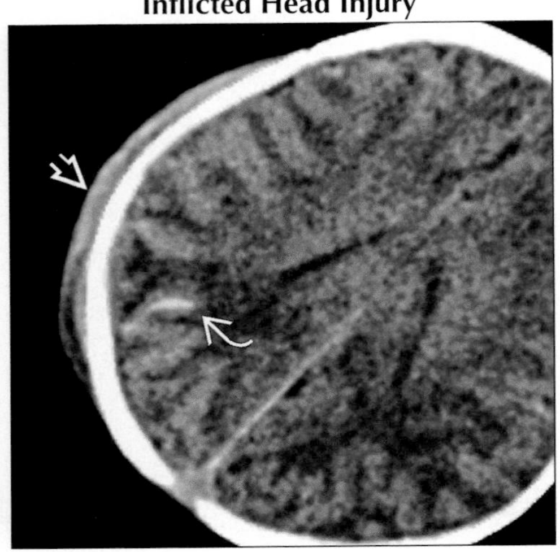

*(**Left**) Axial NECT shows subdural collections ➔ higher in attenuation than CSF, with a focal hyperattenuating area ➔, presumably acute blood. Bright tentorial blood is noted ➔. Gray-white matter differentiation was suspected to be diminished; correlation with follow-up was recommended. (**Right**) Axial NECT shows the same child 8 hours later. Gray-white differentiation is indistinct; the sulci are effaced. In contrast, the basal ganglia ➔ are preserved.*

Inflicted Head Injury

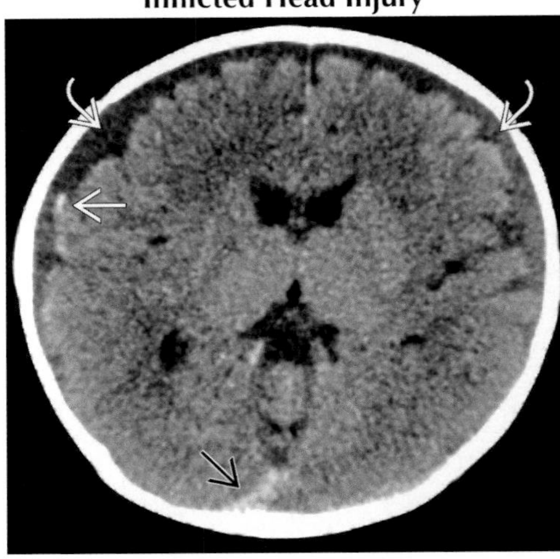

Inflicted Head Injury

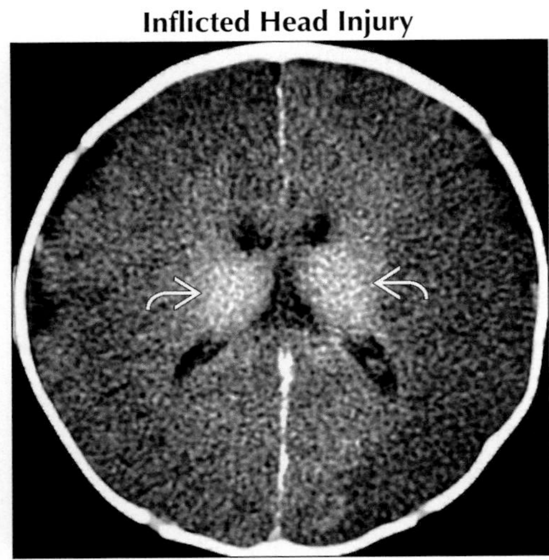

*(**Left**) Frontal radiograph shows a smooth, thin periosteal reaction ➔ extending along only the diaphysis. This is typically seen in ages 2-4 months & is often, not always, symmetric. It was not seen on follow-up 10 days later. (**Right**) Frontal radiograph shows a proximal right humeral fracture ➔ in an infant with a complex medical history, including multivisceral transplant. The bones are severely osteopenic. This should not be confused with child abuse.*

Physiologic Periosteal Reaction (Mimic)

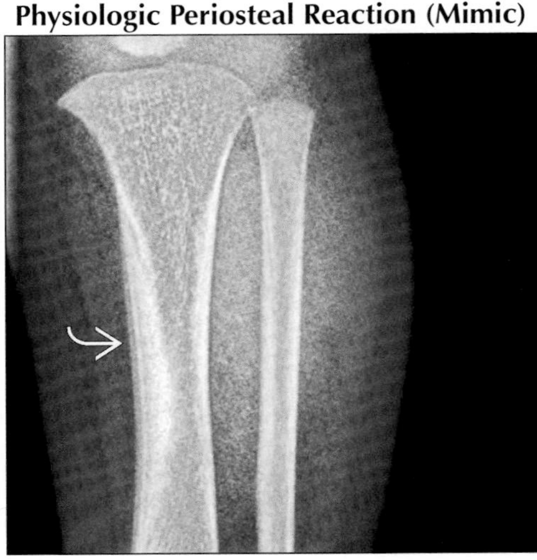

Nutritional Deficiency (Mimic)

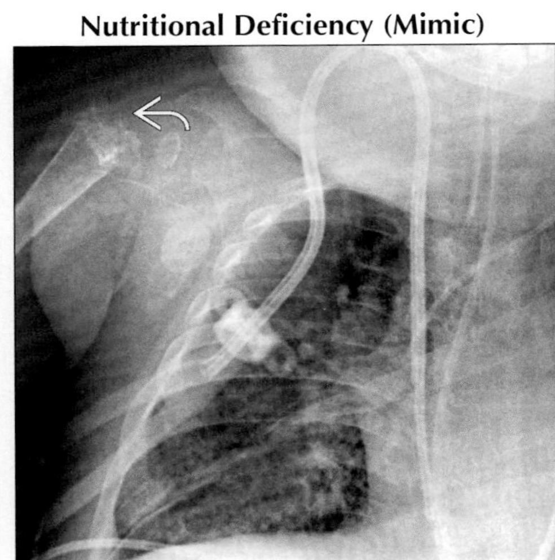

Infection (Mimic)

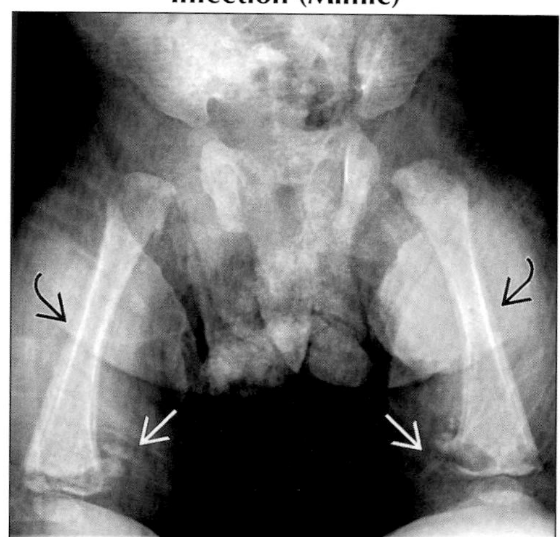

Osteogenesis Imperfecta (Mimic)

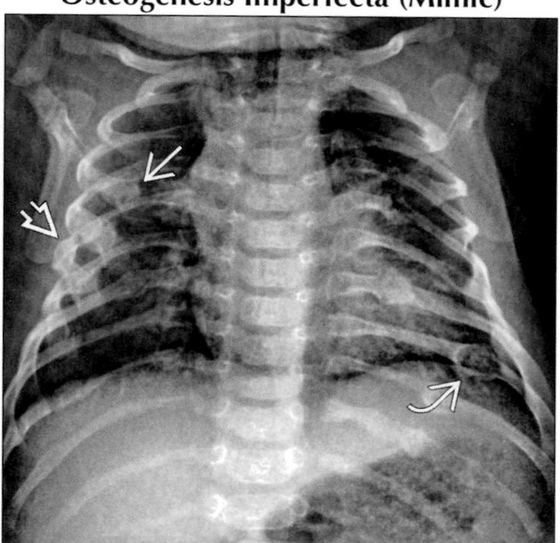

(Left) *Frontal radiograph shows a 10-week-old child with bilateral destructive metaphyseal lesions ➔ and thick periosteal reaction ↷. The RPR of both the mother and child was positive, and the liver enzymes were normal.* ***(Right)*** *Frontal radiograph shows numerous anterior ➔, posterior ↷, and lateral ⇨ fractures of thin, dysplastic-appearing ribs in this 2-month-old child found to have osteogenesis imperfecta. Not all fractures are indicated with arrows.*

Small Bone Fractures

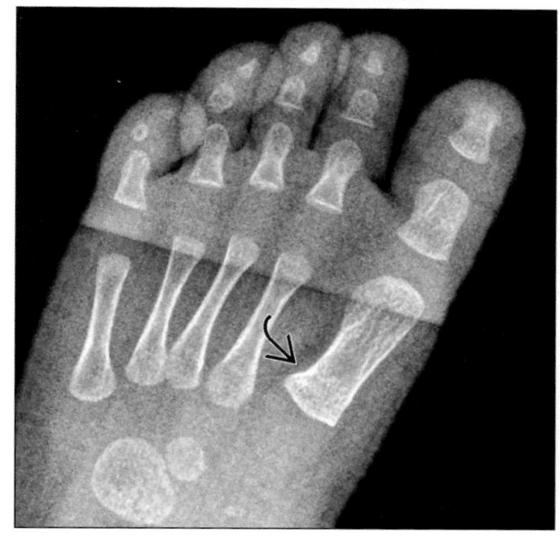

Spinous Process Fractures

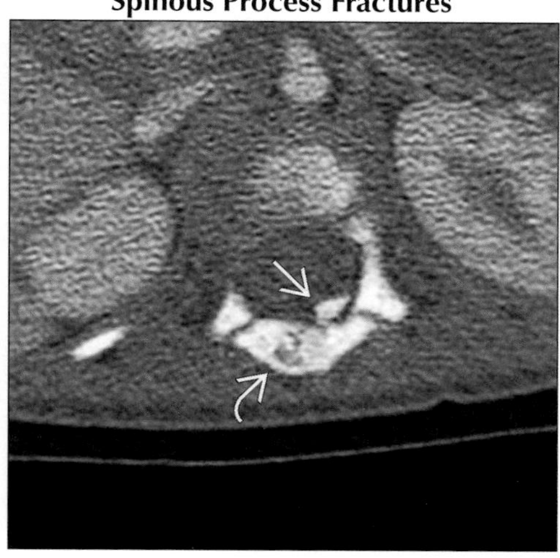

(Left) *AP radiograph shows subtle buckle deformity at the base of the 1st metatarsal ↷ in a 10-month-old child with multiple acute and healing long bone fractures.* ***(Right)*** *Axial CECT shows a complex fracture that involved the posterior elements of L1 ↷, including the spinous process. Note the bone shards within the spinal canal ➔. This child had multiple long bone fractures and a liver laceration.*

Scapular Fractures

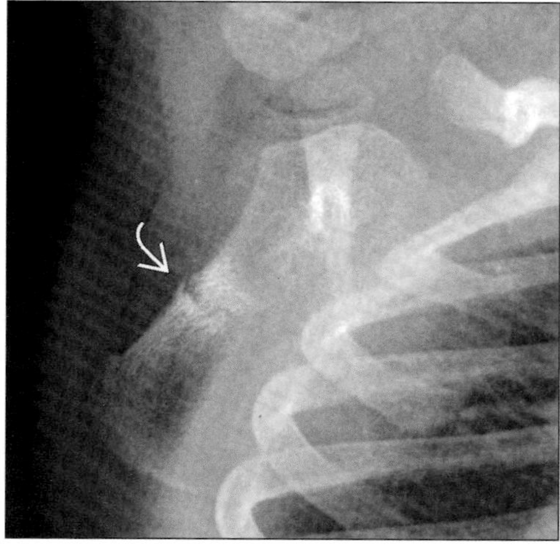

Scapular Fractures

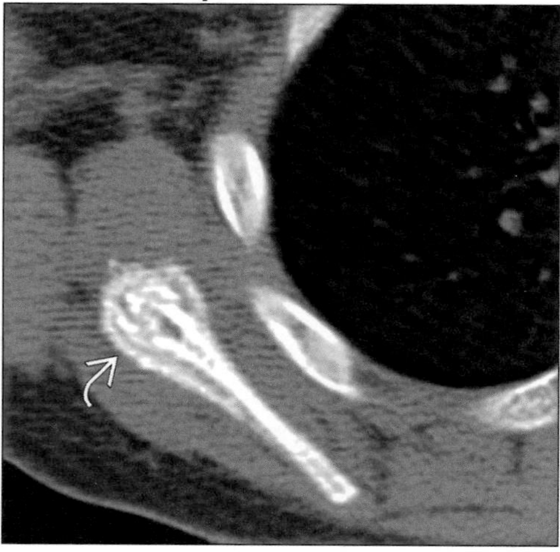

(Left) *Frontal radiograph shows a fracture through the lateral margin of the right scapula ↷ in this 2 year old who presented with unexplained bruising. Scapular injuries are highly specific for child abuse, as they require a great deal of force. A sibling was also discovered to have long bone fractures.* ***(Right)*** *Axial NECT shows the same scapular fracture 11 days later. The periosteal reaction ↷ reflects healing.*

SECTION 6
Brain, Head and Neck

ENLARGED LYMPH NODES IN NECK

DIFFERENTIAL DIAGNOSIS

Common
- Reactive Lymph Nodes
- Suppurative Lymph Nodes
- Hodgkin Lymphoma, Lymph Nodes
- Cat Scratch Disease
- Non-Hodgkin Lymphoma, Lymph Nodes
- Non-TB Mycobacterium, Lymph Nodes

Less Common
- Metastatic Neuroblastoma
- Post-Transplant Lymphoproliferative Disorder
- Differentiated Thyroid Carcinoma, Nodal

Rare but Important
- Systemic Metastases, Nodal
- Langerhans Histiocytosis, Nodal

ESSENTIAL INFORMATION

Helpful Clues for Common Diagnoses
- **Reactive Lymph Nodes**
  - Key facts
    - "Reactive" implies benign
    - Response to infection/inflammation, acute or chronic
    - Any H&N nodal group
  - Imaging
    - Enlarged well-defined oval-shaped nodes with variable contrast enhancement
    - ± cellulitis: Common with bacterial infection
    - Cellulitis is usually absent in non-TB *Mycobacterium* (NTM)
    - ± edema in adjacent muscles (myositis)
    - ± necrosis: Bacterial, NTM, & cat scratch
- **Suppurative Lymph Nodes**
  - Key facts
    - Pus within node = intranodal abscess
    - If untreated, rupture ⇒ soft tissue abscess
  - Imaging
    - If thick enhancing walls + central hypodensity, suspect drainable abscess (phlegmon may have similar appearance)
    - Associated cellulitis: Common in bacterial infection, absent in NTM
    - Associated nonsuppurative adenopathy
    - ± thickening of muscles (myositis)
- **Hodgkin Lymphoma, Lymph Nodes**
  - Key facts
    - B-cell origin; histology shows Reed-Sternberg cells
    - Most commonly involves cervical and mediastinal lymph nodes
    - Extranodal disease uncommon
    - Tumors are EBV positive in up to 50%
  - Imaging
    - Cannot distinguish Hodgkin lymphoma (HL) from non-Hodgkin lymphoma (NHL)
    - Round nodal masses with variable contrast enhancement, ± necrotic center
    - Single or multiple nodal chains
    - Calcification uncommon (unless treated)
    - FDG PET (or Ga-67) scans for staging and evaluating response to treatment
- **Cat Scratch Disease**
  - Key facts
    - Usually self limited
    - Tender or painful regional lymphadenopathy
    - 70-90 % present in fall or early winter
    - 4/5 of patients are < 21 years old
    - Scratch or bite may precede development of adenopathy by 1-4 weeks
    - *Bartonella henselae* most common pathogen
  - Imaging
    - Homogeneous or necrotic lymphadenopathy
- **Non-Hodgkin Lymphoma, Lymph Nodes**
  - Key facts
    - Extranodal disease more common in NHL than HL
  - Imaging
    - Cannot distinguish NHL from HL
    - Single dominant node or multiple enlarged nonnecrotic nodes
    - Non-nodal lymphatic disease: Palatine, lingual, or adenoid tonsils
    - Non-nodal extralymphatic: Paranasal sinus, skull base, and thyroid gland
- **Non-TB Mycobacterium, Lymph Nodes**
  - Key facts
    - *M. avium-intracellulare* (MAI), *M. scrofulaceum, M. kansasii*
    - Usually nontender lymphadenopathy
  - Imaging
    - Necrotic lymphadenopathy common
    - Lack of surrounding cellulitis

ENLARGED LYMPH NODES IN NECK

Helpful Clues for Less Common Diagnoses

- **Metastatic Neuroblastoma**
  - Key facts
    - Most cervical involvement with neuroblastoma is metastatic
  - Imaging
    - Large lymph nodes, rarely necrotic
    - ± bilateral skull base metastasis common
    - ± enhancing masses with aggressive bone erosion
- **Post-Transplant Lymphoproliferative Disorder**
  - Key facts
    - Spectrum: Benign hyperplasia to lymphoma
    - Most common in patients who are EBV seronegative prior to transplant
    - More common after heart or lung than after kidney transplant
    - Children > > > > adults
    - Abdomen, chest, allograft, H&N, CNS
  - Imaging
    - Cervical lymphadenopathy
    - Adenotonsillar hypertrophy; may lead to upper airway obstruction
    - ± sinusitis, otitis media
- **Differentiated Thyroid Carcinoma, Nodal**
  - Key facts
    - Nodal spread common in papillary, distant spread common in follicular
    - 3x more common in women
    - Presents in 3rd and 4th decade; occasionally in adolescents, rare in young children
  - Imaging
    - Variable: Small to large nodes; homogeneous or heterogeneous; hemorrhagic or cystic necrosis
    - Focal calcifications and solid foci of enhancement may be present

Helpful Clues for Rare Diagnoses

- **Systemic Metastases, Nodal**
  - Key facts
    - In children, primary malignancy is usually known
    - Neuroblastoma most common; other primary malignancies such as testicular carcinoma, hepatoblastoma, chordoma
    - Supraclavicular metastasis suggests chest or abdominal primary
  - Imaging
    - Single or multiple enlarged nodes
    - ± necrosis
- **Langerhans Histiocytosis, Nodal**
  - Key facts
    - Focal, localized, or systemic disease
    - Unifocal > > multifocal
    - Skeletal involvement most common, adenopathy with systemic disease
  - Imaging
    - In acute disseminated disease (Letterer-Siwe), diffuse lymphadenopathy
    - + hepatosplenomegaly, skin rash, marrow failure, and pulmonary disease

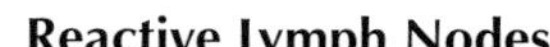

Reactive Lymph Nodes

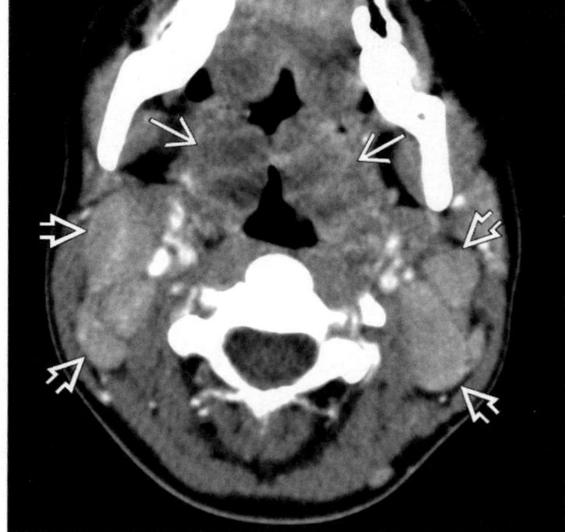

Axial CECT shows enlarged palatine tonsils ➡ and reactive cervical lymph nodes ➡ in a teenager with mononucleosis.

Reactive Lymph Nodes

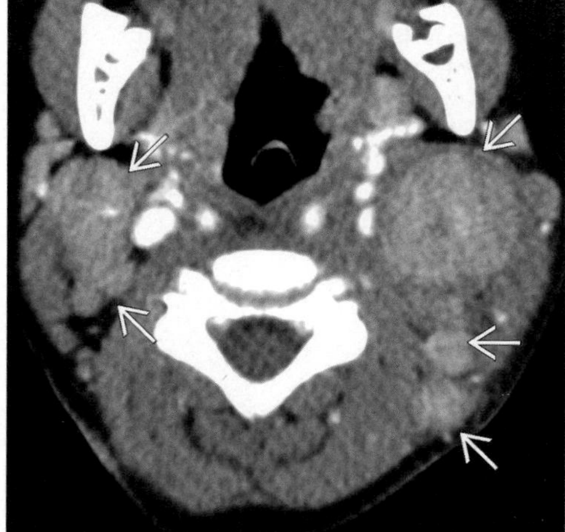

Axial CECT demonstrates left greater than right cervical adenopathy ➡ in a child with a throat swab positive for beta-hemolytic Streptococcus group A.

ENLARGED LYMPH NODES IN NECK

(Left) Axial CECT shows a well-defined, low-attenuation retropharyngeal abscess ➔ (secondary to a suppurative left lateral retropharyngeal lymph node) and nonsuppurative bilateral cervical adenopathy ⇨. (Right) Axial CECT reveals a well-defined, rim-enhancing, low-attenuation intranodal abscess ➔ and significant soft tissue edema in the adjacent subcutaneous fat ⇨.

Suppurative Lymph Nodes

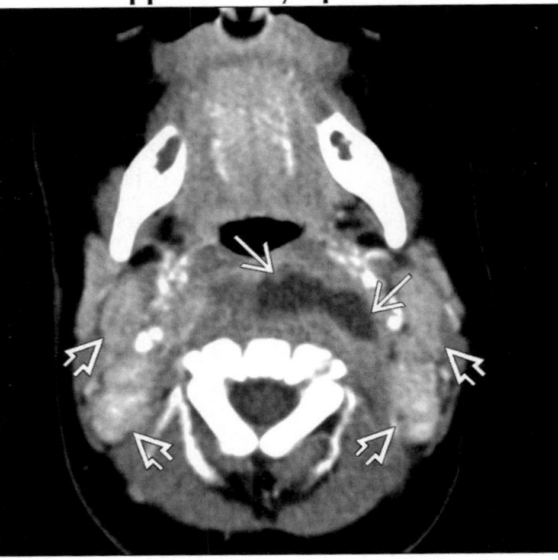

Suppurative Lymph Nodes

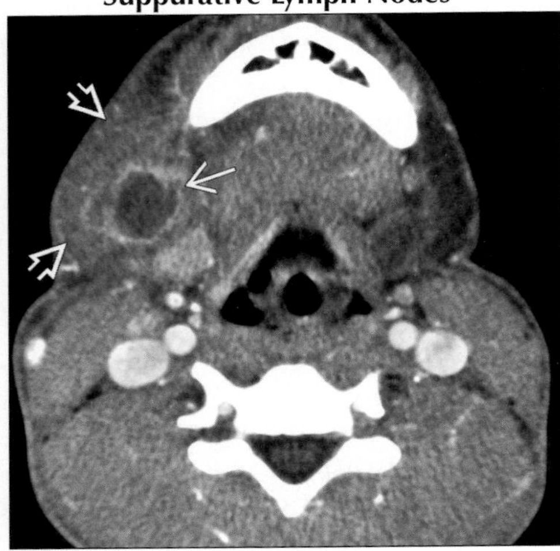

(Left) Axial CECT clearly defines a large moderately enhancing level IV cervical node ➔ along with a level V node ⇨ in a teenager with Hodgkin lymphoma. (Right) Axial CECT demonstrates marked enlargement of the relatively low-attenuation right cervical lymph nodes ➔ in another teenager with Hodgkin lymphoma.

Hodgkin Lymphoma, Lymph Nodes

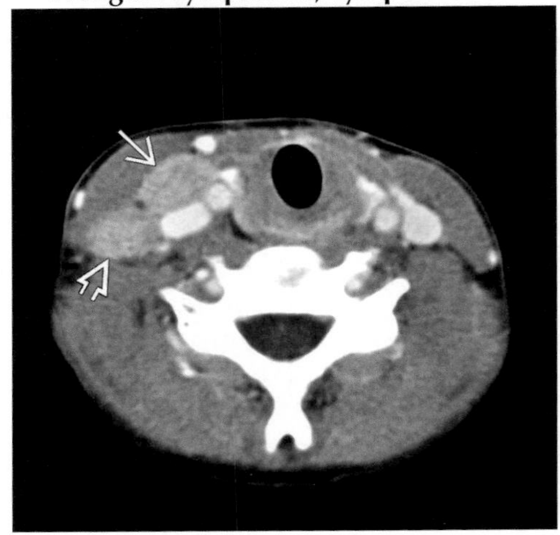

Hodgkin Lymphoma, Lymph Nodes

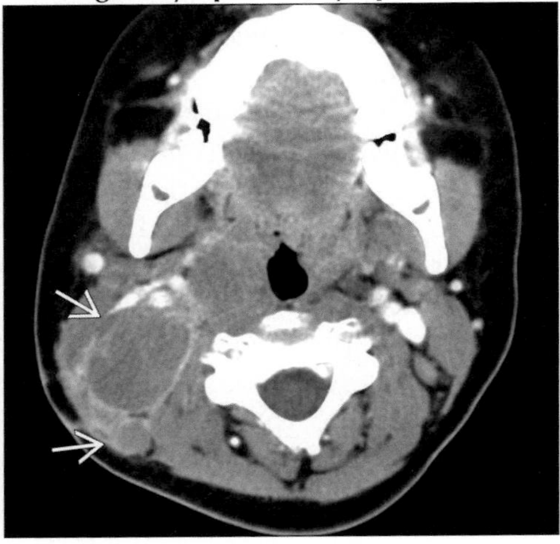

(Left) Axial CECT shows an ill-defined nodal mass ➔ with a small central area of necrosis ⇨, adjacent to the left submandibular gland ➚. There is no significant surrounding soft tissue edema. (Right) Axial CECT clearly defines bilateral, symmetric enlargement of nonnecrotic cervical lymph nodes ➔ in a patient with T-cell lymphoma.

Cat Scratch Disease

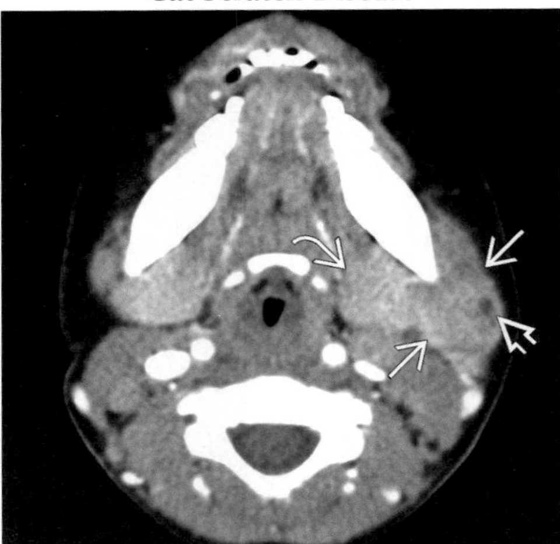

Non-Hodgkin Lymphoma, Lymph Nodes

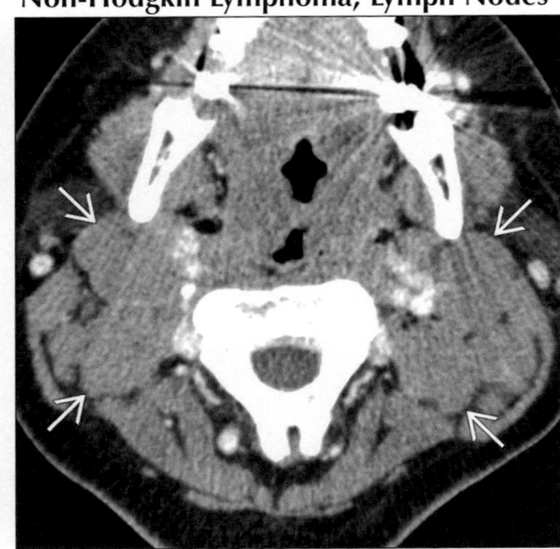

Non-TB Mycobacterium, Lymph Nodes

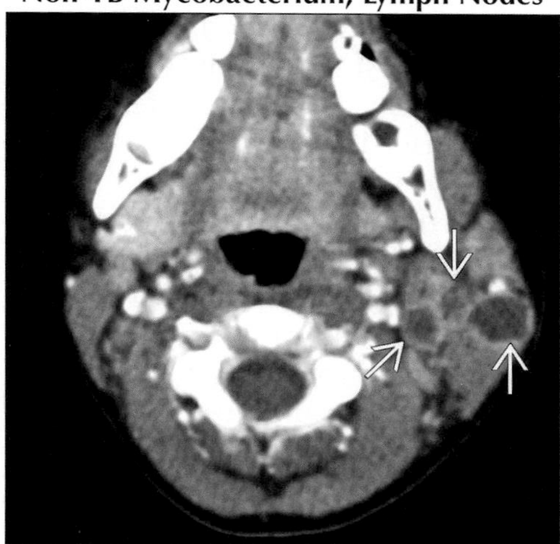

Metastatic Neuroblastoma

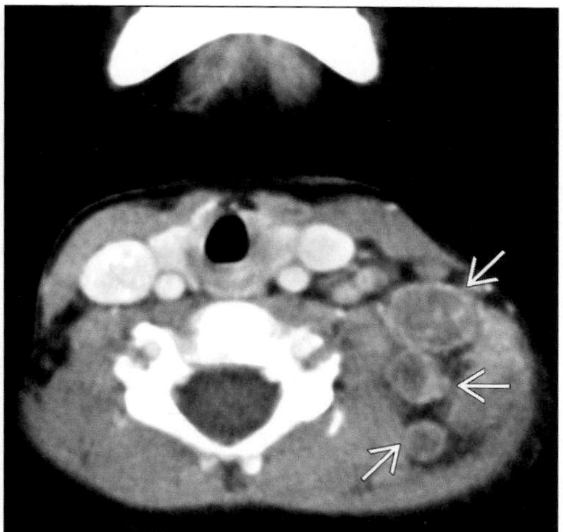

*(**Left**) Axial CECT shows left-sided necrotic cervical lymph nodes ➔ without edema of the adjacent fat. This toddler presented with a left neck mass, without fever or elevated white blood cell count. The Mycobacterium avium intracellulare was isolated from the excision specimen. (**Right**) Axial CECT demonstrates several low-attenuation left supraclavicular metastatic lymph nodes ➔ in a child with known neuroblastoma.*

Post-Transplant Lymphoproliferative Disorder

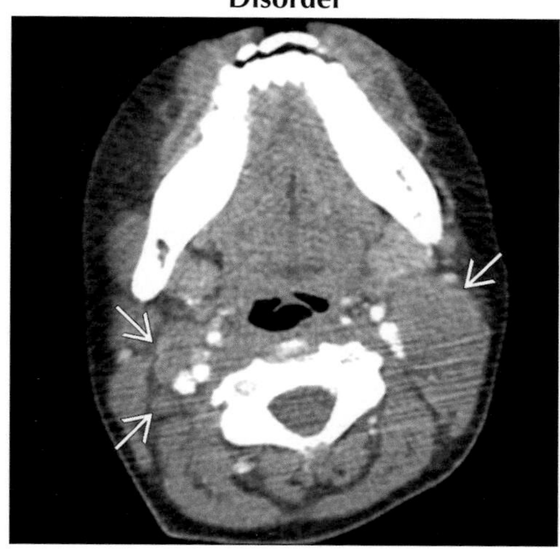

Differentiated Thyroid Carcinoma, Nodal

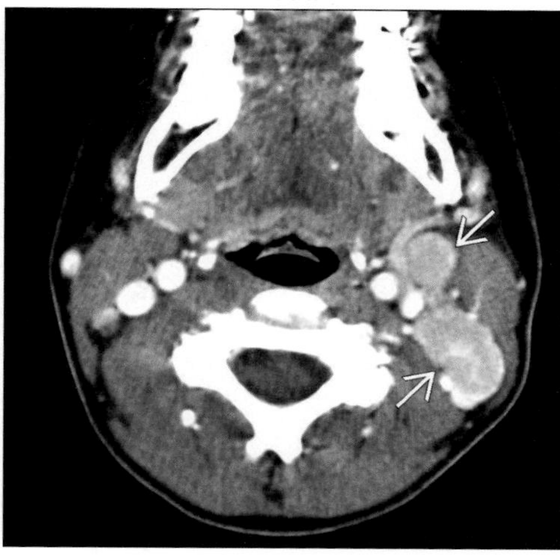

*(**Left**) Axial CECT shows left greater than right cervical adenopathy ➔ in a 10-year-old patient with a prior renal transplant. (**Right**) Axial CECT shows diffusely enhancing left cervical nodes ➔ in a teenager who presented with a left-sided neck mass that proved to be metastatic thyroid carcinoma.*

Systemic Metastases, Nodal

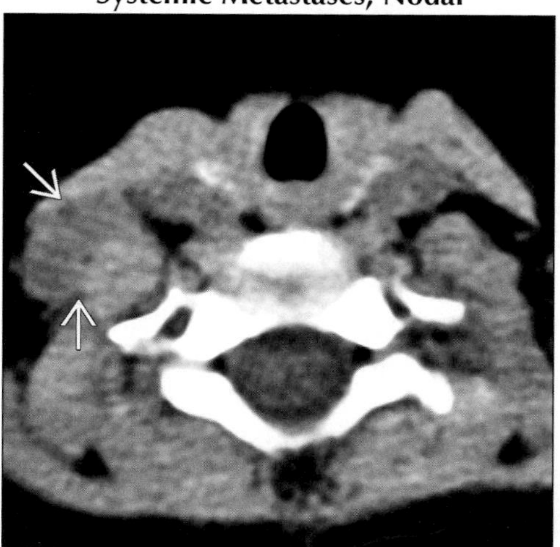

Langerhans Histiocytosis, Nodal

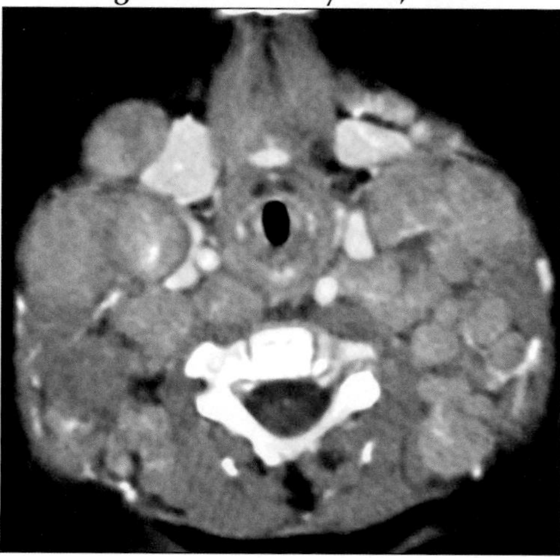

*(**Left**) Axial CECT demonstrates a left supraclavicular metastatic nodal mass ➔ in a child with metastatic chordoma. (**Right**) Axial CECT reveals too numerous to count, massively enlarged anterior and posterior cervical lymph nodes in a child with extensive Langerhans cell histiocytosis.*

SOLID NECK MASS IN NEONATE

DIFFERENTIAL DIAGNOSIS

Common
- Fibromatosis Colli
- Reactive Lymph Nodes
- Infantile Hemangioma

Less Common
- Neurofibromatosis Type 1
- Teratoma

Rare but Important
- Langerhans Cell Histiocytosis, General
- Metastatic Neuroblastoma
- Fibromatosis
- Primary Cervical Neuroblastoma
- Cervical Thymus

ESSENTIAL INFORMATION

Helpful Clues for Common Diagnoses
- **Fibromatosis Colli**
  - Key facts
    - Synonyms: Sternocleidomastoid (SCM) tumor of infancy, congenital muscular torticollis
    - Increased incidence in breech presentation and difficult deliveries
    - Present with neck mass ± torticollis, usually within 1st 2 weeks of life
    - Ultrasound preferred imaging modality
  - Imaging
    - Large SCM muscle, focal or diffuse
    - Almost always unilateral
    - Variable echogenicity, attenuation, signal intensity; heterogeneous contrast enhancement on MR
    - No associated adenopathy
    - No extramuscular extension of mass
- **Reactive Lymph Nodes**
  - Key facts
    - "Reactive" implies benign etiology
    - Acute or chronic
    - Any H&N nodal group
    - Response to infection/inflammation
  - Imaging
    - Enlarged oval-shaped lymph nodes
    - Variable enhancement, usually mild
    - ± enlargement of lingual, faucial, or adenoid hypertrophy
    - ± stranding of adjacent fat (cellulitis)
    - ± edema in adjacent muscles (myositis)
    - ± suppurative nodes or abscess
- **Infantile Hemangioma**
  - Key facts
    - Vacular neoplasm, NOT malformation
    - Usually not well seen at birth, more apparent within 1st few weeks of life
    - Proliferative phase: 1st year of life
    - Involuting phase: 1-5 years
    - Involuted usually by 5-7 years
    - GLUT-1: Specific immunohistochemical marker expressed in all 3 phases of infantile hemangioma; also expressed in placenta, fetal, and embryonic tissue
    - Congenital hemangioma: Rare variant, present at birth or on prenatal imaging (fetal hemangioma); 2 subtypes, rapidly involuting (RICH) shows involution by 8-14 months, noninvoluting (NICH)
  - Imaging
    - Proliferative: Solid, intensely enhancing mass with intralesional high-flow vessels
    - Involutional: Fatty infiltration, ↓ size
    - PHACES syndrome: Posterior fossa abnormalities, hemangiomas, arterial anomalies, cardiovascular defects, eye abnormalities, sternal clefts

Helpful Clues for Less Common Diagnoses
- **Neurofibromatosis Type 1**
  - Key facts
    - Carotid space, perivertebral space (brachial plexus) common
    - Localized, diffuse, or plexiform
    - Single or multiple
  - Imaging
    - Localized: Well-circumscribed, smooth, solid masses with variable enhancement
    - Diffuse: Plaque-like thickening of skin with poorly defined linear branching lesion in subcutaneous fat
    - Plexiform: Lobulated, tortuous, rope-like expansion in major nerve distribution; "tangle of worms" appearance
- **Teratoma**
  - Key facts
    - Contains all 3 germ layers
    - Mature or immature, rarely malignant in neonate
  - Imaging
    - Large, heterogeneous mass
    - Frequently with fat and calcium
    - Solid and cystic components

Helpful Clues for Rare Diagnoses

- **Langerhans Cell Histiocytosis, General**
  - Key facts
    - Acute disseminated form (Letterer-Siwe) occurs in children < 1 year
    - Acute onset of hepatosplenomegaly, rash, lymphadenopathy, marrow failure
    - Skeletal involvement may be absent
  - Imaging
    - Large nonspecific cervical lymph nodes
    - Hepatosplenomegaly
- **Metastatic Neuroblastoma**
  - Key facts
    - Most cervical disease is metastatic from retroperitoneal primary lesion
    - Metastatic cervical disease more common in older children
  - Imaging
    - Large metastatic lymph nodes
    - Bilateral skull base metastasis common
    - Skull base metastases: Enhancing masses with osseous erosion ± intracranial or intraorbital extension
- **Fibromatosis**
  - Key facts
    - Synonyms: Desmoid or aggressive fibromatosis, infantile fibromatosis, extraabdominal desmoid tumor
    - Benign soft tissue tumor arising from musculoaponeurotic structures
    - Tendency to infiltrate adjacent tissues
    - Recurrence common
    - Does not metastasize
    - Identified at all ages
    - In infants, more common in retroperitoneum and extremity
  - Imaging
    - Well-defined or poorly marginated, infiltrative mass
    - Often trans-spatial enhancing mass
    - ± erosion of adjacent bone
- **Primary Cervical Neuroblastoma**
  - Key facts
    - < 5% are primary cervical lesions
    - In general, < 1 year = better prognosis
    - Young children may present with opsoclonus-myoclonus
  - Imaging findings
    - Solid mass closely associated with carotid sheath space
    - Calcifications common
    - Foraminal or intraspinal extension
- **Cervical Thymus**
  - Key facts
    - Remnants along thymopharyngeal duct
  - Imaging findings
    - Mildly enhancing soft tissue mass
    - Small dot-dash echoes on ultrasound, similar to mediastinal thymus

Fibromatosis Colli

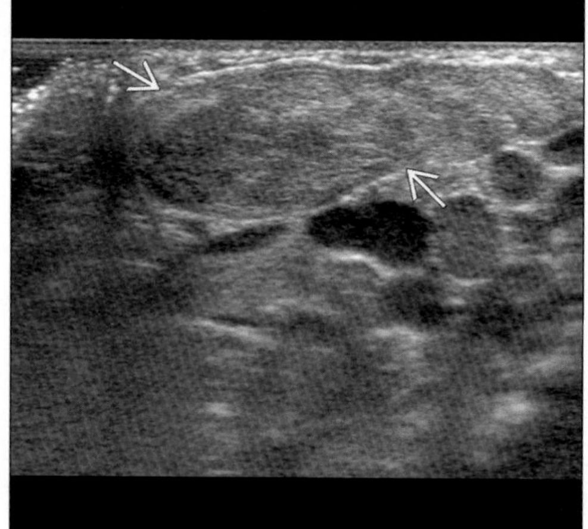

Longitudinal ultrasound shows fusiform enlargement of the left sternocleidomastoid muscle ➔ in a 2 month old with fibromatosis colli.

Fibromatosis Colli

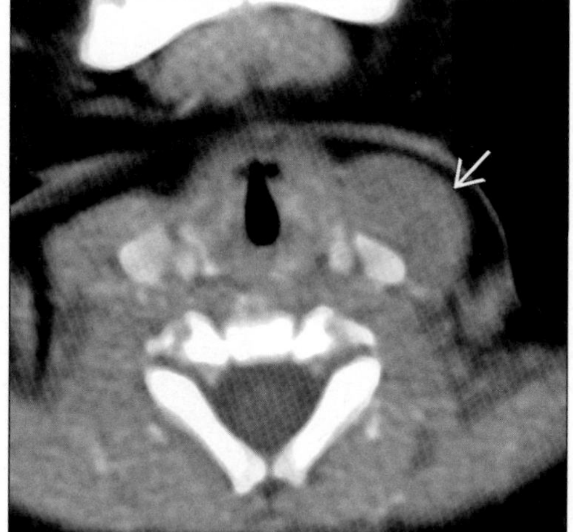

Axial CECT demonstrates diffuse enlargement of the left sternocleidomastoid muscle ➔ in a neonate after a difficult birth with palpable neck mass and torticollis.

SOLID NECK MASS IN NEONATE

Reactive Lymph Nodes

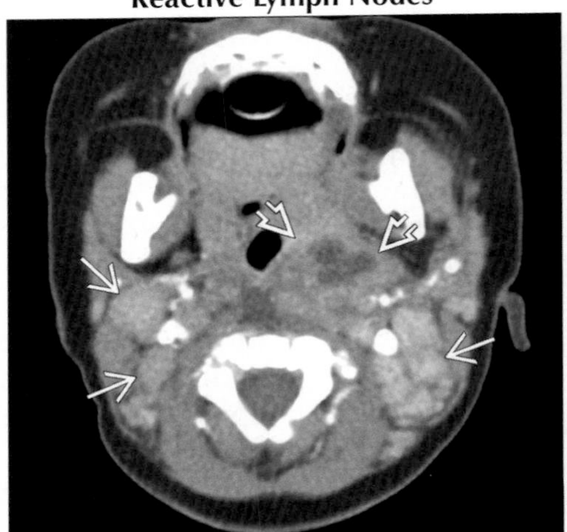

Reactive Lymph Nodes

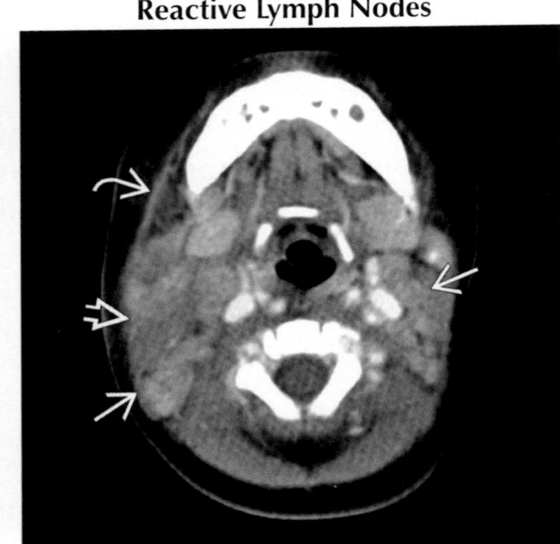

(Left) *Axial CECT in a 4-month-old boy shows bilateral nonsuppurative cervical lymph nodes and a large phlegmonous inflammatory mass in the left lateral retropharyngeal space.* ***(Right)*** *Axial CECT reveals bilateral cervical adenopathy with surrounding stranding of the fat (cellulitis) and thickening of the right platysma muscle (myositis). There is also nonenhancing fluid surrounding the right sternocleidomastoid muscle.*

Infantile Hemangioma

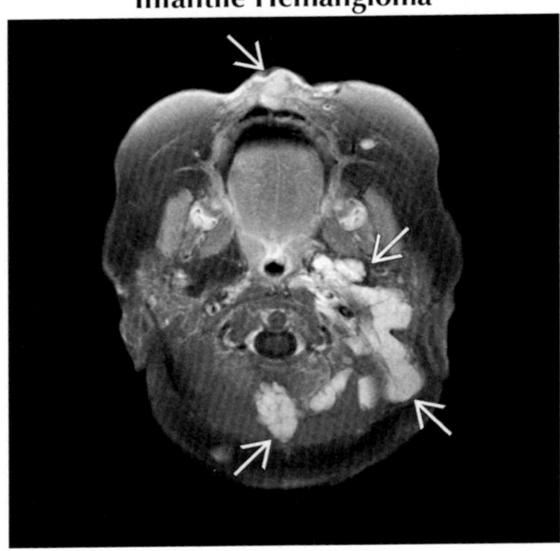

Infantile Hemangioma

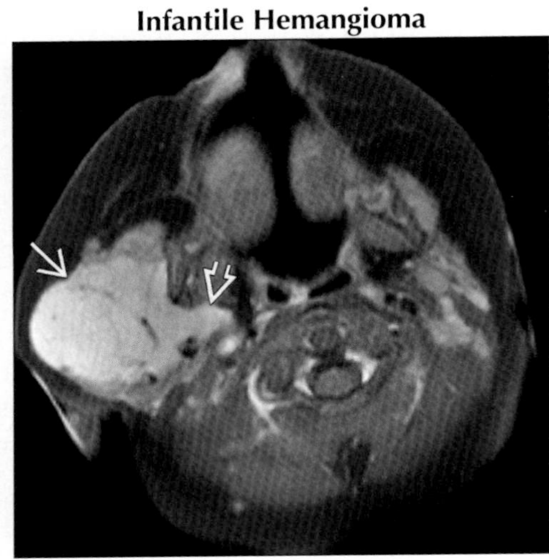

(Left) *Axial T2WI FS MR shows multiple enhancing hemangiomas in an infant with PHACES syndrome (posterior fossa malformations, hemangiomas, arterial anomalies, coarctation of the aorta and cardiac defects, eye abnormalities, and sternal clefting).* ***(Right)*** *Axial T1WI C+ FS MR reveals diffuse enlargement and intense enhancement of parotid hemangioma. Note the lesion is holoparotid, involving both the superficial and deep lobes.*

Neurofibromatosis Type 1

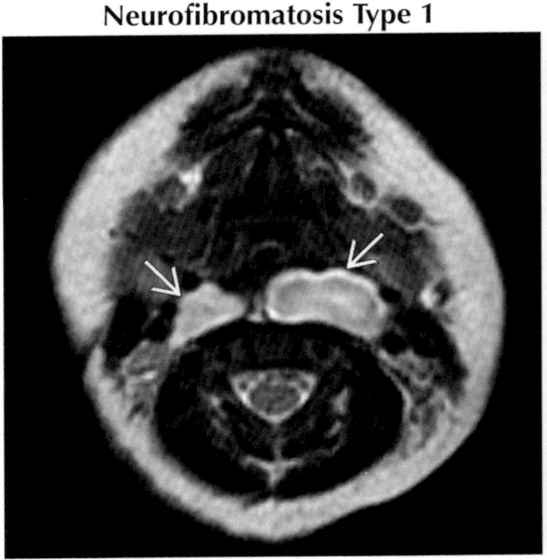

Teratoma

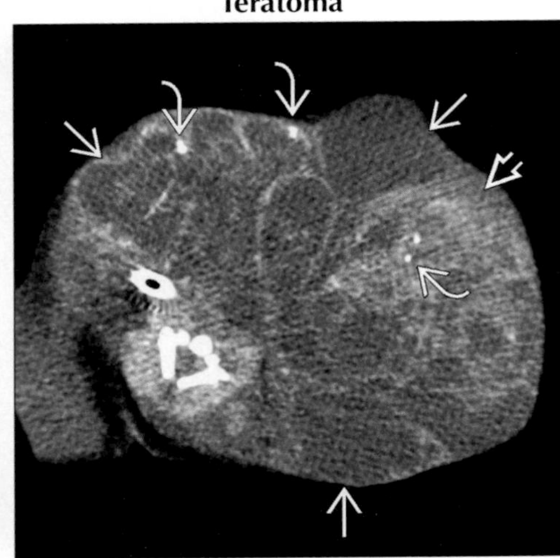

(Left) *Axial T2WI MR depicts bilateral, hyperintense, carotid sheath neurofibromas that extend medially from the carotid sheath into the retropharyngeal space.* ***(Right)*** *Axial CECT shows a large heterogeneous trans-spatial neck mass in a 6-day-old infant. Some areas are cystic, others are more solid, and there are small foci of calcifications, consistent with congenital teratoma.*

Langerhans Cell Histiocytosis, General

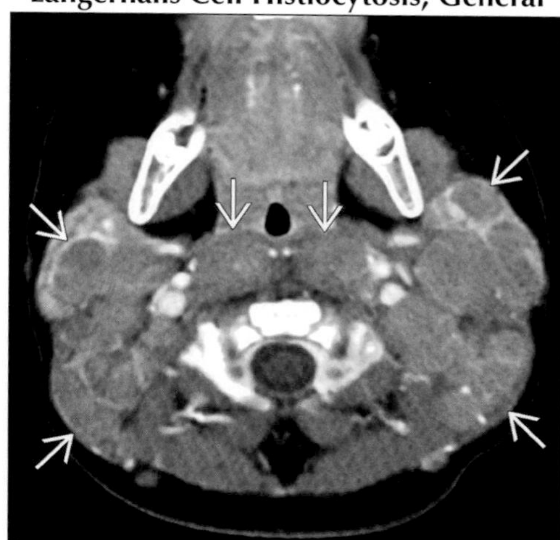

Metastatic Neuroblastoma

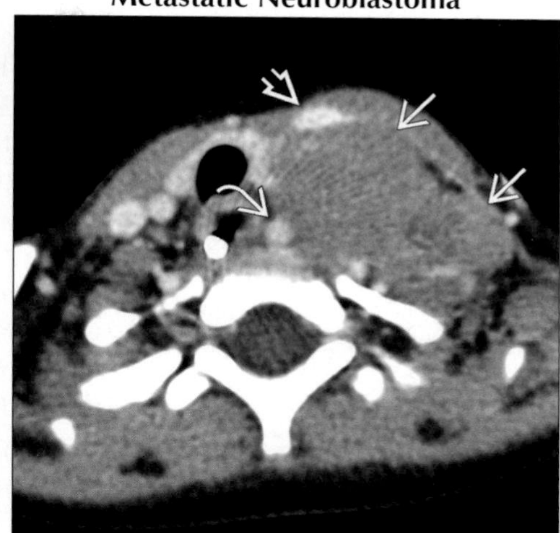

*(**Left**) Axial CECT shows massive bilateral cervical adenopathy in all nodal groups ➡ in an 8-month-old boy with an acute disseminated form of Langerhans cell histiocytosis. (**Right**) Axial CECT demonstrates a large conglomerate of metastatic left cervical lymph nodes in a girl with primary adrenal neuroblastoma ➡. The left jugular vein ➡ is displaced anteriorly, and the left carotid artery ➡ is deviated posteromedially.*

Fibromatosis

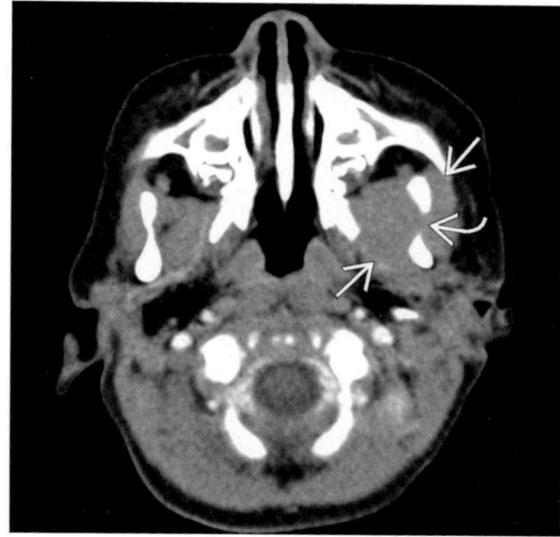

Primary Cervical Neuroblastoma

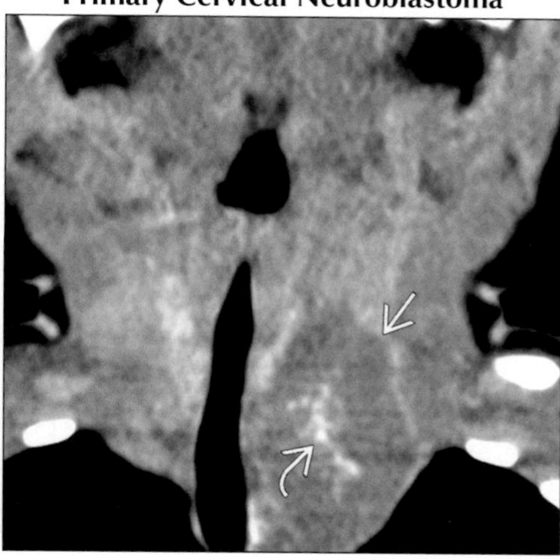

*(**Left**) Axial CECT shows a soft tissue attenuation mass in the left masticator space ➡ with smooth thinning of the left mandible ramus ➡. The imaging diagnosis of possible sarcoma was replaced by surgical pathologic diagnosis of fibromatosis. (**Right**) Coronal CECT reveals a well-defined, low-attenuation, left paratracheal neuroblastoma ➡ with central irregular calcifications ➡ in a 1-year-old girl who presented with ataxia, opsoclonus-myoclonus.*

Primary Cervical Neuroblastoma

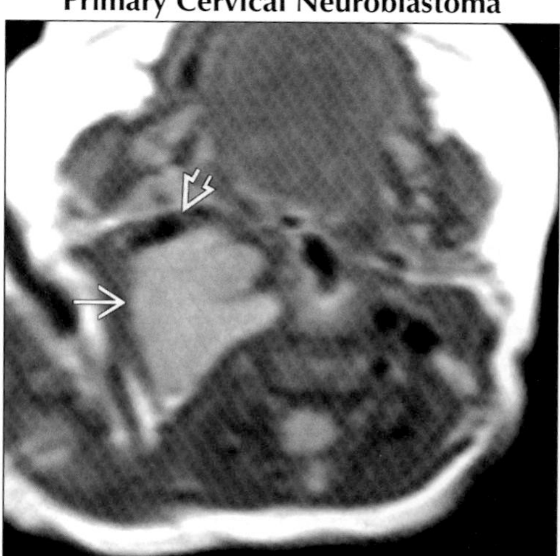

Cervical Thymus

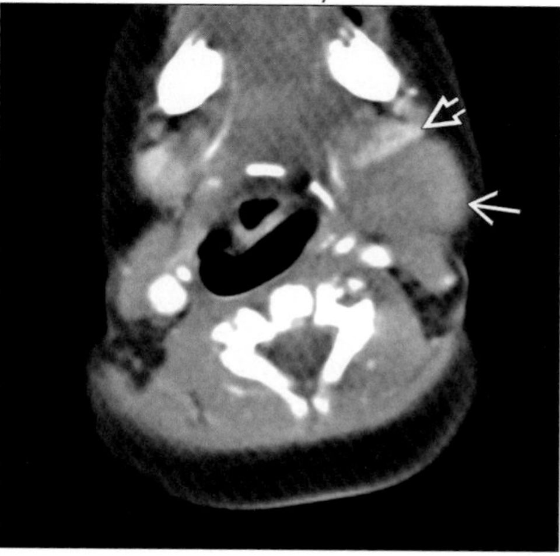

*(**Left**) Axial PD FSE MR reveals a well-defined left carotid sheath primary cervical neuroblastoma ➡ without intraspinal extension. Notice the anterior displacement of the carotid artery and internal jugular vein ➡. (**Right**) Axial CECT shows a well-defined, intermediate-attenuation, left anterior neck mass ➡ in a 3 month old with pathologically proven cervical thymus. The left submandibular gland ➡ is flattened anteriorly.*

SOLID NECK MASS IN A CHILD

DIFFERENTIAL DIAGNOSIS

Common
- Reactive Lymph Nodes
- Hodgkin Lymphoma, Lymph Nodes
- Infantile Hemangioma
- Neurofibromatosis Type 1
- Non-Hodgkin Lymphoma, Lymph Nodes

Less Common
- Lipoma
- Metastatic Neuroblastoma
- Differentiated Thyroid Carcinoma, Nodal

Rare but Important
- Pilomatrixoma
- Primary Cervical Neuroblastoma
- SCCa, Nodes
- Rhabdomyosarcoma
- Cervical Thymus

ESSENTIAL INFORMATION

Helpful Clues for Common Diagnoses
- **Reactive Lymph Nodes**
  - Key facts
    - "Reactive" implies benign etiology
    - Acute or chronic; any H&N nodal group
    - Response to infection/inflammation
  - Imaging
    - Enlarged oval-shaped lymph nodes
    - ± enlargement of lingual, faucial, or adenoidal hypertrophy
    - ± stranding of adjacent fat (cellulitis)
    - ± edema in adjacent muscles (myositis)
    - ± suppurative nodes or abscess
    - Variable enhancement, usually mild
- **Hodgkin Lymphoma, Lymph Nodes**
  - Key facts
    - B-cell origin; histology shows Reed-Sternberg cells
    - Cervical & mediastinal nodes common
    - Waldeyer ring or extranodal < 1%
    - Tumors EBV positive in up to 50%
  - Imaging
    - Cannot distinguish Hodgkin from non-Hodgkin lymphoma
    - Homogeneous lobulated nodal masses
    - Single or multiple nodal chain
    - Variable contrast enhancement
    - Necrotic center may be present
- **Infantile Hemangioma**
  - Key facts
    - True vascular neoplasm
    - Usually not present at birth; typically presents in 1st few months of life
    - Rapid growth and spontaneous involution typical
  - Imaging
    - Solid, avidly enhancing mass
    - Intralesional high-flow vessels
    - Fatty infiltration during involution
    - PHACES syndrome: **P**osterior fossa abnormalities, **h**emangiomas, **a**rterial abnormalities, **c**ardiovascular defects, **e**ye abnormalities, **s**ternal clefts
- **Neurofibromatosis Type 1**
  - Key facts
    - Carotid space, perivertebral space (brachial plexus) common
    - Localized, diffuse, or plexiform
    - Single or multiple
  - Imaging
    - Localized: Well-circumscribed, smooth, solid masses with variable enhancement
    - Diffuse: Plaque-like thickening of skin with poorly defined linear branching lesion in subcutaneous fat
    - Plexiform: Lobulated, tortuous, rope-like expansion in major nerve distribution; "tangle of worms" appearance
- **Non-Hodgkin Lymphoma, Lymph Nodes**
  - Key facts
    - All nodal chains involved
    - 30% extranodal: Lymphatic (palatine or lingual tonsil and adenoids) or extralymphatic (paranasal sinuses, skull base, and thyroid)
  - Imaging
    - Cannot distinguish non-Hodgkin from Hodgkin lymphoma
    - Single dominant node or multiple nonnecrotic enlarged nodes

Helpful Clues for Less Common Diagnoses
- **Lipoma**
  - Key facts: Any space, may be trans-spatial
  - Imaging
    - Homogeneous fat density (CT) or signal (MR) without significant enhancement
    - If enhancement, suspect liposarcoma
- **Metastatic Neuroblastoma**
  - Key facts
    - Most cervical disease is metastatic
  - Imaging

- Large lymph nodes, rarely necrotic
- Bilateral skull base metastasis common
- Enhancing masses with aggressive osseous erosion and intracranial/intraorbital extension

- **Differentiated Thyroid Carcinoma, Nodal**
  - Key facts
    - Nodal spread common in papillary, distant spread common in follicular
    - 3x more common in women
    - Usually 3rd & 4th decade, occasionally in adolescents, rare in young children
  - Imaging
    - Variable: Small to large, "reactive" in appearance or heterogeneous, hemorrhagic, or cystic necrosis
    - Focal calcifications and solid foci of enhancement may be present

Helpful Clues for Rare Diagnoses

- **Pilomatrixoma**
  - Key facts
    - Calcifying epithelioma of Malherbe
    - Usually benign in children
  - Imaging
    - Enhancing mass in subcutaneous fat
    - Variable calcification, adherent to skin
- **Primary Cervical Neuroblastoma**
  - Key facts
    - < 5% of neuroblastomas are primary cervical lesions
    - Range from immature neuroblastoma to mature, benign ganglioneuroma
  - Imaging
    - Well-defined solid mass closely associated with carotid sheath
    - Intraspinal extension rare
    - Calcifications may be present
- **SCCa, Nodes**
  - Key facts
    - Unknown primary SCCa rare in children
    - Nasopharyngeal carcinoma with adenopathy may occur in teenagers
  - Imaging
    - Enlarged, round nodes
    - May be heterogeneous ± multiple confluent nodes
- **Rhabdomyosarcoma**
  - Key facts
    - Most common location in H&N is parameningeal (middle ear, paranasal sinus, nasopharynx)
    - Intracranial extension in up to 55% of parameningeal lesions
  - Imaging
    - Soft tissue mass, variable enhancement
    - Bone erosion or nonaggressive bone remodeling
    - Cervical adenopathy may be associated
- **Cervical Thymus**
  - Key facts: Thymic remnants along path of thymopharyngeal duct
  - Imaging: Mildly enhancing soft tissue mass along path of thymopharyngeal duct

Reactive Lymph Nodes

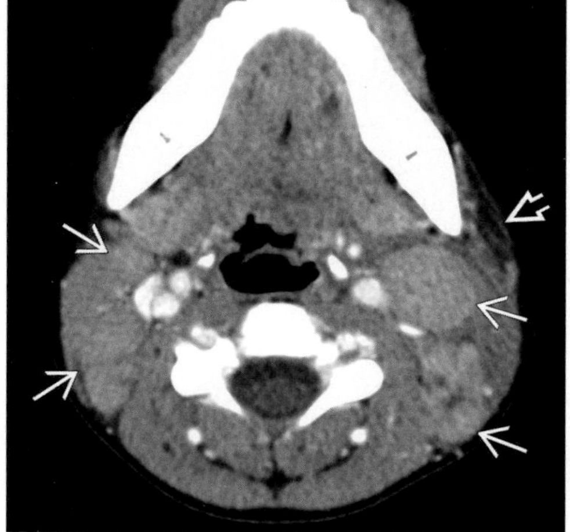

Axial CECT shows left greater than right, nonnecrotic, reactive cervical adenopathy ➡ and mild overlying soft tissue edema ➡ in a toddler with an elevated white blood cell count.

Hodgkin Lymphoma, Lymph Nodes

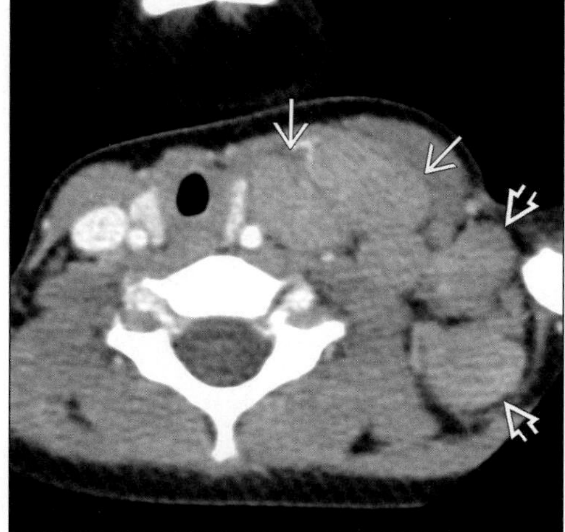

Axial CECT demonstrates multiple large supraclavicular cervical lymph nodes in a 4 year old with Hodgkin lymphoma. Both the internal jugular ➡ and spinal accessory ➡ chain nodes are involved.

SOLID NECK MASS IN A CHILD

Infantile Hemangioma

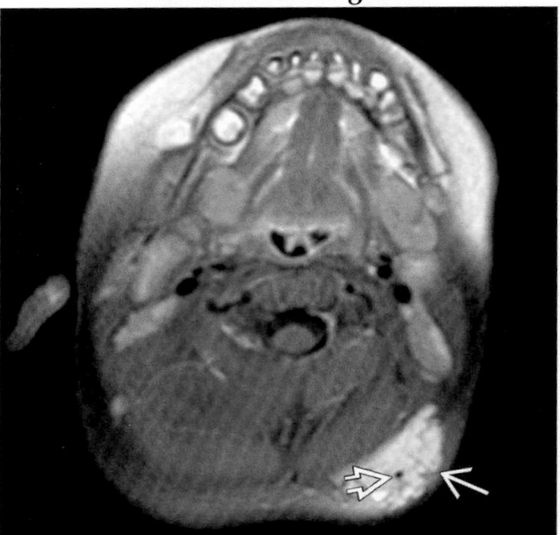

Infantile Hemangioma

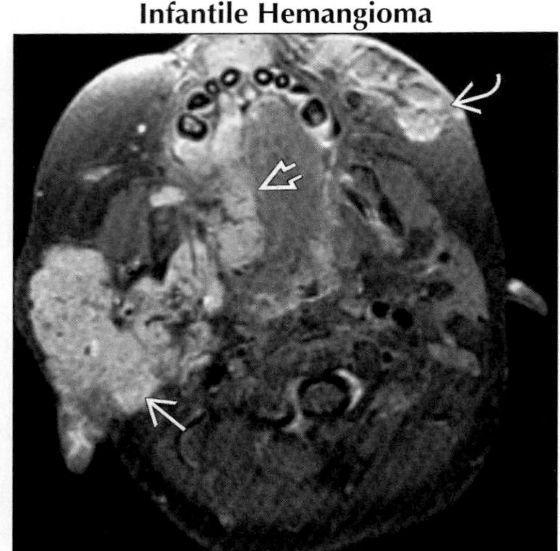

(Left) *Axial T1WI C+ FS MR reveals a homogeneously enhancing, lobulated infantile hemangioma ➡ in the posterior left subcutaneous fat with a single flow void ⇨, consistent with a high-flow intralesional vessel, typical of hemangioma.* ***(Right)*** *Axial T1WI C+ FS MR shows multiple enhancing infantile hemangiomas in the right parotid gland ➡, right sublingual space ⇨, and left cheek ↪ in a patient with PHACES syndrome.*

Neurofibromatosis Type 1

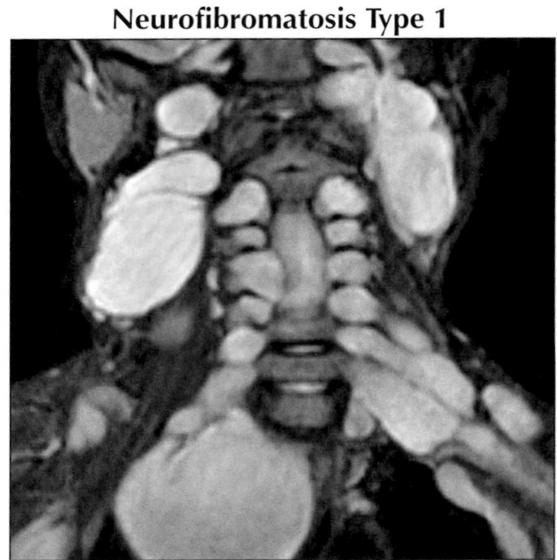

Non-Hodgkin Lymphoma, Lymph Nodes

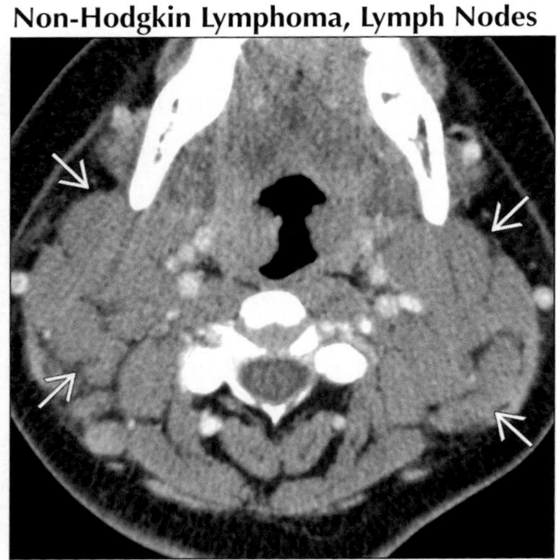

(Left) *Coronal STIR MR demonstrates multiple bilateral neurofibromas involving the neck, neural foramina, cervical canal, brachial plexus, and thoracic inlet in a young child with neurofibromatosis type 1.* ***(Right)*** *Axial CECT reveals multiple bilateral internal jugular chain lymph nodes ➡ in a teenager with T-cell lymphoblastic lymphoma.*

Lipoma

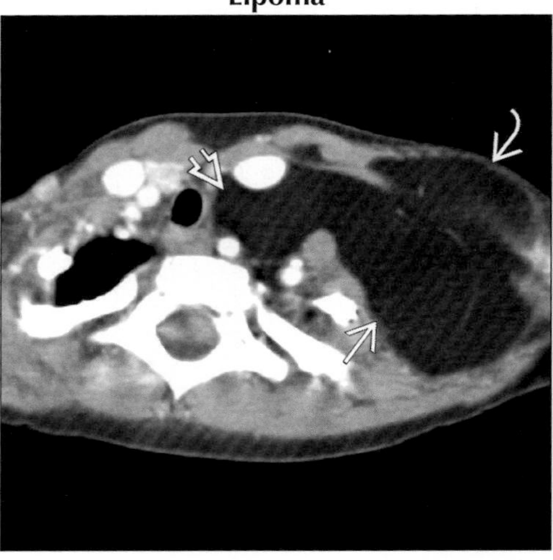

Metastatic Neuroblastoma

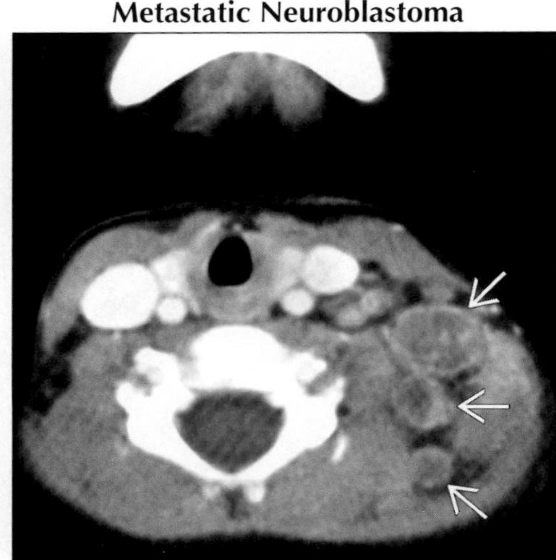

(Left) *Axial CECT shows a trans-spatial left infrahyoid neck mass. The lipoma involves the carotid ⇨, posterior cervical ➡, and superficial ↪ spaces of the infrahyoid neck.* ***(Right)*** *Axial CECT reveals multiple partially necrotic left spinal accessory metastatic lymph nodes ➡ secondary to primary adrenal neuroblastoma.*

Differentiated Thyroid Carcinoma, Nodal

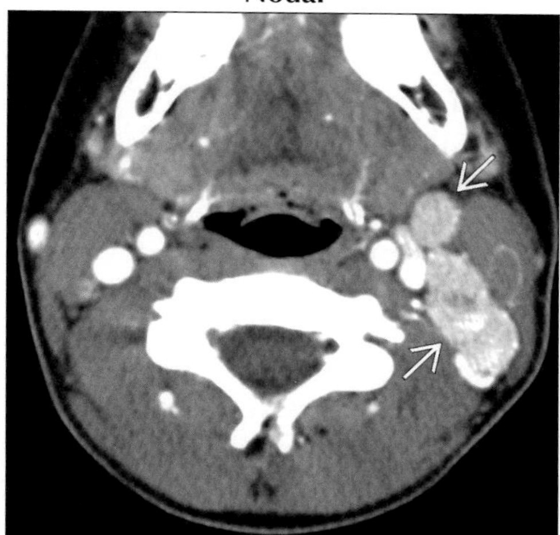

Pilomatrixoma

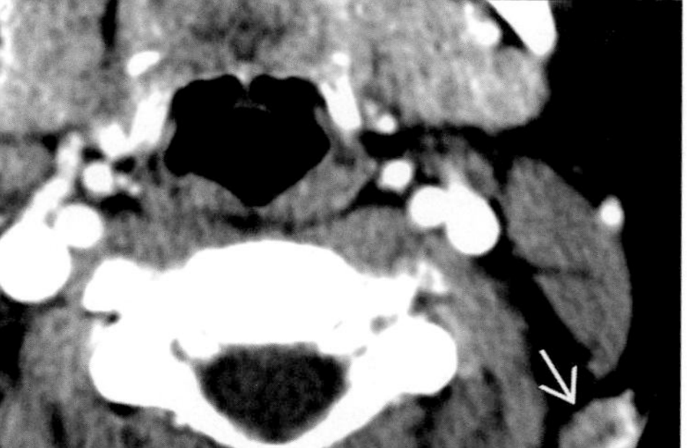

(Left) *Axial CECT demonstrates high-attenuation calcified metastatic papillary thyroid carcinoma nodal metastases ➡. Solid enhancing, cystic, or calcified components in neck nodes suggest differentiated thyroid carcinoma primary.* ***(Right)*** *Axial CECT reveals a well-defined, partially calcified pilomatrixoma ➡ in the subcutaneous fat of the left posterior neck, adherent to the skin ➡.*

Primary Cervical Neuroblastoma

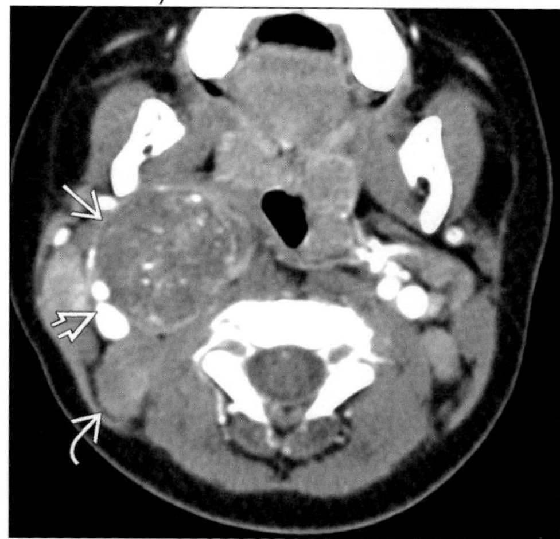

SCCa, Nodes

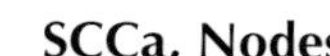

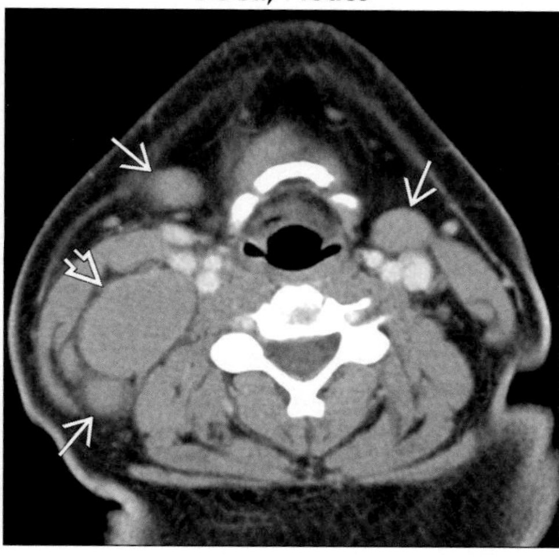

(Left) *Axial NECT reveals a well-defined round mass ➡ with speckled intrinsic calcifications that deviates the carotid space laterally ➡. This proved to be a ganglioneuroblastoma, a mixture of neuroblastoma and ganglioneuroma. Note nodal metastasis ➡.* ***(Right)*** *Axial CECT shows multiple enlarged, nonnecrotic cervical lymph nodes ➡; the largest ➡ is deep to sternocleidomastoid muscle at level of hyoid bone in a teenager with metastatic nasopharyngeal carcinoma.*

Rhabdomyosarcoma

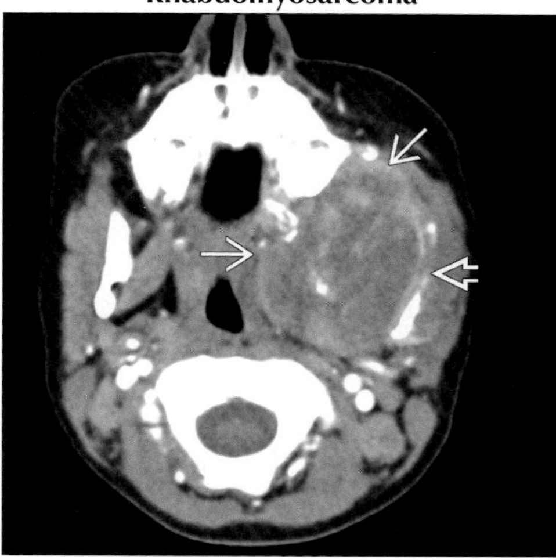

Cervical Thymus

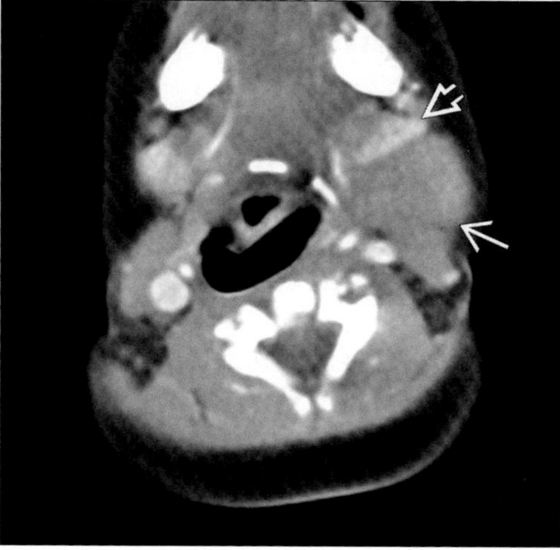

(Left) *Axial CECT reveals a large heterogeneous left masticator space mass ➡ destroying the left mandible ➡ in a 3 year old with rhabdomyosarcoma.* ***(Right)*** *Axial CECT demonstrates an intermediate-attenuation, solid-appearing mass ➡ posterior to the left submandibular gland ➡. Surgical pathology found the mass to be ectopic thymus.*

CYSTIC NECK MASS IN A CHILD

DIFFERENTIAL DIAGNOSIS

Common
- Suppurative Lymph Nodes
- Abscess
- Thyroglossal Duct Cyst
- Lymphatic Malformation
- Ranula
- 2nd Branchial Cleft Cyst

Less Common
- 1st Branchial Cleft Cyst
- Thymic Cyst

Rare but Important
- Dermoid and Epidermoid
- Teratoma

ESSENTIAL INFORMATION

Helpful Clues for Common Diagnoses
- **Suppurative Lymph Nodes**
  - Key facts
    - Pus in lymph node = intranodal abscess
  - Imaging
    - Thick enhancing nodal walls with central hypodensity
    - Edema in surrounding fat (cellulitis)
    - ± thickening of muscles (myositis)
    - Associated nonsuppurative adenopathy
    - Nontuberculous mycobacterial adenitis lacks surrounding inflammatory changes
- **Abscess**
  - Key facts
    - Conglomeration of suppurative nodes or rupture of node ⇒ extranodal abscess
    - Superficial abscesses: Anterior or posterior cervical or submandibular space
    - Deep neck abscesses: Retropharyngeal, parapharyngeal, or tonsillar; may grow rapidly ⇒ airway compromise, ± mediastinal extension
    - If anterior to left thyroid lobe, think 4th branchial apparatus anomaly
    - Exclude dental infection and salivary gland calculus as cause of H&N infection
  - Imaging
    - Wide prevertebral soft tissue = cellulitis and edema ± frank abscess
    - False-positive in children if neck not in extended position
    - Rim-enhancing mass with low-attenuation center; majority drainable pus, up to 25% may be phlegmon without drainable pus
    - Edema in surrounding fat (cellulitis), ± thickening of muscles (myositis), occasionally air in abscess cavity
- **Thyroglossal Duct Cyst**
  - Key facts
    - Remnant of thyroglossal duct, anywhere from foramen cecum at base of tongue to thyroid bed in infrahyoid neck
    - Treatment = resect cyst, tract, and midline hyoid bone (Sistrunk procedure)
  - Imaging
    - Cyst with minimal rim enhancement
    - At hyoid > suprahyoid = infrahyoid
    - Most in suprahyoid neck are midline; may be paramidline in infrahyoid neck
    - Infrahyoid embedded in strap muscles
    - May contain hyperechoic debris without hemorrhage or infection
    - Increased enhancement and surrounding inflammatory change when infected
    - ± nodularity or calcifications if associated thyroid carcinoma (adults)
- **Lymphatic Malformation**
  - Key facts
    - Congenital vascular malformation
    - Variably sized lymphatic channels
    - Present at birth
    - Grows with child
    - Hemorrhage ⇒ sudden increase in size
  - Imaging
    - Unilocular or multilocular; macrocystic or microcystic
    - 1 space or trans-spatial
    - Only septations enhance, unless associated with venous malformation
    - Lack high-flow vessels on flow sensitive MR sequences and angiography
    - Fluid-fluid levels
- **Ranula**
  - Key facts
    - Simple = postinflammatory retention cyst with epithelial lining; arising in sublingual gland or minor salivary gland, in sublingual space (SLS)
    - Diving = extravasation pseudocyst when ruptures out of SLS into submandibular space (SMS)

- Imaging
  - Simple = well-defined cyst in SLS
  - Diving = cyst in SLS and SMS; if SLS component collapsed ⇒ "tail"
- **2nd Branchial Cleft Cyst**
  - Key facts
    - Characteristic location = at or inferior to angle of mandible, posterolateral to submandibular gland, lateral to carotid space, and anteromedial to sternocleidomastoid muscle (SCM)
    - Uncommon locations = parapharyngeal space, beaking in between internal and external carotid artery, anterior surface of infrahyoid carotid space
  - Imaging
    - Well-defined unilocular cyst in typical location
    - No significant contrast enhancement unless infected

Helpful Clues for Less Common Diagnoses

- **1st Branchial Cleft Cyst**
  - Key facts
    - Remnant of 1st branchial apparatus
    - In or superficial to parotid gland, around pinna or external auditory canal
    - May extend to angle of mandible
    - Proximity to facial nerve important for surgical planning
  - Imaging
    - Well-defined nonenhancing cyst; contrast-enhancing wall with surrounding inflammation if infected
- **Thymic Cyst**
  - Key facts
    - Remnant of thymopharyngeal duct
    - 3rd branchial pouch remnant
    - Wall contains Hassall corpuscles
  - Imaging
    - Cystic neck mass along course of thymopharyngeal duct
    - ± solid enhancing thymic tissue
    - Closely associated with carotid sheath
    - May be connected to mediastinal thymus
    - Rarely ruptures into parapharyngeal space

Helpful Clues for Rare Diagnoses

- **Dermoid and Epidermoid**
  - Key facts
    - Dermoid: Epithelial and dermal elements
    - Epidermoid: Epithelial elements only
  - Imaging
    - Well-defined cyst filled with fluid = dermoid OR epidermoid
    - Well-defined cyst with fatty material, mixed fluid ± calcification = dermoid
- **Teratoma**
  - Key facts
    - All 3 germ cell lines
    - Mature, immature, and malignant
  - Imaging
    - Fat, calcium, cystic, and solid components

Suppurative Lymph Nodes

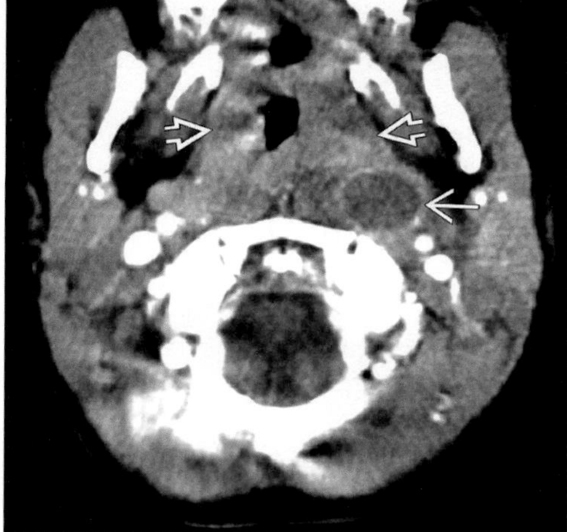

Axial CECT demonstrates a well-defined, rim-enhancing, suppurative left lateral retropharyngeal lymph node ➡ in a patient with pharyngitis. Note the swollen palatine tonsils ➡.

Suppurative Lymph Nodes

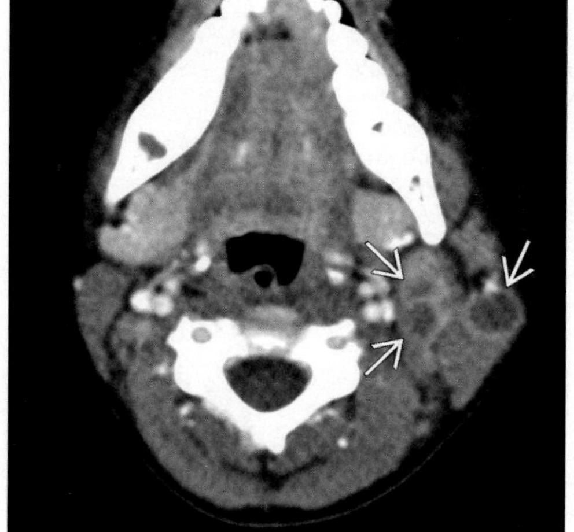

Axial CECT shows multiple necrotic left-sided cervical lymph nodes ➡, without inflammatory changes in the adjacent fat, in a 2 year old with mycobacterium avium intracellulare.

CYSTIC NECK MASS IN A CHILD

*(**Left**) Axial CECT reveals a large, multiloculated abscess with a fairly well-defined rim of contrast enhancement in the left parapharyngeal →, deep parotid →, and oropharyngeal mucosal → spaces in a 10-month-old girl with a persistent neck mass, despite oral antibiotics. (**Right**) Axial CECT demonstrates a well-defined, rim-enhancing, low-attenuation abscess → in the right palatine tonsil. Note the normal size of the left palatine tonsil →.*

Abscess

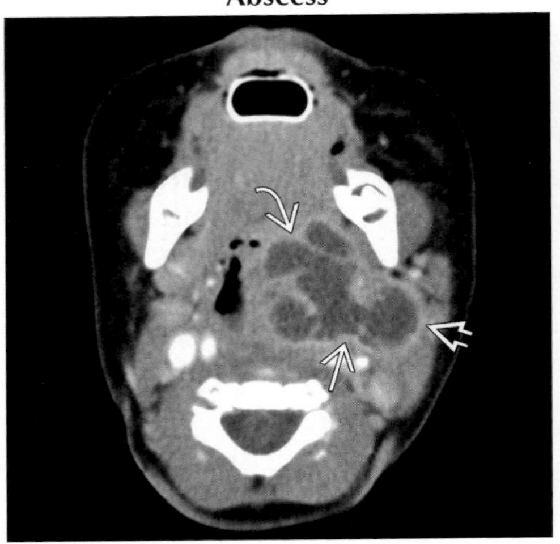

Abscess

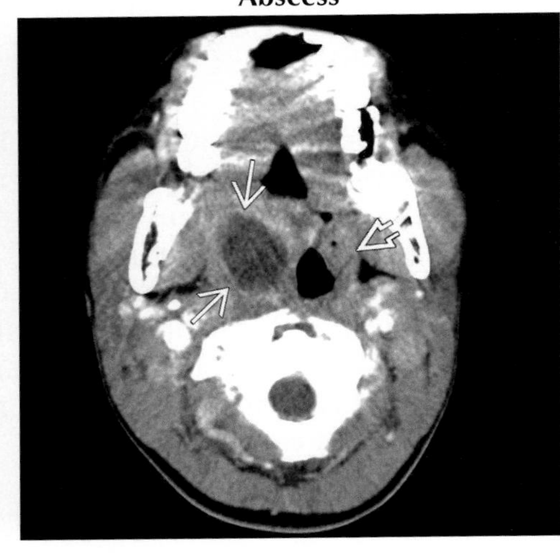

*(**Left**) Axial CECT shows a sharply marginated, nonenhancing infrahyoid thyroglossal duct cyst → embedded in the left strap muscles. The paramedian location of infrahyoid TGDC is characteristic. (**Right**) Sagittal CECT reveals an infected thyroglossal duct cyst → along the inferior margin of the hyoid bone → with significant surrounding inflammatory changes → and posterior rupture of the purulent material to the region of the aryepiglottic folds →.*

Thyroglossal Duct Cyst

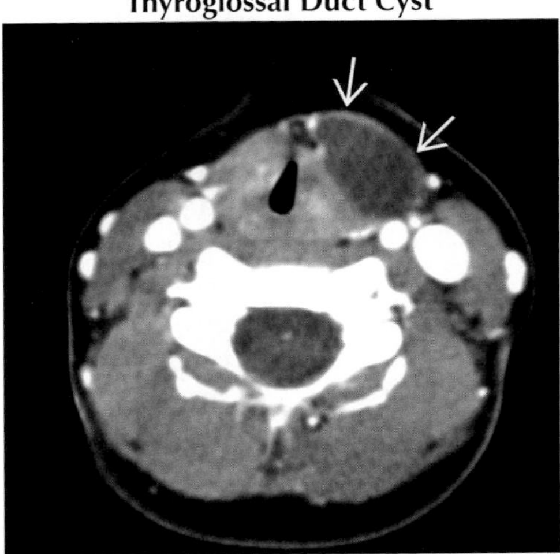

Thyroglossal Duct Cyst

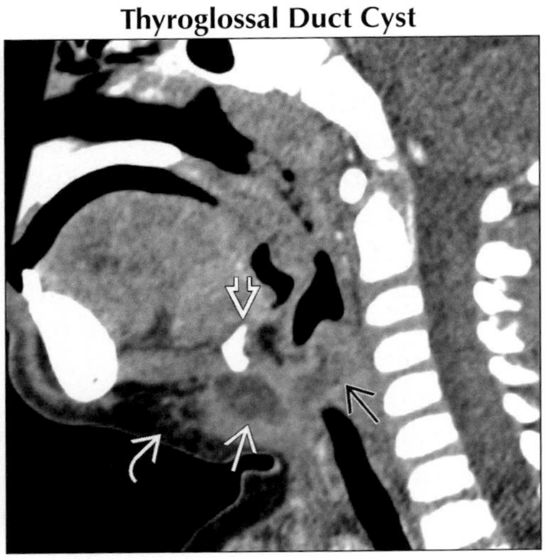

*(**Left**) Axial T1WI MR shows a multiloculated macrocystic lymphatic malformation →. A fluid-fluid level → in the medial locule is secondary to recent hemorrhage. (**Right**) Axial T2WI FS MR reveals the dependent blood products as the inferior component of fluid-fluid levels within 2 locules of the multiloculated, macrocystic lymphatic malformation →.*

Lymphatic Malformation

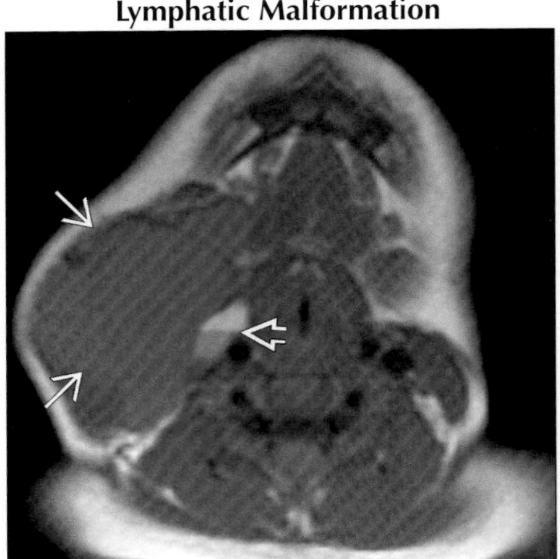

Lymphatic Malformation

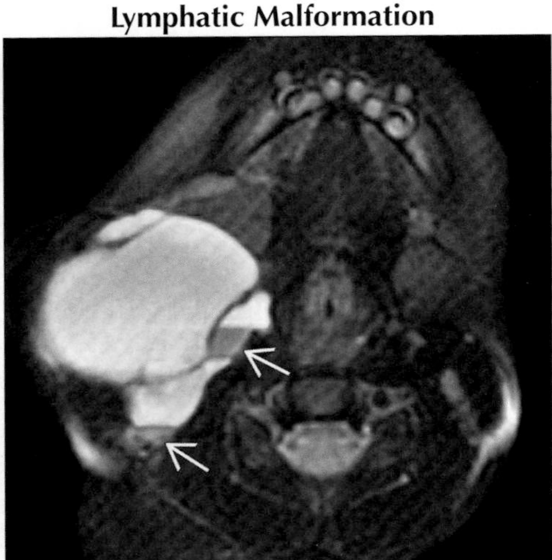

Ranula

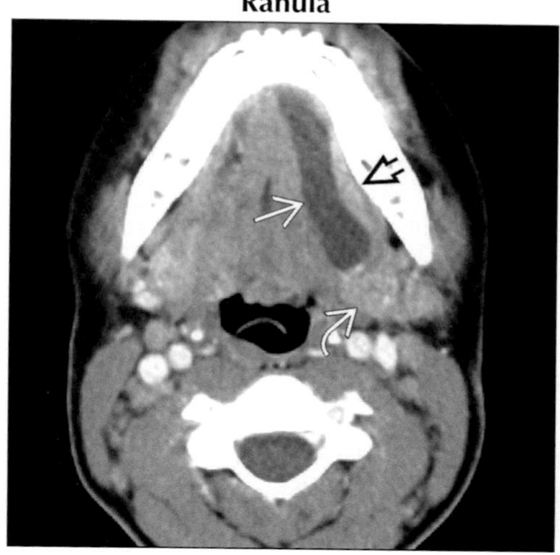

2nd Branchial Cleft Cyst

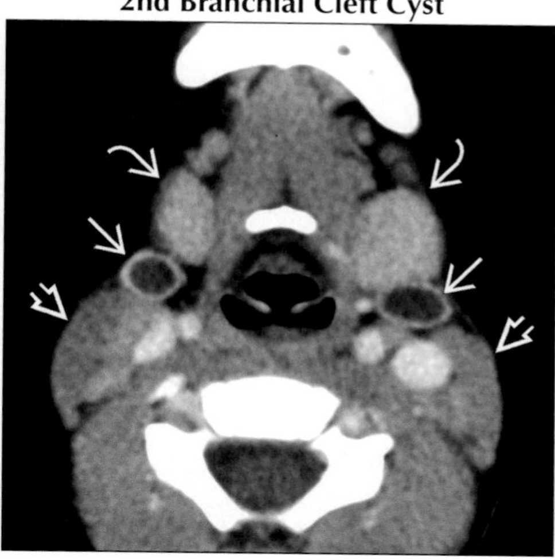

(Left) *Axial CECT in a patient with a sublingual mass shows a low-attenuation, nonenhancing ranula ➔. This is a simple ranula as it is confined to the sublingual space. Note also the submandibular gland ➔ and mylohyoid muscle ➔.* ***(Right)*** *Axial CECT in a child with branchiootorenal syndrome shows small bilateral 2nd branchial cleft cysts ➔ anterior to the sternocleidomastoid muscles ➔ and posterior to the submandibular glands ➔.*

1st Branchial Cleft Cyst

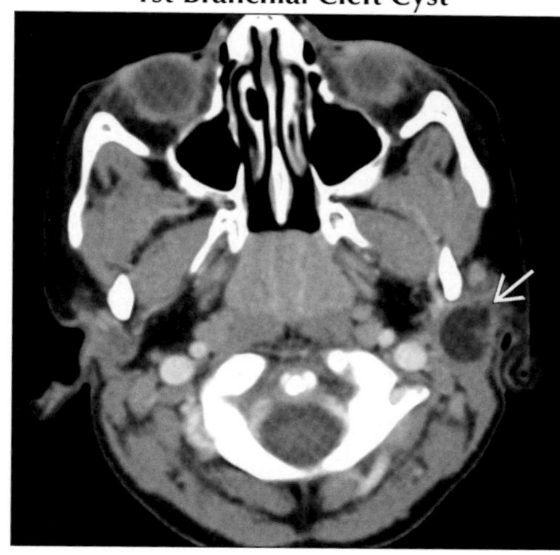

Thymic Cyst

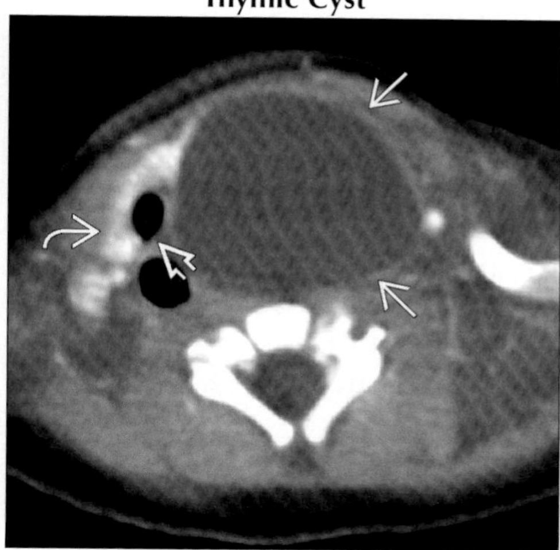

(Left) *Axial CECT shows a low-attenuation, nonenhancing cyst within the left parotid gland in a child with an intraparotid 1st branchial apparatus cyst ➔.* ***(Right)*** *Axial CECT demonstrates a large simple thymic cyst in the left anterior neck ➔, significantly deviating the airway ➔ and thyroid gland ➔ to the right. In this patient, the cyst extended from the skull base to the upper mediastinum.*

Dermoid and Epidermoid

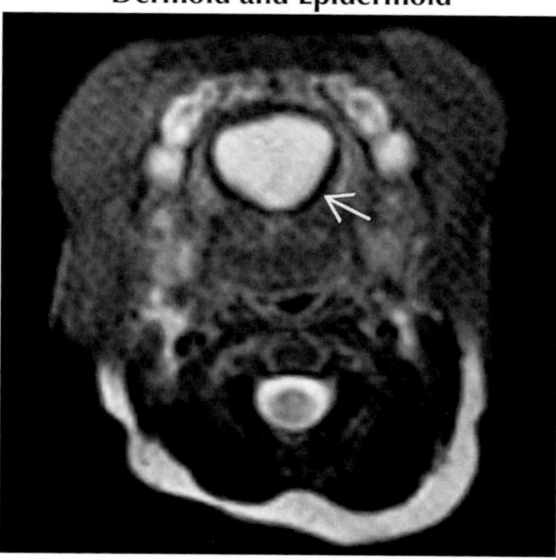

Teratoma

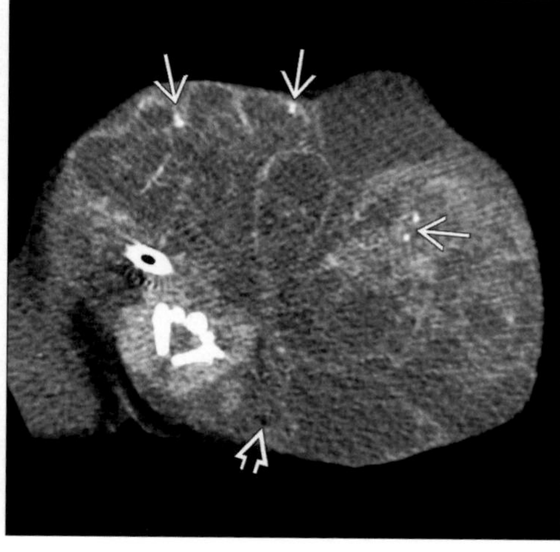

(Left) *Axial T2WI MR shows a hyperintense midline dermoid cyst in the floor of the mouth ➔. Histology showed the cyst lined by squamous epithelium and contained skin, adnexal structures, respiratory epithelium, and gastric epithelium.* ***(Right)*** *Axial CECT reveals a large, multiloculated cystic mass anterior to the vertebral body in an infant with congenital teratoma. The lesion contains only tiny foci of fat ➔ and several foci of calcification ➔.*

TRANS-SPATIAL MASS

DIFFERENTIAL DIAGNOSIS

Common
- Abscess
- Lymphatic Malformation
- Venous Malformation
- Infantile Hemangioma
- Neurofibromatosis Type 1
- Rhabdomyosarcoma

Less Common
- Lipoma
- Thymic Cyst
- 4th Branchial Anomaly

Rare but Important
- Teratoma
- Fibromatosis

ESSENTIAL INFORMATION

Key Differential Diagnosis Issues
- Trans-spatial: Multiple contiguous spaces

Helpful Clues for Common Diagnoses
- **Abscess**
  - Key facts
    - Signs and symptoms of infection
    - May be in deep soft tissues of neck
    - May present with airway impingement
    - 75% drainable pus; 25% phlegmonous, nondrainable inflammatory tissue
  - Imaging
    - Low-attenuation, rim-enhancing mass
    - Retropharyngeal edema common
    - May extend via danger space into mediastinum
- **Lymphatic Malformation**
  - Key facts
    - Most common cystic neck mass with spontaneous hemorrhage
    - Sudden increase in size secondary to hemorrhage or viral respiratory infection
  - Imaging
    - Unilocular or multilocular; macrocystic or microcystic; 1 space or trans-spatial
    - Insinuates morphology
    - Only septations enhance, unless associated with venous malformation
    - Lack high-flow vessels on flow-sensitive MR sequences and angiography
    - Fluid-fluid levels secondary to intralesional hemorrhage common
- **Venous Malformation**
  - Key facts
    - Lobulated soft tissue mass; variably sized venous channels with phleboliths
    - Mass increases in size with Valsalva, crying, or bending over
  - Imaging
    - Intermediate attenuation/hyperintense T2 with variable contrast enhancement
    - No high flow vessels
- **Infantile Hemangioma**
  - Key facts
    - Neoplasm with spontaneous proliferation and involution
    - Present within 1st few weeks of life; usually not present at birth
    - May be multiple (PHACES syndrome)
  - Imaging
    - Lobulated mass, intense enhancement
    - High-flow intralesional vessels
- **Neurofibromatosis Type 1**
  - Key facts
    - Localized neurofibroma (NF), diffuse NF, plexiform NF (PNF), or malignant peripheral nerve sheath tumor (PNST)
    - If multiple or plexiform, think NF1
  - Imaging
    - May be hypoattenuating on CT
    - Localized: Well-circumscribed, fusiform, solid masses and moderate enhancement ± dumbbell-shaped extension into neural foramina
    - Diffuse NF: Plaque-like subcutaneous lesion with poorly defined infiltrating margins, moderate enhancement
    - Plexiform NF: Lobulated, tortuous, rope-like enlargement in major nerve distribution; resembles "tangle of worms"
    - Malignant PNST: Benign vs. malignant difficult to differentiate on imaging; consider malignant if ≥ 5 cm, intensely enhancing with infiltrative margins
- **Rhabdomyosarcoma**
  - Key facts
    - Sites: Orbit, nasopharynx, temporal bone, sinonasal, cervical neck
  - Imaging
    - Soft tissue mass with variable contrast enhancement ± bone erosion
    - Coronal post-contrast fat-saturated T1 images best for intracranial extension

Helpful Clues for Less Common Diagnoses

- **Lipoma**
  - Key facts
    - Benign neoplasm, mature fat
  - Imaging
    - Well-circumscribed homogeneous mass of fat attenuation and signal intensity
    - Small minority of lesions will have a nonfatty soft tissue component
    - Any space of neck
    - Single space or trans-spatial
    - Imaging cannot differentiate between lipoma and low-grade liposarcoma
- **Thymic Cyst**
  - Key facts
    - Remnant of thymopharyngeal duct, 3rd branchial pouch remnant
    - Wall contains Hassall corpuscles
  - Imaging
    - Cystic neck mass along course of thymopharyngeal duct ± solid enhancing thymic tissue
    - Close association with carotid sheath
    - May be connected to mediastinal thymus directly or by fibrous cord
    - Rarely extends to skull base; may rupture into parapharyngeal space
- **4th Branchial Anomaly**
  - Key facts
    - Presents with recurrent thyroiditis or anterior neck abscess secondary to sinus tract extending from apex of pyriform sinus to lower anterior neck
  - Imaging
    - Cyst or abscess anterior to left thyroid lobe with associated thyroiditis
    - Barium swallow or post barium swallow CT may show sinus tract extending from apex of pyriform sinus to anterior lower neck

Helpful Clues for Rare Diagnoses

- **Teratoma**
  - Key facts
    - All 3 germ cell lines
    - Mature, immature, and malignant
  - Imaging
    - Fat, calcium, cyst, and solid components
- **Fibromatosis**
  - Key facts
    - Synonyms: Desmoid fibromatosis, extraabdominal desmoid fibromatosis, infantile fibromatosis
    - Histologically benign fibroproliferative disorder with potentially aggressive clinical course and invasive growth
    - Associated with Gardner syndrome
  - Imaging
    - Poorly marginated trans-spatial mass
    - Moderate post-contrast enhancement
    - ± bone erosion or invasion

Abscess

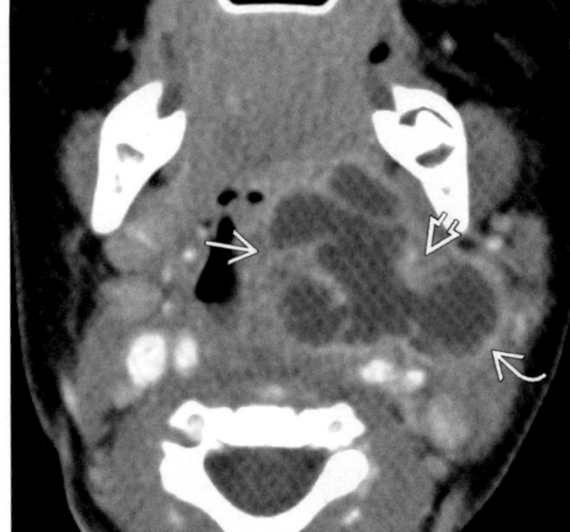

Axial CECT shows a large, multilobulated, rim-enhancing abscess arising from the left palatine tonsil ➡, spreading into the parapharyngeal space ⇨ with extension to the deep parotid space ↪.

Lymphatic Malformation

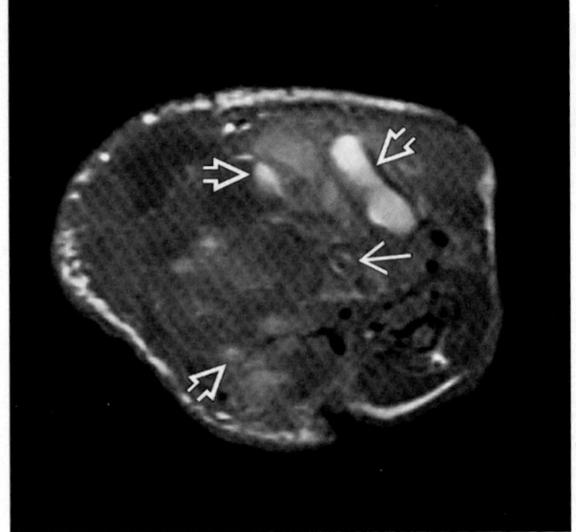

Axial T1WI MR shows an infiltrative, multiloculated, macrocystic neck lymphatic malformation, anterior to the suprastomal trachea ➡. Cysts contain hyperintense T1 signal fluid from hemorrhage ⇨.

TRANS-SPATIAL MASS

*(**Left**) Axial T1WI C+ FS MR reveals a well-defined, lobulated, heterogeneously enhancing venous malformation involving the right masseter ➔ and medial pterygoid ➔ muscles. Note focal signal voids secondary to phleboliths in both the deep and superficial component ➔. (**Right**) Axial CECT shows a lobulated, heterogeneously enhancing venous malformation ➔ in the left cheek with a moderate amount of fat and multiple variably sized phleboliths ➔.*

Venous Malformation

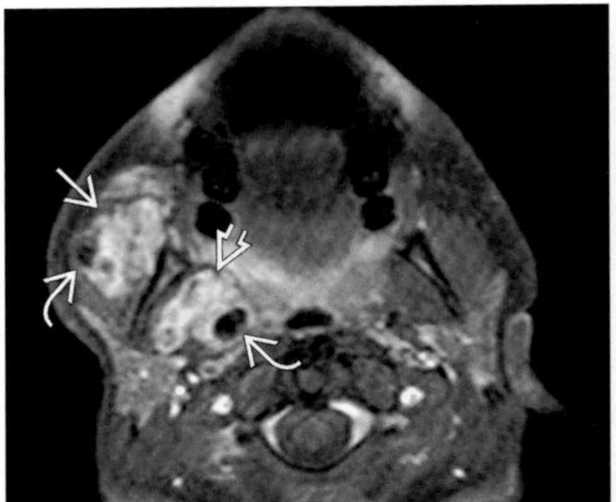

Venous Malformation

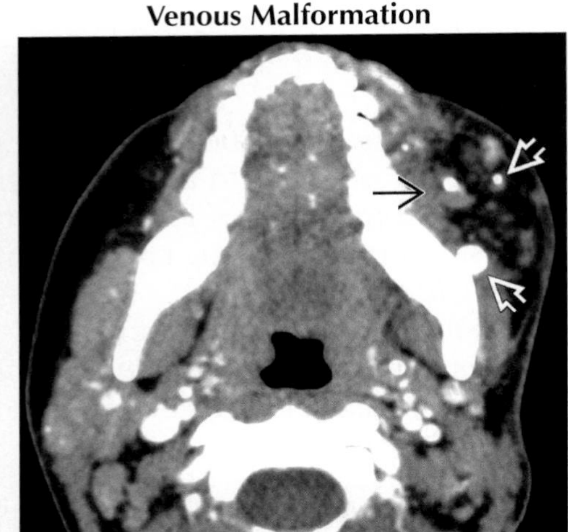

*(**Left**) Axial T1WI C+ FS MR demonstrates a homogeneously enhancing infantile hemangioma involving the left carotid space ➔, posterior cervical space of the neck ➔, and the left submandibular space ➔. (**Right**) Axial CECT shows an infiltrative low-attenuation plexiform neurofibroma involving the retropharyngeal space ➔ and the left carotid space ➔ and extending between the compressed left pyriform sinus and hyoid bone ➔.*

Infantile Hemangioma

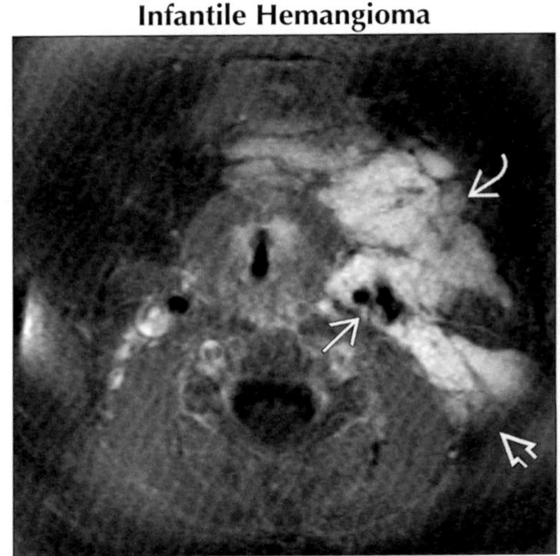

Neurofibromatosis Type 1

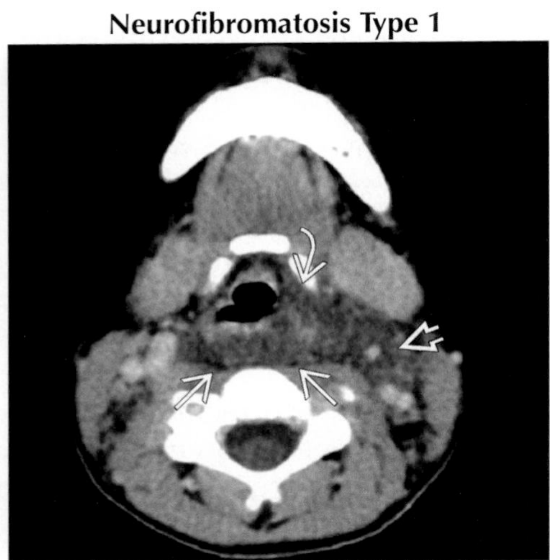

*(**Left**) Axial STIR MR reveals an infiltrative hyperintense plexiform neurofibroma involving the retropharyngeal space ➔, the left carotid space ➔, and parapharyngeal space ➔. Plexiform neurofibroma signals neurofibromatosis 1. (**Right**) Axial T2WI FS MR shows a large heterogeneously enhancing rhabdomyosarcoma involving the left masticator space ➔ and deep parotid space ➔. Note the rhabdomyosarcoma erodes the mandible ➔.*

Neurofibromatosis Type 1

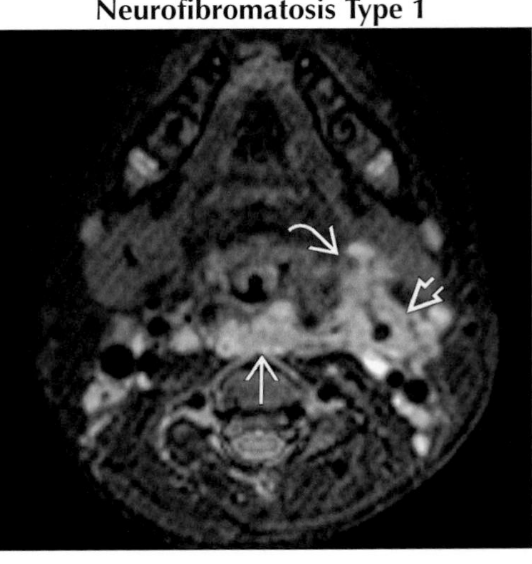

Rhabdomyosarcoma

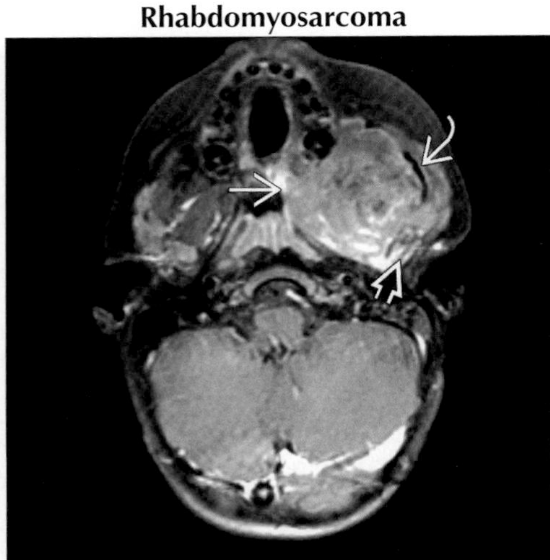

Lipoma

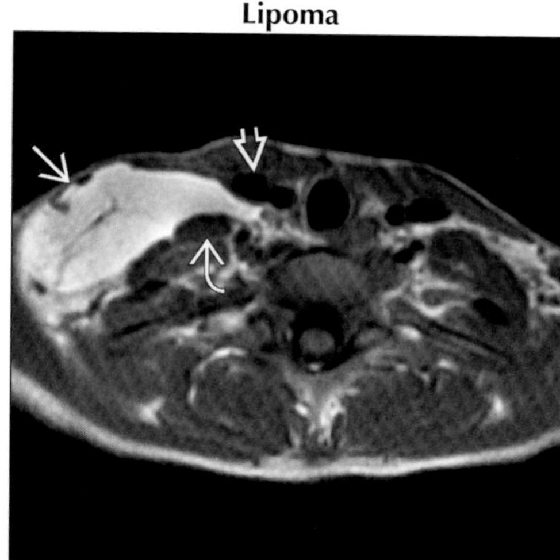

Thymic Cyst

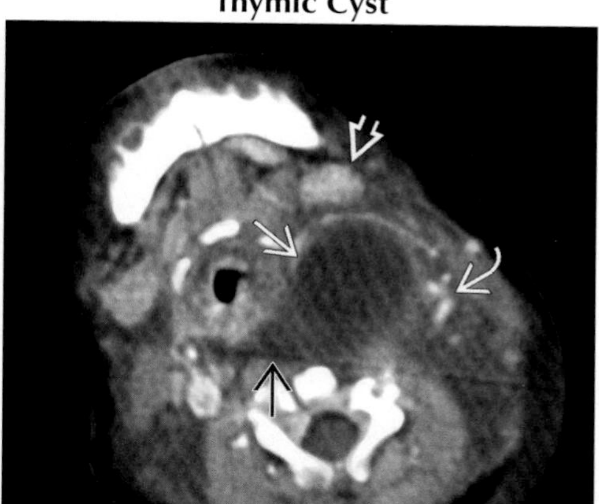

*(**Left**) Axial T1WI MR demonstrates a well-defined right posterior cervical space lipoma → insinuating between the internal jugular vein → and the anterior scalene muscle →, resulting in mild leftward deviation of the trachea. (**Right**) Axial CECT reveals a large thymic cyst → posterior to the left submandibular gland →, anteromedial to the carotid vessels →, and extending to the retropharyngeal space →.*

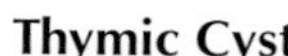

Thymic Cyst

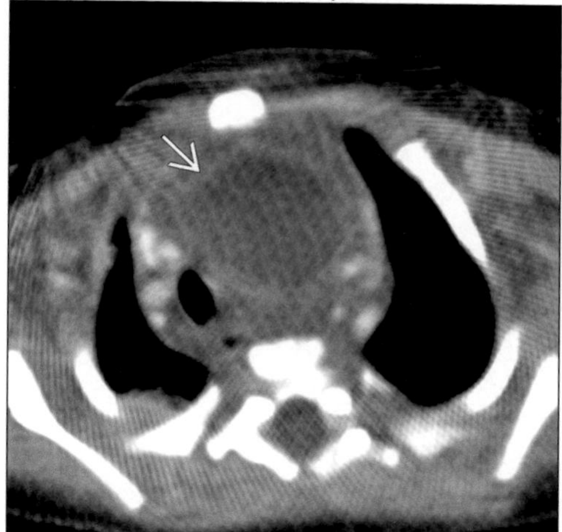

4th Branchial Anomaly

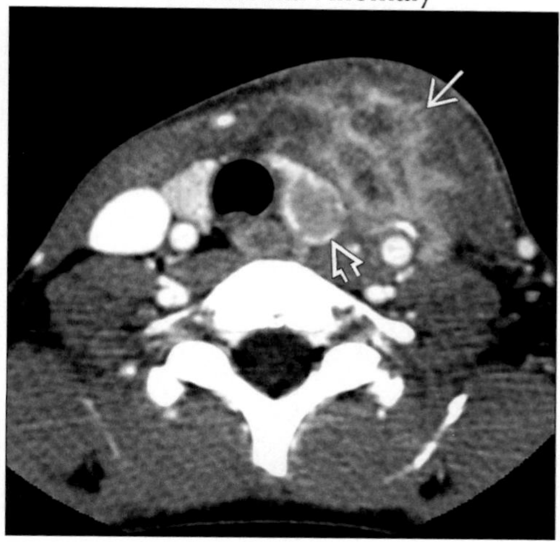

*(**Left**) Axial CECT demonstrates a well-defined thymic cyst in the superior mediastinum → that is contiguous with a cyst in the left neck (not shown). (**Right**) Axial CECT reveals a heterogeneously enhancing inflammatory mass → anterior to the left thyroid lobe, which contains a focal area of decreased enhancement consistent with focal thyroiditis →. Both are secondary to a 4th branchial pouch remnant (pyriform apex sinus tract).*

Teratoma

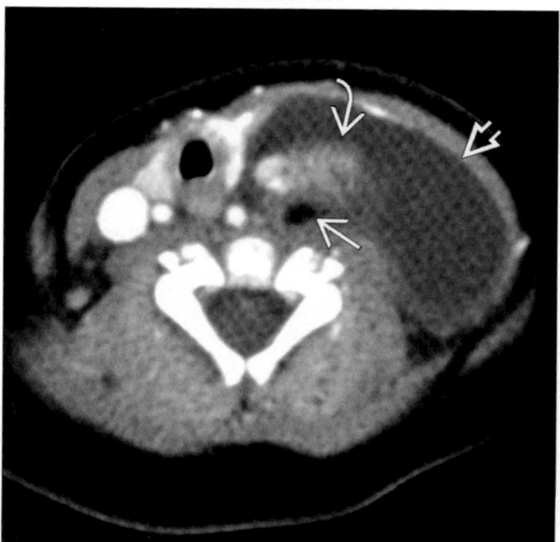

Fibromatosis

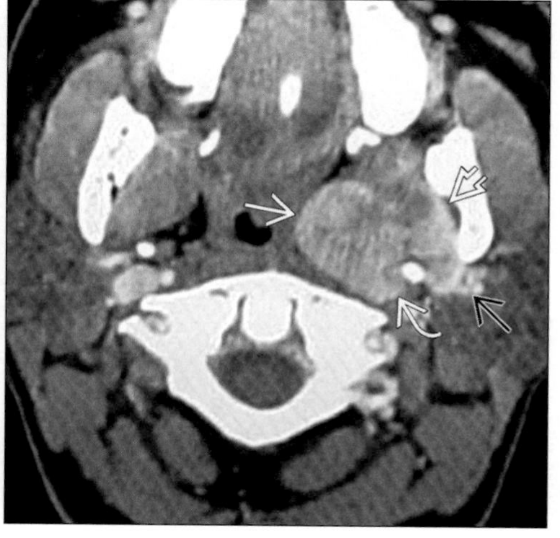

*(**Left**) Axial CECT shows a low-attenuation trans-spatial benign cystic teratoma that contains fat →, as well as cystic → and solid → components. The visceral, carotid, and posterior cervical spaces are all affected. (**Right**) Axial CECT reveals an enhancing trans-spatial mass of the left parapharyngeal space →, masticator space →, carotid space →, and deep parotid space →. Pathologic diagnosis of fibromatosis was made in this patient with Gardner syndrome.*

AIR-CONTAINING LESIONS IN NECK

DIFFERENTIAL DIAGNOSIS

Common
- General Trauma
- Retropharyngeal Space (RPS) Abscess

Less Common
- Laryngocele
- Esophago-Pharyngeal Diverticulum

Rare but Important
- 4th Branchial Anomaly
- Lateral Cervical Esophageal Diverticulum
- Spontaneous Cervical Emphysema

ESSENTIAL INFORMATION

Helpful Clues for Common Diagnoses
- **General Trauma**
  - Key facts: Esophageal, pharyngeal, laryngeal, or superficial trauma
  - Imaging: Extraluminal air in neck ± laryngeal, hyoid, or facial fractures
- **Retropharyngeal Space (RPS) Abscess**
  - Key facts: Posterior to pharyngeal mucosal space, anterior to prevertebral space
  - Imaging: Extranodal purulent fluid in RPS ± air in or adjacent to fluid collection ± extension to mediastinum

Helpful Clues for Less Common Diagnoses
- **Laryngocele**
  - Key facts: Lateral saccular cyst, laryngeal mucocele
  - Imaging: Air ± air-filled level
    - Internal laryngocele in paraglottic space
    - Mixed laryngocele in paraglottic and submandibular spaces
- **Esophago-Pharyngeal Diverticulum**
  - Key facts: Zenker diverticulum = mucosal-lined outpouching of posterior hypopharynx
  - Imaging: Air-filled pouch posterior; usually extends left of esophagus

Helpful Clues for Rare Diagnoses
- **4th Branchial Anomaly**
  - Key facts: 4th pharyngeal pouch remnant
    - Extends from apex of pyriform sinus to lower neck, anterior to left thyroid lobe
    - Present with recurrent thyroiditis or anterior neck abscess
  - Imaging
    - Abscess anterior to left thyroid lobe ± intrinsic inflammatory change in ipsilateral thyroid lobe
    - Inflamed pyriform sinus apex
    - Lack of aeration of pyriform sinus apex
- **Lateral Cervical Esophageal Diverticulum**
  - Key facts: Mucosal-lined outpouching lateral to cervical esophagus
  - Imaging: Air-filled pouch lateral to cervical esophagus
- **Spontaneous Cervical Emphysema**
  - Key facts: No history of vomiting, trauma, asthma, or other inciting event
  - Imaging: Pneumomediastinum and cervical emphysema

General Trauma

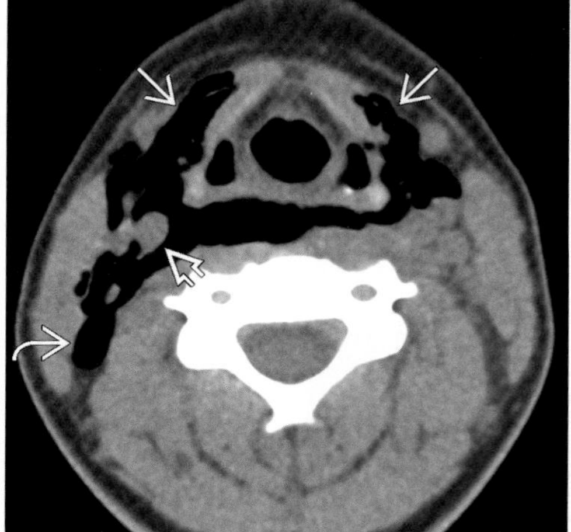

Axial CECT shows extensive air nearly surrounding the larynx ➡, surrounding the right carotid vessels ➡, and in the posterior triangle of the neck ➡ in a child who was thrown from a horse.

General Trauma

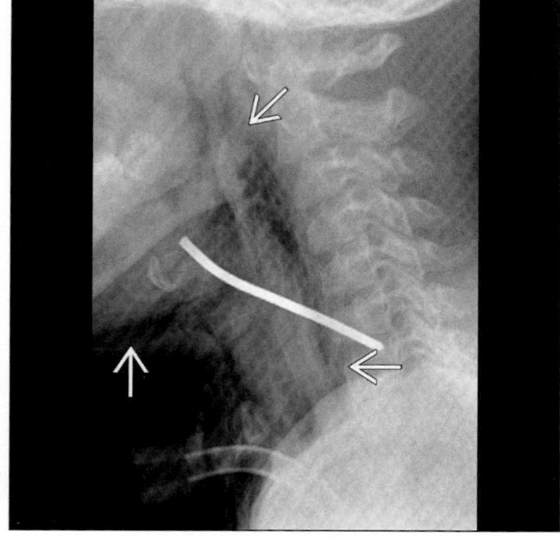

Lateral radiograph shows extensive subcutaneous and deep soft tissue air ➡ in a child who suffered direct penetrating injury from a piece of clothes hangar thrown from under a lawnmower.

Retropharyngeal Space (RPS) Abscess

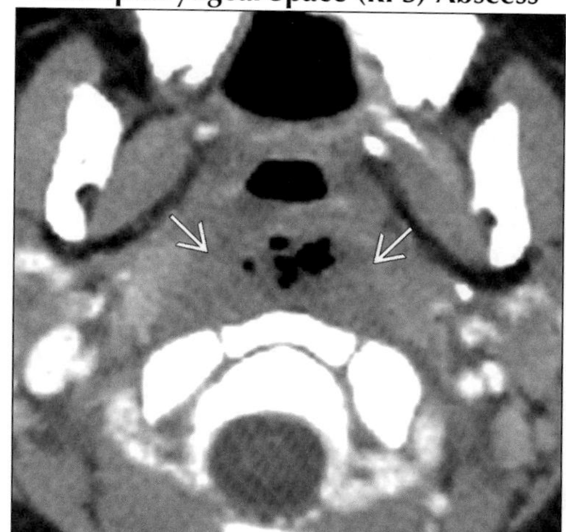

Laryngocele

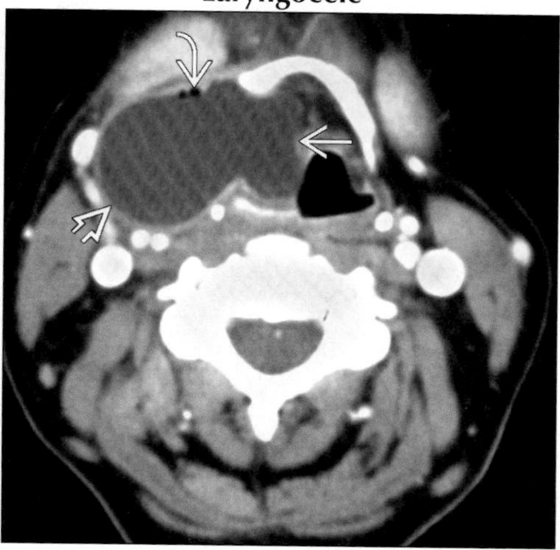

(Left) *Axial CECT shows bubbles of gas within edematous retropharyngeal soft tissues ➔ secondary to abscess.* ***(Right)*** *Axial CECT shows mixed laryngocele involving both the paraglottic space ➔ and the anterior neck ➔. The mass is primarily fluid-filled, but contains small bubbles of gas anteriorly ➔.*

Esophago-Pharyngeal Diverticulum

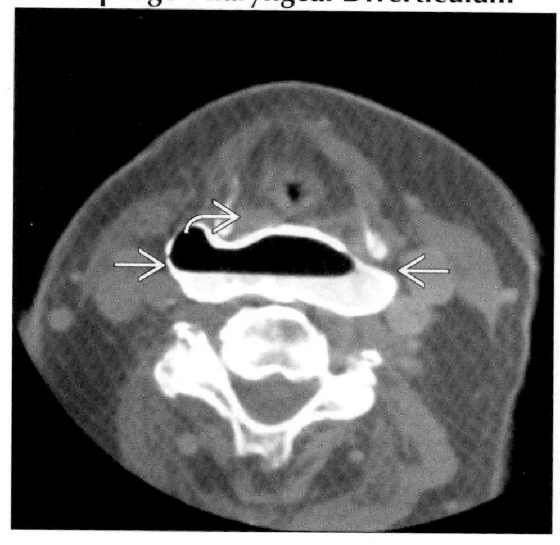

4th Branchial Anomaly

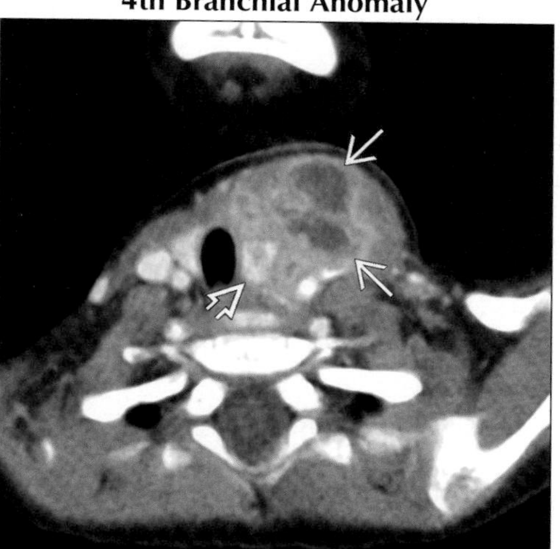

(Left) *Axial NECT shows barium layering within the air-filled space ➔, displacing the pharynx anteriorly ➔, a variant of Zenker diverticulum.* ***(Right)*** *Axial CECT shows a large, irregularly shaped, heterogeneously enhancing abscess ➔ in the left neck, anterior to the left thyroid lobe ➔, in a teenager with recurrent infections secondary to pyriform sinus tract, a 4th pharyngeal pouch remnant.*

Lateral Cervical Esophageal Diverticulum

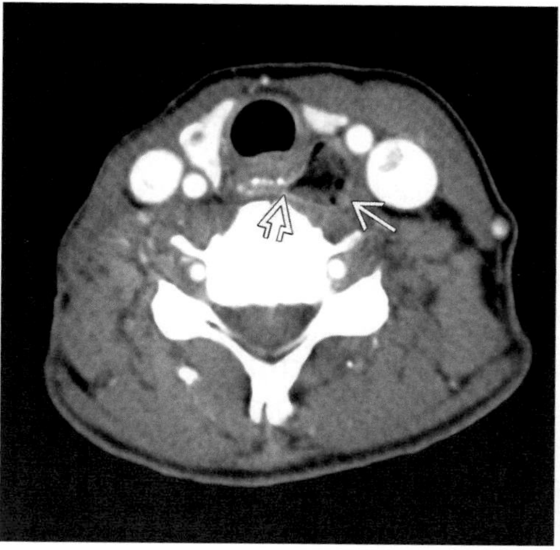

Spontaneous Cervical Emphysema

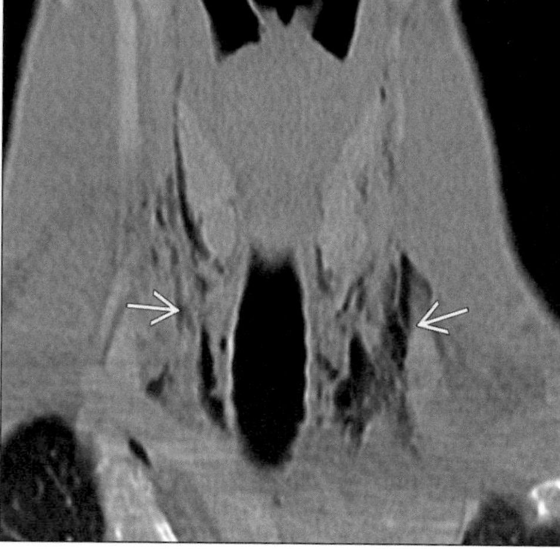

(Left) *Axial CECT demonstrates a connection ➔ between the lateral esophageal wall and a lateral cervical diverticulum ➔. The diverticulum is air and debris-filled.* ***(Right)*** *Coronal CECT shows extensive cervical emphysema ➔ in a teenager with a history of neck fullness and chest pain. No history of trauma, asthma, vomiting, or other event that may have caused rupture of the trachea or esophagus.*

MACROCEPHALY

DIFFERENTIAL DIAGNOSIS

Common
- Benign Extracranial Collections of Infancy
- Hydrocephalus
- Child Abuse

Less Common
- Neurofibromatosis Type 1
- Vein of Galen Aneurysmal Malformation

Rare but Important
- Tay-Sachs Disease
- Alexander Disease
- Canavan Disease
- Krabbe Disease
- Leigh Syndrome

ESSENTIAL INFORMATION

Key Differential Diagnosis Issues
- Measurement of head circumference is part of typical well child check
  - Macrocrania is defined as head circumference > 95th percentile
- Determinants of head circumference: Brain size, cerebral spinal fluid volume, and subdural spaces

Helpful Clues for Common Diagnoses
- **Benign Extracranial Collections of Infancy**
  - a.k.a. benign hydrocephalus of infancy or external hydrocephalus
  - Characterized by excess cerebral spinal fluid (CSF) in subarachnoid space and macrocephaly
    - Excess fluid is more abundant overlying frontal lobes
  - Often family history of macrocephaly
  - Normal long-term development and no additional risk for hydrocephalus
  - Extraaxial collection resolves by age 2
- **Hydrocephalus**
  - Incidence has declined along with decrease of open neural tube defects
  - 2 main types: Communicating and noncommunicating
    - Communicating: Overproduction or underresorption of CSF
    - Obstructive: Intraventricular hemorrhage, aqueductal stenosis, and migrational abnormalities
  - Present with enlarging head, crossing percentiles
    - May have signs of ↑ intracranial pressure
  - Often treated with shunting
- **Child Abuse**
  - Cranial trauma is most common cause of death in abuse
  - Most common cause of head trauma in children < 2 years
  - Mechanism of injury: Shaking and impact
  - Evaluation includes skeletal survey and head CT
  - Findings: Skull fracture, subdural hematomas of different ages, and brain edema

Helpful Clues for Less Common Diagnoses
- **Neurofibromatosis Type 1**
  - Autosomal dominant disorder
  - Affects 1:3,000
  - Characteristic features: Café-au-lait macules, benign neurofibromas, plexiform neurofibromas, and iris hamartomas
  - Neurologic findings: Optic pathway gliomas, seizures, headache, hydrocephalus, and macrocephaly
  - Risk for central nervous system tumors: Astrocytomas, optic pathway gliomas
- **Vein of Galen Aneurysmal Malformation**
  - Account for 1% of all intracranial vascular malformations
    - 30% of vascular intracranial malformations in children
  - Ectatic vascular structure is median prosencephalic vein, not vein of Galen
  - Occurs due to direct communication between arterial network and median prosencephalic vein
  - After birth, increase in blood flow through malformation
    - Up to 80% of left ventricular output may supply brain
    - Leads to increased cardiac output and heart failure
  - Usually associated with other intracranial venous anomalies

Helpful Clues for Rare Diagnoses
- **Tay-Sachs Disease**
  - Autosomal recessive disorder
    - More common in Ashkenazi Jews
  - Cause: Deficiency of β-hexosaminidase

- Characterized by progressive weakness and loss of motor skills beginning at 2-6 months of age
  - Findings: ↑ startle response, hypotonia, hyperreflexia, and cherry red macule
- Progressive neurodegeneration with macrocephaly
  - Macrocephaly due to accumulation of GM2 ganglioside

- **Alexander Disease**
  - Demyelinating disorder characterized by Rosenthal fibers
  - Usually sporadic disorder
  - Types: Infantile, juvenile, and adult
  - Infantile form is most common
    - Characterized by macrocephaly, psychomotor retardation, muscle weakness, pyramidal tract signs, seizures
    - Average age of onset: 6 months
  - Juvenile form characterized by progressive paresis, bulbar signs, and brisk reflexes
    - Average age of onset: 9 years
  - Adult form: Intermittent neurologic disorders similar to multiple sclerosis
  - MR: Frontal lobe demyelination and cysts, ventriculomegaly, and poor gray-white differentiation
- **Canavan Disease**
  - Autosomal recessive disorder
    - More common in Ashkenazi Jews
  - Cause: Inborn error of metabolism, deficiency of aspartoacylase enzyme
    - Leads to increased N-acetyl L-aspartate
  - Characterized by spongy degeneration of brain
  - Findings: Poor head control, macrocephaly, mental retardation, optic atrophy, and seizures
- **Krabbe Disease**
  - Autosomal recessive disorder
  - Characterized by severe myelin loss
  - Cause: Deficiency of lysosomal enzyme galactosylceramidase
  - 2 types: Early infantile or late onset
    - Most common: Early infantile (90%)
- **Leigh Syndrome**
  - Mitochondrial disorder
  - Progressive central nervous system decline due to necrotizing lesions in basal ganglia, diencephalon, cerebellum, or brainstem
  - Caused by deficiency of coenzyme Q or pyruvate dehydrogenase
  - Onset: Infancy and early childhood
  - Symptoms: Psychomotor retardation, nystagmus, ophthalmoparesis, ataxia, optic atrophy, dysphagia, weakness, hypotonia
    - Acute respiratory failure is common
  - MR: Characteristic bilateral symmetric T2WI hyperintensities in basal ganglia, thalamus, substantia nigra
    - Cerebellum, spinal cord, or cerebral white matter can also be affected
    - Cortical atrophy is also present

Benign Extracranial Collections of Infancy

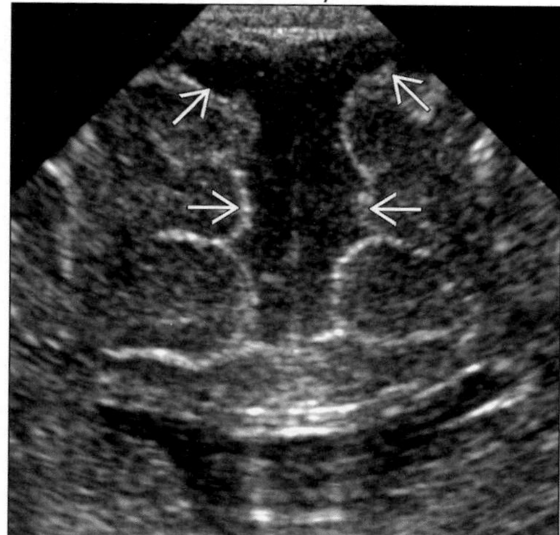

Coronal ultrasound of the head shows prominence of the extraaxial fluid spaces along the convexity and falx ➔. This is a characteristic location for benign extraaxial collections of infancy.

Benign Extracranial Collections of Infancy

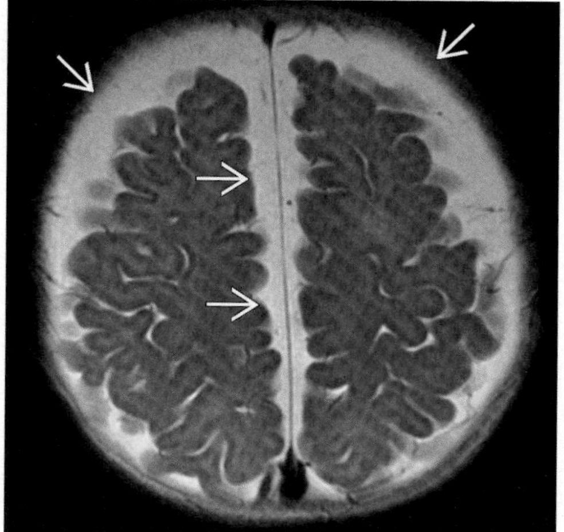

Axial T2WI MR shows prominence of the extraaxial fluid collections frontally and along the falx ➔. Patients with benign extraaxial fluid collections have no neurologic deficits.

MACROCEPHALY

Hydrocephalus

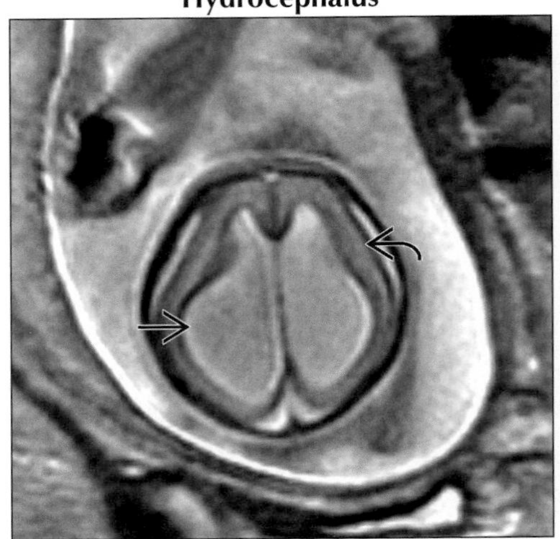

Hydrocephalus

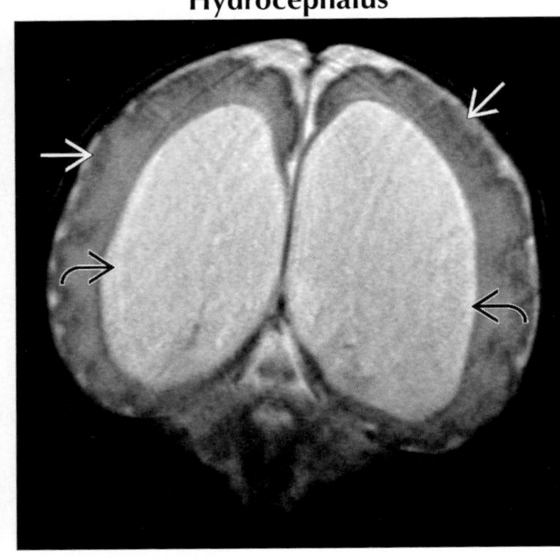

*(**Left**) Axial T2WI MR of a fetus shows marked enlargement of the lateral ventricles ➔ and thinning of the cerebrum ➔. Patients with hydrocephalus can present with macrocephaly and signs of increased intracranial pressure. (**Right**) Coronal T2WI MR shows marked enlargement of the lateral ventricles ➔ and thinning of the cerebrum ➔. Hydrocephalus can either be communicating or noncommunicating. It is often treated with shunting.*

Child Abuse

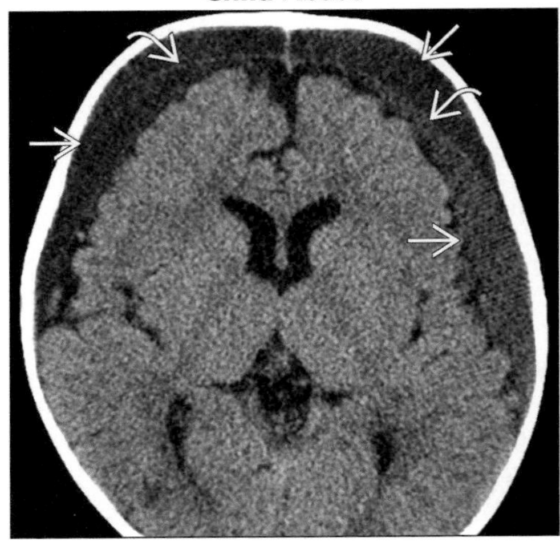

Child Abuse

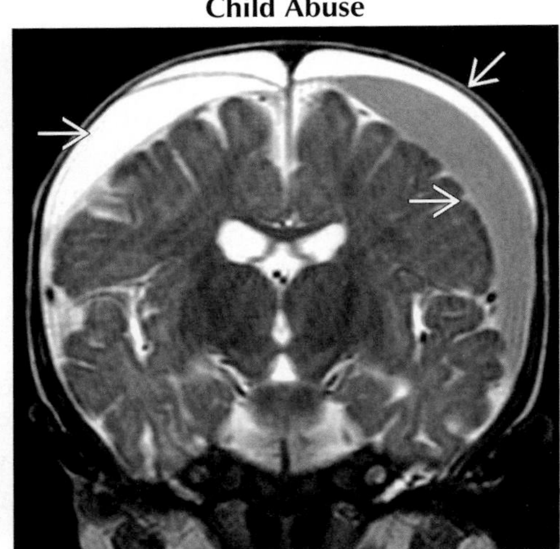

*(**Left**) Axial NECT shows multiple bilateral subdural collections of different densities ➔. A thin membrane separates the collections on each side ➔. Subdural hematomas of different ages are suggestive of abuse. (**Right**) Coronal T2WI MR shows multiple subdural hematomas of different ages ➔. Head trauma is the most common cause of death in child abuse, and abuse is the most common cause of head trauma in children under 2 years of age.*

Vein of Galen Aneurysmal Malformation

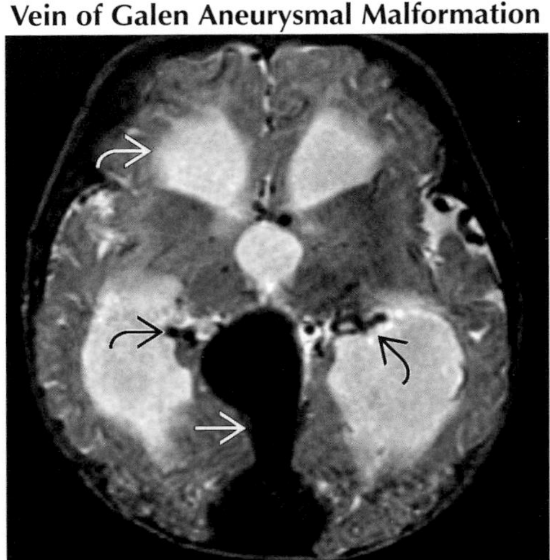

Vein of Galen Aneurysmal Malformation

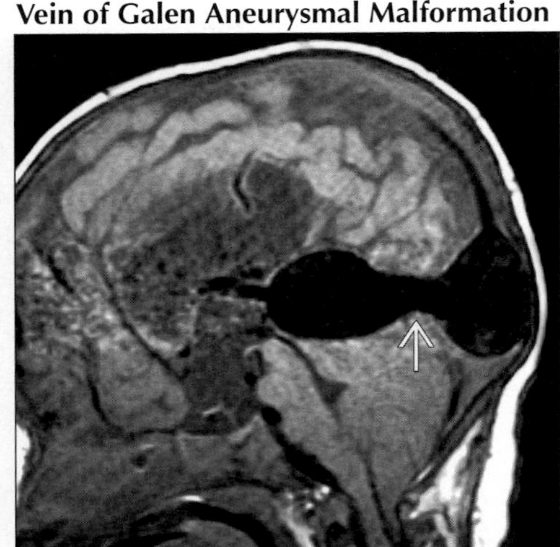

*(**Left**) Axial T2WI MR shows ventriculomegaly ➔ and a massively dilated vein of Galen malformation ➔. There are abnormal arteries bilaterally ➔. Vein of Galen malformations account for 30% of vascular intracranial malformations in children. (**Right**) Sagittal T1WI MR shows a massively dilated vein of Galen malformation ➔. Vein of Galen malformations are due to a direct communication between an arterial network and the medial prosencephalic vein.*

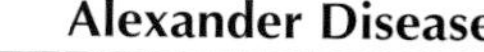

Alexander Disease

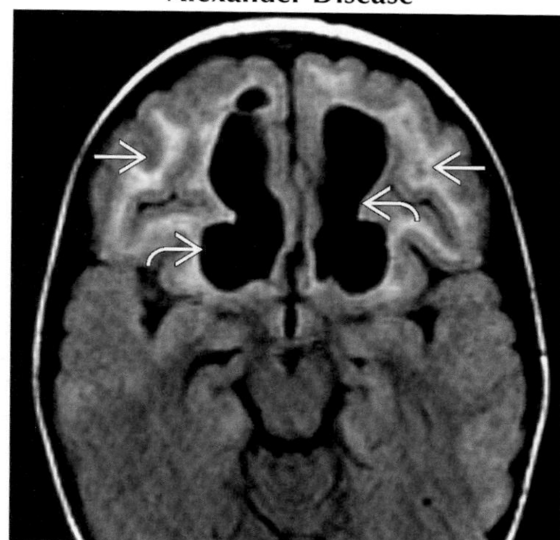

Alexander Disease

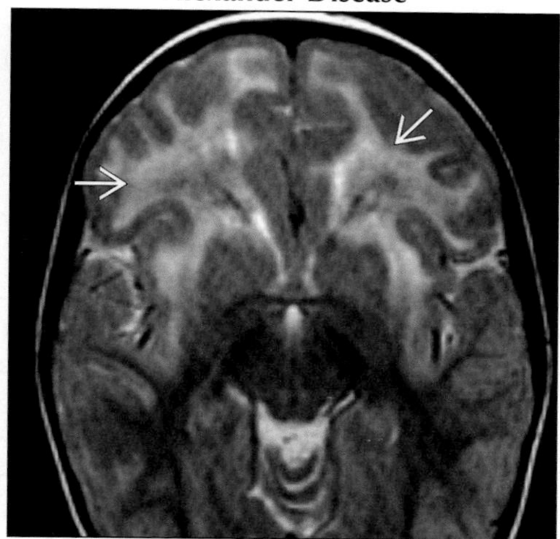

(Left) *Axial FLAIR MR shows abnormal myelination → in the bifrontal region with large bifrontal cysts ↪. Alexander disease is a demyelinating disorder characterized by Rosenthal fibers.* ***(Right)*** *Axial T2WI MR shows abnormal increased signal due to demyelination in the bilateral frontal lobes →. On MR, Alexander disease is characterized by frontal lobe demyelination and cysts. Ventriculomegaly and poor gray-white differentiation can also be present.*

Canavan Disease

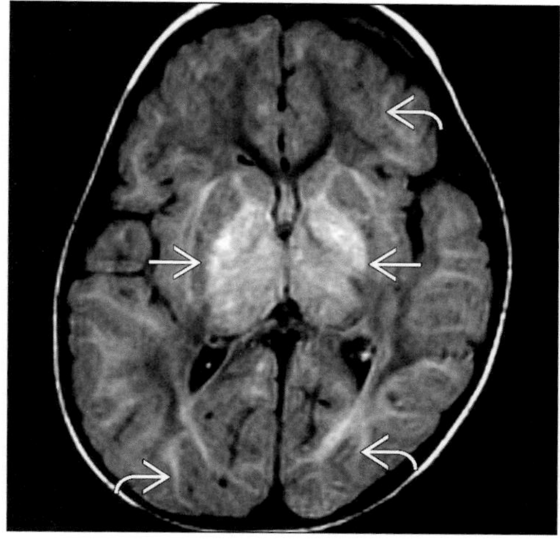

Krabbe Disease

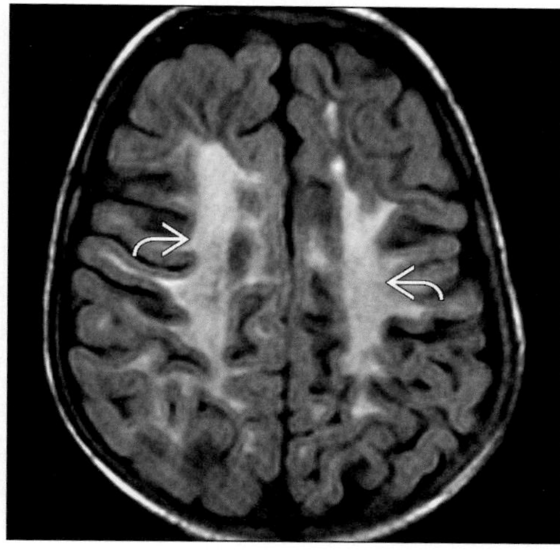

(Left) *Axial FLAIR MR shows abnormal increased signal in the basal ganglia → and subcortical U fibers ↪. Canavan disease is caused by a deficiency of the aspartoacylase enzyme, which leads to increased N-acetyl L-aspartate.* ***(Right)*** *Axial FLAIR MR shows increased signal in the centrum semiovale bilaterally ↪. The subcortical U fibers are spared. Krabbe disease is caused by a deficiency in the lysosomal enzyme galactosylceramidase.*

Leigh Syndrome

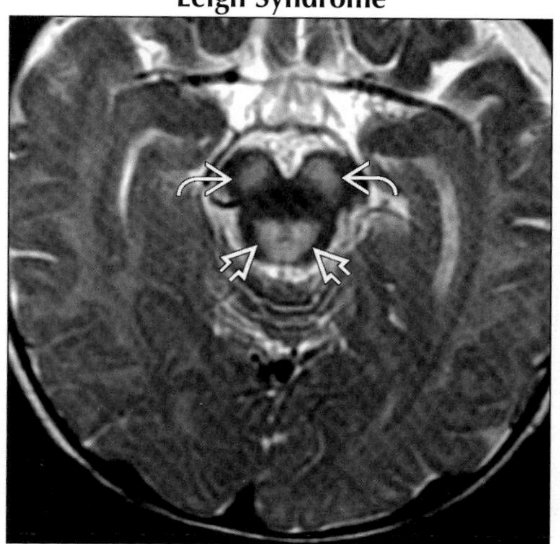

Leigh Syndrome

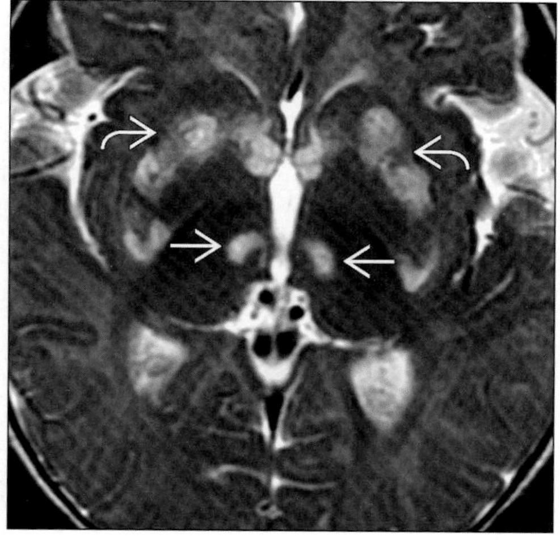

(Left) *Axial T2WI MR shows symmetric increased signal in the substantia nigra ↪ and periaqueductal gray matter ⇨. Leigh disease is a mitochondrial disorder characterized by necrotizing lesions in the basal ganglia, diencephalon, cerebellum, or brainstem.* ***(Right)*** *Axial T2WI MR shows symmetric abnormal increased signal in the basal ganglia ↪ and thalamus →. Leigh syndrome is caused by a deficiency of coenzyme Q or pyruvate dehydrogenase.*

MICROCEPHALY

DIFFERENTIAL DIAGNOSIS

Common

- Secondary/Acquired from
  - Hypoxic Ischemic Encephalopathy
  - TORCH Infections
  - Nonaccidental Trauma
  - Meningitis
  - Fetal Alcohol Syndrome

Less Common

- Primary/Genetic with
  - Gyral Simplification
  - Cortical Dysplasia
  - Midline Anomaly
  - Cerebellar Hypoplasia
  - Hypomyelination

Rare but Important

- Microlissencephaly
- Pseudo-TORCH
  - Aicardi-Goutières
- Progeroid Syndromes
  - Cockayne

ESSENTIAL INFORMATION

Key Differential Diagnosis Issues

- Was head circumference ever normal?
- Decreased cranio-facial ratio on sagittal view helpful, tape measure best
- Do not disregard nonaccidental trauma as cause of small head

Helpful Clues for Common Diagnoses

- **Hypoxic Ischemic Encephalopathy**
  - Perinatal or birth asphyxia (asphyxia neonatorium)
  - Patterns helpful, even if no history
  - Profound: Atrophy, gliosis
    - Posterior putamen
    - Lateral thalami
    - Rolandic cortex
  - Prolonged progressive
    - Typical watershed encephalomalacia
  - Mixed
    - Features of both, ± calcified thalami
- **TORCH Infections**
  - Cytomegalovirus (CMV) (common) and rubella (rare, today) most likely to have microcephaly
  - Toxo, CMV, HIV, and rubella may have intracranial Ca++, which may help in determining underlying etiology
    - CMV: Parenchymal or periventricular Ca++
    - HIV: Basal ganglia and subcortical calcifications
    - Toxo: Parenchymal or periventricular Ca++
  - Rubella and HSV cause lobar brain destruction/encephalomalacia
  - CMV may also have cortical dysplasia, periventricular Ca++, hypomyelination
- **Nonaccidental Trauma**
  - History is crucial
    - Majority of abuse in children < 1 year old
    - Most common in children 2-6 months old
    - After trauma: Subarachnoid and subdural hemorrhages are common
    - Subdural hemorrhage over convexity, interhemispheric, overlying tentorium
    - Caution in attempting to determine age of subdural hemorrhage
  - BUT look for evidence of trauma/fractures on ALL available films
  - Brain imaging of microcephaly
    - Global atrophy or hemiatrophy
    - Hemosiderin
- **Meningitis**
  - Early infancy: Group B strep most damaging
    - Hypothalamus
    - Chiasm
    - Inferior basal ganglia
    - Diffuse cortex, often asymmetric
- **Fetal Alcohol Syndrome**
  - Microcephaly
    - By tape measure
    - Or MR volumetrics
    - Anomalies may occur, but not specific
  - Diffusion tensor imaging (DTI) reported to show abnormal connectivity

Helpful Clues for Less Common Diagnoses

- **Gyral Simplification**
  - Small, grossly normal brain
  - Looks like "small but perfect" brain
  - Corpus callosum may appear thick, lack isthmus
- **Cortical Dysplasia**
  - Any severe, diffuse dysplasia

- Lissencephaly
- Pachygyria
- **Midline Anomaly**
  - Holoprosencephaly
    - Most severe are smallest
  - Agenesis of corpus callosum
    - Assess corpus callosum presence, size, shape
    - Is there isthmus?
- **Cerebellar Hypoplasia**
  - In multiple syndromes
    - Olivopontocerebellar degeneration
    - Spinocerebellar ataxia
    - Carbohydrate deficient glycoprotein syndrome type 1a
  - May be clue to rare disorders
    - Microlissencephaly
    - *TUBA1A* mutations: Lissencephaly PLUS cerebellar hypoplasia
  - Assess degree of deficiency
    - Fastigial recess, primary fissure
    - Degree of vermian lobulation
    - Tegmento-vermian angle (is the inferior 4th ventricle open?)
- **Hypomyelination**
  - May be a clue to rare disorders
    - Early onset West syndrome with cerebral hypomyelination and reduced white matter
    - 3-phosphoglycerate dehydrogenase deficiency
    - Progressive encephalopathy, edema, hypsarrhythmia, optic atrophy (PEHO)

Helpful Clues for Rare Diagnoses

- **Microlissencephaly**
  - Z-shaped brainstem
  - Callosal agenesis
  - Surface often totally smooth
  - Very small brain
- **Pseudo-TORCH**
  - **Aicardi-Goutières**
    - CMV-like: Ca++
    - Hypomyelinaton
    - Atrophy
    - Autosomal recessive, important to diagnose
    - Elevated CSF α-interferon
    - Early onset: *TREX1* mutation
    - Late onset: *RNASEH2B* mutation
- **Progeroid Syndromes**
  - **Cockayne**
    - Cachectic dwarfism with mental retardation
    - Disorder of DNA repair: Several mutations known, but lack phenotype-genotype correlation
    - Facies & neuroimaging progressive
    - Basal ganglia/dentate Ca++
    - Demyelination
    - Atrophy

Hypoxic Ischemic Encephalopathy

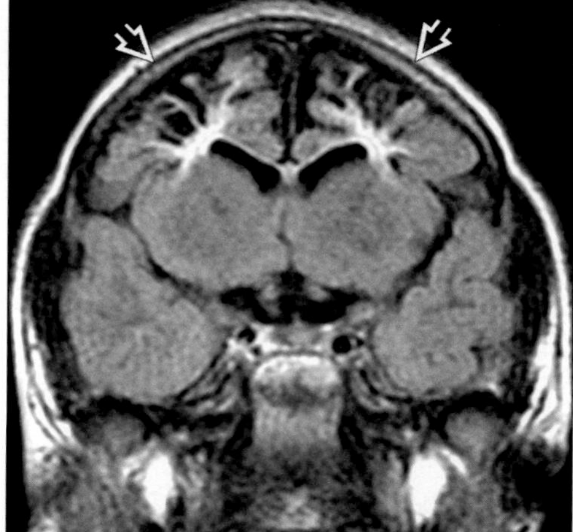

Coronal FLAIR MR shows cystic encephalomalacia ➡ in the border zone distribution in this 3 year old with a history of peripartum prolonged partial asphyxia.

Hypoxic Ischemic Encephalopathy

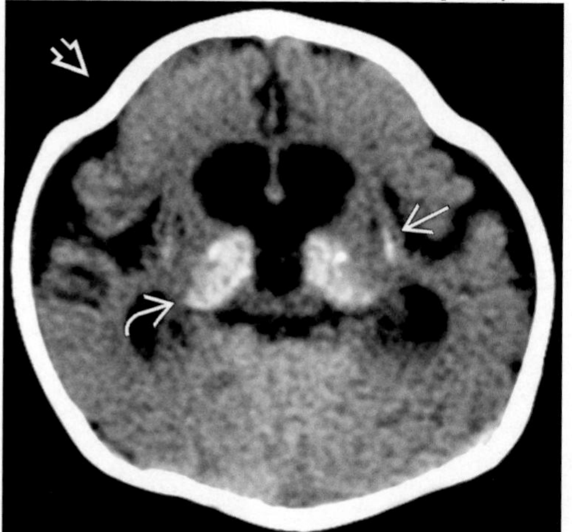

Axial NECT in a 3-month-old infant shows fusion of the coronal sutures ➡ due to severe brain volume loss, shrunken and calcified putamina ➡ and thalami ➡ following severe mixed HIE.

MICROCEPHALY

TORCH Infections

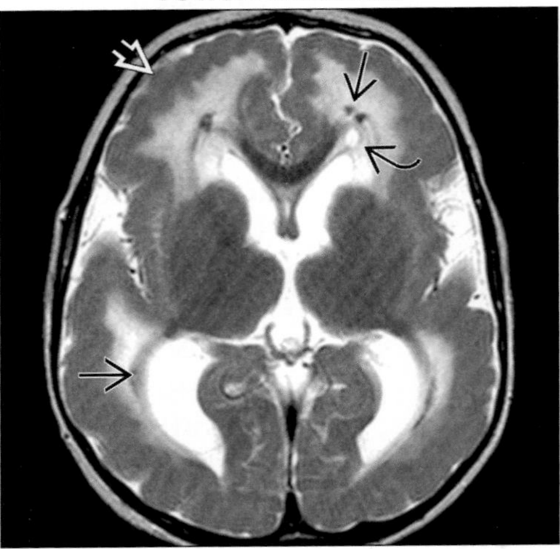

TORCH Infections

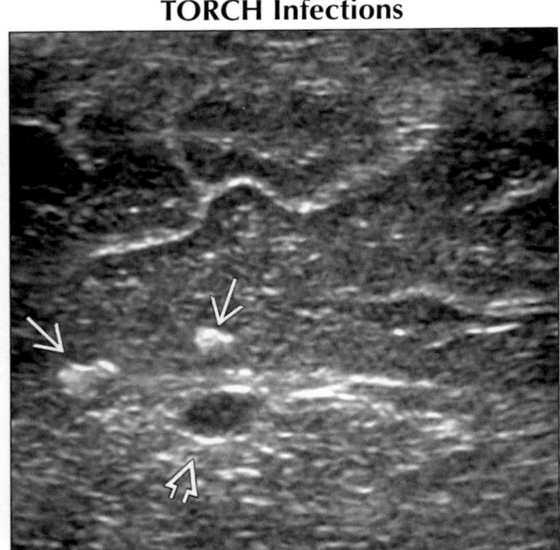

*(**Left**) Axial T2WI MR shows diffuse white matter increased signal, periventricular calcifications →, periventricular cysts →, and diffuse frontal lobe polymicrogyria → in an infant with confirmed cytomegalovirus. (**Right**) Sagittal ultrasound shows periventricular calcifications, seen here as foci of increased echogenicity →. Note the periventricular cyst → in this patient with confirmed congenital cytomegalovirus.*

Nonaccidental Trauma

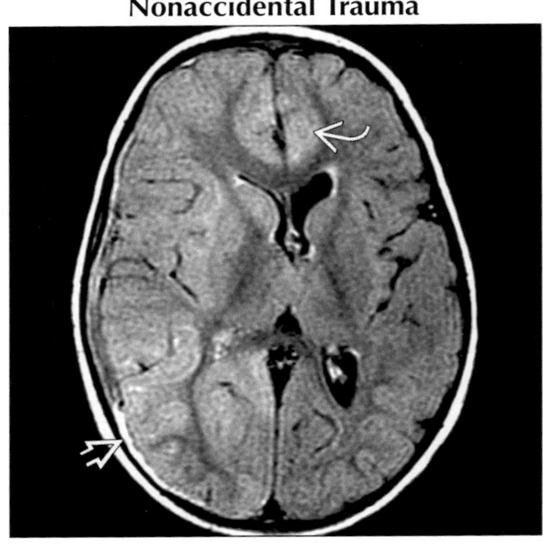

Nonaccidental Trauma

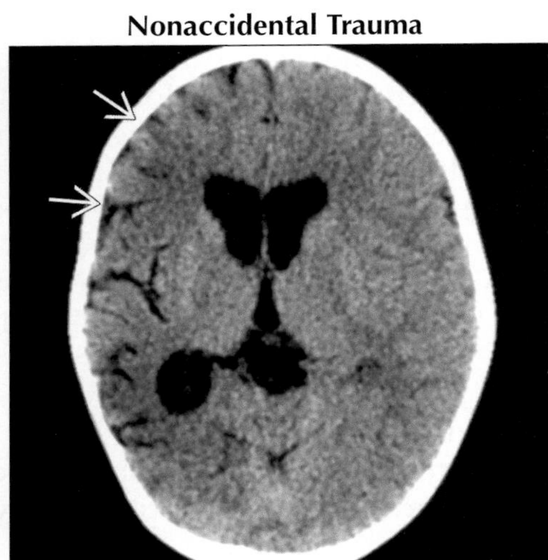

*(**Left**) Axial FLAIR MR shows diffuse right hemispheric swelling and signal increase, left mesial frontal edema →, and a right pancake subdural hematoma →. There is shift of midline structures and compression of the ipsilateral lateral ventricle. (**Right**) Axial NECT on follow-up in the same child, whose head circumference is falling below normal, shows right hemispheric volume loss and sulcal widening →.*

Meningitis

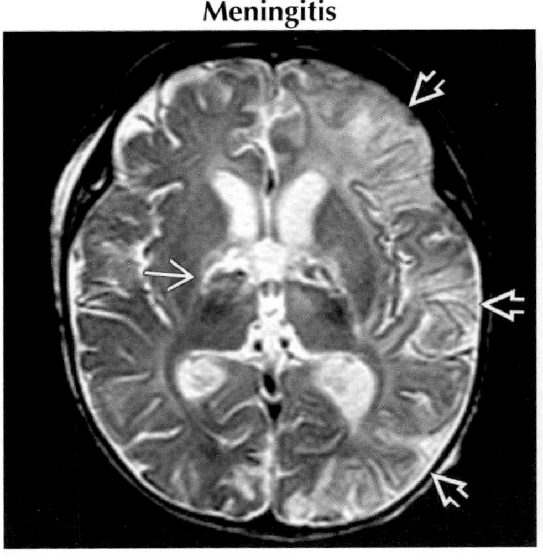

Meningitis

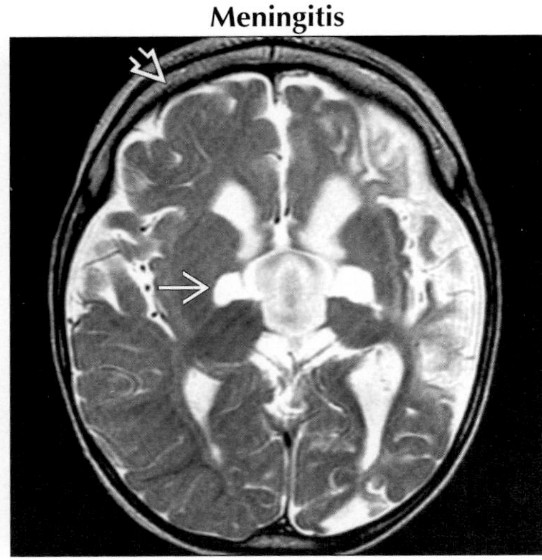

*(**Left**) Axial T2WI MR during the subacute phase of recovery following neonatal group B strep meningitis shows global volume loss. The left hemisphere → is more affected than the right, although both are involved. Focal necrosis of the globus pallidi → and hypothalamus is present. (**Right**) Axial T2WI MR in the same infant during the chronic phase shows calvarial thickening → and global, but asymmetric, volume loss. Cavitary globus pallidus → changes are now seen.*

Fetal Alcohol Syndrome

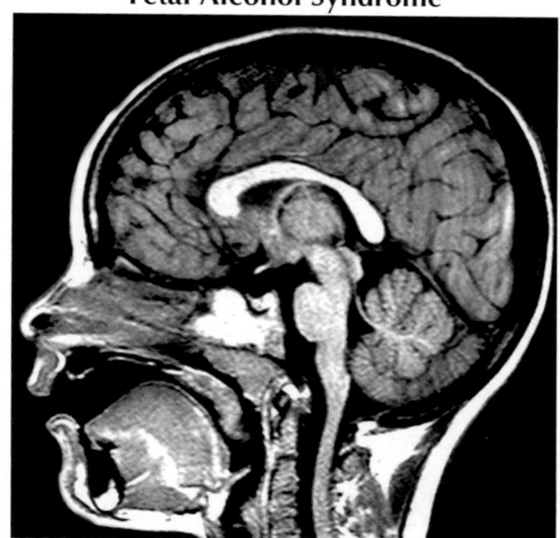

Fetal Alcohol Syndrome

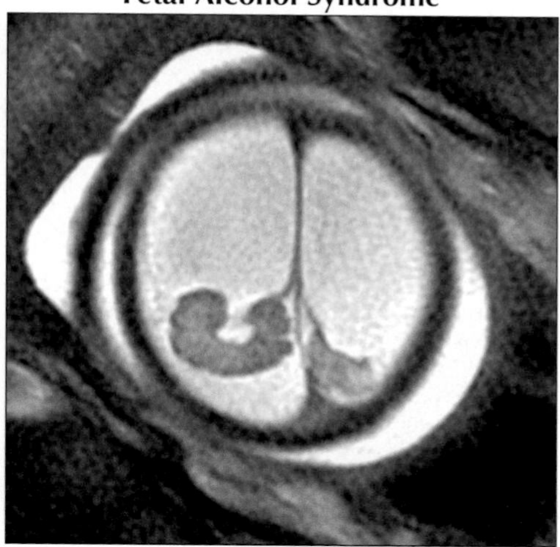

(Left) *Sagittal T1WI MR in a 3 year old with FAS and microcephaly shows only a decreased cranio-facial ratio. Microcephaly in fetal alcohol syndrome is easily confirmed by tape measure, as routine anatomic imaging is usually normal. Volumetrics and DTI do, however, show abnormalities.* ***(Right)*** *Axial T2WI MR in a 39-week fetus shows a few cerebral remnants. Hydranencephaly in this fetus follows exposure to alcohol, smoking, and polydrug abuse.*

Gyral Simplification

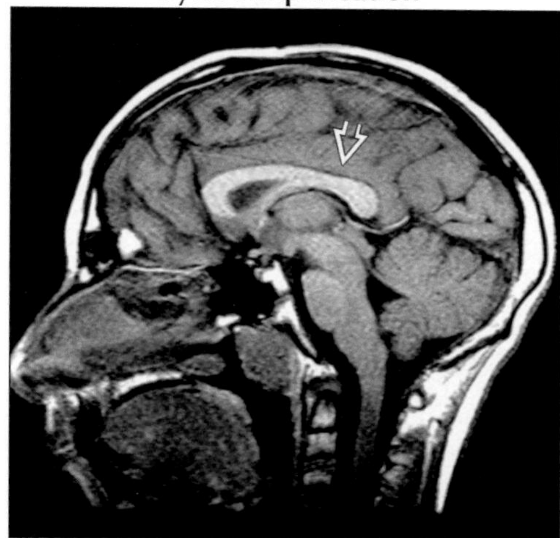

Gyral Simplification

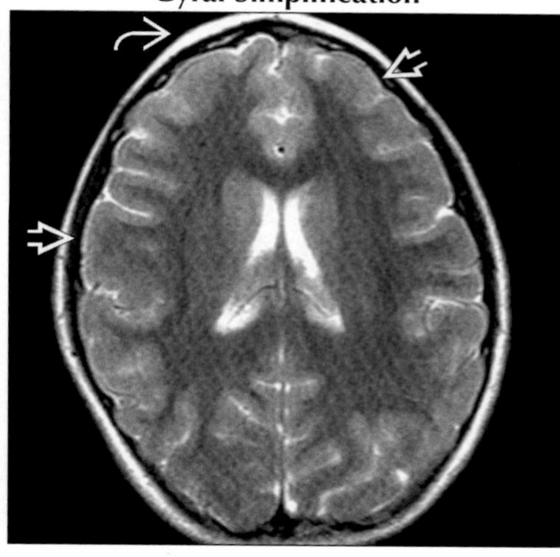

(Left) *Sagittal T1WI MR shows a decreased cranio-facial ratio and lack of a callosal isthmus ➡. The brainstem and cerebellum are normal.* ***(Right)*** *Axial T2WI MR shows a relatively normal-appearing brain. However, closer perusal reveals mild trigonocephaly ➡ and generalized gyral simplification ➡. The myelin maturation is normal.*

Cortical Dysplasia

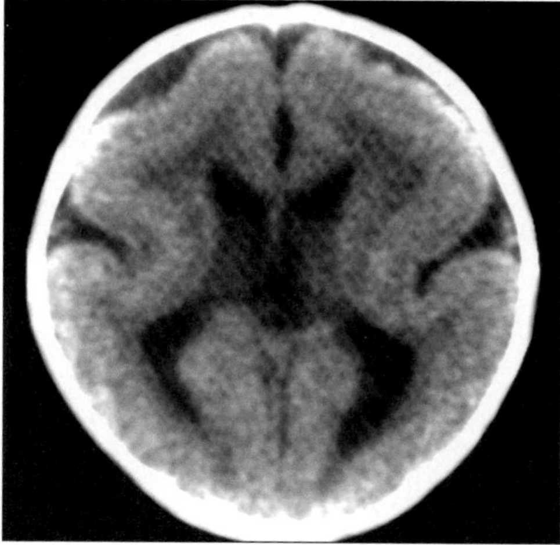

Cortical Dysplasia

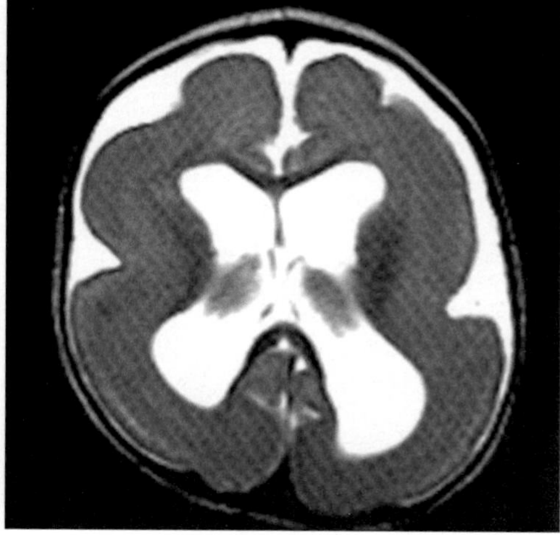

(Left) *Axial NECT shows a thick cortex with thin outer layer, sparse cell layer, and thick inner band of gray matter. Primitive sylvian fissures and very shallow sulci are present.* ***(Right)*** *Axial T2WI MR in another child shows a similar appearance to the previous image.*

MICROCEPHALY

(Left) Sagittal T2WI MR in an infant with severe microcephaly shows absence of the corpus callosum, cortex crossing the midline ➾, fused deep gray structures ➞, and a large dorsal cyst ➞. There is also a single central incisor ➞. (Right) Axial T2WI MR again shows the large dorsal cyst. There is a monoventricle ➞, gray matter crossing the midline ➾ and a primitive fused hippocampus ➞.

Midline Anomaly

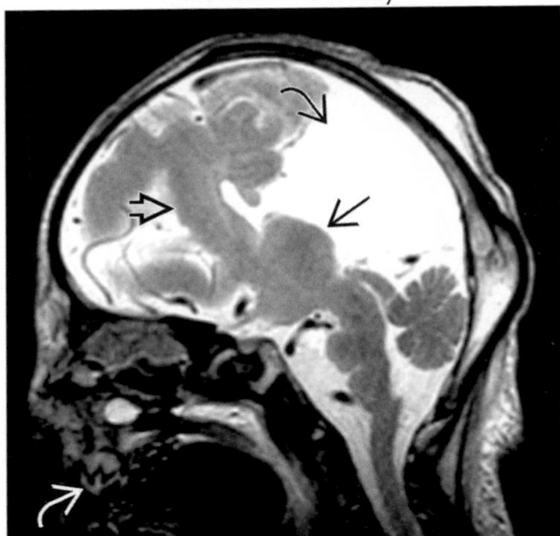

Midline Anomaly

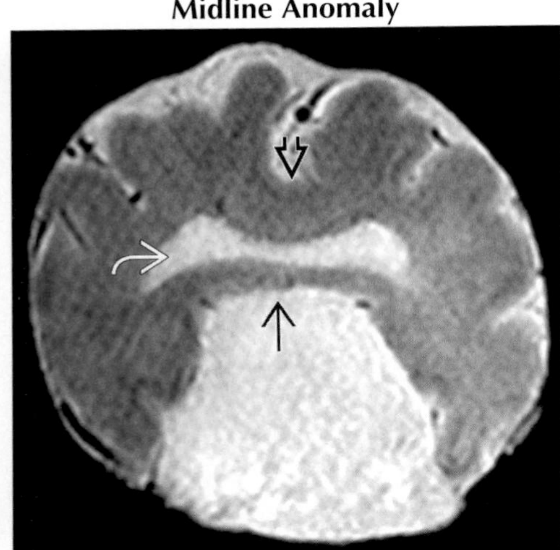

(Left) Sagittal T1WI MR shows mildly hypoplastic vermis with prominent surrounding CSF. The fastigial recess, primary fissure, and vermian lobulation are present. (Right) Sagittal T2WI MR shows upward rotation of severely hypoplastic vermis in an infant with callosal agenesis, microcephaly, and only primitive sulcation ➞. Fastigial crease and primary fissure are seen. Vermian lobulation is simplified. The mesencephalon is "angled" but not Z-shaped.

Cerebellar Hypoplasia

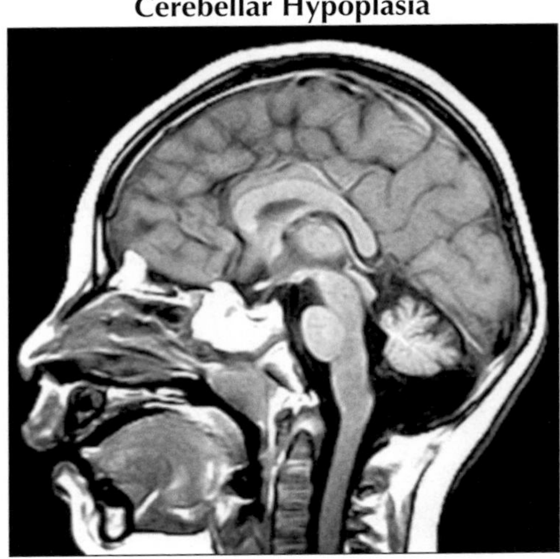

Cerebellar Hypoplasia

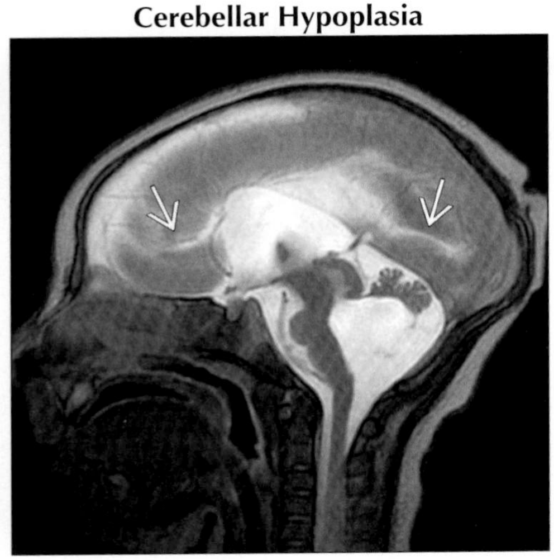

(Left) Sagittal T1WI MR shows a very thin corpus callosum ➾ in this microcephalic infant. (Right) Axial T2WI MR shows corresponding severe hypomyelination.

Hypomyelination

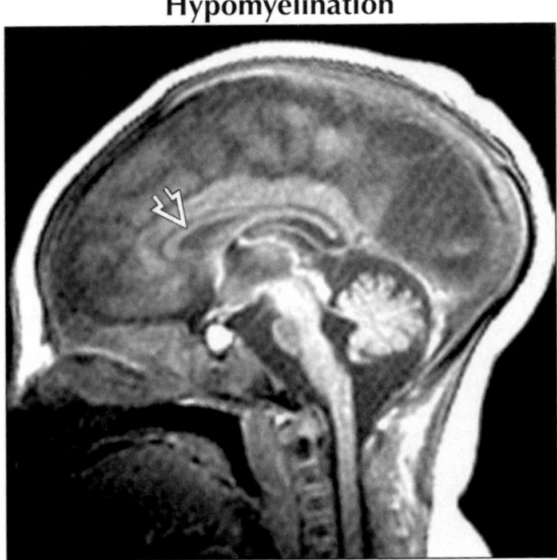

Hypomyelination

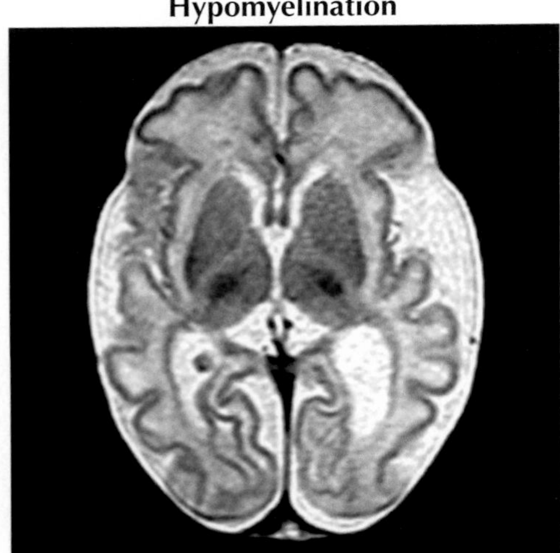

Microlissencephaly

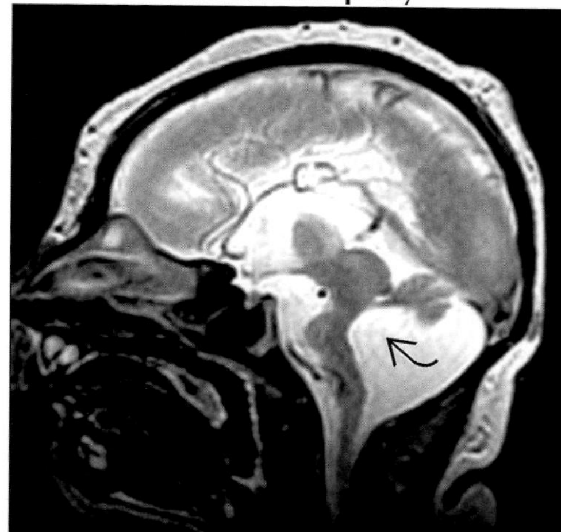

Microlissencephaly

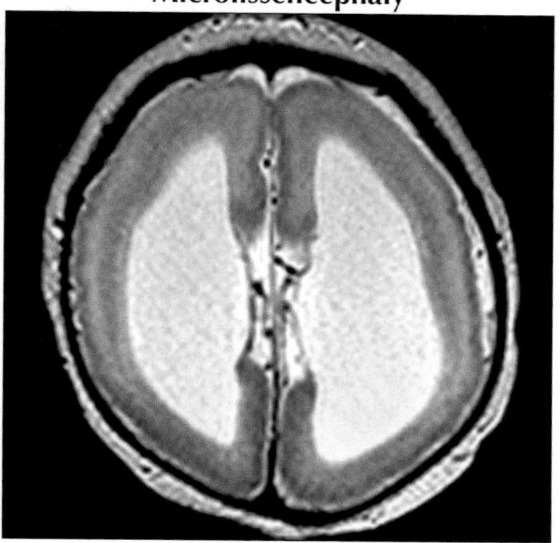

(Left) *Sagittal T2WI MR shows a Z-shaped brainstem and severe cerebellar hypoplasia. Note the open inferior 4th ventricle ➔, microcephaly, callosal agenesis, and a smooth cortical surface.* ***(Right)*** *Axial T2WI MR shows a complete lack of cerebral gyral formation in the same child.*

Aicardi-Goutières

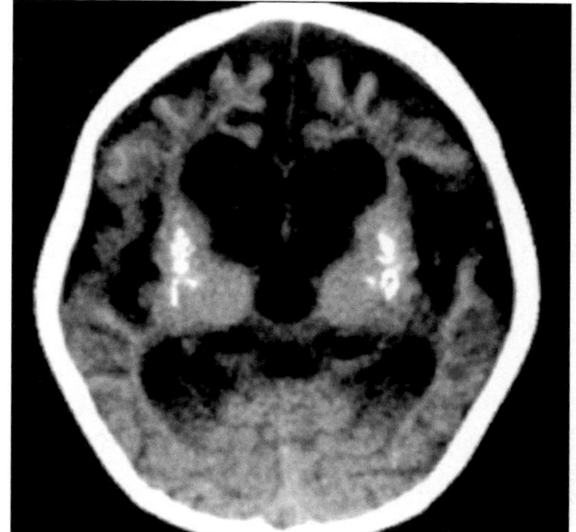

Aicardi-Goutières

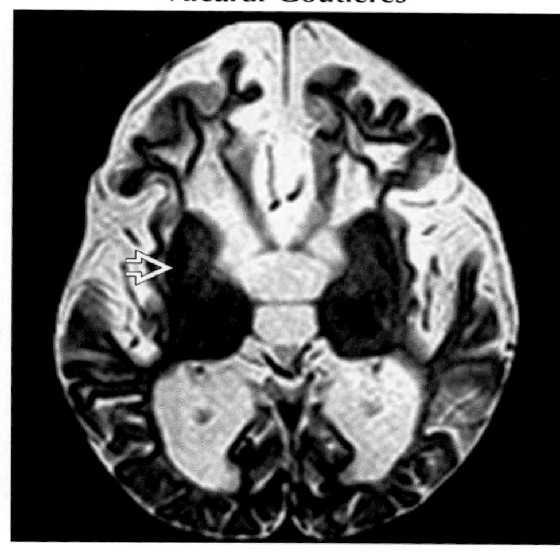

(Left) *Axial NECT in this infant shows TORCH-like calcifications within the basal ganglia.* ***(Right)*** *Axial T2WI MR shows hypomyelination and severe atrophy in the same patient. Calcifications ➔ are relatively occult on MR in this child.*

Cockayne

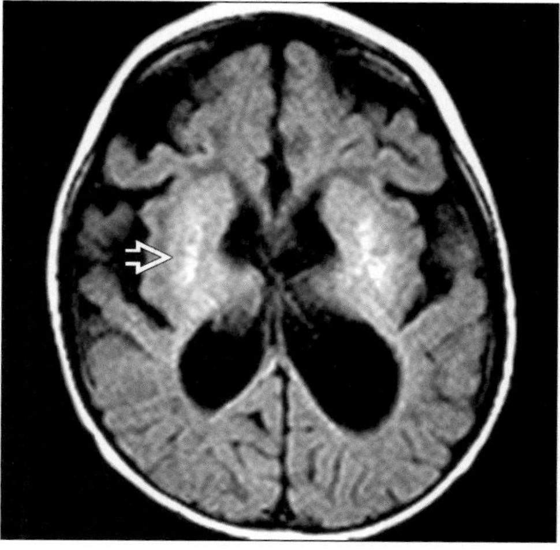

Cockayne

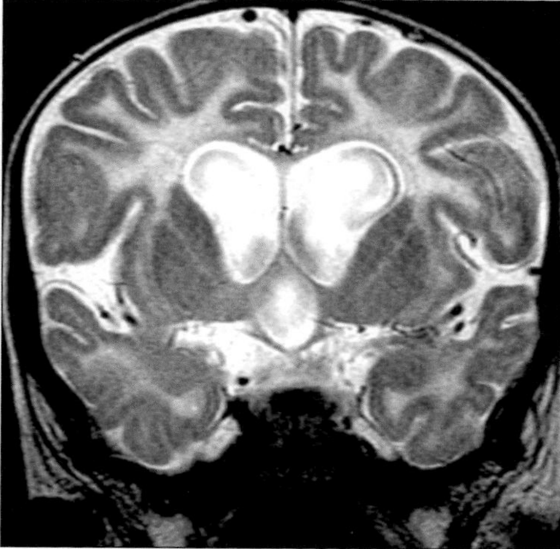

(Left) *Axial T1WI MR shows volume loss, hypomyelination, and hazy increased signal intensity of the basal ganglia ➔, representing calcification.* ***(Right)*** *Coronal T2WI MR shows volume loss and hypomyelination in the same child. These findings became more apparent with serial imaging.*

LEUKOCORIA

DIFFERENTIAL DIAGNOSIS

Common
- Retinoblastoma

Less Common
- Retinal Detachment
- Retinopathy of Prematurity
- Persistent Hyperplastic Primary Vitreous
- Coats Disease
- Coloboma
- Congenital Cataract

Rare but Important
- Toxocariasis, Orbit
- Ocular Melanoma, Amelanotic
- Retinal Dysplasia

ESSENTIAL INFORMATION

Helpful Clues for Common Diagnoses
- **Retinoblastoma**
  - Key facts
    - Primary retinal malignancy, PNET type
    - Most common childhood ocular tumor
    - 60% sporadic; 40% inherited
    - *RB1* gene mutation
  - Imaging
    - Punctate, speckled, or flocculent calcification in > 90%
    - Strong enhancement
    - Retinal detachment not unusual
    - Unilateral in 75%
    - Look for coincident contralateral, suprasellar, or pineal tumor in patients with inherited disease

Helpful Clues for Less Common Diagnoses
- **Retinal Detachment**
  - Key facts
    - Separation between inner sensory retina and outer pigmented epithelium
    - Myriad etiologies, including vascular, inflammatory, neoplastic, congenital, traumatic, and other processes
    - 3 mechanisms: Rhegmatogenous (tear), tractional (adhesions), and exudative (tumor or inflammation)
  - Imaging
    - Detached retina bulges toward vitreous, with underlying biconvex collection
    - Leaves of retina converge at optic disk, resulting in "V" contour
    - Signal varies depending on content
    - Often bloody or proteinaceous fluid
    - Hyperdense on CT
    - Hyperintense on most MR sequences
- **Retinopathy of Prematurity**
  - Key facts
    - Synonym: Retrolental fibroplasia
    - Fibrovascular proliferation of immature retina, presumably related to hyperoxia of extrauterine NICU environment
  - Imaging
    - Microphthalmia
    - Retinal detachment common, often with blood-fluid levels
    - Ca++ rare except in advanced stages
- **Persistent Hyperplastic Primary Vitreous**
  - Key facts
    - Primary vitreous = fetal ocular hyaloid vascular tissue
    - Normally regresses at 7 months gestation
    - Bilateral lesions typically syndromic, e.g., Norrie and Warburg syndromes
  - Imaging
    - Small globe
    - Hyperdense tissue in globe on CT
    - Hyperintense on T1WI and T2WI
    - Enhancing retrolental hyaloid remnant
    - Retinal detachment common
- **Coats Disease**
  - Key facts
    - Underlying lesion is retinal telangiectasia
    - Subretinal exudate causes retinitis and subsequent detachment
  - Imaging
    - Retinal detachment is *sine qua non*
    - Hyperdense exudate on CT
    - Hyperintense on T1WI and T2WI
    - Occasionally calcifies (~ 10%)
- **Coloboma**
  - Key facts
    - Defect of embryonic ocular cleft
    - Syndromic associations (e.g., CHARGE)
    - Morning glory anomaly is variation
    - Excavated defect on funduscopy
  - Imaging
    - May occur anywhere in eye; defects at disc are visible on imaging
    - Defect at optic nerve head with outpouching of vitreous
    - May be associated with microphthalmia &/or secondary cyst

- **Congenital Cataract**
  - Key facts
    - Opacification of lens that presents from birth to 6 months of age
    - Bilateral cataracts often syndromic, including genetic, metabolic, infectious, gestational, and other processes
  - Imaging
    - Best seen with direct visualization
    - Shape and location of lesion indicate timing and etiology of insult
    - Often limited to central portion of lens

Helpful Clues for Rare Diagnoses

- **Toxocariasis, Orbit**
  - Key facts
    - *Toxocara canis/cati* (dog/cat roundworm)
    - Larvae migrate to eye from intestine
    - Sclerosing endophthalmitis with small eosinophilic abscess
  - Imaging
    - Uveoscleral thickening and nodularity
    - Subretinal exudate at site of larval infiltration, with variable hyperintensity
- **Ocular Melanoma, Amelanotic**
  - Key facts
    - Primary uveal tract malignancy
    - Most common adult ocular tumor
  - Imaging
    - US for initial evaluation and surveillance
    - MR or CT to assess retrobulbar invasion
    - Less intrinsic T1 signal when amelanotic
    - Moderate enhancement
    - Retinal detachment common
- **Retinal Dysplasia**
  - Key facts
    - Associated with congenital syndromes
  - Imaging
    - Retinal detachment, hyperintense fluid
    - Variably enhancing dysplastic tissue

Alternative Differential Approaches

- Calcification
  - Calcification present
    - Retinoblastoma (> 90%)
    - Late inflammatory or traumatic changes
  - Calcification absent
    - Persistent hyperplastic primary vitreous
    - Coats disease
    - Retinopathy of prematurity
    - Coloboma
    - Toxocariasis
- Globe size
  - Enlarged globe
    - Coloboma, except with microphthalmia
  - Normal globe size
    - Retinoblastoma, except bulky tumor
    - Retinal detachment
    - Coats disease
    - Toxocariasis
  - Small globe
    - Persistent hyperplastic primary vitreous
    - Retinopathy of prematurity
    - Coloboma with microphthalmia

Retinoblastoma

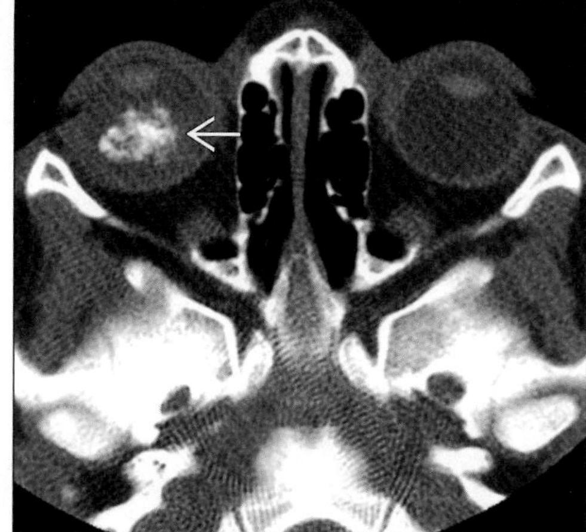

Axial NECT shows dense flocculent calcification ➔ centrally within an intraocular mass in the right eye of a child.

Retinoblastoma

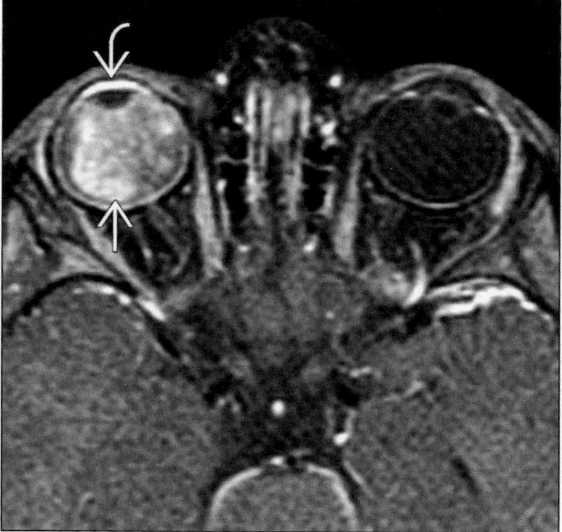

Axial T1WI C+ MR reveals a bulky enhancing tumor ➔ that fills and slightly enlarges the right eye of a child. Enhancement in the anterior chamber ➔ is a poor prognostic sign.

LEUKOCORIA

(Left) *Graphic shows a detached retina in the right eye ➡. The retinal attachment at the optic nerve head results in the characteristic "V" shape. By comparison, choroidal detachment typically has a lenticular contour, as demonstrated in the left eye ➡.* ***(Right)*** *Axial T2WI MR shows a retinal detachment ➡ at the lateral aspect of the right eye. Detachment is often related to an underlying lesion, such as the ocular melanoma ➡ present in this patient.*

Retinal Detachment

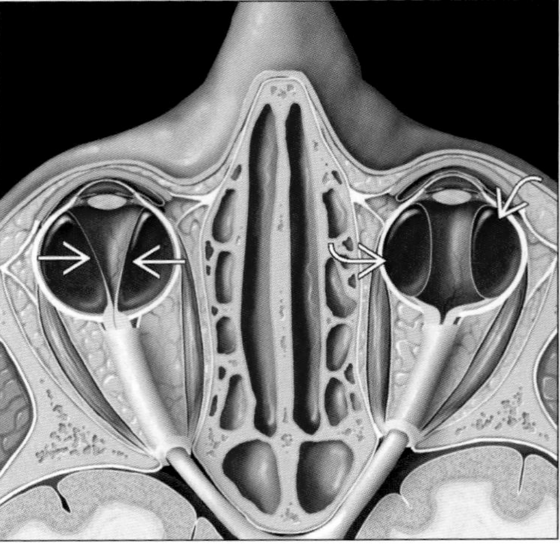

Retinal Detachment

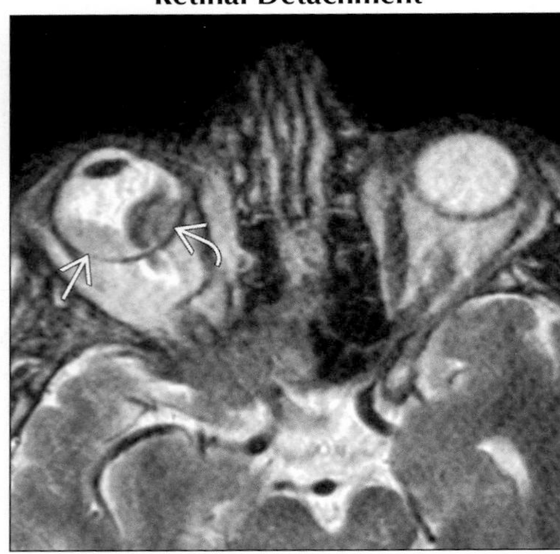

(Left) *Axial T2WI FS MR shows bilateral small globes with a heterogeneous signal. Blood-fluid level is evident on the right ➡. Peripheral low signal on the left represents calcification ➡ due to advanced disease.* ***(Right)*** *Axial CECT shows enhancing tissue ➡ behind the lens of the left eye, representing persistent primary vitreous. A remnant of the hyaloid artery is seen as intense linear enhancement ➡.*

Retinopathy of Prematurity

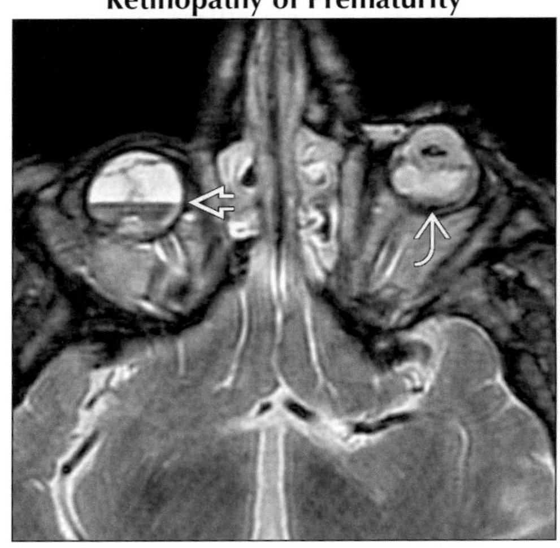

Persistent Hyperplastic Primary Vitreous

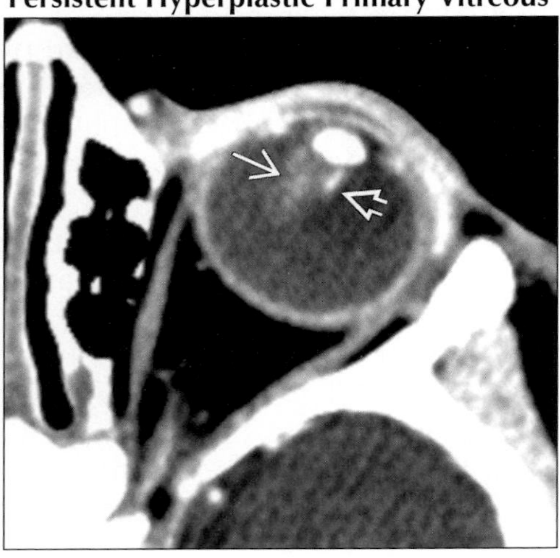

(Left) *Axial T1WI C+ MR shows triangular retrolental enhancing tissue ➡ and stalk-like hyaloid remnant ➡ representing failure of involution of embryonic fibrovascular tissue. The contour of this tissue has been described as resembling a "martini glass."* ***(Right)*** *Axial NECT shows ill-defined hyperdensity in the posterior aspect of the left globe ➡, representing subretinal exudate. A vague V-shaped contour of the vitreous ➡ is typical of retinal detachment.*

Persistent Hyperplastic Primary Vitreous

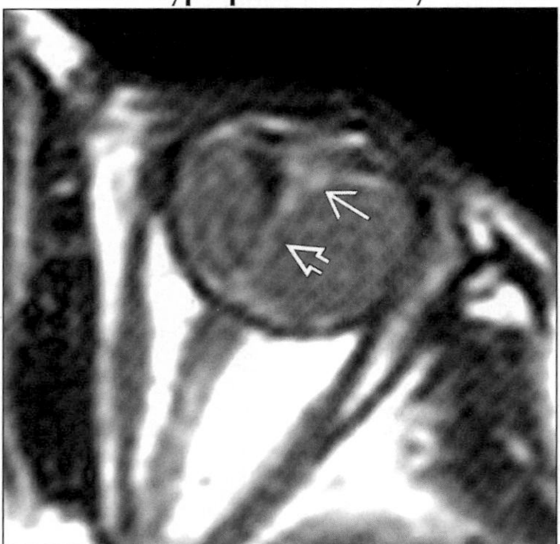

Coats Disease

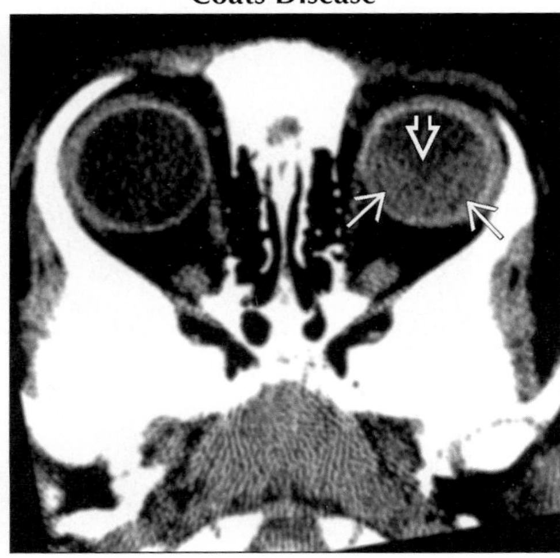

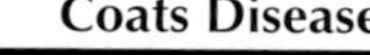

Coats Disease

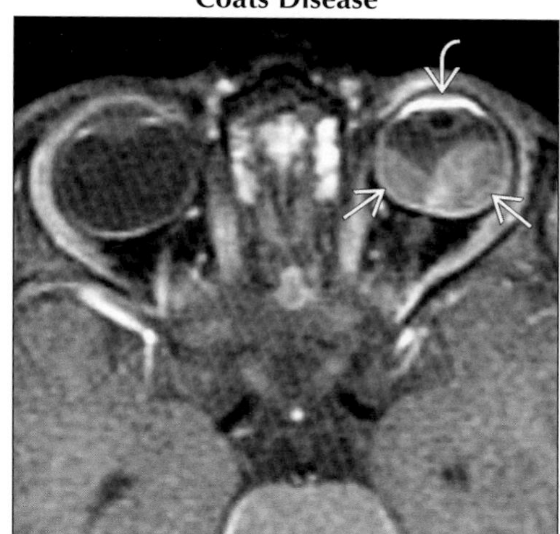

Coloboma

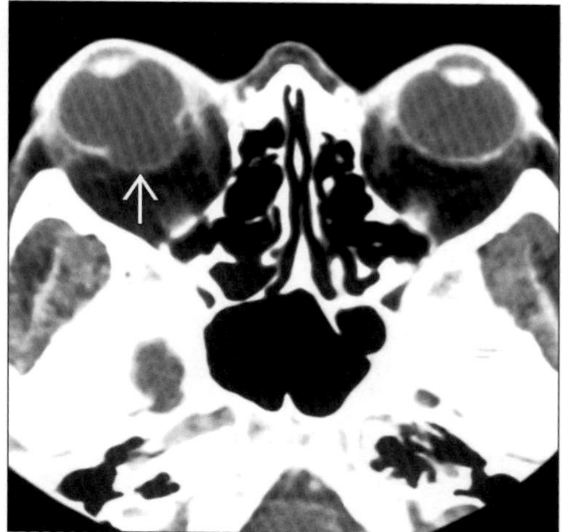

(Left) *Axial T1WI C+ FS MR shows moderately hyperintense subretinal exudates involving the left eye. Anterior hyperintensity probably relates to anterior chamber cholesterolosis.* ***(Right)*** *Axial NECT shows an optic disc coloboma, seen as a dehiscence of the posterior globe through a broad defect centered at the location of the optic nerve head.*

Congenital Cataract

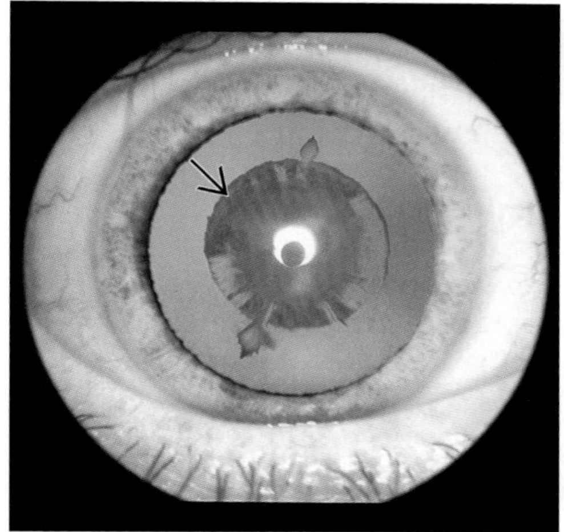

Toxocariasis, Orbit

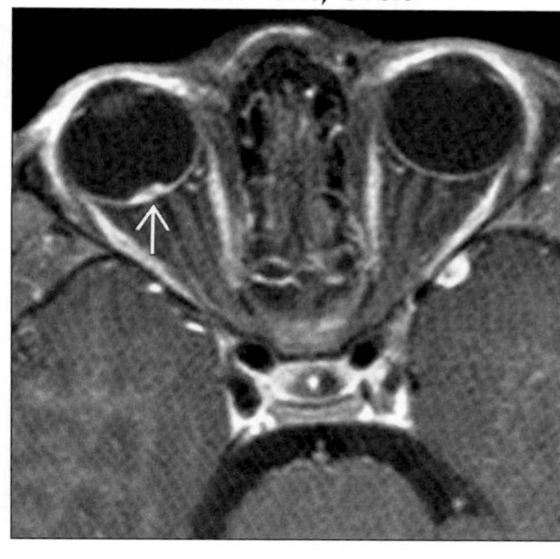

(Left) *Clinical photograph shows opacity of the central portion of the lens corresponding to the fetal nucleus, with relatively clear surrounding cortex.* ***(Right)*** *Axial T1WI C+ FS MR shows ocular toxocariasis manifesting as uveoscleral nodularity in the posterior aspect of the right globe. Hyperintensity is attributable to intrinsic signal of subretinal effusion and associated enhancement.*

Ocular Melanoma, Amelanotic

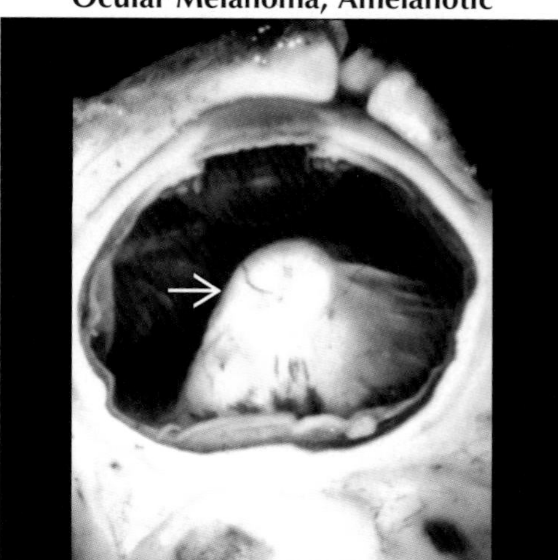

Retinal Dysplasia

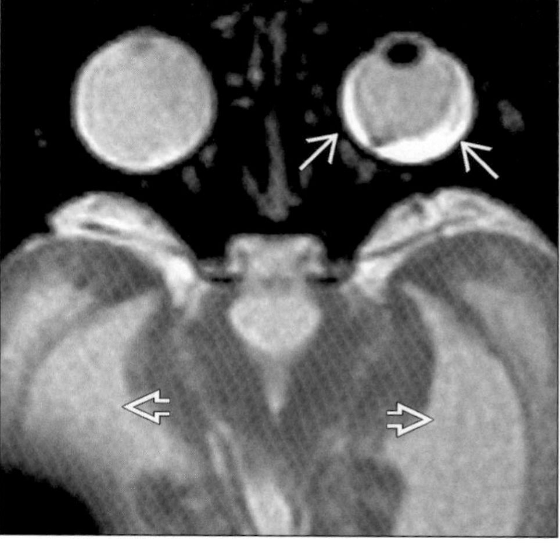

(Left) *Gross pathology shows a large exophytic mass projecting into the vitreous from the posterior aspect of the eye. Melanoma was confirmed histologically, but the mass is largely without pigmentation.* ***(Right)*** *Axial T2WI MR in a newborn with Walker-Warburg syndrome shows peripheral T2 hyperintensity of the left globe, indicating retinal dysplasia and associated subretinal hemorrhage. Note the presence of marked ventriculomegaly.*

RAPIDLY DEVELOPING PROPTOSIS

DIFFERENTIAL DIAGNOSIS

Common
- Abscess, Subperiosteal, Orbit
- Infantile Hemangioma, Orbit
- Lymphatic Malformation, Orbit

Less Common
- Trauma, Orbit
- Idiopathic Orbital Inflammatory Disease (Pseudotumor)
- Rhabdomyosarcoma
- Metastatic Neuroblastoma

Rare but Important
- Langerhans Histiocytosis
- Lymphoproliferative Lesions, Orbit
- Traumatic Carotid-Cavernous Fistula

ESSENTIAL INFORMATION

Helpful Clues for Common Diagnoses
- **Abscess, Subperiosteal, Orbit**
  - Key facts
    - Pus between orbital wall and periosteum
    - Almost always associated with sinusitis
    - Anywhere in orbit, especially adjacent to ethmoid sinusitis
    - Brain MR if intracranial complication of sinusitis suspected
  - Imaging
    - Lentiform, rim-enhancing extraconal fluid collection (phlegmon or abscess)
    - ± air-fluid level = drainable pus
    - Usually with preseptal cellulitis and deviation of extraocular muscle (EOM)
    - ± edematous intraconal or extraconal fat, enlargement of EOMs (myositis)
- **Infantile Hemangioma, Orbit**
  - Key facts
    - Vascular neoplasm, NOT malformation
    - Not well seen at birth; more apparent within 1st few weeks of life
    - Proliferating phase: 1st year
    - Involuting phase: 1-5 years
    - Involuted phase: 5-7 years
    - GLUT-1: Specific immunohistochemical marker expressed in all 3 phases of infantile hemangioma
    - Congenital hemangioma: Rare variant, present at or before birth
    - 2 subtypes of congenital hemangioma = rapidly involuting (RICH) and noninvoluting (NICH)
    - RICH shows involution by 8-14 months
  - Imaging
    - Proliferating phase: Solid, intensely enhancing mass with high-flow vessels
    - Involuting phase: Fat infiltration, ↓ size
    - May be part of PHACES syndrome: **P**osterior fossa abnormalities, **h**emangiomas, **a**rterial anomalies, **c**ardiovascular defects, **e**ye abnormalities, **s**ternal clefts
- **Lymphatic Malformation, Orbit**
  - Key facts
    - Congenital vascular malformation
    - Lymphatic channels of varying sizes
    - Present at birth, grows with child
    - Hemorrhage or respiratory infection causes sudden ↑ in size with resultant rapidly developing proptosis
    - Intracranial vascular anomalies present in ~ 2/3 of patients with periorbital lymphatic malformation
  - Imaging
    - Uni- or multilocular; macrocystic or microcystic
    - Intra- ± extraconal location
    - Only septations enhance, unless mixed venolymphatic malformation
    - Fluid-fluid levels best seen on MR

Helpful Clues for Less Common Diagnoses
- **Trauma, Orbit**
  - Key facts
    - Metallic foreign bodies (FB) most dense
    - Glass more dense than bone
    - Wood: Very low density (~ air density) → soft tissue density as it resorbs serum
    - Living plant material ~ soft tissue density
  - Imaging
    - FB, bone fragments, &/or adjacent hematoma ⇒ proptosis
    - ± globe rupture, intraocular FB, intracranial injury
- **Idiopathic Orbital Inflammatory Disease (Pseudotumor)**
  - Key facts
    - Benign inflammatory process with fibrosis ⇒ painful proptosis
  - Imaging
    - Myositic: Most common subtype

- Diffuse enlargement and enhancement of EOMs, including tendinous insertions
- Lacrimal: Enlargement and enhancement
- Anterior: Thickening and enhancement of sclera ± choroid, ± involvement of retrobulbar fat, nerve, or sheath
- Diffuse: Intra- ± extraconal, may be mass-like, usually without globe deformity or bone erosion
- Apical: Enhancing orbital apex mass, extension through fissures

- **Rhabdomyosarcoma**
  - Key facts
    - H&N sites: Orbit, parameningeal (middle ear, paranasal sinus, nasopharynx), and all other H&N sites
  - Imaging
    - Soft tissue mass, variable enhancement
    - ± bone erosion
    - ± intracranial or sinus extension
- **Metastatic Neuroblastoma**
  - Key facts
    - Most common malignant tumor in children < 1 year of age
    - Majority of primary tumors retroperitoneal adrenal origin
  - Imaging
    - Soft tissue mass + aggressive bone erosion and spiculated periosteal reaction
    - When bilateral, frequently involves lateral orbital walls
    - ± intracranial extension

Helpful Clues for Rare Diagnoses

- **Langerhans Histiocytosis**
  - Key facts
    - In H&N: Orbit, maxilla, mandible, temporal bone, cervical spine, skull
  - Imaging
    - Enhancing soft tissue mass with smooth osseous erosion
- **Lymphoproliferative Lesions, Orbit**
  - Key facts
    - Includes NHL and lymphoid hyperplasia (benign polyclonal reactive hyperplasia and indeterminate atypical hyperplasia)
  - Imaging
    - Diffuse or focal masses
    - Homogeneous enhancing soft tissue mass anywhere in orbit
- **Traumatic Carotid-Cavernous Fistula**
  - Key facts
    - Direct fistula between cavernous ICA and cavernous sinus
    - Secondary to trauma, venous thrombosis, or aneurysm
  - Imaging
    - Proptosis + large superior ophthalmic vein, cavernous sinus, and EOMs
    - "Dirty" orbital fat related to edema

Abscess, Subperiosteal, Orbit

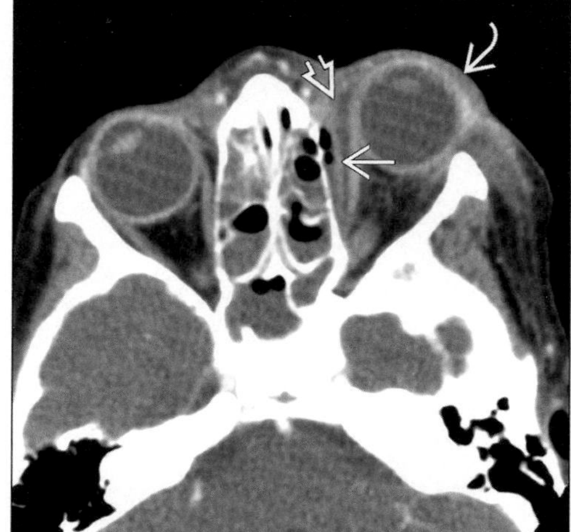

Axial CECT shows an elliptical subperiosteal abscess with an air-fluid level ➔ in the medial left orbit with extraconal edema ➔, medial rectus muscle deviation, proptosis, and preseptal soft tissue edema ➔.

Abscess, Subperiosteal, Orbit

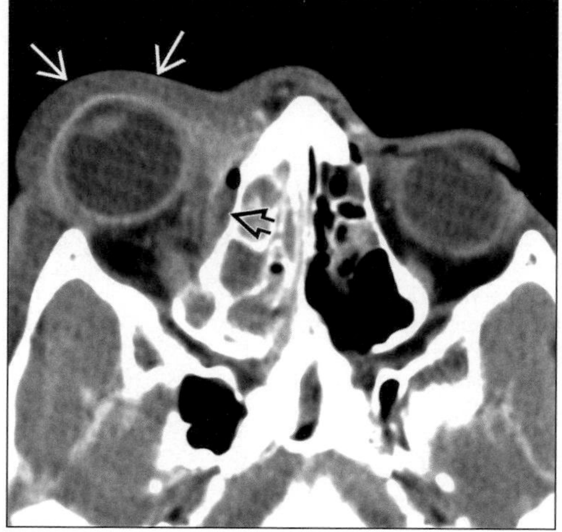

Axial CECT reveals significant right-sided ethmoid sinusitis, preseptal cellulitis ➔, proptosis, and a small air-fluid level within a medial extraconal subperiosteal abscess ➔.

RAPIDLY DEVELOPING PROPTOSIS

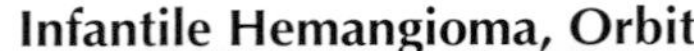

Infantile Hemangioma, Orbit | **Infantile Hemangioma, Orbit**

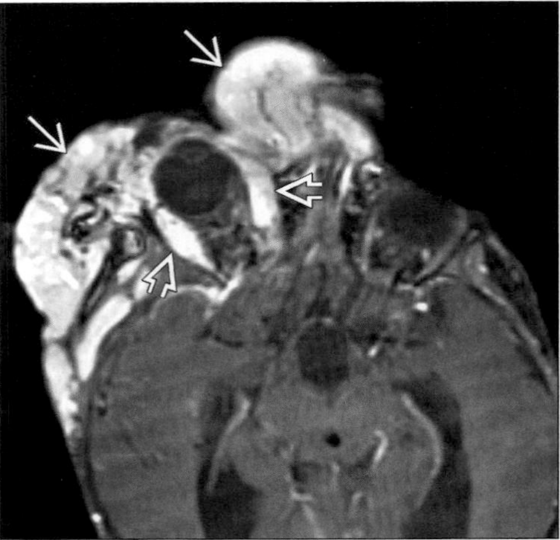

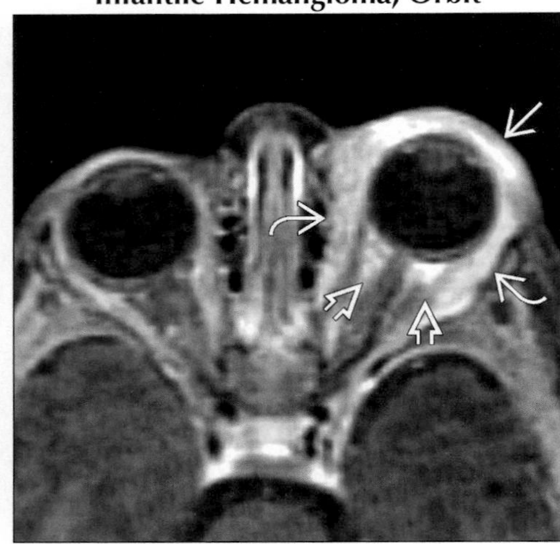

(Left) *Axial T1WI C+ FS MR shows a large, intensely enhancing infantile hemangioma → involving the right orbit, face, and nose with postseptal extension → resulting in proptosis. Solid, intensely enhancing mass with high-flow vessels indicates that the lesion is in the proliferating phase.* ***(Right)*** *Axial T1WI C+ FS MR defines the preseptal →, postseptal intra- → and extraconal → extension of an infantile hemangioma. Note the resultant proptosis.*

Lymphatic Malformation, Orbit | **Lymphatic Malformation, Orbit**

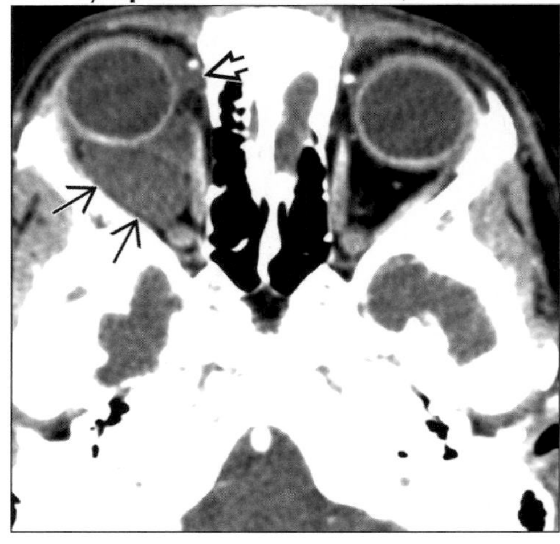

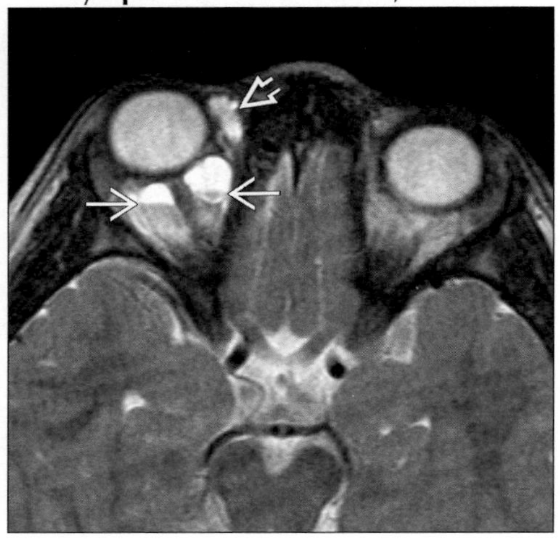

(Left) *Axial CECT demonstrates a multilobular cystic-appearing intraconal right orbital lymphatic malformation → with small anteromedial postseptal component →.* ***(Right)*** *Axial T2WI MR in the same patient better defines the mass as a large intraconal macrocystic lymphatic malformation with fluid-fluid levels → secondary to intralesional hemorrhage. Note the smaller extraconal component anteromedially →. Acutely developing proptosis resulted.*

Trauma, Orbit | **Trauma, Orbit**

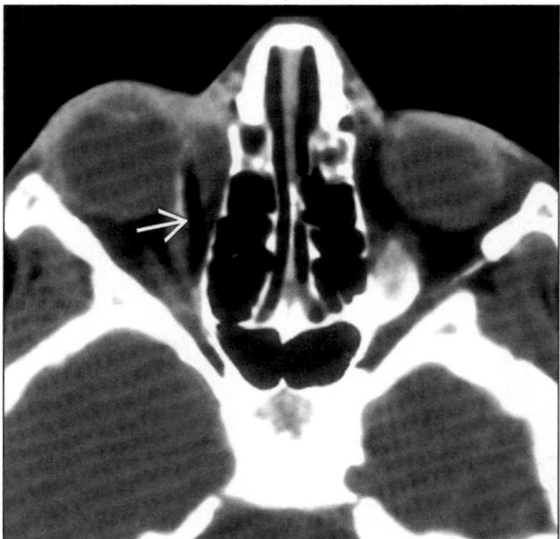

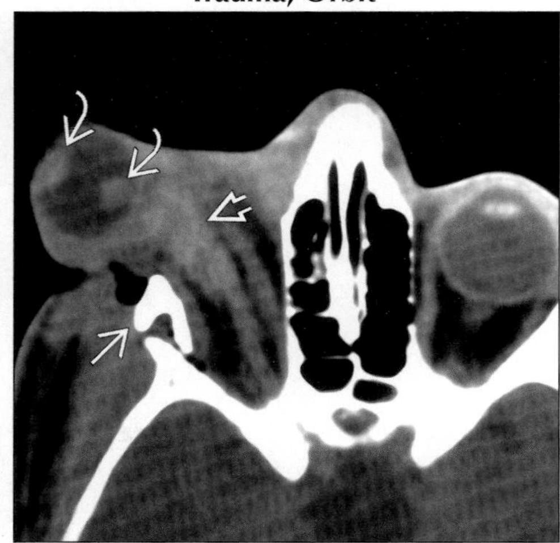

(Left) *Axial NECT reveals mild right proptosis secondary to the penetration of the medial extraconal space by air that contains a twig →. Care must be taken not to confuse wooden foreign bodies with air or fat.* ***(Right)*** *Axial NECT shows depressed lateral wall fracture fragments → and orbital hemorrhage →, leading to severe proptosis and near complete traumatic enucleation of the small right globe with shattered fragments of lens →.*

RAPIDLY DEVELOPING PROPTOSIS

Idiopathic Orbital Inflammatory Disease (Pseudotumor)

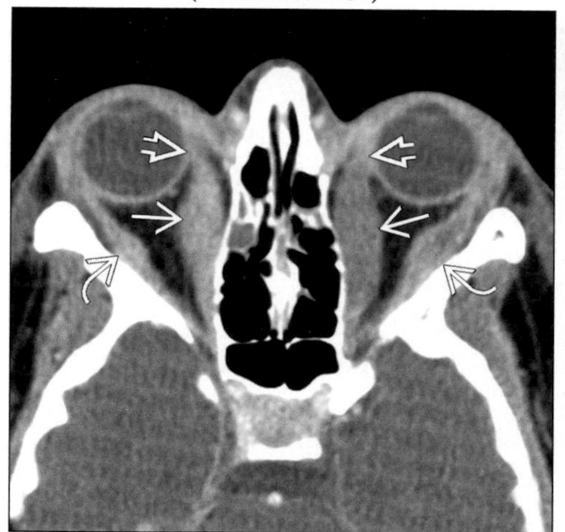

Idiopathic Orbital Inflammatory Disease (Pseudotumor)

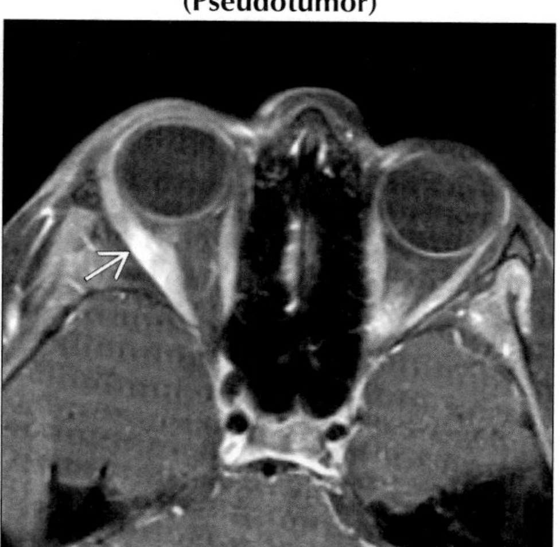

*(**Left**) Axial CECT shows diffuse enlargement of bilateral medial → and, to a lesser extent, lateral rectus muscles →, including involvement of the tendinous insertions →. This child presented with painful proptosis. Biopsy showed idiopathic orbital inflammatory disease. (**Right**) Axial T1WI C+ FS MR reveals diffuse enlargement and increased enhancement of the lateral rectus muscle →. This child presented with mild pain and proptosis.*

Rhabdomyosarcoma

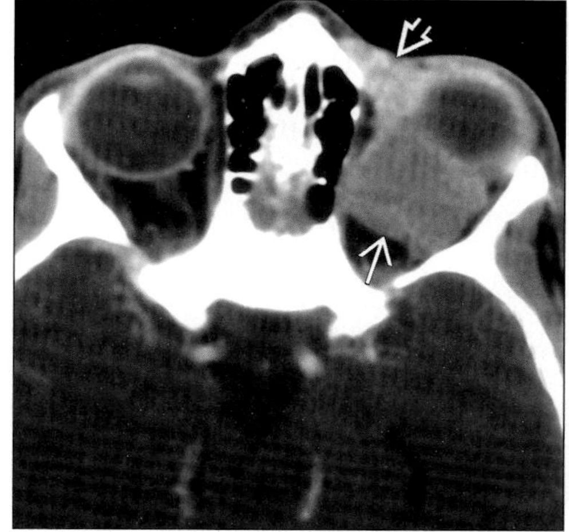

Langerhans Histiocytosis

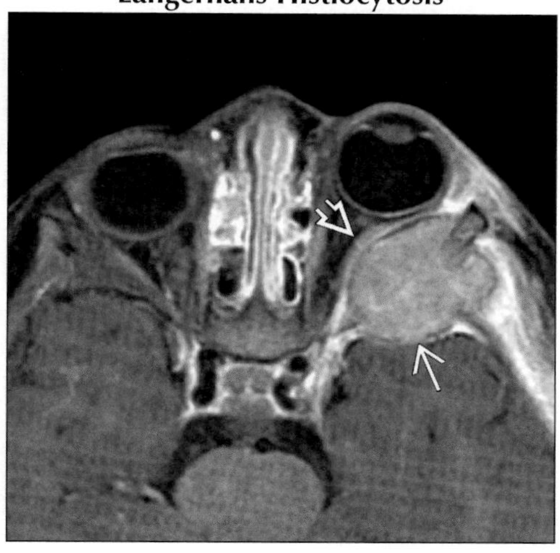

*(**Left**) Axial CECT depicts an enhancing retrobulbar rhabdomyosarcoma → that spreads into the preseptal area medially →. Note the mild associated proptosis. (**Right**) Axial T1 C+ FS MR defines the cause of this child's left proptosis as a large, well-defined, moderately enhancing, expansile mass in the sphenoid wing with orbital → and intracranial → extension. Biopsy specimen showed Langerhans cell histiocytosis.*

Lymphoproliferative Lesions, Orbit

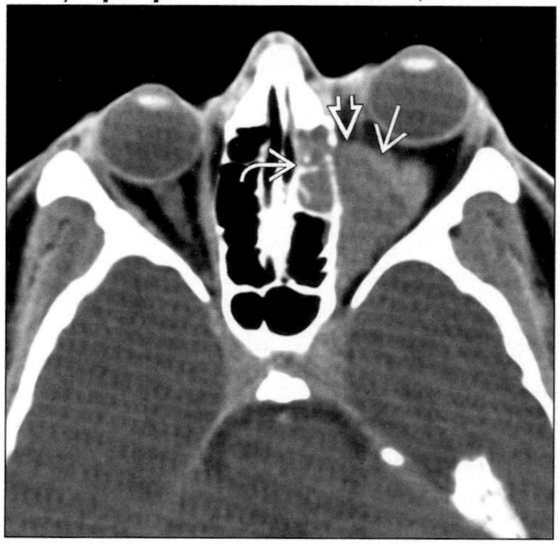

Traumatic Carotid-Cavernous Fistula

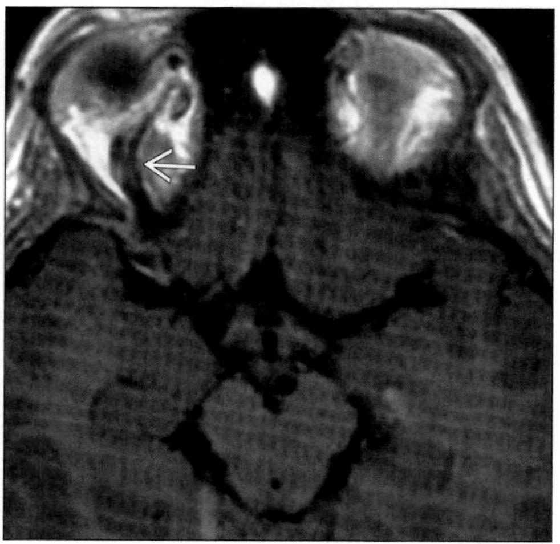

*(**Left**) Axial CECT demonstrates an intraconal → and extraconal → left orbital mass with ethmoid extension →. This non-Hodgkin lymphoma explains this teenager's proptosis and periorbital ecchymosis. (**Right**) Axial T1 C+ MR reveals a large left superior ophthalmic vein → in a child with post-traumatic carotid-cavernous fistula. This child's proptosis presented 2 years after skull base fractures.*

OCULAR LESION

DIFFERENTIAL DIAGNOSIS

Common
- Retinoblastoma
- Persistent Hyperplastic Primary Vitreous
- Retinopathy of Prematurity
- Congenital Cataract

Less Common
- Coats Disease
- Coloboma
- Toxocariasis, Orbit
- Congenital Microphthalmos

Rare but Important
- Retinal Astrocytoma
- Norrie Disease
- Walker-Warburg Syndrome

ESSENTIAL INFORMATION

Helpful Clues for Common Diagnoses

- **Retinoblastoma**
  - Key facts: Malignant tumor arising from neuroectodermal cells of retina
    - Classified as primitive neuroectodermal tumor (PNET)
    - Most common intraocular tumor of childhood
    - Most common cause of leukocoria
    - Rare trilateral or quadrilateral form involves bilateral globes + pineal, or pineal + suprasellar tumor
  - Imaging
    - Unilateral (70-75%)
    - CT: Punctate or speckled calcified intraocular mass
    - MR: T1 mildly hyperintense, T2 moderately hypointense (cf. vitreous); moderate to marked heterogeneous enhancement
- **Persistent Hyperplastic Primary Vitreous**
  - Key facts: Congenital lesion due to incomplete regression of embryonic vitreous and blood supply
    - 2nd most common cause of leukocoria
  - Imaging
    - Hyperdense or hyperintense small globe
    - No calcification
    - Retrolental enhancing soft tissue, classically with "martini glass" shape
    - Associated retinal detachments common
- **Retinopathy of Prematurity**
  - Key facts: Occurs due to prolonged exposure to supplemental oxygen in premature infants
    - Premature birth interrupts normal vasculogenesis ⇒ incomplete vascularization of retina ⇒ hypoxia ⇒ abnormal neovascularization
  - Imaging
    - Usually bilateral
    - Hyperdense globe ± abnormal retrolental soft tissue
    - Early: Microphthalmia
    - Advanced: Vitreal calcification
- **Congenital Cataract**
  - Key facts: Lens opacification
    - Most are sporadic and unilateral
    - ~ 20% familial
    - ~ 17% associated with systemic disease or syndrome: Trisomy 21, craniofacial syndromes, diabetes, etc.
  - Imaging
    - Small, hypodense lens
    - Lens may assume spherical shape (spherophakia), differentiating from acquired cataract

Helpful Clues for Less Common Diagnoses

- **Coats Disease**
  - Key facts: Primary retinal vascular anomaly with retinal telangiectasis and exudative retinal detachment
    - Unilateral in 80-90% of patients
    - Most patients male
  - Imaging
    - Advanced stages may appear to obliterate vitreous
    - CT: Mild diffusely and homogeneously hyperdense vitreous without calcification
    - MR: Retinal detachment with nonenhancing T1 and T2 hyperintense subretinal exudate
- **Coloboma**
  - Key facts: Defect in ocular tissue involving structures of embryonic cleft
    - Bilateral > unilateral
  - Imaging
    - Focal defect of posterior globe with outpouching of vitreous
    - Defect at optic nerve head insertion with funnel-shaped excavation
- **Toxocariasis, Orbit**

- Key facts: Eosinophilic granuloma caused by infection of larval nematode *Toxocara cani* or *cati*
- Imaging
  - CT: Diffuse hyperdensity in vitreous ± discrete mass; no calcification
  - MR: Enhancing, variable T1 hypo/isointense, T2 iso/hyperintense retrolental or vitreous mass

- **Congenital Microphthalmos**
  - Key facts: Corneal diameter of < 11 mm and anteroposterior diameter of globe < 20 mm at birth
    - Isolated
    - Or associated with craniofacial anomalies, coloboma, persistent hyperplastic primary vitreous, retinopathy of prematurity
  - Imaging
    - Overall volume and dimension of globe < unaffected side or comparison normal
    - Simple microphthalmia: Structurally normal small eye or complex with associated findings, as above

Helpful Clues for Rare Diagnoses

- **Retinal Astrocytoma**
  - Key facts: Retinal astrocytic hamartoma is ocular manifestation of tuberous sclerosis complex
  - Imaging
    - Enhancing exophytic juxtapapillary or epipapillary retinal mass
    - Mass may be multifocal ± bilateral
    - Rarely may occur in isolation without tuberous sclerosis complex
- **Norrie Disease**
  - Key facts: X-linked recessive syndrome of retinal malformation, deafness, and mental retardation
  - Imaging
    - Bilateral hyperdense vitreous
    - Small anterior chamber
    - Small lens without calcification
    - May have associated retrolental mass, retinal detachment, microphthalmia, optic nerve atrophy
- **Walker-Warburg Syndrome**
  - Key facts: Also known as HARD+E
    - **H**ydrocephaly
    - **A**gyria
    - **R**etinal **d**etachment
    - ± **e**ncephalocele
  - Imaging
    - Bilateral retinal detachment
    - Vitreous ± subretinal hemorrhage
    - Associated hydrocephalus, agyria/dysgenesis of cerebral and cerebellar gray and white matter

Retinoblastoma

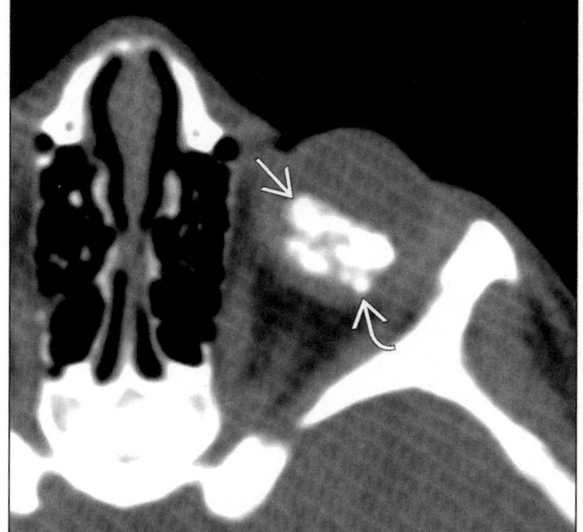

Axial NECT shows coarse calcifications typical of retinoblastoma in the posterior segment of the globe ➔ involving the vitreous body, as well as the choroidal-retinal layers ➔.

Retinoblastoma

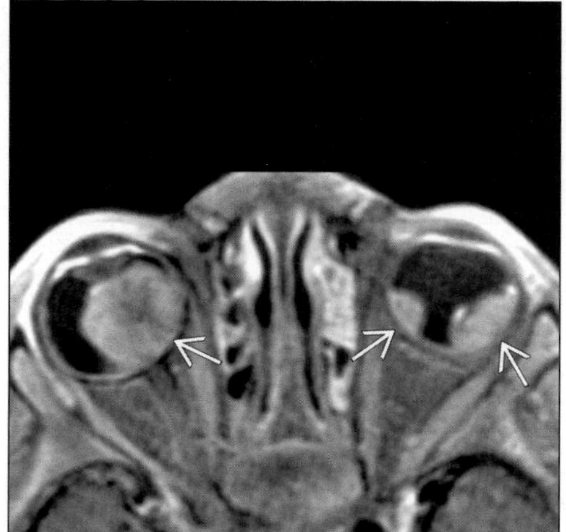

Axial T1WI FS MR shows bilateral enhancing retinal masses ➔ extending into the vitreous but not extending beyond the sclera into the optic nerve or intraconal orbit.

OCULAR LESION

(**Left**) *Axial T2WI FS MR reveals a hypointense retrolental "martini glass"-shaped mass with associated fluid-fluid levels in the vitreous body and a subretinal effusion.* (**Right**) *Axial CECT demonstrates an enhancing retrolental embryonic fibrovascular tissue and right small globe (microphthalmia).*

Persistent Hyperplastic Primary Vitreous

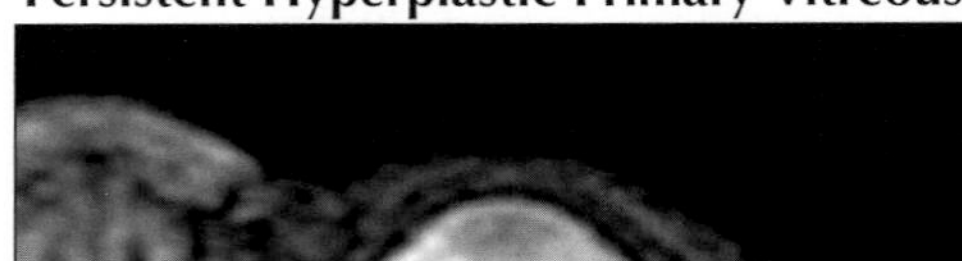

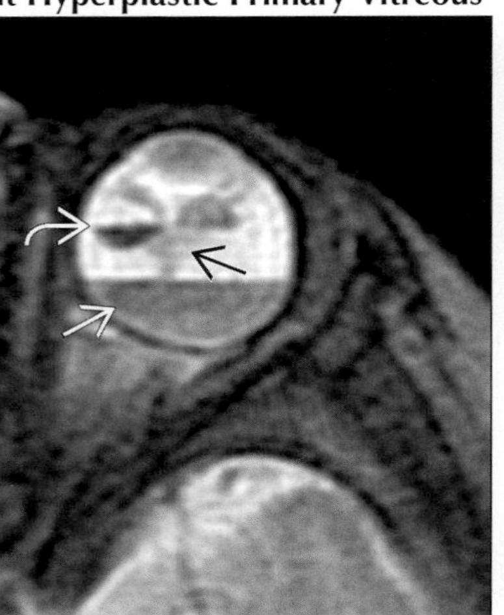

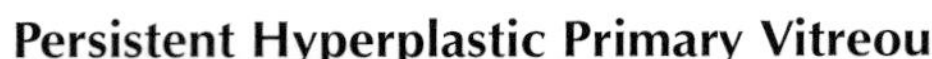

Persistent Hyperplastic Primary Vitreous

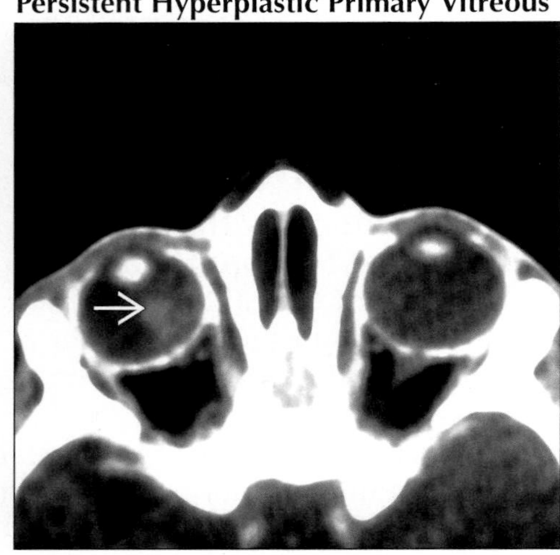

(**Left**) *Axial CECT shows a small left globe with dense peripheral calcifications. Both lenses are also calcified. The right globe shows more punctate scattered calcifications and fluid-fluid level, indicating retinal detachment.* (**Right**) *Axial T2WI MR in the same patient reveals fluid-fluid level and peripheral low signal intensity from dense calcification. Note the deformed, low signal intensity calcified lens.*

Retinopathy of Prematurity

Retinopathy of Prematurity

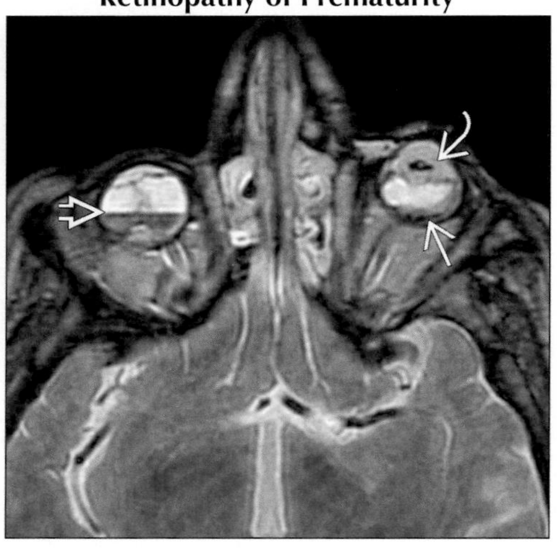

(**Left**) *Axial CECT in a child with leukocoria shows significant thinning and loss of density from the right lens with increased depth of the anterior chamber compared to the opposite normal left globe.* (**Right**) *Axial NECT depicts diffuse homogeneous hyperdense vitreous of the left globe in a child with no history of trauma or surgery. Coats disease as a primary retinal vascular anomaly with retinal telangiectasis caused this exudative retinal detachment.*

Congenital Cataract

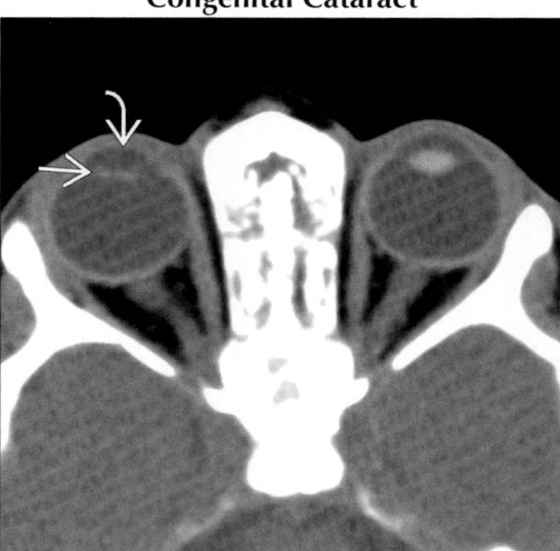

Coats Disease

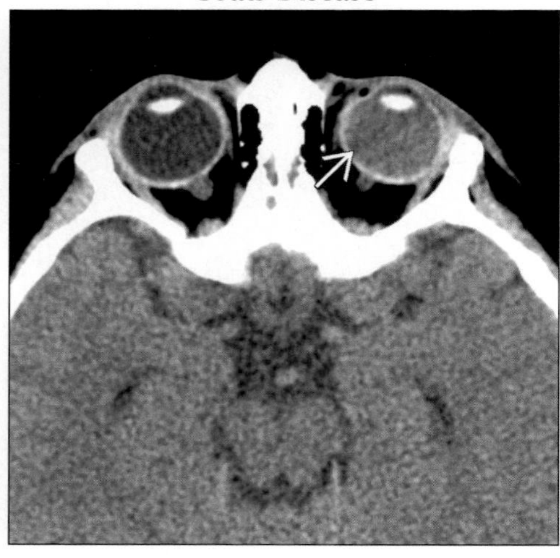

Coloboma

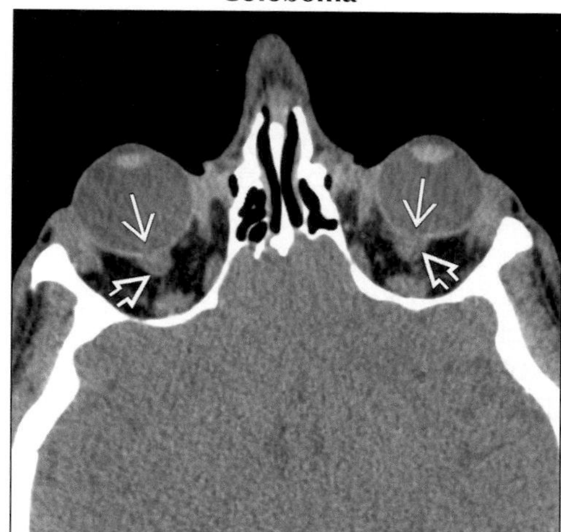

Toxocariasis, Orbit

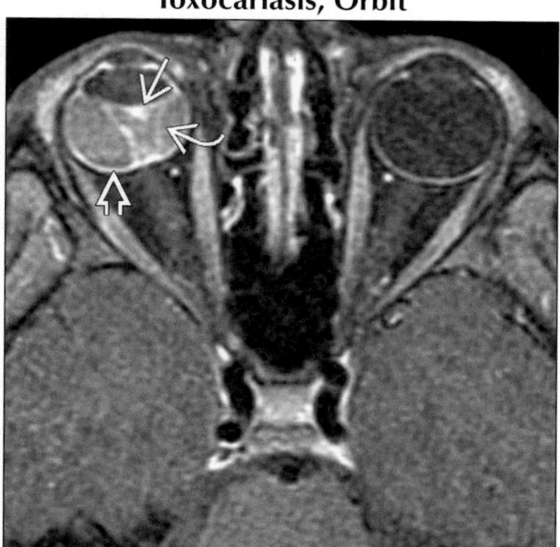

*(**Left**) Axial NECT shows a defect in the posterior globes bilaterally ➡ with outpouching of the vitreous ⇨. (**Right**) Axial T1WI C+ FS MR demonstrates hyperintensity of the right globe vitreous with an enhancing retrolental mass ⇨, retinal detachments ➡, with retinal and scleral nodules ⇨.*

Congenital Microphthalmos

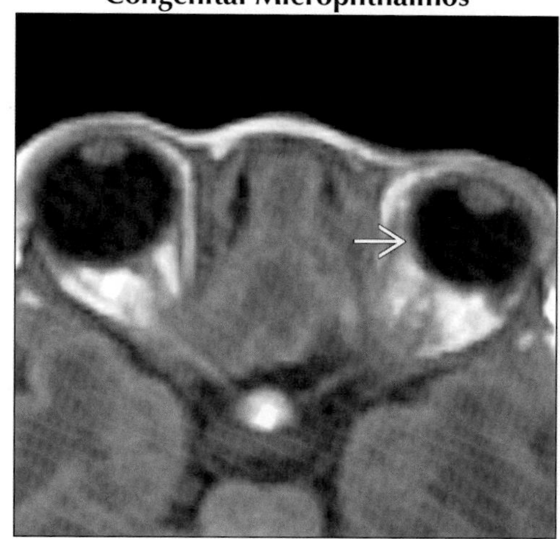

Retinal Astrocytoma

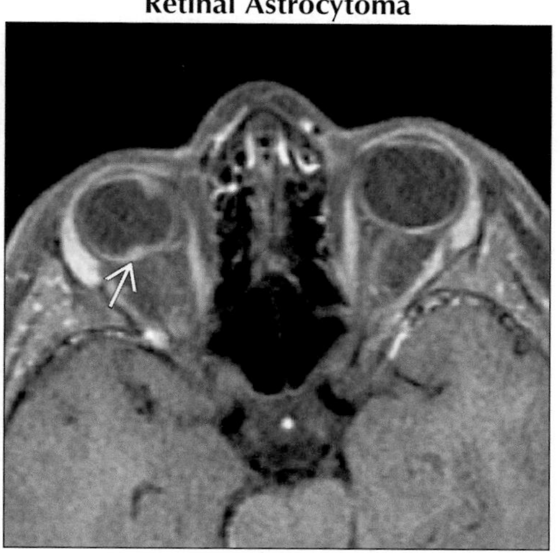

*(**Left**) Axial T2WI MR shows an asymmetrically small left globe ➡ with otherwise normal lens, vitreous body, and choroidal-retinal layers. (**Right**) Axial T1 C+ FS MR reveals an enhancing nodular retinal astrocytoma ➡ at the optic nerve head in a child with tuberous sclerosis.*

Norrie Disease

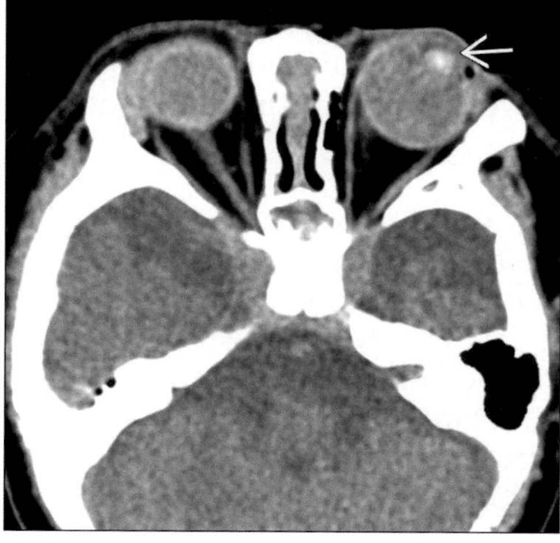

Walker-Warburg Syndrome

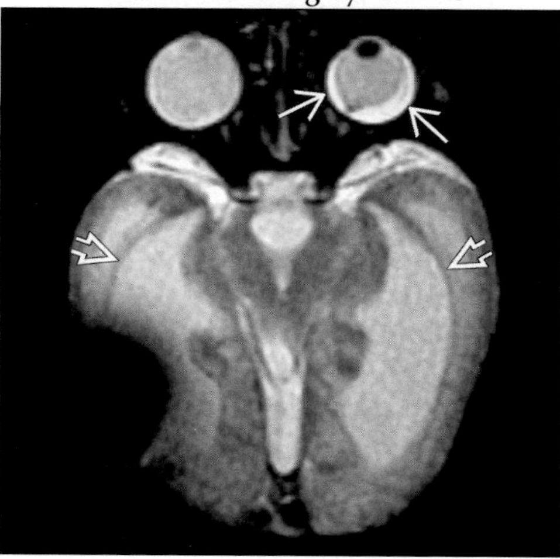

*(**Left**) Axial NECT shows bilateral abnormal increase in globe density. Left globe and orbit are enlarged with decrease in size of anterior chamber ➡. Norrie disease is diagnosed clinically when grayish-yellow fibrovascular masses are found in globes of an infant. (**Right**) Axial T2WI MR reveals a rim of T2 hyperintensity along the posterior left globe ➡, suggestive of retinal dysplasia ± subretinal hemorrhage. Note the marked lateral ventricle dilatation ⇨.*

MICROPHTHALMOS

DIFFERENTIAL DIAGNOSIS

Common
- Trauma, Orbit
- Retinopathy of Prematurity (ROP)
- Retinal Detachment (RD)
- Coloboma

Less Common
- Persistent Hyperplastic Primary Vitreous (PHPV)
- Congenital Microphthalmos

Rare but Important
- Infection, Other Pathogen, Orbit
- Toxocariasis, Orbit

ESSENTIAL INFORMATION

Helpful Clues for Common Diagnoses
- **Trauma, Orbit**
  - Key facts
    - Any trauma may lead to globe rupture
  - Imaging
    - Small globe ± ocular hemorrhage or detachment ± gas within globe
    - If foreign body: BB common; wood may be air or intermediate attenuation
    - Posterior scleral rupture may lead to deep anterior chamber
- **Retinopathy of Prematurity (ROP)**
  - Retrolental fibroplasia
  - Key facts
    - Vasculoproliferative disorder in low birth weight premature infants
    - Secondary to exposure to supplemental O_2
  - Imaging
    - Noncalcified, retrolental mass = retinal detachment
    - Bilateral microphthalmia, hyperdense globe ± calcification as late findings
- **Retinal Detachment (RD)**
  - Key facts
    - 3 potential spaces/ocular detachments
    - Posterior hyaloid (between posterior hyaloid membrane and inner sensory retina)
    - Subretinal (between inner sensory retina and outer retinal pigmented epithelium)
    - Posterior choroidal (between choroid and sclera)
    - Ocular detachments occur in trauma, persistent hyperplastic primary vitreous (PHPV), ROP, ocular masses, Coats disease, or infection
  - Imaging
    - Retinal detachment = V-shaped density
    - Total retinal detachment may simulate persistent hyperplastic primary vitreous
- **Coloboma**
  - Key facts
    - Normal or small globe size
    - Gap or defect of ocular tissue; may involve any structures of embryonic cleft
    - Optic disc coloboma (ODC): Defect confined to optic disc
    - Choroidoretinal coloboma (CRC): Separate from or extends beyond disc, arises from globe wall
    - Morning glory disc anomaly (MGDA): Central tuft of glial tissue within defect
    - Peripapillary staphyloma (PPS): Congenital scleral defect at optic nerve head; nearly all unilateral
  - Imaging
    - Focal outpouching of vitreous
    - Bilateral or unilateral
    - Usually with microphthalmos, rarely with macrophthalmos
    - ± optic tract and chiasm atrophy
    - Retrobulbar colobomatous cyst may communicate with globe
    - Sclera enhances, glial tuft in MGDA may enhance
    - Rarely dystrophic calcification at margins
    - ± other abnormalities if associated with syndromes (Meckel, Walker-Warburg, Aicardi, CHARGE), basal cephaloceles, midline facial clefting

Helpful Clues for Less Common Diagnoses
- **Persistent Hyperplastic Primary Vitreous (PHPV)**
  - Key facts
    - Remnants of primary vitreous and primitive hyaloid artery (failure of involution) occur along course of Cloquet canal: Anterior, posterior, or both (most common)
    - 2nd most common cause of leukocoria after retinoblastoma

- Sporadic, unilateral; bilateral more common in association with syndromes (Walker-Warburg, Norrie)
- Imaging
  - Noncalcified, tubular, cylindrical, or triangular-shaped enhancing tissue within vitreous compartment
  - Microphthalmos, retinal detachment ± ↑ attenuation of entire vitreous body common
  - Small dysplastic lens and shallow anterior chamber with anterior involvement

- **Congenital Microphthalmos**
  - Key facts
    - Microphthalmia = eye < 2/3 normal size, or < 16 mm axial dimension
    - Anophthalmia: Complete absence of globe or only vestigial remnant
  - Imaging
    - Small globe; unilateral or bilateral
    - ± intracranial structural abnormalities (more common in bilateral)
    - ± coloboma or cyst

Helpful Clues for Rare Diagnoses

- **Infection, Other Pathogen, Orbit**
  - Key facts
    - Viral (herpes simplex, herpes zoster, CMV, rubella, rubeola, mumps, EBV)
    - Bacterial (syphilis, Lyme, brucellosis, cat scratch, *E. coli*)
    - Fungal (candidiasis) or parasitic (*Toxocara canis*)
    - Most patients are not imaged
    - Most treated without sequelae of microphthalmia
  - Imaging
    - Thickened, enhancing sclera (scleritis)
    - Thickened, enhancing uvea (uveitis)
    - ↑ attenuation/signal of vitreous secondary to ↑ protein ± uveitis ± ocular detachment in endophthalmitis
    - Endophthalmitis: Intraocular infectious or inflammatory process involving vitreous cavity or anterior chamber
- **Toxocariasis, Orbit**
  - Key facts
    - Inflammatory response to nematode *Toxocara canis* causes chorioretinitis
    - Granulomatous inflammation surrounds dead larvae
    - May appear as focal posterior or peripheral retinal granuloma
    - Most commonly unilateral
  - Imaging
    - Focal or diffuse thickening and enhancement of globe
    - Retinal detachment may be associated
    - ↑ attenuation/intensity of vitreous possible

Other Essential Information

- End-stage damage to globe from any cause may ⇒ phthisis bulbi (calcified, small globe)

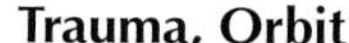
Trauma, Orbit

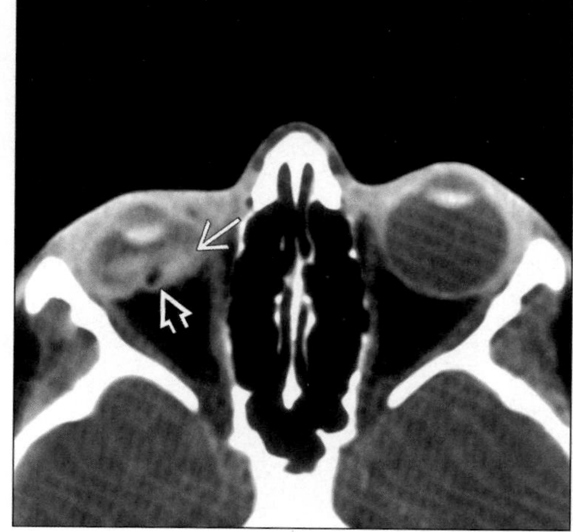

Axial NECT shows rupture of the right globe with decreased volume of vitreous cavity and high attenuation, consistent with hemorrhage ➔. Note also a small posterior bubble of gas ⇨.

Trauma, Orbit

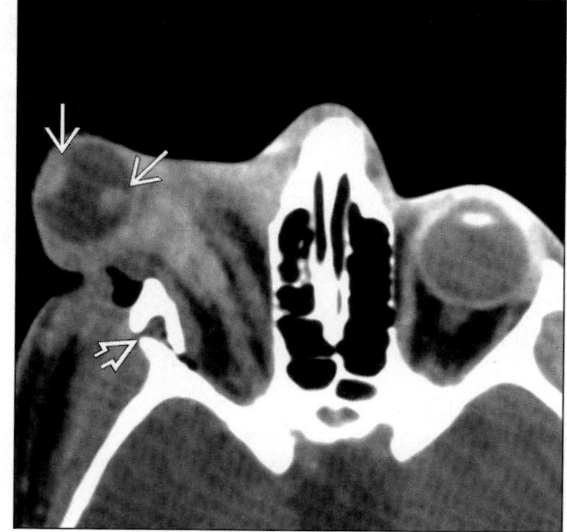

Axial NECT shows shattered pieces of lens ➔ within a small right globe. Also note the near complete post-traumatic enucleation from orbital wall fractures ⇨ in this patient with severe head trauma.

MICROPHTHALMOS

(Left) *Axial CECT shows bilateral microphthalmia with increased attenuation secondary to chronic retinal detachment.* ***(Right)*** *Axial T2WI MR in an infant born prematurely demonstrates bilateral microphthalmia with hyperintense proteinaceous fluid nearly obliterating the vitreous cavity.*

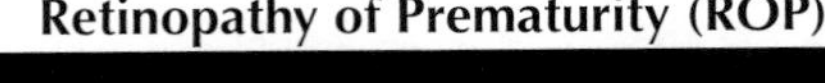

Retinopathy of Prematurity (ROP)

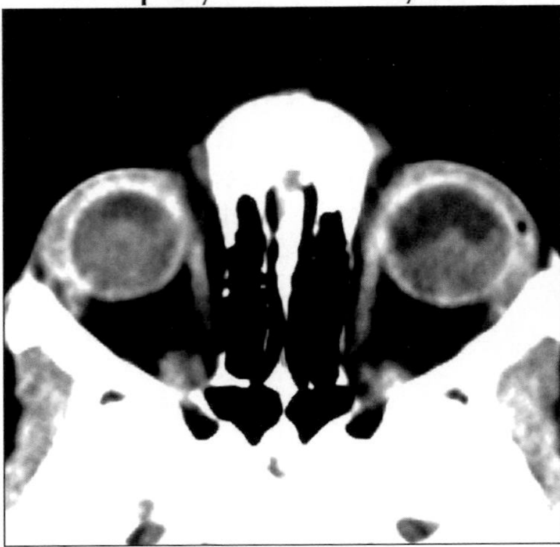

Retinopathy of Prematurity (ROP)

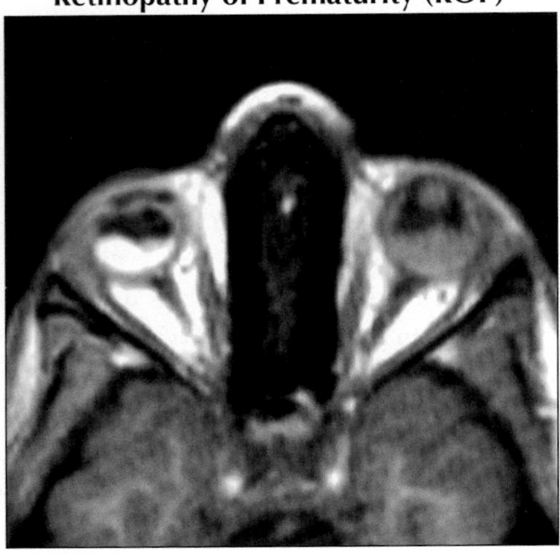

(Left) *Axial FLAIR MR reveals a small hyperintense right globe with near complete retinal detachment →, obliterating the vitreous cavity.* ***(Right)*** *Axial T1 C+ FS MR reveals a large right colobomatous cyst → projecting off the posterior aspect of a microphthalmic globe ⇨.*

Retinal Detachment (RD)

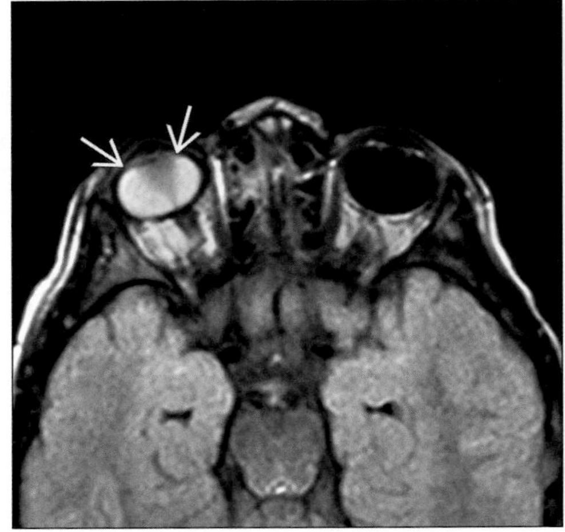

Coloboma

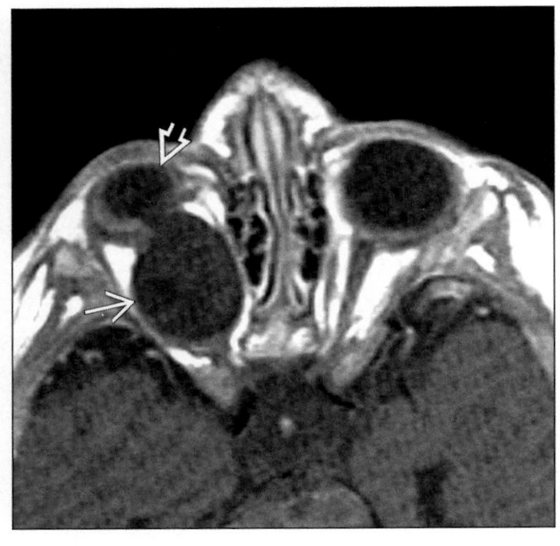

(Left) *Axial NECT shows bilateral microphthalmia with bilateral optic disc colobomas →. Note the large left-sided retrobulbar colobomatous cyst ⇨.* ***(Right)*** *Axial T2WI MR reveals a small globe with a fluid level in the posterior vitreous → and a linear hypointense structure ⇨ extending from the posterior aspect of the lens to the optic nerve head. This linear structure represents the persistent Cloquet canal in a patient with Walker-Warburg syndrome.*

Coloboma

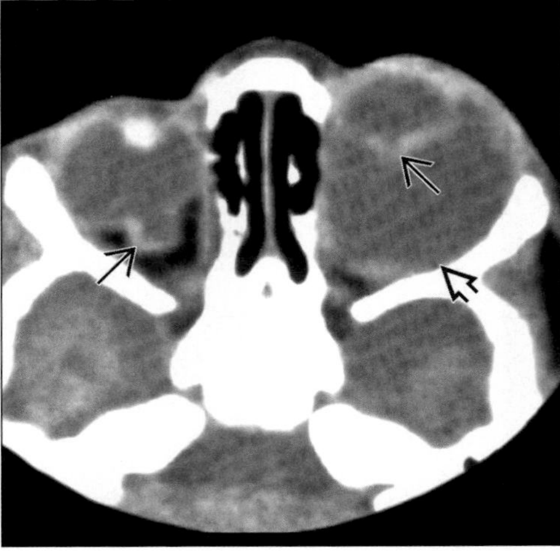

Persistent Hyperplastic Primary Vitreous (PHPV)

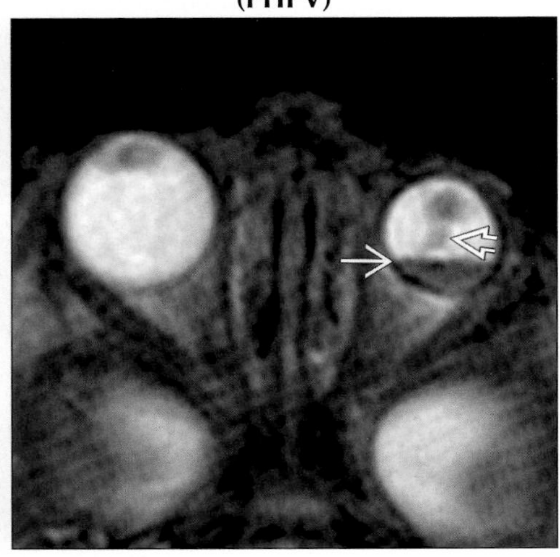

MICROPHTHALMOS

Congenital Microphthalmos

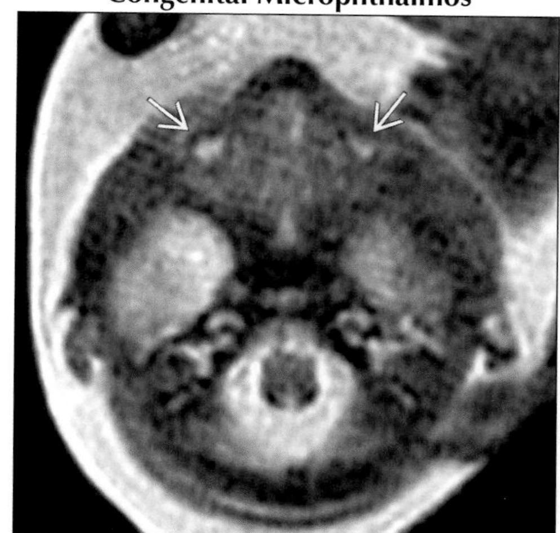

Congenital Microphthalmos

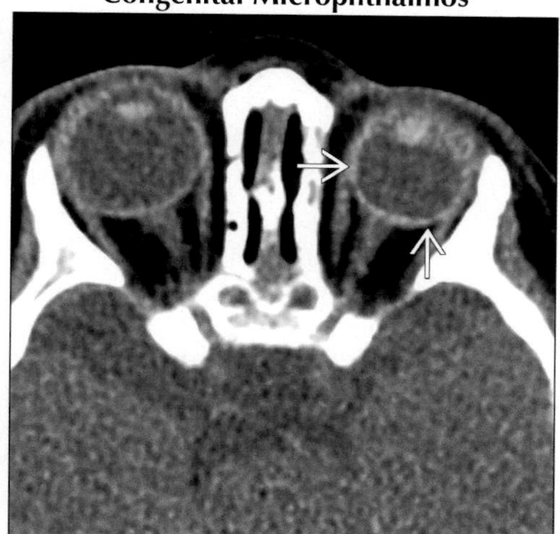

*(**Left**) Axial T2WI MR in a 27-week fetus demonstrates severe bilateral microphthalmia →. (**Right**) Axial NECT in a 7-month-old child demonstrates moderate left-sided microphthalmia →.*

Congenital Microphthalmos

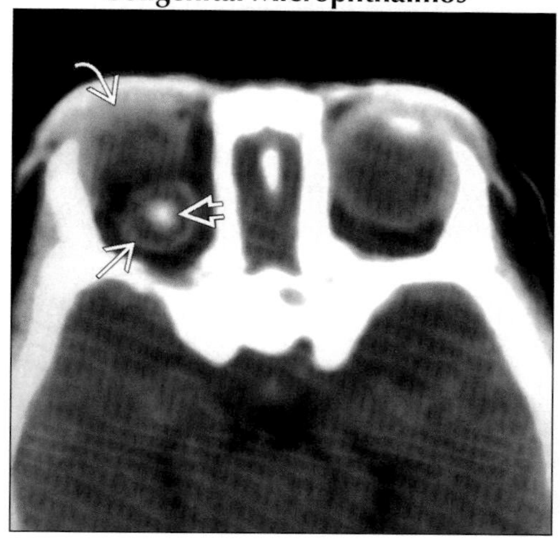

Congenital Microphthalmos

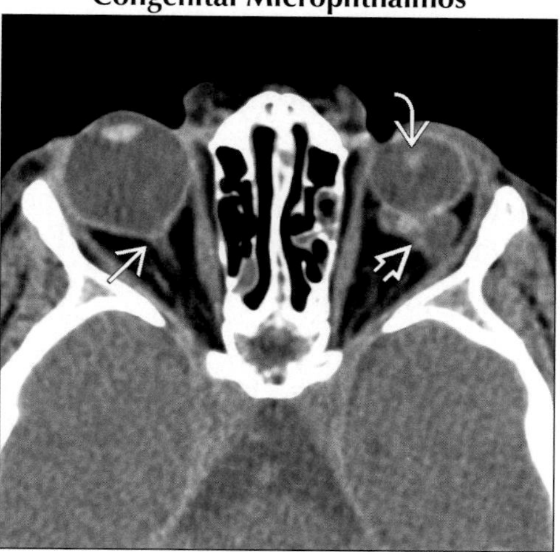

*(**Left**) Axial NECT reveals a small microphthalmic right globe → with a malpositioned lens → and a large anterior cyst →. (**Right**) Axial NECT demonstrates a deformed right globe with a small optic disc coloboma → and a small microphthalmic left globe with multiple small posterior colobomatous cysts →. Notice also the small left lens →.*

Infection, Other Pathogen, Orbit

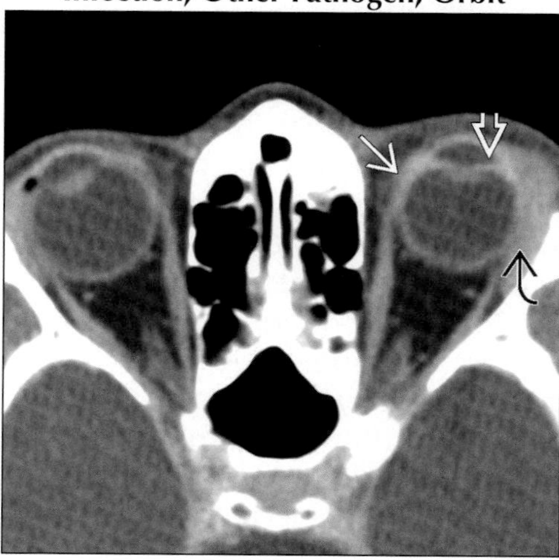

Toxocariasis, Orbit

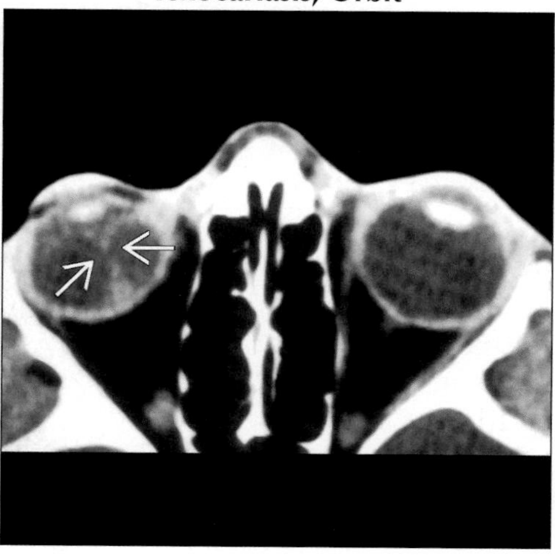

*(**Left**) Axial CECT shows thick, enhancing sclera → and ciliary body → in association with a mild decrease in the size of the left globe and enlargement of the left lacrimal gland → in a patient with nonspecific scleritis and uveitis. (**Right**) Axial NECT shows small right globe with complete retinal detachment → secondary to toxocariasis.*

MACROPHTHALMOS

DIFFERENTIAL DIAGNOSIS

Common
- Staphyloma
- Neurofibromatosis Type 1

Less Common
- Acquired Glaucoma
- Congenital Glaucoma

Rare but Important
- Congenital Myopia
- Sturge-Weber Syndrome
- Congenital Cystic Eye
- Coloboma with Macrophthalmia

ESSENTIAL INFORMATION

Key Differential Diagnosis Issues
- Elongated globe in anteroposterior (AP) dimension may be secondary to myopia, staphyloma, or coloboma
- Diffuse enlargement of globe in AP and transverse dimension = buphthalmos ("ox eye" or "cow eye")
  - Buphthalmos may be present in congenital glaucoma, neurofibromatosis type 1 (NF1), Sturge-Weber, acquired glaucoma

Helpful Clues for Common Diagnoses
- **Staphyloma**
  - Key facts
    - Thinning and stretching of scleral-uveal layers of globe
    - Progressive myopia (nearsightedness) results in posterior staphyloma
    - Posterior staphyloma may also occur in glaucoma, connective tissue disorders, scleritis, necrotizing infection, or trauma
    - Anterior staphyloma may occur if infection or inflammation ⇒ corneal thinning
  - Imaging
    - Elongated globe, thinning of posterior wall, unilateral or bilateral
- **Neurofibromatosis Type 1**
  - Key facts
    - Congenital neurocutaneous syndrome
    - Mutation of gene on chromosome 17
    - Orbitofacial abnormalities in NF1 typically unilateral
    - Plexiform neurofibroma (PNF) diagnostic
    - Up to 50% with facial and eyelid involvement have ipsilateral glaucoma
  - Imaging
    - Buphthalmos
    - Thickening of uveal and scleral layer; anterior rim enlargement
    - PNF orbit and skull base + sphenoid bony dysplasia ⇒ enlargement of orbital foramina and middle cranial fossa ⇒ herniation of intracranial contents into orbit ⇒ pulsatile exophthalmos
    - ± enlargement, tortuosity, and enhancement of optic nerve glioma

Helpful Clues for Less Common Diagnoses
- **Acquired Glaucoma**
  - Key facts
    - Leading cause of blindness in African-Americans and 2nd leading cause of blindness worldwide
    - > 4,000,000 Americans have glaucoma; only 1/2 know they have it
    - Risk factors: African-American, > 60 years, family member with glaucoma, Hispanic, Asian, high myopia, diabetes mellitus, hypertension, trauma
    - Primary open angle > > angle closure
    - Diagnosis by tonometry (measures intraocular pressure), ophthalmoscopy (may show evidence of optic nerve atrophy), visual field tests (lose peripheral vision 1st), or gonioscopy (measure angle between iris and cornea)
  - Imaging
    - Less plasticity in globe of adults; therefore buphthalmos and deep anterior chamber uncommon
- **Congenital Glaucoma**
  - Key facts
    - Incidence 1:5,000-1:10,000 live births; boys > > girls; bilateral in majority
    - Present at birth; usually diagnosed within 1st year of life
    - Clinical: Large eyes, excessive tearing, cloudy cornea, and light sensitivity
    - Obstruction to flow of aqueous humor from anterior chamber ⇒ elevated intraocular pressure, enlargement of globe and deep anterior chamber
    - Normal mean anterior chamber depth: 3 mm; in congenital glaucoma, mean anterior chamber depth: 6.3 mm

- Complications: Subluxated lens, optic nerve atrophy
- Imaging
  - Enlarged AP dimension of globe
  - Deep anterior chamber

Helpful Clues for Rare Diagnoses

- **Congenital Myopia**
  - Key facts
    - Idiopathic globe enlargement (AP dimension) ⇒ convergence of light anterior to retina (nearsightedness)
  - Imaging
    - Increased AP dimension of oval-shaped globe, unilateral or bilateral
- **Sturge-Weber Syndrome**
  - Key facts
    - Sporadic congenital disorder of fetal cortical vein development ⇒ progressive venous occlusion and chronic venous ischemia
    - Up to 30% of patients have glaucoma
  - Imaging
    - Contrast enhancement at site of choroidal angioma ⇒ ↑ intraocular pressure, glaucoma, and buphthalmos
    - ± retinal telangiectatic vessels, scleral angioma, iris heterochromia
    - Serpentine leptomeningeal contrast enhancement of pial angiomatosis (80% unilateral)
    - Enlarged ipsilateral choroid plexus
    - Cortical calcification with parenchymal volume loss
- **Congenital Cystic Eye**
  - Key facts
    - Synonym: Anophthalmos with cyst
    - Secondary to failure of involution of primary optic nerve vesicle early in embryologic development ⇒ cyst formation rather than a globe
    - Cyst filled with proliferating glial tissue, may ⇒ complex cyst
  - Imaging
    - Large malformed cyst within orbit, without identifiable lens
    - ± complex solid-appearing components
- **Coloboma with Macrophthalmia**
  - Key facts
    - Gap or defect of ocular tissue, usually with microphthalmia, rarely with macrophthalmia
    - Colobomatous macrophthalmia with microcornea syndrome: Autosomal dominant inheritance; gene linked to region of 2p23-p16
  - Imaging
    - Axial enlargement of globe
    - Myopia and microcornea
    - Inferonasal iris coloboma
    - Chorioretinal coloboma

Staphyloma

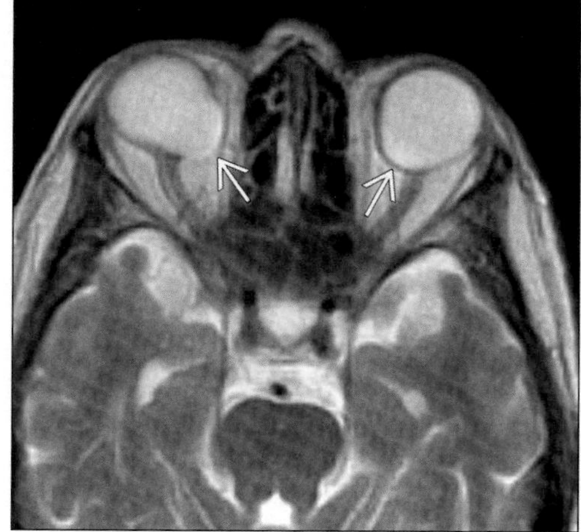

Axial T2WI MR shows bilateral longitudinal extension of the globes ➔ caused by degenerative weakness of the posterior sclera.

Staphyloma

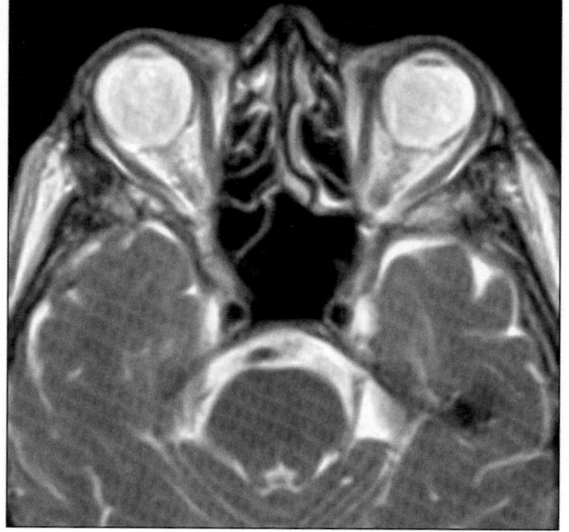

Axial T2WI MR demonstrates mild elongation of both globes in a patient with staphyloma.

MACROPHTHALMOS

(**Left**) *Axial NECT reveals mild enlargement of the right globe with bilateral lens dislocation in an adult with Marfan syndrome.* (**Right**) *Axial T1 C+ MR shows severe sphenoid dysplasia ➔, plexiform neurofibroma ➲, marked proptosis, and buphthalmos ➲.*

Staphyloma

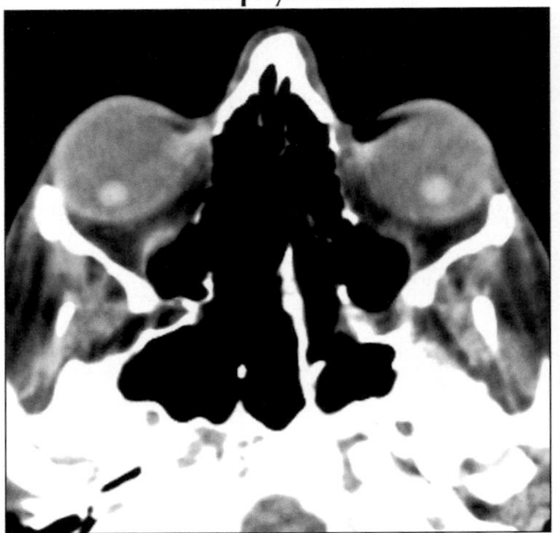

Neurofibromatosis Type 1

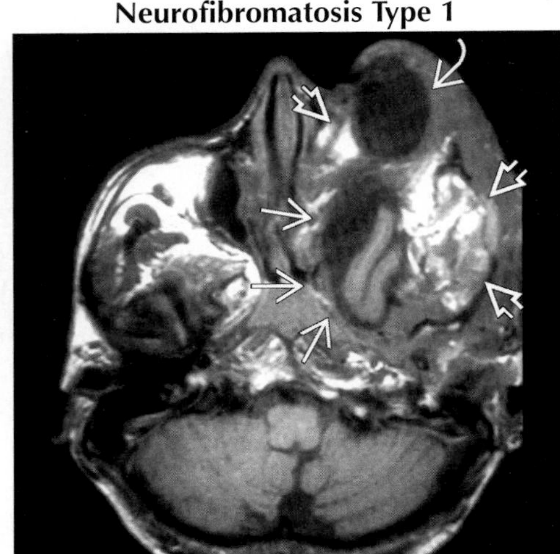

(**Left**) *Axial T2WI MR demonstrates sphenoid wing dysplasia ➔ and infiltrative nodular hyperintense plexiform neurofibroma ➲ causing distortion of the orbit, proptosis, and buphthalmos ➲.* (**Right**) *Axial CECT shows right buphthalmos, dysplastic right sphenoid bone ➔, and plexiform neurofibroma that involves the right cavernous sinus ➲ and orbit ➲.*

Neurofibromatosis Type 1

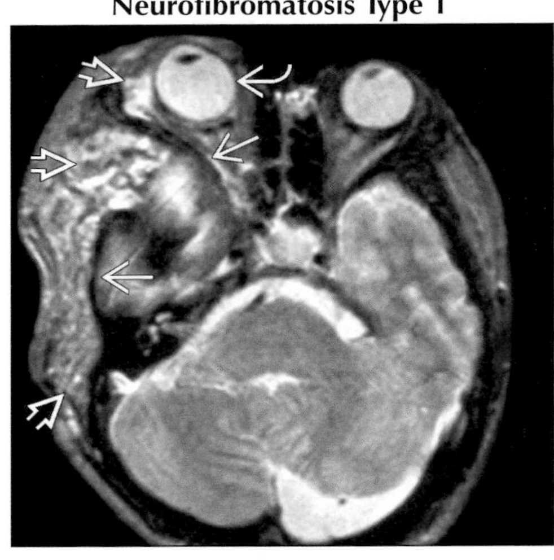

Neurofibromatosis Type 1

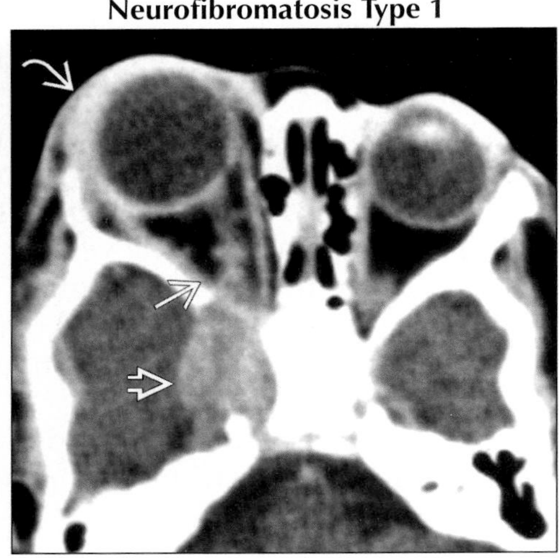

(**Left**) *Axial T2WI FS MR reveals enlargement of the right globe ➔ with minimal asymmetry in the depth of the right anterior chamber.* (**Right**) *Axial T1WI MR demonstrates bilateral globe enlargement with increased depth of the anterior chambers ➔.*

Congenital Glaucoma

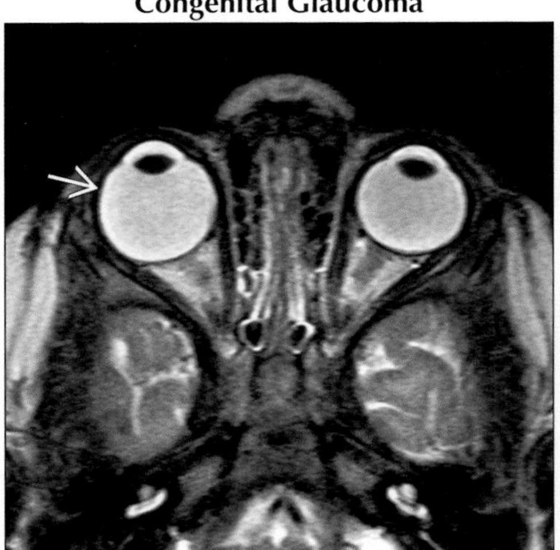

Congenital Glaucoma

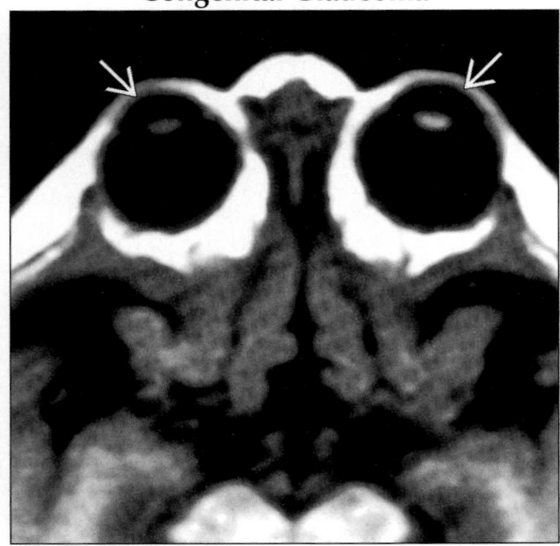

MACROPHTHALMOS

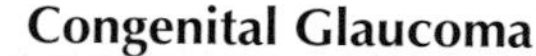

Congenital Glaucoma

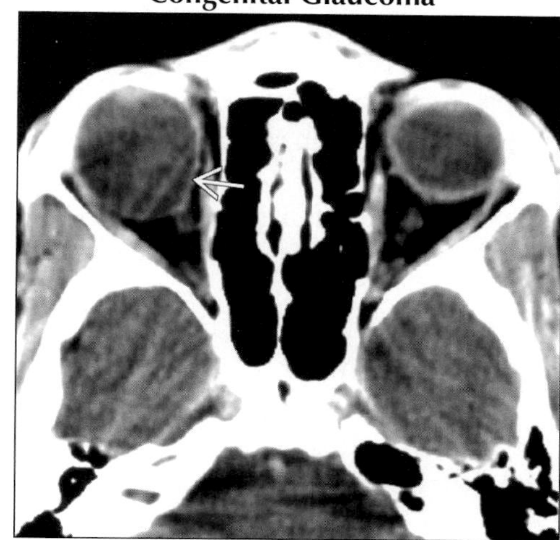

Congenital Myopia

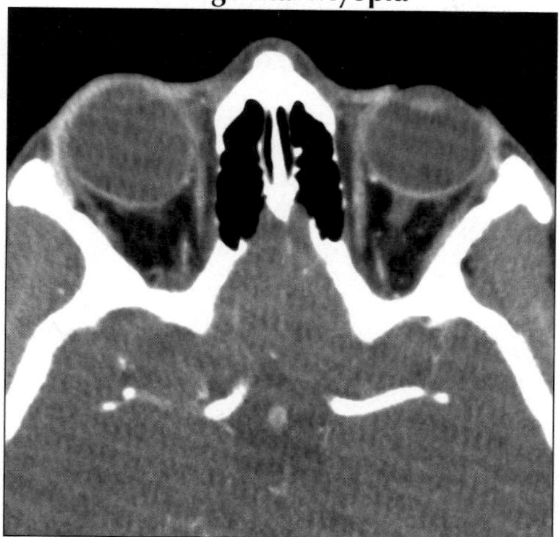

(Left) *Axial CECT in this patient with congenital glaucoma reveals an elongated right globe → (buphthalmos).* ***(Right)*** *Axial CECT shows an enlarged right globe in a patient with congenital myopia.*

Sturge-Weber Syndrome

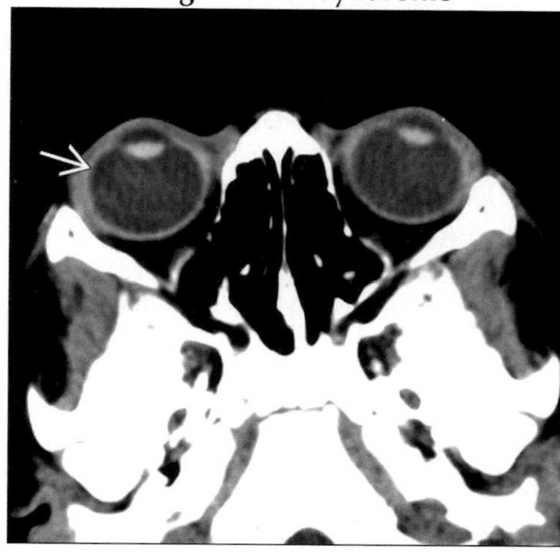

Sturge-Weber Syndrome

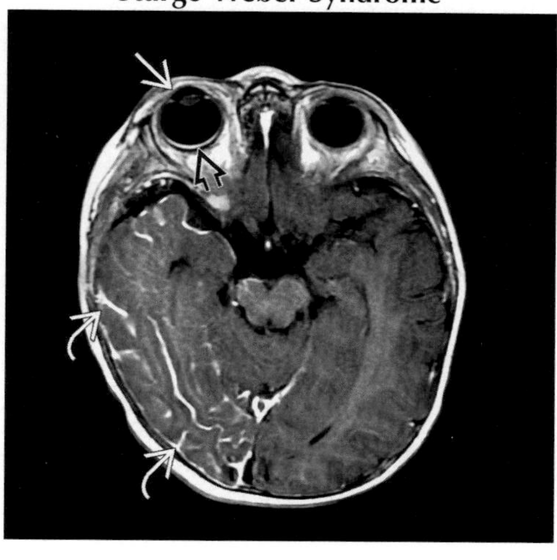

(Left) *Axial NECT shows subtle enlargement of the right globe →, without visualized angioma, in a child with Sturge-Weber syndrome.* ***(Right)*** *Axial T1WI C+ MR shows enlargement of the right globe, deep anterior chamber →, mild thickening and contrast enhancement of choroidal angioma ⇨, and diffuse abnormal leptomeningeal enhancement throughout the small right cerebral hemisphere ↪.*

Congenital Cystic Eye

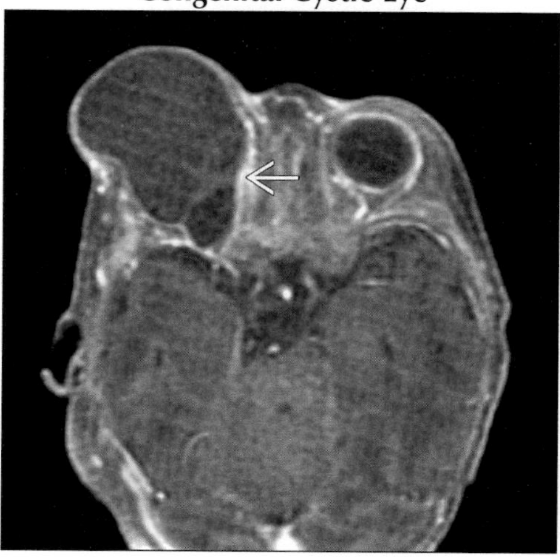

Coloboma with Macrophthalmia

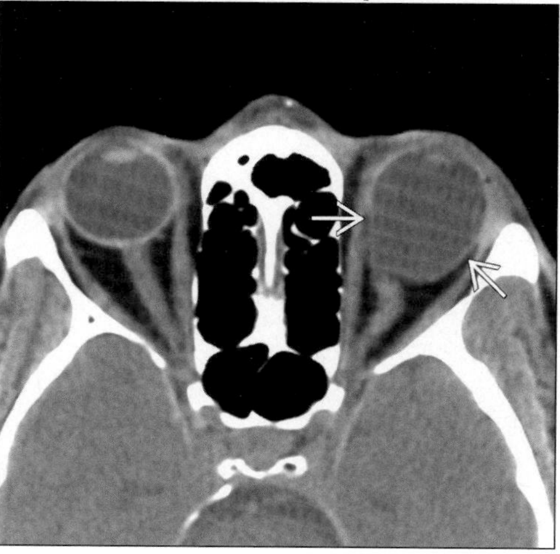

(Left) *Axial T1 C+ FS MR shows a large cystic mass in the right orbit with complex elements posteromedially →, without an identifiable lens.* ***(Right)*** *Axial NECT reveals a broad-based coloboma defect → involving the large left globe.*

OPTIC NERVE SHEATH LESION

DIFFERENTIAL DIAGNOSIS

Common
- Optic Neuritis
- Optic Pathway Glioma

Less Common
- Idiopathic Orbital Inflammatory Disease (Pseudotumor)
- Lymphoproliferative Lesions, Orbit
- Sarcoidosis, Orbit

Rare but Important
- Meningioma, Optic Nerve Sheath

ESSENTIAL INFORMATION

Helpful Clues for Common Diagnoses
- **Optic Neuritis**
  - Key facts: Inflammatory, autoimmune, infectious, post-radiation
    - Acute vision loss, unilateral (70%)
  - Imaging: Enhancement, minimal enlargement, focal or diffuse
- **Optic Pathway Glioma**
  - Key facts: Pilocytic astrocytoma
    - 30-40% have neurofibromatosis type 1
  - Imaging: Tubular enlargement and tortuosity of intraorbital optic nerve
    - Optic nerve, chiasm, tract &/or optic radiations, variable enhancement

Helpful Clues for Less Common Diagnoses
- **Idiopathic Orbital Inflammatory Disease (Pseudotumor)**
  - Key facts: Painful, anterior subtype of IOID
    - Isolated or with other subtypes of IOID (myositic, lacrimal, diffuse, or apical)
  - Imaging: Irregular nerve sheath thickening and enhancement
- **Lymphoproliferative Lesions, Orbit**
  - Key facts: Leukemia or lymphoma (low-grade small B-cell, large B-cell, Burkitt, or T-cell)
  - Imaging: Optic nerve sheath/complex enhancement ± solid mass anywhere in orbit
- **Sarcoidosis, Orbit**
  - Key facts: Noncaseating granulomas
    - Lacrimal gland, EOMs, optic nerve/sheath complex, intraconal/extraconal space, or uvea/sclera
  - Imaging: Enhancing soft tissue mass or enlargement and enhancement of any involved orbital structure

Helpful Clues for Rare Diagnoses
- **Meningioma, Optic Nerve Sheath**
  - Key facts: Benign tumor from arachnoid "cap" cells within optic nerve sheath
    - Rare in children, minority have neurofibromatosis type 2
  - Imaging: "Tram track" = tumor enhancement or calcification on either side of optic nerve
    - Moderate to marked enhancement
    - "Perioptic cyst" = ↑ CSF surrounding optic nerve, between tumor and globe

Optic Neuritis

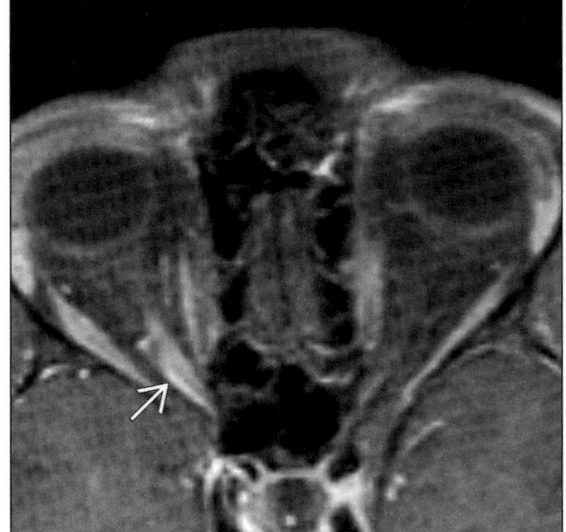

Axial T1WI C+ FS MR shows fusiform enhancement of a minimally enlarged right optic nerve ➔.

Optic Pathway Glioma

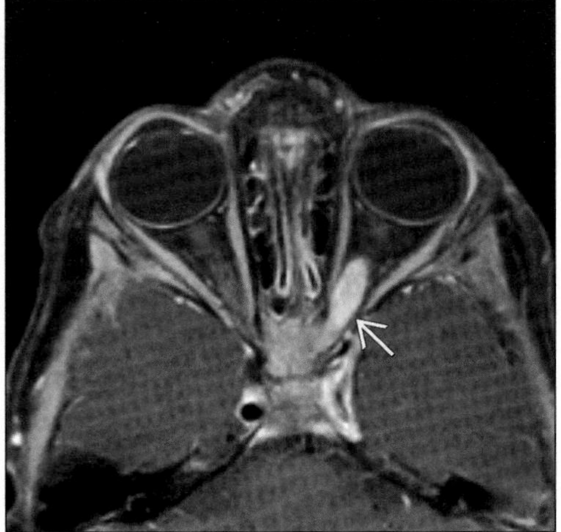

Axial T1WI C+ FS MR shows marked enhancement of an enlarged left optic nerve ➔ in a child with NF1. Absent flow void in the left intracavernous carotid artery is secondary to prior aneurysm embolization.

Optic Pathway Glioma

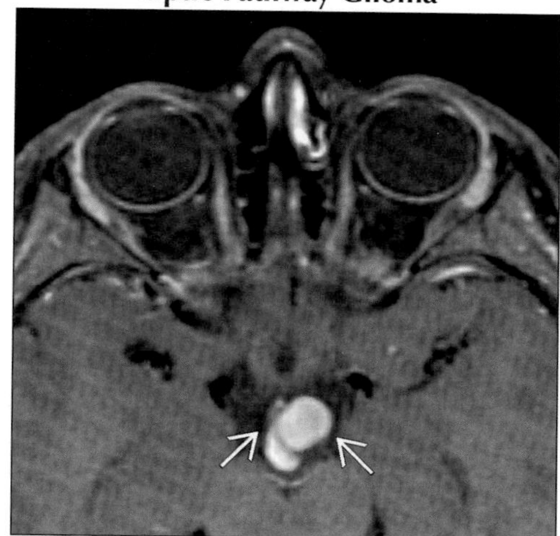

Idiopathic Orbital Inflammatory Disease (Pseudotumor)

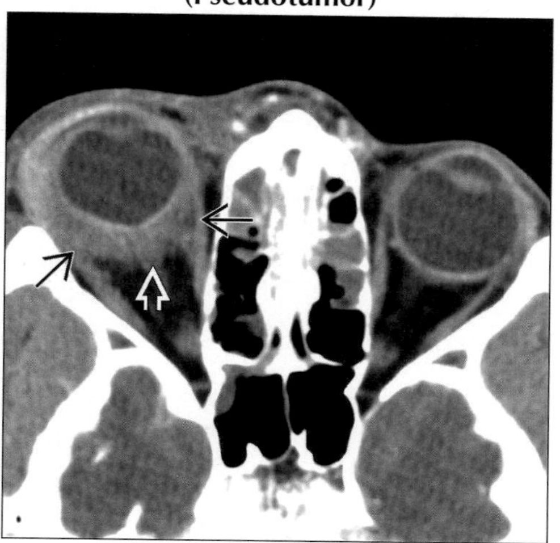

(Left) *Axial T1WI C+ FS MR shows a lobulated, intensely enhancing mass involving the optic chiasm ➡.* ***(Right)*** *Axial CECT shows diffuse, ill-defined soft tissue ➔ surrounding and deforming the posterior aspect of the left globe and distal intraorbital optic nerve ➡.*

Idiopathic Orbital Inflammatory Disease (Pseudotumor)

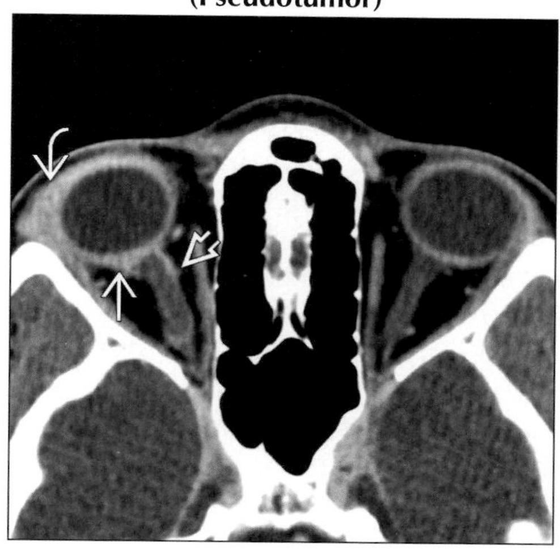

Lymphoproliferative Lesions, Orbit

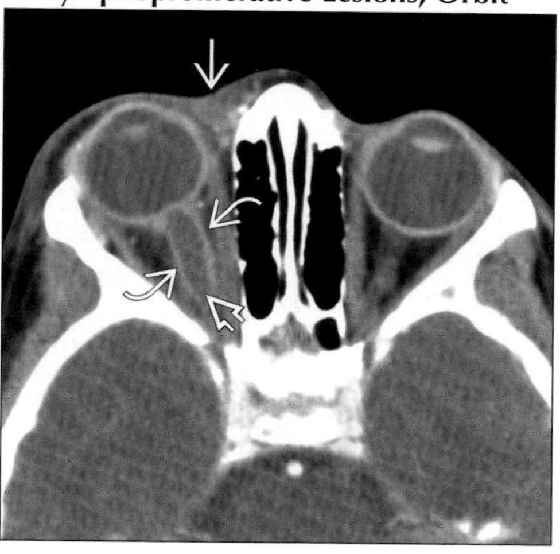

(Left) *Axial CECT shows minimal periscleral soft tissue ➡ surrounding the right globe, abnormal enhancement surrounding the intraorbital right optic nerve ➡, and a prominent right lacrimal gland ➡.* ***(Right)*** *Axial CECT in a child with leukemia shows minimal right preseptal soft tissue swelling ➡, mild enlargement of the intraorbital right optic nerve ➡, and diffuse abnormal contrast enhancement of the optic nerve sheath ➡.*

Sarcoidosis, Orbit

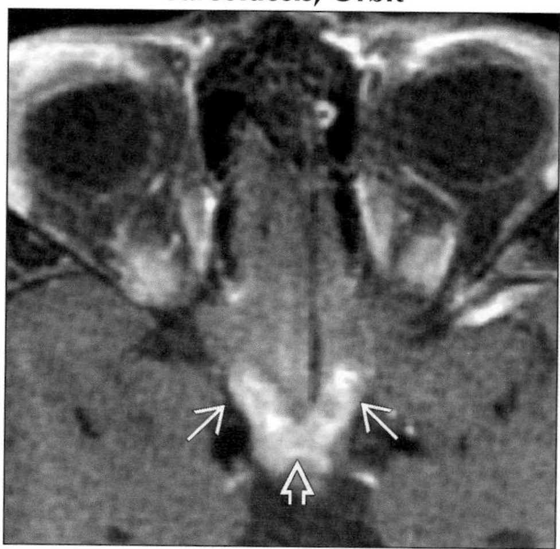

Meningioma, Optic Nerve Sheath

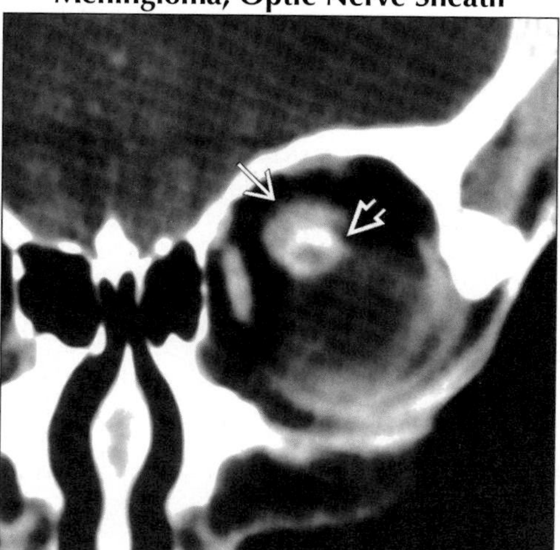

(Left) *Axial T1WI C+ FS MR shows bilateral enhancement of the prechiasmatic optic nerves ➡ and optic chiasm ➡ in a child with neurosarcoidosis.* ***(Right)*** *Coronal CECT shows a mildly enhancing mass ➡ and mild, diffuse, peripheral enhancement of the optic nerve sheath ➡. (Courtesy G. Snowden, MD.)*

SINONASAL ANATOMIC VARIANTS

DIFFERENTIAL DIAGNOSIS

Common

- Nasal Septal Deviation
- Agger Nasi Cell
- Nasal Septal Spur
- Concha Bullosa
- Infraorbital Ethmoid (Haller) Cell
- Paradoxical Middle Turbinate

Less Common

- Pneumatized Anterior Clinoid Process
- Fovea Ethmoidalis, Asymmetric (Low)
- Pneumatized Uncinate Process
- Frontal Cells
- Pneumatized Crista Galli
- Supraorbital Ethmoid Cell
- Dehiscent Lamina Papyracea

Rare but Important

- Sphenoethmoidal (Onodi) Cell
- Carotid Artery, Sphenoid Dehiscence

ESSENTIAL INFORMATION

Key Differential Diagnosis Issues

- Anatomic variants are rule rather than exception
- Multiple variants often present in same patient, so identify and report them!
- Variants may make patients prone to recurrent inflammatory disease and may increase risk of complications during functional endoscopic sinus surgery (FESS)

Helpful Clues for Common Diagnoses

- **Nasal Septal Deviation**
  - Most common variant; often associated with previous trauma
    - Deviates from midline or S-shaped
    - Impact on nasal airway patency depends on overall nasal cavity width
  - Measure maximum deviation from midline
- **Agger Nasi Cell**
  - Present in > 85% (really a variant?); most anterior extramural ethmoid air cell
  - Located anterior to frontal recess; at level of lacrimal sac or head of middle turbinate on coronal CT
- **Nasal Septal Spur**
  - Nearly always associated with septal deviation; often at ethmoid-vomer junction
  - Document direction and length of spur; bony or cartilaginous; contact with lateral nasal wall structures or septum?
- **Concha Bullosa**
  - Pneumatization of conchal turn of middle turbinate; may narrow middle meatus
  - Can be diseased with mucosal thickening, fluid, retention cysts, osteoma
  - Inferior pneumatization is uncommon
- **Infraorbital Ethmoid (Haller) Cell**
  - Air cell located along inferior surface of orbital floor (antral roof)
    - ↑ risk of orbital injury during FESS
  - Variable size; often bilateral; can narrow infundibulum and be diseased
- **Paradoxical Middle Turbinate**
  - Concavity of turbinate concha directed toward septum
    - Diffuse or focal; variable size; often club-shaped
  - Can narrow middle meatus and be diseased

Helpful Clues for Less Common Diagnoses

- **Pneumatized Anterior Clinoid Process**
  - Position lateral to optic nerve ↑ risk of injury during sphenoid surgery
- **Fovea Ethmoidalis, Asymmetric (Low)**
  - Low position ↑ risk of skull base complication during ethmoidectomy
    - Resulting in CSF leak
    - Encephalocele
    - Parenchymal brain injury
  - Report measurement of asymmetry in millimeters in dictation
- **Pneumatized Uncinate Process**
  - May narrow either infundibulum or middle meatus
- **Frontal Cells**
  - Located anterior to frontal recess (above agger nasi cell) or within frontal sinus; 4 types (Bent classification); ↑ incidence of these cells with other variants (concha bullosa); types 3 and 4 may be associated with ↑ disease in frontal sinus
    - Type 1: Single cell above agger nasi
    - Type 2: Tier of 2 or more cells above agger nasi
    - Type 3: Single large cell above agger nasi that extends superiorly into frontal recess

- Type 4: Cell located completely within frontal sinus
- **Pneumatized Crista Galli**
  - Drains into 1 of frontal sinuses or frontal recess; mucocele formation and subsequent infection (mucopyocele)
    - ↑ risk of anterior cranial fossa infection
- **Supraorbital Ethmoid Cell**
  - Cell within orbital plate of frontal bone; posterior to frontal sinus and frontal recess
    - Best delineated on axial imaging
- **Dehiscent Lamina Papyracea**
  - Post-traumatic or congenital
  - Orbital fat or medial rectus muscle may herniate into ethmoid labyrinth
  - ↑ risk for orbital injury during FESS

Helpful Clues for Rare Diagnoses

- **Sphenoethmoidal (Onodi) Cell**
  - Pneumatization of posterior ethmoid cell superior to optic nerve
    - Optic nerve at ↑ risk during posterior ethmoidectomy
  - Best seen on axial imaging
    - Look for horizontal septation on coronal images between this cell superiorly and sphenoid sinus inferiorly
- **Carotid Artery, Sphenoid Dehiscence**
  - Absence of bony covering over internal carotid artery; artery bulges into sphenoid sinus lumen; artery at ↑ risk for injury during sphenoid sinus surgery
  - Better delineated on axial imaging

Other Essential Information

- Anatomic variations can also be categorized based on location or anatomic structure involved
  - Frontal region variants
  - Ethmoid region variants
  - Middle turbinate variants
  - Uncinate variants
  - Sphenoethmoidal region variants
  - Nasal septal variants
- Additional variants not mentioned above
  - Variable pneumatization
    - Aplasia, hypoplasia, hyperpneumatization
  - Intersinus septal cell
    - Located within septum between frontal sinuses
  - Fusion of uncinate to middle turbinate, lamina papyracea, or skull base
  - Pneumatization of vertical lamella of middle turbinate
  - Septal recess
    - Cell within posterior nasal septum
  - Sphenoid sinus septations inserting on carotid canal
  - Pneumatization of dorsum sella

Nasal Septal Deviation

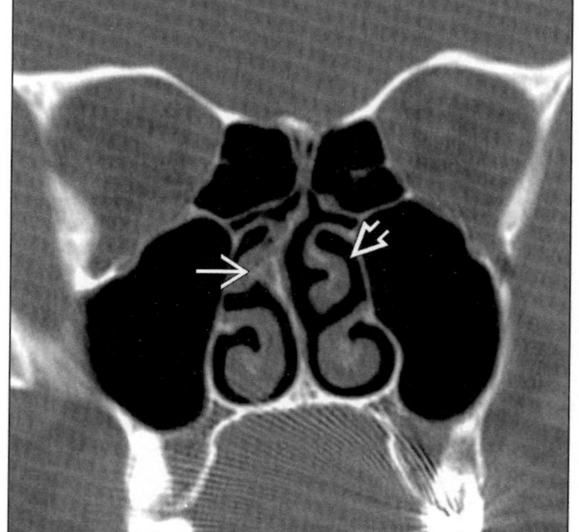

Coronal bone CT shows deviation of the nasal septum to the right with a small bony spur ➡. Also note the paradoxical curvature of the middle turbinate ➡ on the left side.

Agger Nasi Cell

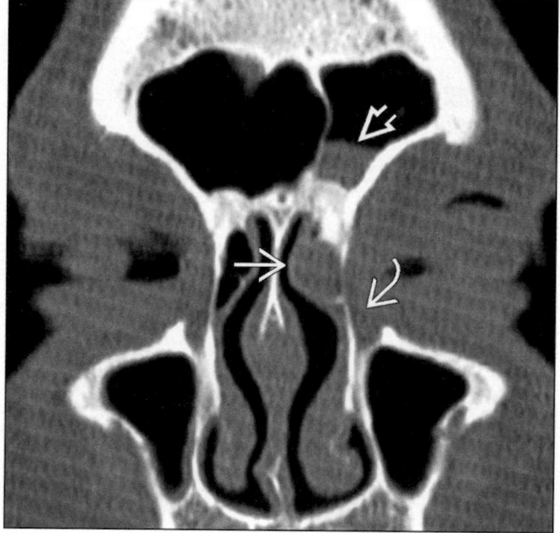

Coronal bone CT shows opacified agger nasi air cell ➡ on the left with additional left frontal mucosal sinus disease ➡. This air cell is seen on the same coronal slice as the lacrimal sac ➡.

SINONASAL ANATOMIC VARIANTS

(Left) *Coronal bone CT shows broad-based bony nasal septal spur directed toward the left with superolateral displacement of the middle turbinate.* ***(Right)*** *Coronal bone CT shows the pneumatized left middle turbinate (concha bullosa). Also note the septal deviation, pneumatized uncinate, and low left fovea ethmoidalis.*

Nasal Septal Spur

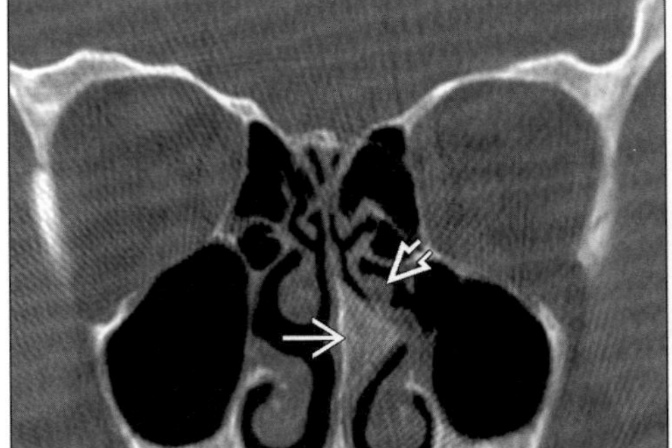

Concha Bullosa

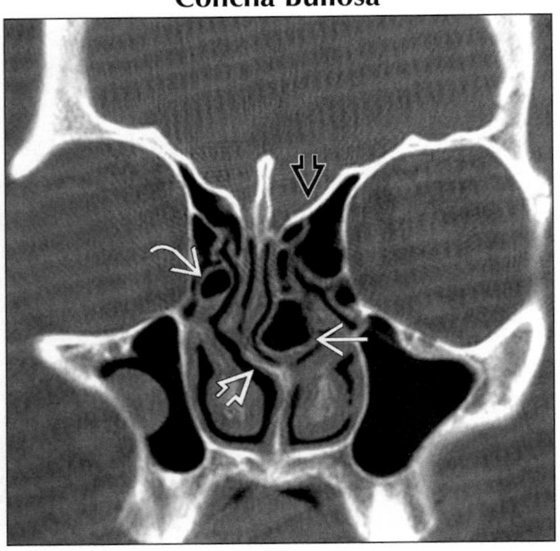

(Left) *Coronal bone CT reveals a large infraorbital Haller cell on the right. The cell narrows the infundibulum. Note the infraorbital nerve location lateral to the air cell.* ***(Right)*** *Coronal bone CT shows bilateral paradoxical curvature of the middle turbinates. The concavity of the conchae is directed toward the nasal septum. This patient had sinusitis at the time of imaging.*

Infraorbital Ethmoid (Haller) Cell

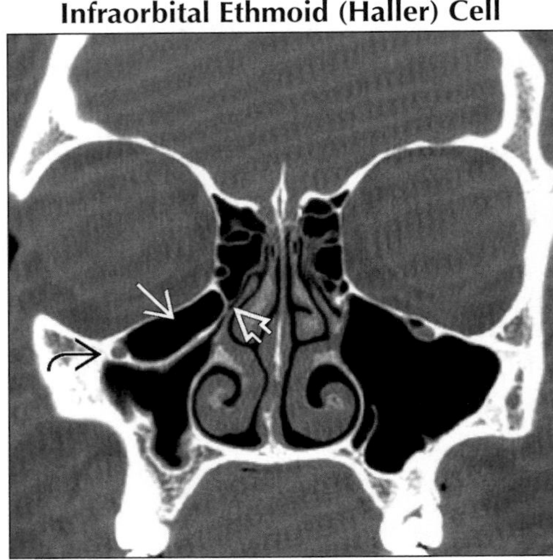

Paradoxical Middle Turbinate

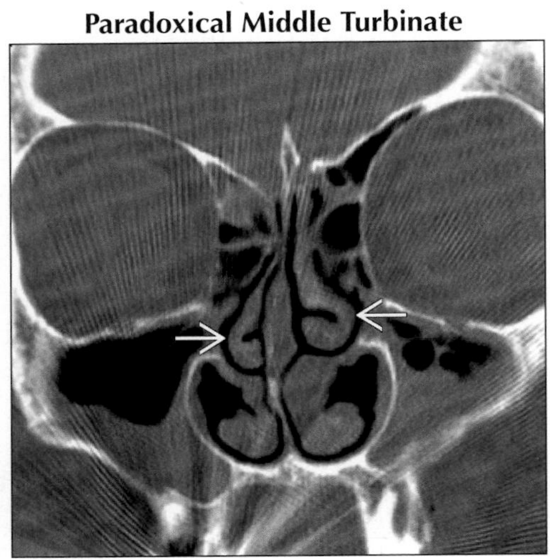

(Left) *Axial bone CT demonstrates a well-aerated air cell within the left anterior clinoid process. The optic nerve and internal carotid artery lie medial to this air cell.* ***(Right)*** *Coronal bone CT shows asymmetry in the position of the fovea ethmoidalis with the left inferior in position compared to the right sinus. Infundibular pattern disease is seen on the left with a maxillary air-fluid level.*

Pneumatized Anterior Clinoid Process

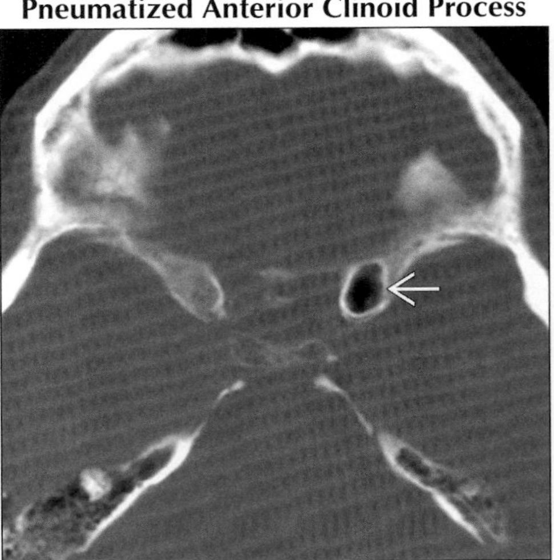

Fovea Ethmoidalis, Asymmetric (Low)

Pneumatized Uncinate Process

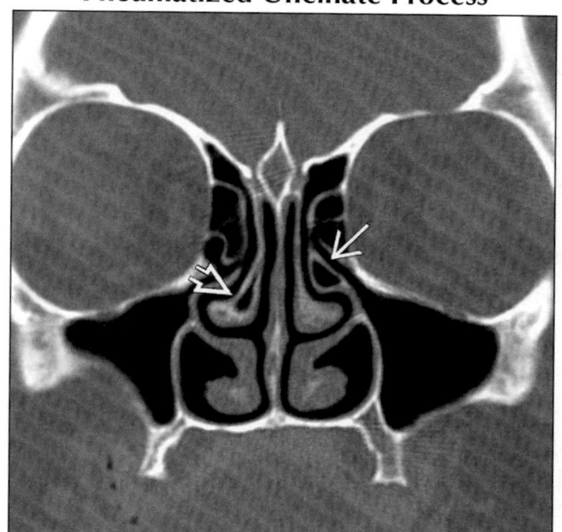

Frontal Cells

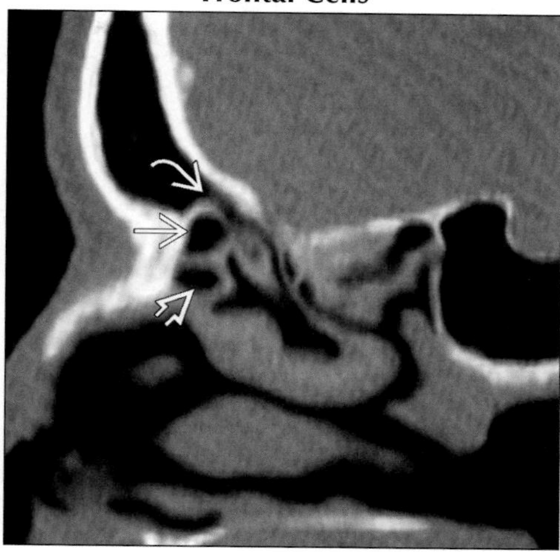

(Left) Coronal bone CT demonstrates an air cell within the left uncinate process ➡. A small concha bullosa is incidentally noted on the right ➡. *(Right)* Sagittal bone CT reveals a type 1 frontal cell ➡ superior to the agger nasi air cell ➡. The cell is located anterior to the frontal recess and, in this case, is at the level of the frontal ostium ➡ .

Pneumatized Crista Galli

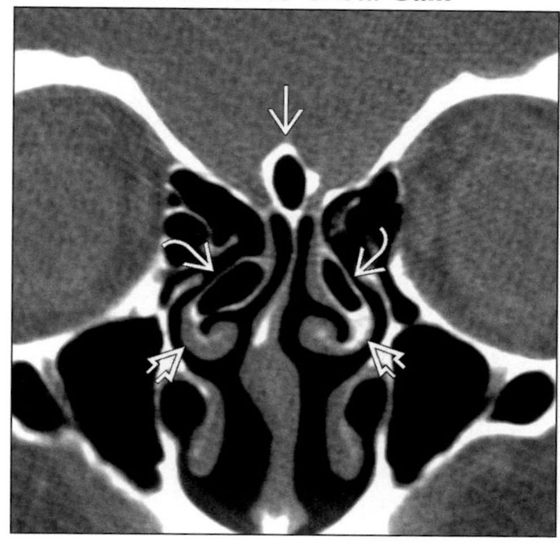

Supraorbital Ethmoid Cell

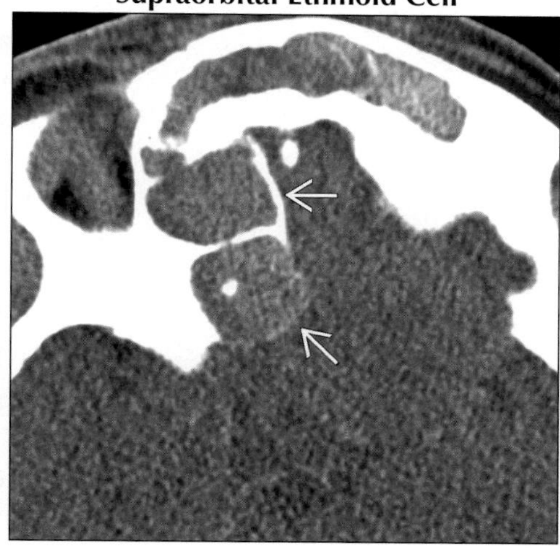

(Left) Coronal bone CT shows pneumatization of crista galli ➡. Note the paradoxical curvature of the middle turbinates ➡ and pneumatization of the vertical lamellae ➡. *(Right)* Axial NECT shows 2 expanded opacified supraorbital ethmoid air cells ➡ in a patient with sinonasal polyposis. Note the position of these air cells posterior to the frontal sinus.

Dehiscent Lamina Papyracea

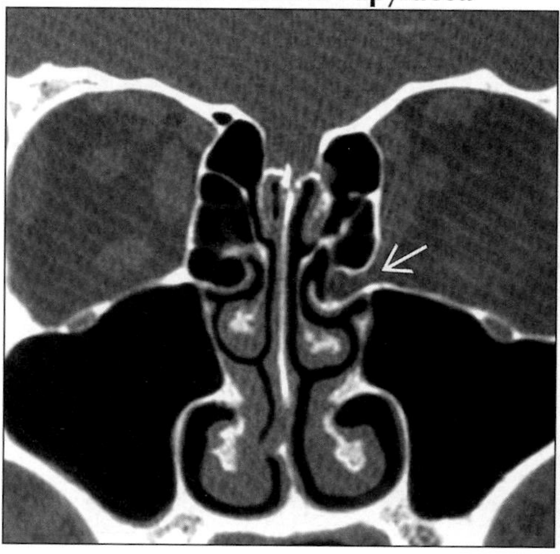

Sphenoethmoidal (Onodi) Cell

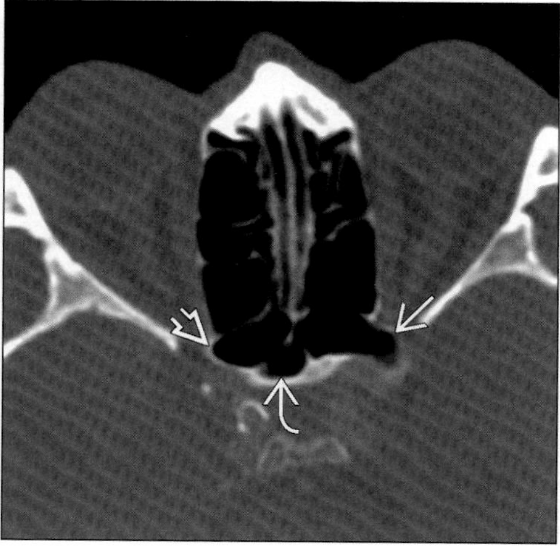

(Left) Coronal bone CT demonstrates dehiscence of the left lamina papyracea ➡ inferiorly with herniation of extraconal orbital fat through the defect into the ethmoid region. *(Right)* Axial bone CT shows a left sphenoethmoidal cell ➡ extending over the optic canal. A smaller cell is seen on the right ➡. Note the position of these cells superior to the sphenoid sinus ➡.

CONGENITAL MIDLINE NASAL LESION

DIFFERENTIAL DIAGNOSIS

Common
- Nasal Dermal Sinus
- Frontoethmoidal Cephalocele
- Sinonasal Hemangioma
- Nasal Choanal Atresia

Less Common
- Nasal Glioma

Rare but Important
- Pyriform Aperture Stenosis

ESSENTIAL INFORMATION

Key Differential Diagnosis Issues
- Nasal dermal sinus and cephalocele: Intracranial extension and associated cysts/dermoids are important to identify at imaging
- MR is best imaging tool to evaluate extent of dermal sinuses and cephaloceles
- CT is modality of choice for evaluating bony narrowing in choanal atresia and pyriform aperture stenosis

Helpful Clues for Common Diagnoses
- **Nasal Dermal Sinus**
  - Clinical clue: Pit may be present along nasal dorsum
  - CT/MR: Fluid density or signal intensity tract from nasal tip to enlarged foramen cecum traversing nasal septum
    - Bifid crista galli may be present
  - Associated craniofacial anomalies possible
- **Frontoethmoidal Cephalocele**
  - Clinical clue: Nasoglabellar or intranasal mass that may change in size with crying
  - MR: Extension of meninges, CSF, and brain tissue through bony defect in cribriform plate or between frontal and nasal bones
- **Sinonasal Hemangioma**
  - Clinical clue: Soft, reddish mass; capillary type most common; often arises from nasal septum
  - MR: Well-defined mass; T2 hyperintense; diffusely enhancing
- **Nasal Choanal Atresia**
  - Clinical: Respiratory distress in newborn if bilateral; later presentation if unilateral
  - CT: Membranous or bony; unilateral or bilateral; thickened posterior vomer

Helpful Clues for Less Common Diagnoses
- **Nasal Glioma**
  - Clinical clues: Subcutaneous blue or red mass on nasal dorsum (extranasal type); polypoid submucosal mass (intranasal type)
  - MR: Intra- or extranasal soft tissue mass
    - MR signal typically NOT similar to brain parenchyma; no connection to intracranial contents

Helpful Clues for Rare Diagnoses
- **Pyriform Aperture Stenosis**
  - Anterior nasal bony stenosis
  - Look for central megaincisor and midline intracranial anomalies

Nasal Dermal Sinus

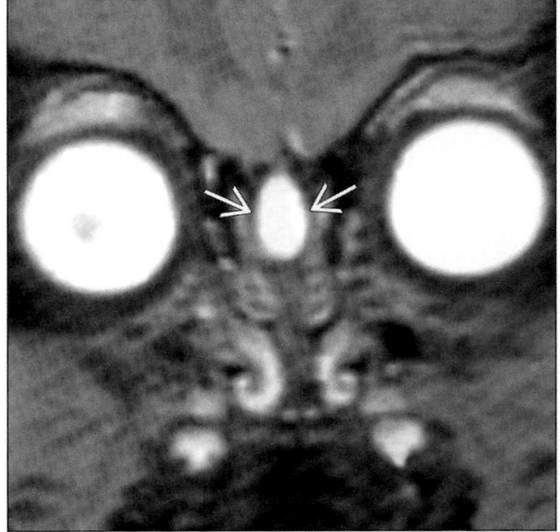

Coronal T2WI MR shows a portion of a nasal dermal sinus that extended from the skull base to the nasal tip. This image shows the hyperintense, fluid-filled sinus ➔ within the septum.

Frontoethmoidal Cephalocele

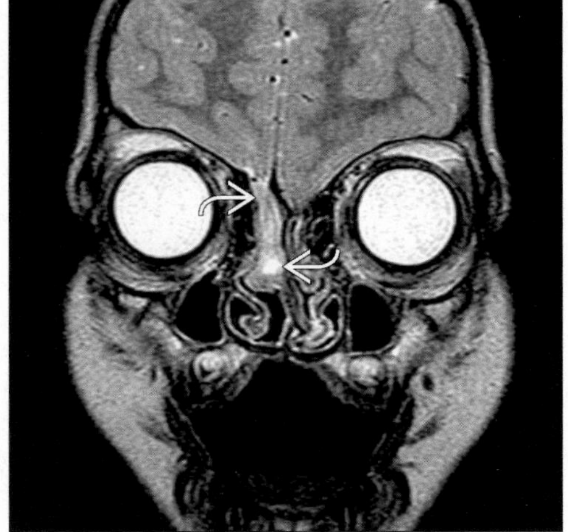

Coronal T2WI MR shows a cephalocele ➔ extending from the anterior fossa through a skull base defect into the right nasal cavity. The meninges contain CSF and dysplastic brain tissue.

Frontoethmoidal Cephalocele

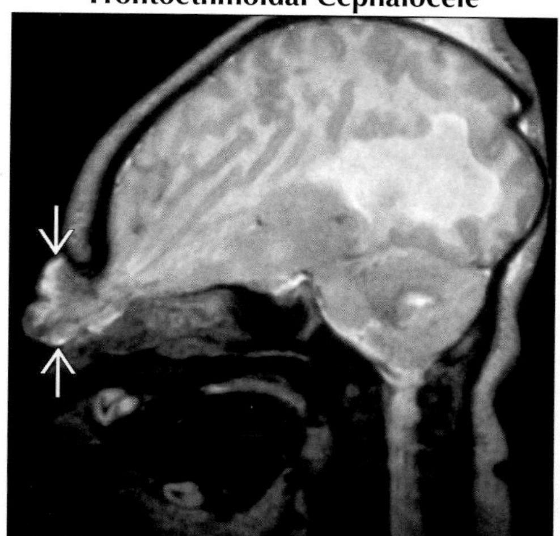

Sinonasal Hemangioma

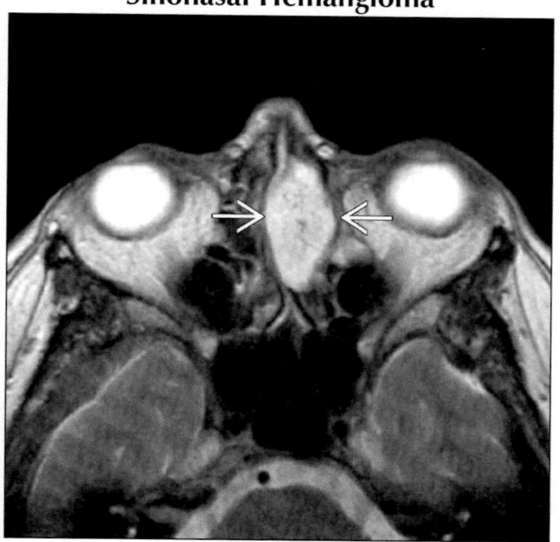

*(**Left**) Sagittal T2WI MR shows a frontonasal type of cephalocele. Herniation of brain parenchyma ➡ through the fonticulus frontalis results from lack of fusion of the frontal and nasal bones. (**Right**) Axial T2WI MR shows a well-defined soft tissue mass in the left nasal cavity ➡. Hyperintense signal on this T2-weighted sequence is a characteristic feature of hemangiomas.*

Nasal Choanal Atresia

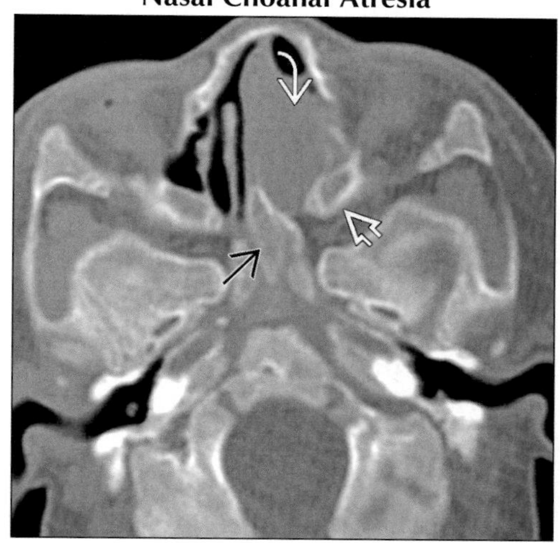

Nasal Glioma

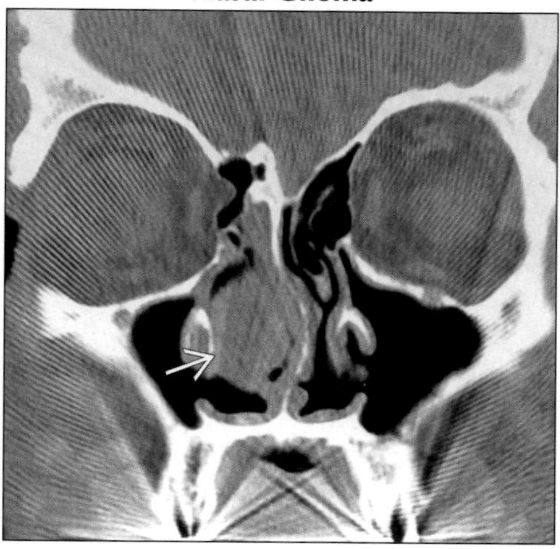

*(**Left**) Axial bone CT shows unilateral choanal atresia with soft tissue in the left nasal cavity ➡ and narrowing of the left choana. The vomer is thickened ➡ and opposes the left maxilla ➡. (**Right**) Coronal bone CT shows a "missed" intranasal glioma ➡ in an adult patient with a history of cephalocele repair. The anterior skull base is intact on this image.*

Nasal Glioma

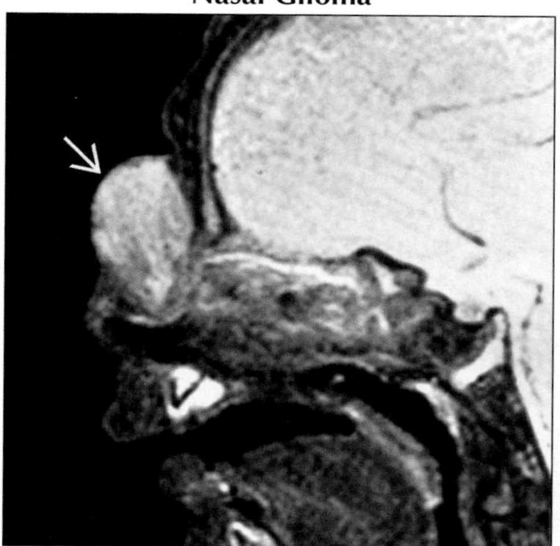

Pyriform Aperture Stenosis

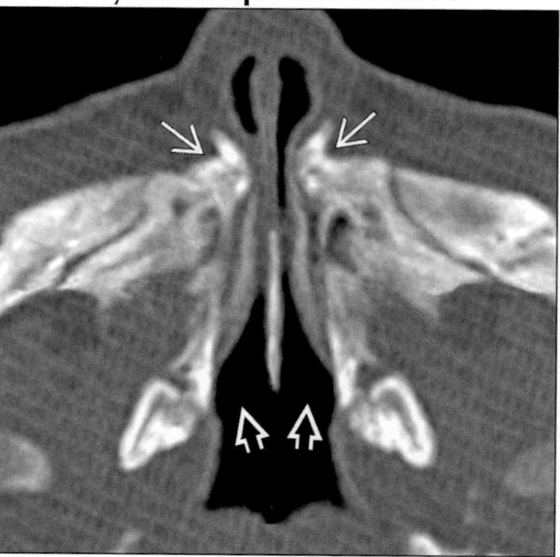

*(**Left**) Sagittal T2WI MR shows an extranasal glioma over the nasal bridge anterior to the expected location of the fused frontal and nasal bones ➡. (**Right**) Axial bone CT shows pyriform aperture stenosis in a newborn as a result of overgrowth of the nasal processes of the maxilla ➡ but no associated membranous atresia ➡.*

NASAL OBSTRUCTION

DIFFERENTIAL DIAGNOSIS

Common
- Nasolacrimal Duct Cyst
- Nasal Choanal Atresia

Less Common
- Nasal Dermal Sinus
- Frontoethmoidal Cephalocele
- Nasal Glioma
- Sinonasal Hemangioma
- Prominent/Asymmetric Tonsillar Tissue

Rare but Important
- Pyriform Aperture Stenosis
- Rhabdomyosarcoma

ESSENTIAL INFORMATION

Key Differential Diagnosis Issues
- Bilateral nasal cavity lesions in newborn produce respiratory distress as newborns are obligate nasal breathers
- Unilateral lesions that do not cause respiratory distress may present later in childhood

Helpful Clues for Common Diagnoses
- **Nasolacrimal Duct Cyst**
  - Inferior meatus location produces nasal obstruction
  - Well-defined cystic lesion below inferior turbinate; dilated nasolacrimal duct
- **Nasal Choanal Atresia**
  - Stenosis > atresia; unilateral:bilateral (2:1); bony (90%) and membranous (10%)
  - CT: Posterior nasal cavity narrowed by thickened vomer and medialized maxilla; soft tissue or bony plate occludes choanae

Helpful Clues for Less Common Diagnoses
- **Nasal Dermal Sinus**
  - Fluid-filled cyst or sinus tract from foramen cecum to nasal tip; within midline septum; bifid crista galli
- **Frontoethmoidal Cephalocele**
  - Nasoethmoidal form presents as intranasal mass; may enlarge with crying; intracranial connection
- **Nasal Glioma**
  - Well-defined soft tissue mass with no connection intracranially
  - MR: Signal typically not similar to brain and may enhance
- **Sinonasal Hemangioma**
  - Enhancing lesion along anterior nasal septum; T2 hyperintense
- **Prominent/Asymmetric Tonsillar Tissue**
  - Midline nasopharyngeal soft tissue

Helpful Clues for Rare Diagnoses
- **Pyriform Aperture Stenosis**
  - Bony narrowing of anterior nasal passageway
  - Associated maxillary central megaincisor and midline intracranial anomalies
- **Rhabdomyosarcoma**
  - Aggressive soft tissue malignancy; rare in newborn

Nasolacrimal Duct Cyst

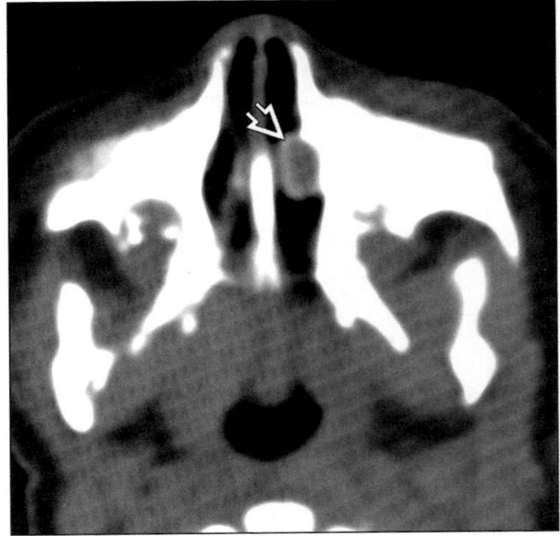

Axial NECT shows a mucoid-density nasolacrimal duct cyst ➡ at the level of the inferior meatus. Because this was a unilateral lesion, the infant did not present in respiratory distress.

Nasal Choanal Atresia

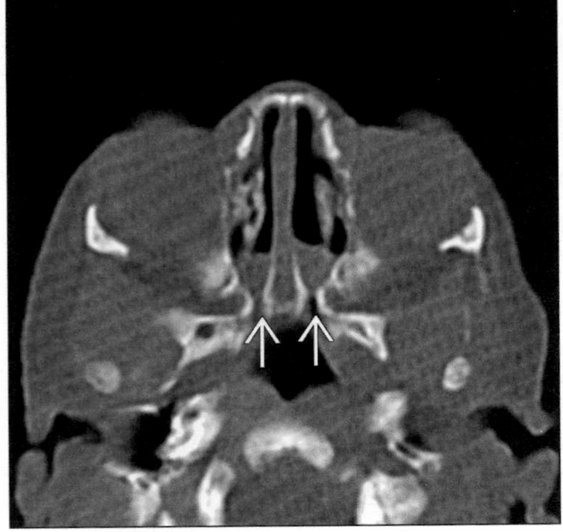

Axial bone CT shows bilateral membranous atresia with bony stenosis ➡. Note the very small choanae and fluid layering in the nasal cavity. This newborn was in respiratory distress.

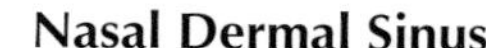

Nasal Dermal Sinus

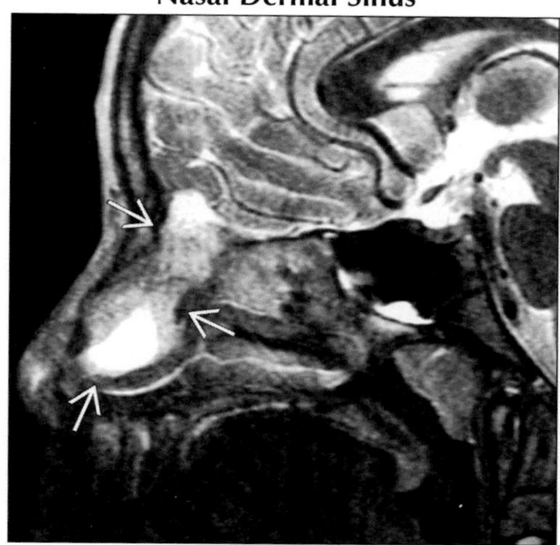

Frontoethmoidal Cephalocele

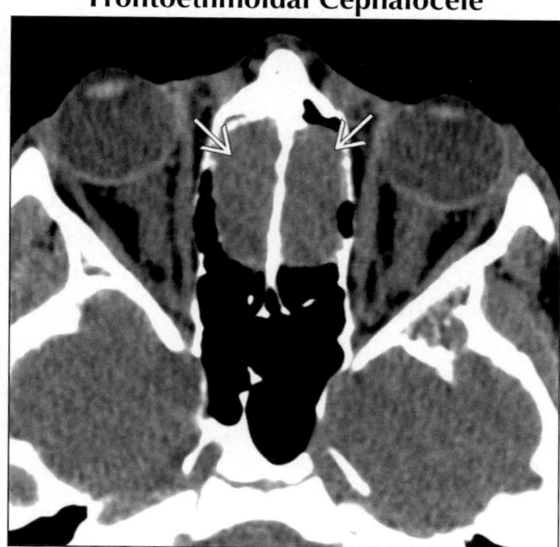

***(Left)** Sagittal T2WI MR shows a sinus tract ➔ extending from a widened foramen cecum in the anterior skull base towards the nasal tip. The lesion is hyperintense, consistent with fluid. **(Right)** Axial NECT shows bilateral frontoethmoidal encephaloceles of the nasoethmoidal type ➔. These cephaloceles protrude through the cribriform plates into the nasal cavity and ethmoid region.*

Nasal Glioma

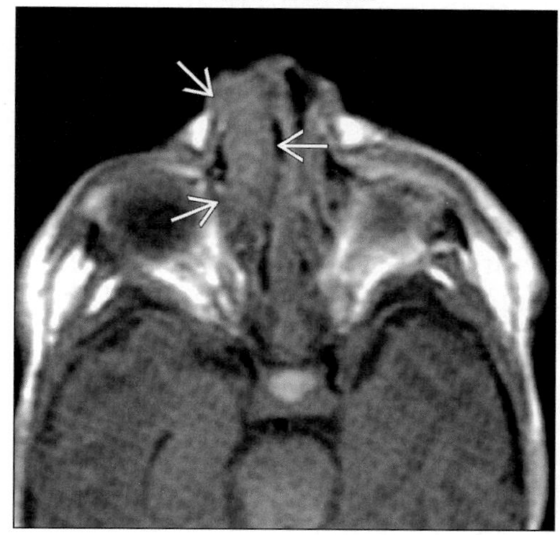

Sinonasal Hemangioma

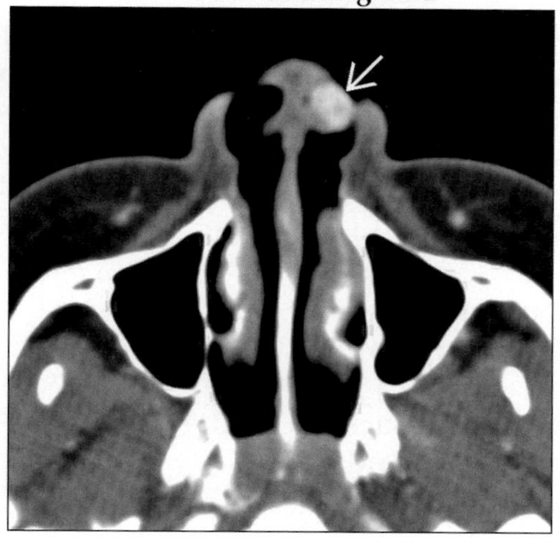

***(Left)** Axial T1WI MR shows a nasal cavity mass ➔ in an infant obstructing the nasal airway. This intranasal glioma is isointense to brain on this sequence, but that is not always the case. **(Right)** Axial CECT shows an small enhancing capillary hemangioma in the left nasal vestibule ➔. The lesion was clinically visible within the nostril.*

Pyriform Aperture Stenosis

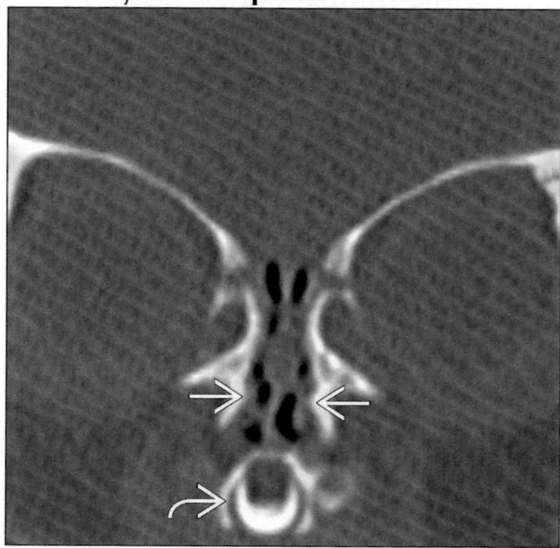

Rhabdomyosarcoma

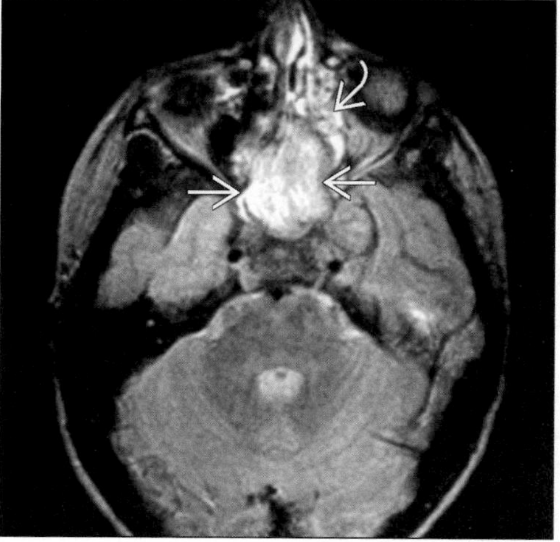

***(Left)** Coronal bone CT shows marked narrowing of the anterior nasal passage (pyriform aperture) ➔ and the associated finding of an unerupted central "megaincisor" ➔. **(Right)** Axial FLAIR MR shows a hyperintense mass ➔ in the nasopharynx extending into the posterior nasal cavity with obstructed left ethmoid sinus secretions ➔.*

SENSORINEURAL HEARING LOSS IN A CHILD

DIFFERENTIAL DIAGNOSIS

Common
- Large Endolymphatic Sac Anomaly (IP-2)
- Fractures, Temporal Bone
- Semicircular Canal Dysplasia
- Labyrinthine Ossificans

Less Common
- Labyrinthitis
- Cochlear Nerve Deficiency
- Cystic Cochleovestibular Anomaly (IP-1)
- Lipoma, CPA-IAC

Rare but Important
- Common Cavity, Inner Ear
- Cochlear Aplasia, Inner Ear
- Labyrinthine Aplasia
- Vestibular Schwannoma
- Schwannoma, Facial Nerve, CPA-IAC

ESSENTIAL INFORMATION

Key Differential Diagnosis Issues
- History is important
  - In setting of fluctuating or "cascading" sensorineural hearing loss (SNHL) in child who could hear at birth (without history of meningitis)
    - Look for large vestibular aqueduct ± cochlear dysplasia and modiolar deficiency on CT
    - Look for enlarged endolymphatic sac and duct with cochlear dysplasia and modiolar deficiency on MR
  - Trauma: Look for fracture involving inner ear structures ± pneumolabyrinth on CT
  - Genetic disorders: In CHARGE, Alagille, Waardenburg, Crouzon or Apert syndrome, look for semicircular canal (SCC) dysplasia
  - Prior meningitis
    - Look for labyrinthine ossificans on CT
    - Look for enhancement or replacement of high T2 intensity with low T2 intensity within structures of membranous labyrinth on MR (depends on timing of imaging)
- Best imaging tool
  - Thin-section T-bone CT identifies many congenital inner ear anomalies
  - High-resolution T2 MR imaging identifies large endolymphatic sac, cochlear dysplasia; best to show cochlear nerve aplasia/hypoplasia
  - Contrast MR best evaluates schwannoma, acute labyrinthitis, and lipoma

Helpful Clues for Common Diagnoses
- **Large Endolymphatic Sac Anomaly (IP-2)**
  - Most common congenital anomaly of inner ear found by imaging
  - Vestibular aqueduct on CT ≥ 1.5 mm bony transverse dimension
    - Newer literature suggests ≥ 2 mm at operculum or ≥ 1 mm at midpoint
  - Look for associated cochlear dysplasia, modiolar deficiency, vestibule &/or SCC dysplasia
  - Additional diagnosis information
    - Avoidance of contact sports or other activities that may lead to head trauma is recommended in children with IP-2 anomaly
    - Genetic testing for Pendred syndrome is becoming increasingly recommended in children with IP-2 anomaly
    - Up to 15% of all patients with IP-2 will have Pendrin gene = Pendred syndrome, with severe profound bilateral SNHL; 50% with goiter and 50% of those with goiter, will be hypothyroid
- **Fractures, Temporal Bone**
  - Thin-section T-bone CT (0.625-1 mm)
  - Transverse or longitudinal fracture may cross inner ear structures, ± pneumolabyrinth
- **Semicircular Canal Dysplasia**
  - Spectrum of abnormalities: 1 or more of SCC dysmorphic, hypoplastic, or aplastic
  - Unilateral or bilateral: Bilateral more common in syndromic form
  - Most common is short, dilated lateral SCC and vestibule forming single cavity
  - Look for associated cochlear dysplasia, oval window atresia, and ossicular anomalies
  - CHARGE syndrome
    - Bilateral absence of all SCCs
    - Associated anomalies: Small vestibule, absent cochlear nerve aperture ("isolated cochlea"), oval window atresia (± overlying tympanic segment of CN7), choanal atresia, coloboma

- ○ Lateral SCC last to form embryologically, therefore if lateral SSC is normal, posterior superior should be normal
  - ▪ Except if obliterated by labyrinthine ossificans or hypoplastic in Waardenburg and Alagille syndrome
- **Labyrinthine Ossificans**
  - ○ Synonyms: Labyrinthitis ossificans, labyrinthine ossification, chronic labyrinthitis, ossifying labyrinthitis
  - ○ Acute inflammatory response results in fibrous and then osseous replacement of membranous labyrinth
    - ▪ May involve cochlea ± vestibule ± semicircular canals
  - ○ Bilateral in meningogenic form (meningitis) and in hematogenic form (blood-borne infections)
    - ▪ Unilateral in tympanogenic form (middle ear infection)
  - ○ T-bone CT: High-attenuation bone deposition in formerly fluid-filled membranous labyrinth
  - ○ T2 MR: Focal or diffuse low intensity replaces high intensity fluid, with apparent "enlargement" of modiolus if cochlea is involved
  - ○ T1 C+: Enhancement of involved membranous labyrinth structures in early stage, may persist into ossifying stages

Helpful Clues for Less Common Diagnoses

- **Labyrinthitis**
  - ○ Subacute inflammation of fluid-filled inner ear structures
  - ○ T-bone CT: Normal in early phases, may progress to labyrinthine ossificans
  - ○ T2 MR: Low intensity replaces normal fluid signal within membranous labyrinth structures
  - ○ T1 C+: Mild to moderate enhancement
- **Cochlear Nerve Deficiency**
  - ○ Very small or absent cochlear nerve with small IAC
- **Cystic Cochleovestibular Anomaly (IP-1)**
  - ○ Cochlea and vestibule form bilobed cyst
- **Lipoma, CPA-IAC**
  - ○ Fatty lesion of CPA, IAC ± inner ear

Helpful Clues for Rare Diagnoses

- **Common Cavity, Inner Ear**
  - ○ Cystic cochlea and vestibule form a common cavity ± SCC absence or dysplasia
- **Cochlear Aplasia, Inner Ear**
  - ○ Absent cochlea
- **Labyrinthine Aplasia**
  - ○ Absent membranous labyrinth
- **Vestibular Schwannoma**
  - ○ Enhancing lesion ± cysts in CPA-IAC
  - ○ Rare in children
- **Schwannoma, Facial Nerve, CPA-IAC**
  - ○ Enlarged labyrinthine segment CN7 canal with enhancing tubular mass in CPA-IAC and labyrinthine segment of CN7
  - ○ Rare in children

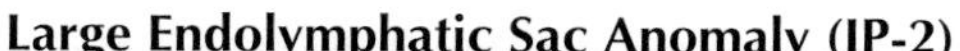

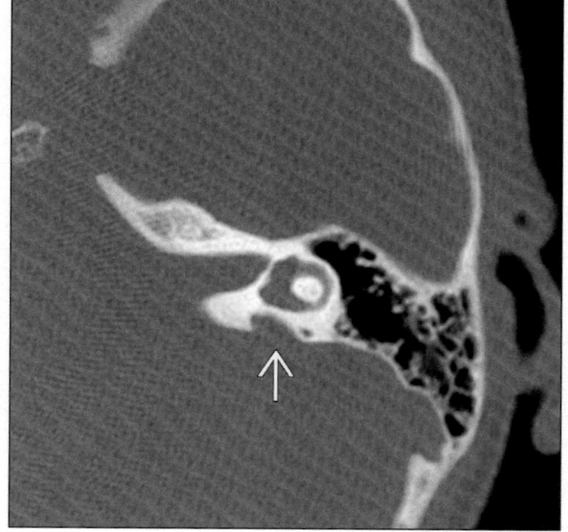

Axial bone CT shows enlargement of the left vestibular aqueduct ➔.

Large Endolymphatic Sac Anomaly (IP-2)

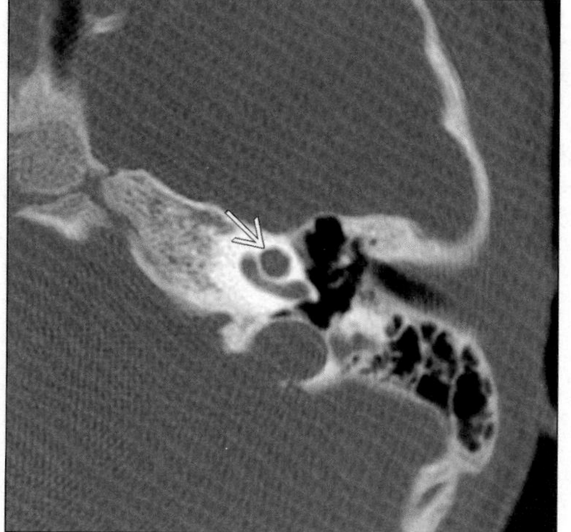

Axial bone CT shows associated incomplete partitioning of the left cochlea ➔.

SENSORINEURAL HEARING LOSS IN A CHILD

(**Left**) *Axial bone CT shows a longitudinal temporal bone fracture ➡ with associated pneumolabyrinth ➡.* (**Right**) *Coronal oblique bone CT shows a transverse temporal bone fracture ➡ with associated pneumolabyrinth and gas in the vestibule ➡ and lateral semicircular canal.*

Fractures, Temporal Bone

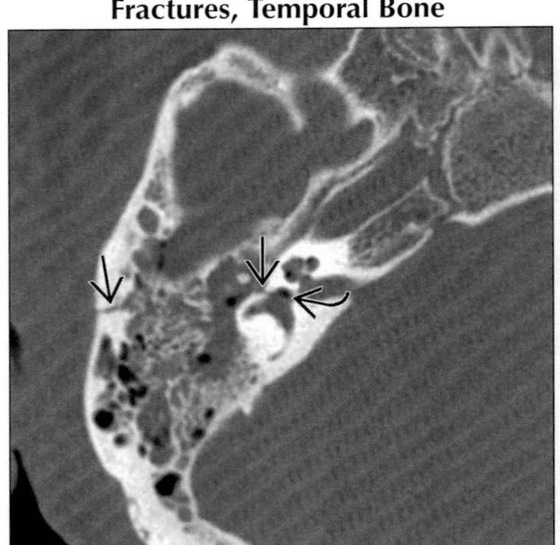

Fractures, Temporal Bone

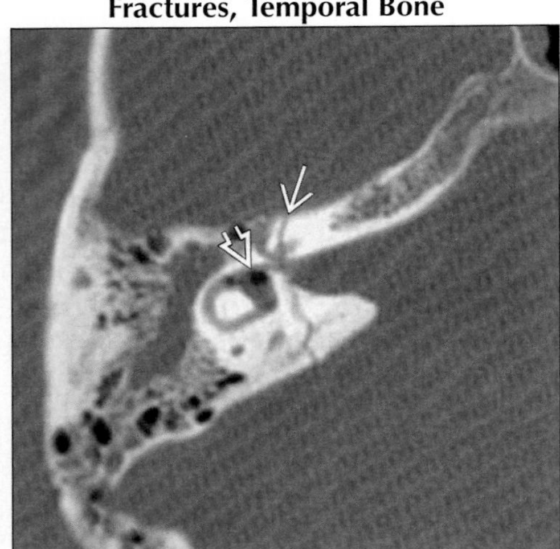

(**Left**) *Axial bone CT shows severe hypoplasia of the right IAC ➡ and hypoplasia of the vestibule and semicircular canals with only a small remnant ➡.* (**Right**) *Axial bone CT shows lack of the normal right cochlear aperture ➡ and severe hypoplasia of the vestibule and SCCs ➡ in a patient with CHARGE syndrome.*

Semicircular Canal Dysplasia

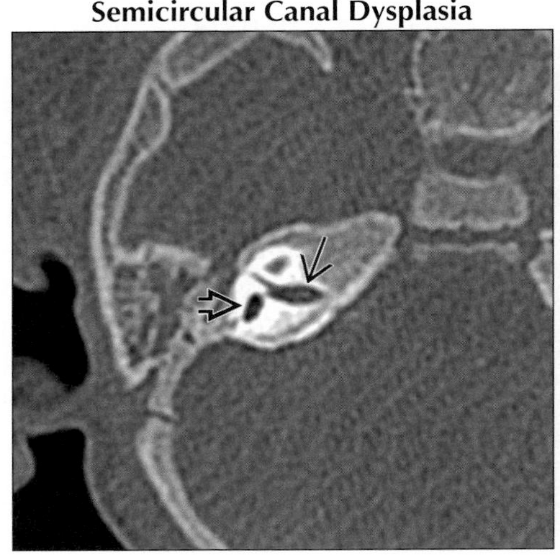

Semicircular Canal Dysplasia

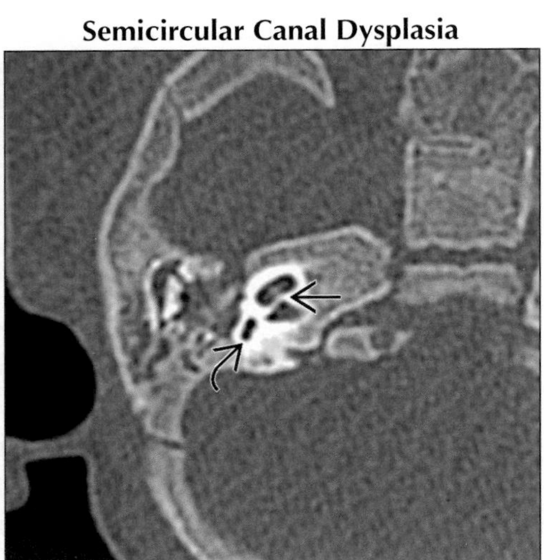

(**Left**) *Axial bone CT shows osseous replacement of the vestibule and right lateral semicircular canals ➡.* (**Right**) *Axial bone CT shows complete osseous replacement of the right cochlea ➡. Notice the presence of the normal right cochlear promontory, convex laterally ➡.*

Labyrinthine Ossificans

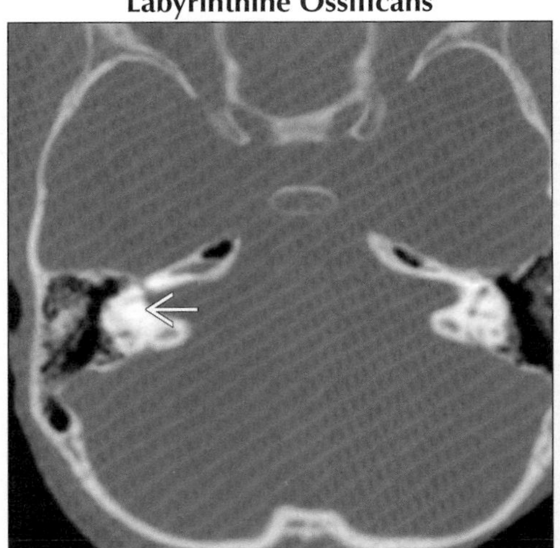

Labyrinthine Ossificans

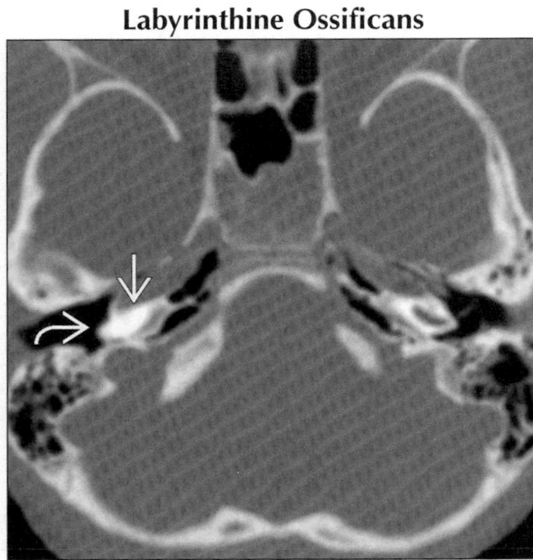

Labyrinthitis

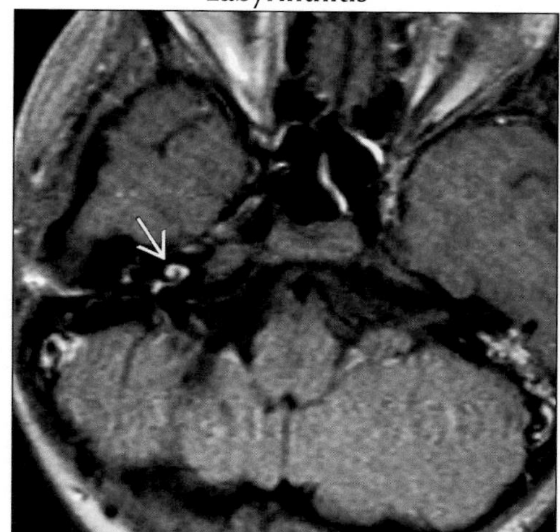

Labyrinthitis

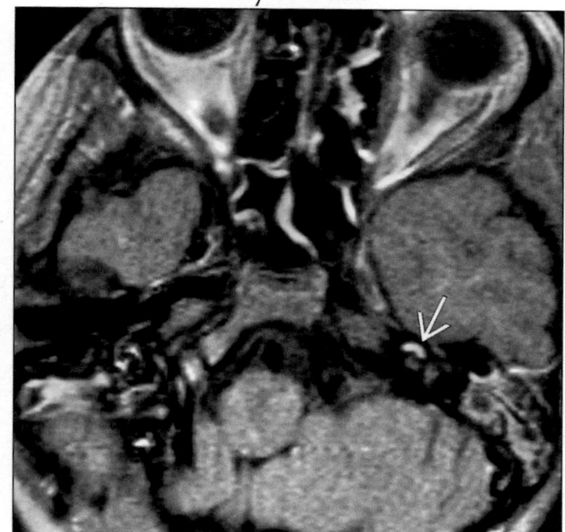

(Left) *Axial T1 C+ FS MR shows abnormal enhancement of the right cochlea ➡ in this patient with Cogan syndrome.* ***(Right)*** *Axial T1WI C+ FS MR shows abnormal enhancement of the left cochlea ➡ in this patient with Cogan syndrome.*

Labyrinthitis

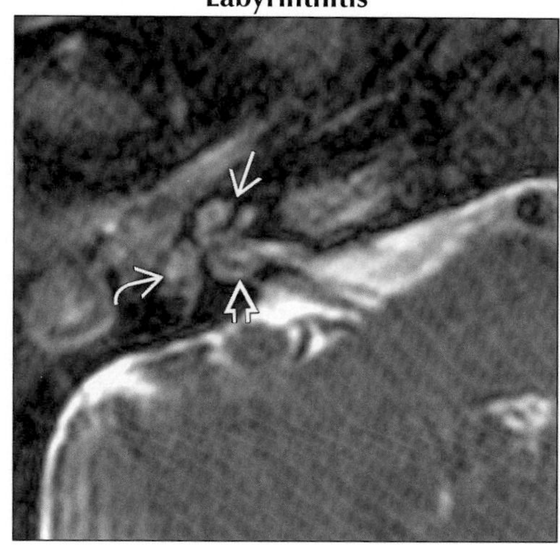

Labyrinthitis

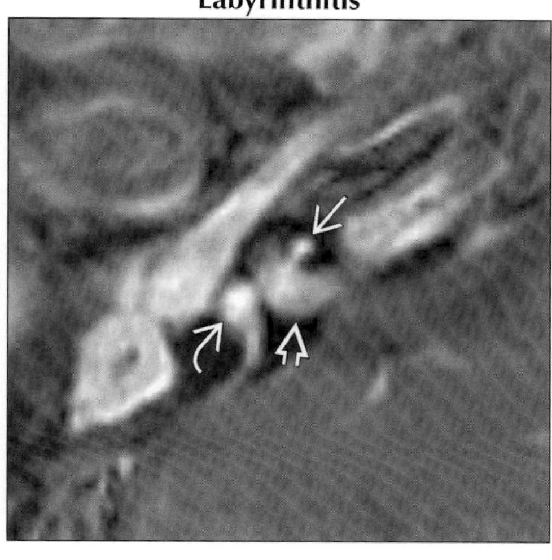

(Left) *Axial T2WI FS MR shows corresponding loss of hyperintense T2 signal in the cochlea ➡, vestibule ➡, and internal auditory canal ➡.* ***(Right)*** *Axial T1WI C+ FS MR shows abnormal contrast enhancement in the middle ear, mastoid, cochlea ➡, vestibule ➡, and internal auditory canal ➡ secondary to actinomycosis labyrinthitis.*

Cochlear Nerve Deficiency

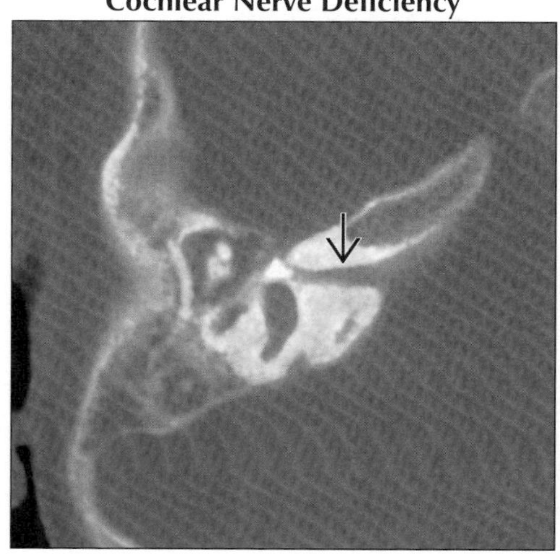

Cochlear Nerve Deficiency

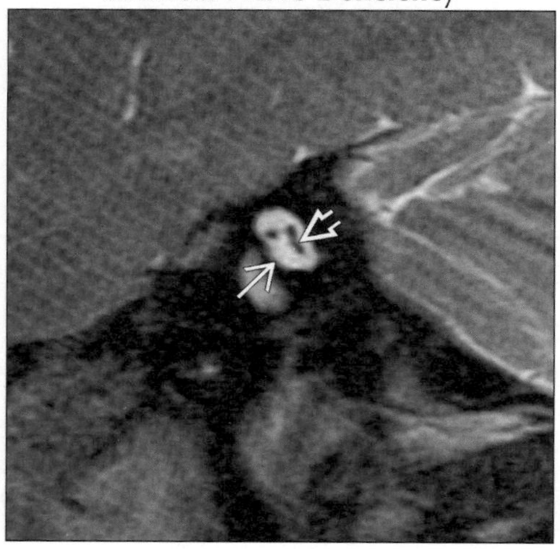

(Left) *Axial bone CT reveals hypoplastic right IAC ➡ related to right cochlear nerve deficiency.* ***(Right)*** *Longitudinal oblique T2WI MR shows an absent cochlear nerve on the left ➡ in association with a small internal auditory canal. The superior and inferior vestibular nerves are connected ➡.*

SENSORINEURAL HEARING LOSS IN A CHILD

(Left) *Axial T2WI MR shows a tiny right IAC ➔ and nonvisualization of the cochlear nerve.* **(Right)** *Sagittal oblique T2WI MR shows nonvisualization of cochlear nerve ➔ in association with a small internal auditory canal. CN8 and CN7 formation in the IAC area provides the IAC formation stimulation.*

Cochlear Nerve Deficiency

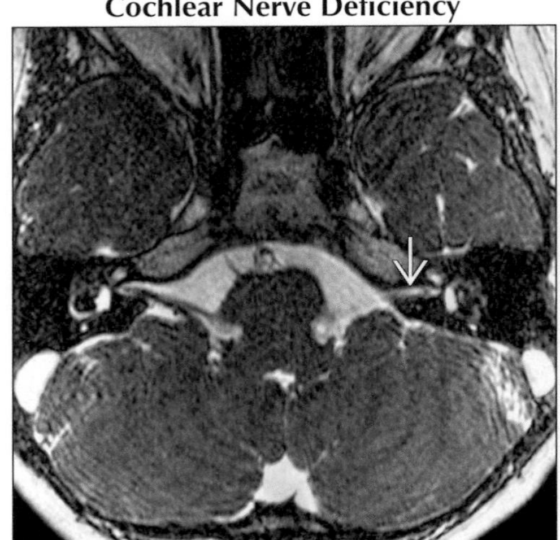

Cochlear Nerve Deficiency

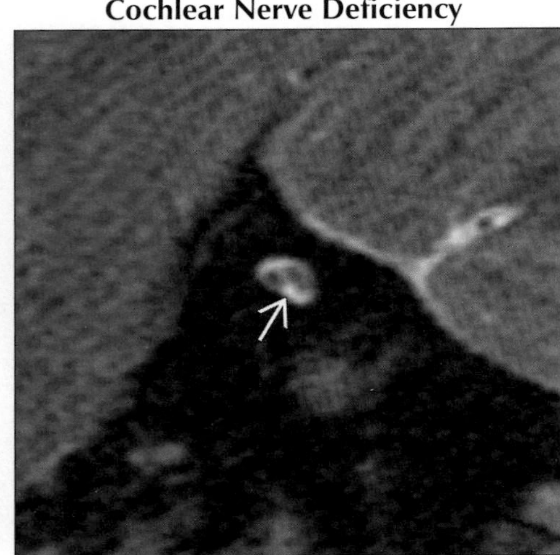

(Left) *Axial bone CT shows the typical CT appearance of cystic cochleovestibular anomaly. The vestibule is enlarged ➔.* **(Right)** *Axial bone CT shows that the cochlea is featureless ➔ and without a definable modiolus.*

Cystic Cochleovestibular Anomaly (IP-1)

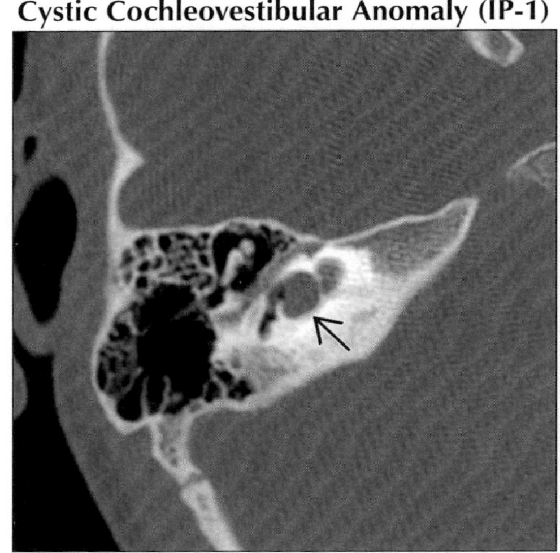

Cystic Cochleovestibular Anomaly (IP-1)

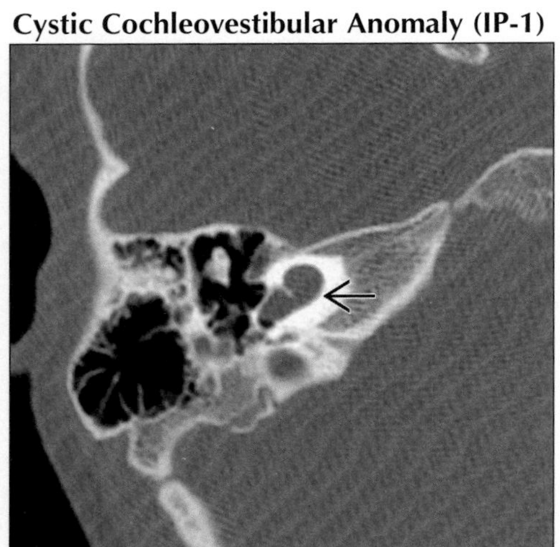

(Left) *Axial NECT shows the typical CT appearance of a small lipoma in the left CPA cistern ➔.* **(Right)** *Coronal T1WI MR shows a hyperintense lipoma in the left CPA cistern ➔.*

Lipoma, CPA-IAC

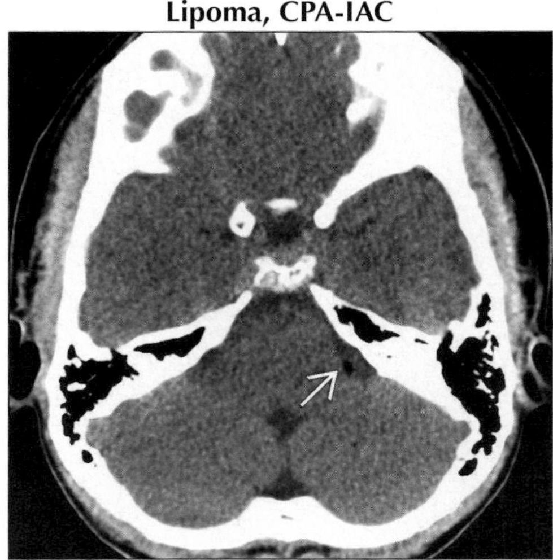

Lipoma, CPA-IAC

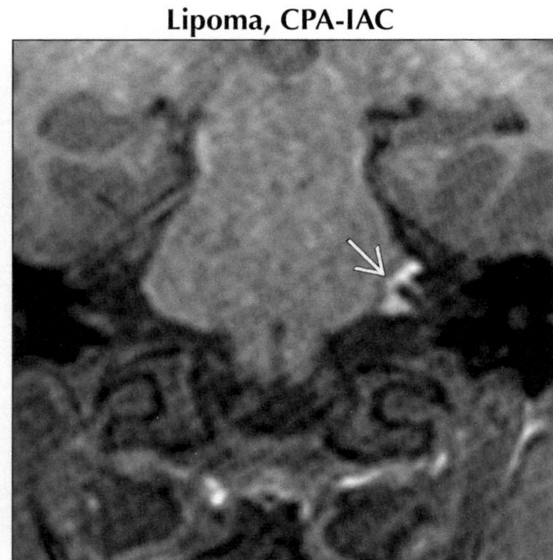

Cochlear Aplasia, Inner Ear

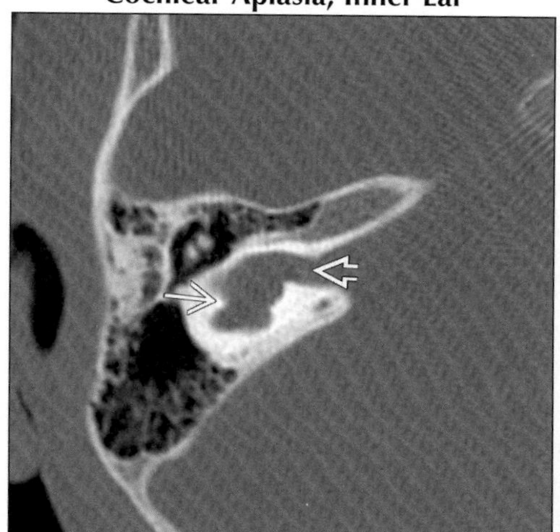

Labyrinthine Aplasia

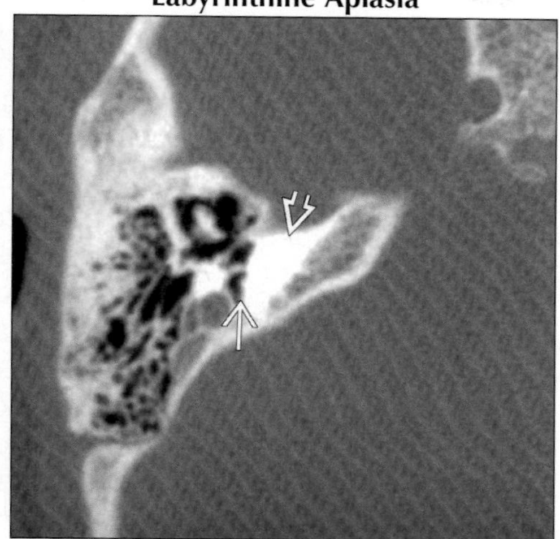

*(**Left**) Axial bone CT demonstrates a dysplastic vestibule ➡ that communicates with a small IAC through a broad gap at the IAC fundus ➡. There is no cochlea anterior to the vestibule. (**Right**) Axial bone CT shows that the otic capsule is featureless ➡ and without definable labyrinthine structures. The lateral wall is flat ➡, indicating congenital absence rather than acquired ossificans.*

Vestibular Schwannoma

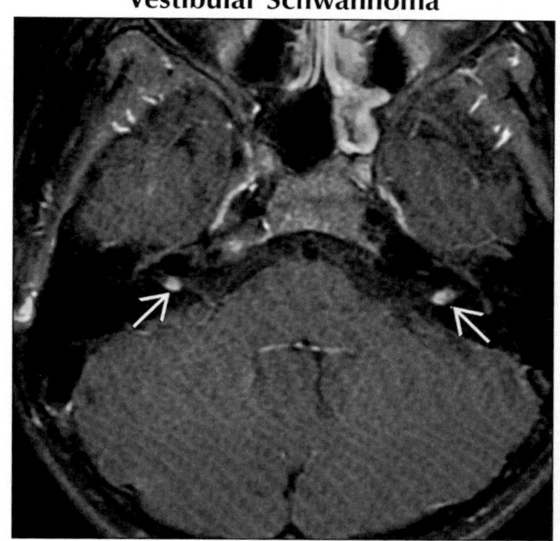

Vestibular Schwannoma

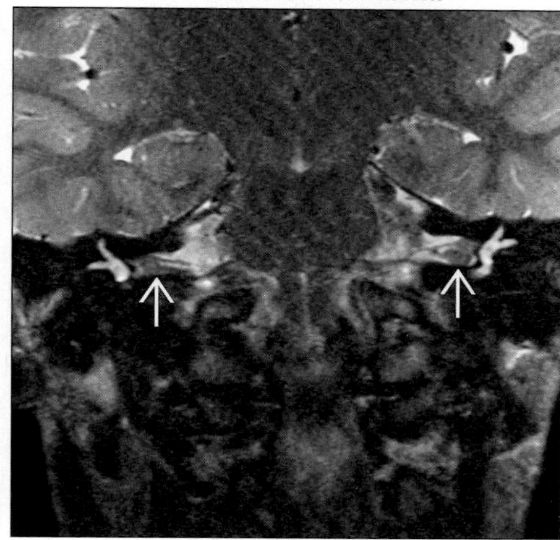

*(**Left**) Axial T1 C+ FS MR shows enhancement of small bilateral vestibular schwannomas ➡. (**Right**) Coronal T2WI MR shows hypointense masses ➡ in the inferior aspect of the IACs consistent with vestibular nerve origin.*

Schwannoma, Facial Nerve, CPA-IAC

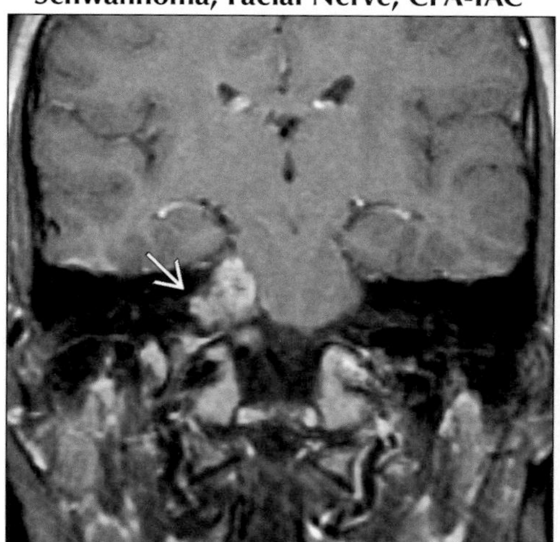

Schwannoma, Facial Nerve, CPA-IAC

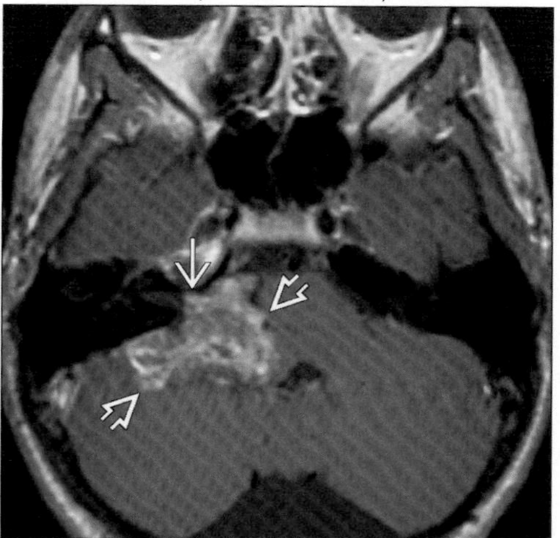

*(**Left**) Coronal T1WI C+ MR shows a large, heterogeneously enhancing mass in the CPA cistern and proximal internal auditory canal ➡. (**Right**) Axial T1 C+ MR shows variant appearance of a heterogeneously enhancing extraaxial mass ➡ in the right CPA with extension into the porous acusticus of the right IAC ➡.*

NORMAL SKULL BASE VENOUS VARIANTS

DIFFERENTIAL DIAGNOSIS

Common
- Jugular Foramen Asymmetry
- Jugular Bulb Pseudolesion
- Pterygoid Venous Plexus Asymmetry
- Transmastoid Emissary Vein
- Asymmetric Posterior Condylar Canal

Less Common
- High Jugular Bulb
- Jugular Bulb Diverticulum
- Dehiscent Jugular Bulb
- Asymmetric Sphenoidal Emissary Vein (of Vesalius)

Rare but Important
- Foramen Cecum
- Petrosquamosal Emissary Vein

ESSENTIAL INFORMATION

Key Differential Diagnosis Issues
- Intracranial venous flow must exit through skull base foramina
- Normal structures may be asymmetric
- Normal variants may be uni- or bilateral
- Variants may be mistaken for masses, especially jugular foramen pseudolesion
  - MR pitfall results from variable signal intensity secondary to venous flow
  - Normal CECT ± normal bone CT clarifies
- Asymmetric or enlarged veins may be sign of pathology

Helpful Clues for Common Diagnoses
- **Jugular Foramen Asymmetry**
  - Key facts
    - Jugular veins usually asymmetric in size
    - Exaggerated asymmetry may result in larger side mimicking mass
    - More often MR pitfall
  - Imaging
    - MR: Unilateral high signal and enhancement
    - Look for ipsilateral enlarged transverse sinus
    - CECT: Normal jugular enhancement
    - Bone CT: Preservation of normal foraminal contours
- **Jugular Bulb Pseudolesion**
  - Key facts
    - Turbulent venous flow creates MR pitfall
    - Asymmetric signal mimics pathology
  - Imaging
    - MR: Typically high signal intensity and avid enhancement
    - MRV or coronal T1 C+ usually clarify jugular bulb as normal
    - CECT: Normal jugular enhancement
    - Bone CT: Preservation of normal foraminal contours
- **Pterygoid Venous Plexus Asymmetry**
  - Key facts
    - Unilateral prominence of deep facial veins that drain from cavernous sinus
    - Often incidental finding
    - Asymmetry may be pathological: Increased venous flow with caroticocavernous fistula
  - Imaging
    - CT: Curvilinear enhancement in medial masticator &/or parapharyngeal space
    - MR: Enhancement or flow voids in deep face, but no mass effect
    - Normal signal intensity of adjacent masticator muscles
- **Transmastoid Emissary Vein**
  - Key facts
    - Transverse sinus to posterior auricular or occipital veins
    - Large veins may be pathological
    - Skull base dysplasia with small jugular foramina (e.g., achondroplasia)
    - Emissary and suboccipital veins "replace" jugular veins and are surgical hazard
  - Imaging
    - CECT: Enhancement of veins traversing mastoid bone
    - Bone CT: Smooth well-corticated channels through bone
- **Asymmetric Posterior Condylar Canal**
  - Key facts
    - Synonym: Condyloid canal
    - Posterolateral to hypoglossal canal
    - Important channel for venous flow with atretic jugular veins
    - Contents: Meningeal branch of ascending pharyngeal artery; emissary vein from sigmoid sinus to suboccipital veins
  - Imaging
    - Bone CT: Well-corticated venous channel
    - CECT/MR C+: Venous enhancement

Helpful Clues for Less Common Diagnoses

- **High Jugular Bulb**
  - Key facts
    - Usually incidental finding
    - May be associated with pulsatile tinnitus
  - Imaging
    - Axial bone CT: Bulb at level of cochlea
    - Coronal bone CT: Medial ± inferior to semicircular canals
    - MR: May be mistaken for unilateral mass because of high signal
    - MRV or coronal T1 C+ should clarify
- **Jugular Bulb Diverticulum**
  - Key facts
    - Normal variant, incidental finding
    - May be associated with pulsatile tinnitus
  - Imaging
    - Bone CT: Best evaluated in coronal plane
    - Small "pouch" projecting from superior aspect of jugular bulb
    - MR: May be mistaken for temporal bone mass because of high signal
    - MRV or coronal T1 C+ should clarify
- **Dehiscent Jugular Bulb**
  - Key facts
    - Otoscopy: "Vascular" middle ear mass
    - May be associated with pulsatile tinnitus
    - Absence of bony covering between jugular bulb and middle ear cavity
  - Imaging
    - CT: Absence of bony plate over jugular bulb at posterior hypotympanum
- **Asymmetric Sphenoidal Emissary Vein (of Vesalius)**
  - Key facts
    - Synonym: Sphenoid emissary foramen
    - Transmits emissary vein from cavernous sinus to pterygoid venous plexus
    - Enlargement is pathological if ↑ venous flow from caroticocavernous fistula or tumor direct invasion
  - Imaging
    - May be partially assimilated with ovale or may be duplicated
    - Bone CT: Located medial to anterior aspect foramen ovale; usually < 2 mm

Helpful Clues for Rare Diagnoses

- **Foramen Cecum**
  - Key facts
    - Usually closes during embryogenesis
    - Contains vein from sup sagittal sinus
    - Large foramen can be pathological
    - Suspect anterior neuropore anomaly
  - Imaging
    - Bone CT: Midline anterior to crista galli
    - Usually < 2 mm
- **Petrosquamosal Emissary Vein**
  - Key facts
    - Embryonic venous remnant
    - Connects transverse sinus and retromandibular vein
  - Imaging
    - Bone CT: Vertical channel, ≤ 4 mm
    - Posterior to TMJ, anterior to EAC

Jugular Foramen Asymmetry

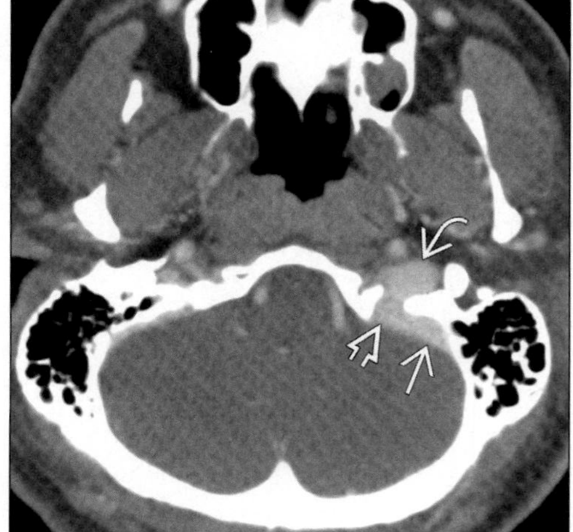

Axial CECT shows a normal left jugular foramen, though larger compared to the right. Note the left sigmoid sinus ➡, jugular foramen ➡, and internal jugular vein ➡ are all significantly larger than the right.

Jugular Foramen Asymmetry

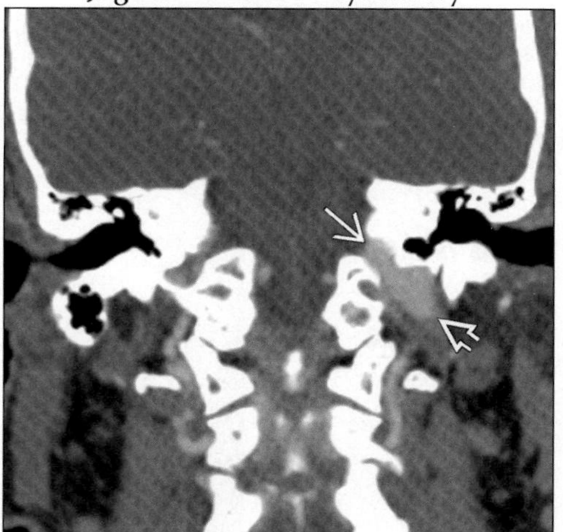

Coronal CECT in the same patient reveals the larger left jugular foramen ➡ and internal jugular vein ➡. Such asymmetry is normal and does not imply underlying pathology.

NORMAL SKULL BASE VENOUS VARIANTS

*(**Left**) Axial T2WI FS MR performed during work-up of a possible metastatic disease reveals asymmetric hyperintensity in the right skull base ➔, which was intermediate intensity on T1 & enhanced with gadolinium (not shown). (**Right**) Axial CECT in the same patient reveals normal enhancement of the right sigmoid sinus ➔ & jugular bulb ⇨ with normal foraminal contour. MR finding is attributed to turbulent venous flow in jugular foramen, not metastatic tumor.*

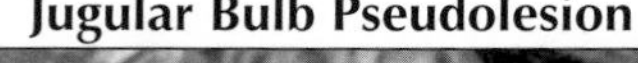

Jugular Bulb Pseudolesion

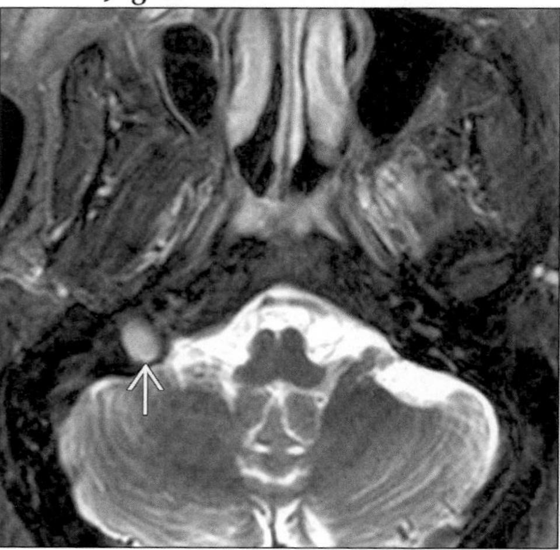

Jugular Bulb Pseudolesion

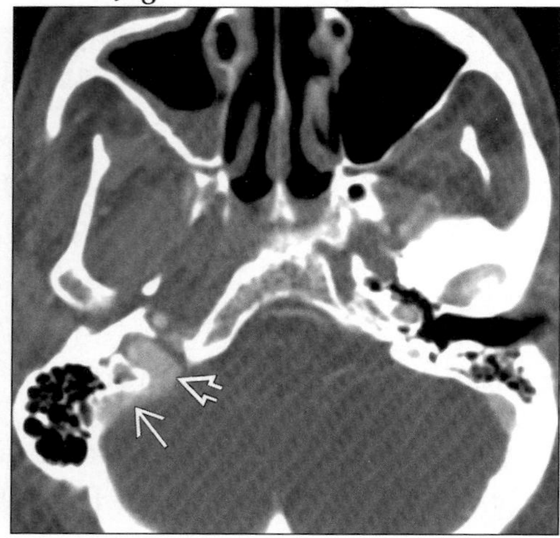

*(**Left**) Axial CECT reveals curvilinear enhancement of the pterygoid venous plexus (PVP) bilaterally in the deep face. The right PVP ⇨ has several linear vessels while the left ↪ has a more prominent mass-like appearance. (**Right**) Coronal CECT in the same patient again shows asymmetry of the pterygoid plexus vessels ⇨ in deep face. It also better illustrates the curvilinear vascular appearance of the plexus, confirming that this is not a true mass.*

Pterygoid Venous Plexus Asymmetry

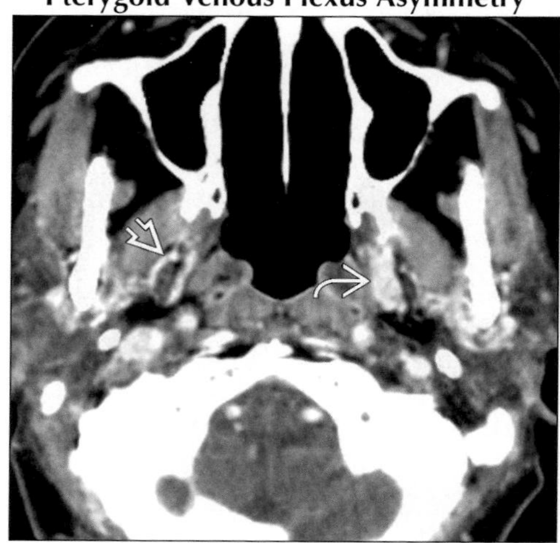

Pterygoid Venous Plexus Asymmetry

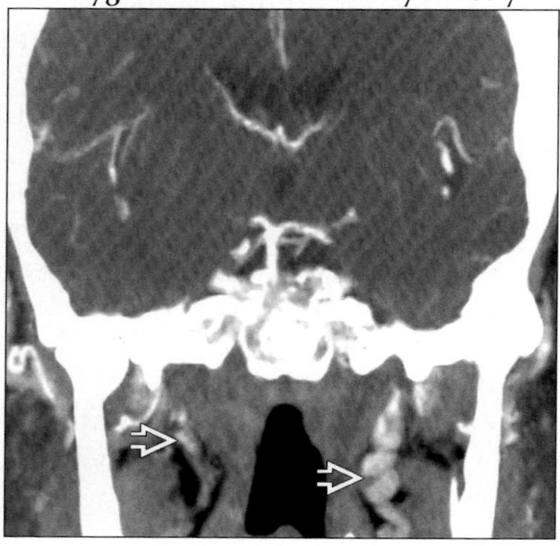

*(**Left**) Axial bone CT demonstrates a right transmastoid emissary vein ➔ coursing from the transverse sinus through the bone adjacent to the occipital suture ↪. Portions of the left emissary vein are also evident ⇨. (**Right**) Sagittal bone CT reformat shows a well-corticated linear venous channel ➔ extending through the posterior mastoid bone, adjacent to occipital suture ↪.*

Transmastoid Emissary Vein

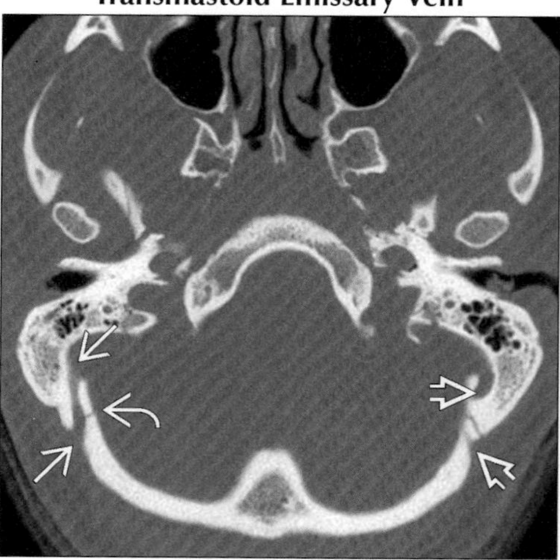

Transmastoid Emissary Vein

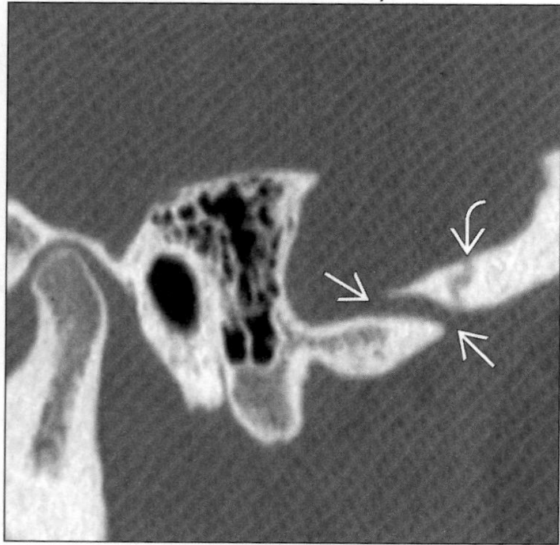

Asymmetric Posterior Condylar Canal

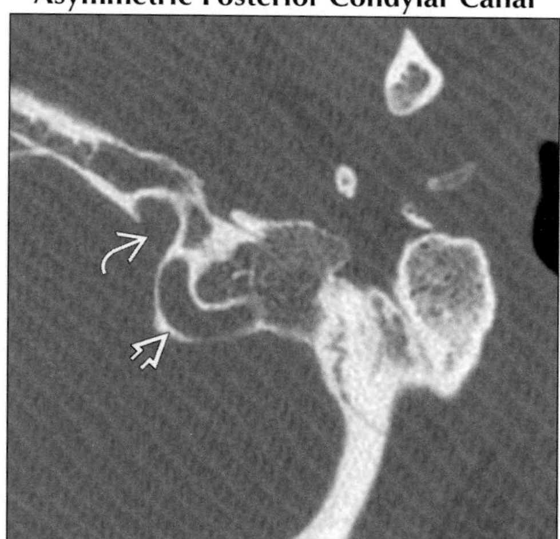

Asymmetric Posterior Condylar Canal

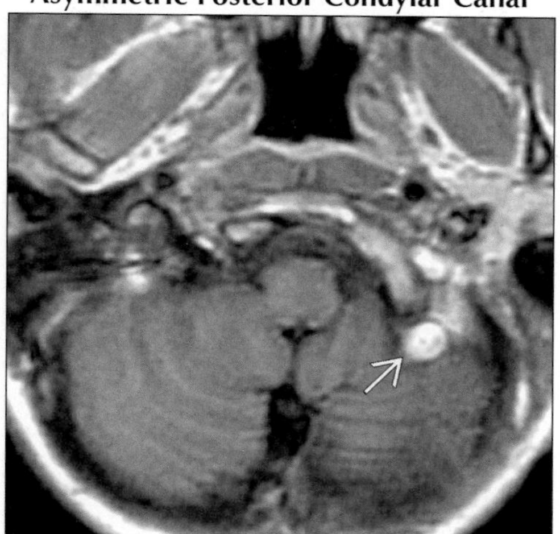

(Left) *Axial bone CT through inferior temporal bone demonstrates a well-defined venous channel through the left skull base* → *posterolateral to the left hypoglossal canal* →*, which is also known as the anterior condylar canal.* ***(Right)*** *Axial T1 C+ MR in a different patient shows asymmetric focal enhancement in the inferior skull base* →*, representing a normal but prominent left posterior condylar vein.*

High Jugular Bulb

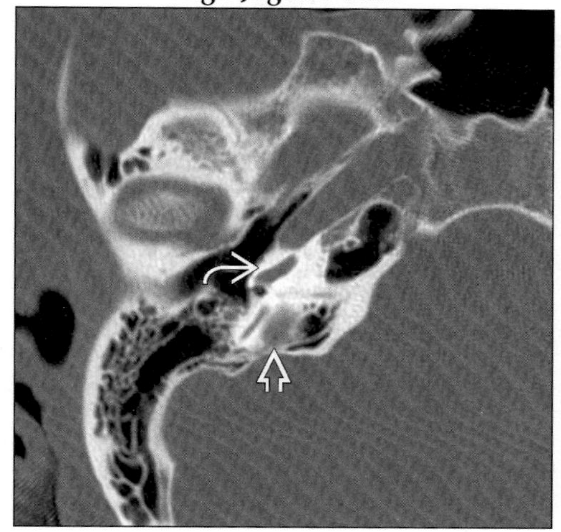

High Jugular Bulb

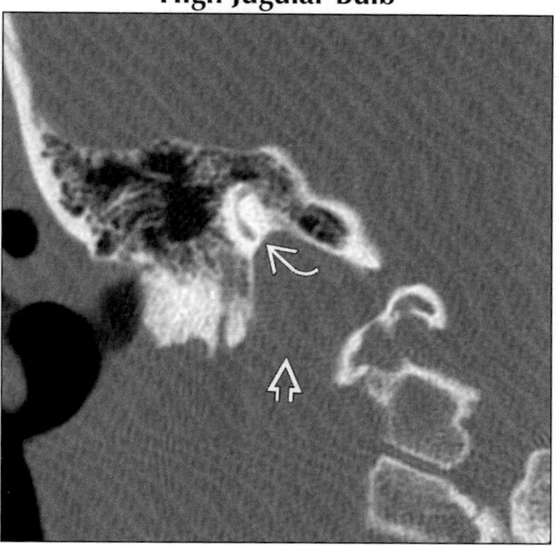

(Left) *Axial bone CT through the temporal bone at the level of the basal turn of the cochlea* → *demonstrates focal rounded lucency* → *immediately medial to the posterior semicircular canal.* ***(Right)*** *Coronal bone CT in the same patient reveals an enlarged right jugular foramen* → *at this level. The large foramen is "scalloping" the inferomedial margin of hyperdense otic capsule bone* → *that contains membranous labyrinth.*

Jugular Bulb Diverticulum

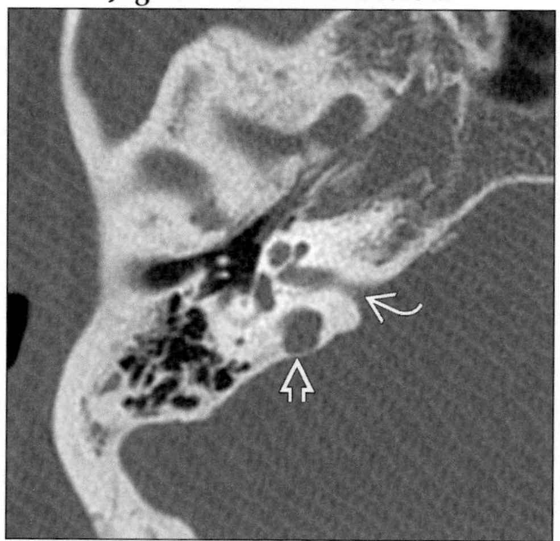

Jugular Bulb Diverticulum

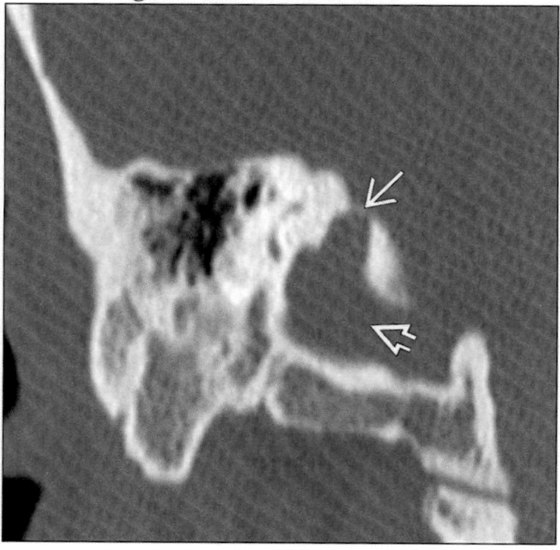

(Left) *Axial bone CT demonstrates well-defined lucency* → *in the posteromedial aspect of the right temporal bone at the level of the internal auditory canal* →*.* ***(Right)*** *Coronal bone CT reformat reveals this to be a focal diverticulum of the jugular bulb* →*, which extends superomedially from the normal-sized jugular foramen* →*. The overlying bone is intact.*

NORMAL SKULL BASE VENOUS VARIANTS

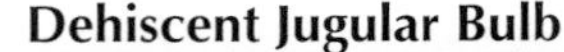

Dehiscent Jugular Bulb

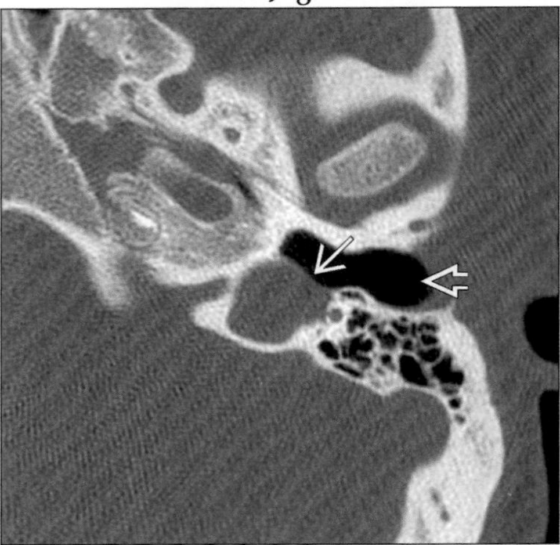

Dehiscent Jugular Bulb

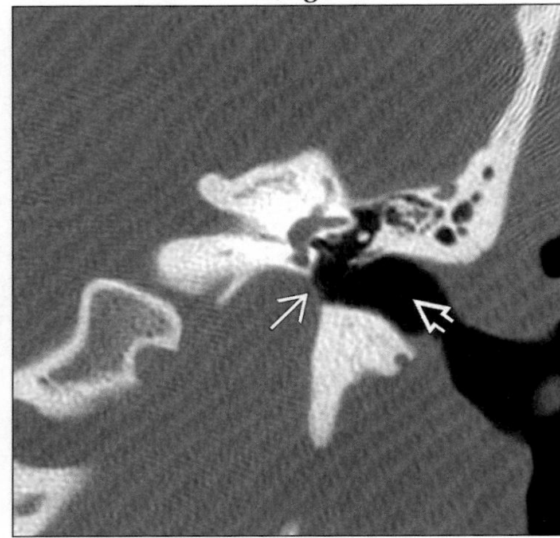

(Left) *Axial bone CT through the left temporal bone and external auditory canal demonstrates a prominent jugular bulb without apparent bony covering to separate it from the middle ear cavity .* ***(Right)*** *Coronal bone CT through the external auditory canal in the same patient again demonstrates the jugular bulb "peeking" into the hypotympanum. The dehiscent jugular bulb can also be thought of as a lateral jugular bulb diverticulum.*

Dehiscent Jugular Bulb

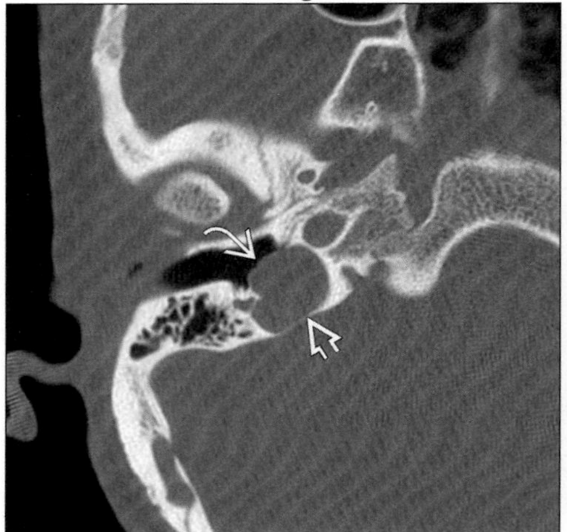

Dehiscent Jugular Bulb

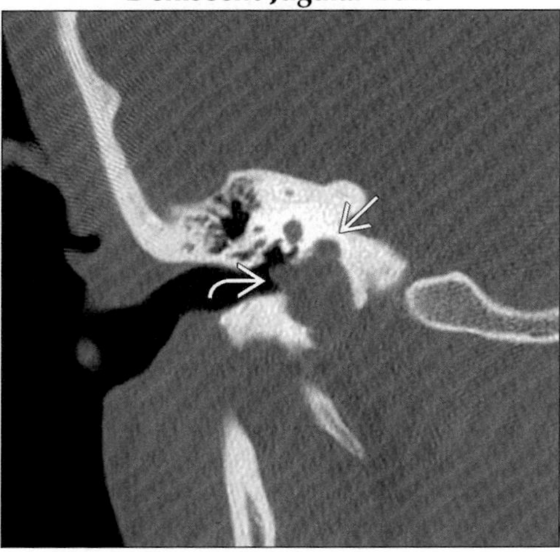

(Left) *Axial bone CT demonstrates a very large right jugular bulb , which also appears to "herniate" into the hypotympanum . No overlying bony covering is evident; hence, the bulb is described as dehiscent.* ***(Right)*** *Coronal bone CT in the same patient reveals the bulb to have 2 diverticula: A lateral diverticulum into the middle ear cavity and a medial superior jugular bulb diverticulum , which also creates a high jugular bulb.*

Asymmetric Sphenoidal Emissary Vein (of Vesalius)

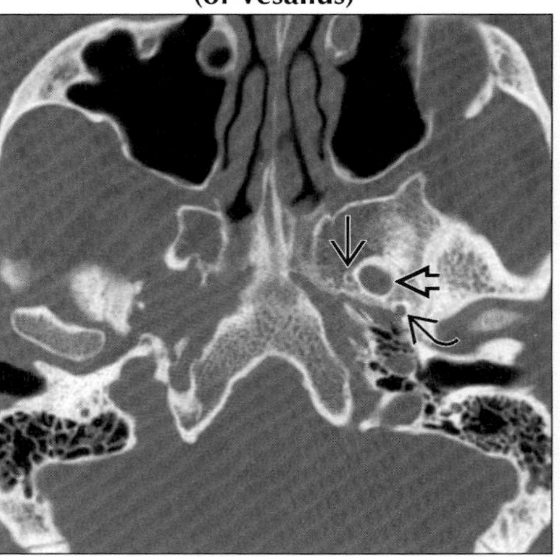

Asymmetric Sphenoidal Emissary Vein (of Vesalius)

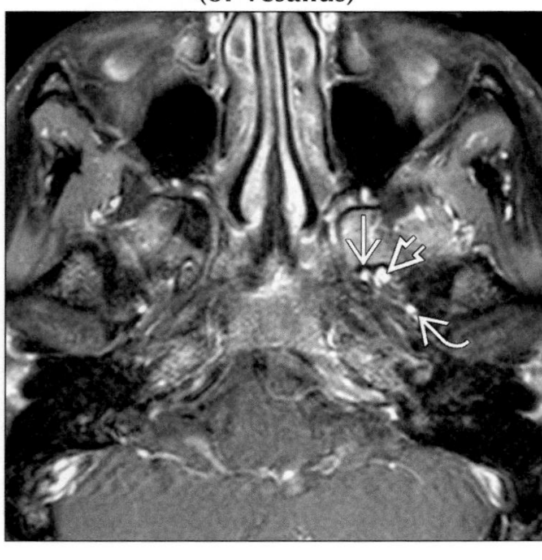

(Left) *Axial bone CT through the skull base shows a small foramen of Vesalius just medial to the foramen ovale . The foramen ovale and spinosum are readily identified by searching for a "stiletto heel footprint."* ***(Right)*** *Axial T1 C+ FS MR shows normal enhancement of the foramen spinosum (middle meningeal artery), foramen ovale , and foramen of Vesalius . The latter 2 carry emissary veins to the pterygoid venous plexus.*

Asymmetric Sphenoidal Emissary Vein (of Vesalius)

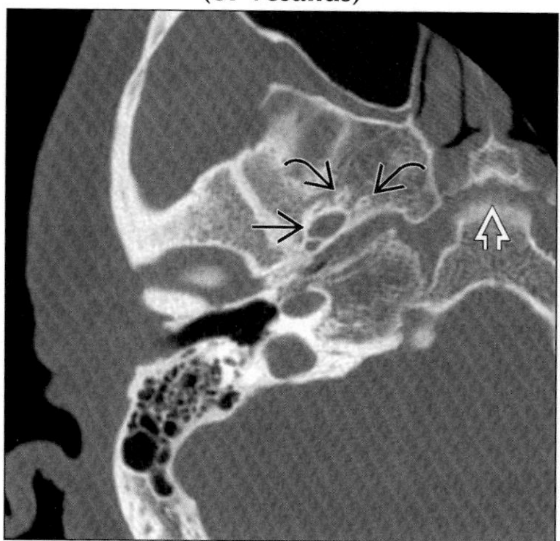

Asymmetric Sphenoidal Emissary Vein (of Vesalius)

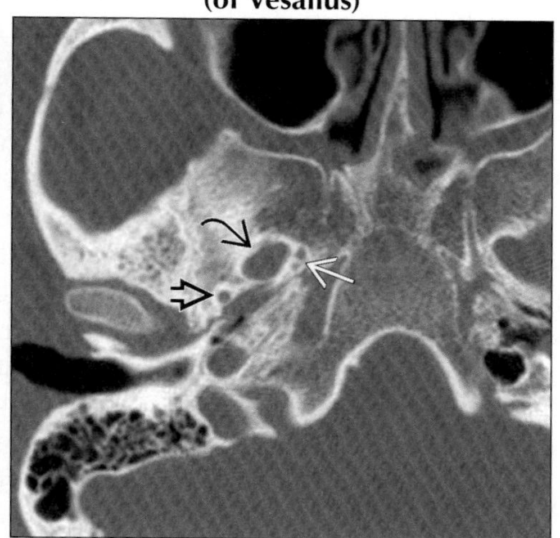

(Left) *Axial bone CT through the right skull base in a child reveals 2 small foramina ➢ anteromedial to the foramen ovale ➔, indicating duplicated right foramina of Vesalius. Note the expected lack of fusion of the sphenooccipital synchondrosis ➡.* ***(Right)*** *Axial bone CT shows a normal-caliber foramen ovale ➢ and spinosum ➡. Notice the 2 small foramina of Vesalius ➔ just medial to the anterior margin of the foramen ovale.*

Foramen Cecum

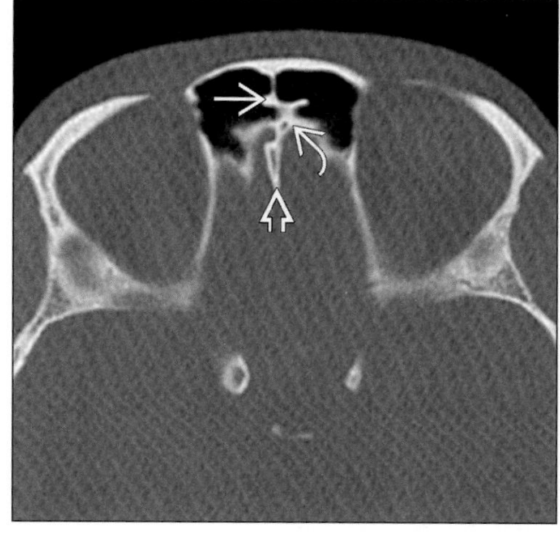

Foramen Cecum

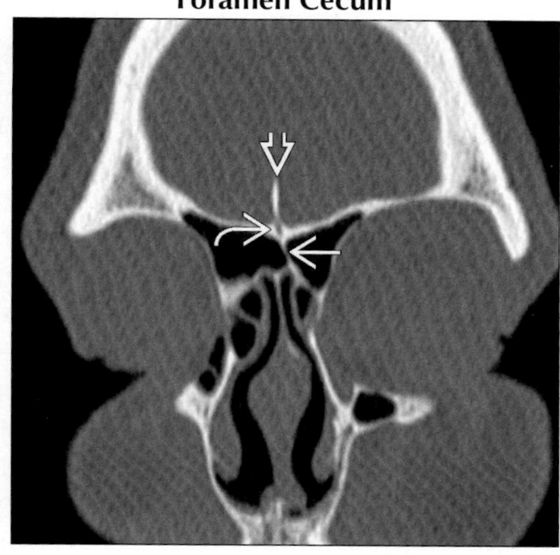

(Left) *Axial bone CT in an adult patient demonstrates a small foramen cecum ➢ anterior to the crista galli ➡. This venous channel courses anteroinferiorly through the anterior skull base to the frontal intersinus septum ➔.* ***(Right)*** *Coronal reformat through the anterior fossa in the same patient shows the location of a small persistent foramen cecum ➢ at the anterior limit of the crista galli ➡ and coursing toward the intersinus septum ➔. The vein drains to the nasal cavity.*

Petrosquamosal Emissary Vein

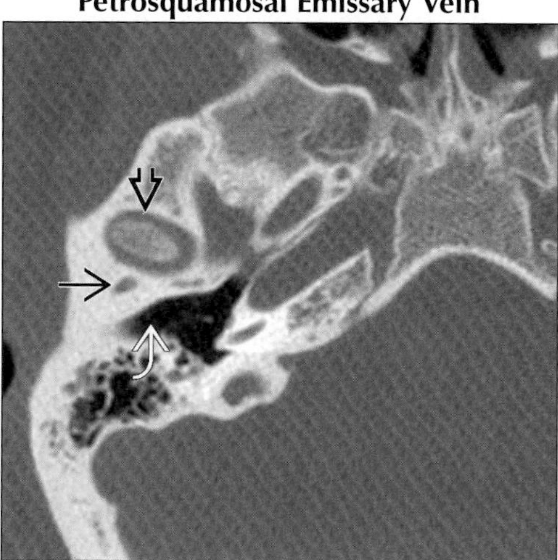

Petrosquamosal Emissary Vein

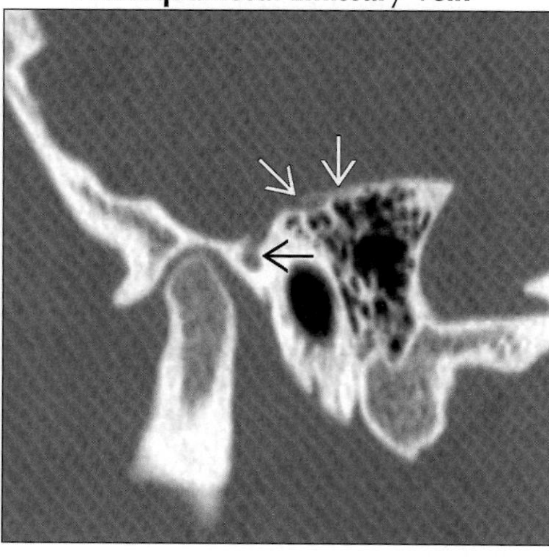

(Left) *Axial bone CT shows the vertical component of the emissary vein ➔ as it descends through the temporal bone posterior to the TMJ ➡ and anterior to the external auditory canal ➢.* ***(Right)*** *Sagittal bone CT reformat reveals the distal course of the emissary vein ➔ posterior to TMJ as it exits down through the skull base. The more proximal aspect of the venous channel is also seen ➔ coursing through the lateral aspect of the petrous bone from the transverse sinus.*

CONGENITAL ANOMALIES OF THE SKULL BASE

DIFFERENTIAL DIAGNOSIS

Common
- Internal Jugular Vein Asymmetry
- Jugular Bulb Diverticulum
- Chiari 1
- Chiari 2
- Neurofibromatosis Type 1

Less Common
- Aberrant Internal Carotid Artery
- Persistent Stapedial Artery
- Carotid Artery, Sphenoid Migration
- Agenesis Internal Carotid Artery

Rare but Important
- Craniostenoses
- 4th Occipital Sclerotome Anomalies
- Persistent Craniopharyngeal Canal
- Medial Basal Canal (Basilaris Medianus)
- Chiari 3

ESSENTIAL INFORMATION

Helpful Clues for Common Diagnoses
- **Internal Jugular Vein Asymmetry**
  - Key facts: Right internal jugular vein (IJV) dominant in 68-75%
    - Left IJV commonly smaller than right
    - IJV asymmetry < in larger cranial vault
  - Imaging
    - Most commonly seen normal asymmetry: Right sigmoid sinus, jugular bulb, and IJV larger than left
    - Increased signal of left IJV due to compression of left brachiocephalic vein during respiratory cycle
- **Jugular Bulb Diverticulum**
  - Key facts: Asymptomatic normal variant
  - Imaging
    - Coronal best: Bone CT, MRV, or T1 C+
    - "Pouch" projects from jugular bulb
    - High signal on MR may simulate mass
- **Chiari 1**
  - Key facts: Mismatch between posterior fossa size and cerebellar tissue
  - Imaging
    - Low-lying pointed (not rounded) peg-like cerebellar tonsils
    - Tonsils project below (≥ 5 mm) OR are impacted in foramen magnum
    - 4th occipital sclerotome anomalies in > 50% ⇒ small occipital enchondral skull
- **Chiari 2**
  - Key facts
    - 100% with neural tube closure defect
  - Imaging
    - Small bony posterior fossa
    - "Scalloped" petrous pyramid
    - "Notched" clivus
    - Low-lying tentorium/torcular
    - Large funnel-shaped foramen magnum
- **Neurofibromatosis Type 1**
  - Key facts: Neurocutaneous disorder
    - Characterized by diffuse neurofibromas, intracranial hamartomas, benign and malignant neoplasms
  - Imaging
    - Progressive sphenoid wing dysplasia
    - Enlarged optic foramina and fissures
    - Foramen magnum and skull base defects

Helpful Clues for Less Common Diagnoses
- **Aberrant Internal Carotid Artery**
  - Key facts: Displaced ICA courses through middle ear
  - Imaging
    - Enters posterior middle ear through enlarged inferior tympanic canaliculus
    - Courses anteriorly across cochlear promontory
    - Joins horizontal carotid canal through dehiscent carotid plate
    - Absent carotid foramen & vertical segment of petrous ICA
    - Look for associated persistent stapedial artery (PSA) in 30%
- **Persistent Stapedial Artery**
  - Key facts
    - Embryologic stapedial artery persists
    - PSA becomes middle meningeal artery
  - Imaging
    - Enlarged CN7 canal
    - Small canaliculus leaving carotid canal at genu of vertical and horizontal petrous ICA
    - Absent ipsilateral foramen spinosum
- **Carotid Artery, Sphenoid Migration**
  - Key facts: Seen in skull base syndromes involving enchondral bone
    - Achondroplasia, branchiootorenal syndrome, bicoronal synostoses (Apert, Pfeiffer, Crouzon)
  - Imaging

    - Medial migration of bony carotid artery walls at level of sphenoid
- **Agenesis Internal Carotid Artery**
  - Key facts
    - Isolated or syndromic (PHACES, morning glory, Goldenhar, clefting syndromes)
  - Imaging
    - Absent or hypoplastic vertical and horizontal petrous portions of ICA

Helpful Clues for Rare Diagnoses

- **Craniostenoses**
  - Key facts
    - Syndromic (fibroblastic growth factor, TWIST, and *MSX2* mutations) + nonsyndromic premature osseous obliteration of cranial sutures
  - Imaging
    - Early fusion of occipital sutures surrounding foramen magnum
    - Enchondral skull base: Achondroplasia, syndromic bicoronal synostoses, kleeblattschädel
- **4th Occipital Sclerotome Anomalies**
  - Synonym: Proatlas anomalies
  - Hypocentrum of 4th occipital sclerotome (OS) ⇒ anterior clival tubercle
  - Centrum of 4th OS ⇒ apical cap of dens and apical ligament
  - Ventral portion of neural component of 4th OS ⇒ anterior margin of foramen magnum and occipital condyle
  - Caudal portion of neural component of 4th OS ⇒ lateral atlantal masses and superior posterior arch of atlas
  - Imaging: 4th OSA finding
    - Short clivus and atlas assimilation
    - Craniovertebral bony anomalies
- **Persistent Craniopharyngeal Canal**
  - Key facts
    - Look for associated canal atresia or stenosis, moyamoya, coloboma
  - Imaging
    - Small: Nonpituitary tissue containing remnant channel
    - Large: Contains pituitary gland or frank encephalocele or artery
- **Medial Basal Canal (Basilaris Medianus)**
  - Key facts
    - Notochord remnant cephalic terminus
  - Imaging: Midline clivus
    - Posterior to sphenooccipital synchondrosis
    - Currarino types A-F denote completeness and location of defect
    - Tortuous canal may indent superior or inferior aspect of clivus
- **Chiari 3**
  - Key facts: Intracranial Chiari 2 + meningoencephalocele
    - High cervical meningoencephalocele
  - Imaging
    - Occipital squama defect may involve upper cervical vertebrae
    - Bony features of Chiari 2 in addition

Internal Jugular Vein Asymmetry

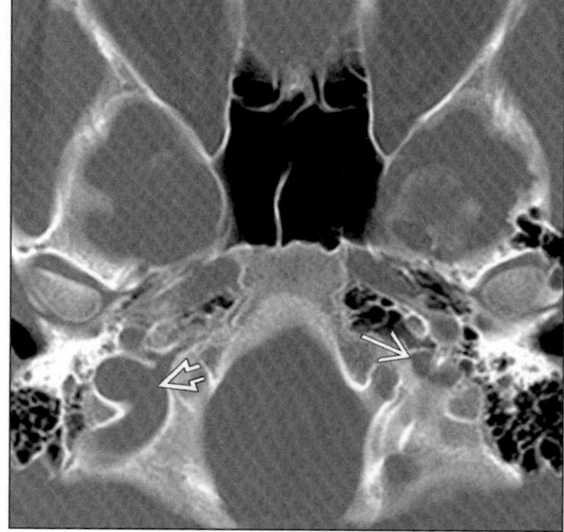

Axial bone CT demonstrates marked asymmetry with the jugular foramen on the right ⮕ larger than the small left jugular foramen ⮕.

Internal Jugular Vein Asymmetry

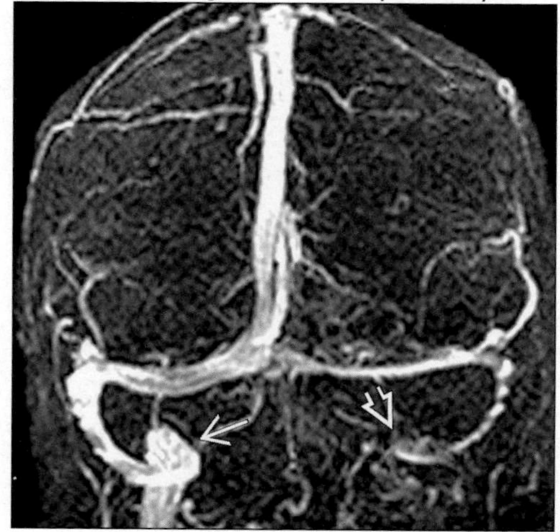

Coronal MRV in the same patient confirms marked asymmetry of the jugular veins. The left ⮕ tapers and is poorly visualized while the right ⮕ is normal in size.

CONGENITAL ANOMALIES OF THE SKULL BASE

*(**Left**) Axial bone CT in a teenager with achondroplasia shows asymmetry of the jugular foramina, both of which are stenosed. (**Right**) Sagittal MRV in a different patient with achondroplasia reveals severe restriction of the jugular vein at the level of the stenosed jugular foramina. There are excessive venous collaterals in the soft tissues of the neck.*

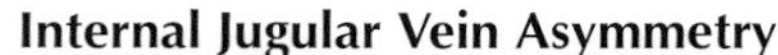

Internal Jugular Vein Asymmetry

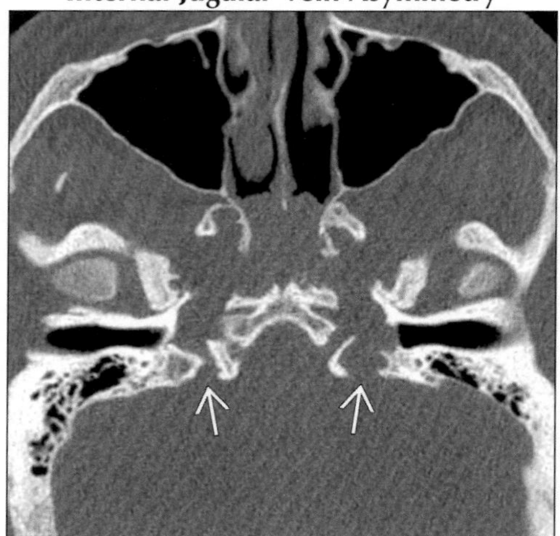

Internal Jugular Vein Asymmetry

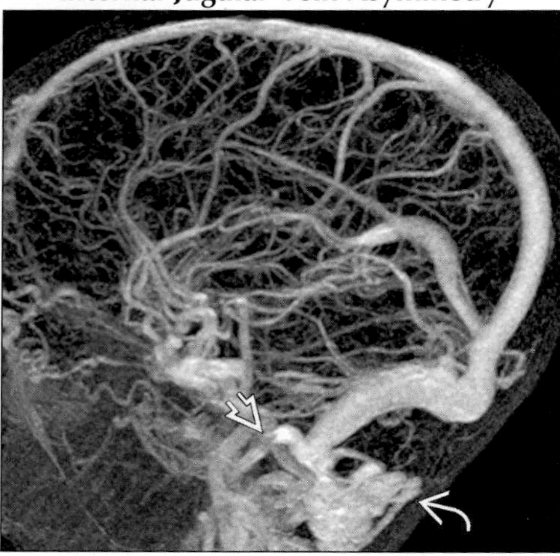

*(**Left**) Coronal bone CT demonstrates a typical cephalad projecting jugular bulb diverticulum. The diverticulum most commonly projects superiorly posterior to the internal auditory canal. (**Right**) Axial bone CT reveals the diverticulum to be located posterior to the internal auditory canal. When the diverticulum is large, axial enhanced T1 MR imaging may appear to have an "enhancing lesion" in this location related to slow flow in the diverticulum.*

Jugular Bulb Diverticulum

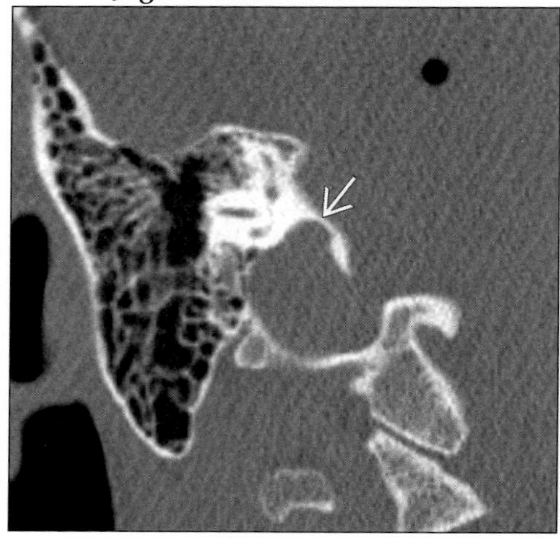

Jugular Bulb Diverticulum

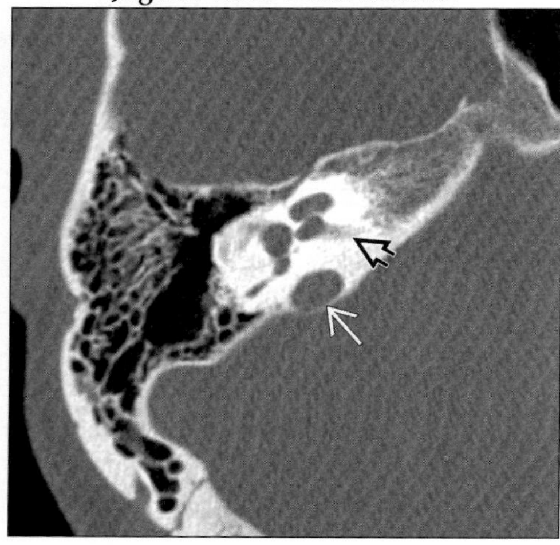

*(**Left**) Sagittal T1WI MR shows marked herniation of the cerebellar tonsils behind the upper cervical spinal cord. There is an associated short scalloped clivus. (**Right**) Sagittal T2WI MR reveals a typical enlarged foramen magnum, herniation of the uvula of the vermis, cascading cerebellar tissue, and a notched clivus. Note also the beaked tectum and the prominent massa intermedia associated with Chiari 2 malformation.*

Chiari 1

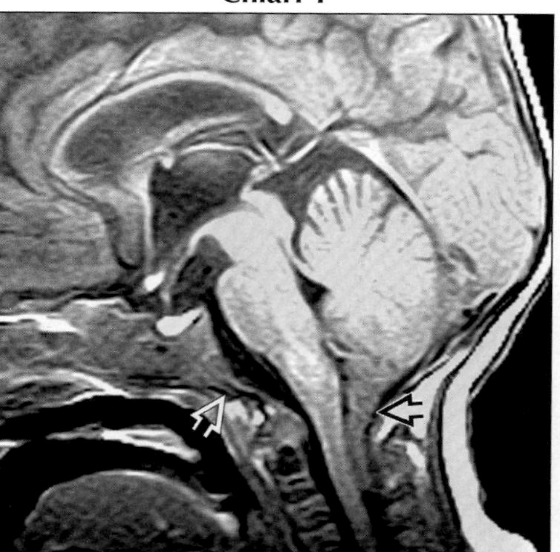

Chiari 2

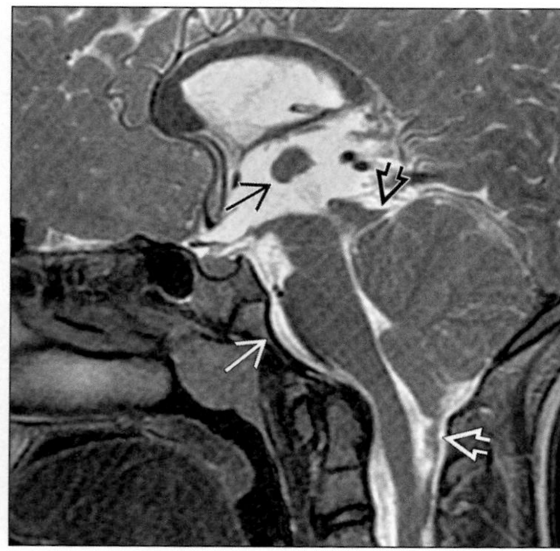

Neurofibromatosis Type 1

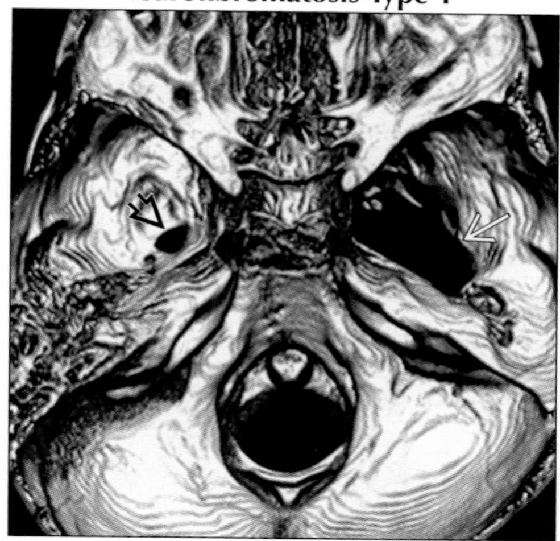

Neurofibromatosis Type 1

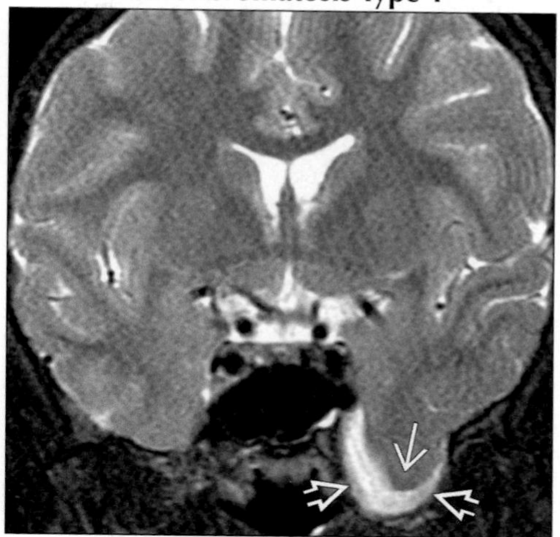

*(**Left**) 3D reformatted CT shows a large defect ➡ of the left middle cranial fossa, centered on the foramen ovale. Note the normal-sized contralateral foramen ovale ⇨. (**Right**) Coronal T2WI MR in the same child shows an encephalocele with herniation of the temporal lobe ➡ and hyperintense cerebral spinal fluid ⇨ through the middle cranial floor defect.*

Aberrant Internal Carotid Artery

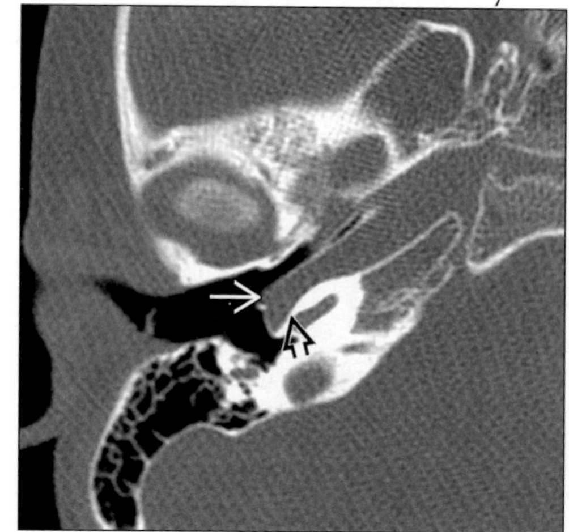

Aberrant Internal Carotid Artery

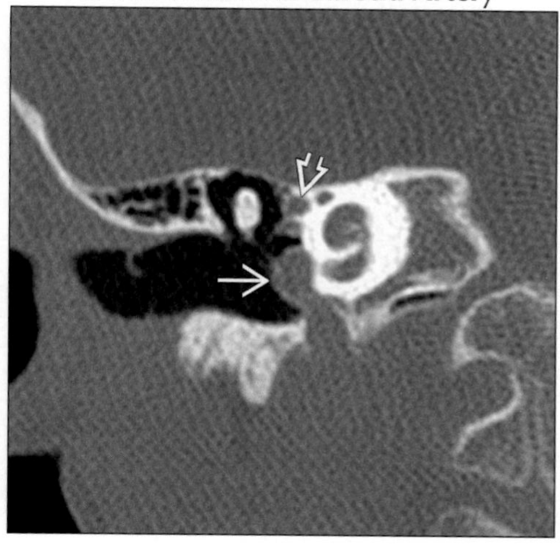

*(**Left**) Axial bone CT demonstrates an aberrant internal carotid artery ➡ traversing the middle ear cavity over the cochlear promontory ⇨. (**Right**) Coronal bone CT shows the aberrant internal carotid artery ➡ extending through the medial floor of the hypotympanum to overlie the cochlear promontory, inferior and lateral to the cochlea. The enlarged anterior tympanic CN7 canal ⇨ suggests that the persistent stapedial artery is present.*

Persistent Stapedial Artery

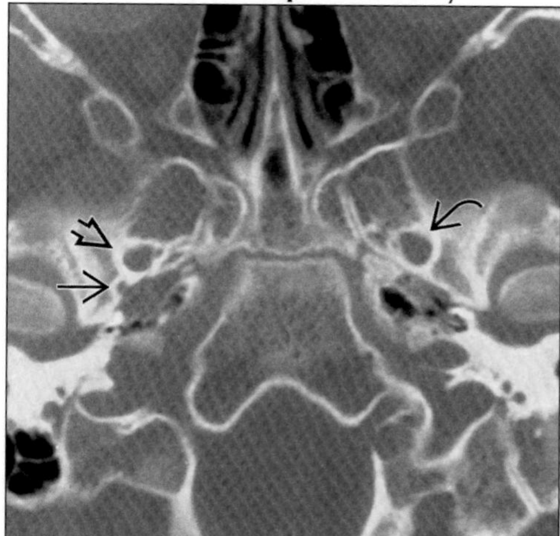

Persistent Stapedial Artery

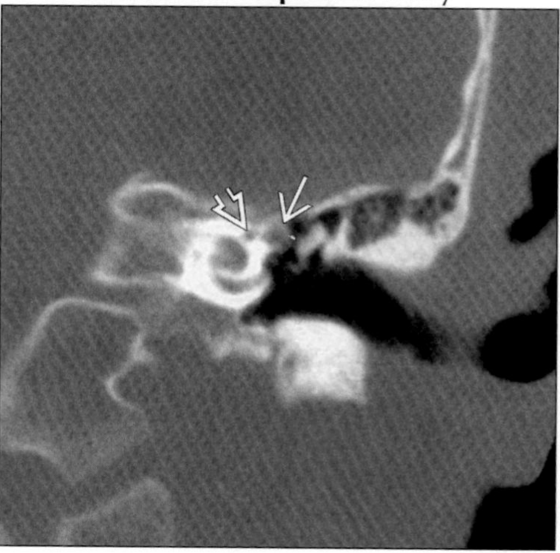

*(**Left**) Axial bone CT shows a persistent stapedial artery in the absence of an aberrant internal carotid artery. Side-to-side comparison shows an absent left foramen spinosum with a normal left foramen ovale ↗. Note the normal right foramen ovale ⇨ and foramen spinosum →. (**Right**) Coronal bone CT demonstrates an enlarged anterior tympanic segment of the facial nerve canal ➡ lateral to the normal labyrinthine segment ⇨.*

CONGENITAL ANOMALIES OF THE SKULL BASE

(Left) Axial bone CT in a child with achondroplasia shows marked medial deviation of the internal carotid arteries ➡. The bony covering remains, although indenting the posterior wall of the sphenoid sinus. (Right) Axial bone CT reveals a normal-sized right horizontal petrous internal carotid artery canal ➡ and atretic left carotid canal ➡. Notice the prominent craniopharyngeal canal ➡ in this child with morning glory syndrome.

Carotid Artery, Sphenoid Migration

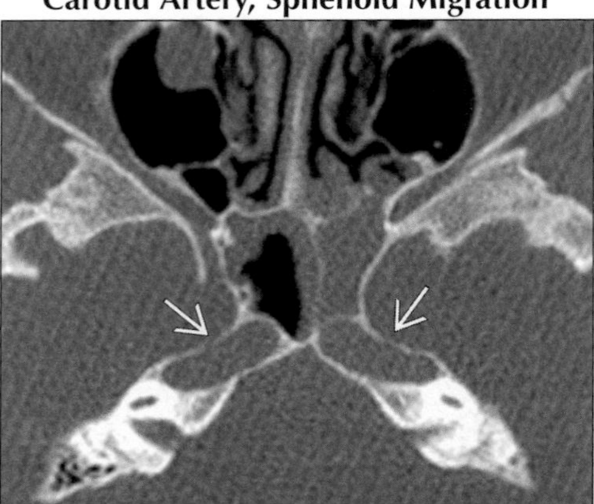

Agenesis Internal Carotid Artery

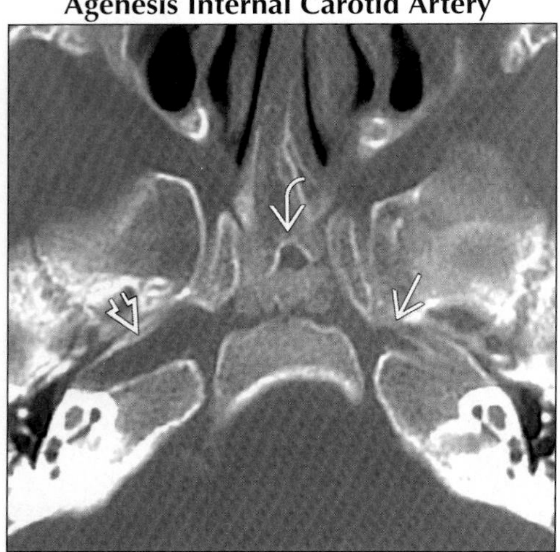

(Left) 3D reformatted CT in a newborn shows patency of the anterior ➡ and posterior ➡ intraoccipital sutures. The foramen ovale ➡ are symmetric. (Right) 3D reformatted CT in another newborn, this one with a disorder of enchondral cartilage, shows a deformed foramen magnum due to fusion of the sutures. There is hypertrophy of the internal occipital crest ➡. Note also the distortion of the left foramen ovale ➡.

Craniostenoses

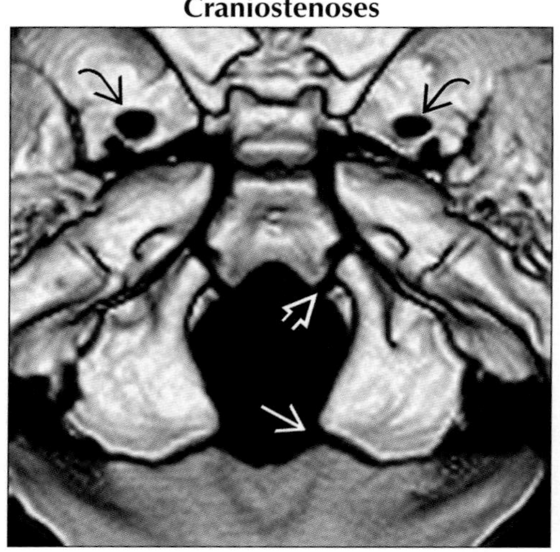

Craniostenoses

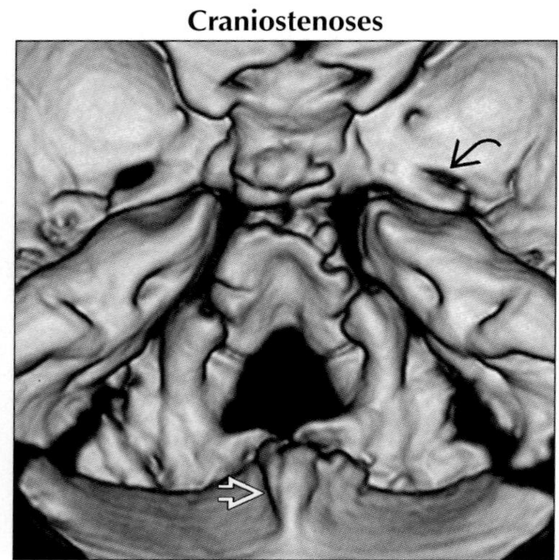

(Left) Axial NECT demonstrates absence of the clivus ➡ and an anomalous odontoid ➡ in an infant with severe anomalies of the skull base. (Right) Sagittal T1WI MR shows a pituitary gland ➡ "pointing" to a persistent craniopharyngeal canal ➡. Multiple midline anomalies are associated. The brainstem is thin, and the inferior 4th ventricle is open ➡. The anterior corpus callosum is thin ➡, and there is no anterior commissure.

4th Occipital Sclerotome Anomalies

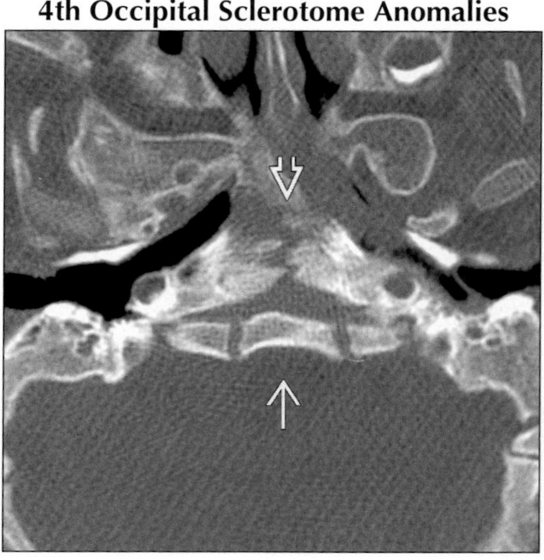

Persistent Craniopharyngeal Canal

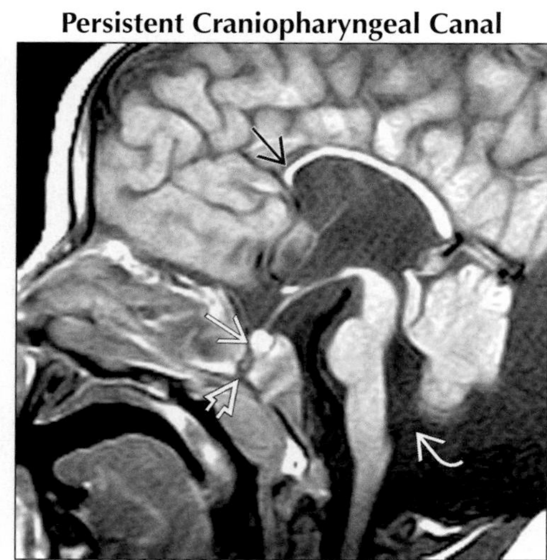

Persistent Craniopharyngeal Canal

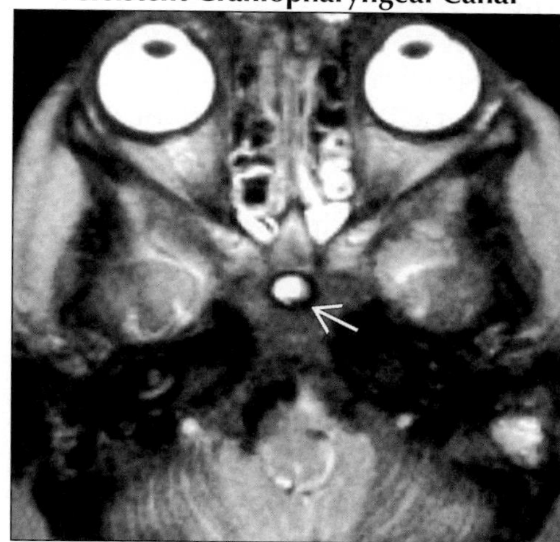

Persistent Craniopharyngeal Canal

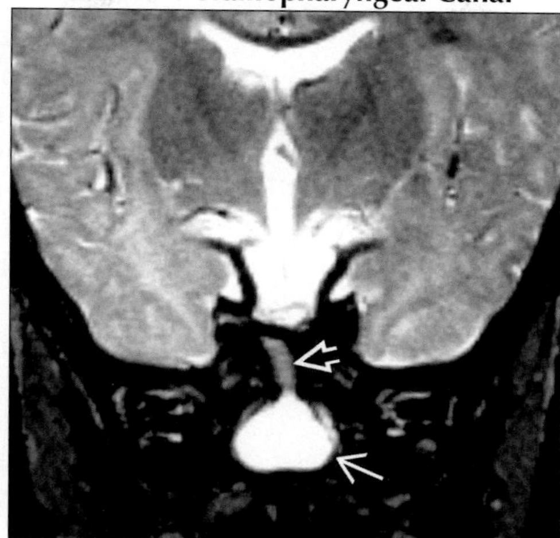

(Left) *Axial T2WI MR in a child with sphenoidal encephalocele reveals cerebrospinal fluid and pituitary tissue ➡ within the enlarged craniopharyngeal canal. This canal may contain fibrous tissue, CSF, pituitary tissue, and occasionally an artery.* ***(Right)*** *Coronal PD FSE FS MR shows a sphenoidal encephalocele ➡ projecting through a persistent craniopharyngeal canal ⇨ into the pharynx. The pituitary gland is in the tissue signal within the canal.*

Medial Basal Canal (Basilaris Medianus)

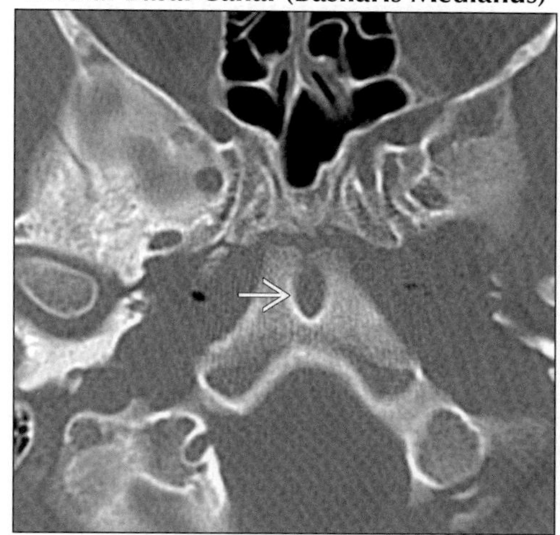

Medial Basal Canal (Basilaris Medianus)

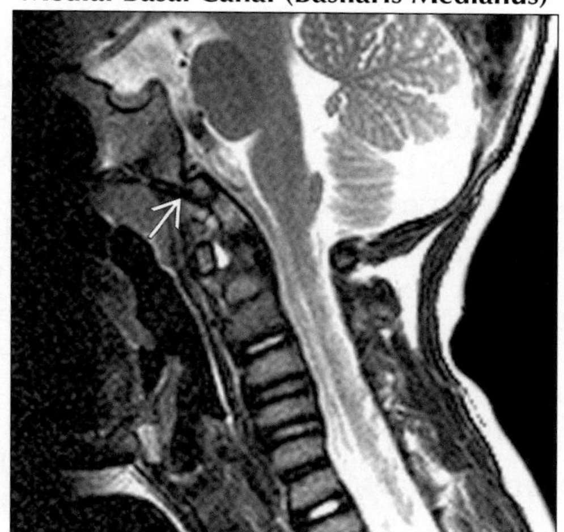

(Left) *Axial NECT demonstrates an incidental incomplete midline defect ➡ in the inferior aspect of the clivus.* ***(Right)*** *Sagittal T2WI MR in another child shows a complete defect ➡ traversing the clivus. Defects may be on the anterior or the posterior clival surface and may be through-and-through or incomplete.*

Chiari 3

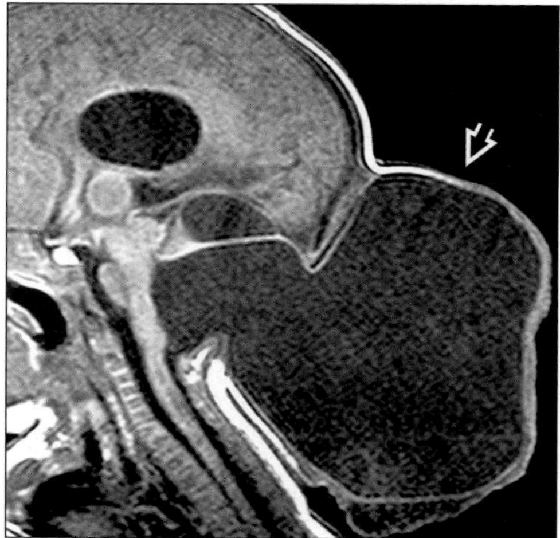

Chiari 3

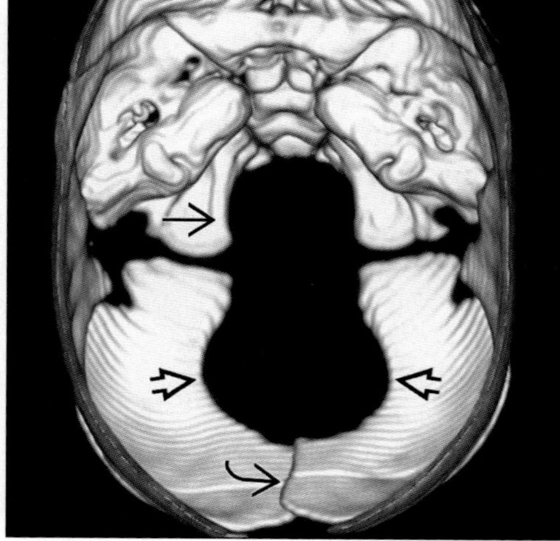

(Left) *Sagittal T1WI MR in a newborn shows a very large posterior encephalocele ⇨ involving the foramen magnum and supraoccipital bone.* ***(Right)*** *3D reformatted CT in the same patient reveals a large bone defect ⇨ communicating with the foramen magnum →. There is an additional midline overlapping suture ↪ splitting the supraoccipital bone.*

SKULL BASE FORAMINAL OR FISSURAL VARIANTS

DIFFERENTIAL DIAGNOSIS

Common

- Jugular Foramen Asymmetry
- Glossopharyngeal Canal

Less Common

- Petromastoid Canal
- Asymmetric Sphenoidal Emissary Vein (of Vesalius)
- Persistent Craniopharyngeal Canal
- Medial Basal Canal (Basilaris Medianus)
- Internal Auditory Canal Hypoplasia
- Enlarged Emissary Vein, Transmastoid
- Asymmetric Posterior Condylar Vein

Rare but Important

- Enlarged Inferior Tympanic Canaliculus
- Absent Foramen Spinosum
- Innominate Canal
- Accessory Foramen Ovale

ESSENTIAL INFORMATION

Key Differential Diagnosis Issues

- Normal variants may be uni- or bilateral
- When normal structures are asymmetric, this may be normal variation or sign of pathology
- Many are incidental findings
- Imaging strategy
  - CT: Best defines or clarifies variants
  - MR: Often source of pitfalls

Helpful Clues for Common Diagnoses

- **Jugular Foramen Asymmetry**
  - Key facts
    - Common developmental asymmetry of jugular foramen
  - Imaging
    - CT: Smooth cortical bone surrounds enlarged jugular foramen
    - MR: Various flow phenomena may result in misinterpretation of mass lesion
- **Glossopharyngeal Canal**
  - Key facts
    - 30% have partial or complete canal
    - Glossopharyngeal nerve (CN9) enters canal prior to jugular foramen
  - Imaging
    - CT: Small funnel-shaped canal leading to anterior portion of jugular foramen (pars nervosa)
    - MR: High-resolution T2 may show CN9

Helpful Clues for Less Common Diagnoses

- **Petromastoid Canal**
  - Key facts
    - Synonyms: Subarcuate canaliculus
    - From posterior CPA to mastoid air cells
    - Canal passes between and below crura of superior semicircular canal
    - Vestige of neonatal subarcuate fossa
    - Contents: Subarcuate artery and vein; branch of AICA or labyrinthine artery
    - In infant, subarcuate artery pseudolesion may confound radiologist
  - Imaging
    - If seen in adult: ≤ 1 mm curvilinear canal below superior semicircular canal
    - May be ≥ 2 mm in young children; subarachnoid space association may mimic lesion
- **Asymmetric Sphenoidal Emissary Vein (of Vesalius)**
  - Key facts
    - Transmits emissary vein from cavernous sinus to pterygoid venous plexus
    - May enlarge with ↑ venous flow from caroticocavernous fistula
  - Imaging
    - Located medial to anterior aspect of foramen ovale; usually < 2 mm
    - May be partially assimilated with ovale or may be duplicated
- **Persistent Craniopharyngeal Canal**
  - Key facts
    - Synonym: Trans-sphenoidal canal; persistent hypophyseal canal
    - Considered embryologic remnant of vascular channel
    - Site of trans-sphenoidal cephalocele
  - Imaging
    - Bone CT: Midline sphenoid, < 1.5 mm
    - Anterior to sphenooccipital synchondrosis
- **Medial Basal Canal (Basilaris Medianus)**
  - Key facts
    - Considered remnant of cephalic end of notochord
    - Rarely enlarged to form basal cephalocele
  - Imaging
    - Midline sphenoid; < 1.5 mm
    - Posterior to sphenooccipital synchondrosis

SKULL BASE FORAMINAL OR FISSURAL VARIANTS

- **Internal Auditory Canal Hypoplasia**
  - Key facts
    - Contents: CN7 and CN8
    - Hypoplasia from congenital absence or deficiency of CN8
    - Associated with inner ear malformations
    - Normal canal diameter: 4-8 mm
  - Imaging
    - CT: Small caliber IAC, < 4 mm
    - MR: High-resolution imaging may show deficient CN8
- **Enlarged Emissary Vein, Transmastoid**
  - Key facts
    - Connects transverse sinus to posterior auricular or occipital veins
    - Enlargement may be associated with small jugular foramen (JF)
  - Imaging
    - Horizontal canal through posteromedial mastoid bone adjacent to occipital suture
- **Asymmetric Posterior Condylar Vein**
  - Key facts
    - Contents: Emissary vein from sigmoid sinus to suboccipital veins; meningeal branch of ascending pharyngeal artery
    - Enlargement associated with small JF
  - Imaging
    - Well-corticated curvilinear channel

Helpful Clues for Rare Diagnoses

- **Enlarged Inferior Tympanic Canaliculus**
  - Key facts
    - Normally transmits Jacobsen nerve (inferior tympanic branch of CN9)
    - Aberrant internal carotid artery (ICA) enters middle ear through this
  - Imaging
    - Aberrant ICA widens canaliculus to reach cochlear promontory
    - CTA or MRA to confirm aberrant ICA
- **Absent Foramen Spinosum**
  - Key facts
    - Normally transmits middle meningeal artery (MMA)
    - May be absent if MMA arises from ophthalmic artery or replaced by persistent stapedial artery (PSA)
    - Foramen rarely duplicated when MMA has anterior and posterior branches
  - Imaging
    - Foramen normally < 3 mm
    - Posterolateral to foramen ovale
    - Look for PSA and aberrant ICA
- **Innominate Canal**
  - Key facts
    - Synonym: Canal of Arnold
    - Contains lesser petrosal nerve
  - Imaging
    - Between foramen ovale and spinosum
    - Usually ≤ 2 mm
- **Accessory Foramen Ovale**
  - Key facts
    - Contains accessory meningeal artery
  - Imaging
    - Lateral to foramen ovale; < 2 mm
    - May be partially assimilated with ovale resulting in posterolateral groove

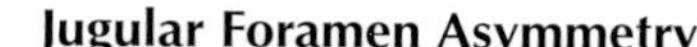

Jugular Foramen Asymmetry

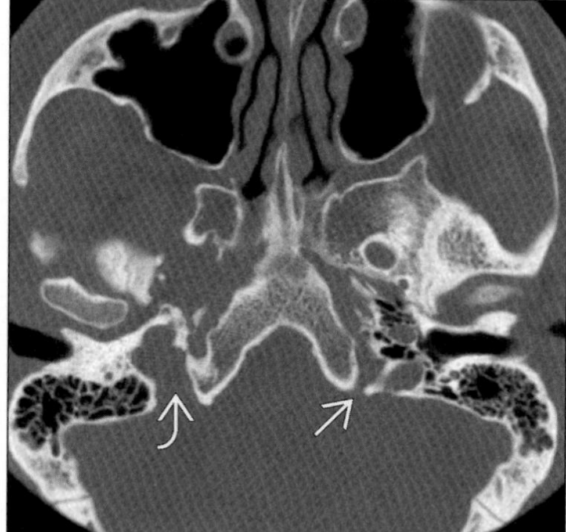

Axial bone CT through the low skull base demonstrates asymmetry of jugular foramina with the left foramen ➡ much smaller compared to the right ➡. This is a normal finding and does not indicate pathology.

Glossopharyngeal Canal

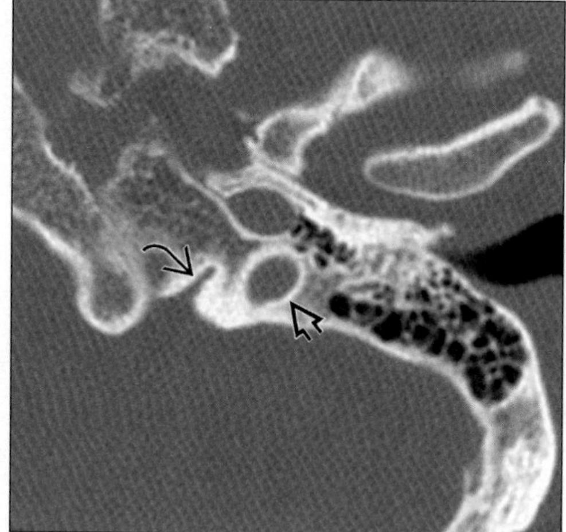

Axial bone CT demonstrates a funnel-shaped canal ➡ inferior to the level of the internal auditory canal. The canal connects inferiorly to the anterior portion of the jugular foramen ➡ (pars nervosa).

SKULL BASE FORAMINAL OR FISSURAL VARIANTS

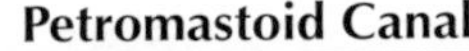

Petromastoid Canal

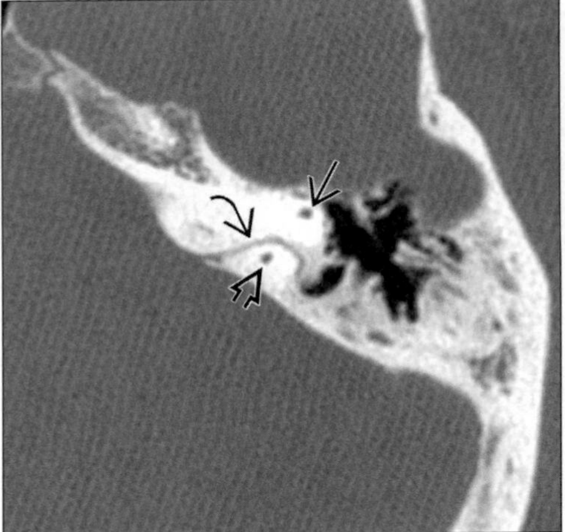

Petromastoid Canal

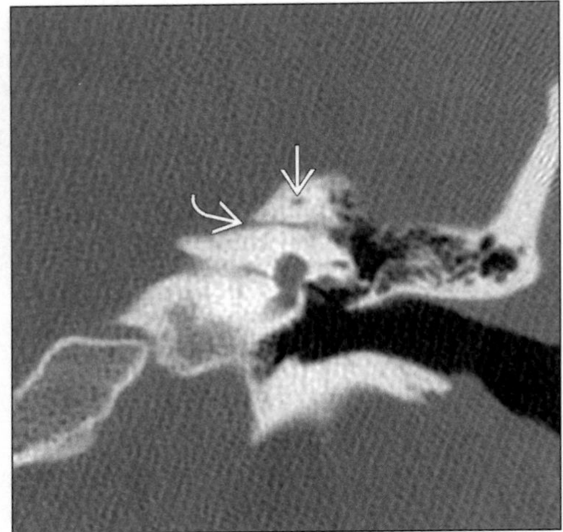

(Left) *Axial bone CT in an adult patient demonstrates a curvilinear thin channel coursing through the left petrous temporal bone between the posterior and anterior crura of the superior semicircular canal.* ***(Right)*** *Coronal bone CT reveals a petromastoid canal coursing laterally from the posterior cerebellopontine angle to the mastoid air cells. The canal courses beneath the superior semicircular canal.*

Asymmetric Sphenoidal Emissary Vein (of Vesalius)

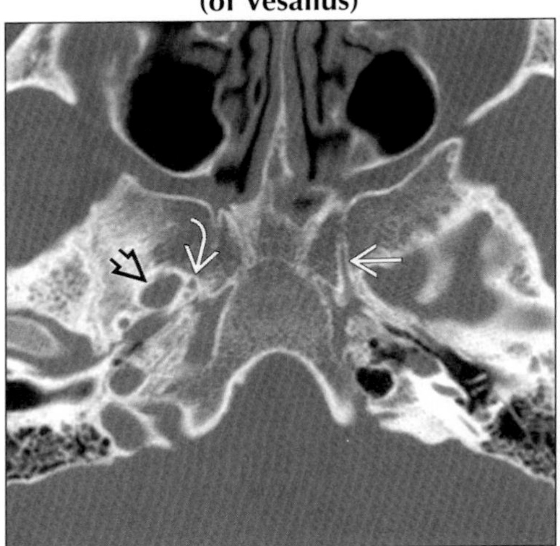

Persistent Craniopharyngeal Canal

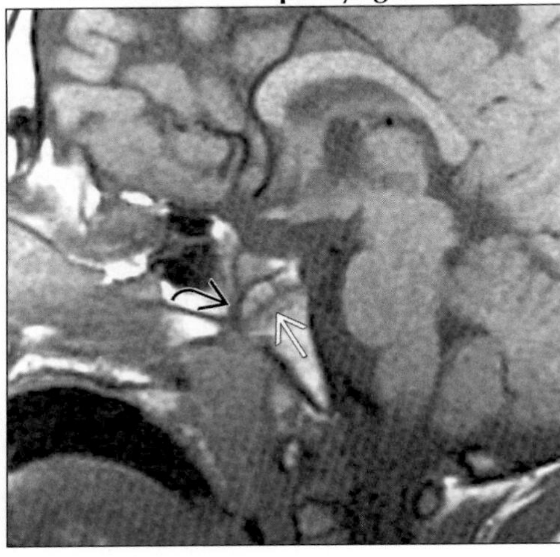

(Left) *Axial bone CT shows 2 small foramina of Vesalius at anteromedial margin of the right foramen ovale. The left skull base shows anteromedial contour of the foramen ovale and vidian canal but no accessory foramina.* ***(Right)*** *Sagittal T1WI MR in a child shows a small well-corticated canal from the inferior aspect of the sella to the inferior aspect of the sphenoid bone. This craniopharyngeal canal is anterior to nonfused sphenooccipital synchondrosis.*

Medial Basal Canal (Basilaris Medianus)

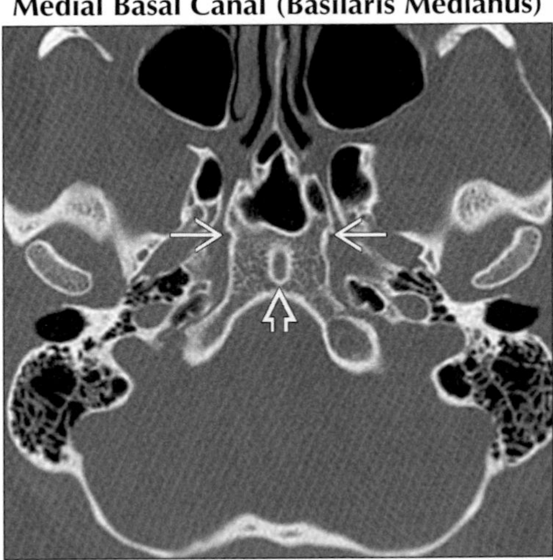

Internal Auditory Canal Hypoplasia

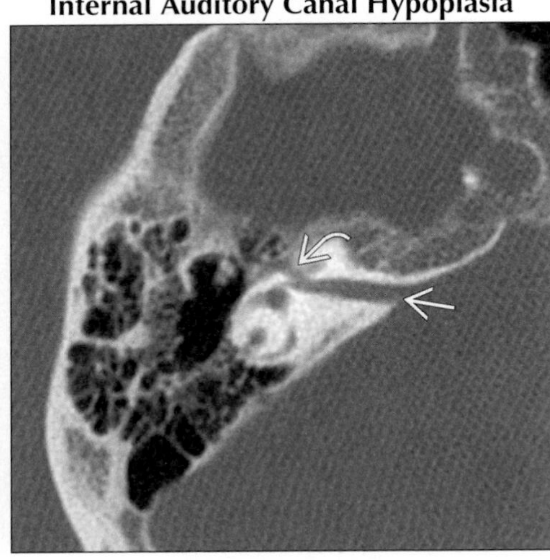

(Left) *Axial bone CT demonstrates a well-defined, midline keyhole-shaped foramen in the posterior aspect of the sphenoid (basisphenoid). This is posterior to the location of the sella and posterior to the site of fused sphenooccipital synchondrosis.* ***(Right)*** *Axial bone CT shows a small internal auditory canal in an adult with a history of congenital hearing loss. Even without measuring caliber, IAC is only slightly larger than caliber of labyrinthine segment of CN7.*

Enlarged Emissary Vein, Transmastoid

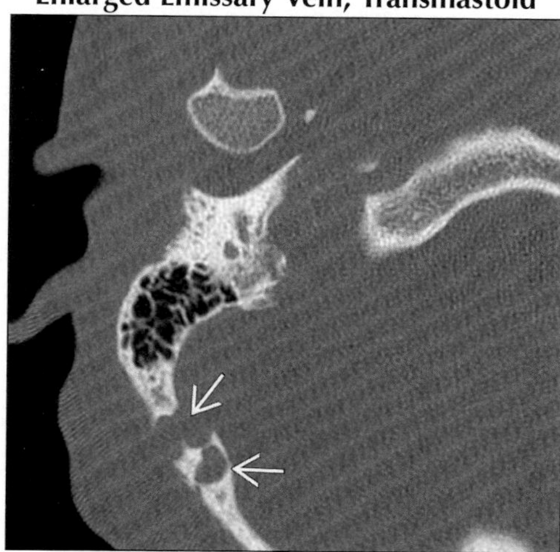

Asymmetric Posterior Condylar Vein

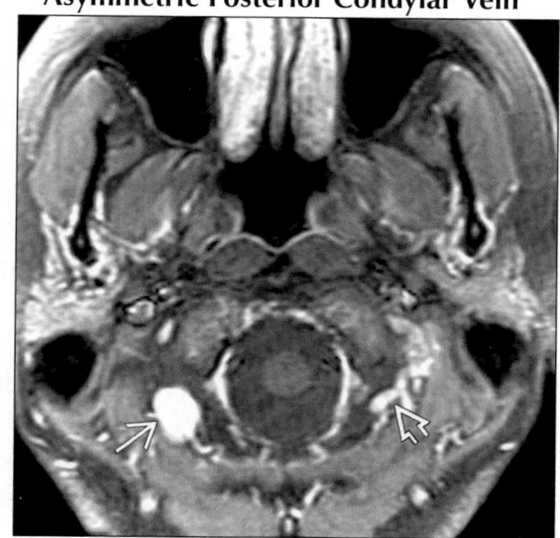

(Left) *Axial NECT reveals multiple transmastoid emissary vein canals ➡ connecting the transverse sinus to the occipital veins.* ***(Right)*** *Axial T1 C+ FS MR demonstrates nodular enhancement just below the right skull base ➡ with more linear enhancement seen on the contralateral side ➡, which clearly appears vascular. Both are posterior condylar veins, and this asymmetry is a normal finding.*

Enlarged Inferior Tympanic Canaliculus

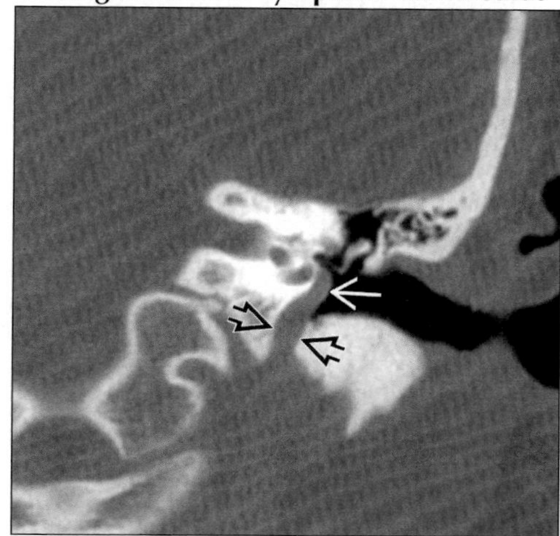

Absent Foramen Spinosum

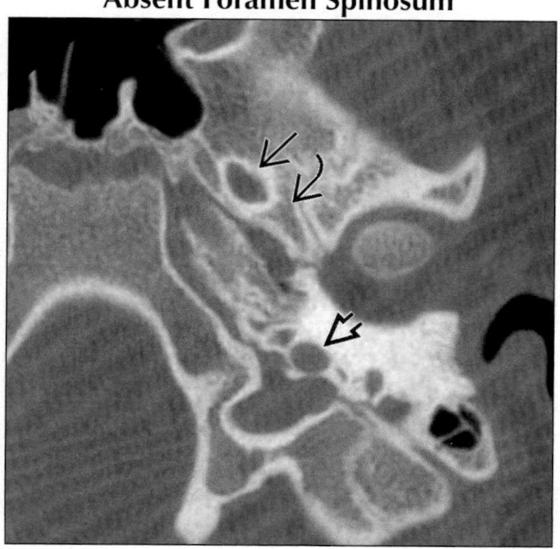

(Left) *Coronal bone CT shows an enlarged inferior tympanic canaliculus ➡ secondary to an aberrant internal carotid artery ➡.* ***(Right)*** *Axial bone CT in the same patient shows an enlarged inferior tympanic canaliculus ➡. Note the additional finding of an absent ipsilateral foramen spinosum ➡ posterior to the foramen ovale ➡, indicating that a persistent stapedial artery is present.*

Innominate Canal

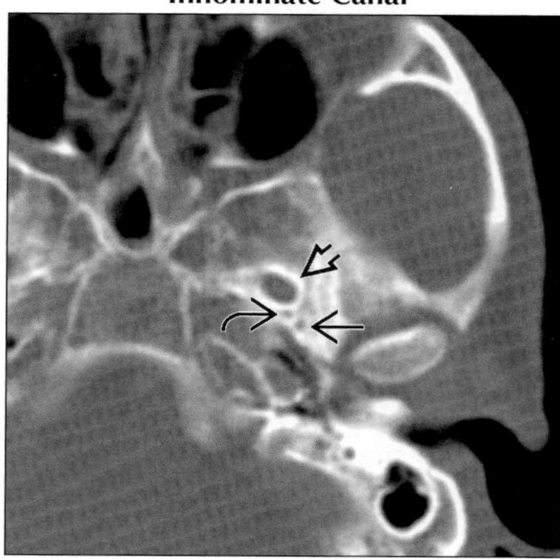

Accessory Foramen Ovale

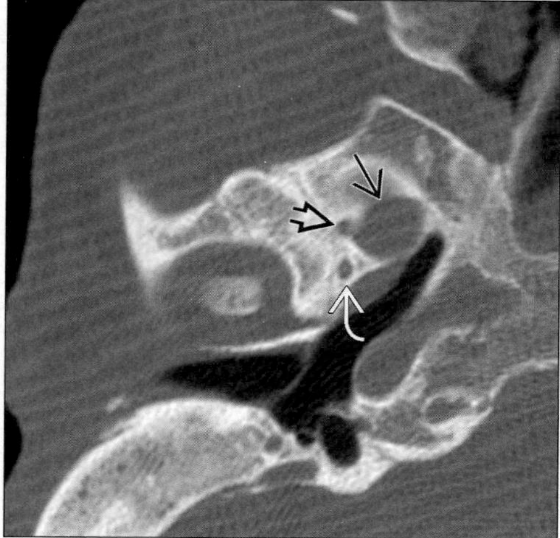

(Left) *Axial bone CT demonstrates a tiny innominate canal ➡ anterior to the foramen spinosum ➡ and posterior to the foramen ovale ➡. This was an incidental unilateral variant.* ***(Right)*** *Axial bone CT shows an incidental unilateral small accessory foramen ➡ at the lateral margin of the foramen ovale ➡. The foramen spinosum containing the middle meningeal artery appears normal ➡.*

MIDDLE EAR LESION

DIFFERENTIAL DIAGNOSIS

Common
- Chronic Otitis Media (COM)
- Acquired Cholesteatoma, Pars Flaccida
- Congenital Cholesteatoma, Middle Ear

Less Common
- Acute Otomastoiditis (AOM) with Coalescent Otomastoiditis
- Acquired Cholesteatoma, Pars Tensa
- Cholesterol Granuloma, Middle Ear
- COM with Tympanosclerosis
- COM with Ossicular Erosions

Rare but Important
- Rhabdomyosarcoma, Middle Ear
- Langerhans Histiocytosis, T-Bone
- Dehiscent Jugular Bulb
- Aberrant Internal Carotid Artery

ESSENTIAL INFORMATION

Key Differential Diagnosis Issues
- Otoscopic findings often provide critical clues to precise diagnosis of middle ear lesion in child
  - Presence or absence of tympanic membrane (TM) rupture important
    - Pars tensa &/or flaccida acquired cholesteatoma has ruptured TM
  - Color and location of retrotympanic mass may be key to imaging diagnosis

Helpful Clues for Common Diagnoses
- **Chronic Otitis Media (COM)**
  - Otoscopy: Thickened tympanic membrane
  - Bone CT: Linear, sporadic middle ear-mastoid tissue; mastoid air cells may be underpneumatized
- **Acquired Cholesteatoma, Pars Flaccida**
  - Otoscopy: Rupture or retraction pocket affecting pars flaccida portion of tympanic membrane
  - Bone CT: Nondependent soft tissue filling Prussak space with ossicle and/or bony wall erosions
    - Possible complications: Tegmen tympani, lateral semicircular canal, facial nerve canal dehiscence
- **Congenital Cholesteatoma, Middle Ear**
  - Otoscopy: White mass behind intact TM
  - Bone CT: Smooth, well-circumscribed soft tissue mass filling middle ear; often medial to ossicle chain
    - Ossicle erosion often absent
    - Mastoid pneumatization often normal

Helpful Clues for Less Common Diagnoses
- **Acute Otomastoiditis (AOM) with Coalescent Otomastoiditis**
  - Otoscopy: Bulging, inflamed tympanic membrane
  - Bone CT: Complete middle ear-mastoid opacification with mastoid trabecular breakdown
    - **Hint**: Look on soft tissue windows for adjacent postauricular abscess or epidural abscess
- **Acquired Cholesteatoma, Pars Tensa**
  - Otoscopy: Ruptured pars tensa portion of TM
  - Bone CT: Meso- and hypotympanic soft tissue mass often extending posteriorly or medially
- **Cholesterol Granuloma, Middle Ear**
  - Otoscopy: Blue-black material behind intact TM
  - Bone CT: Middle ear soft tissue mass with minimal bony erosion
  - MR: High T1 and high T2 signal of material in middle ear (ME)
    - **Hint**: Old blood in cholesterol granuloma creates T1 shortening
- **COM with Tympanosclerosis**
  - Otoscopy: Opaque, calcified tympanic membrane
  - Bone CT: Postinflammatory calcifications may affect ossicles, ligaments or TM
- **COM with Ossicular Erosions**
  - Otoscopy: Thickened TM without normal ossicle impressions
  - Bone CT: Linear middle ear and mastoid air cell opacifications with partial ossicle absence
    - Long process of incus-lenticular process and stapes hub most commonly affected

Helpful Clues for Rare Diagnoses
- **Rhabdomyosarcoma, Middle Ear**
  - Otoscopy: EAC "polyp"
  - Bone CT: Destructive middle ear mass that often affects EAC, ossicles, surrounding bones, overlying dura
- **Langerhans Histiocytosis, T-bone**

- Otoscopy: Postauricular mass common
- Bone CT: Unilateral or bilateral (30%) destructive T-bone lesions affecting middle ear secondarily
  - Mastoid air cell more commonly affected than petrous apex or inner ear
- **Dehiscent Jugular Bulb**
  - Otoscopy: Blue lesion behind posteroinferior quadrant of TM
  - Bone CT: Dehiscent sigmoid plate projects jugular bulb into posteroinferior middle ear cavity
- **Aberrant Internal Carotid Artery**
  - Otoscopy: Reddish mass passes across inferior half of TM
  - Bone CT: Tubular lesion passes into posteroinferior middle ear cavity through enlarged inferior tympanic canaliculus
    - Aberrant ICA passes out of middle ear cavity anteroinferiorly by accessing posterolateral margin of horizontal petrous internal carotid artery

Other Essential Information

- Best imaging tool for middle ear lesion in child: T-bone CT without contrast
  - Thin-section, fat-saturated MR only used for further evaluation of larger lesions involving inner ear, floor middle cranial fossa or sigmoid sinus-posterior fossa
- Tumor or tumor-like lesions to consider in middle ear of child
  - Rhabdomyosarcoma and Langerhans cell histiocytosis
  - May be difficult to tell these 2 lesions apart
  - **Rhabdomyosarcoma, Middle Ear**
    - Unilateral; centered in middle ear cavity; may present with EAC "polyp"
  - **Langerhans Histiocytosis, T-Bone**
    - May be bilateral; centered around middle ear cavity, especially in mastoid; may present as postauricular mass

Alternative Differential Approaches

- Otoscopic exam findings vs. diagnosis
  - White middle ear (ME) mass with associated ruptured or retracted pars flaccida TM
    - Acquired cholesteatoma, pars flaccida
  - White ME mass with associated ruptured pars tensa TM
    - Acquired cholesteatoma, pars tensa
  - White ME mass behind intact TM
    - Congenital cholesteatoma, middle ear
  - Blue-black ME mass behind intact TM
    - Cholesterol granuloma, middle ear
  - Red ME mass behind inferior half of intact TM
    - Aberrant internal carotid artery
  - Blue ME mass behind posteroinferior intact TM
    - Dehiscent jugular bulb

Chronic Otitis Media (COM)

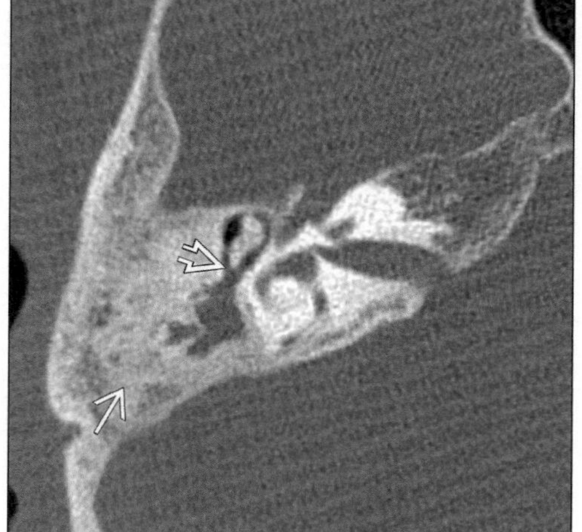

Axial bone CT shows inflammatory debris in the posterior epitympanum ➡ and mastoid antrum with underpneumatization of the mastoid ➡ consistent with the diagnosis of chronic otitis media.

Acquired Cholesteatoma, Pars Flaccida

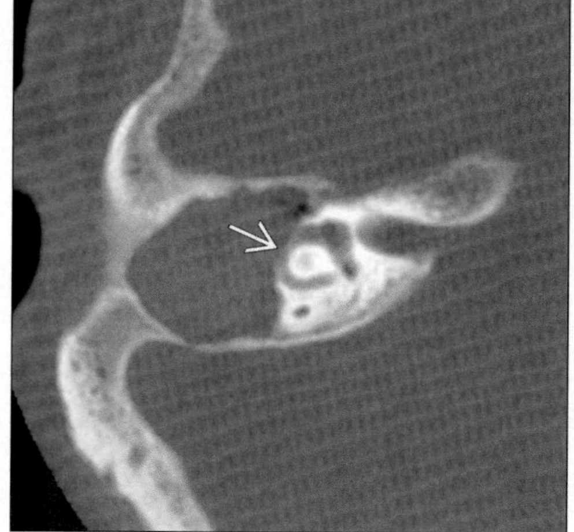

Axial bone CT shows large epitympanic and mastoid cholesteatoma causing dehiscence of the lateral semicircular canal ➡. Notice scalloping enlargement of the mastoid cavity and ossicle destruction.

MIDDLE EAR LESION

(Left) *Axial bone CT reveals a smooth soft tissue mass → filling the anterior mesotympanum medial to ossicle chain. Subtle anterior bony wall erosion is associated →.* **(Right)** *Axial bone CT shows infection of the mastoid has resulted in the confluence of air cells → and destruction of the mastoid cortex →, resulting in TMJ infection with erosion of mandibular condyle →.*

Congenital Cholesteatoma, Middle Ear

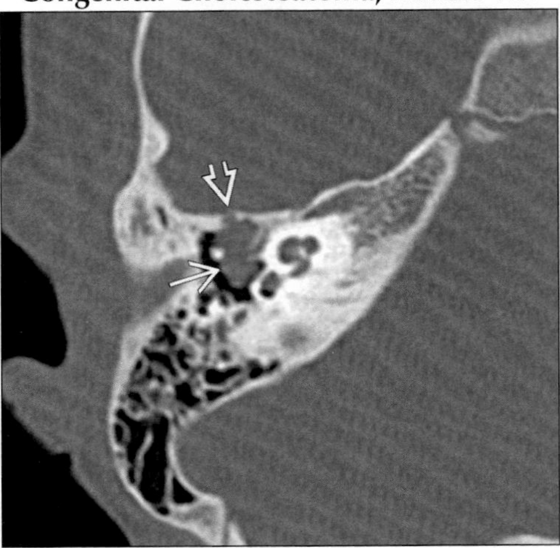

Acute Otomastoiditis (AOM) with Coalescent Otomastoiditis

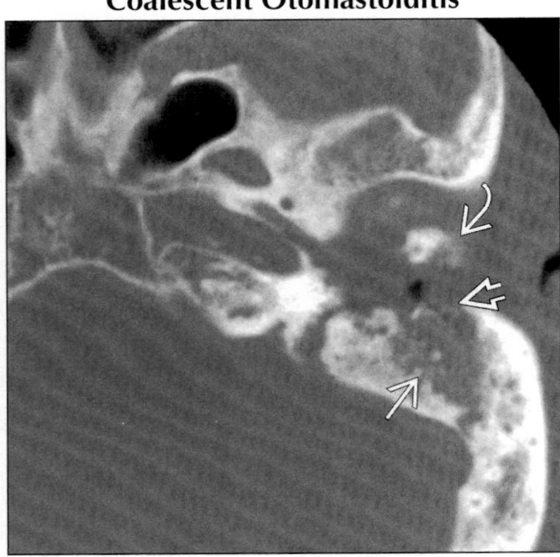

(Left) *Axial bone CT shows a middle ear soft tissue mass → medial to ossicles with a short process of incus erosion and sparing of the Prussak space →. Otoscopy shows perforation in pars tensa TM.* **(Right)** *Axial T1WI MR shows high signal material in the middle ear → and mastoid → cavities. High T1 in cholesterol granuloma is probably secondary to a mixture of old blood and high protein.*

Acquired Cholesteatoma, Pars Tensa

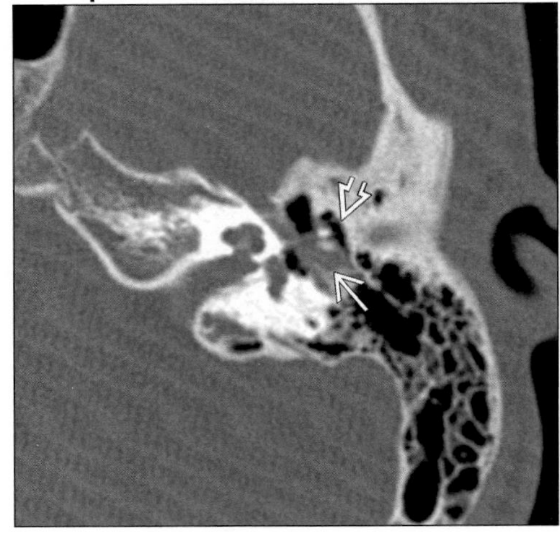

Cholesterol Granuloma, Middle Ear

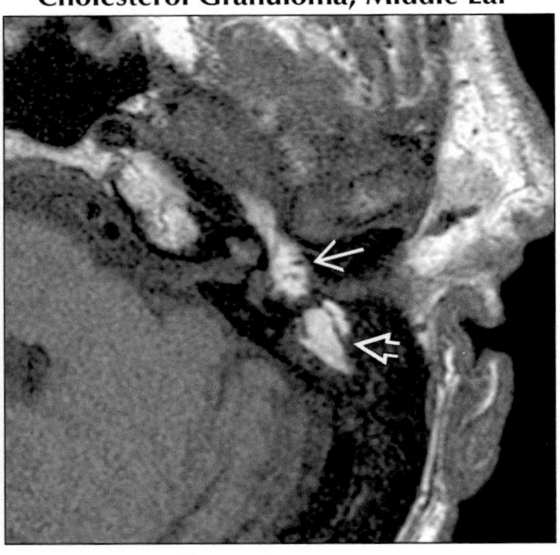

(Left) *Axial bone CT reveals multiple calcified foci → in inflammatory debris surrounding the ossicles in the epitympanum. Underpneumatized mastoid is a common finding of chronic otitis media.* **(Right)** *Axial bone CT shows absence of the distal incus-lenticular process as well as the hub of the stapes →. Notice also the linear stranding in the middle ear cavity from chronic otomastoiditis.*

COM with Tympanosclerosis

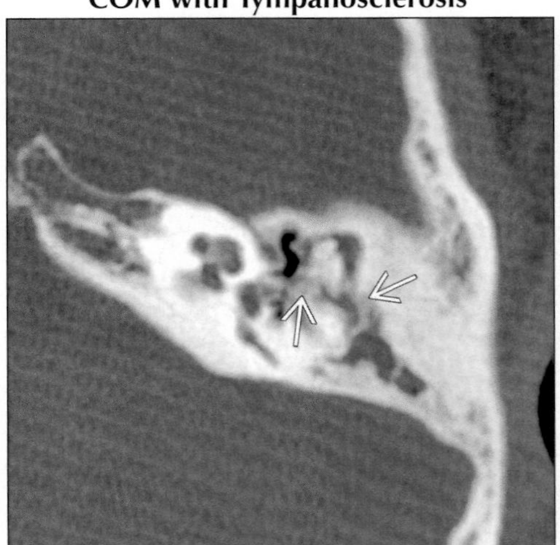

COM with Ossicular Erosions

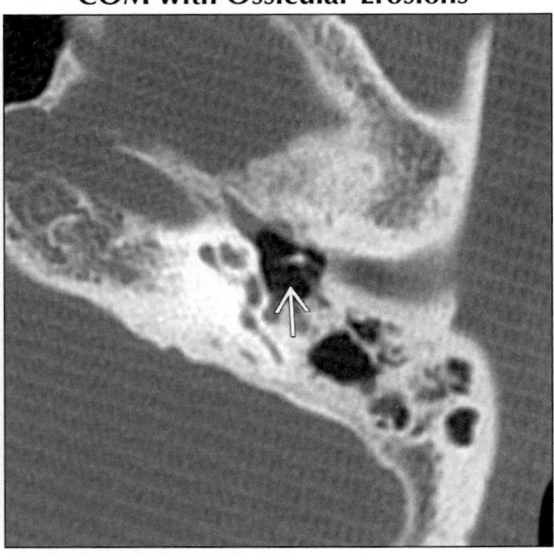

Rhabdomyosarcoma, Middle Ear

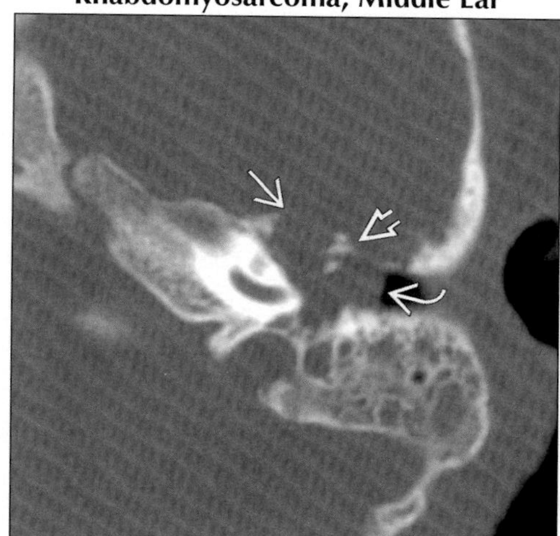

Langerhans Histiocytosis, T-Bone

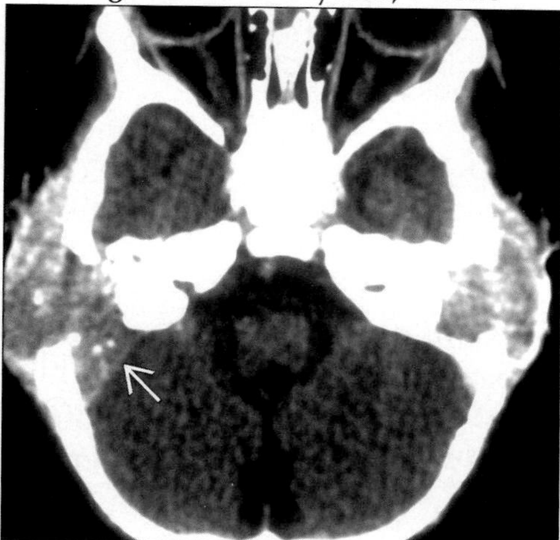

(Left) Axial bone CT demonstrates a destructive mass in the middle ear with loss of anterior bony wall ➔ and ossicular chain erosion ➔. Otoscopic exam showed an EAC "polyp" ➔. *(Right)* Axial CECT shows bilateral enhancing masses in the middle ear and mastoid as well as external ears. Note that on the right the lesion has dehisced the sigmoid plate, involving the posterior fossa ➔.

Dehiscent Jugular Bulb

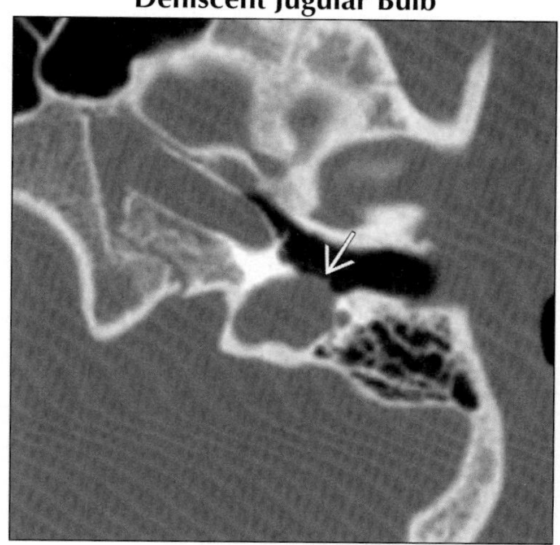

Dehiscent Jugular Bulb

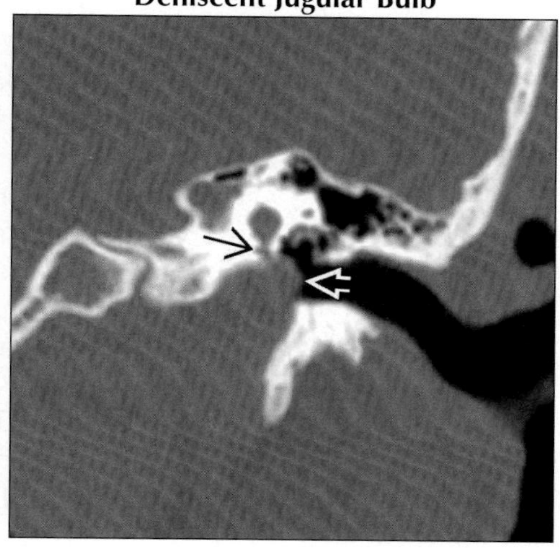

(Left) Axial bone CT reveals a large jugular bulb with a dehiscent lateral margin ➔. The protruding jugular bulb reaches the posteroinferior tympanic membrane where it is visible on otoscopy as a blue lesion. *(Right)* Coronal bone CT reveals a dehiscent jugular bulb projecting superolateral into the middle ear cavity. Note that it "leans" on the tympanic membrane ➔ and fills the round window niche ➔.

Aberrant Internal Carotid Artery

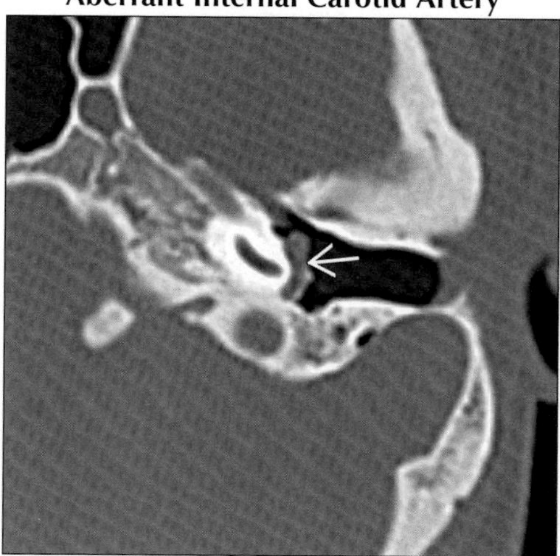

Aberrant Internal Carotid Artery

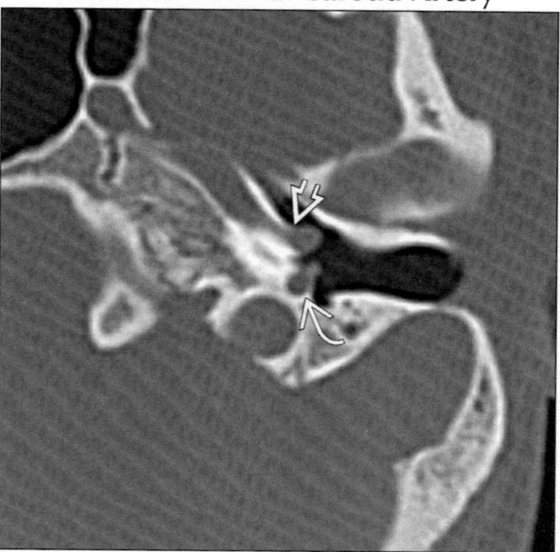

(Left) Axial bone CT demonstrates a tubular lesion ➔ on the cochlear promontory in the middle ear. Do not mistake this lesion for paraganglioma. The tubular appearance is the key to diagnosis. *(Right)* Axial bone CT shows an aberrant internal carotid artery entering the middle ear via an enlarged inferior tympanic canaliculus ➔ and exiting through the horizontal petrous ICA canal ➔.

PETROUS APEX LESION

DIFFERENTIAL DIAGNOSIS

Common
- Asymmetric Marrow, Petrous Apex
- Trapped Fluid, Petrous Apex
- Cholesterol Granuloma, Petrous Apex
- Primary or Metastatic Disease

Less Common
- Cephalocele, Petrous Apex
- Meningioma, T-Bone
- Fibrous Dysplasia, T-Bone
- Schwannoma, Trigeminal, Skull Base
- Cholesteatoma, Petrous Apex
- Chondrosarcoma, Skull Base
- Langerhans Histiocytosis, Skull Base
- Apical Petrositis
- Mucocele, Petrous Apex

ESSENTIAL INFORMATION

Key Differential Diagnosis Issues
- Best imaging tool
  - CT and MR are complementary
    - Bone CT to evaluate petrous apex (PA) "bony" expansion or destruction
    - MR for lesion tissue analysis; characteristic signal per diagnosis
- Beware confusing high T1 MR signal in trapped fluid with PA cholesterol granuloma
  - When protein content is high, T1 signal may be high
  - In absence of bony expansion on CT, lesion should be considered trapped fluid

Helpful Clues for Common Diagnoses
- **Asymmetric Marrow, Petrous Apex**
  - Asymmetric pneumatization makes contralateral fatty marrow conspicuous
  - CT findings
    - Nonexpansile fat density PA
  - MR findings
    - High T1 normal fatty marrow
- **Trapped Fluid, Petrous Apex**
  - Remote otomastoiditis leaves behind PA air cell fluid of variable protein content
  - CT findings
    - Opacified air cells, trabeculae present
  - MR findings
    - Low T1, high T2 signal
- **Cholesterol Granuloma, Petrous Apex**
  - Chronic otitis media; pneumatized PA with recurrent hemorrhage
  - CT findings
    - Smooth, expansile margins
    - Larger lesions affect clivus, jugular tubercle, ICA
  - MR findings
    - High T1 and T2 signal in expanded PA
- **Primary or Metastatic Disease**
  - Rhabdomyosarcoma (primary or mets), neuroblastoma
  - Metastasis occurs late in the disease process
    - Dx of primary disease is usually known
  - Radiographic appearance is variable

Helpful Clues for Less Common Diagnoses
- **Cephalocele, Petrous Apex**
  - Incidental PA lesion where Meckel cave appears herniated into subjacent PA
  - CT findings
    - Expansile ovoid lesion
  - MR findings
    - Low T1, high T2 "pseudopod" from Meckel cave to PA; nonenhancing
- **Meningioma, T-Bone**
  - CT findings
    - Permeative
    - Sclerotic or hyperostotic bony changes
  - MR findings
    - Dural-based mass invades PA with avid contrast-enhancement, dural tail
- **Fibrous Dysplasia, T-Bone**
  - Bone disorder of younger women (< 30 years) with progressive replacement of normal marrow by mixture of fibrous tissue and disorganized trabeculae
    - Active phase: Cystic
    - Least active/burned out: Sclerotic
  - CT findings
    - Expansile bone lesion with mixed ground-glass/sclerotic and cystic components sparing otic capsule
  - MR findings
    - Low T1 and T2 signal, foci of enhancement common
- **Schwannoma, Trigeminal, Skull Base**
  - Larger trigeminal nerve schwannoma involves preganglionic segment as it passes into Meckel cave
  - CT findings
    - Smooth PA remodeling of inferior porus trigeminus margin
  - MR findings

- Homogeneously enhancing tubular mass
- Intramural cysts when large

- **Cholesteatoma, Petrous Apex**
  - Congenital or acquired PA cholesteatoma
  - CT findings
    - Smooth, expansile, low-density lesion
  - MR findings
    - Low T1, high T2
    - Nonenhancing PA lesion with restricted diffusion on DWI
- **Chondrosarcoma, Skull Base**
  - Originates from petrooccipital fissure
  - CT findings
    - Characteristic chondroid matrix in 50%, invasive bony changes
  - MR findings
    - T2 high signal, mixed enhancement
- **Langerhans Histiocytosis, Skull Base**
  - Langerhans histiocytes proliferation forming lytic sites in skull and skull base
  - Peds
    - Onset at 1 year; multifocal < 5 years
  - CT findings
    - Lytic lesion with beveled margins
  - MR findings
    - Avidly enhancing soft tissue mass
- **Apical Petrositis**
  - Fever, retroorbital pain, diplopia, otorrhea
  - CT findings
    - Bony destructive changes
  - MR findings
    - Enhancing thick dura, PA pus does not enhance
- **Mucocele, Petrous Apex**
  - Mimics cholesteatoma; no DWI restriction
  - CT findings
    - Expansile, smooth margined lesion
  - MR findings
    - T1 low, T2 high signal fluid, nonenhancing

Alternative Differential Approaches

- Destructive PA lesions
  - Metastasis
  - Chondrosarcoma
  - Apical petrositis
- Nondestructive, expansile PA lesions
  - Cholesteatoma
  - Cholesterol granuloma
  - Schwannoma
  - Mucocele
  - Aneurysm
- Nondestructive, nonexpansile PA lesions
  - Trapped fluid
  - Asymmetric bone marrow
- Enhancing PA lesions
  - Schwannoma
  - Chondrosarcoma
  - Langerhans cell histiocytosis
  - Apical petrositis
- Marked bone marrow expansion
  - Fibrous dysplasia
- High T1 and T2 signal
  - Cholesterol granuloma
  - High-protein trapped fluid

Asymmetric Marrow, Petrous Apex

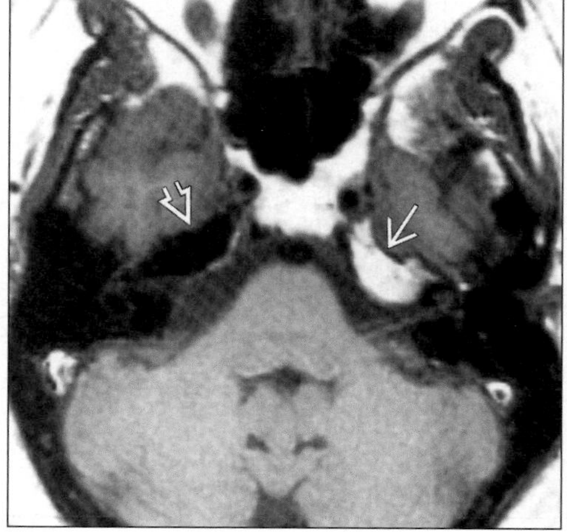

Axial T1WI MR shows high signal intensity fatty marrow in the left petrous apex ➔ without expansile or destructive changes. The contralateral aerated right petrous apex lacks signal ➔.

Trapped Fluid, Petrous Apex

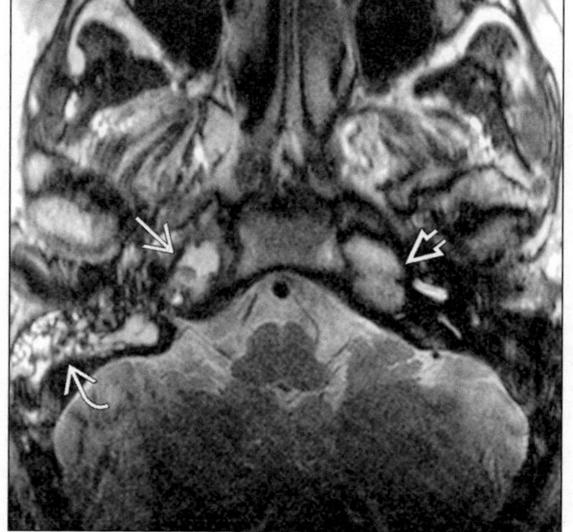

Axial T2WI MR shows high right petrous apex signal, ➔ consistent with fluid. Signal in the left PA ➔ is fat intensity, similar to adjacent marrow. Right mastoid fluid is noted ➔.

PETROUS APEX LESION

(Left) Axial T1WI MR shows a high signal expansile cholesterol granuloma of the petrous apex ➡. (Right) Axial NECT shows a lytic right petrous apex lesion ➡ with destruction of the posterior wall of the middle cranial fossa and anterior margin of the carotid canal.

Cholesterol Granuloma, Petrous Apex

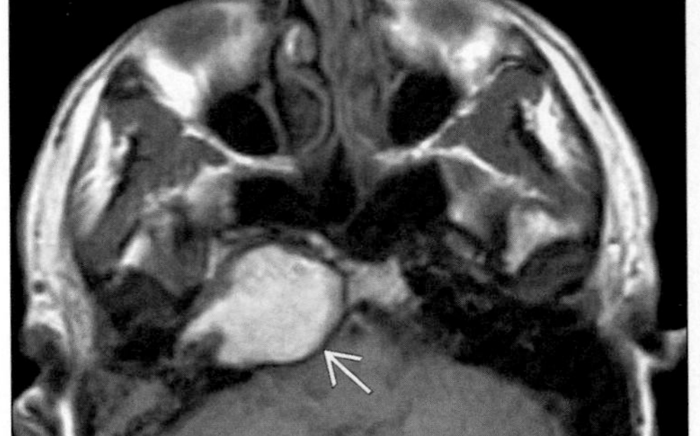

Primary or Metastatic Disease

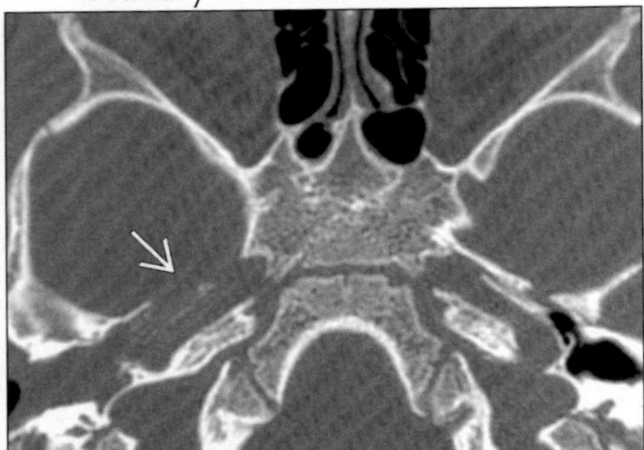

(Left) Coronal NECT in the same child shows a destructive right petrous apex lesion ➡. This lesion was pathologically proven to be primary parameningeal rhabdomyosarcoma. Rhabdomyosarcomas are the most common primary lesion of the PA. (Right) Axial bone CT reveals benign osseous expansion of the anterior left petrous apex ➡, posterior to the left Meckel cave, typical of petrous apex cephalocele.

Primary or Metastatic Disease

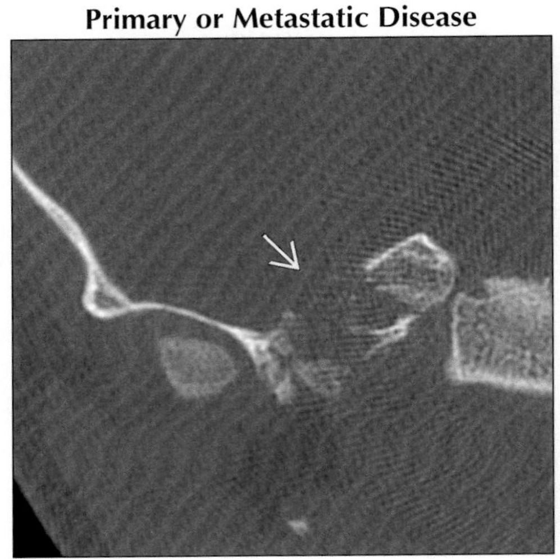

Cephalocele, Petrous Apex

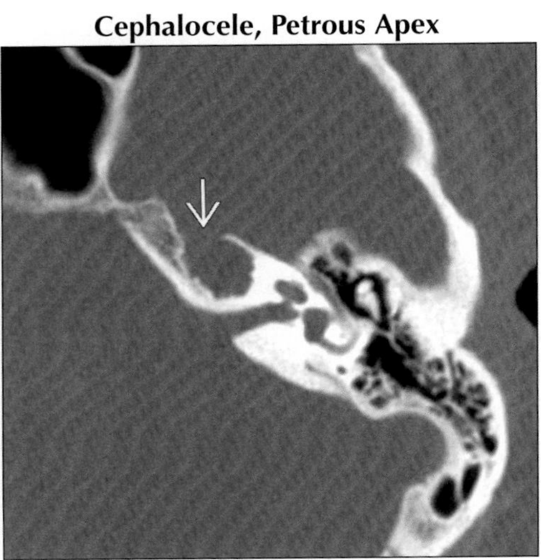

(Left) Axial bone CT shows a high-attenuation dural-based mass in the CPA cistern ➡. Note that the tumor passes through the petrous apex and inferior inner ear bone to access the middle ear ➡. (Right) Axial bone CT demonstrates the characteristic expansile ground-glass appearance of the inner ear ➡ and petrous apex ➡ areas of the temporal bone. The vestibular aqueduct is engulfed ➡.

Meningioma, T-Bone

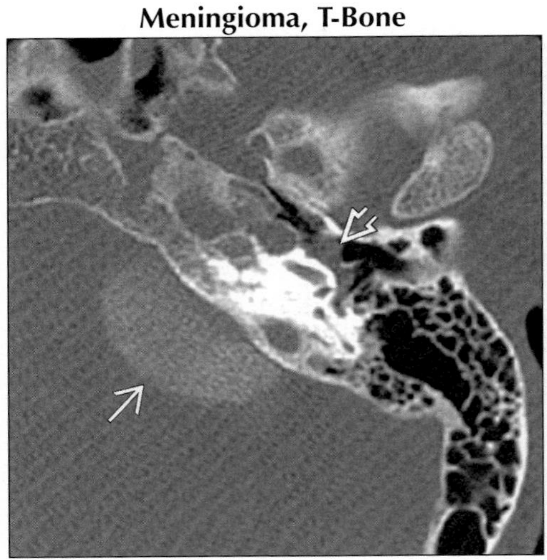

Fibrous Dysplasia, T-Bone

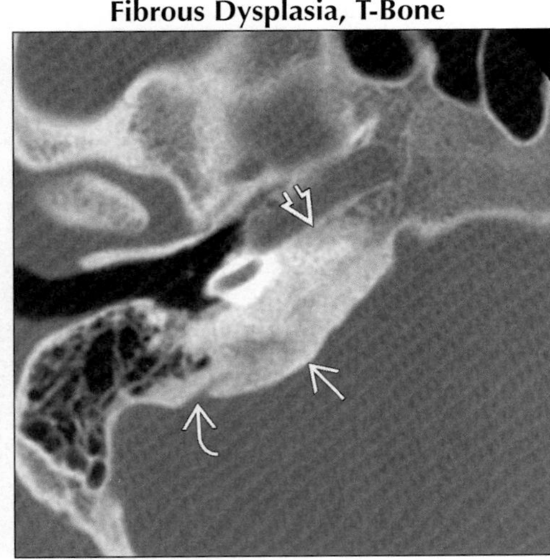

Schwannoma, Trigeminal, Skull Base

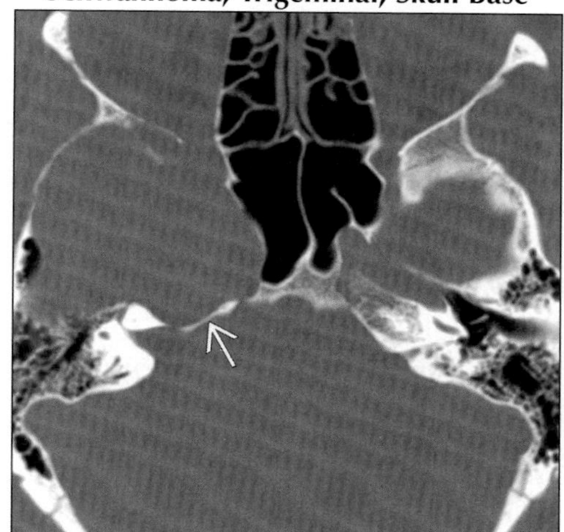

Cholesteatoma, Petrous Apex

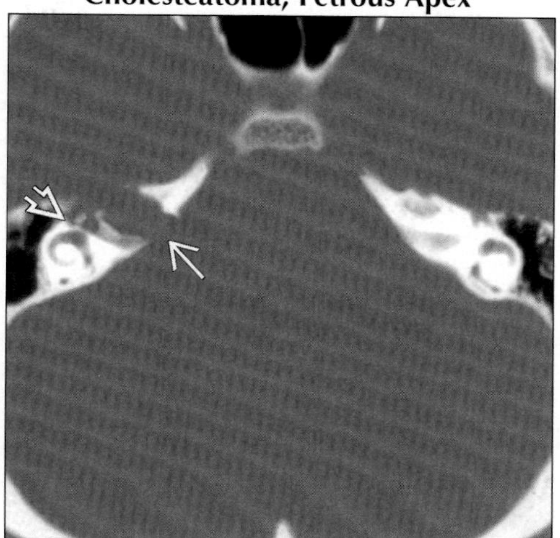

(Left) *Axial bone CT reveals remodeling ➡ of the inferior margin of the porus trigeminus of the Meckel cave from a large trigeminal schwannoma, affecting the preganglionic segment and Meckel cave portion of CN5.* ***(Right)*** *Axial bone CT shows a smooth, expansile lesion in the right petrous apex ➡ with bony erosion of the adjacent cochlea ➡.*

Chondrosarcoma, Skull Base

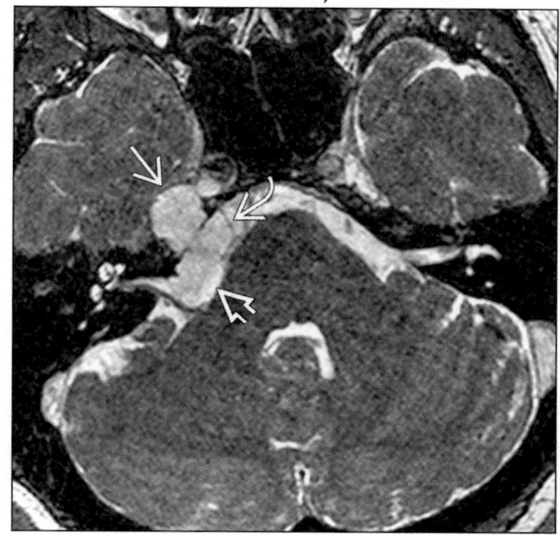

Langerhans Histiocytosis, Skull Base

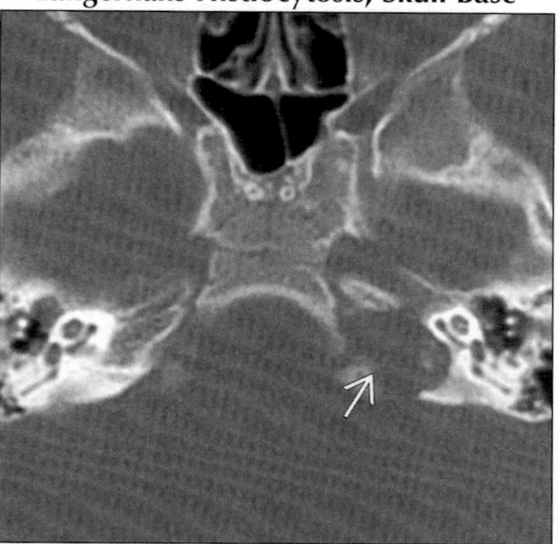

(Left) *Axial T2WI MR 2 mm slice shows high signal chondrosarcoma extending up from the petrooccipital fissure into the petrous apex ➡ and CPA cistern ➡. Note CN6 in the anterior CPA cistern ➡.* ***(Right)*** *Axial bone CT shows a lytic lesion in the left petrous apex ➡ in a child. As rhabdomyosarcoma in this area is centered in middle ear, Langerhans cell histiocytosis is the 1st choice here.*

Apical Petrositis

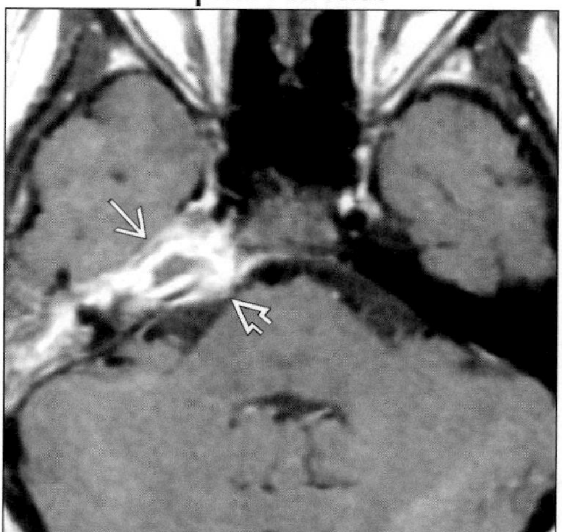

Mucocele, Petrous Apex

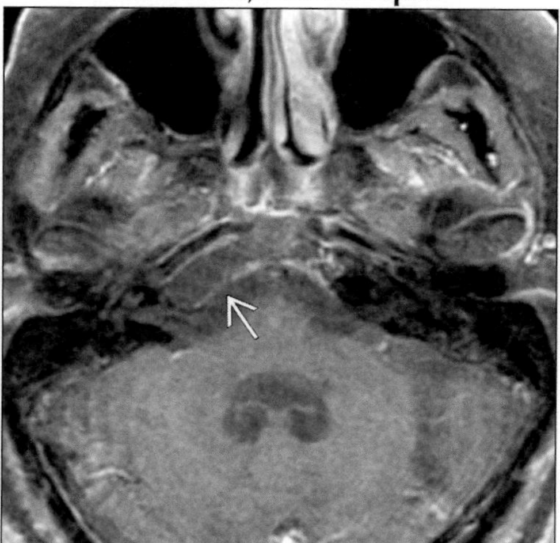

(Left) *Axial T1WI C+ MR reveals abnormal enhancement ➡ around a nonenhancing focus of pus in the petrous apex. Note the associated dural enhancement and thickening ➡.* ***(Right)*** *Axial T1WI C+ FS MR reveals that the expansile right petrous apex mucocele ➡ does not enhance. It lacks MR DWI restriction, which differentiates this lesion from cholesteatoma.*

INNER EAR LESION IN A CHILD

DIFFERENTIAL DIAGNOSIS

Common
- Fracture, T-Bone
- Large Endolymphatic Sac Anomaly (IP-2)
- Labyrinthine Ossificans
- Subarcuate Artery Pseudolesion

Less Common
- Semicircular Canal Dysplasia, CHARGE Syndrome
- Labyrinthitis
- Intralabyrinthine Hemorrhage

Rare but Important
- Cystic Cochleovestibular Anomaly (IP-1)
- Aplasia-Hypoplasia, Cochlear Nerve Canal
- Common Cavity, Inner Ear
- Cochlear Aplasia, Inner Ear
- Osteogenesis Imperfecta, T-Bone
- Branchiootorenal Syndrome, Inner Ear
- X-Linked Mixed Hearing Loss Anomaly
- Labyrinthine Aplasia

ESSENTIAL INFORMATION

Key Differential Diagnosis Issues
- Congenital lesions in differential diagnosis
  - Congenital deafness has imaging diagnosis associated < 50%
  - If imaging diagnosis is found, large endolymphatic sac anomaly (incomplete partition type 2) is most common diagnosis discovered
  - All other inner ear congenital lesions that can be diagnosed by imaging are rare
- Imaging recommendations in childhood sensorineural hearing loss (SNHL)
  - Begin with T-bone CT
  - Add high-resolution T2 MR in axial and oblique sagittal plane when cochlear implant under consideration
    - Define IAC size, integrity of cochlear nerve canal, presence of cochlear nerve

Helpful Clues for Common Diagnoses
- **Fracture, T-Bone**
  - Complex T-bone fractures may involve inner ear structures
  - T-bone CT: Fracture line crosses inner ear ± pneumolabyrinth
- **Large Endolymphatic Sac Anomaly (IP-2)**
  - Clinical clues: Bilateral congenital SNHL that appears in child with cascading hearing loss pattern
  - Most common congenital imaging abnormality
  - CT: Enlarged bony vestibular aqueduct + mild cochlear dysplasia
  - MR: Enlarged endolymphatic sac + mild cochlear aplasia (modiolar deficiency, bulbous apical turn, scala vestibuli larger than scala tympani)
- **Labyrinthine Ossificans**
  - Clinical clues: Child develops profound SNHL after episode of meningitis or middle ear infection
  - Healing of suppurative labyrinthitis may result in osteoneogenesis within inner ear fluid spaces
  - CT: Ossific plaques impinges on inner ear fluid spaces
    - Define as cochlear and noncochlear for cochlear implant evaluation
  - MR: High-resolution T2 shows encroachment on membranous labyrinthine fluid spaces
- **Subarcuate Artery Pseudolesion**
  - Asymptomatic normal variant that disappears in 1st 2 years of life
  - CT: Prominent canal passes beneath superior semicircular canal arch
  - MR: Conspicuous high signal canal on T2 imaging underneath superior semicircular canal

Helpful Clues for Less Common Diagnoses
- **Semicircular Canal Dysplasia, CHARGE Syndrome**
  - Clinical clues: Colobomata, heart defects, choanal atresia, retardation, genitourinary problems, ear abnormalities
  - CT: Bilateral semicircular canal absence, small vestibules, oval window atresia, cochlear nerve canal atresia
  - MR: Cochlear nerve absence
- **Labyrinthitis**
  - Clinical clue: Acute onset vertigo, hearing loss ± facial nerve paralysis
  - CT: Acute phase normal
  - MR: Often normal; if positive, diffuse enhancement of inner ear fluid spaces most common presentation
- **Intralabyrinthine Hemorrhage**

- Clinical clue: May be idiopathic or post-traumatic
- CT: Normal unless associated with trauma
- MR: High T1 signal in inner ear fluid

Helpful Clues for Rare Diagnoses

- **Cystic Cochleovestibular Anomaly (IP-1)**
  - Inner ear morphology: Inner ear looks like tilted "snowman" configuration on axial image
  - CT: Cochlea and vestibule cystic; bony vestibular aqueduct usually normal
  - MR: Both cochlea and vestibule are cystic; endolymphatic sac usually normal
- **Aplasia-Hypoplasia, Cochlear Nerve Canal**
  - CT: Complete or partial bony narrowing of base of cochlear nerve canal
  - MR: Fluid in cochlear nerve canal completely or partially replaced by low signal bone
    - Cochlear nerve absent if aplasia of cochlear nerve canal
- **Common Cavity, Inner Ear**
  - Inner ear morphology: Inner ear looks like single cyst
  - CT: Single cyst with semicircular canals and vestibular aqueduct blended in
  - MR: Single inner ear fluid-filled cyst
- **Cochlear Aplasia, Inner Ear**
  - CT: Cochlea absent with variable deformity of vestibule, semicircular canals and vestibular aqueduct
  - MR: Absent cochlea and cochlear nerve
- **Osteogenesis Imperfecta, T-Bone**
  - Clinical clues: Blue sclera; mild form develops deafness by age 40 years
  - Imaging same as cochlear otosclerosis
  - CT: Active disease shows lucent foci in otic capsule surrounding cochlea
  - MR: Active disease shows enhancing foci in otic capsule
- **Branchiootorenal Syndrome, Inner Ear**
  - Clinical clues: Auricular deformity, prehelical pits, mixed hearing loss, branchial fistulae and renal abnormalities
  - Genetics: 40% with clinical manifestations have mutations of *EYA1* gene on chromosome 8q13.3
  - CT: Hypoplastic apical turn of cochlea, medial deviation of facial nerve, funnel-shaped IAC and patulous eustachian tube
- **X-Linked Mixed Hearing Loss Anomaly**
  - Clinical clues: Male child with bilateral mixed conductive and SNHL
    - Open communication between IAC CSF pressure and cochlear fluid creates perilymphatic hydrops with "gusher" resulting if stapes disturbed
  - CT: Cochlear nerve canal is enlarged with no modiolus
    - Labyrinthine and anterior tympanic facial nerve canal may be enlarged
    - Oval window atresia may be present
- **Labyrinthine Aplasia**
  - CT and MR: Inner ear structures and IAC absent

Fracture, T-Bone

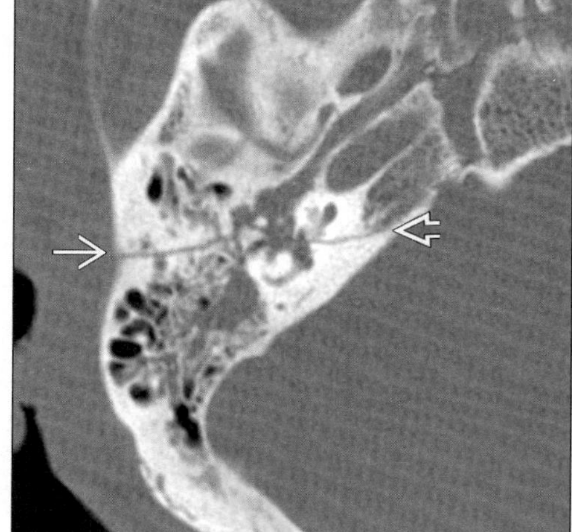

Axial bone CT shows a longitudinal fracture traversing the mastoid ➔, ossicles (note malleus head slightly separated from short process incus), oval window, and inner ear ➔.

Large Endolymphatic Sac Anomaly (IP-2)

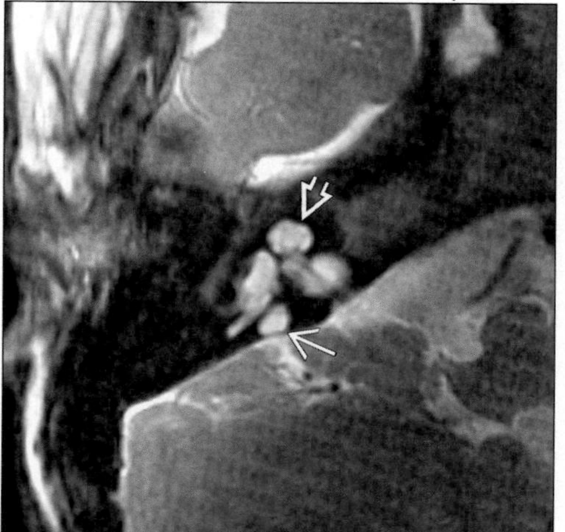

Axial T2WI MR reveals a large endolymphatic sac ➔ associated with significant cochlear dysplasia ➔ characterized by modiolar absence and cystic morphology.

INNER EAR LESION IN A CHILD

*(**Left**) Axial bone CT reveals labyrinthine ossificans affecting the basal turn of the cochlea ➔. Notice the bony encroachment on the cochlear fluid space extends to the round window niche ➔. (**Right**) Axial bone CT shows prominent but normal subarcuate artery canal and associated subarachnoid space ➔ passing under the superior semicircular canal arch ➔ prior to its involution.*

Labyrinthine Ossificans

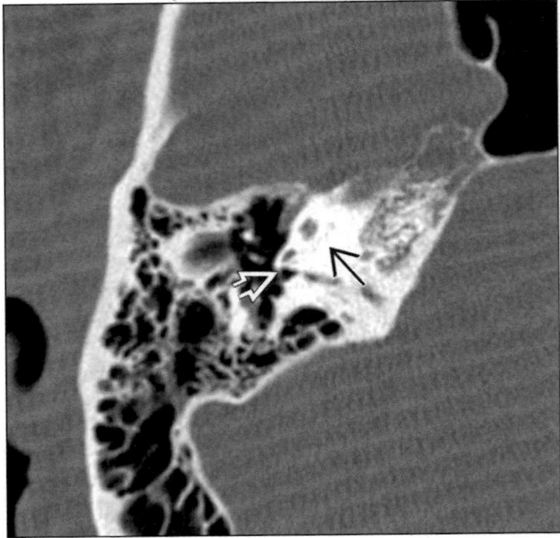

Subarcuate Artery Pseudolesion

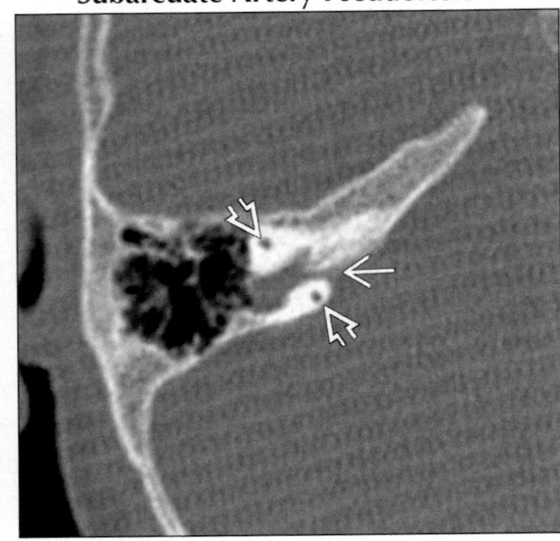

*(**Left**) Axial bone CT shows CHARGE-related absent semicircular canals associated with oval window atresia. The "bare vestibule" has a characteristic small, slightly elongated shape ➔. (**Right**) Axial T1 C+ MR reveals acute otomastoiditis ➔ with secondary suppurative labyrinthitis. The cochlear membranous labyrinth enhances ➔ from being infected by the middle ear pathogens.*

Semicircular Canal Dysplasia, CHARGE Syndrome

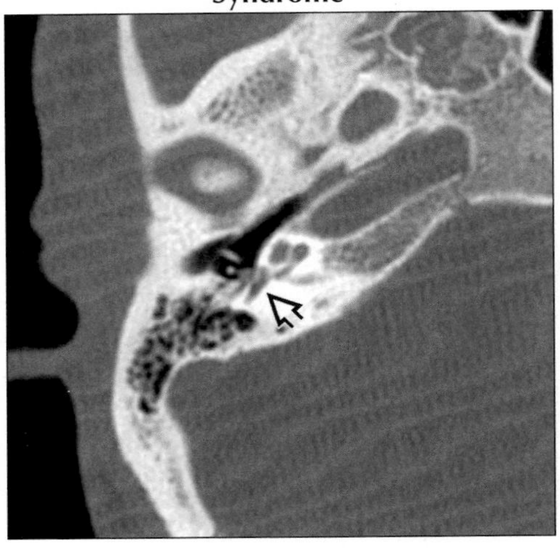

Labyrinthitis

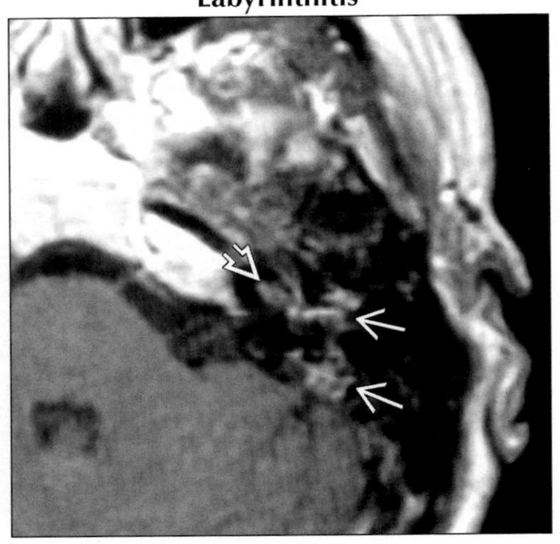

*(**Left**) Axial MRA source image shows high signal blood in ear vestibular ➔ and cochlear ➔ fluid space. Acute sensorineural hearing loss and vertigo heralded this intralabyrinthine bleed. (**Right**) Axial bone CT shows a grossly abnormal inner ear. Both the cochlea ➔ and the vestibule ➔ are cystic, hence the name cystic cochleovestibular anomaly.*

Intralabyrinthine Hemorrhage

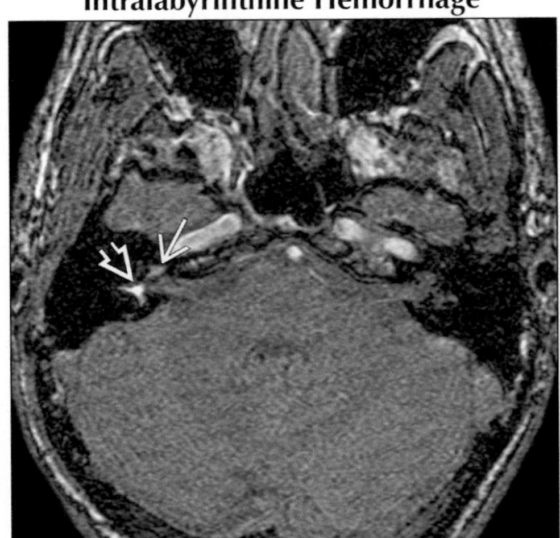

Cystic Cochleovestibular Anomaly (IP-1)

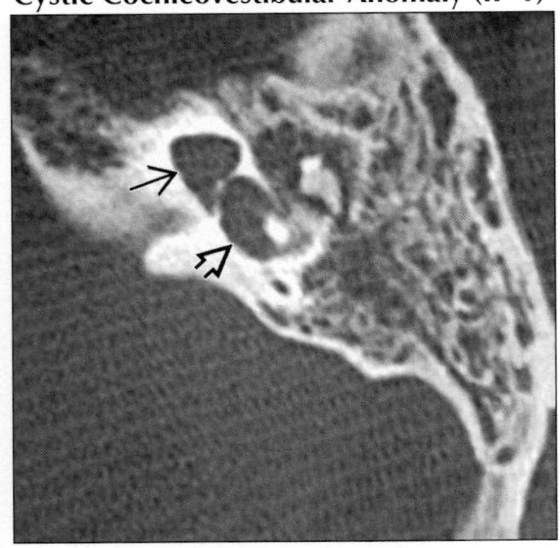

Aplasia-Hypoplasia, Cochlear Nerve Canal

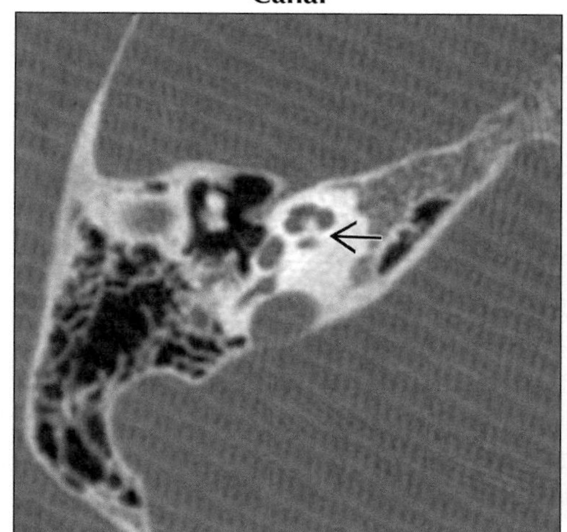

Common Cavity, Inner Ear

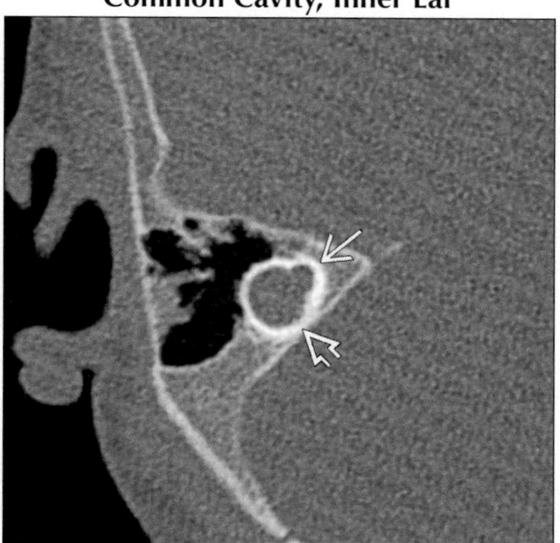

(Left) Axial bone CT demonstrates a bony bar ➔ across the cochlea base separating it from the IAC fundus. Given the cochlear nerve canal is absent, no cochlear nerve is present in this lesion. *(Right)* Axial bone CT shows a multilobular inner common cavity with a large vestibular ➔ and a small cochlear ➔ component.

Cochlear Aplasia, Inner Ear

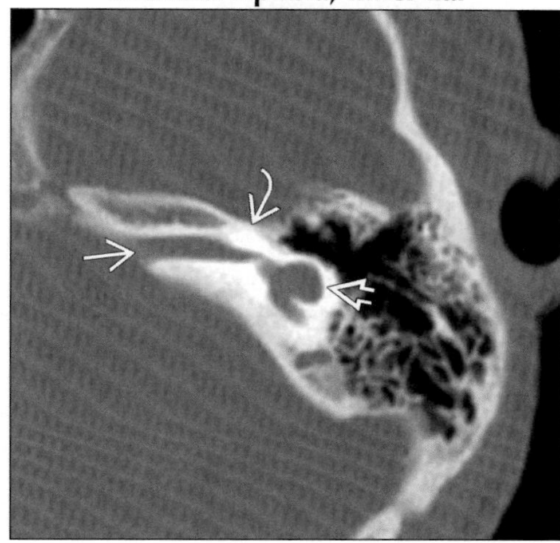

Osteogenesis Imperfecta, T-Bone

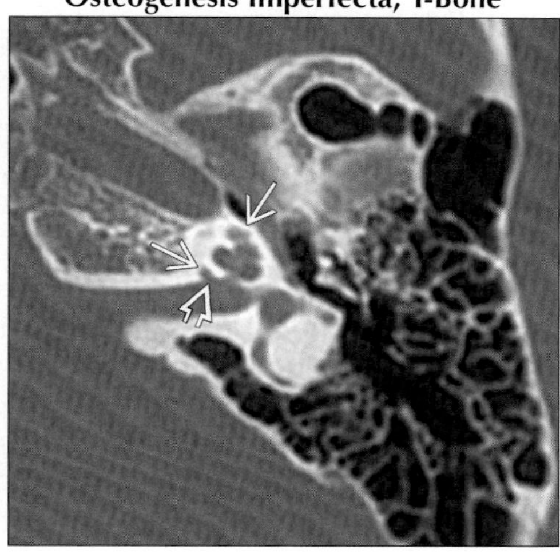

(Left) Axial bone CT reveals a small internal auditory canal ➔, dysplastic vestibule-semicircular canals ➔ and absent cochlea ➔. Absent cochlea implies absent cochlear nerve. *(Right)* Axial bone CT shows multiple lucent foci ➔ in the bony labyrinth. Notice that the active focus medial to the cochlea appears to communicate with the internal auditory canal ➔.

Branchiootorenal Syndrome, Inner Ear

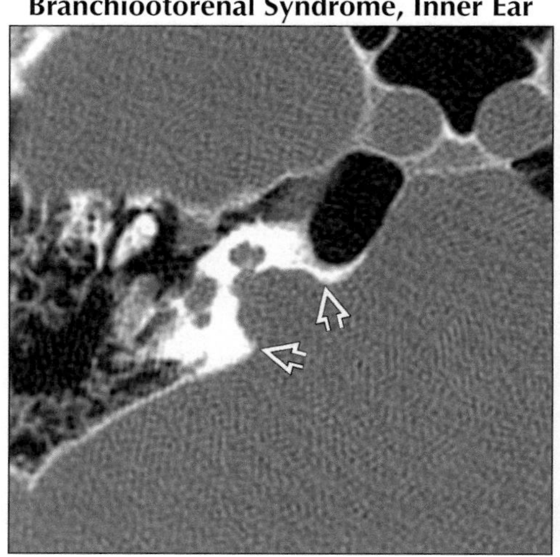

X-Linked Mixed Hearing Loss Anomaly

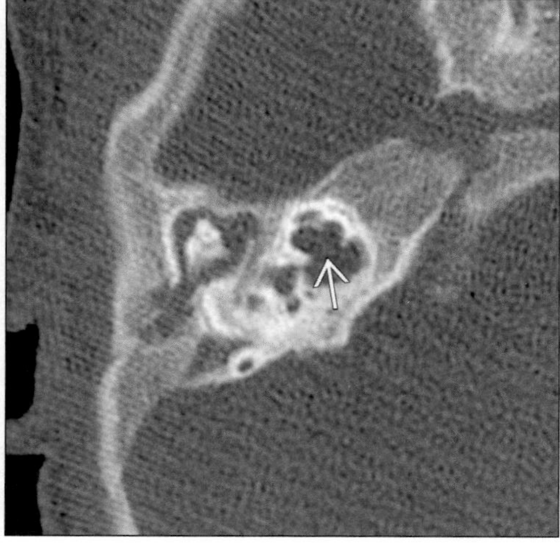

(Left) Axial bone CT shows a widely flared internal auditory canal ➔ suggestive of this diagnosis. A medialized labyrinthine segment of the facial nerve (not shown) is also seen in this lesion. *(Right)* Axial bone CT shows an enlarged cochlear nerve canal ➔ which allows direct communication between the IAC and the cochlea. Note also that the modiolus is absent.

CISTERN, SUBARACHNOID SPACE NORMAL VARIANT

DIFFERENTIAL DIAGNOSIS

Common
- Cavum Septi Pellucidi (CSP)
- Mega Cisterna Magna
- Flow-Related MR Artifacts
- Enlarged Subarachnoid Spaces

Less Common
- Cavum Velum Interpositum (CVI)
- Enlarged Optic Nerve Sheath

Rare but Important
- Blake Pouch Cyst
- Liliequist Membrane

ESSENTIAL INFORMATION

Key Differential Diagnosis Issues
- Normal variants have CSF density/intensity
- Important to recognize normal variants and not mistake for more ominous pathology

Helpful Clues for Common Diagnoses
- **Cavum Septi Pellucidi (CSP)**
  - Elongated finger-shaped CSF collection between frontal horns of lateral ventricles
  - Posterior continuation between fornices often associated (cavum vergae)
- **Mega Cisterna Magna**
  - Enlarged cisterna magna communicates freely with 4th ventricle and basal cisterns
  - Large posterior fossa
  - Normal vermis
  - Cistern crossed by falx cerebelli, tiny veins
  - Occipital bone may appear scalloped
- **Flow-Related MR Artifacts**
  - CSF flow artifact is common in basal cisterns, ventricles
  - Commonly seen on FLAIR MR
  - Artifact often extends outside skull
- **Enlarged Subarachnoid Spaces**
  - Idiopathic enlargement of subarachnoid spaces (SAS) during 1st year of life
  - Increased head circumference (> 95%)
  - Resolves without therapy by 12-24 months

Helpful Clues for Less Common Diagnoses
- **Cavum Velum Interpositum (CVI)**
  - Triangular-shaped CSF space between bodies of lateral ventricles, below fornices, above 3rd ventricle
  - Often elevates, splays fornices and causes inferior displacement of internal cerebral veins and 3rd ventricle
- **Enlarged Optic Nerve Sheath**
  - May occur as normal variant
  - Occurs in idiopathic intracranial hypertension (pseudotumor cerebri), NF1

Helpful Clues for Rare Diagnoses
- **Blake Pouch Cyst**
  - Failure of regression of Blake pouch cyst causes compression of basal cisterns
  - Free communication of 4th ventricle with prominent inferior CSF space
- **Liliequist Membrane**
  - Thin arachnoid membrane separates suprasellar, interpeduncular, and prepontine cisterns

Cavum Septi Pellucidi (CSP)

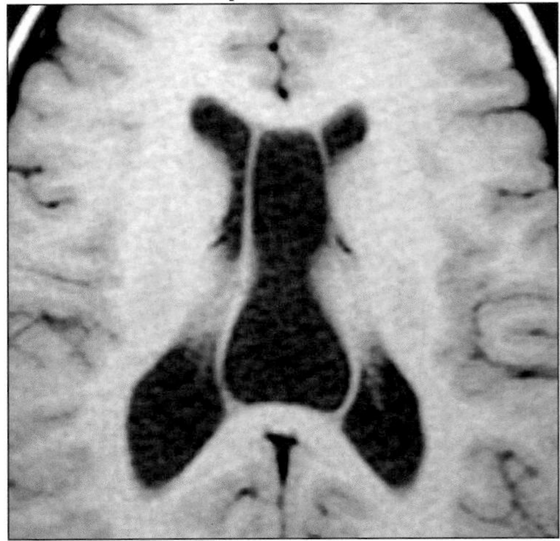

Axial T1WI MR shows a cavum septi pellucidi with posterior extension into a cavum vergae, seen as a CSF-signal collection that lies between the bodies of the lateral ventricles.

Mega Cisterna Magna

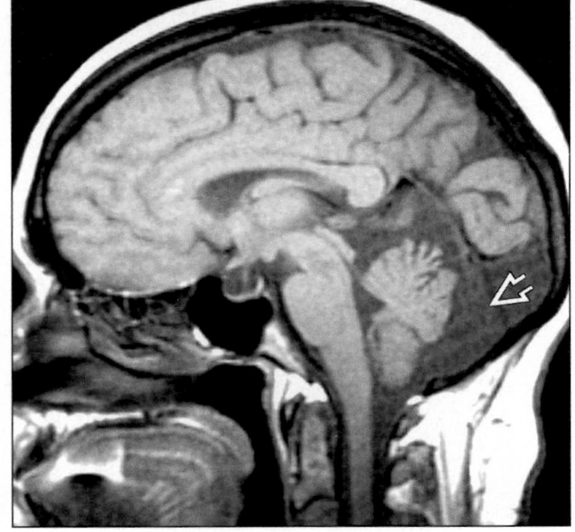

Sagittal T1WI MR shows a prominent retrocerebellar CSF space ➡, a mega cisterna magna. This normal variant requires no treatment. Note the normal vermis and 4th ventricle.

Mega Cisterna Magna

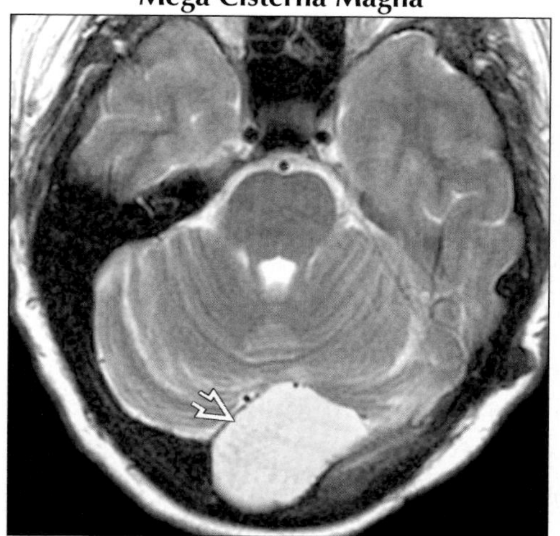

Flow-Related MR Artifacts

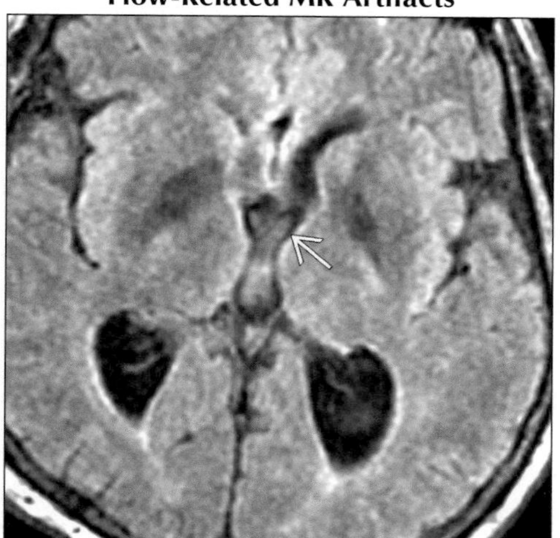

*(**Left**) Axial T2WI MR shows a mega cisterna magna ➡ with scalloping and remodeling of the adjacent occipital bone, likely related to CSF pulsation. (**Right**) Axial FLAIR MR shows a flow artifact in the 3rd ventricle and foramen of Monro ➡, which can mimic a mass. This artifact is often seen on FLAIR MR and can be confirmed on spin-echo sequences (T1).*

Enlarged Subarachnoid Spaces

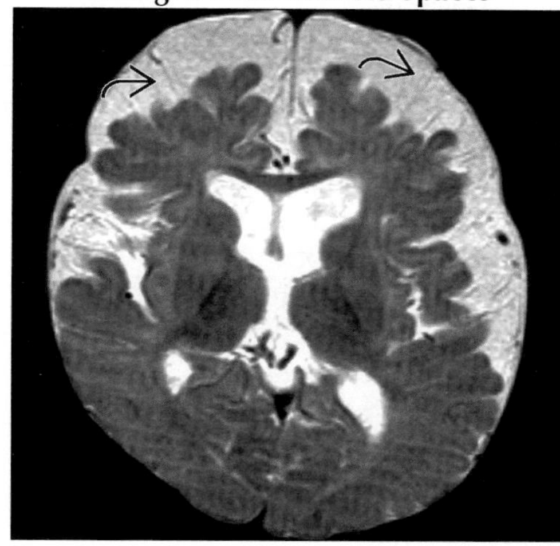

Cavum Velum Interpositum (CVI)

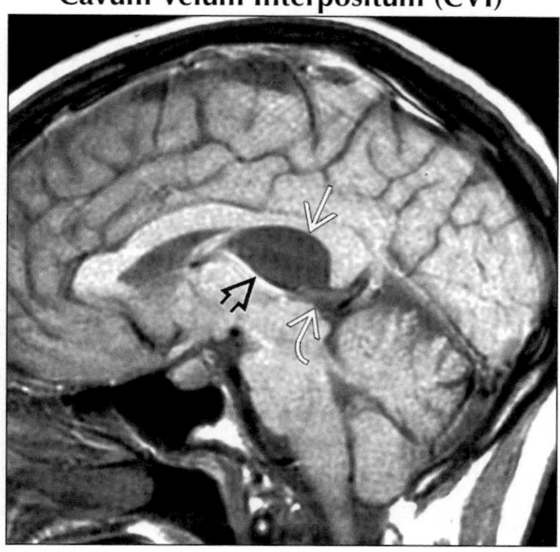

*(**Left**) Axial T2WI MR shows marked enlargement of the frontal CSF spaces. Flow-voids due to traversing veins ➡ are seen, confirming that these are enlarged subarachnoid spaces and not subdural or epidural collections. This condition typically resolves without therapy. (**Right**) Sagittal T1WI MR shows a CVI ➡ that flattens the internal cerebral veins ➡ and compresses the quadrigeminal cistern ➡. Inferior displacement of the 3rd ventricle is also typical.*

Enlarged Optic Nerve Sheath

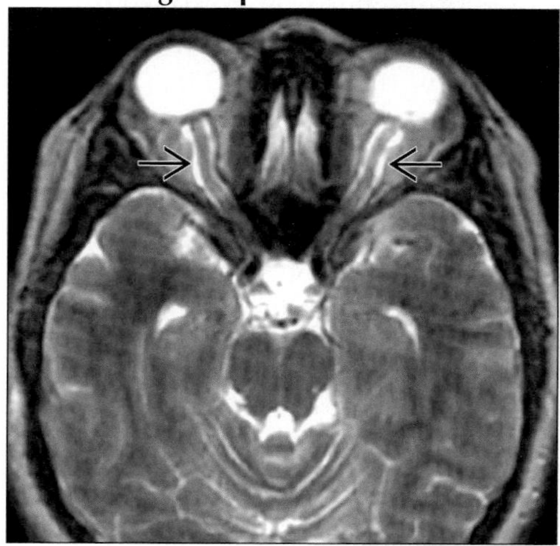

Blake Pouch Cyst

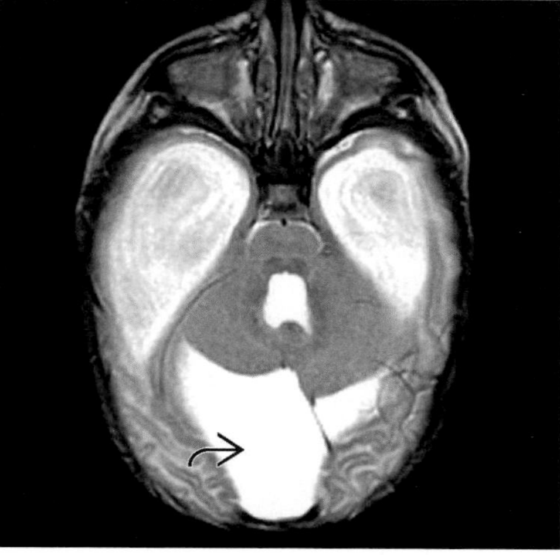

*(**Left**) Axial T2WI MR shows prominent, dilated optic nerve sheaths ➡ and flattened orbits. While patulous optic nerve sheaths can occur as a normal variant, the imaging findings together with clinical presentation are consistent with idiopathic intracranial hypertension. (**Right**) Axial T2WI MR shows an enlarged posterior fossa and Blake pouch cyst ➡. The vermis is typically rotated but normal in these patients.*

INTRACRANIAL HEMORRHAGE

DIFFERENTIAL DIAGNOSIS

Common
- Cerebral Contusion
- Germinal Matrix Hemorrhage
- Diffuse Axonal Injury (DAI)
- Cavernous Malformation

Less Common
- Arteriovenous Malformation
- Venous Thrombosis
- Acute Hypertensive Encephalopathy, PRES

Rare but Important
- Coagulopathies and Blood Dyscrasias
- Herpes Encephalitis
- Hemorrhagic Neoplasms
- Cerebral Infarction, Subacute

ESSENTIAL INFORMATION

Helpful Clues for Common Diagnoses
- **Cerebral Contusion**
  - Key facts
    - Post-traumatic
    - Accidental or nonaccidental
  - Imaging findings
    - Parenchymal hemorrhage: GM and contiguous subcortical WM
    - Typically adjacent to irregular bony protuberance or dural fold
    - Anterior inferior frontal and temporal lobes most common
    - ± surrounding edema
    - ± ST swelling, SDH, SAH, EDH, fracture
    - ± mass effect and herniation
    - Contrecoup injury opposite impact site, frequently more severe than coup injury
    - Coronal reformats very helpful
- **Germinal Matrix Hemorrhage**
  - Key facts
    - Usually < 32 weeks; GA < 1,500 grams
    - Rare > 34 weeks gestational age
    - Rupture of germinal matrix capillaries due to alterations in CBF, ↑ in CVP, coagulopathy, capillary fragility, deficient vascular support, ↑ fibrinolysis
  - Imaging findings
    - Hemorrhage in subependymal region, usually caudothalamic notch (grade 1)
    - ± intraventricular hemorrhage (grade 2)
    - ± ventriculomegaly (grade 3)
    - ± cerebral hemorrhage (grade 4)
    - ± cerebellar parenchymal hemorrhage
    - US: Initial imaging modality of choice
- **Diffuse Axonal Injury (DAI)**
  - Key facts
    - Secondary to trauma-induced axonal stretching
    - Usually high-velocity MVA
    - Hemorrhagic and nonhemorrhagic
  - Imaging findings
    - CT: Frequently normal
    - MR: Punctate hemorrhages at GW junction > corpus callosum, deep GM, and brainstem
    - GRE/SWI for optimal imaging
    - ± diffusion restriction
- **Cavernous Malformation**
  - Key facts
    - a.k.a. cavernomas
    - Benign collections of closely apposed vascular spaces ("caverns")
    - May enlarge, regress, or form de novo
    - Sporadic > > familial (autosomal dominant with variable penetrance)
  - Imaging findings
    - Hemorrhages of different ages
    - "Popcorn ball" appearance with mixed hyper/hypointense blood in locules
    - Hypointense hemosiderin rim on T2WI
    - ± surrounding edema if acute
    - GRE/SWI for optimal imaging
    - Minimal or no CE of lesion
    - ± adjacent enhancing DVA

Helpful Clues for Less Common Diagnoses
- **Arteriovenous Malformation**
  - Key facts
    - Vascular malformation with AV shunting; no intervening capillary bed
    - Supratentorial > > > infratentorial
    - Usually solitary; multiple in HHT
    - Spetzler-Martin scale estimates surgical risk: Size (small, medium, large), location (noneloquent or eloquent area), and venous drainage (superficial or deep)
  - Imaging findings
    - Enlarged arteries and draining veins
    - "Honeycomb" of flow voids
    - ± calcification
    - ± hemorrhage
    - ± surrounding high signal gliosis
- **Venous Thrombosis**
  - Cortical vein &/or dural sinus thrombosis

- Patchy cortical/subcortical hemorrhages
- Temporal lobe hemorrhage: Think vein of Labbe thrombus

- **Acute Hypertensive Encephalopathy, PRES**
  - Key facts
    - Posterior reversible encephalopathy syndrome (PRES)
    - Abnormal cerebrovascular autoregulation
    - Present with headache, seizure, and altered mental status
    - Associated with hypertension, uremic encephalopathies, drug toxicity, tumor lysis syndrome, and sepsis with shock
  - Imaging findings
    - Multifocal edema in posterior parietal, occipital lobes > basal ganglia > brainstem
    - Frequently bilateral but asymmetric
    - Restricted diffusion uncommon
    - Hemorrhage in minority of lesions, may only be petechial hemorrhage on MR

Helpful Clues for Rare Diagnoses

- **Coagulopathies and Blood Dyscrasias**
  - HUS, TTP, DIC, thrombocytopenia, vitamin K deficiency
    - Supratentorial and parenchymal hemorrhage most common
  - Anticoagulation complications
    - Mixed-density hemorrhages, ± fluid-fluid levels, unclotted blood, hemorrhage may be hypoechoic on US
    - Diligent search for hemorrhage in patients on ECMO
- **Herpes Encephalitis**
  - Key facts
    - Reactivation in non-neonate, immunocompetent patient = HSV-1
    - Neonatal disease: HSV-2 = 85% peripartum transmission
  - Imaging findings
    - **HSV-1:** Edema in limbic system = temporal lobes, insula, subfrontal area, cingulate gyri
    - Typically bilateral but asymmetric
    - Rarely effects midbrain and pons
    - ± patchy contrast enhancement
    - ± petechial hemorrhage, usually in subacute phase
    - **HSV-2:** Early edema and diffusion abnormality
    - WM, GM (cortical and BG), temporal lobe, brainstem, CB ± watershed
    - Hemorrhage less common than with HSV-1
- **Hemorrhagic Neoplasms**
  - Glioblastoma multiforme: Necrosis and hemorrhage common, may be multifocal
  - Leukemia (± dural sinus thrombosis), primary CNS lymphoma in HIV/AIDS
  - Other neoplasms before or after radiation therapy
- **Cerebral Infarction, Subacute**
  - Hemorrhagic transformation 2-3 days after arterial infarction uncommon in children

Cerebral Contusion

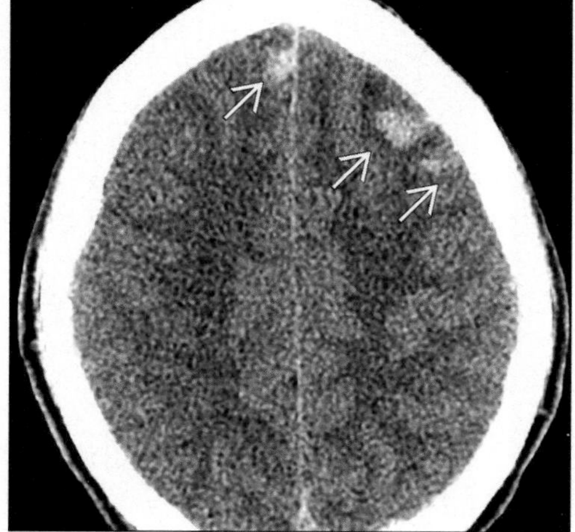

Axial NECT shows multiple hemorrhagic frontal lobe contusions ➡ adjacent to the left frontal bone and anterior falx.

Germinal Matrix Hemorrhage

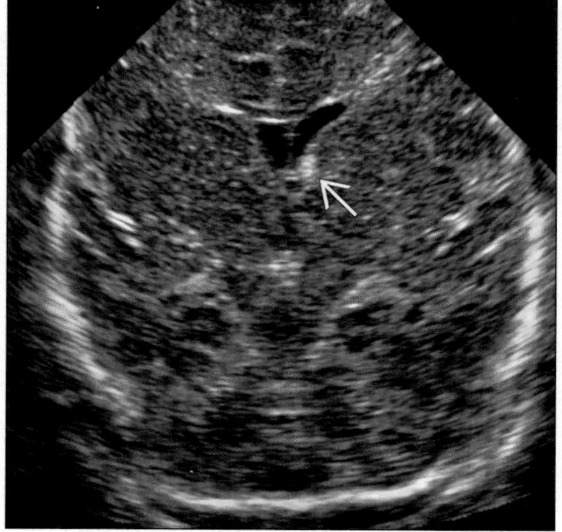

Coronal ultrasound shows left caudothalamic notch grade 1 germinal matrix hemorrhage ➡.

INTRACRANIAL HEMORRHAGE

*(**Left**) Axial NECT shows minimal prominence of the lateral ventricles and sulci, without intraparenchymal hemorrhage. CT is frequently normal in the setting of DAI. (**Right**) Axial GRE MR in the same patient shows multiple foci of hemorrhage secondary to DAI, involving the gray-white junction ➔, right thalamus ➔, and corpus callosum ➔.*

Diffuse Axonal Injury (DAI)

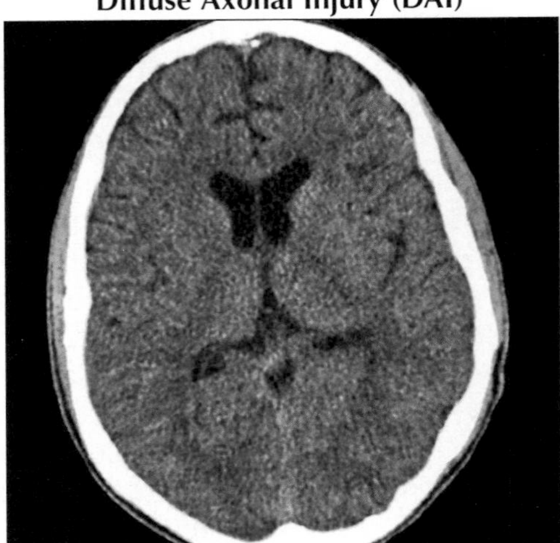

Diffuse Axonal Injury (DAI)

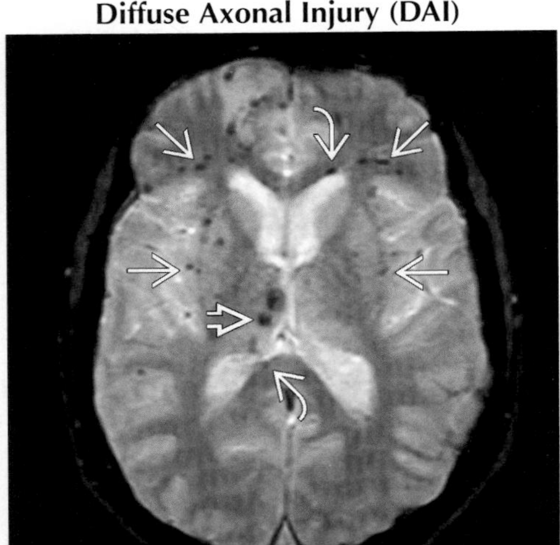

*(**Left**) Axial NECT demonstrates a focal area of high attenuation ➔ in the left frontal lobe white matter, with ill-defined margins, punctate foci of higher attenuation ➔, and without surrounding edema or mass effect. (**Right**) Axial T1WI MR shows the typical "popcorn" appearance ➔ of a subacute hemorrhage, with minimal adjacent edema ➔.*

Cavernous Malformation

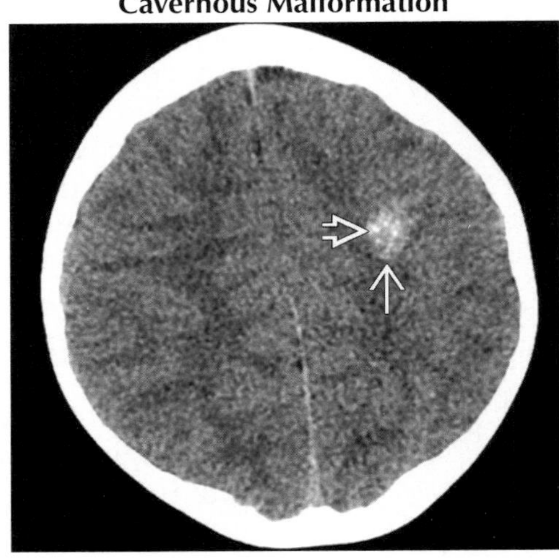

Cavernous Malformation

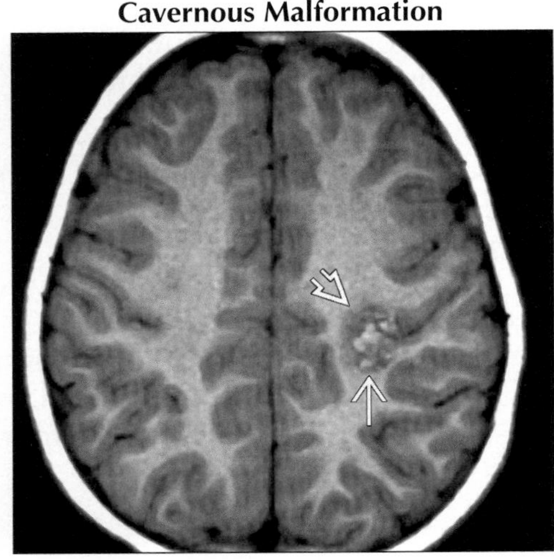

*(**Left**) Axial NECT shows a large left frontal lobe hematoma ➔ with mild surrounding edema, mass effect, left-to-right shift of midline ➔, and minimal 3rd ventricle hemorrhage ➔. (**Right**) Axial T2WI MR in the same patient shows a lobulated area of flow voids at the periphery of the hematoma ➔, which were proven to represent prominent draining veins on conventional angiography. Notice also the prominent left perimesencephalic vein ➔.*

Arteriovenous Malformation

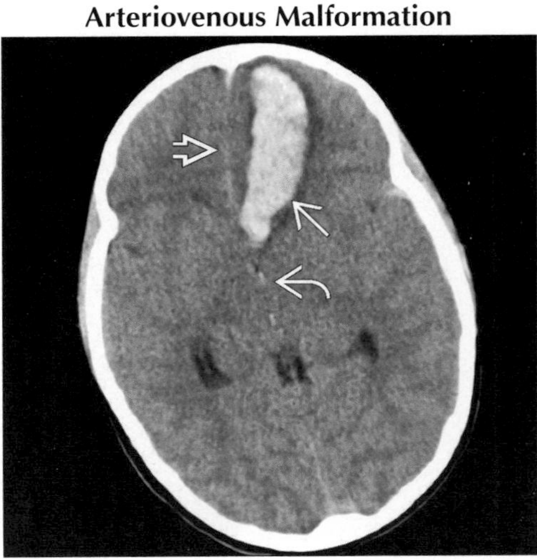

Arteriovenous Malformation

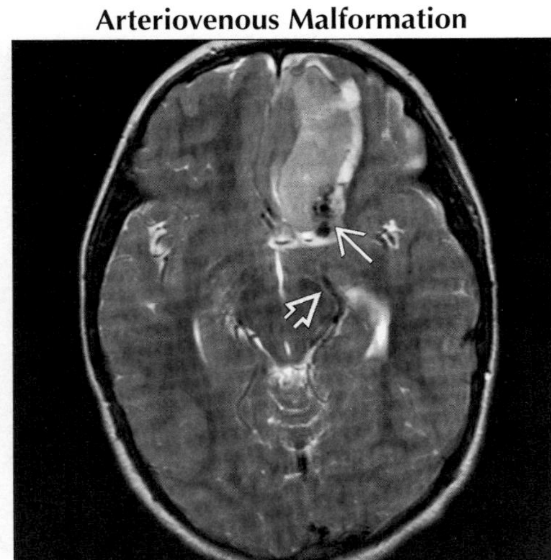

Venous Thrombosis

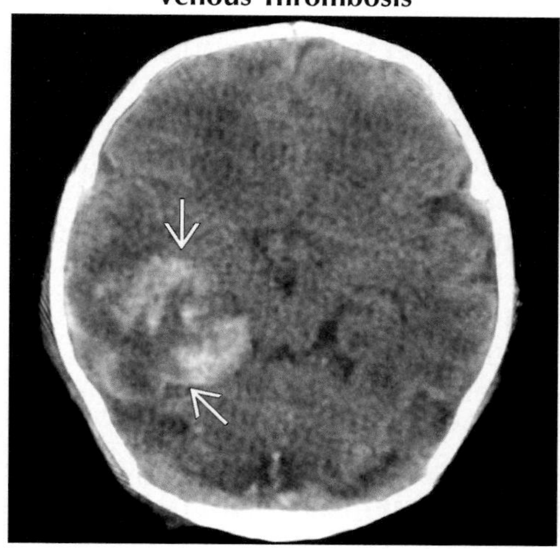

Acute Hypertensive Encephalopathy, PRES

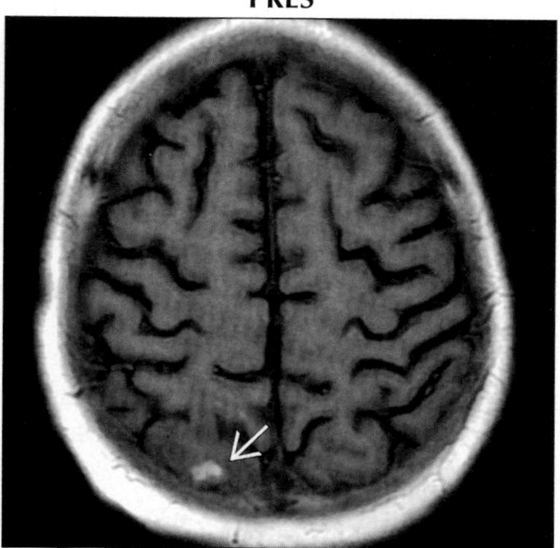

(Left) *Axial NECT shows the typical location of parenchymal hemorrhage in the posterior right temporal lobe ➡, secondary to vein of Labbe thrombosis in a neonate.* ***(Right)*** *Axial FLAIR MR shows a small hemorrhagic focus in the right parietal lobe ➡ with mild edema, in a child who had multiple other areas of nonhemorrhagic vasogenic edema in the posterior circulation and watershed territories (not shown), secondary to hypertensive encephalopathy.*

Coagulopathies and Blood Dyscrasias

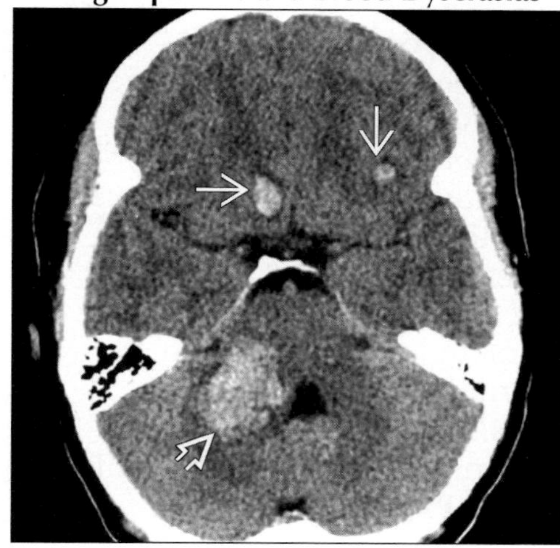

Herpes Encephalitis

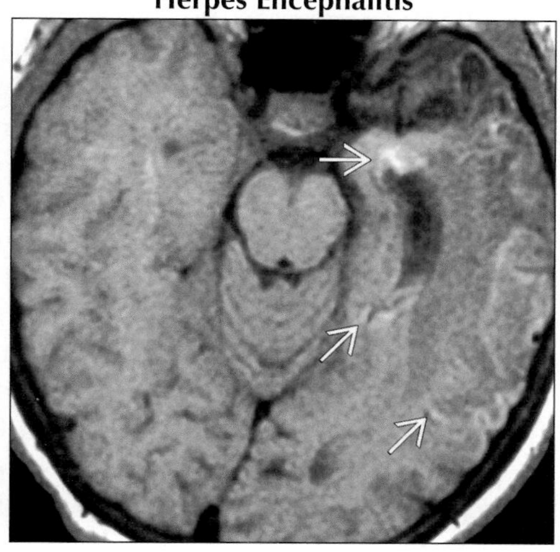

(Left) *Axial NECT shows multiple spontaneous hemorrhages in the frontal lobes ➡ and right brachium pontis ➡ in a child with severe thrombocytopenia and ALL. Differential diagnosis includes hemorrhagic leukemic infiltrates.* ***(Right)*** *Axial T1WI MR shows T1 hyperintense petechial hemorrhage in the left temporal lobe ➡.*

Herpes Encephalitis

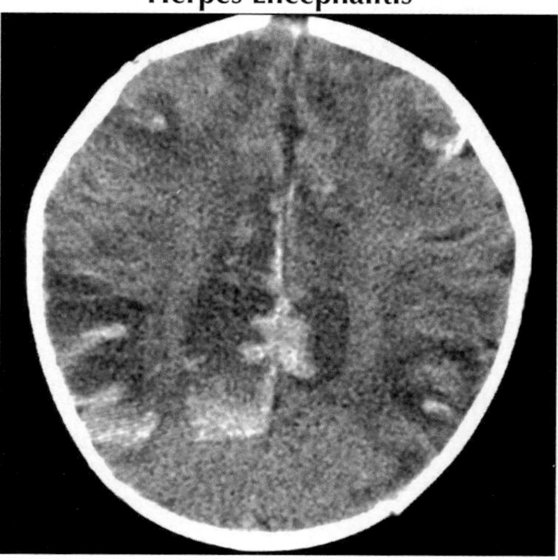

Hemorrhagic Neoplasms

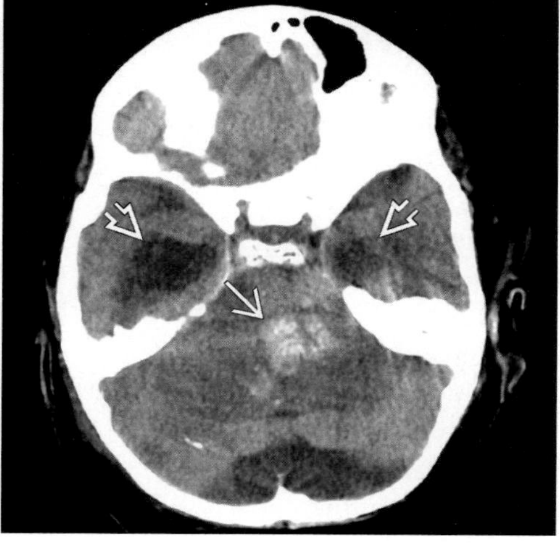

(Left) *Axial NECT shows multifocal cortical hemorrhage with surrounding edema in the bilateral frontal and parietal lobes in a neonate with hemorrhagic encephalitis secondary to HSV-2.* ***(Right)*** *Axial NECT shows heterogeneous hemorrhage ➡ within a large pontine glioma, in a child who had previously been treated with radiation therapy. Also note the obstructive hydrocephalus ➡.*

LATERAL VENTRICULAR MASS

DIFFERENTIAL DIAGNOSIS

Common
- Choroid Plexus Cyst
- Intraventricular Hemorrhage (IVH)

Less Common
- Subependymal Giant Cell Astrocytoma
- Ependymal Cyst
- Choroid Plexus Papilloma

Rare but Important
- Choroid Plexus Carcinoma
- Meningioma
- Langerhans Cell Histiocytosis
- Central Neurocytoma
- Subependymoma
- Ependymoma

ESSENTIAL INFORMATION

Helpful Clues for Common Diagnoses
- **Choroid Plexus Cyst**
  - Key facts
    - Most common intraventricular mass in children and adults
    - Any age; adults > > children
    - Frequently bilateral
    - Usually incidental; rarely large enough to ⇒ obstructive hydrocephalus
    - Lateral ventricle > > > 3rd ventricle
  - Imaging findings
    - Cyst within or attached to choroid plexus
    - CE cyst wall and surrounding choroid
    - Hyperintense FLAIR and DWI common
    - ± irregular peripheral calcifications
    - Xanthogranuloma = laden degenerative cyst; more common in adults
- **Intraventricular Hemorrhage (IVH)**
  - Key facts
    - 2° to germinal matrix hemorrhage, trauma, tumor, or vascular malformation
  - Imaging findings
    - Intraventricular hemorrhage initially hyperechoic and hyperdense
    - ± dependent fluid-fluid level
    - ± clotted blood adherent to choroid plexus
    - May → ventriculitis &/or hydrocephalus
    - Post-traumatic IVH: Frequently with SAH, and usually sequelae of severe injury

Helpful Clues for Less Common Diagnoses
- **Subependymal Giant Cell Astrocytoma**
  - Key facts
    - Present in 15% of patients with tuberous sclerosis complex
  - Imaging findings
    - Heterogeneously enhancing mass near foramen of Monro
    - ± calcifications
    - + intraparenchymal hamartomas
    - ± obstructive hydrocephalus
    - ± globe hamartomas
    - Enhancement alone does not allow discrimination from hamartoma
    - Growth suggests subependymal giant cell astrocytoma rather than hamartoma
    - MRS: Less than expected ↓ NAA due to neuronal elements in tumor
- **Ependymal Cyst**
  - Key facts
    - Synonym: Neuroepithelial cyst
    - Congenital, benign ependymal-lined cyst
    - Intraventricular, central WM of temporoparietal and frontal lobes, subarachnoid space, mesencephalon
  - Imaging findings
    - Lateral ventricle > > > 3rd and 4th ventricle
    - Nonenhancing, thin-walled cyst
    - Round or multiseptated
    - Similar to CSF on all imaging
    - ± hyperintensity on T2WI and FLAIR
- **Choroid Plexus Papilloma**
  - Key facts
    - Lateral > 3rd and 4th ventricle in children
    - 4th ventricle most common site in adults
    - Usually < 1 year of age at diagnosis
    - Males > > > females
    - Rarely bilateral
    - Usually present with hydrocephalus secondary to obstruction, CSF overproduction by tumor or hemorrhage ⇒ impaired CSF resorption
    - Differentiation from choroid plexus carcinoma is histologic, not radiologic
  - Imaging findings
    - CT: Lobulated, isodense, or hyperdense
    - ± punctate foci calcification
    - T2 hypointense center
    - Intense contrast enhancement

- MRS: Absent NAA and Cr/PhCr peak, increased lactate secondary to necrosis, not necessarily more aggressive
- ± CSF metastases

Helpful Clues for Rare Diagnoses

- **Choroid Plexus Carcinoma**
  - Key facts
    - ≈ always in lateral ventricle
    - Usually 3-5 years of age
    - Males = females
    - Usually present with hydrocephalus ± focal neurological deficits related to local brain invasion
  - Imaging findings
    - Heterogeneous mass with irregular margins + parenchymal invasion ± surrounding edema
    - Cysts, hemorrhage, and necrosis common
    - MRS: Absent NAA and Cr/PhCr peak; higher choline peak than papilloma + increased lactate
    - ± CSF metastasis
- **Meningioma**
  - Key facts
    - Lateral ventricle atrium most common site; left > right
    - Uncommon in children; consider NF2
    - Pediatric meningiomas: More frequently large, cystic, rapidly growing, and malignant vs. adult disease
  - Imaging findings
    - Lobular, intensely enhancing intraventricular mass
    - ± calcification ± cysts, hemorrhage
    - Heterogeneity or indistinct margins favor higher degrees of malignancy
- **Langerhans Cell Histiocytosis**
  - CNS involvement = pituitary infundibulum, parenchymal, dural, or choroid plexus
  - Marked T2 and FLAIR hypointensity, intense contrast enhancement
- **Central Neurocytoma**
  - Key facts: Arise from septum pellucidum
    - Primarily in young adults
  - Imaging findings
    - "Bubbly" mass with heterogeneous CE
    - Well-defined, lobulated mass
    - Necrosis and cysts common
- **Subependymoma**
  - Key facts: Middle-aged and elderly
  - Imaging findings
    - Nonenhancing mass
    - Inferior 4th ventricle and frontal horns of lateral ventricles most common locations
- **Ependymoma**
  - Key facts
    - 4th ventricle > > lateral ventricles
    - Supratentorial, usually in periventricular white matter
  - Imaging findings
    - Ca++ common ± cysts, hemorrhage, necrosis
    - Variable CE of cyst walls & solid portion

Choroid Plexus Cyst

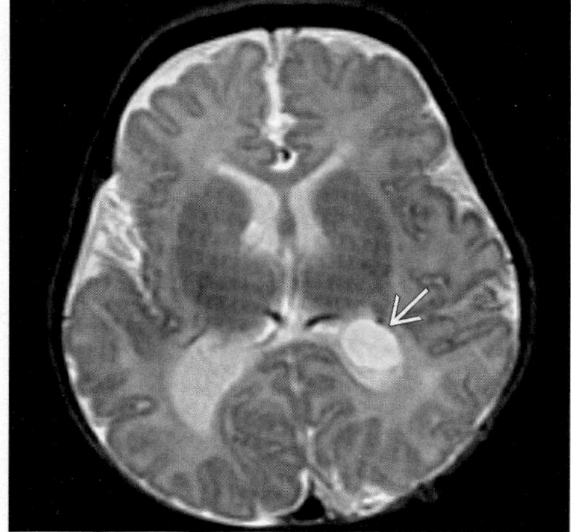

Axial T2WI MR shows a mildly hyperintense, incidental choroid plexus cyst ➔ in the atrium of the left lateral ventricle.

Intraventricular Hemorrhage (IVH)

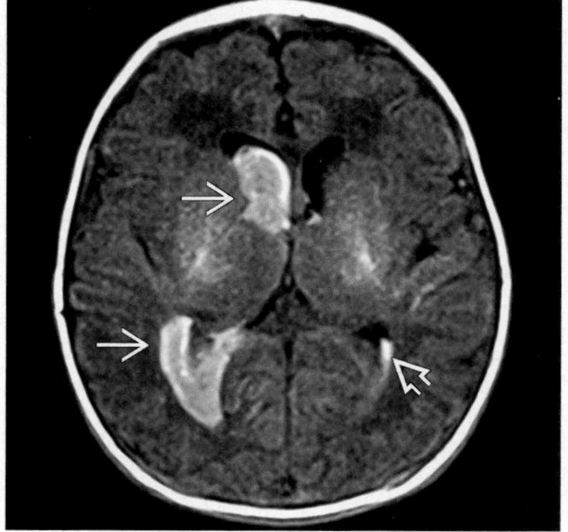

Axial T1WI FS MR shows hyperintense subacute hemorrhage filling the right lateral ventricle ➔, with a small amount of hemorrhage in the occipital horn of the left lateral ventricle ➔.

LATERAL VENTRICULAR MASS

Intraventricular Hemorrhage (IVH)

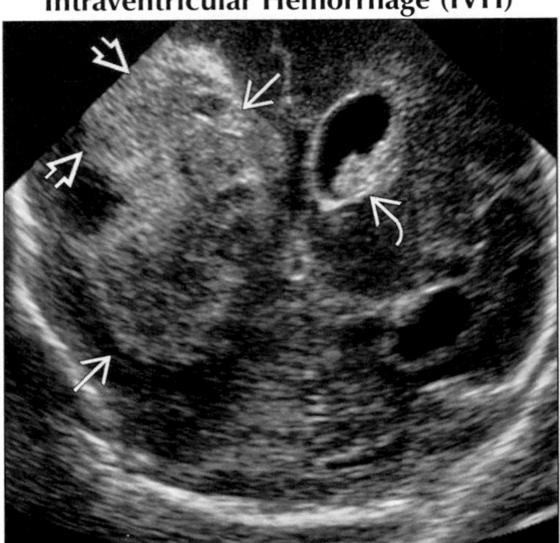

Subependymal Giant Cell Astrocytoma

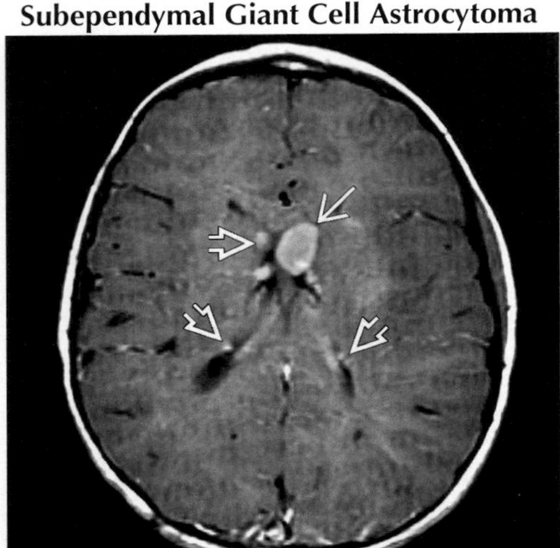

(Left) *Coronal ultrasound shows extensive cast of clot filling and distending the right lateral ventricle →, grade IV intracranial hemorrhage →, and left germinal matrix hemorrhage → in this 9-day-old, 26-week-premature infant.* ***(Right)*** *Axial T1 C+ MR demonstrates an enhancing mass → in the anterior horn of the left lateral ventricle, without ventricular obstruction, and several smaller subependymal hamartomas →.*

Ependymal Cyst

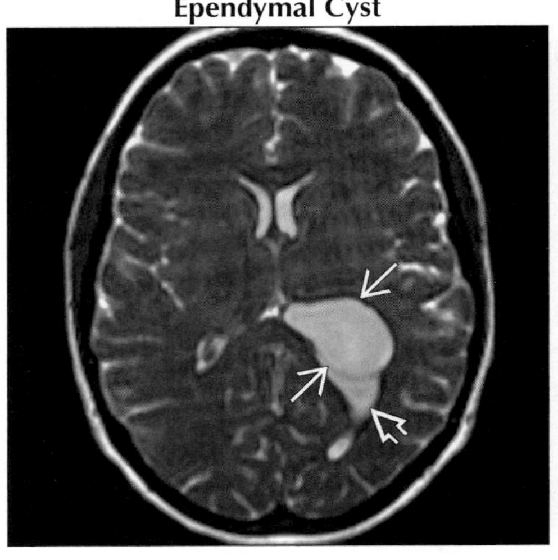

Choroid Plexus Papilloma

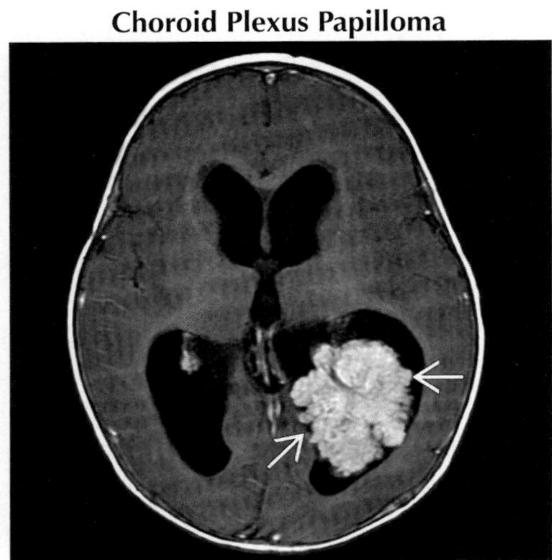

(Left) *Axial GRE MR image shows a simple-appearing intraventricular cyst → obstructing the left occipital horn →.* ***(Right)*** *Axial T1WI C+ MR shows a large, lobulated, intensely enhancing mass arising from the choroid plexus in the atrium of the left lateral ventricle →. There is ventriculomegaly secondary to overproduction of CSF.*

Choroid Plexus Carcinoma

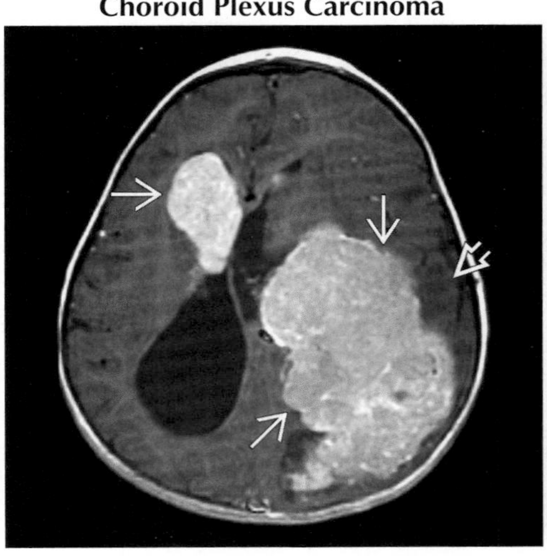

Choroid Plexus Carcinoma

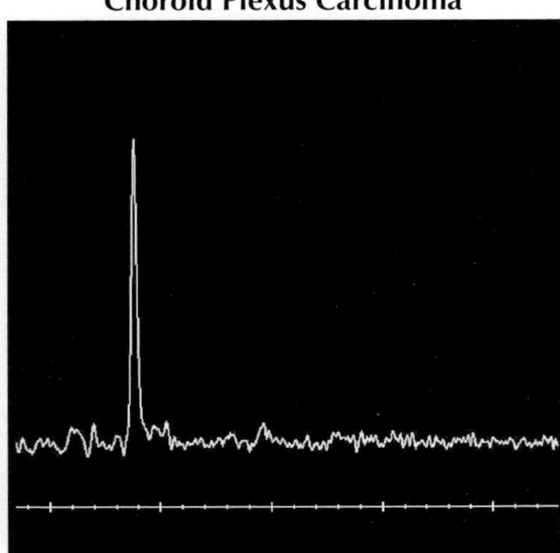

(Left) *Axial T1WI C+ FS MR shows large, enhancing masses in the left more than right lateral ventricles →. The appearance of the margins of the lesion on the left, with edema in the adjacent temporal lobe →, suggests parenchymal invasion.* ***(Right)*** *MRS long echo shows complete absence of creatine/phosphocreatine and NAA peaks, with a single dominant choline peak, typical of choroid plexus carcinoma.*

Meningioma

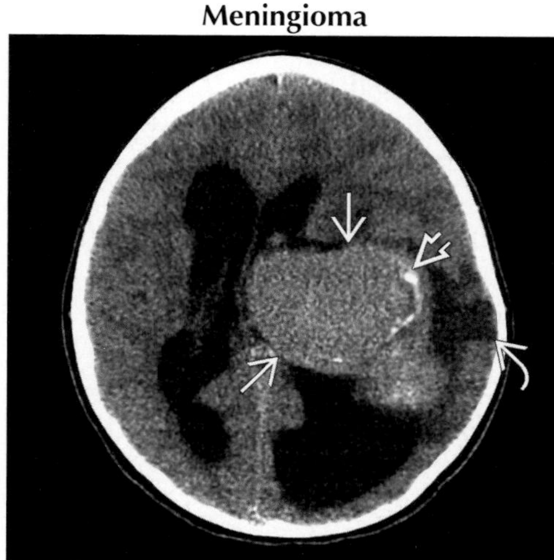

Meningioma

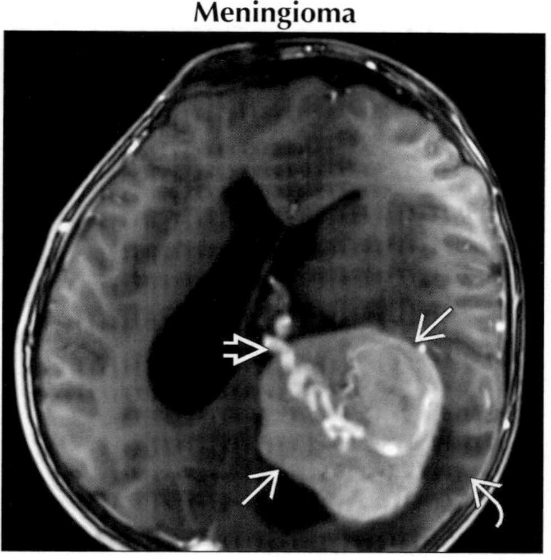

(Left) Axial NECT shows a large intermediate- to high-attenuation intraventricular mass ➔ with peripheral calcifications ➔, mild inciting edema in the adjacent parenchyma ➔, and ventriculomegaly. (Right) Axial T1 C+ MR shows a large, intensely enhancing intraventricular mass ➔ with a large draining vein ➔ and mild parenchymal edema ➔.

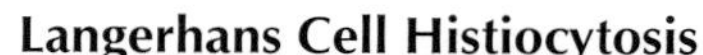

Langerhans Cell Histiocytosis

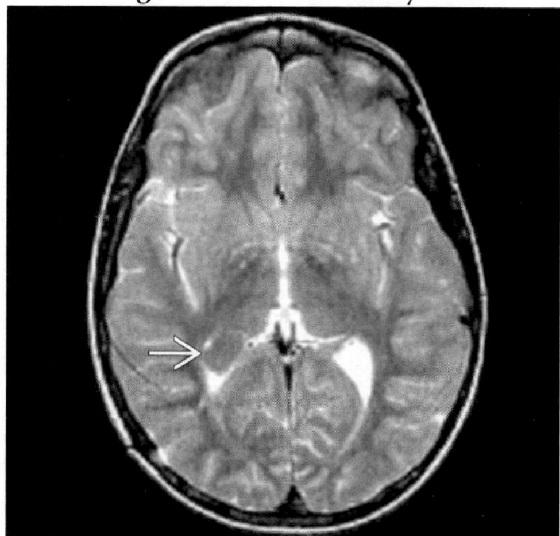

Langerhans Cell Histiocytosis

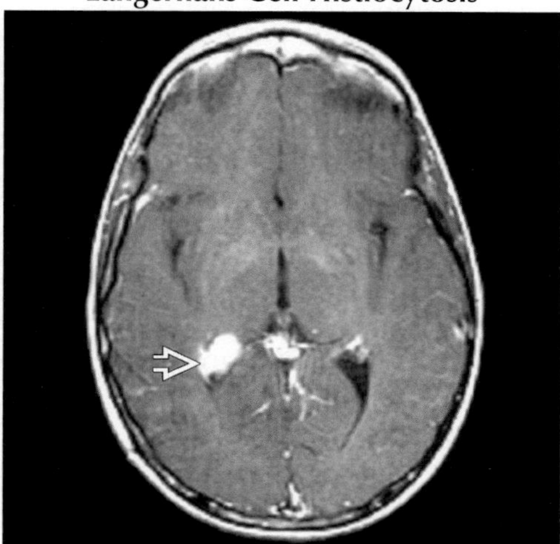

(Left) Axial T2WI MR shows a hypointense choroid plexus mass within the right lateral ventricle ➔. (Right) Axial T1WI C+ MR shows intense enhancement of the choroid plexus mass ➔ in a patient who also had nonenhancing bilateral cerebellar white matter lesions and supratentorial enhancing parenchymal lesions (not shown).

Central Neurocytoma

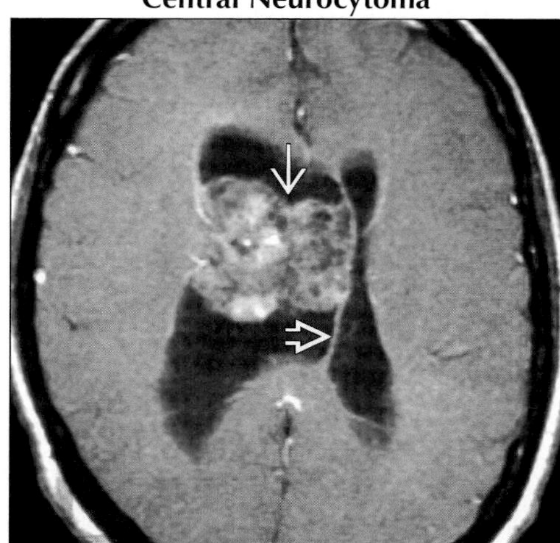

Subependymoma

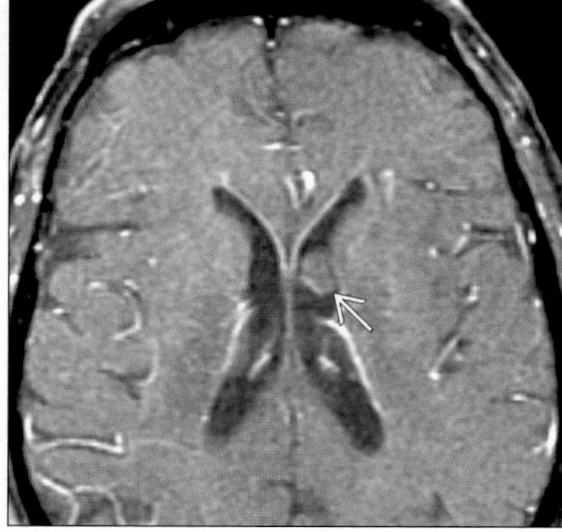

(Left) Axial T1 C+ MR in an adult patient shows a typical "bubbly," heterogeneously enhancing lateral ventricular mass ➔, with mild ventricular enlargement and leftward bowing of the septum pellucidum ➔. (Right) Axial T1 C+ FS MR shows a small, nonenhancing mass ➔ in the anterior horn of the left lateral ventricle in an adult.

ABNORMAL SHAPE/CONFIGURATION OF CORPUS CALLOSUM

DIFFERENTIAL DIAGNOSIS

Common

- Normal Variant
- Callosal Dysgenesis
- Callosotomy
- Neoplasm
  - Lipoma
  - Glioblastoma Multiforme
  - Lymphoma, Primary CNS
- Decreased White Matter Volume
  - Hypomyelination
  - Periventricular Leukomalacia
  - HIE, Term
  - Chronic Cerebral Infarction
  - Diffuse Axonal Injury (DAI)
  - Multiple Sclerosis
  - Radiation and Chemotherapy
- Obstructive Hydrocephalus

Less Common

- Holoprosencephaly
- Holoprosencephaly Variants

Rare but Important

- Hypertensive Intracranial Hemorrhage

ESSENTIAL INFORMATION

Key Differential Diagnosis Issues

- Normal corpus callosum (CC) varies in thickness, shape
- Isolated callosal dysgenesis not common
  - Look for 2nd lesion
  - Associated CNS anomalies in > 50%
    - Heterotopia
    - Cortical dysplasia
    - Noncallosal midline anomalies
    - Abnormal brainstem or cerebellum
- If not congenital, history crucial!

Helpful Clues for Common Diagnoses

- **Normal Variant**
  - Size, shape, thickness of normal corpus callosum vary
    - Splenium, genu are largest parts of corpus callosum
    - Narrowing between body, splenium ("isthmus") is normal
    - Dorsal surface of fully developed, normally myelinated corpus callosum often "wavy"
  - Immature corpus callosum is thin
    - Premyelination
    - Gradually thickens with progressive myelination
- **Callosal Dysgenesis**
  - One or all segments absent
    - Rostrum, splenium most likely deficient
    - Remnants vary in size, shape, configuration
  - "Micro" corpus callosum
    - Small, but well-formed
    - Often syndromic
  - "Mega" corpus callosum
    - Isthmus usually absent
    - Megalencephalic (bulky white matter)
    - Or small to normal brain (syndromic)
- **Callosotomy**
  - Surgical disruption
    - Focal: Approach to 3rd ventricle or suprasellar tumor
    - Diffuse: Surgery for intractable seizures
  - Best seen on sagittal or coronal MR
- **Neoplasm**
  - Can be benign/focal or malignant/diffusely infiltrating
  - **Lipoma**
    - 40-50% of interhemispheric fissure
    - Almost always located in subarachnoid space; blood vessels and cranial nerves course through lipoma; high surgical morbidity → surgery rarely indicated
    - Common in callosal dysgenesis
    - Can be bulky, mass-like ("tubonodular" type, usually associated with corpus callosum agenesis; may extend through choroidal fissures into lateral ventricles)
    - Thin mass curving around corpus callosum body/splenium ("curvilinear" type, corpus callosum present but may be dysgenetic)
    - Midline lipomas may be part of more general midline developmental disorder
  - **Glioblastoma Multiforme**
    - Most commonly seen in adults, can occur in adolescents (rare)
    - "Butterfly" glioma
    - Central necrosis + thick irregular rim enhancement
  - **Lymphoma, Primary CNS**
    - Hyperdense on NECT
    - Strong, uniform enhancement
- **Decreased White Matter Volume**

- Many causes (congenital, acquired)
- All may result in focal or diffuse callosal thinning
- **Hypomyelination**
  - Chromosomal, inborn errors of metabolism
- **Periventricular Leukomalacia**
  - Premature infant
  - Increased echogenicity ± loss of normal architecture on ultrasound head
  - May see cavitation, periventricular cysts
  - Reduced volume of periventricular white matter
  - Corpus callosal thinning most commonly in posterior body and splenium
  - "Scalloped" lateral ventricles
- **HIE, Term**
  - Term infant with profound partial asphyxia → WM/cortex damaged
- **Chronic Cerebral Infarction**
  - Axonal loss → focal/diffuse thinning of corpus callosum
- **Diffuse Axonal Injury (DAI)**
  - 20% involve corpus callosum (splenium, undersurface of posterior body)
- **Multiple Sclerosis**
  - Chronic, late

- **Obstructive Hydrocephalus**
  - Acute
    - Corpus callosum stretched, bowed upward
    - Forniceal columns bowed downward
  - Chronic
    - Post-shunt encephalomalacia
    - Sequela of acute callosal impingement against falx

Helpful Clues for Less Common Diagnoses

- **Holoprosencephaly**
  - Corpus callosum absent in alobar holoprosencephaly
    - Large dorsal "cyst" often present
    - Monoventricle
    - "Pancake" anterior cerebral tissue
  - Semilobar may have residual splenium
    - Frontal fusion and hypoplasia
    - Caudate head fusion
    - Splenium may be present
  - Lobar
    - Genu may or may not be present
    - Absent anterior midline falx and fissure
    - Gray matter often crosses with genu
- **Holoprosencephaly Variants**
  - Middle interhemispheric variant
    - a.k.a. syntelencephaly
    - Splenium, genu present, body deficient
    - Middle corpus callosum body "dips"
    - Gray matter crosses at dip
    - If severe, add bilateral perisylvian polymicrogyria

Helpful Clues for Rare Diagnoses

- **Hypertensive Intracranial Hemorrhage**
  - Corpus callosum is rare primary site

Normal Variant

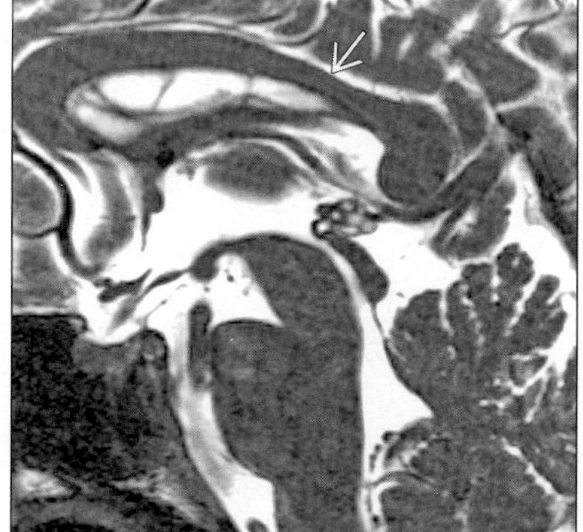

Sagittal T1WI FS MR with a close-up view of the corpus callosum shows normal "wavy" dorsal surface. Note the focal thinning along the posterior body ➔, a common normal finding.

Normal Variant

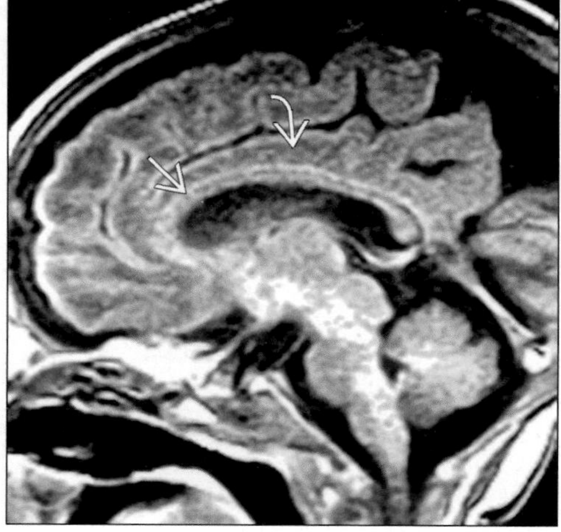

Sagittal T1WI MR shows a normal neonatal corpus callosum ➔, thin due to age-appropriate lack of myelin maturation. The cingulate gyrus ➔ is normal.

ABNORMAL SHAPE/CONFIGURATION OF CORPUS CALLOSUM

(Left) Sagittal T1WI MR shows callosal agenesis. Note the radial array of paracentral gyri "pointing" to the 3rd ventricle, as well as the absence of identifiable cingulate gyrus. Hippocampal commissure is visualized posteriorly ➡. (Right) Coronal T2WI MR shows the absence of crossing callosal fibers, the presence of Probst bundles ➡, and vertical hippocampi ⇨.

Callosal Dysgenesis

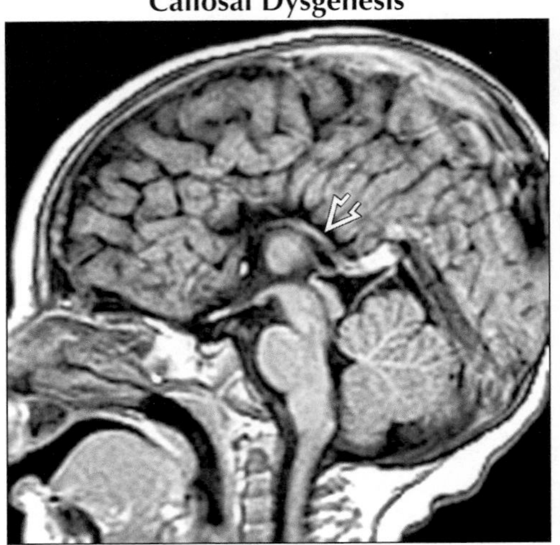

Callosal Dysgenesis

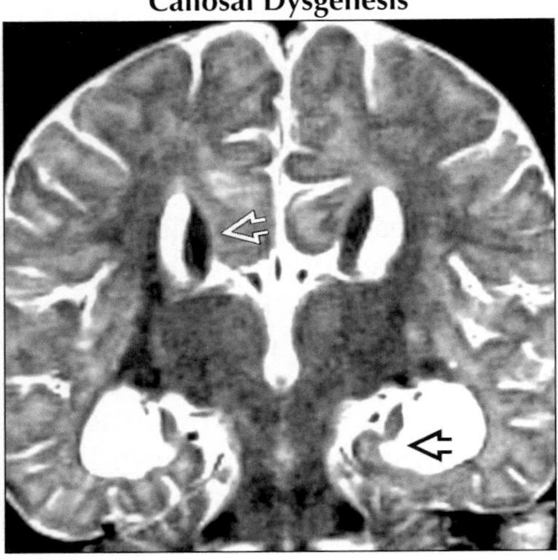

(Left) Sagittal T1WI MR shows only a residual genu ➡ of the corpus callosum, with absence of the body and splenium and truncation of the rostrum. (Right) Sagittal T1WI MR shows absent rostrum, small deformed genu, thick body ➡, and absent splenium in this child with Chiari 2. Note the prominent massa intermedia ➡, inferiorly beaked tectum ➡, and caudally displaced 4th ventricle.

Callosal Dysgenesis

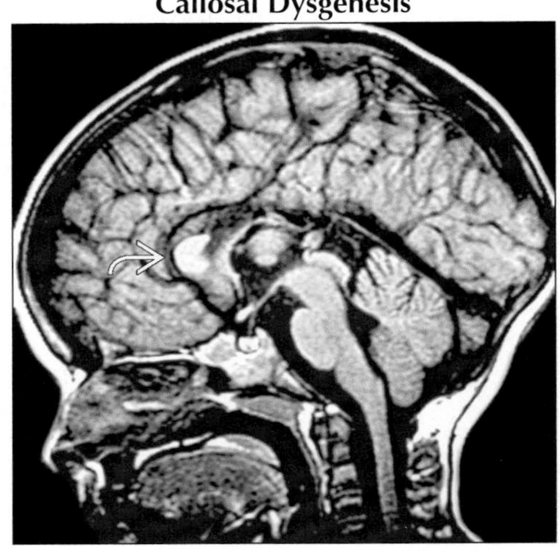

Callosal Dysgenesis

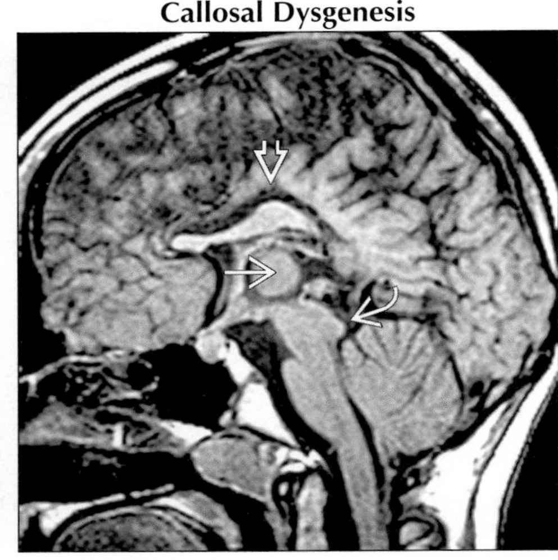

(Left) Sagittal T1WI MR in a child with severe microcephaly shows a short, thick corpus callosum ➡. Note the normal narrowing (isthmus) at the junction of the body; the splenium is absent. Actual callosal volume is small. (Right) Sagittal T1WI MR shows a focal defect at the junction of the genu and body of the corpus callosum ➡, the site of surgical approach to this child's suprasellar tumor ➡.

Callosal Dysgenesis

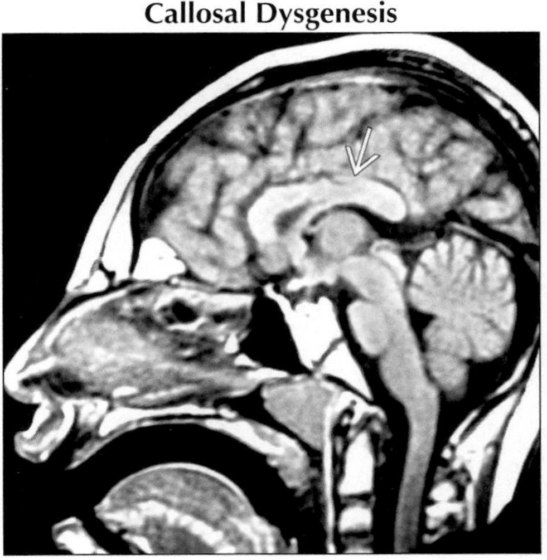

Callosotomy

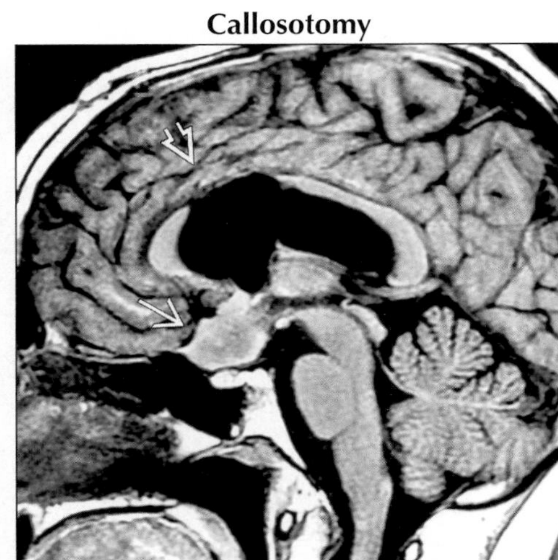

ABNORMAL SHAPE/CONFIGURATION OF CORPUS CALLOSUM

Lipoma

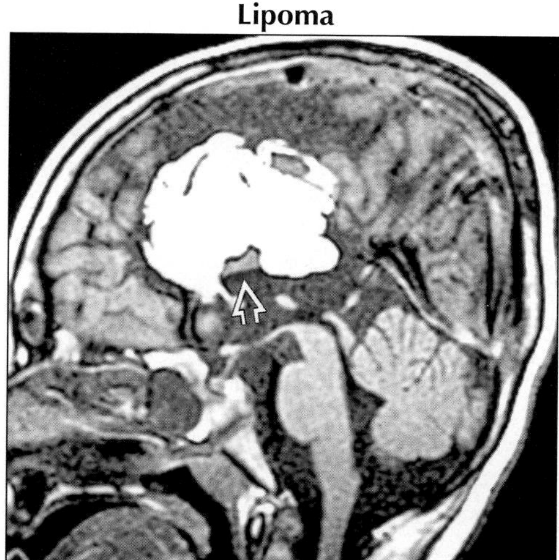

Glioblastoma Multiforme

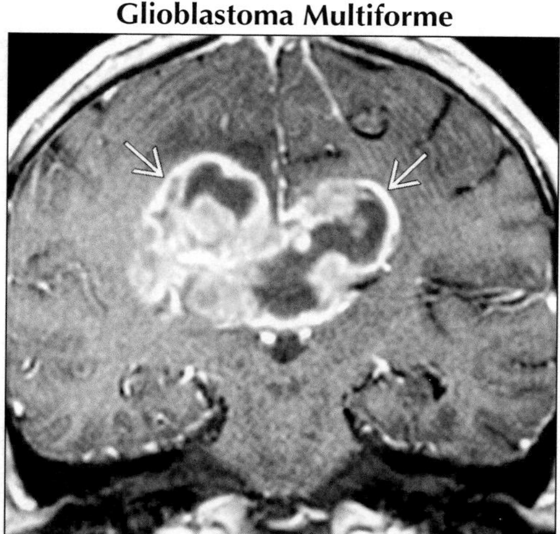

*(**Left**) Sagittal T1WI MR shows a large midline lipoma and a small remnant of the body of the corpus callosum. (**Right**) Coronal T1 C+ MR shows classic "butterfly" glioblastoma multiforme of the corpus callosum. Central necrosis with an irregular rind of enhancing tumor is typical.*

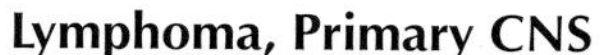

Lymphoma, Primary CNS

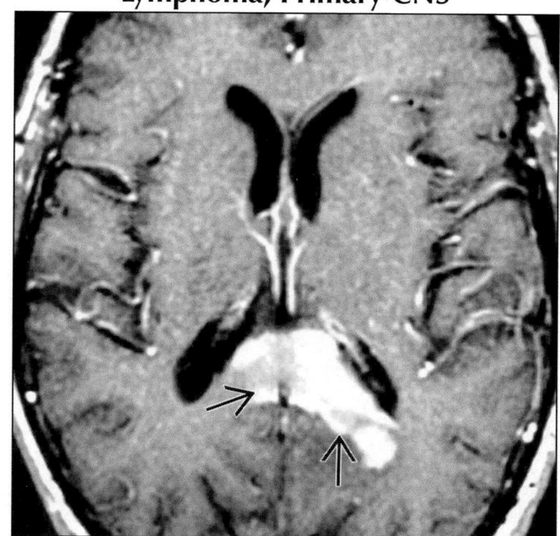

Periventricular Leukomalacia

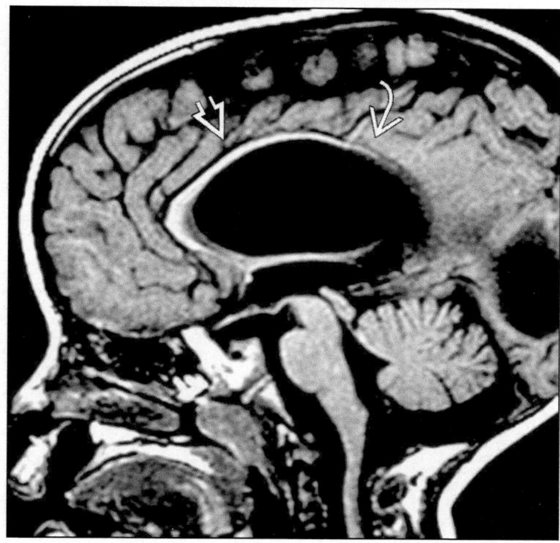

*(**Left**) Axial T1WI C+ MR shows primary CNS lymphoma involving the splenium of the corpus callosum. Gadolinium enhancement shows avid, solid enhancement of a splenial tumor and extension into adjacent parenchymal white matter. (**Right**) Sagittal T1WI MR shows marked callosal thinning and atrophy in a child whose hydrocephalus follows unilateral grade 4 intraventricular hemorrhage. Note more severe callosal volume loss posteriorly.*

Periventricular Leukomalacia

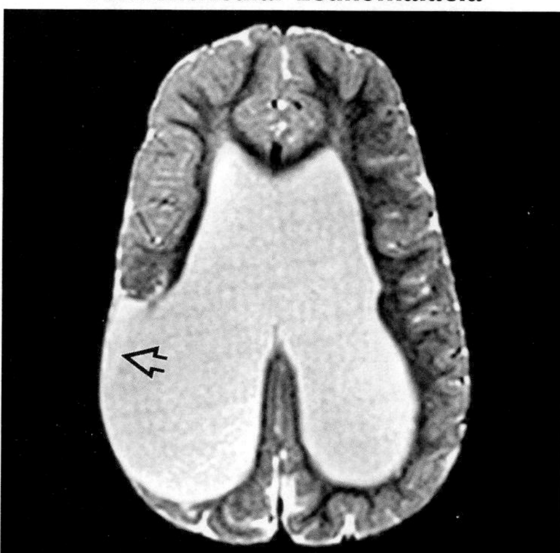

Periventricular Leukomalacia

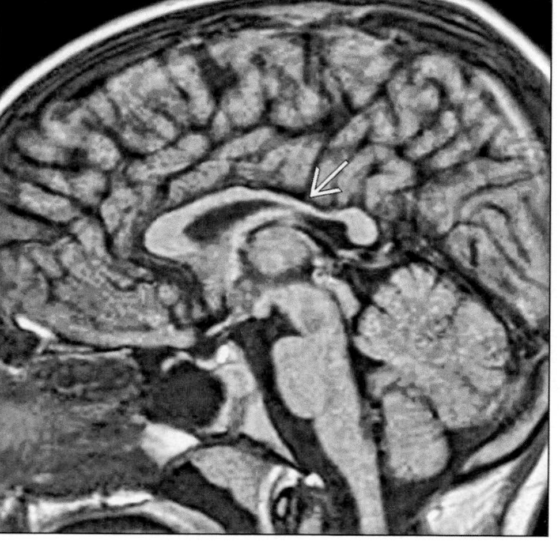

*(**Left**) Axial T2WI MR in the same child shows marked loss of periventricular white matter, septal destruction, and focal porencephaly at the site of a prior grade 4 hemorrhage. Posterior white matter loss correlates with focal corpus callosum atrophy. (**Right**) Sagittal T1WI MR shows diffuse thinning of the posterior corpus callosum. The thinning of the corpus callosum is secondary to loss of commissural fibers, damaged by periventricular leukomalacia.*

ABNORMAL SHAPE/CONFIGURATION OF CORPUS CALLOSUM

(Left) *Sagittal T1WI MR shows focal thinning of the body and splenium of the corpus callosum, following neonatal parietooccipital ischemia and gliosis from a combination of hypoxic ischemic encephalopathy and hypoglycemia.* **(Right)** *Coronal T2WI MR shows parietal ulegyria and marked thinning of the corpus callosum at the psalterium.*

Chronic Cerebral Infarction

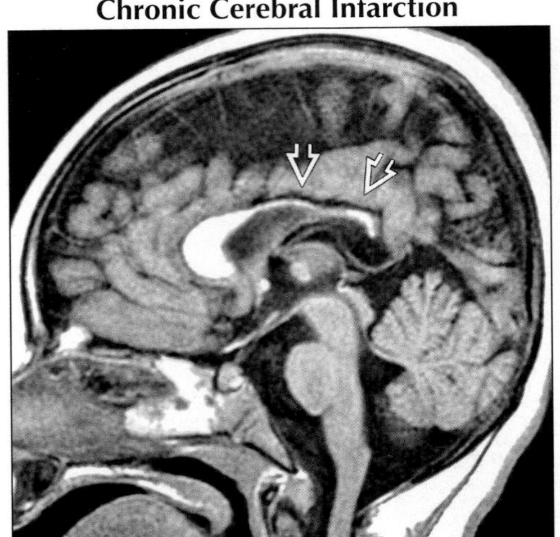

Chronic Cerebral Infarction

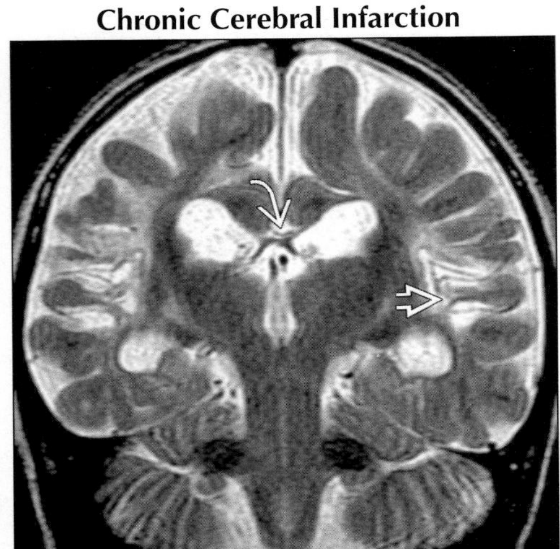

(Left) *Sagittal T1WI MR shows swelling and signal loss of the expected region of the isthmus of the corpus callosum due to shear injury.* **(Right)** *Axial FLAIR MR shows abnormal signal of crossing callosal fiber tracts following traumatic shear injury.*

Diffuse Axonal Injury (DAI)

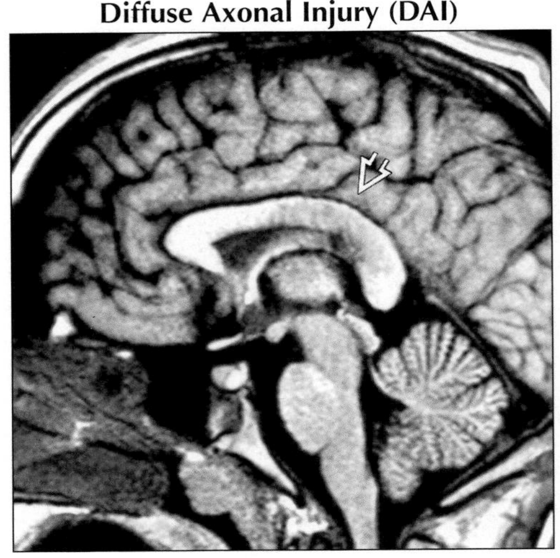

Diffuse Axonal Injury (DAI)

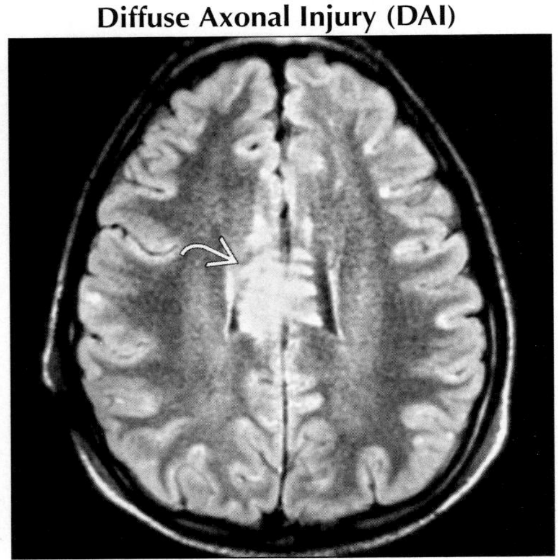

(Left) *Sagittal FLAIR MR shows multiple hyperintense foci in the corpus callosum as well as a large pontine lesion. The isthmus (posterior body) of the corpus callosum is thinned more than normally because of axonal loss from multiple centrum semiovale lesions.* **(Right)** *Sagittal T1WI MR shows diffuse thinning of the rostrum, genu, and body of the corpus callosum following treatment for acute lymphocytic leukemia.*

Multiple Sclerosis

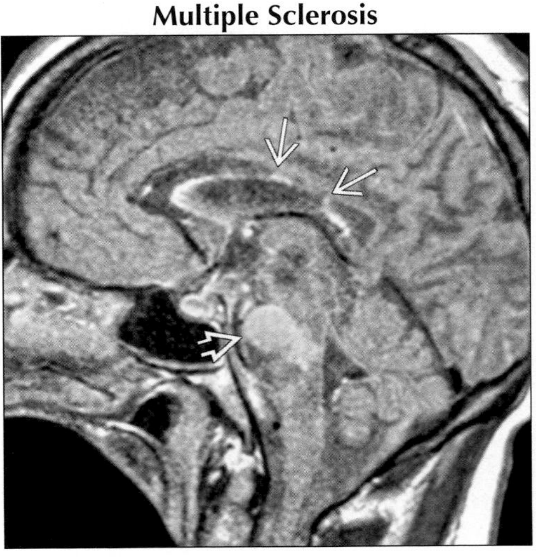

Radiation and Chemotherapy

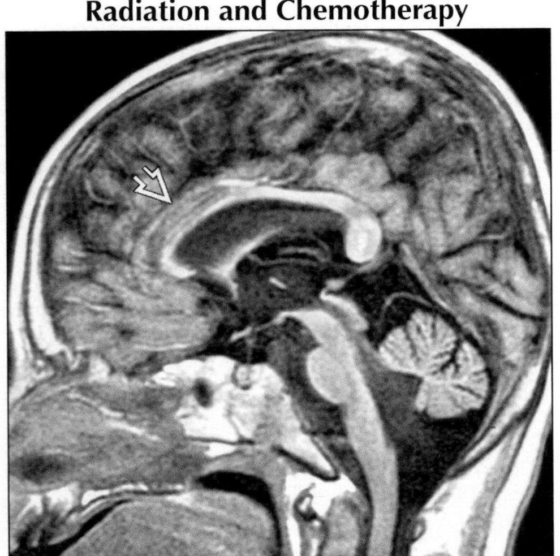

Obstructive Hydrocephalus

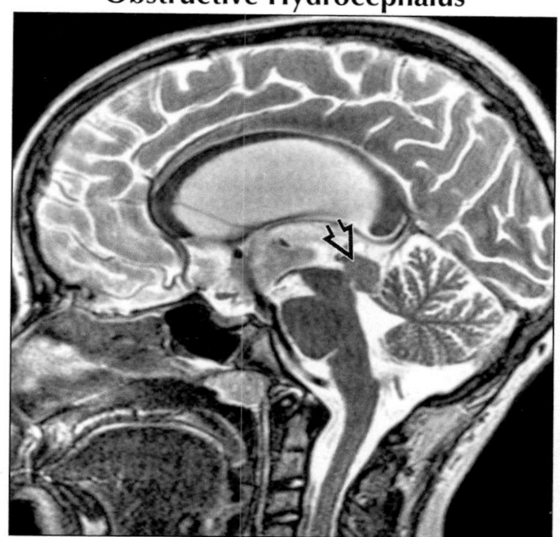

Holoprosencephaly

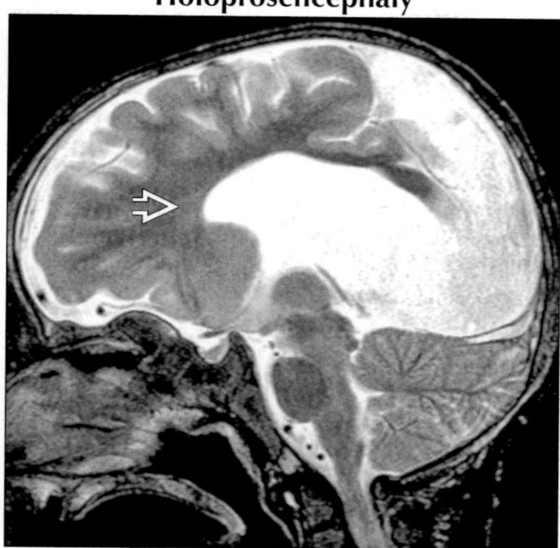

(Left) *Sagittal T2WI MR shows mild stretching and thinning of the corpus callosum due to hydrocephalus. There is obstruction of the aqueduct of Sylvius by a tectal glioma* ➩. *(Right)* *Sagittal T2WI MR shows the absence of corpus callosum. White matter* ➩ *traverses the midline, although not in compact bundle form. There is a large dorsal cyst. Note the lack of vermian primary fissure due to associated rhombencephalosynapsis.*

Holoprosencephaly

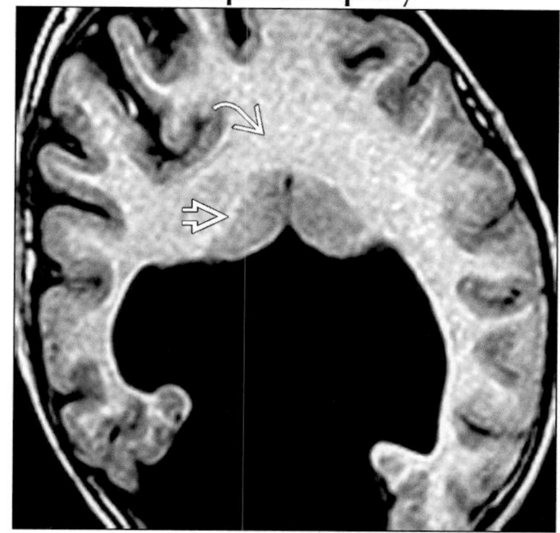

Holoprosencephaly Variants

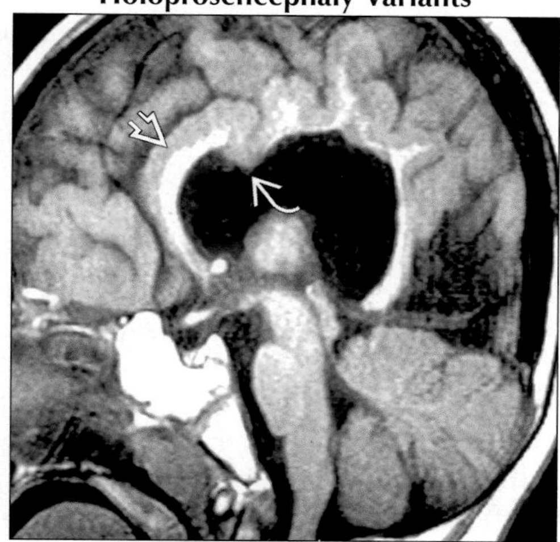

(Left) *Axial T1WI MR shows the lack of midline fissure. White matter* ➩ *is in continuity along the midline. Basal ganglia* ➩ *approximate each other.* *(Right)* *Sagittal T1WI MR shows both white and gray matter* ➩ *crossing midline anterior and posterior to the "dip"* ➩ *in the corpus callosum where only gray matter traverses. This is a middle interhemispheric variant (syntelencephaly).*

Holoprosencephaly Variants

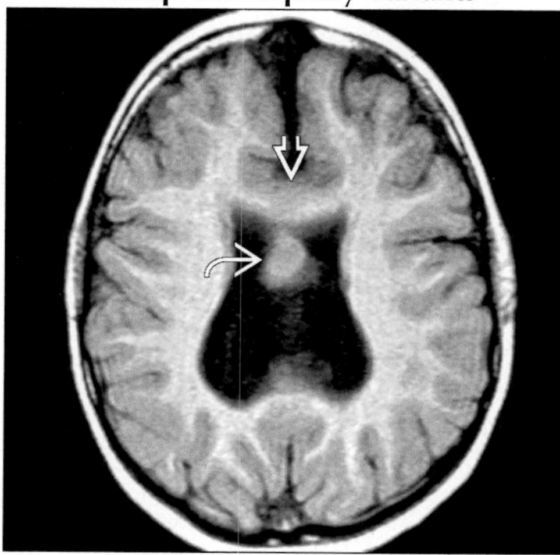

Hypertensive Intracranial Hemorrhage

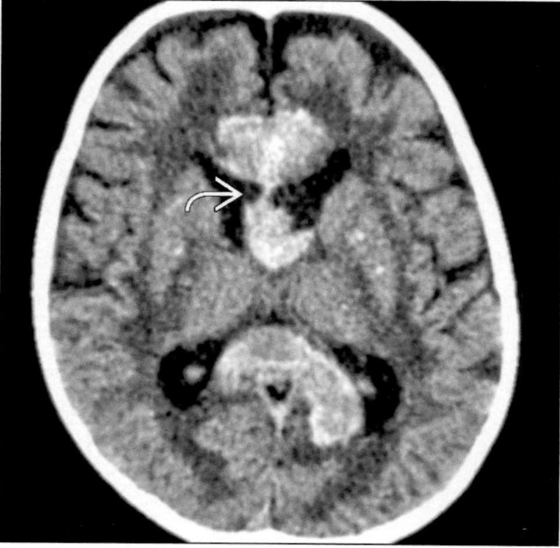

(Left) *Axial T1WI MR in the same patient shows gray-white matter traversing together* ➩ *in the expected location of the splenium. Gray matter protrudes* ➩ *into the ventricular system. Septum pellucidum is absent.* *(Right)* *Axial NECT shows extensive hemorrhage into the genu and splenium of the corpus callosum, with extension along the septal leaflets* ➩ *and into the ventricles in this child following cardiac transplant.*

THIN CORPUS CALLOSUM

DIFFERENTIAL DIAGNOSIS

Common
- Normal Variant
- Immature Brain
- Encephalomalacia
- Multiple Sclerosis
- White Matter Injury of Prematurity
- Callosal Dysgenesis
- Callosectomy/Callosotomy
- Obstructive Hydrocephalus

Less Common
- Hypomyelination
- Injury (Any Cause)

Rare but Important
- Susac Syndrome
- Holoprosencephaly
- Inherited Metabolic Disorders
- Hereditary Spastic Paraplegia with Thin Corpus Callosum (HSP-TCC)

ESSENTIAL INFORMATION

Key Differential Diagnosis Issues
- Diffuse corpus callosum (CC) thinning can be normal
  - Newborn (immature brain)
- Abnormally thin CC can be inherited or acquired
  - Broad spectrum of congenital malformations, inherited metabolic disorders can all result in thin CC
  - Check history for trauma, surgery, ischemia-infarction
- Thin CC, normal signal hyperintensity
  - Normal variant, immature brain
  - Secondary to hemispheric white matter (WM) volume loss
  - Dysgenesis
- Thin CC, abnormal signal intensity
  - Hypomyelination or demyelinating disease (chronic MS, Susac syndrome)
  - Injury (trauma, ischemia, radiation, toxic-metabolic insult)
  - Obstructive hydrocephalus

Helpful Clues for Common Diagnoses
- **Normal Variant**
  - Focal thinning of corpus callosum at "isthmus" (junction between posterior body, splenium) is normal
  - Sagittal section slightly off-midline can make corpus callosum appear mildly thinned
- **Immature Brain**
  - Hemispheric WM in newborn unmyelinated, corpus callosum thin and hypointense on T1WI
  - As myelination progresses, corpus callosum thickens, becomes hyperintense on T1WI
    - Corpus callosum splenium at 4 months
    - Corpus callosum genu at 6 months
    - By 8 months, corpus callosum essentially like an adult's
- **Encephalomalacia**
  - Holohemispheric WM volume loss, regardless of etiology, causes diffuse corpus callosum thinning
  - Focal WM loss can cause focal corpus callosum thinning
- **Multiple Sclerosis**
  - Look for T2/FLAIR hyperintense lesions along callososeptal interface
  - Ependymal "dot-dash" sign along callosoventricular border occurs early
  - Longstanding MS with decreased hemispheric WM volume results in thinned corpus callosum
- **White Matter Injury of Prematurity**
  - Corpus callosum thinning secondary to periventricular white matter infarction
  - Posterior corpus callosum disproportionately affected
- **Callosal Dysgenesis**
  - Hypoplasia or absence of part or all of corpus callosum
    - Rostrum, splenium most likely deficient
    - Remnants vary in size, shape, and configuration
  - Most common abnormality associated with other malformations
    - Chiari 2 malformation
    - Heterotopias
    - Interhemispheric lipoma
    - Cephaloceles
- **Callosectomy/Callosotomy**
  - History important!
  - Surgical disruption
  - Look for surgical changes of craniotomy, ventriculostomy
- **Obstructive Hydrocephalus**

- Causes 2 kinds of corpus callosum abnormalities: Stretching and intrinsic signal abnormality
- As lateral ventricles enlarge, corpus callosum is stretched, appears thinned
  - Look for associated signal abnormality in corpus callosum (sagittal T2WI/FLAIR best)
- Post-shunt decompression may show corpus callosum thinning, signal abnormality
  - Can appear bizarre, causing horizontal hyperintense "streaks" in corpus callosum on axial imaging
  - Can extend into periventricular WM
  - Theories: Impingement of corpus callosum against falx cerebri with resulting ischemia or axonal stretch

Helpful Clues for Less Common Diagnoses

- **Hypomyelination**
  - Undermyelination, delayed myelin maturation
  - Diminished/absent WM myelination for age
  - Can be primary or secondary to other pathology
- **Injury (Any Cause)**
  - Trauma (e.g., axonal injury, radiation-induced leukoencephalopathy)
  - Ischemia

Helpful Clues for Rare Diagnoses

- **Susac Syndrome**
  - M < F
  - Classic triad
    - Encephalopathy (headache, confusion, memory loss)
    - Vision problems (retinal artery occlusions)
    - Hearing loss
  - Always involves corpus callosum
    - Central > callososeptal interface lesions
    - Middle callosal "holes" (subacute/chronic)
- **Holoprosencephaly**
  - Many variants; often affect corpus callosum
- **Inherited Metabolic Disorders**
  - Focal or diffuse atrophy
    - Focal: X-linked adrenoleukodystrophy
    - Diffuse: Many
- **Hereditary Spastic Paraplegia with Thin Corpus Callosum (HSP-TCC)**
  - HSP-TCC is 1 of many hereditary spastic paraplegias
    - Autosomal recessive with *SPG11* gene mutations on chromosome 15q13-15
    - Progressive neurodegenerative disorder
  - Clinical
    - Slow ↑ spastic paraparesis
    - Adolescent-onset cognitive decline
    - Pseudobulbar dysfunction
  - Imaging
    - Thin corpus callosum (especially genu, body) with progressive atrophy
    - Cerebral, cerebellar atrophy often associated

Immature Brain

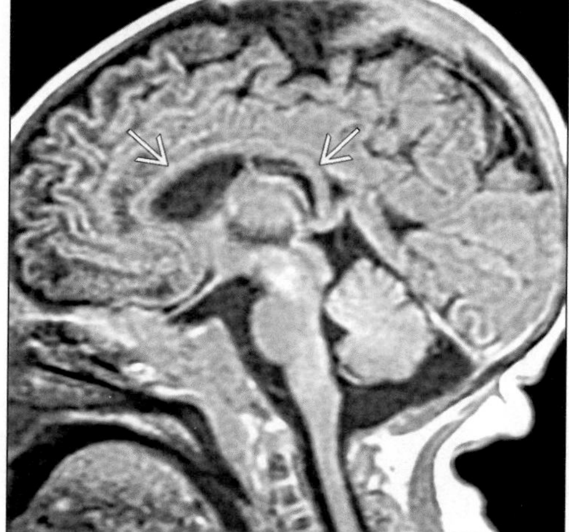

Sagittal T1WI MR in a term infant imaged at 2 days of age shows a thin corpus callosum ➔ with no discernible myelination. This is the normal appearance of an immature, largely unmyelinated brain.

Immature Brain

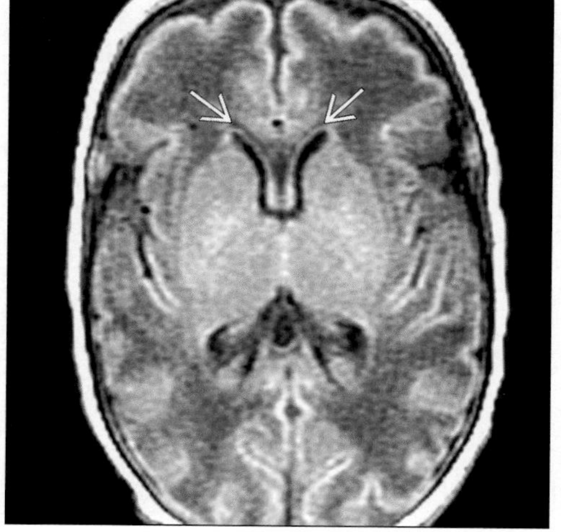

Axial T1WI MR in 32-week-gestation premature infant shows a very thin corpus callosum genu ➔, reflecting total lack of hemispheric myelination.

THIN CORPUS CALLOSUM

*(**Left**) Axial DWI MR in a newborn shows extensive diffusion restriction of the left hemisphere following perinatal stroke. Acute axonal degeneration of the corpus callosum is present. (**Right**) Coronal T2WI MR at follow-up shows a large area of cystic encephalomalacia and a very thin corpus callosum.*

Encephalomalacia

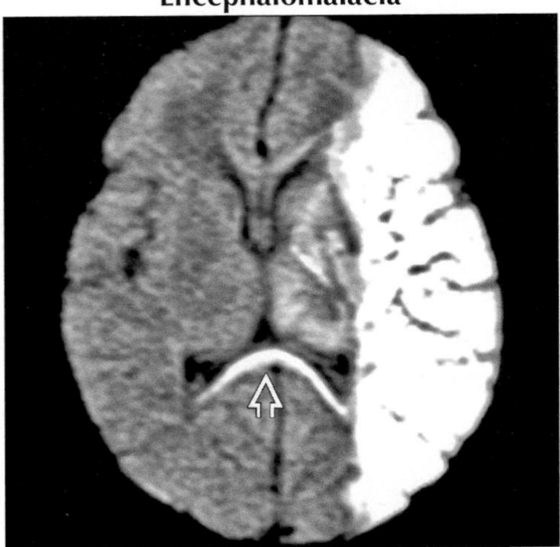

Encephalomalacia

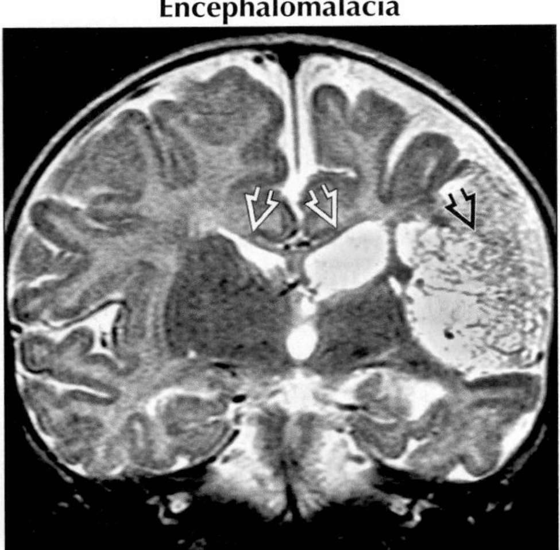

*(**Left**) Sagittal DWI MR in a neonate with group B strep meningitis shows multifocal brain ischemia. There is diffusion restriction of the corpus callosum due to axonal degeneration. (**Right**) Sagittal T1WI MR in the same child at follow-up imaging shows severe thinning of the corpus callosum.*

Encephalomalacia

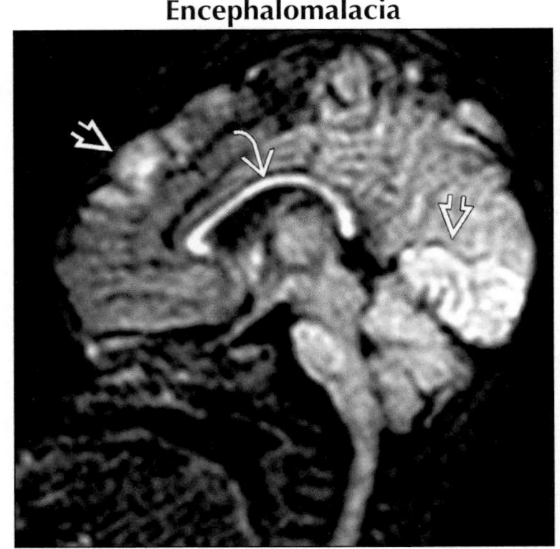

Encephalomalacia

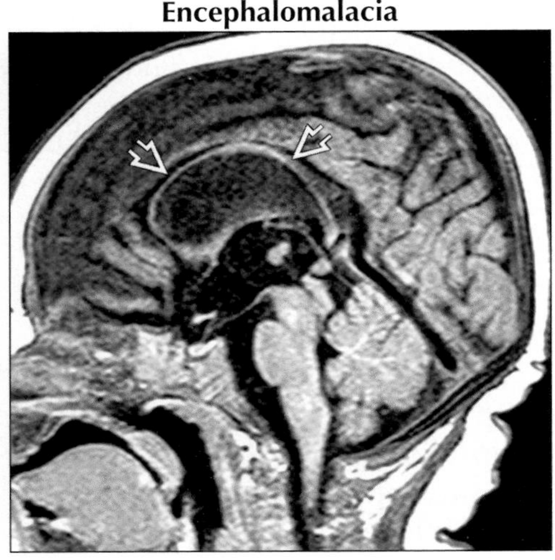

*(**Left**) Sagittal FLAIR MR in a teenager with MS shows severe atrophy of the corpus callosum with increased signal intensity of the corpus callosum, the septal-callosal interface, and the fornix. (**Right**) Axial FLAIR MR shows extensive demyelinating plaques in the same teen.*

Multiple Sclerosis

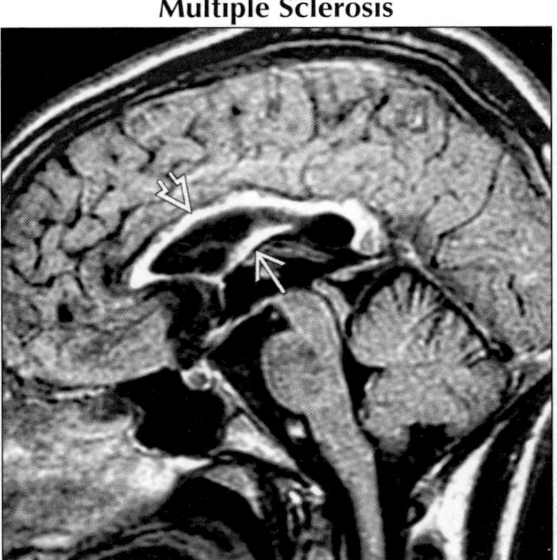

Multiple Sclerosis

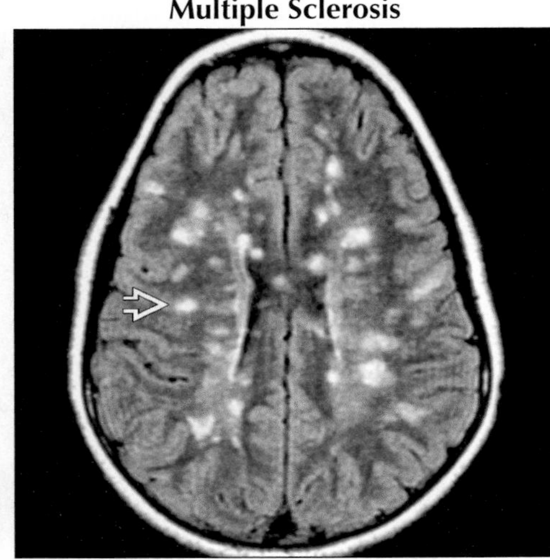

THIN CORPUS CALLOSUM

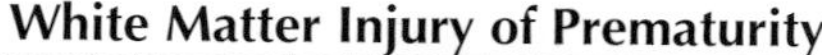

White Matter Injury of Prematurity

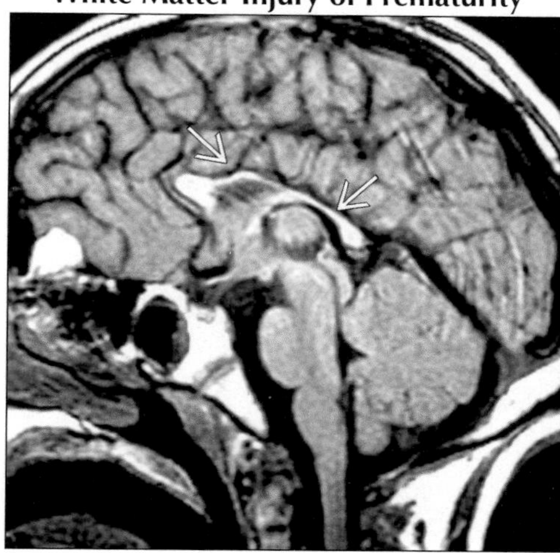

White Matter Injury of Prematurity

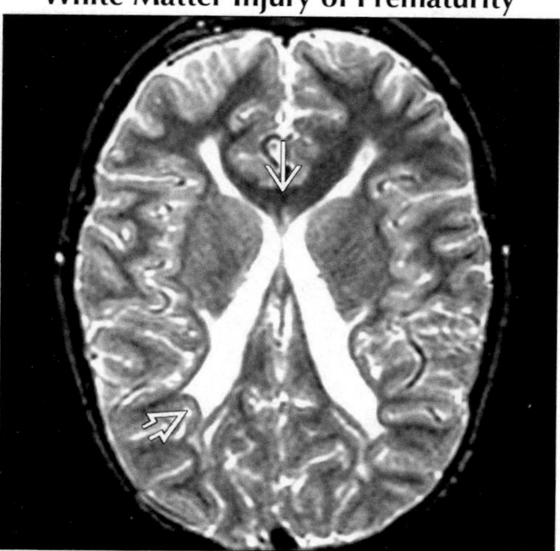

(Left) *Sagittal T1WI MR shows extreme thinning of the corpus callosum ➔ in a child with cerebral palsy and history of premature birth and prolonged stay in NICU.* ***(Right)*** *Axial T2WI MR shows typical scalloping of the ventricles due to indentation by gray matter ⇨. The peritrigonal white matter is severely deficient in this same ex-premature infant with periventricular leukomalacia. Note the relative sparing of genu ➔.*

Callosal Dysgenesis

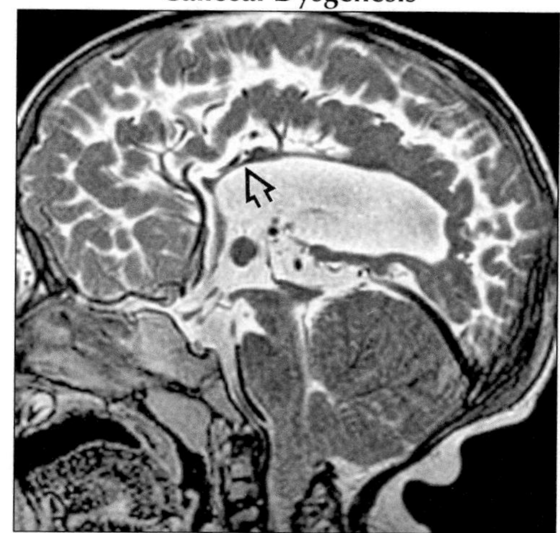

Callosal Dysgenesis

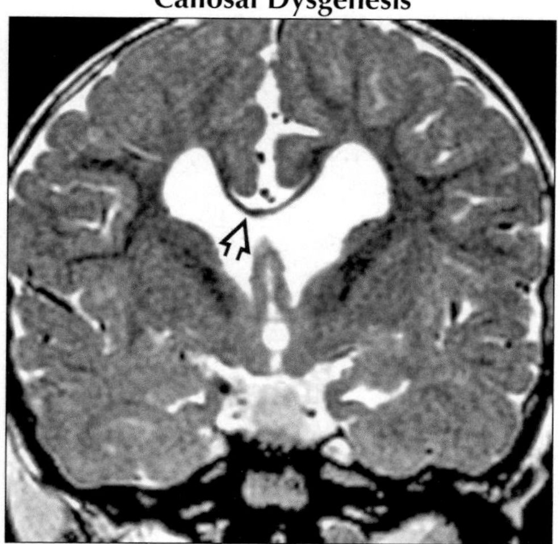

(Left) *Sagittal T1WI MR in a child with Chiari 2 malformation shows a thin, dysgenetic-appearing corpus callosum ⇨.* ***(Right)*** *Coronal T2WI MR shows severe thinning of the dysgenetic corpus callosum ⇨ in the same child with Chiari 2 malformation. Note the absence of the leaflets of the septum pellucidum.*

Callosectomy/Callosotomy

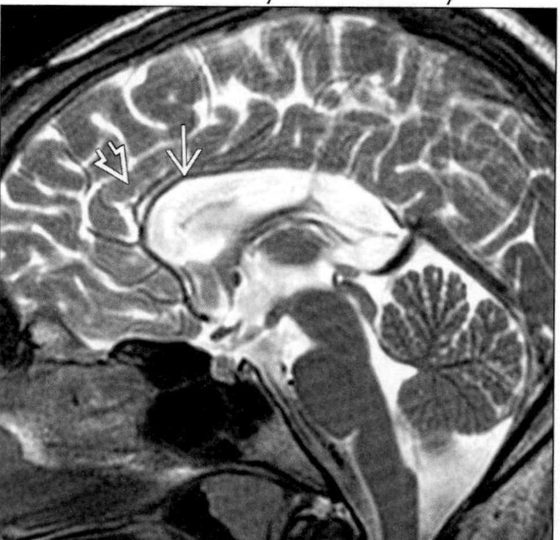

Callosectomy/Callosotomy

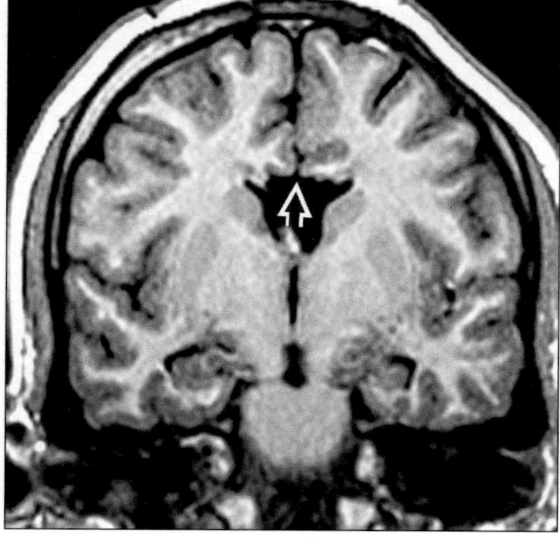

(Left) *Sagittal T2WI MR shows absent midline corpus callosum, post-callosotomy for seizure control. Note the normal cingulate gyrus ⇨ and pericallosal artery ➔.* ***(Right)*** *Coronal T1WI MR shows a large callosotomy defect ⇨ in the same child in treatment of intractable epilepsy due to Lennox-Gastaut syndrome.*

THIN CORPUS CALLOSUM

(Left) *Sagittal T2WI MR in patient with longstanding aqueductal stenosis ➡ shows thinned, stretched corpus callosum with some hyperintensity posteriorly ➡. Note hyperdynamic CSF with "flow voids" ➡.* **(Right)** *Sagittal T1WI MR shows a very thin corpus callosum ➡ with hypomyelination and minimal T1 shortening ➡ indicative of minimal myelination in the splenium. Other images showed a striking lack of myelination in this 5-month-old infant.*

Obstructive Hydrocephalus

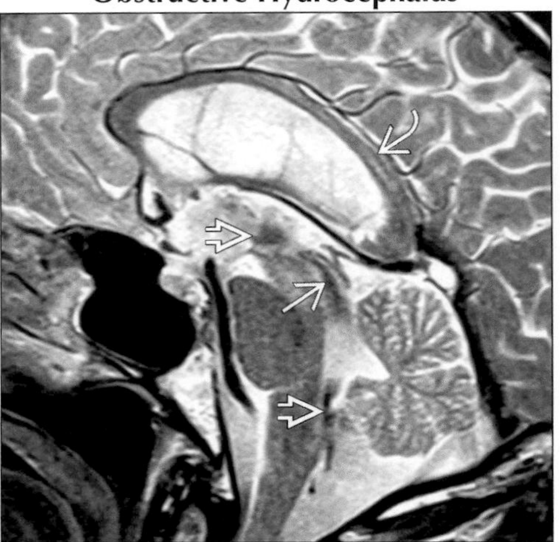

Hypomyelination

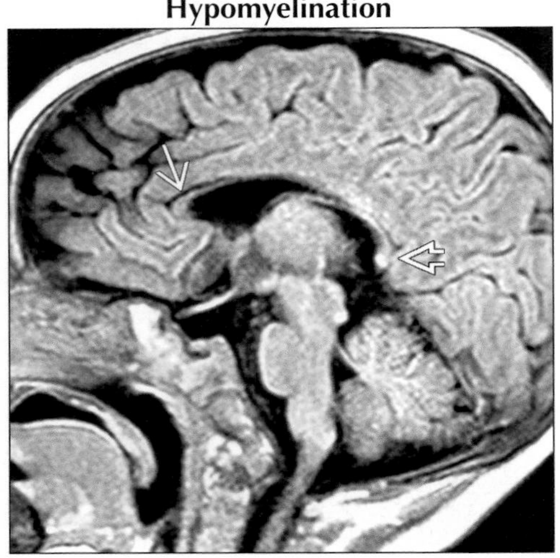

(Left) *Sagittal T1WI MR shows thinned body splenium of the corpus callosum ➡ following neonatal parietooccipital ischemia from a combination of HIE and hypoglycemia.* **(Right)** *Axial T2WI MR in the same infant reflects sequelae of HIE and hypoglycemia. There is extensive posterior atrophy. The genu ➡ of the corpus callosum is normal in size, and the splenium is severely atrophied ➡.*

Injury (Any Cause)

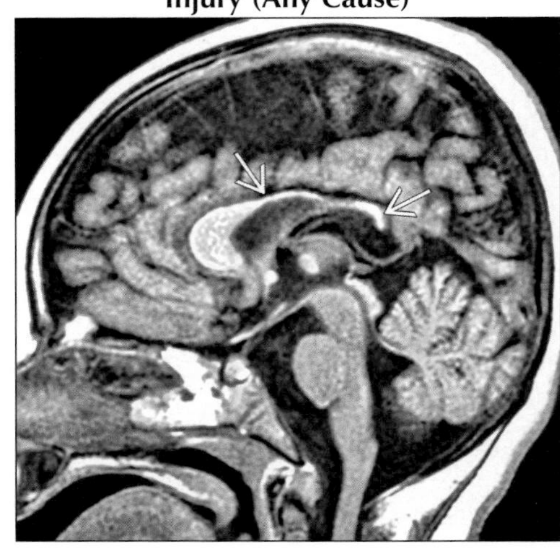

Injury (Any Cause)

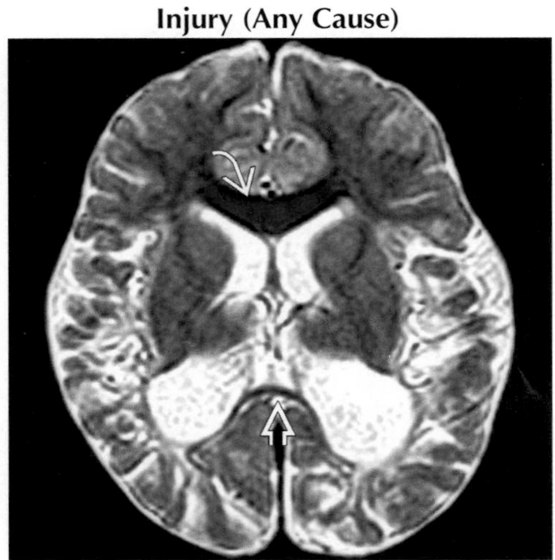

(Left) *Sagittal T1WI MR shows thinning ➡ of the posterior corpus callosal body in this 8-year-old child who had a history of cerebral palsy.* **(Right)** *Sagittal FLAIR MR shows a moderately thinned corpus callosum with multiple hyperintensities, especially in the middle and posterior segments ➡. Note several middle callosal "holes" ➡, characteristic for Susac syndrome.*

Injury (Any Cause)

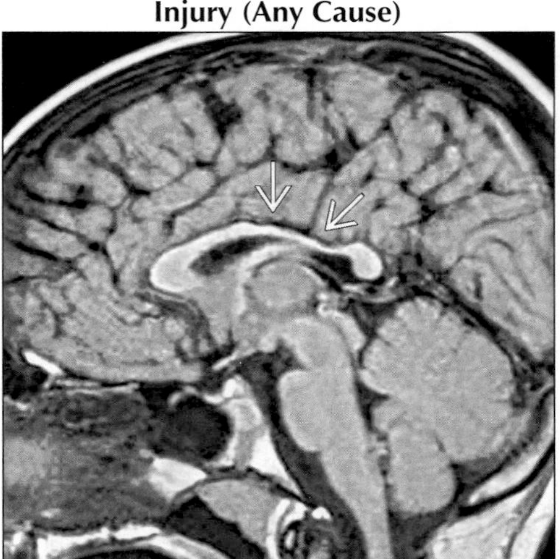

Susac Syndrome

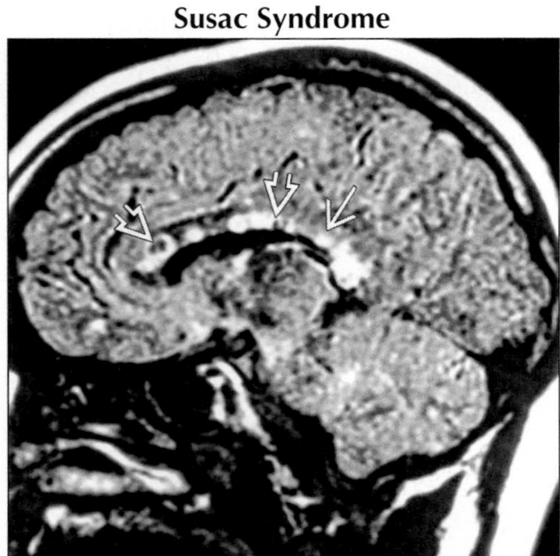

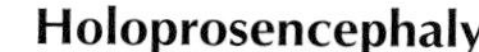

Holoprosencephaly

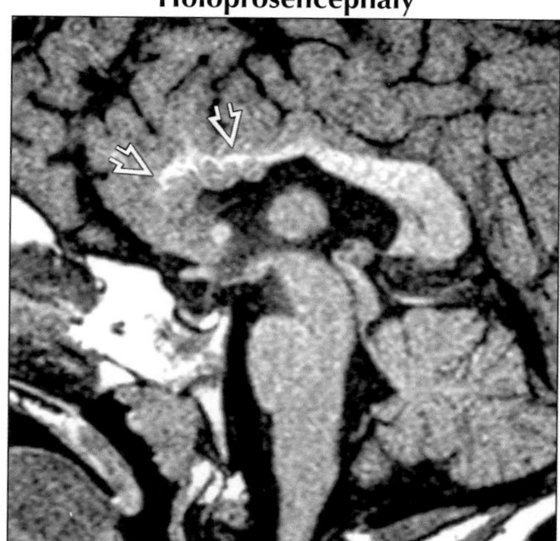

Holoprosencephaly

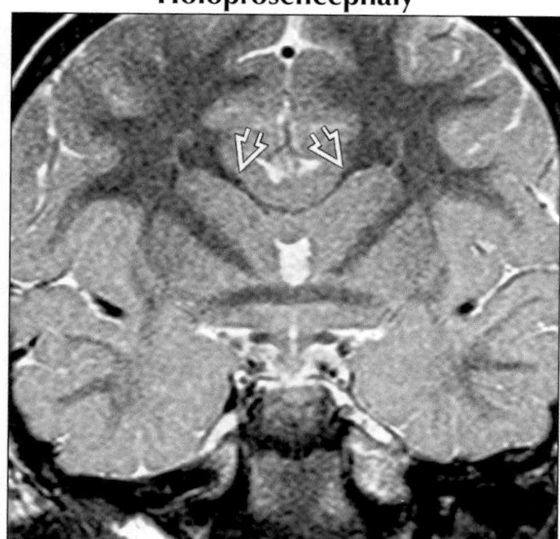

(Left) *Sagittal T1WI MR shows layers of white ➡ and gray matter comprising the anterior corpus callosum in this child with semilobar holoprosencephaly.* ***(Right)*** *Coronal T2WI MR shows layering of white ➡ and gray matter in the expected region of the genu of the corpus callosum in this same child with semilobar holoprosencephaly.*

Inherited Metabolic Disorders

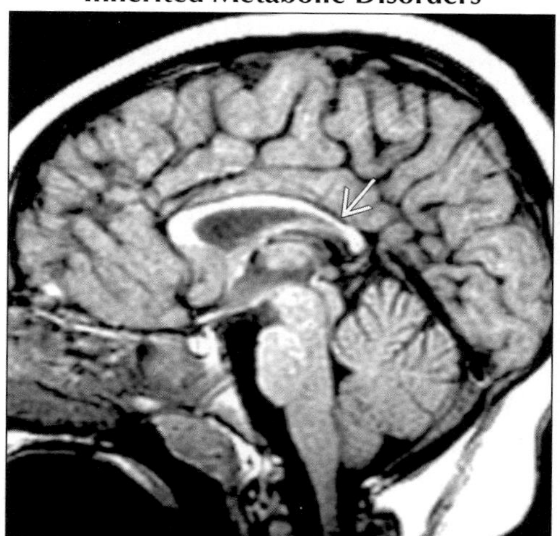

Inherited Metabolic Disorders

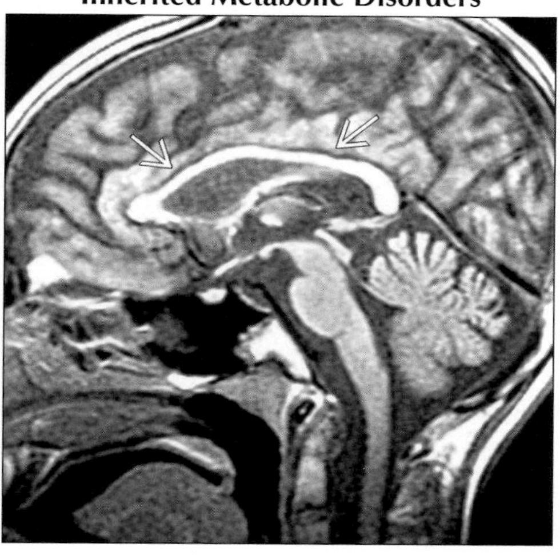

(Left) *Sagittal T1WI MR in a child with urea cycle disorder shows diffuse thinning of the corpus callosum, most striking in the posterior body and splenium ➡.* ***(Right)*** *Axial NECT in a 10 year old with cobalamin C deficiency shows marked volume loss of the body ➡ of the well-myelinated corpus callosum. This finding and hypomyelination (mild in this child) are characteristic of this disorder. It is important to consider this diagnosis, as treatment is available.*

Inherited Metabolic Disorders

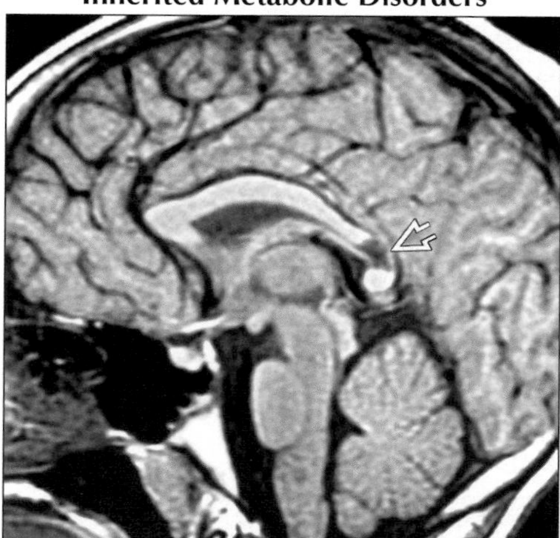

Inherited Metabolic Disorders

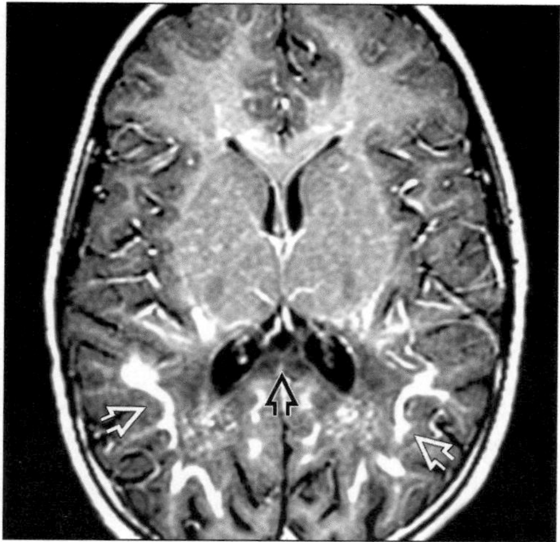

(Left) *Sagittal T1WI MR in a pre-teen boy with symptomatic X-linked adrenoleukodystrophy shows focal thinning ➡ and signal loss in the splenium of the corpus callosum.* ***(Right)*** *Axial T1WI C+ MR in the same child with classic X-linked adrenoleukodystrophy shows enhancement of the leading edge of demyelination ➡ and focal atrophy ⇨ of the splenium of the corpus callosum.*

PERIVENTRICULAR CALCIFICATION

DIFFERENTIAL DIAGNOSIS

Common
- TORCH, General
  - Congenital CMV
  - Congenital Toxoplasmosis
  - Congenital Herpes Encephalitis
  - Congenital HIV
  - Congenital Rubella
- Tuberous Sclerosis Complex

Less Common
- Neurocysticercosis
- Tuberculosis
- Ventriculitis (Chronic)
- Germinal Matrix Hemorrhage

Rare but Important
- Radiation and Chemotherapy
- Pseudo-TORCH
  - Aicardi-Goutières Syndrome
  - Coats-Plus Syndrome

ESSENTIAL INFORMATION

Key Differential Diagnosis Issues
- Look for associations
  - Brain destruction
  - Malformations
  - Other loci of calcification
  - History

Helpful Clues for Common Diagnoses
- **TORCH, General**
  - Classic acronym for congenital infections
    - Caused by transplacental transmission of pathogens
    - **To**xoplasmosis
    - **R**ubella
    - **C**ytomegalovirus
    - **H**erpes
    - All cause parenchymal calcifications
    - Most can cause lenticulostriate mineralization, vasculopathy
    - Some (CMV) cause migrational defects
    - Some (syphilis, herpes) cause meningitis, meningoencephalitis
    - Some (e.g., CMV) cause germinolytic cysts
    - Others (e.g., rubella, HSV) cause striking lobar destruction/encephalomalacia
  - Congenital HIV, syphilis also considered part of TORCH
  - Consider congenital HIV
    - If bilateral symmetric basal ganglia calcifications identified in child > 2 months old
  - If congenital infection is diagnostic consideration, obtain NECT to detect calcifications
- **Congenital CMV**
  - Most common cause of intrauterine infection in USA
  - Timing of infection predicts pattern of damage
  - Hypomyelination
  - Cortical gyral anomalies
  - Microcephaly
  - Symmetric periventricular calcifications in 30-70%
- **Congenital Toxoplasmosis**
  - Periventricular and scattered calcifications
  - Hydrocephalus (colpocephaly-like)
- **Congenital Herpes Encephalitis**
  - Calcification pattern varies in HSV2
    - Asymmetric periventricular
    - Scattered periventricular and deep gray
    - Subcortical white matter and cortex
    - Calcification pronounced in foci of hemorrhagic ischemia
    - Like rubella, rare cause of "stone brain"
  - Brain atrophy or cystic encephalomalacia
    - Focal or diffuse
- **Congenital HIV**
  - Vertical HIV infection
  - Basal ganglia calcifications
  - Atrophy
  - Consider congenital HIV
    - If bilateral symmetric basal ganglia calcifications present and child is > 2 months old
- **Congenital Rubella**
  - Periventricular and scattered calcifications
  - Scattered or hazy basal ganglia calcifications
  - Rarely "stone brain"
    - Extensive gyral calcification
    - Gliosis
  - Micro-infarcts
- **Tuberous Sclerosis Complex**
  - a.k.a. Bourneville disease
  - Classic triad
    - Mental retardation
    - Epilepsy

- Adenoma sebaceum
- Look for cutaneous markers of tuberous sclerosis
- Subependymal nodules
  - Variable-sized periventricular calcifications
- Cortical tubers also calcify

Helpful Clues for Less Common Diagnoses

- **Neurocysticercosis**
  - Best clue: Dot inside cyst
  - Usually convexity subarachnoid space
  - Also gray-white junction, intraventricular
  - Nodular calcified (healed) stage
    - Shrunken calcified nodule
- **Tuberculosis**
  - Best diagnostic clue
    - Basal meningitis
    - Pulmonary tuberculosis
  - Acute
    - Typically basal meningitis
    - ± localized CNS tuberculoma
  - Chronic
    - Residual pachymeningeal
    - ± localized calcifications
  - "Target" sign
    - Calcification surrounded by enhancing rim (not specific)
- **Ventriculitis (Chronic)**
  - Areas of prior hemorrhagic infarction prone to dystrophic calcification
- **Germinal Matrix Hemorrhage**
  - Occasional ependymal, germinal matrix calcific foci

Helpful Clues for Rare Diagnoses

- **Radiation and Chemotherapy**
  - History
  - Mineralizing microangiopathy
- **Pseudo-TORCH**
  - **Aicardi-Goutières Syndrome**
    - "Mendelian mimic of congenital infection"
    - Multifocal punctate calcifications
    - Variable locations including periventricular white matter, basal ganglia, dentate nuclei
    - Elevated CSF interferon (IFN-α)
    - *TREX1* mutations in some
  - **Coats-Plus Syndrome**
    - a.k.a. cerebroretinal microangiopathy with calcifications and cysts
    - Ocular coats: Retinal telangiectasia and exudate
    - CNS small blood vessel calcification
    - Extensive thalamic and gyral calcification
    - Defects of bone marrow and integument
    - Growth failure

Congenital CMV

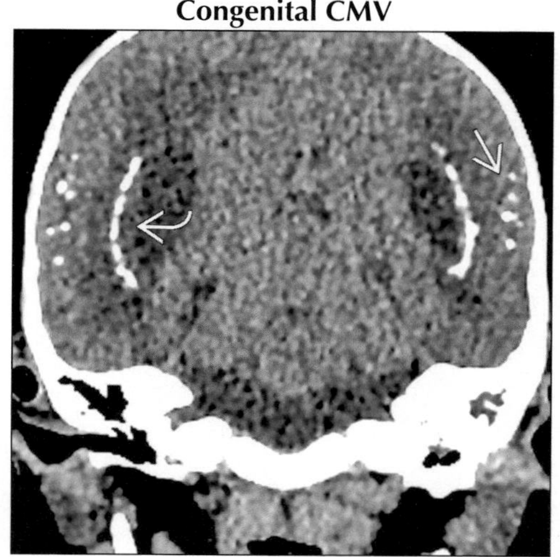

Coronal NECT shows classic findings of TORCH. Note the linear periventricular Ca++ ➔ with scattered Ca++ foci within the cortex ➔ in this deaf child, suggesting prior intrauterine CMV exposure.

Congenital CMV

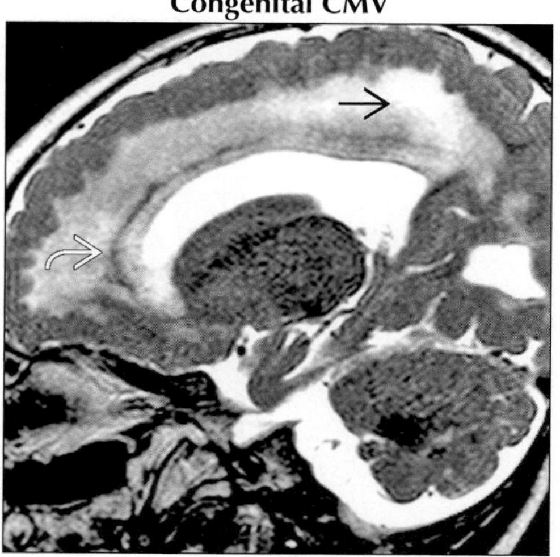

Sagittal T2WI MR shows a thick cortex with small gyri, hyperintense white matter →, and a thin layer of calcification ➔ in the same 18-month-old deaf toddler.

PERIVENTRICULAR CALCIFICATION

(Left) Axial NECT shows basal ganglia ➡ and periventricular calcifications ➡ in a child with typical colpocephalic dilation of the ventricles. (Right) Coronal T2WI MR shows marked ventriculomegaly and loss of the periventricular white matter. The periventricular and basal ganglia calcifications are occult on MR but do involve the right choroid plexus glomus ➡.

Congenital Toxoplasmosis

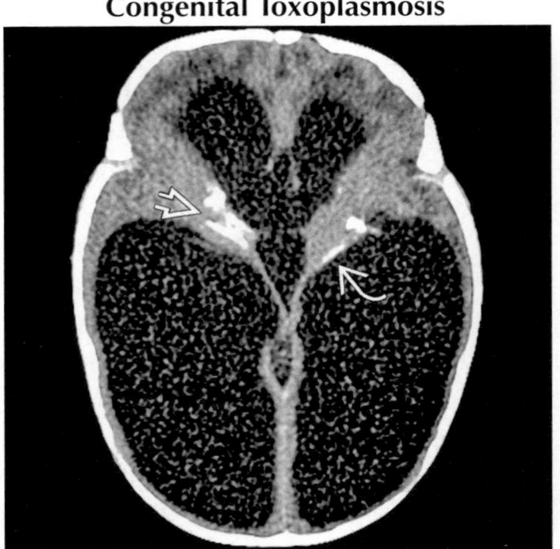

Congenital Toxoplasmosis

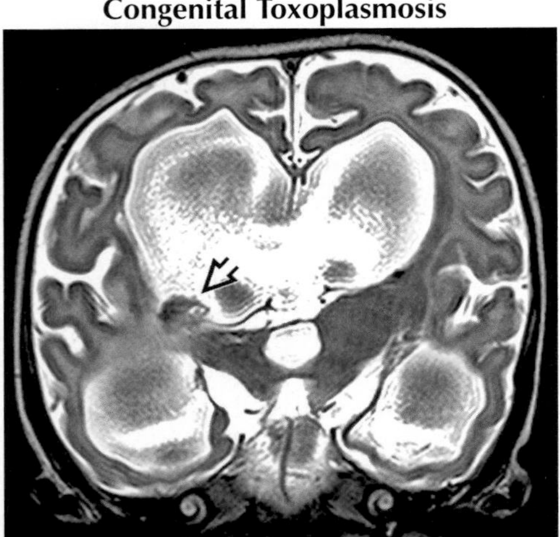

(Left) Axial NECT shows scattered and periventricular calcifications. In this child, there is unilateral left-sided colpocephaly ➡. Note the severe cortical mantle thinning ➡ over the colpocephalic ventricle. (Right) Axial T2 GRE MR shows similar findings, although the calcifications ➡ are not as well visualized.*

Congenital Toxoplasmosis

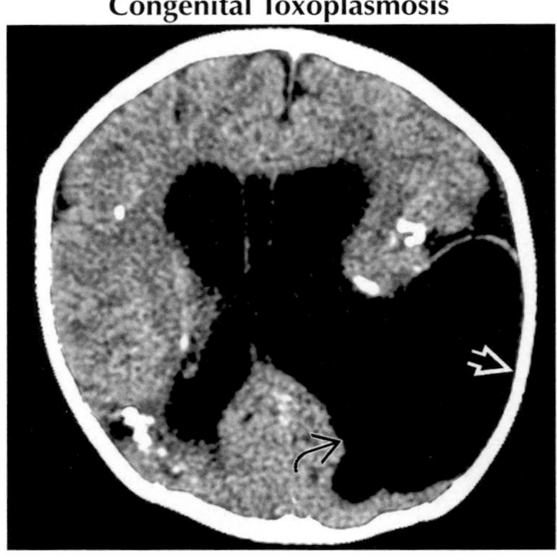

Congenital Toxoplasmosis

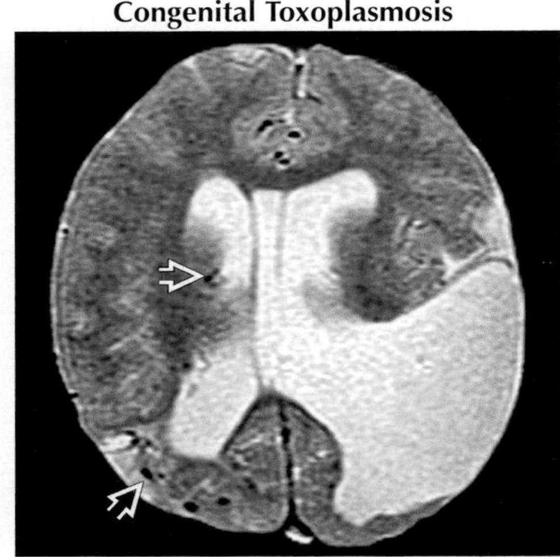

(Left) Axial NECT in a child who survived congenital herpes encephalitis shows scattered parenchymal calcifications ➡. (Right) Axial NECT in the same patient shows calcifications of the infarcted Rolandic cortex ➡. They can be variable, predominantly involving damaged brain.

Congenital Herpes Encephalitis

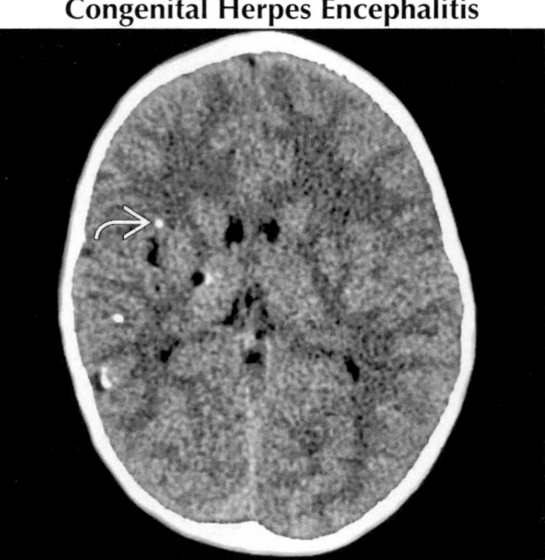

Congenital Herpes Encephalitis

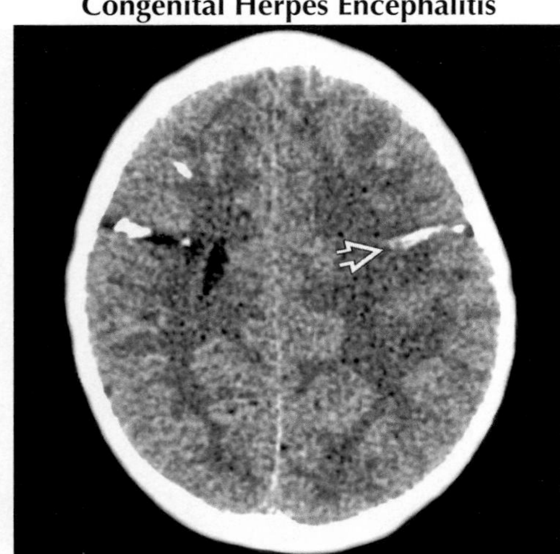

Congenital HIV

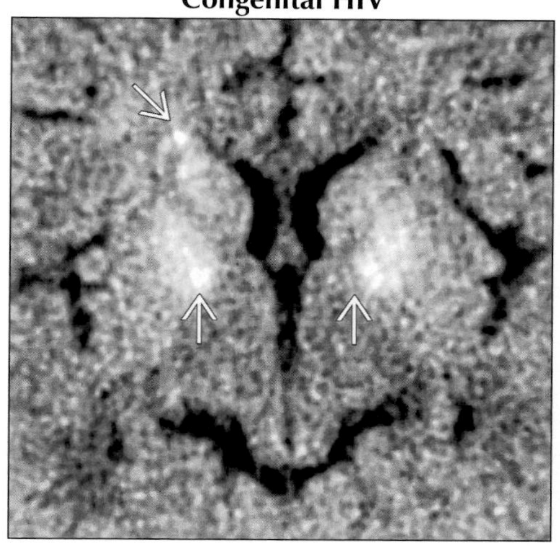

Congenital Rubella

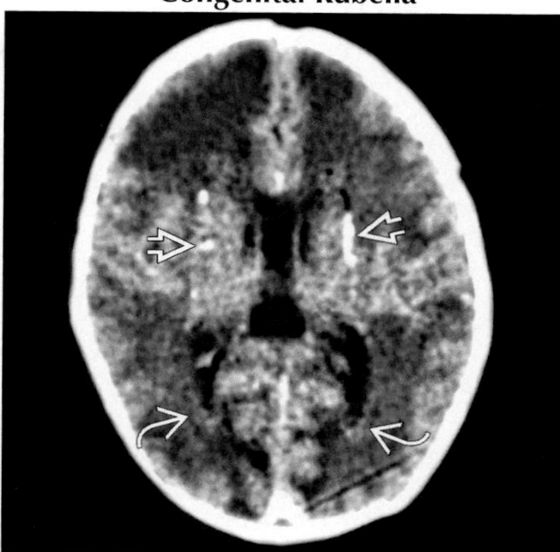

*(**Left**) Axial NECT shows hazy, symmetric basal ganglia calcification ➡ with diffusely prominent sulci and cisterns consistent with volume loss. In this 1 year old, the findings are highly suggestive of congenital HIV. (**Right**) Axial NECT shows basal ganglia calcifications ➡ and diffuse white matter hypointensity. There are faint bilateral subependymal calcifications lining the posterior horns ➡.*

Tuberous Sclerosis Complex

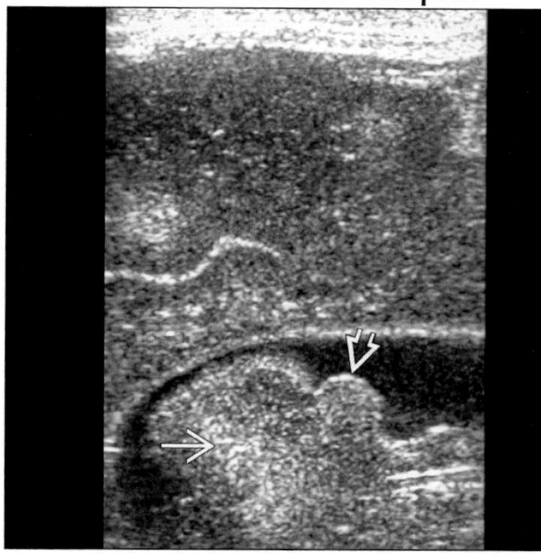

Tuberous Sclerosis Complex

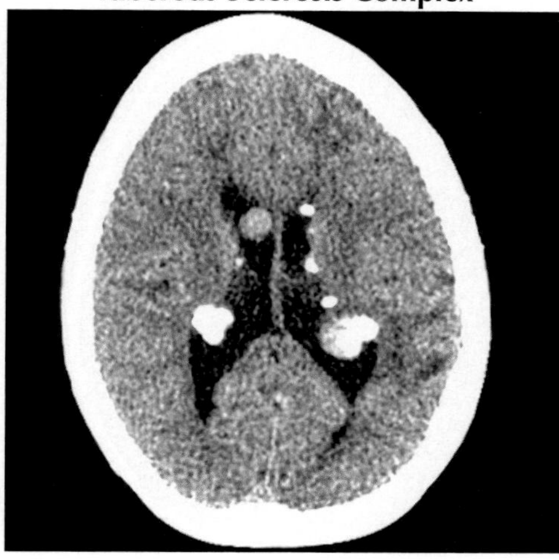

*(**Left**) Longitudinal ultrasound in a child with tuberous sclerosis complex and subependymal giant cell astrocytoma shows a mass indenting the lateral ventricle ➡. The tumor shows increased echogenicity ➡. (**Right**) Axial NECT shows variable calcification in the subependymal nodules. Calcification in these lesions progresses over time.*

Neurocysticercosis

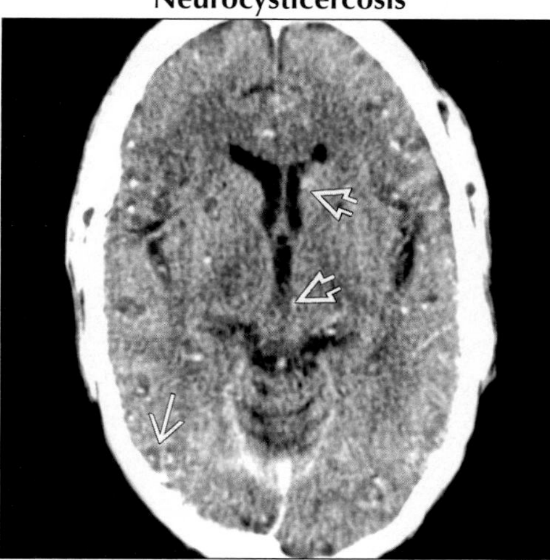

Neurocysticercosis

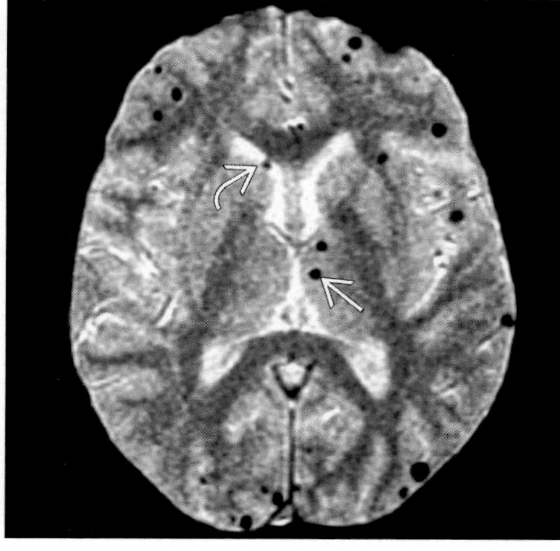

*(**Left**) Axial CECT shows the disseminated "miliary" form of neurocysticercosis (NCC). Note the numerous cysts, each with a hyperdense central "dot" representing scolex ➡. Innumerable small calcific foci, some of which are periventricular ➡, cause the classic "starry sky" appearance of healed NCC. (**Right**) Axial T2* GRE MR show scattered calcifications throughout the brain. A few are in the deep gray structures ➡, and 1 is intraventricular ➡.*

PERIVENTRICULAR CALCIFICATION

(Left) Axial NECT shows nodular calcification ➔ along the posteromedial temporal lobe on the tentorial surface. *(Right)* Axial CECT in the same patient shows the calcification ➔ to be largely obscured by the thick rind of pachymeningeal and leptomeningeal thickening and enhancement ➔.

Tuberculosis

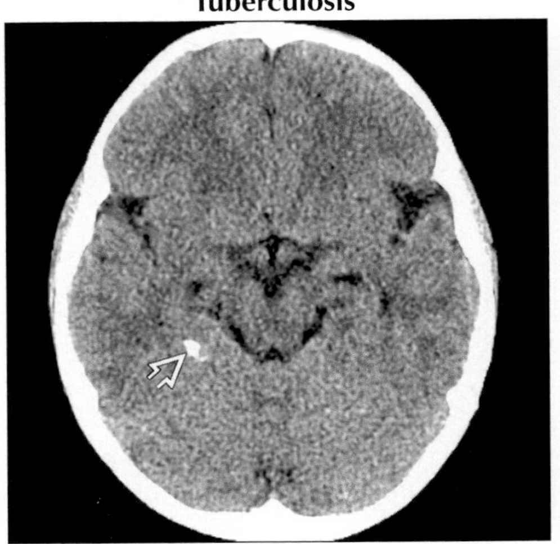

Tuberculosis

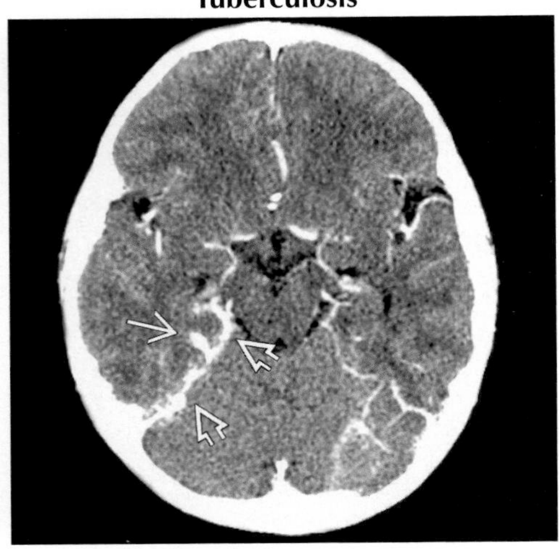

(Left) Axial T1WI MR early in the course of the disease shows hemorrhagic infarction ➔ of the ependyma and subependymal brain. *(Right)* Axial NECT shows subependymal tissue necrosis and calcification in the same areas ➔.

Ventriculitis (Chronic)

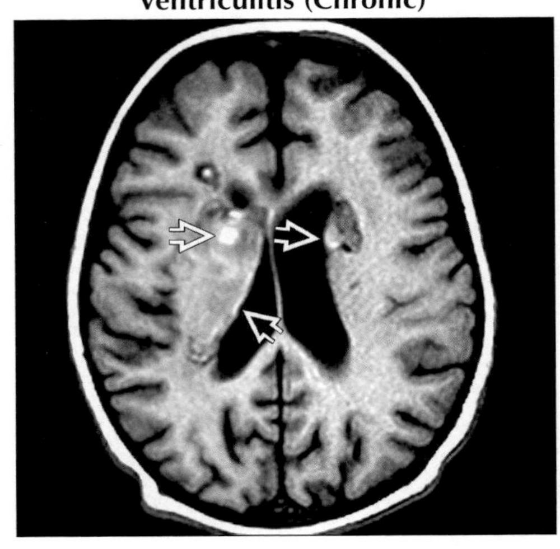

Ventriculitis (Chronic)

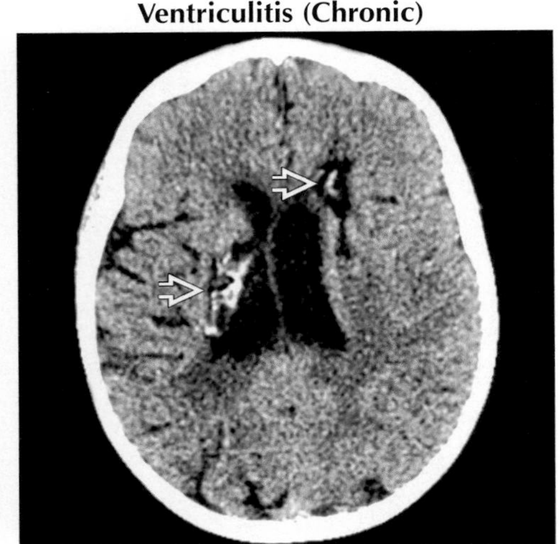

(Left) Axial NECT shows white matter deficiency due to periventricular leukomalacia. The gray matter ➔ nearly approximates the ventricular surface. Small periventricular calcifications ➔ are present at the site of a prior germinal matrix hemorrhage. *(Right)* Axial NECT shows bilateral symmetric calcifications at the gray-white junction ➔ due to mineralizing microangiopathy following radiation and chemotherapy.

Germinal Matrix Hemorrhage

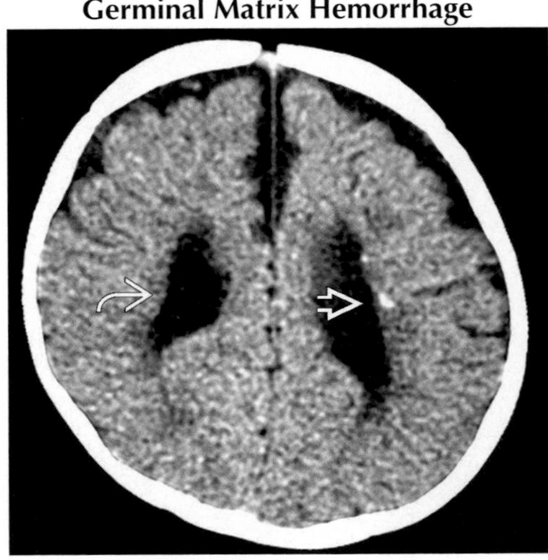

Radiation and Chemotherapy

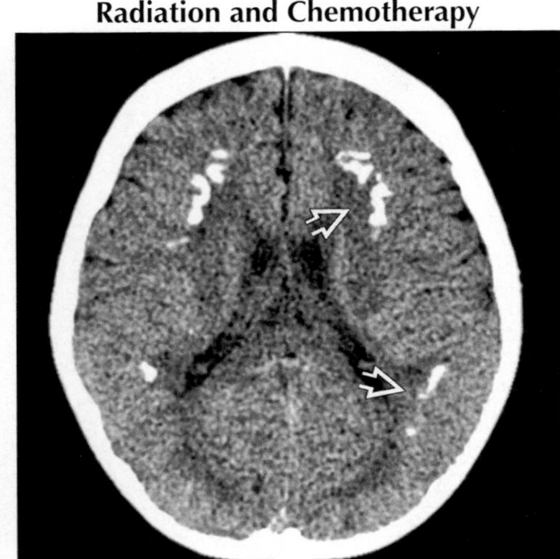

Radiation and Chemotherapy

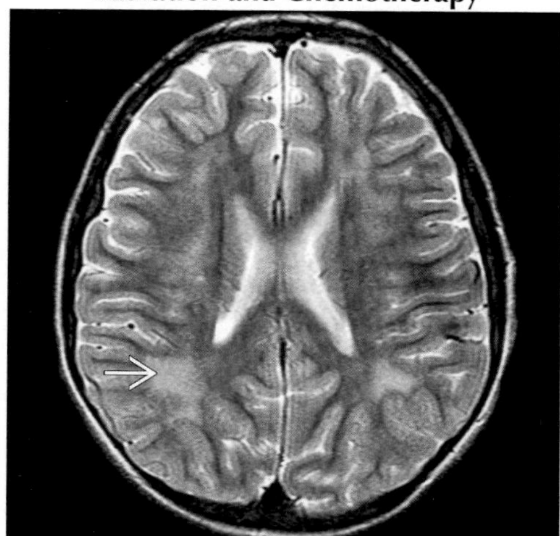

Aicardi-Goutières Syndrome

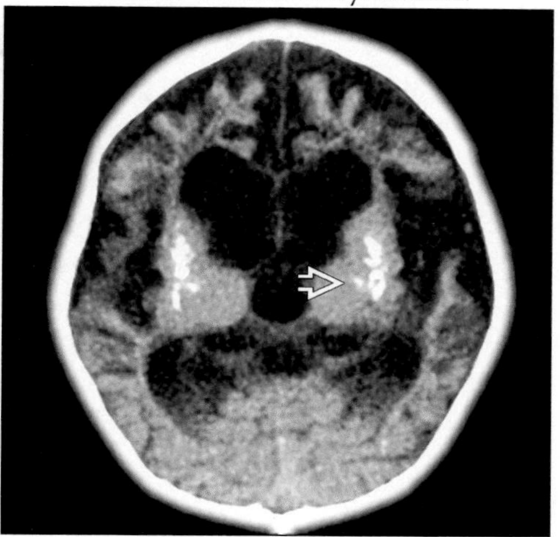

(Left) *Axial T2WI MR from the same patient shows white matter demyelination ➡. The calcifications are occult.* ***(Right)*** *Axial NECT shows brain atrophy and bilateral symmetrical calcifications in the basal ganglia ➡. Extension into the corona radiata (not shown) was also present.*

Aicardi-Goutières Syndrome

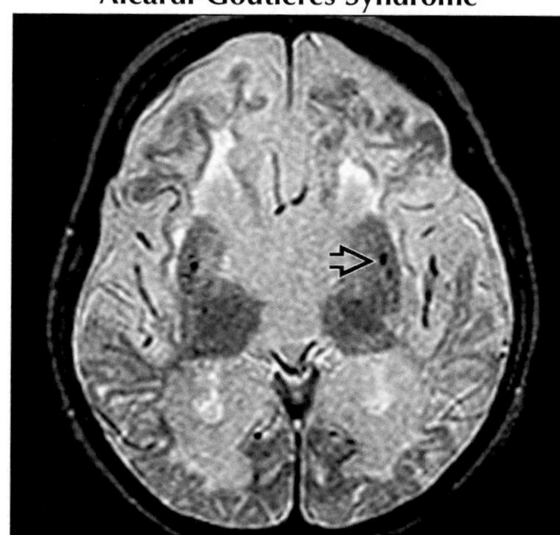

Aicardi-Goutières Syndrome

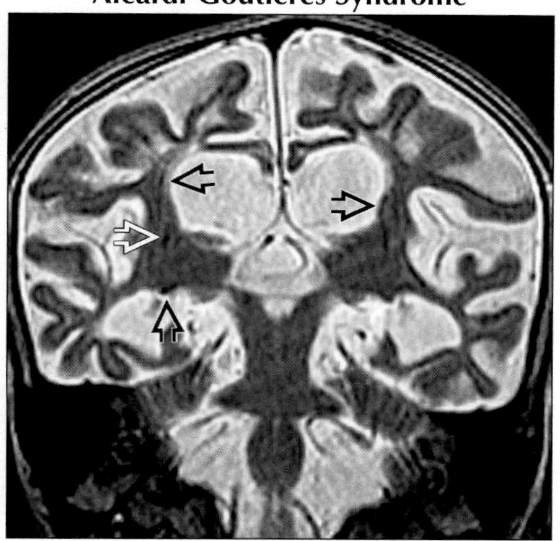

(Left) *Axial PD FSE MR shows extensive abnormal signal of white matter and volume loss of gray and white matter. Faint calcifications ➡ are present, although they are less well seen on MR than on NECT.* ***(Right)*** *Coronal T2WI MR again shows severe volume loss. Faint periventricular calcifications ➡ and basal ganglia calcifications ➡ are present, mimicking the appearance of TORCH infections.*

Coats-Plus Syndrome

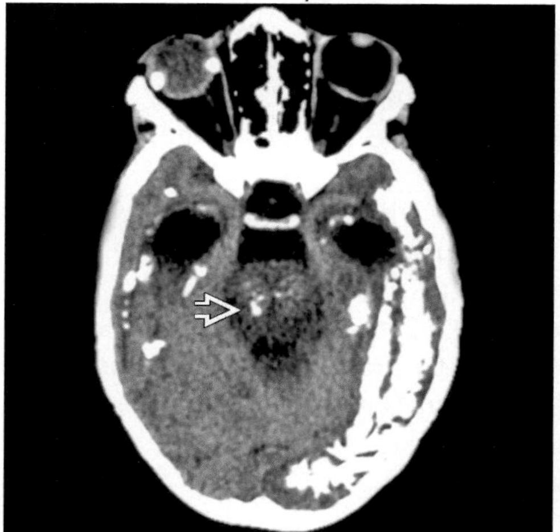

Coats-Plus Syndrome

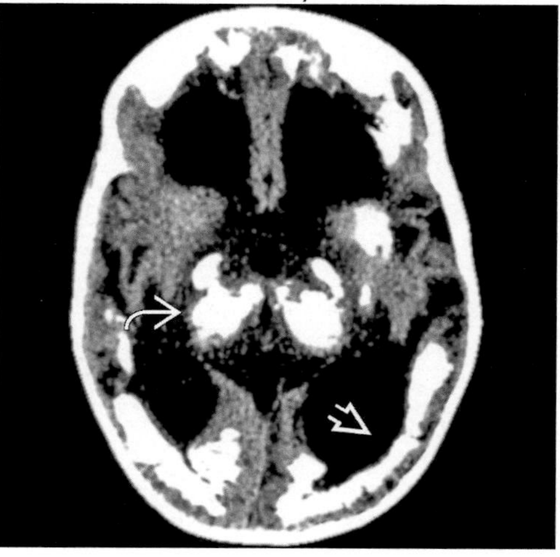

(Left) *Axial NECT shows extensive gyral, brainstem, and periventricular calcifications. The brainstem is also swollen ➡ and low density. Note the postoperative change of the right globe.* ***(Right)*** *Axial NECT shows dense periventricular calcification that extends to involve the sparse subcortical white matter posteriorly ➡, the frontal white matter, cortex, and thalami ➡. The pattern of calcification is typical, although swelling occurs beforehand.*

SUPRASELLAR MASS

DIFFERENTIAL DIAGNOSIS

Common
- Pilocytic Astrocytoma (PA)
- Craniopharyngioma
- Pituitary Hyperplasia (Physiologic)
- Hydrocephalus

Less Common
- Germinoma
- Tuber Cinereum Hamartoma
- Arachnoid Cyst
- Langerhans Cell Histiocytosis
- Pituitary Stalk Anomalies
- Teratoma

Rare but Important
- Lipoma
- Pituitary Macroadenoma
- Dermoid Cyst
- Leukemia
- Pilomyxoid Astrocytoma
- Saccular Aneurysm
- Retinoblastoma (Trilateral)
- Lymphocytic Hypophysitis
- Lymphoma, Primary CNS
- Rathke Cleft Cyst

ESSENTIAL INFORMATION

Key Differential Diagnosis Issues
- Is mass extra- or intraaxial?
- Extraaxial masses arise from pituitary/infundibulum, meninges, vessels
  - If extraaxial mass appears to arise from pituitary/infundibulum, determine origin of mass as precisely as possible
    - Pituitary gland: Think physiologic hyperplasia, hypophysitis, macroadenoma (rare in children)
    - Infundibular stalk: Germinoma, histiocytosis; stalk anomalies, lymphoma, leukemia (rare)
  - Nonpituitary extraaxial masses (normal pituitary gland can usually be identified inferior to lesion)
    - Craniopharyngioma
    - Hydrocephalus
    - Arachnoid cyst
    - Saccular aneurysm
- Intraaxial masses arise from chiasm/hypothalamus/3rd ventricle
  - Optic chiasm/hypothalamus: Pilocytic or pilomyxoid astrocytoma, tuber cinereum hamartoma, lipoma
  - Third ventricle: Hydrocephalus > > neoplasm
- T1 hyperintense suprasellar mass in child? Think craniopharyngioma, lipoma, dermoid, posterior pituitary ectopia

Helpful Clues for Common Diagnoses
- **Pilocytic Astrocytoma (PA)**
  - Most occur in children 5-15 years old
  - Enlarged optic nerve/chiasm/tract
  - Usually solid, iso-/hypointense on T1WI; hyperintense on T2WI, FLAIR
  - Variable enhancement (none to intense)
  - If large, bulky H-shaped mass in infant, may be pilomyxoid variant
- **Craniopharyngioma**
  - 90% Ca++ (globular, rim)
  - 90% cystic (may have multiple)
  - 90% enhance (rim, nodule)
  - Density/signal intensity within cysts/locules varies with content
- **Pituitary Hyperplasia (Physiologic)**
  - Up to 10 mm height, convex superior margin in young menstruating females
  - "Macroadenoma-appearing" mass in child?
    - May be hyperplasia, not tumor (especially prepubescent male)!
- **Hydrocephalus**
  - Enlarged 3rd ventricle (aqueductal stenosis, obstructive hydrocephalus)
  - Anterior recesses protrude inferiorly
  - May enlarge bony sella over time

Helpful Clues for Less Common Diagnoses
- **Germinoma**
  - 50-60% involve pituitary gland/stalk
  - Often presents with diabetes insipidus (DI)
- **Tuber Cinereum Hamartoma**
  - Isosexual precocious puberty > gelastic seizures
  - Pedunculated ("collar button") or sessile mass between infundibular stalk, mamillary bodies
    - Can be tiny (1-2 mm) or giant (3-5 cm)
    - Isointense with gray matter (occasionally slightly hyperintense on FLAIR)
    - Doesn't enhance
- **Arachnoid Cyst**
  - 10% suprasellar
  - Sharply marginated CSF-like cyst

- Sagittal T1- or T2WI shows 3rd ventricle elevated, compressed over cyst
- Suppresses on FLAIR, DWI negative

- **Langerhans Cell Histiocytosis**
  - Child usually < 2 years old
    - May have central DI
  - 10% of LCH cases involve stalk, pituitary gland ± hypothalamus
    - Rare: Choroid plexus, leptomeninges, cerebellar WM, brain parenchyma
  - Look for solitary/multiple lytic skull lesions with "beveled edges"
- **Pituitary Stalk Anomalies**
  - Posterior pituitary ectopia
    - Short stature ± endocrine deficiencies
    - Posterior pituitary "bright spot" missing
    - Mislocated along tuber cinereum
    - Stalk small/absent
  - Duplicated pituitary gland/stalk
    - Endocrinologically normal
    - ± midline facial anomalies
    - Tuber cinereum/mamillary bodies fused
- **Teratoma**
  - Optic chiasm > pineal
  - Ca++, cysts, soft tissue, fat

Helpful Clues for Rare Diagnoses

- **Lipoma**
  - Fatty hypothalamic mass
- **Pituitary Macroadenoma**
  - "Figure of 8" pituitary mass
  - Gland cannot be separated from mass
- **Dermoid Cyst**
  - Fat-like mass ± droplets in CSF
    - Fat suppression sequences confirm
  - 20% Ca++
- **Leukemia**
  - Rare; look for other lesions (sinuses, dura)
- **Pilomyxoid Astrocytoma**
  - Rare variant of PA
  - Large, bulky suprasellar mass in infant
  - May hemorrhage (rare in PA)
- **Saccular Aneurysm**
  - Rare in children (< 2% of all saccular aneurysms occur in pediatric age group)
  - When occur, often large/bizarre
  - Thrombus common
  - Look for residual patent lumen, phase artifact
- **Retinoblastoma (Trilateral)**
  - 3rd tumor in pineal or suprasellar region
- **Lymphocytic Hypophysitis**
  - Adolescent > child
  - May cause DI
  - Can mimic macroadenoma, pituitary apoplexy
- **Lymphoma, Primary CNS**
  - Rare in children
  - Can mimic hypophysitis, germinoma, LCH
- **Rathke Cleft Cyst**
  - Rare in children
  - Cyst in/above pituitary, separate from stalk
  - Rarely calcifies, does not enhance ("claw" of enhancing pituitary tissue may surround mass)
  - Intracystic nodule virtually pathognomonic

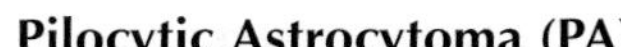

Pilocytic Astrocytoma (PA)

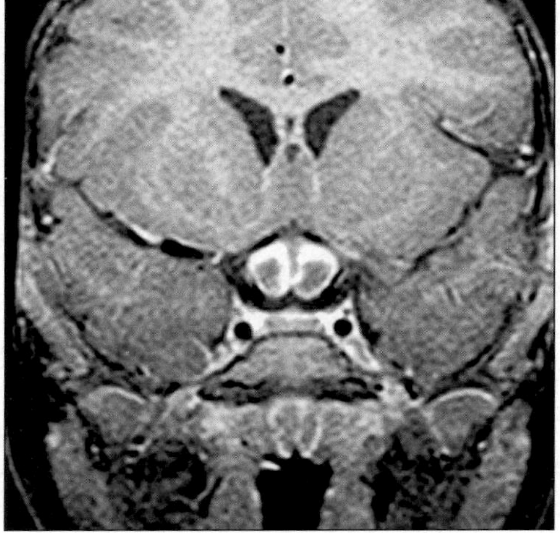

Coronal T1 C+ MR shows chiasmatic glioma. The prechiasmatic optic nerves are expanded and surrounded by enhancing tumor.

Pilocytic Astrocytoma (PA)

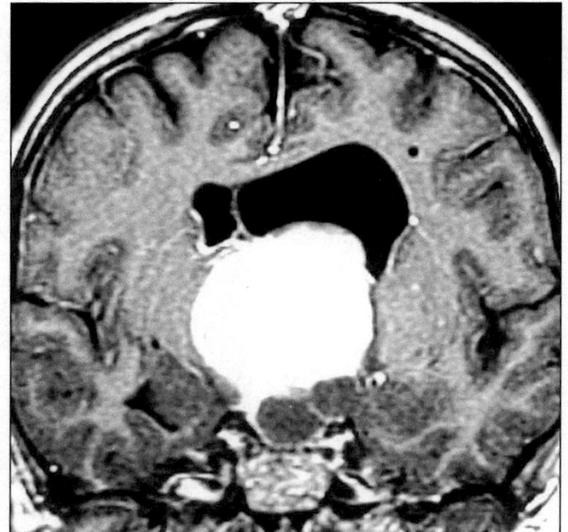

Coronal T1WI C+ MR shows a very large suprasellar pilocytic astrocytoma. This solid and cystic mass involves the suprasellar cistern, the chiasm, the hypothalamus and protrudes into the 3rd ventricle.

SUPRASELLAR MASS

(Left) *Sagittal T1WI MR shows typical cysts of varying signal intensity in the suprasellar cistern, herniating into the 3rd ventricle. There is enlargement of the bony sella and erosion of the dorsum sella ➔.* ***(Right)*** *Coronal T2WI MR shows calcification ➔ at the base of the lesion.*

Craniopharyngioma

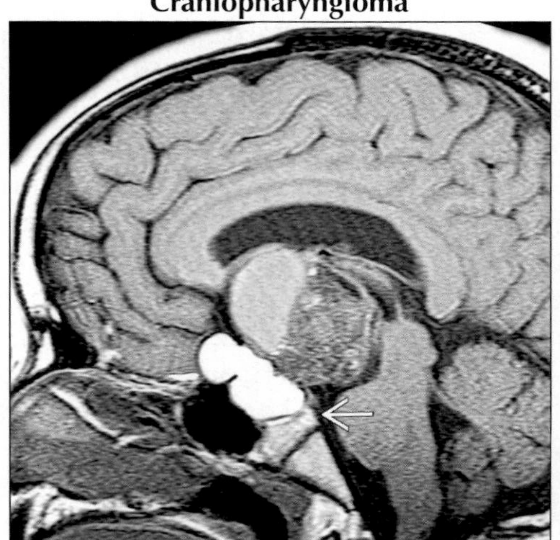

Craniopharyngioma

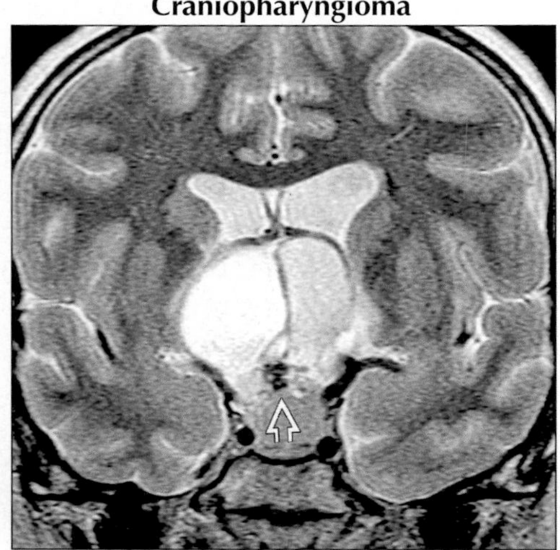

(Left) *Sagittal T1WI C+ MR shows a large pituitary gland ➔ projecting above shallow pituitary fossa following prolonged shunting. Note the associated thickened calvarium ➔.* ***(Right)*** *Sagittal T2WI MR shows typical synchronous suprasellar ➔, pineal ➔ masses in a teen who presented with signs of ↑ intracranial pressure. Note increased signal in body of corpus callosum at site of hippocampal commissure disruption ➔ caused by acute hydrocephalus.*

Pituitary Hyperplasia (Physiologic)

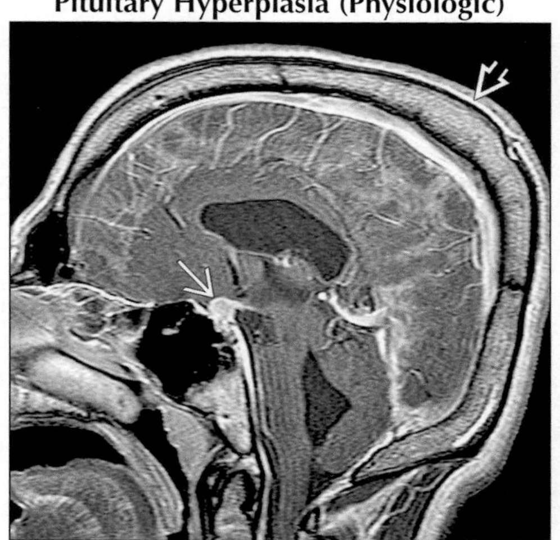

Germinoma

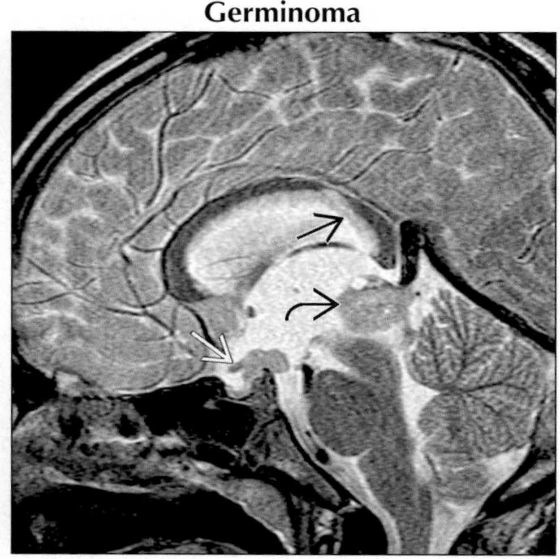

(Left) *Sagittal T1WI C+ MR in the same patient shows inhomogeneous enhancement ➔. The suprasellar mass perches on the dorsum sella; the pineal obstructs the aqueduct.* ***(Right)*** *Sagittal T1WI C+ MR shows a large nonenhancing pedunculated mass ➔ extending from the tuber cinereum between the mamillary bodies and infundibular stalk in a child with gelastic seizures.*

Germinoma

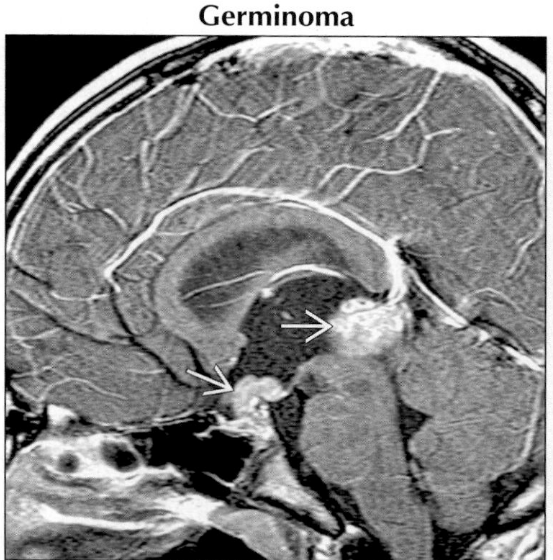

Tuber Cinereum Hamartoma

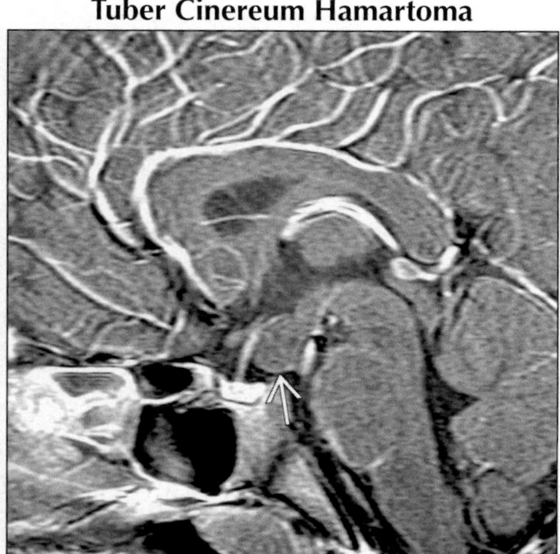

Tuber Cinereum Hamartoma

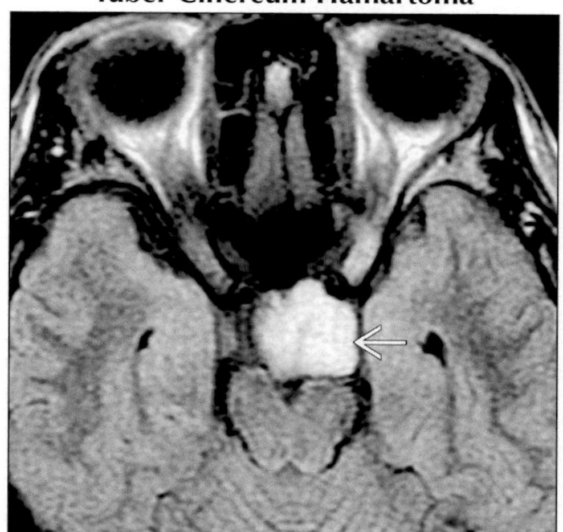

Arachnoid Cyst

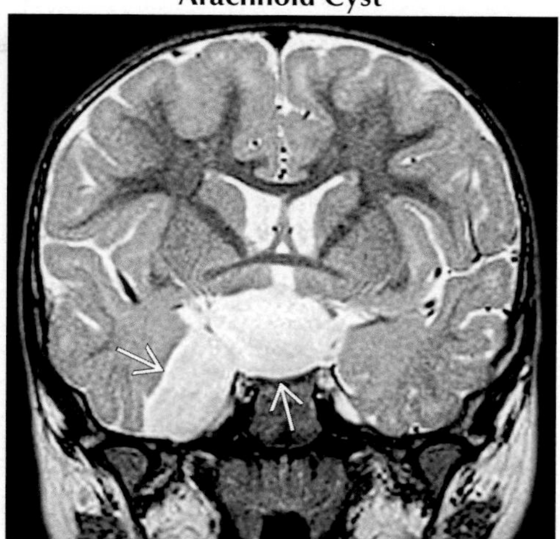

(Left) *Axial FLAIR MR shows mildly increased signal intensity within the hamartoma* ➡*. Unlike small hamartomas, which follow gray matter signal on T2 and FLAIR sequences, large hamartomas may be slightly brighter on FLAIR and T2 than gray matter.* ***(Right)*** *Coronal T2WI MR shows erosion of the dorsum sella, upward displacement of the hypothalamus, and extension into the right middle cranial fossa caused by suprasellar arachnoid cyst* ➡*.*

Langerhans Cell Histiocytosis

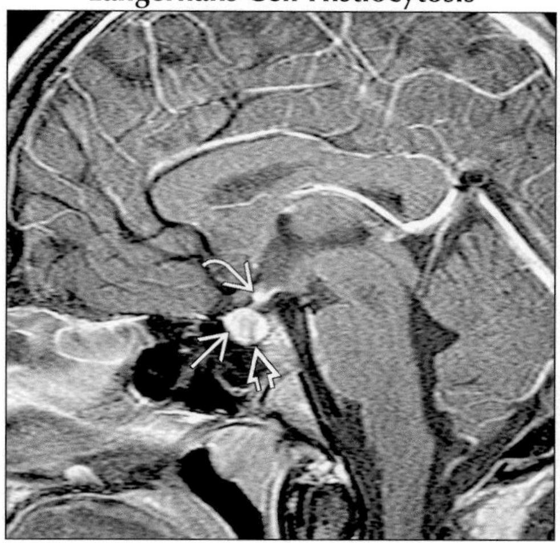

Pituitary Stalk Anomalies

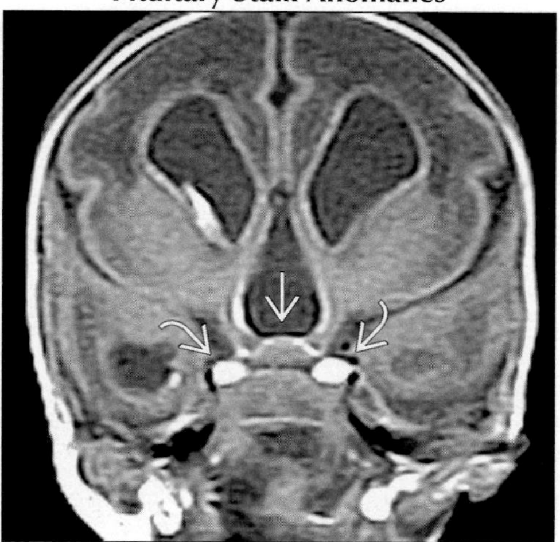

(Left) *Sagittal T1WI C+ MR in a teen shows nodular thickening of infundibular recess* ➡*. Additionally, there is a tiny pars intermedia cyst* ➡*. Note the upwardly convex pituitary gland (normal physiologic hyperplasia)* ➡*.* ***(Right)*** *Coronal T1WI MR shows thickening of the tuber cinereum (tubomammillary fusion)* ➡ *in a child with 2 pituitary glands* ➡ *due to maternal genetics. Both glands are bright on T1WI images in the premature newborn.*

Teratoma

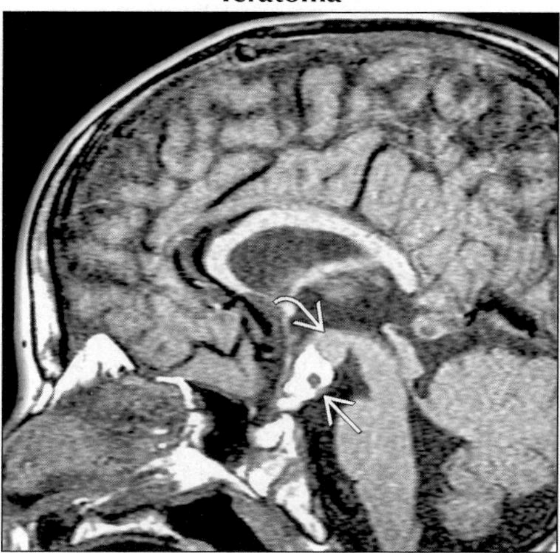

Teratoma

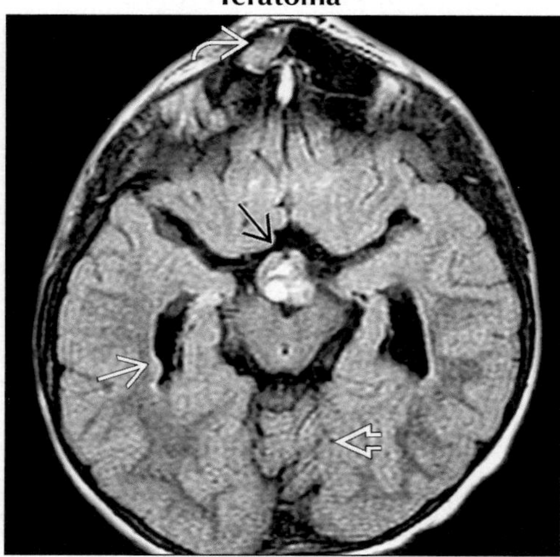

(Left) *Sagittal T1WI MR shows bright fat with a central focus of calcification* ➡*. There is a soft tissue mass* ➡ *in the region of the tuber cinereum in this child who had multiple other congenital anomalies.* ***(Right)*** *Axial FLAIR MR in the same patient shows heterogeneous suprasellar teratoma* ➡*, metopic synostosis* ➡*, and dehiscent tentorium* ➡*. A small nodule of periventricular heterotopia is also seen in the wall of the right temporal horn* ➡*.*

SUPRASELLAR MASS

(Left) Axial T1WI MR shows a multilobed lipoma ➡ in the suprasellar cistern. *(Right)* Sagittal T1WI C+ FS MR in the same patient shows loss of signal in the lipoma ➡ following fat saturation.

Lipoma

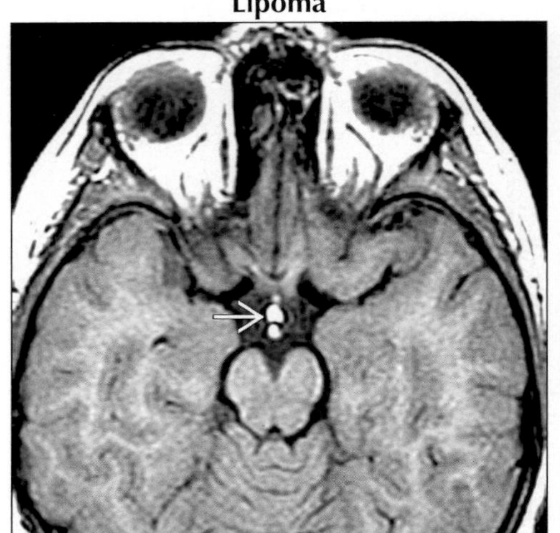

Lipoma

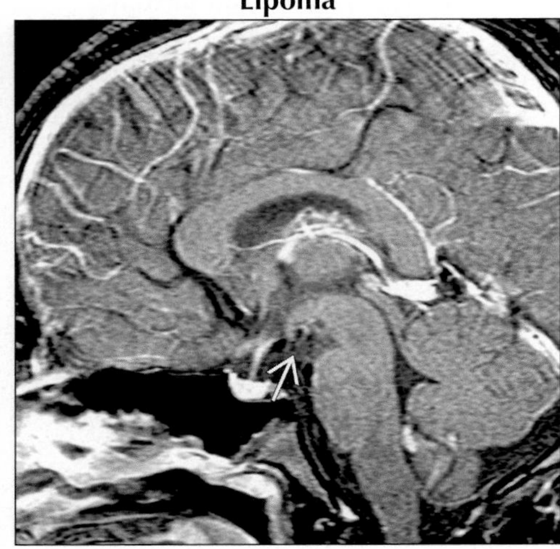

(Left) Sagittal T1WI MR shows a large bilobed sellar and suprasellar ➡ macroadenoma in a teenager with acromegaly. Note also the enlarged frontal sinuses ➡. *(Right)* Coronal T1WI C+ MR shows a fairly homogeneously enhancing macroadenoma ➡ that abuts the cavernous sinus in the same acromegalic teenager. Note the thickened scalp ➡.

Pituitary Macroadenoma

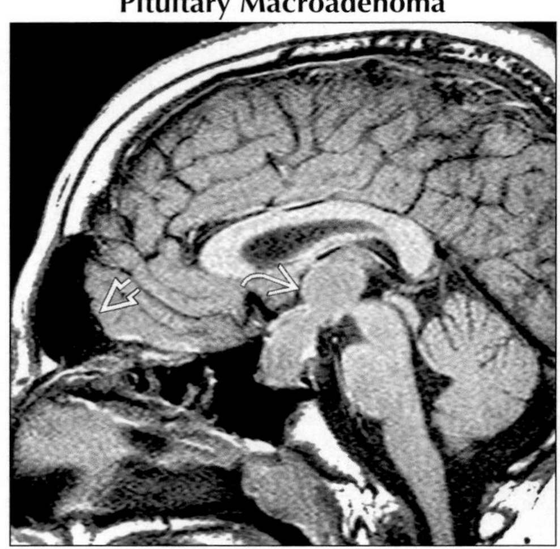

Pituitary Macroadenoma

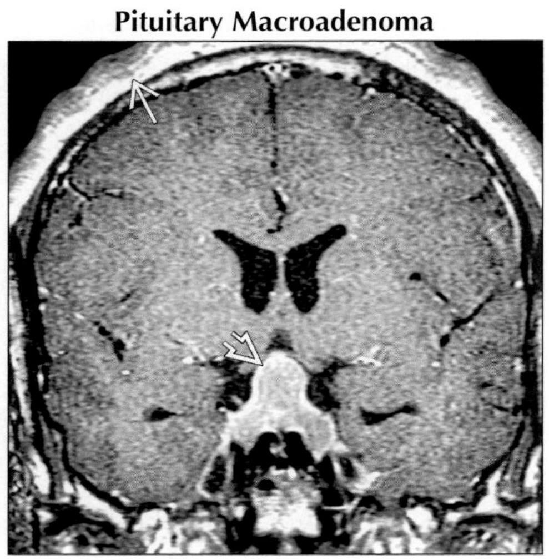

(Left) Sagittal T2WI MR shows a large, very hyperintense, suprasellar pilomyxoid astrocytoma that displaces the mesencephalon posteriorly. *(Right)* Sagittal T2WI FS MR in a newborn shows a large, lobular, thrombosing, suprasellar saccular aneurysm ➡.

Pilomyxoid Astrocytoma

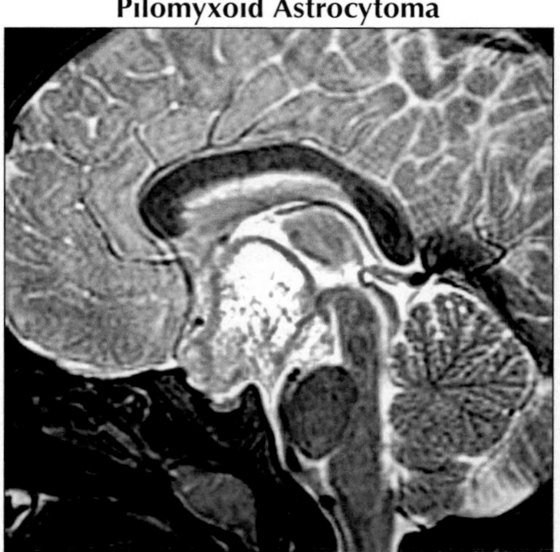

Saccular Aneurysm

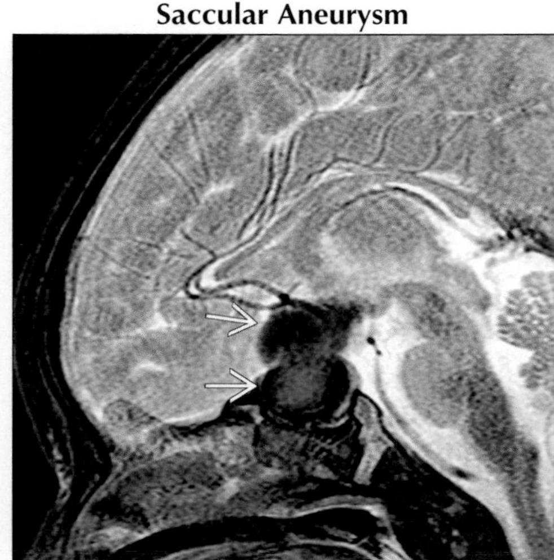

Saccular Aneurysm

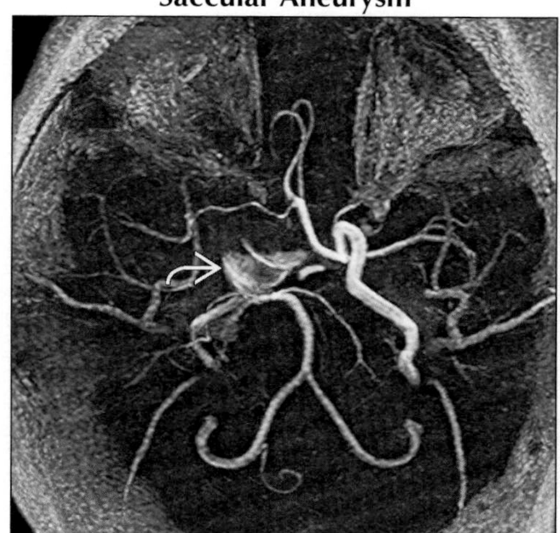

Retinoblastoma (Trilateral)

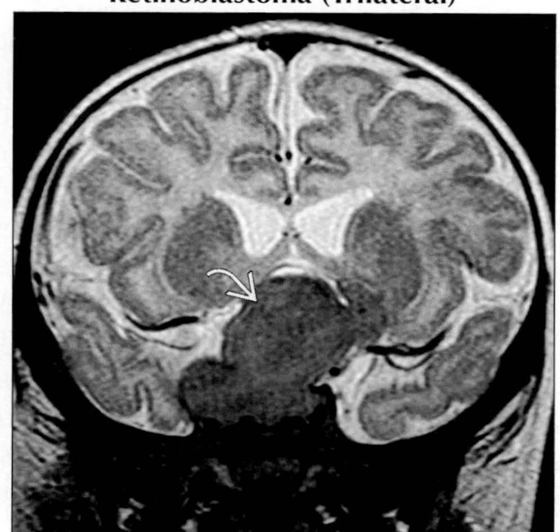

(Left) *Axial MRA shows obliteration of the right distal internal carotid artery and faint increased signal in the posterior* ➡ *aspect of the thrombosing aneurysm.* ***(Right)*** *Coronal T2WI MR shows a large low signal suprasellar mass* ➡ *that abuts the hypothalamus. This patient had ocular retinoblastoma.*

Retinoblastoma (Trilateral)

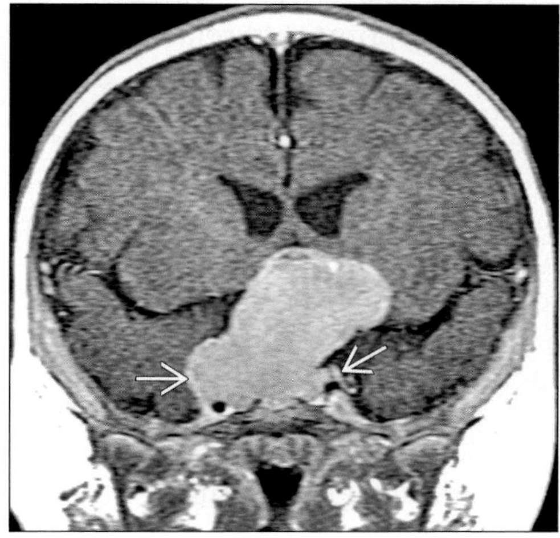

Lymphocytic Hypophysitis

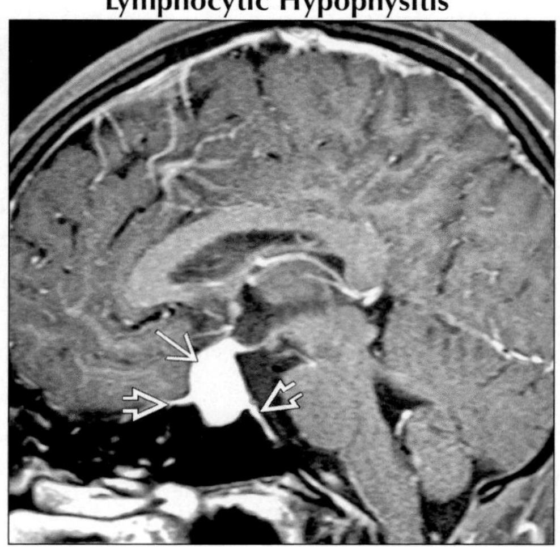

(Left) *Coronal T1WI C+ MR in the same patient shows intense, uniform enhancement. Note the bilateral cavernous sinus invasion* ➡*.* ***(Right)*** *Sagittal T1WI C+ FS MR in a pregnant teenager who developed acute onset of vision problems in the late 3rd trimester shows a large enhancing mass* ➡ *with reactive dural thickening* ➡*. Preoperative diagnosis was macroadenoma.*

Lymphoma, Primary CNS

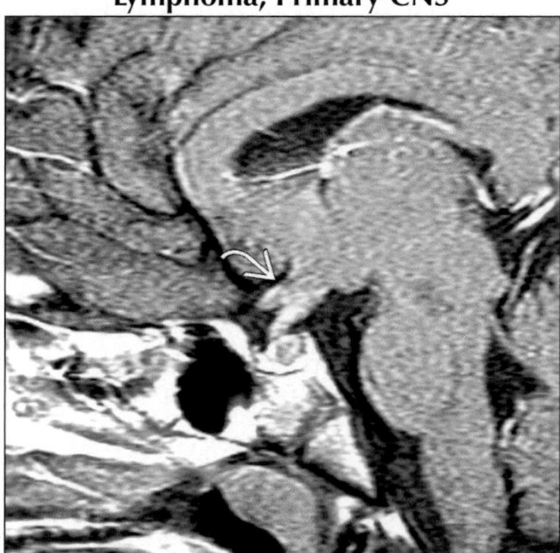

Rathke Cleft Cyst

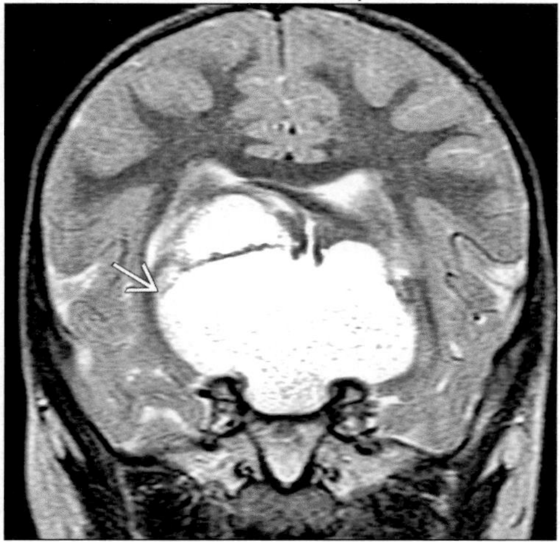

(Left) *Sagittal T1 C+ MR shows thickening* ➡ *and subtle enhancement of the infundibular stalk, chiasm, and tuber cinereum.* ***(Right)*** *Coronal T2WI MR shows a well-delineated suprasellar cyst* ➡*. The pituitary gland and stalk are not seen, and there was no calcification on high-resolution NECT.*

PINEAL MASS

DIFFERENTIAL DIAGNOSIS

Common
- Pineal Cyst

Less Common
- Germinoma
- Teratoma

Rare but Important
- Pineoblastoma
- Retinoblastoma
- Pineocytoma

ESSENTIAL INFORMATION

Helpful Clues for Common Diagnoses
- **Pineal Cyst**
  - Key facts
    - Intrapineal glial-lined cyst, nonneoplastic
    - May form or involute over time
    - Majority 5-10 mm and asymptomatic; may be > 20 mm
    - Rarely ⇒ hemorrhage, acute hydrocephalus, or Parinaud syndrome
    - Incidence of cysts > 5 mm: 11-20 years (3%), 21-30 years (3.4%), 70 years (< 0.5%)
    - If > 1 cm, nodularity, or associated clinical symptoms, recommend short interval follow-up
  - Imaging
    - Well-defined, uni-/multiloculated cyst
    - Posterior to 3rd ventricle, above tectum, below internal cerebral veins
    - If large, may ⇒ flattening of tectum, aqueduct compression, internal cerebral vein elevation
    - T1 and T2WI; Iso- to hyperintense to CSF
    - FLAIR: Usually hyperintense to CSF
    - DWI: Typically isointense to CSF
    - T2* GRE: Occasionally bloom if recent or old hemorrhage
    - ± thin (< 2 mm) rim of enhancement = compressed pineal tissue
    - Rarely nodular enhancement
    - Avoid delayed post-contrast imaging; may show enhancement of cyst contents, making differentiation from tumors impossible

Helpful Clues for Less Common Diagnoses
- **Germinoma**
  - Key facts
    - Tumor of primordial germ cells
    - Most common pineal tumor in children
    - 30-40% of CNS germinomas in pineal region (50-60% suprasellar, up to 14% thalamus and basal ganglia)
    - Males > > females in pineal region
    - Males ≈ females in suprasellar region
    - Present with headache, hydrocephalus, and Parinaud syndrome (paralysis of upward gaze)
  - Imaging
    - Classic well-defined mass "engulfs" pineal gland
    - CT: Iso-/hyperdense to gray matter
    - T1 and T2WI: Iso- to hypointense relative to GM
    - ± hyperintense cysts T2WI
    - FLAIR: Iso- to hypointense relative to gray matter
    - DWI: Restricted diffusion
    - Avid contrast enhancement; "speckled" enhancement common
    - Relatively small lesion may ⇒ ventricular obstruction
    - May engulf or displace pineal Ca++
    - MRS: ↑ choline, ↓ NAA, ± lactate
    - ± enhancing subarachnoid metastases
- **Teratoma**
  - Key facts
    - 2nd most common pineal tumor in children
    - Benign, nongerminomatous germ cell tumor
    - Mature, immature, and malignant types
    - Males > > females pineal and suprasellar region
    - Present with headache, hydrocephalus, and Parinaud syndrome (paralysis of upward gaze)
  - Imaging
    - Heterogeneous pineal region mass with fat, soft tissue, Ca++, and cysts
    - T1WI: ↑ signal from fat, variable signal from Ca++
    - T2WI: Soft tissue iso- to hyperintense
    - FLAIR: ↓ signal intensity from cysts, ↑ signal intensity from solid tissue
    - MRS: ↑ lipid moieties on short echo

- Fat suppression MR helps to confirm fat content
- Difficult to distinguish mature from immature by imaging

- **Pineoblastoma**
  - Key facts
    - Primitive neuroectodermal tumor (PNET) of pineal gland
    - Highly malignant
    - Children > adults
    - Up to 40% in infants
  - Imaging
    - Large (usually > 3 cm) pineal mass
    - Hydrocephalus 2° aqueductal obstruction
    - "Exploded" peripheral Ca++ on CT
    - Extension into 3rd ventricle, thalamus, midbrain, cerebellar vermis common
    - CT: Solid portion hyperdense
    - T1WI: Solid portion iso- to hyperintense relative to GM
    - T2WI: Solid portion iso- to hyperintense relative to GM; mild peritumoral edema common; frequent necrosis; occasional hemorrhage
    - Moderate heterogeneous enhancement
    - MRS: ↑ choline, ↓ NAA
    - CSF spread in up to 40% at time of presentation

Helpful Clues for Rare Diagnoses

- **Retinoblastoma**
  - Key facts
    - Trilateral retinoblastoma = bilateral ocular retinoblastoma + midline intracranial neuroblastic tumor
    - Pineal (80%), suprasellar (20%)
    - Intracranial 3rd tumor usually present 2-3 years after primary ocular tumors
    - Histologically identical to ocular tumors
  - Imaging
    - Enhancing mass + bilateral ocular retinoblastoma
    - DDx = metastatic retinoblastoma
- **Pineocytoma**
  - Key facts
    - Pineal parenchymal tumor
    - Uncommon in children; may occur at any age (mean age 35 years)
    - Males = females
    - Variable natural history from noninvasive slow growing to aggressive with extensive metastases
  - Imaging
    - Well-defined, round, homogeneous mass
    - T1WI: Iso- to hypointense relative to GM
    - T2WI and FLAIR: Iso- to hyperintense
    - Peripheral or central homogeneous enhancement
    - More uniform enhancement than pineoblastoma
    - May be similar to CSF on pre-contrast images, therefore simulate simple pineal cyst
    - Areas of necrosis common in larger lesions

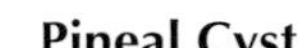

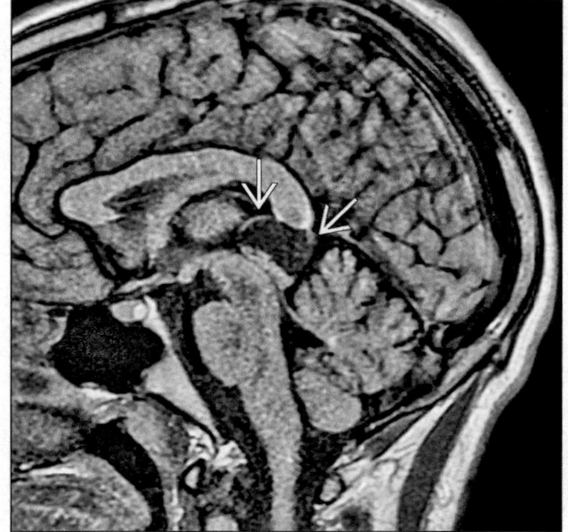

Sagittal T1WI MR shows a moderate-sized, simple-appearing pineal cyst ➔ with mild mass effect on the adjacent tectum. The cyst was incidentally noted on prior head CT after closed head injury.

Pineal Cyst

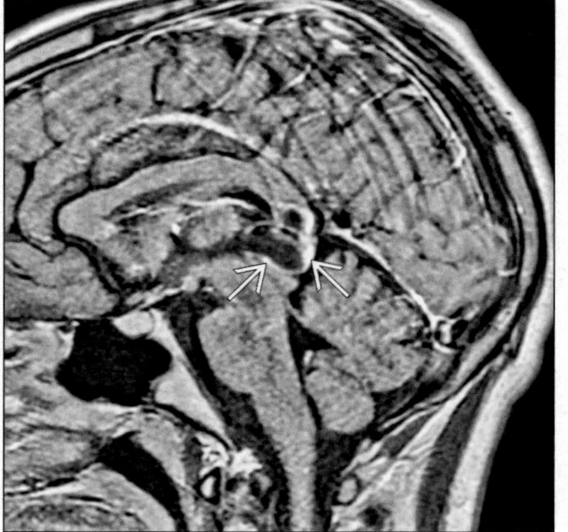

Sagittal T1WI C+ FS MR shows minimal peripheral enhancement ➔ of compressed pineal tissue.

PINEAL MASS

(Left) *Axial NECT shows a large, well-defined hyperdense mass ➔ in the pineal region, causing mild obstructive hydrocephalus ➔. This teenager presented with a headache and diplopia.* **(Right)** *Sagittal T1WI C+ MR shows a large, diffusely enhancing pineal region mass ➔ and enlargement of the 3rd ventricle ➔ secondary to aqueductal obstruction.*

Germinoma

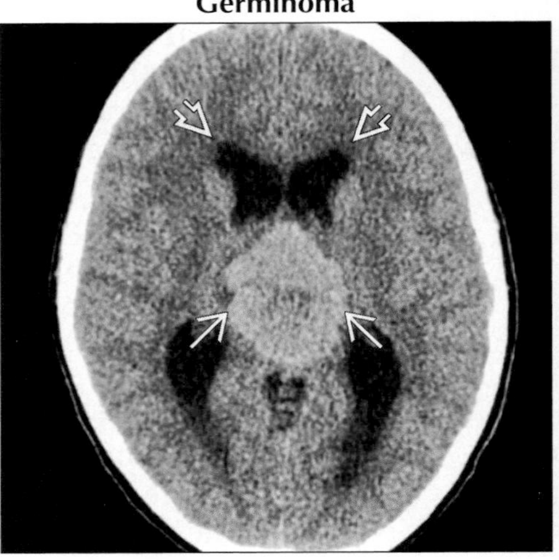

Germinoma

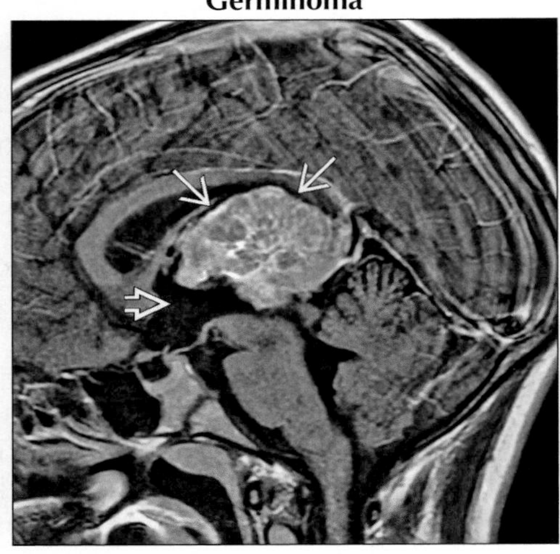

(Left) *Axial T2WI FSE MR in the same patient shows the mass nearly isointense to GM ➔, with mild surrounding edema ➔ and moderate ventriculomegaly ➔.* **(Right)** *Sagittal T1 C+ MR in another patient shows a moderately enhancing mass ➔ compressing the superior colliculus and causing obstructive enlargement of the 3rd ventricle ➔.*

Germinoma

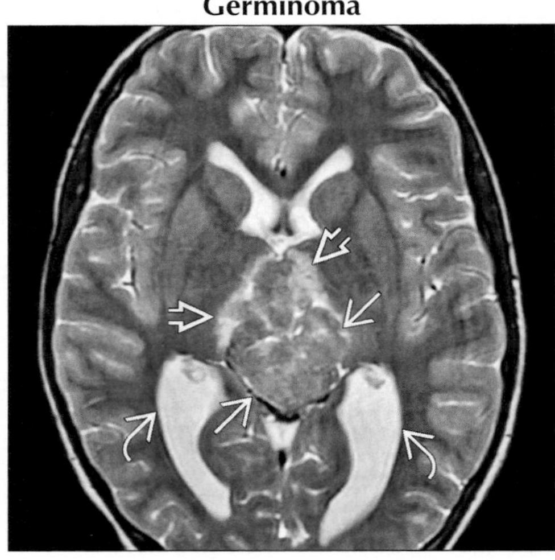

Germinoma

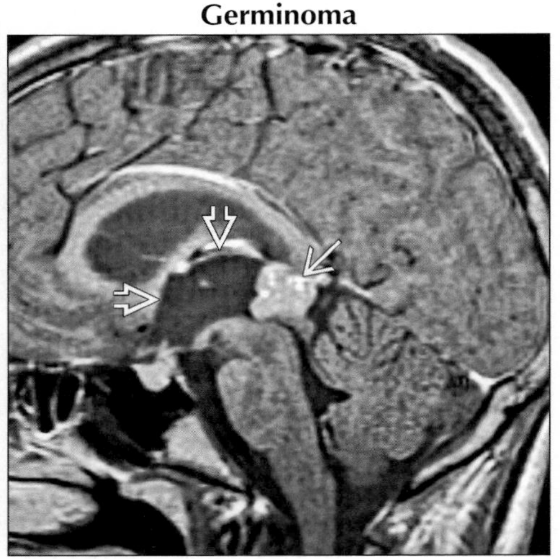

(Left) *Axial T1WI MR shows a large heterogeneous mass with multiple foci of hyperintense fat ➔ causing obstructive hydrocephalus ➔.* **(Right)** *Axial T1 C+ FS MR shows suppression of the foci of fat signal intensity ➔ and heterogeneous contrast enhancement.*

Teratoma

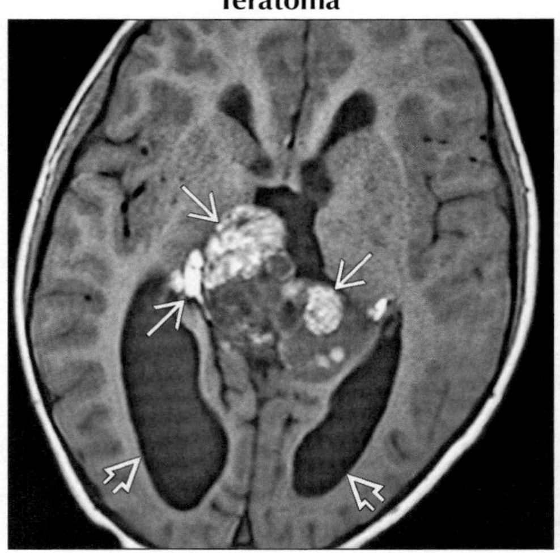

Teratoma

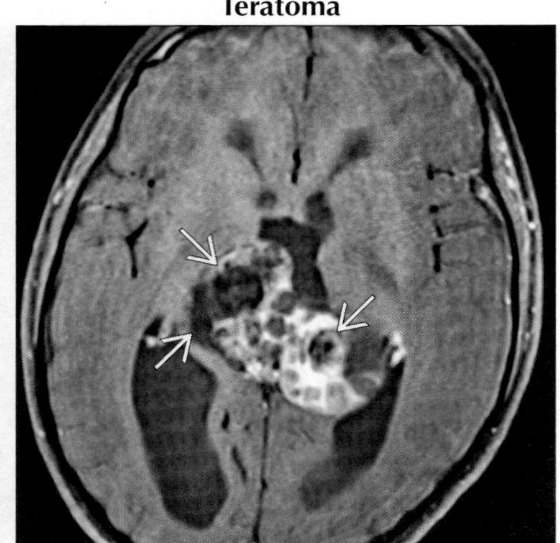

Pineoblastoma

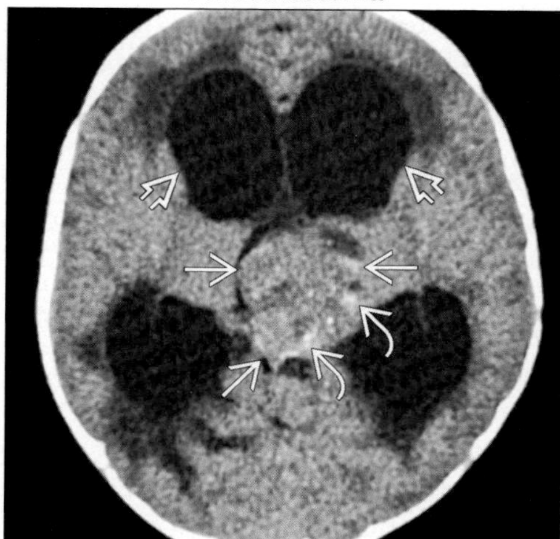

Pineoblastoma

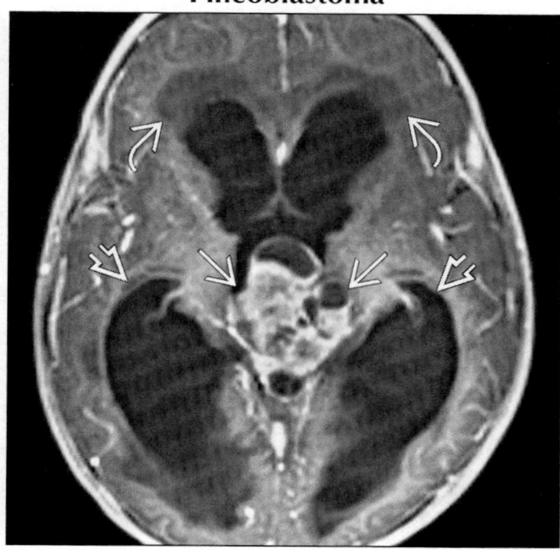

(Left) *Axial NECT shows a moderate-sized, intermediate-attenuation mass → causing significant obstructive hydrocephalus →. Notice the "exploded" peripheral calcifications →. This infant presented with somnolence and gaze abnormality.* ***(Right)*** *Axial T1 C+ MR in the same patient shows intense but heterogeneous enhancement within a large pineal mass →, obstructive hydrocephalus →, and transependymal flow of CSF →.*

Pineoblastoma

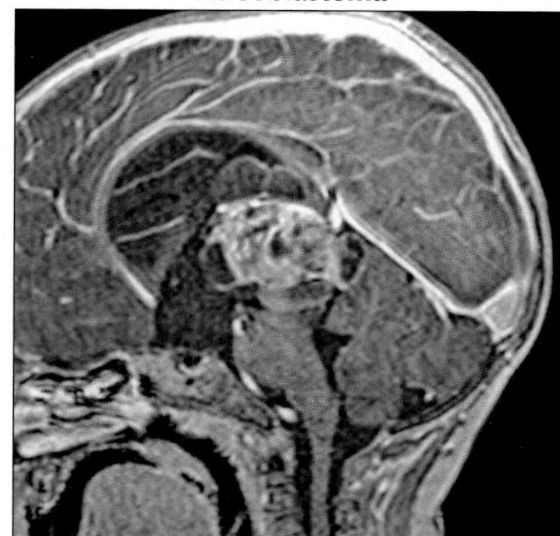

Retinoblastoma

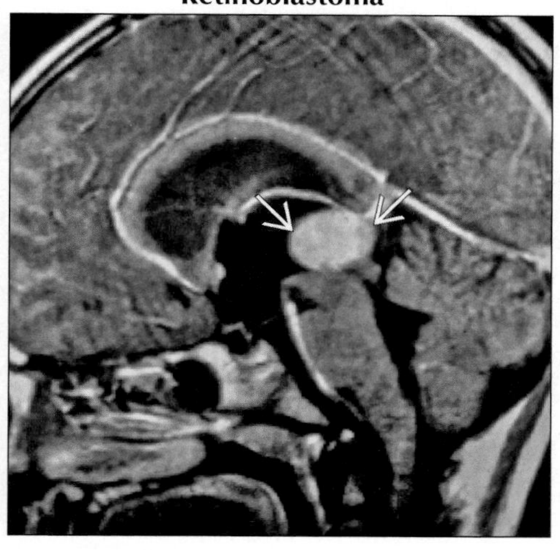

(Left) *Sagittal T1 C+ MR shows heterogeneous contrast enhancement with small focal cysts at the periphery.* ***(Right)*** *Sagittal T1 C+ MR shows an intensely enhancing pineal mass → in a child with diagnosis of bilateral retinoblastoma 2 years prior. Notice the moderate enlargement of the 3rd ventricle secondary to aqueductal obstruction.*

Pineocytoma

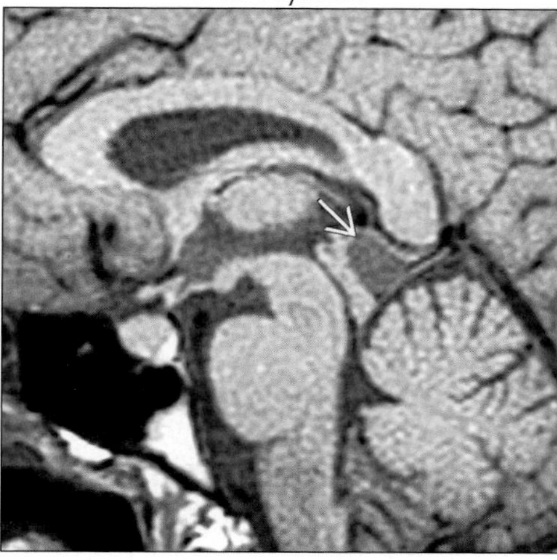

Pineocytoma

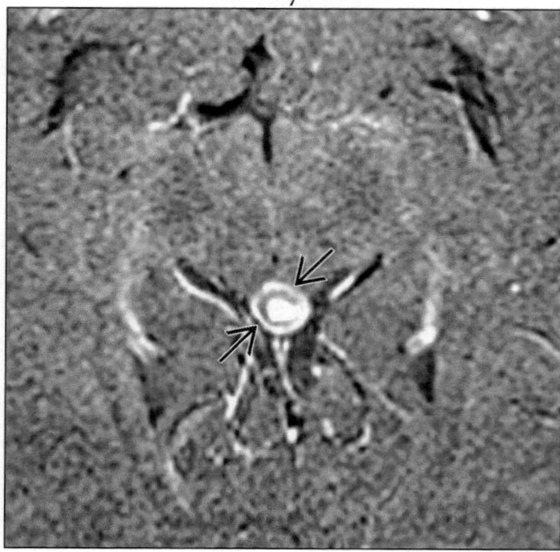

(Left) *Sagittal T1WI MR shows a small cystic pineal region mass → with minimal mass effect on the superior colliculus.* ***(Right)*** *Axial T1 C+ MR shows both peripheral and central enhancement of the pineal mass →.*

BRAIN TUMOR IN NEWBORN/INFANT

DIFFERENTIAL DIAGNOSIS

Common
- Anaplastic Astrocytoma
- Teratoma
- Medulloblastoma (PNET-MB)
- Supratentorial PNET
- Supratentorial Ependymoma
- Choroid Plexus Papilloma

Less Common
- Subependymal Giant Cell Astrocytoma
- Desmoplastic Infantile Ganglioglioma
- Desmoplastic Infantile Astrocytoma
- Glioblastoma Multiforme

Rare but Important
- Choroid Plexus Carcinoma
- Atypical Teratoid-Rhabdoid Tumor
- Neurocutaneous Melanosis (Melanoma/Melanocytoma)
- Pineoblastoma
- Brainstem Glioma, Pediatric
- Medulloepithelioma

ESSENTIAL INFORMATION

Key Differential Diagnosis Issues
- Newborn/infant brain tumors
  - Typically large, bulky, inhomogeneous
  - Supra- > infratentorial (infratentorial more common in older children)

Helpful Clues for Common Diagnoses
- **Anaplastic Astrocytoma**
  - Infiltrating mass, predominantly white matter (WM)
    - Hemispheric WM (frontotemporal)
  - Ca++ rare; heterogeneous on MR
  - No or variable enhancement
    - Ring enhancement, bleed, necrosis, flow voids suggest GBM
- **Teratoma**
  - Midline, supratentorial
  - Small lobular or holocranial
  - Contents
    - Ca++, cysts, fat
    - Enhancing soft tissue
  - Look for associated congenital brain anomalies
- **Medulloblastoma (PNET-MB)**
  - 4th ventricle mass with hydrocephalus
    - Restricts on DWI (best MR clue)
    - Sparse Ca++ ≈ 20%
    - Enhancement usual (may be late/slow)
    - Hemorrhage rare
  - Hypercellularity reflected on imaging
    - Hyperdense (NECT), hypointense (T2)
  - Medulloblastoma with extensive nodularity
    - Subtype with expanded lobular architecture
    - Grape-like enhancement
    - Better prognosis
- **Supratentorial PNET**
  - Large complex mass
    - Restricts on DWI (differentiates from ependymoma)
    - Heterogeneous signal, enhancement
    - Ca++ more common than in posterior fossa PNETs
    - Hemorrhage, necrosis common
  - Hemispheric
    - Mean diameter 5 cm
    - Especially newborn/infants
    - Minimal peritumoral edema
  - Suprasellar
    - Early neuroendocrine, visual disturbances
  - Pineal (pineoblastoma)
    - Hydrocephalus, Parinaud syndrome
- **Supratentorial Ependymoma**
  - Peri/extraventricular > intraventricular
    - Periventricular ependymal rests
    - Large, bulky
    - Ca++ ≈ 50%
    - Variable necrosis, hemorrhage
- **Choroid Plexus Papilloma**
  - CPP: Lobulated intraventricular mass
    - Lateral > 4th > 3rd
    - NECT: Iso- to dense
    - Iso- to slightly hyperintense on T2WI
    - Vividly enhancing
  - Hydrocephalus common

Helpful Clues for Less Common Diagnoses
- **Subependymal Giant Cell Astrocytoma**
  - Enhancing mass near foramen of Monro
  - Found in tuberous sclerosis complex
  - Look for
    - Subependymal Ca++ nodules
    - Tubers (best on FLAIR)
- **Desmoplastic Infantile Ganglioglioma**
  - DIGs often have large cyst
  - Cortically based enhancing tumor nodule

- Enhancing adjacent pia and dura
- **Desmoplastic Infantile Astrocytoma**
  - Similar to (but rarer than) DIG
- **Glioblastoma Multiforme**
  - Bulky irregular enhancing tumor
  - Peritumoral edema, mass effect
  - Hemorrhage, central necrosis, cysts
  - ↑ glucose metabolism, avid FDG accumulation on PET

Helpful Clues for Rare Diagnoses

- **Choroid Plexus Carcinoma**
  - Similar to CPP PLUS
    - Brain invasion
    - Ca++, cysts, bleed
    - Ependymal, subarachnoid space seeding (can be seen with both CPP, CPC)
- **Atypical Teratoid-Rhabdoid Tumor**
  - PNET-MB-like PLUS
    - Metastases at diagnosis more common
    - Cysts, hemorrhage more common
    - Cerebellopontine angle cistern location more common
- **Neurocutaneous Melanosis (Melanoma/Melanocytoma)**
  - Giant or multiple cutaneous melanocytic nevi PLUS
    - Melanosis: Bright T1 amygdala, cerebellum
    - Melanoma: Melanosis + diffuse leptomeningeal enhancement
- **Pineoblastoma**
  - Large heterogeneous pineal region mass
    - Peripheral Ca++
    - Small cysts
    - Inhomogeneous enhancement
  - Invades adjacent structures
    - Corpus callosum, thalamus, midbrain, vermis
  - Hydrocephalus usual at diagnosis
- **Brainstem Glioma, Pediatric**
  - Imaging appearance, prognosis vary with tumor type, location
  - Tectal
    - Pilocytic astrocytoma
    - Clinically indolent course (may cause obstructive hydrocephalus)
    - Variable enhancement/Ca++
  - Focal tegmental mesencephalic
    - Pilocytic astrocytoma
    - Cyst + nodule
    - Surgery, radiation, or chemotherapy
    - Patients generally do well
  - Diffuse pontine glioma
    - Diffusely infiltrating fibrillary astrocytoma
    - Nonenhancing early in course
    - Enhancement with malignant progression
    - Survival generally poor
- **Medulloepithelioma**
  - Rare malignant embryonal brain tumor
  - Young children (< 5 years)
  - Histologic differentiation varies
    - Neuronal, astrocytic, ependymal, melanotic, etc.
  - Imaging appearance reflects variable differentiation

Anaplastic Astrocytoma

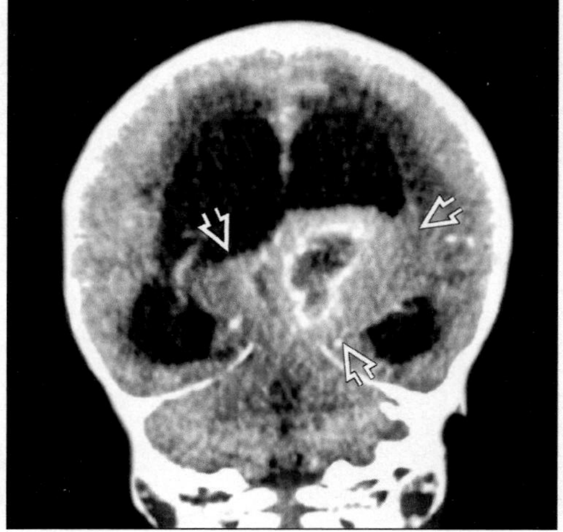

Coronal CECT in this 7 month old shows obstructive hydrocephalus and a large, ill-defined midline mass ➡ with ring enhancement and central necrosis.

Anaplastic Astrocytoma

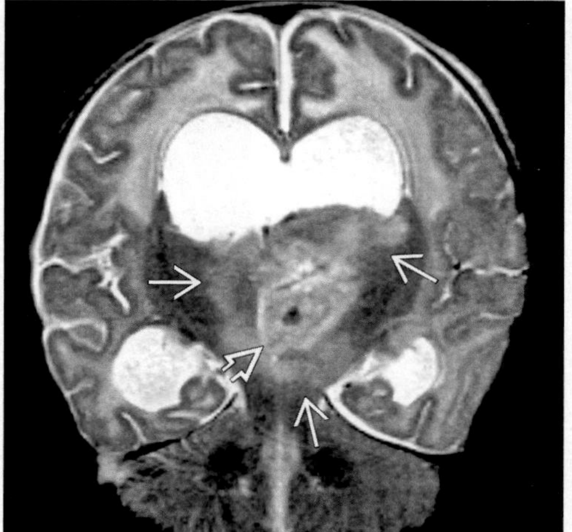

Coronal T2WI MR in same case shows the mass ➡ is extensively infiltrating, with bithalamic and upper midbrain hyperintensity ➡, causing obstructive hydrocephalus with transependymal CSF migration.

BRAIN TUMOR IN NEWBORN/INFANT

Teratoma

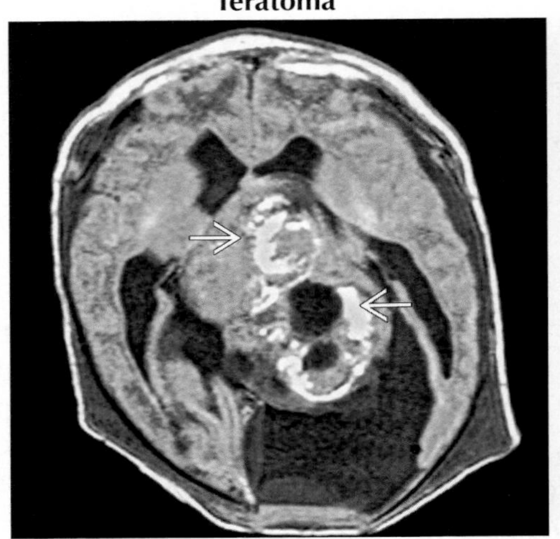

Teratoma

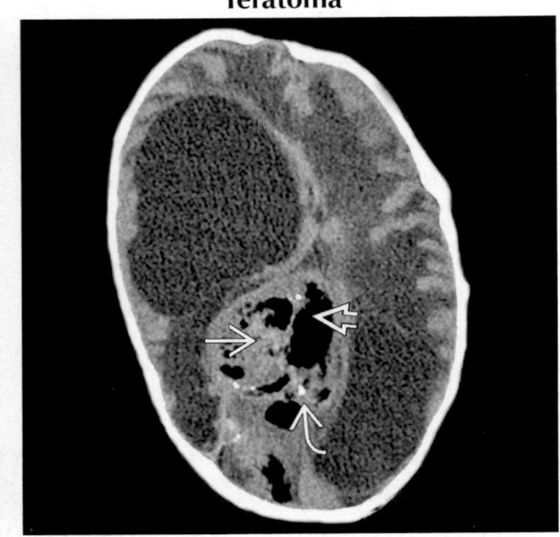

(Left) *Axial T1WI MR in this 7-day-old infant shows T1 bright signal from fat ➔ scattered throughout the lesion.* ***(Right)*** *Axial NECT in the same child at 15 months shows a complicated pineal region mass consisting of fat ➔, solid tissue ➔, and calcification ➔.*

Medulloblastoma (PNET-MB)

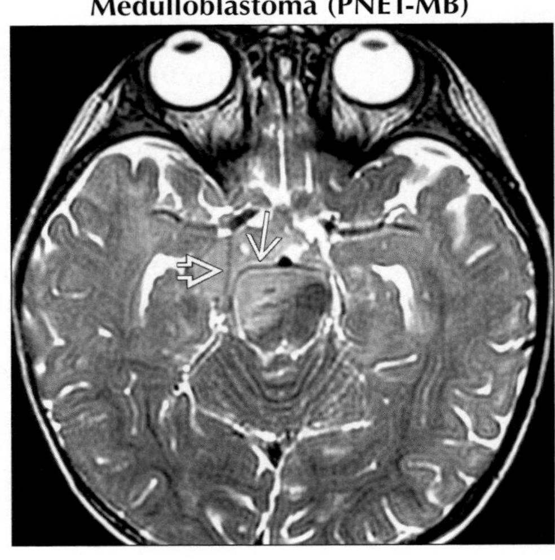

Medulloblastoma (PNET-MB)

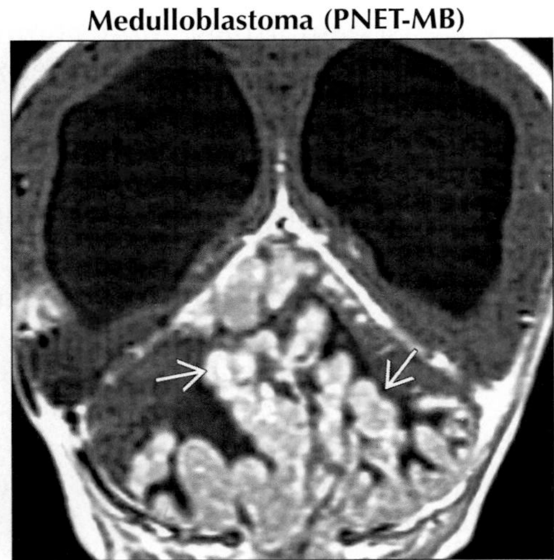

(Left) *Axial T2WI MR in a 4-month-old infant shows an intermediate to low signal mass that splays and encases posterior communicating ➔ and superior cerebellar ➔ arteries.* ***(Right)*** *Coronal T1 C+ MR in this 10 month old shows grape-like nodular enhancement ➔. Medulloblastoma with extensive nodularity is a PNET-MB variant that has somewhat better prognosis.*

Supratentorial Ependymoma

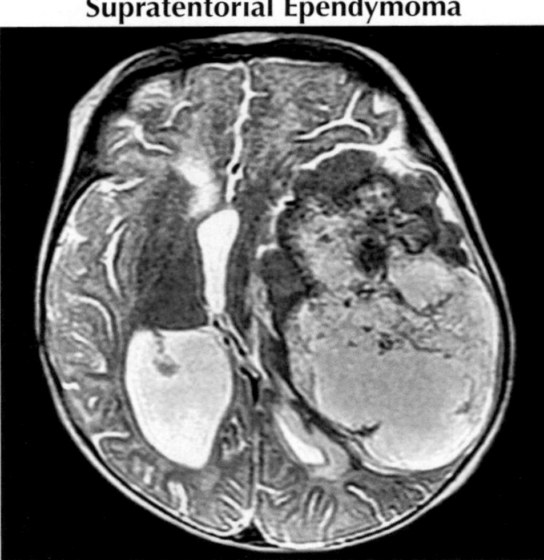

Supratentorial Ependymoma

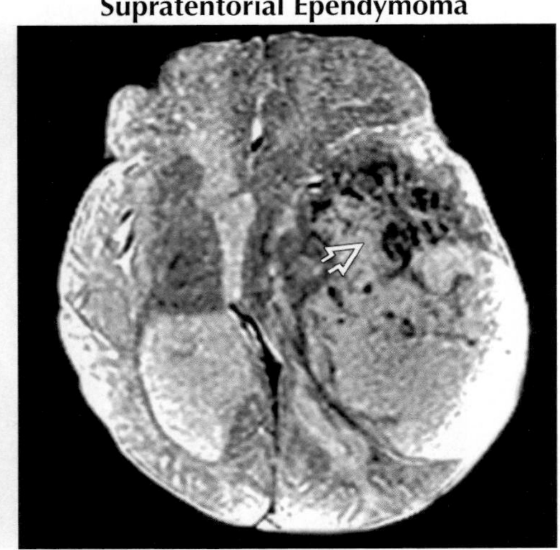

(Left) *Axial T2WI MR in a 12-week-old infant shows a mixed heterogeneity left temporal lobe mass.* ***(Right)*** *Axial T2* GRE MR shows multifocal hemosiderin and calcific foci ➔.*

Choroid Plexus Papilloma

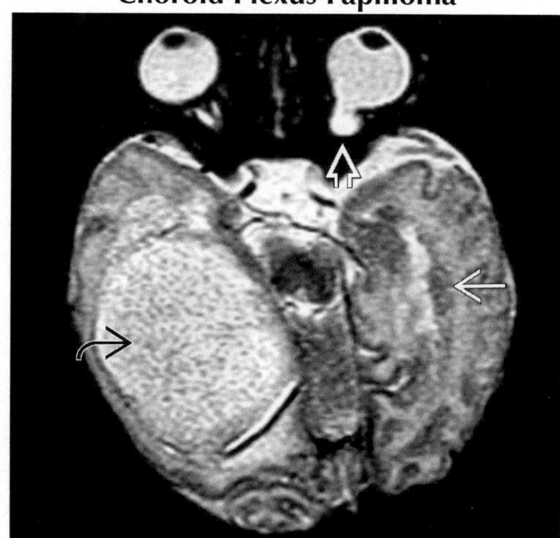

Choroid Plexus Papilloma

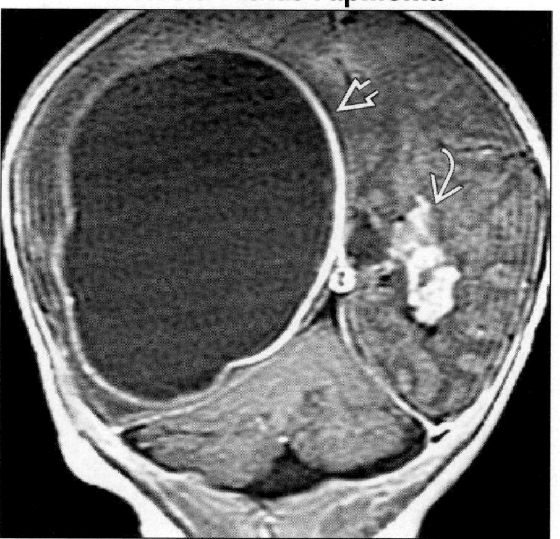

(Left) Axial T2WI MR shows a large cyst, coloboma, and temporal lobe subependymal heterotopia in a 4-day-old girl with Aicardi syndrome. *(Right)* Coronal T1 C+ MR shows bilateral choroid plexus papillomas. The left is bulky and frond-like, while the right is stretched by the associated cyst.

Subependymal Giant Cell Astrocytoma

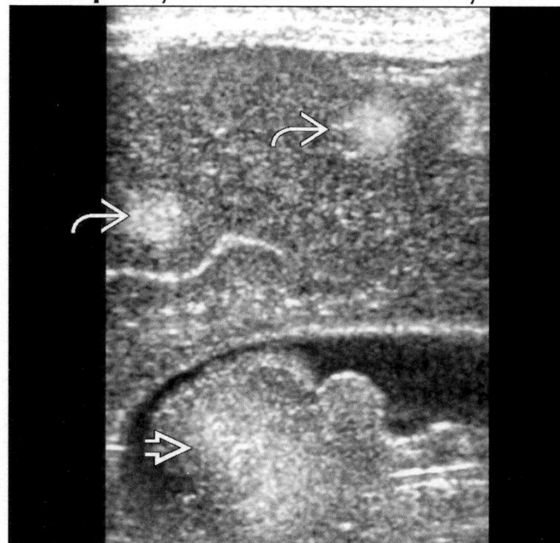

Desmoplastic Infantile Ganglioglioma

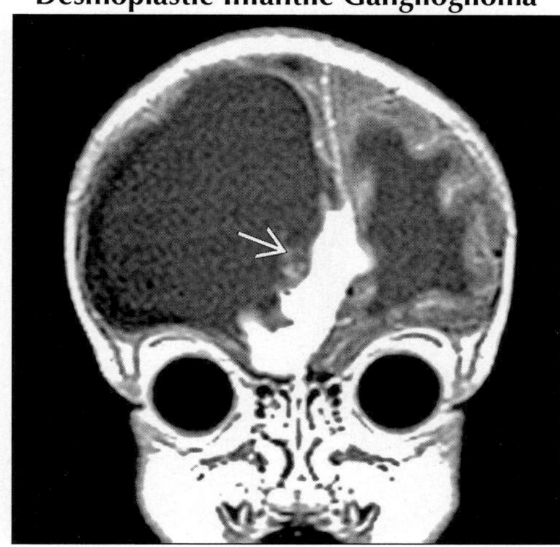

(Left) Longitudinal ultrasound shows a bulky subependymal giant cell astrocytoma at the foramen of Monro in this newborn with cardiac rhabdomyoma and tuberous sclerosis. There are multiple additional tubers on the same image. *(Right)* Coronal T1WI C+ MR in a 7-month-old infant shows a massive right frontal cystic tumor with a solid enhancing component that involves the medial frontal cortex and falx.

Desmoplastic Infantile Astrocytoma

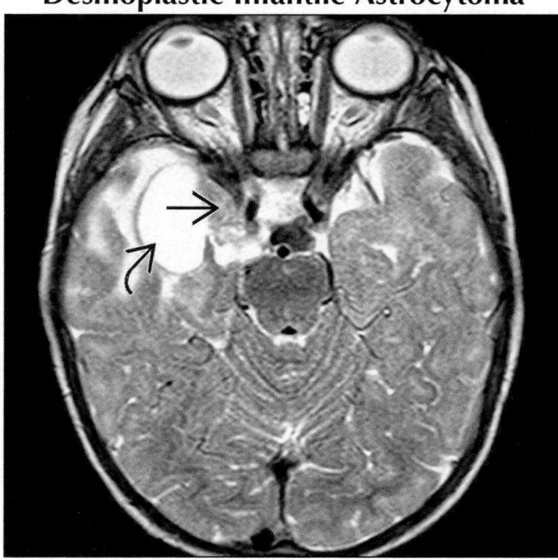

Desmoplastic Infantile Astrocytoma

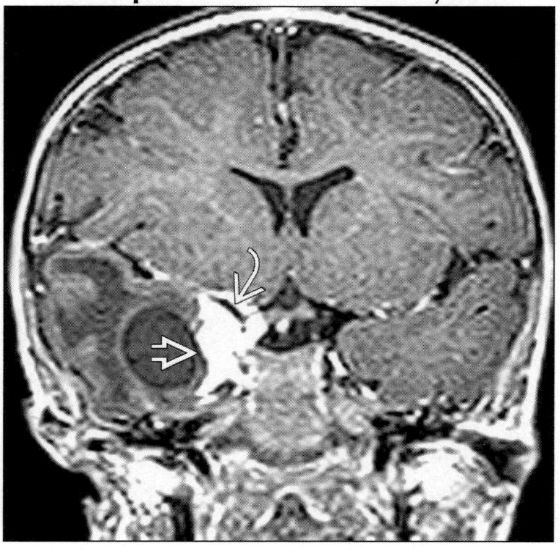

(Left) Axial T2WI MR in a 9-month-old infant shows a right temporal cystic and solid tumor with surrounding edema. *(Right)* Coronal T1 C+ MR in the same infant shows encasement of the right middle cerebral artery by the avidly enhancing solid component of the tumor.

BRAIN TUMOR IN NEWBORN/INFANT

*(**Left**) Axial T2WI MR in this 6-week-old infant shows a markedly heterogeneous bifrontal mass lesion with hemorrhages of various ages →. There is obstruction of both foramina of Monro and enlargement of the lateral ventricular trigones. (**Right**) Axial T1 C+ MR shows extensive enhancement of this tumor.*

Glioblastoma Multiforme

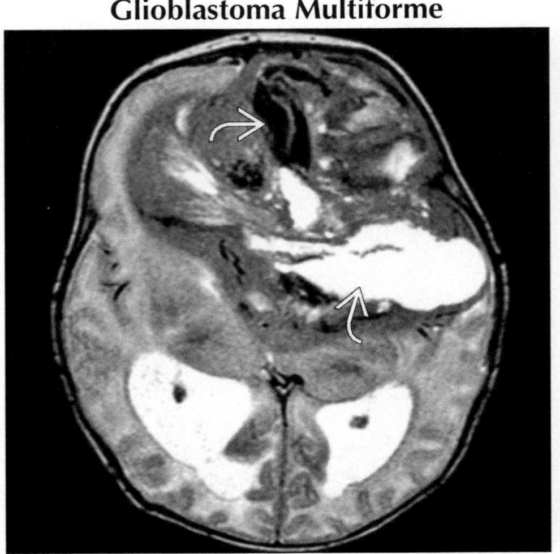

Glioblastoma Multiforme

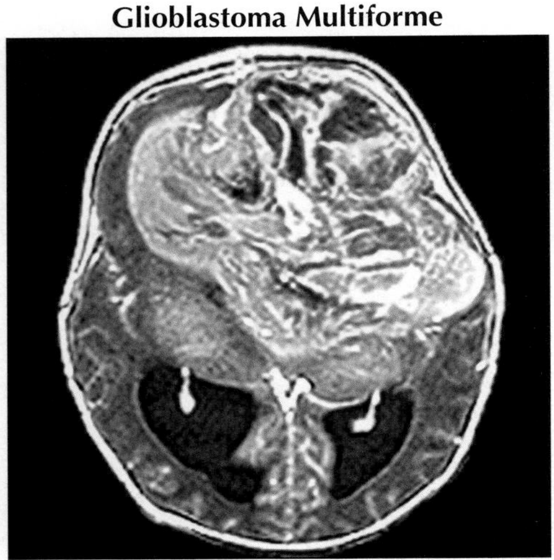

*(**Left**) Axial T1WI C+ MR in this 9-month-old infant shows a large, bulky, avidly enhancing left intraventricular tumor → with invasion of the overlying brain →. There are multiple intraventricular metastases →. (**Right**) Anteroposterior angiography performed as a part of preoperative embolization shows hypervascularity → and multiple areas of contrast puddling →.*

Choroid Plexus Carcinoma

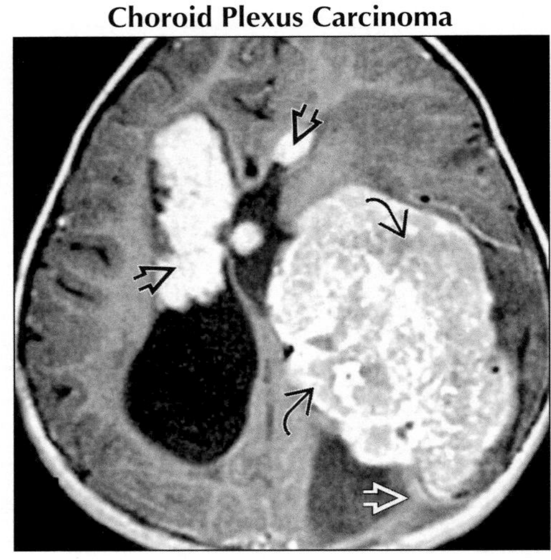

Choroid Plexus Carcinoma

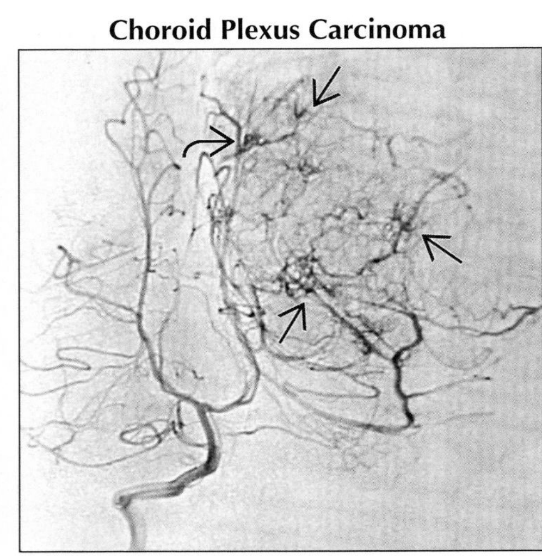

*(**Left**) Sagittal T2WI MR in this 7-month-old infant shows hydrocephalus and a complicated solid and cystic tumor filling the 4th ventricle, supravermian cistern and extending through the tentorial incisura →. (**Right**) Coronal T1 C+ MR in the same 7 month old shows a right frontal metastatic deposit →.*

Atypical Teratoid-Rhabdoid Tumor

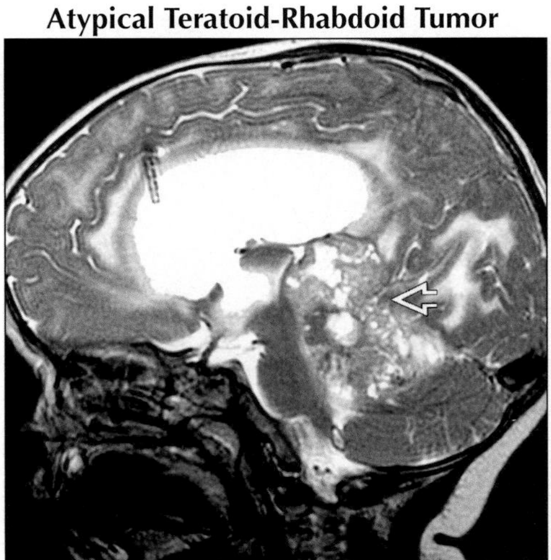

Atypical Teratoid-Rhabdoid Tumor

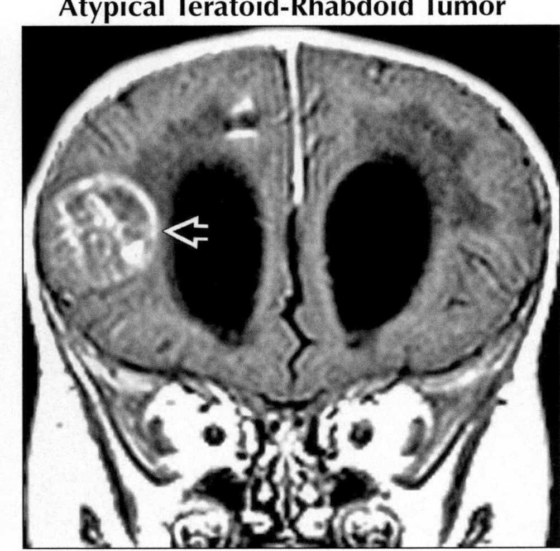

BRAIN TUMOR IN NEWBORN/INFANT

Neurocutaneous Melanosis (Melanoma/Melanocytoma)

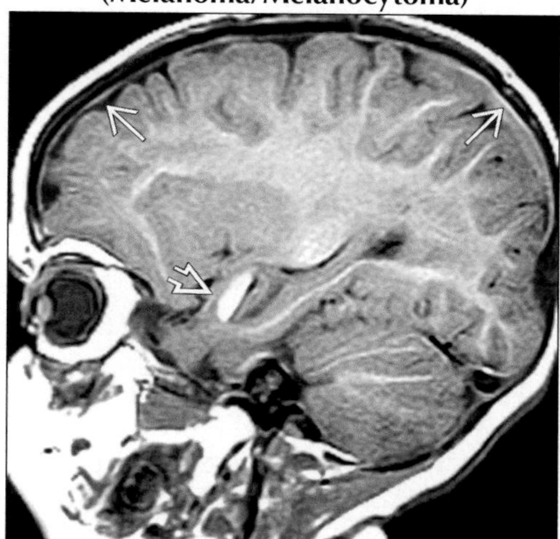

Neurocutaneous Melanosis (Melanoma/Melanocytoma)

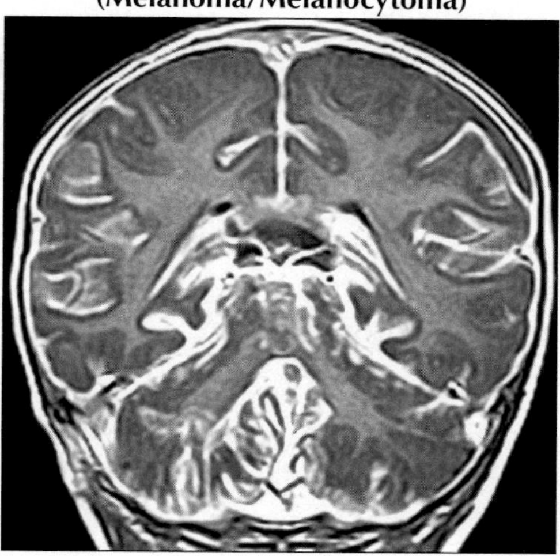

(Left) *Sagittal T1WI MR shows increased signal intensity of the hippocampus ➡ in this 10 month old with a large cutaneous nevus. Pachymeningeal thickening ➡ is present prior to contrast administration.* ***(Right)*** *Coronal T1 C+ MR during the same examination shows diffuse pachy- and leptomeningeal metastatic melanoma.*

Pineoblastoma

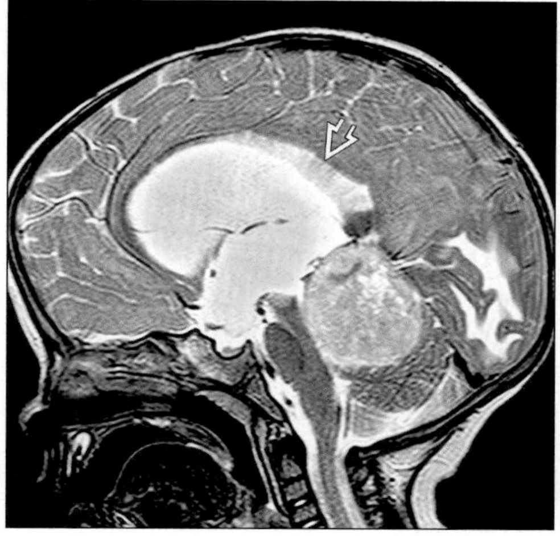

Pineoblastoma

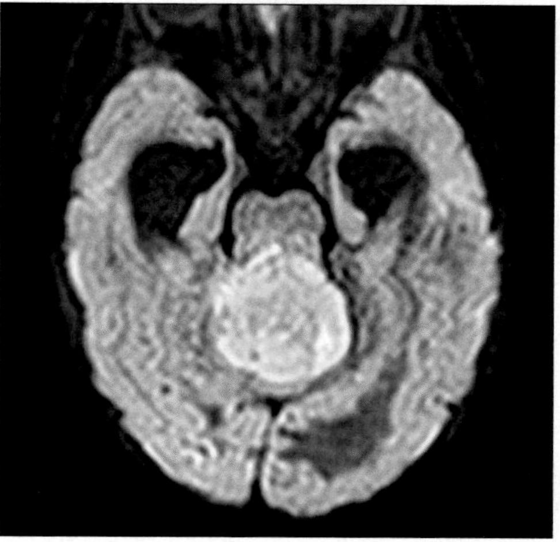

(Left) *Sagittal T2WI MR in a 7-month-old infant shows a mass in the pineal region traversing the tentorial incisura into the supravermian cistern. There is compression of the aqueduct of Sylvius with resultant hydrocephalus. Acute edema along the fiber tracts of the corpus callosum renders a striated pattern ➡.* ***(Right)*** *Axial DWI MR in the same patient shows typical diffusion restriction.*

Brainstem Glioma, Pediatric

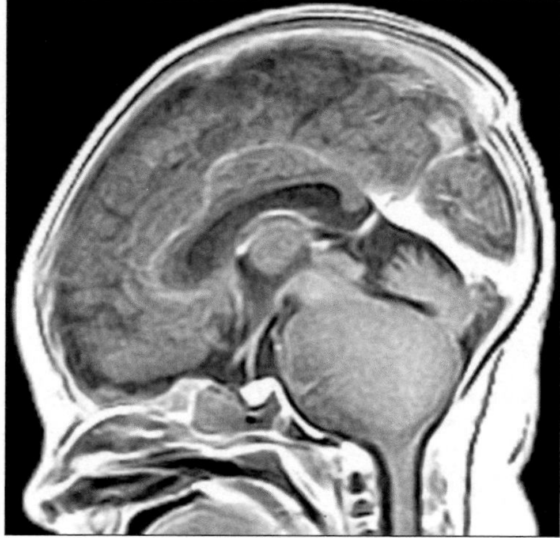

Medulloepithelioma

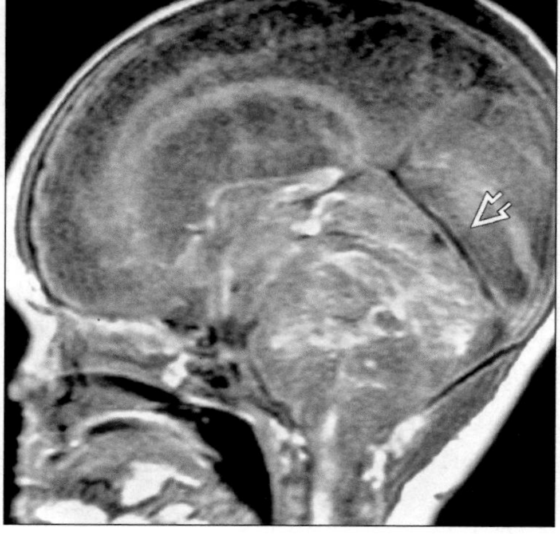

(Left) *Sagittal T1 C+ MR in this newborn shows massive expansion of the pons and medulla by a nonenhancing mass.* ***(Right)*** *Sagittal T1WI MR in a 5-day-old infant shows a massive hemorrhagic tumor replacing and expanding the upper cervical spinal cord, the brainstem, and the cerebellum. The tumor protrudes through the incisura and displaces the straight sinus ➡.*

BRAIN TUMOR IN CHILD > 1 YEAR

DIFFERENTIAL DIAGNOSIS

Common
- Pilocytic Astrocytoma
  - Cerebellar JPA
  - Optic Pathway Glioma
  - Pilomyxoid Astrocytoma (Rare)
- Medulloblastoma (PNET-MB)
- Ependymoma
- Pediatric Brainstem Glioma
- Low-Grade Diffuse Astrocytoma
- Subependymal Giant Cell Astrocytoma
- DNET
- Craniopharyngioma

Less Common
- Germinoma
- Choroid Plexus Papilloma
- Ganglioglioma
- Oligodendroglioma
- Neurofibromatosis Type 2
  - Meningioma
  - Schwannoma
- Pineoblastoma
- Pleomorphic Xanthoastrocytoma
- Anaplastic Astrocytoma
- Glioblastoma Multiforme
- Gliomatosis Cerebri
- Supratentorial PNET
- Teratoma

Rare but Important
- Astroblastoma
- Choroid Plexus Carcinoma
- Atypical Teratoid-Rhabdoid Tumor
- Primary CNS Sarcoma
- Metastases
  - Skull and Meningeal Metastases
  - Parenchymal Metastases
  - Leukemia
  - Metastatic Neuroblastoma
  - Neurocutaneous Melanosis (Melanoma, Melanocytoma)
- Central Neurocytoma
- Dysplastic Cerebellar Gangliocytoma

ESSENTIAL INFORMATION

Key Differential Diagnosis Issues
- Diffusion weighted imaging helpful
- All of the following restrict on DWI
  - PNET-MB
  - Pineoblastoma (pineal PNET)
  - Atypical teratoid-rhabdoid tumor (ATRT)
  - Germinoma
  - Epidermoid
- May present with hemorrhage into tumor
  - Primary CNS sarcoma
  - Supratentorial PNET
  - Neuroblastoma metastatic to brain tissue
  - Pilomyxoid variant of pilocytic astrocytoma

Helpful Clues for Common Diagnoses
- **Pilocytic Astrocytoma**
  - Low density on NECT
  - High signal on T2
- **Medulloblastoma (PNET-MB)**
  - Hyperdense 4th ventricle (V) mass on NECT
  - Restricts on DWI
- **Ependymoma**
  - 60% posterior fossa
    - "Plastic" tumor in 4th ventricle, extrudes through foramina
  - 40% supratentorial
    - Mixed cystic, solid mass with Ca++
- **Pediatric Brainstem Glioma**
  - Location predicts pathology, prognosis
    - Infiltrating pontine glioma worst
- **Low-Grade Diffuse Astrocytoma**
  - Hemispheres, thalami (can be bithalamic), tectum, brainstem (pons, medulla)
    - 50% of brainstem "gliomas" are low grade, diffusely infiltrating astrocytomas
  - Poorly marginated
  - Hypo- on T1WI, hyperintense on T2WI
  - No enhancement
- **Subependymal Giant Cell Astrocytoma**
  - Location at foramina of Monro typical
  - Look for cortical/subcortical tubers
  - Look for subependymal nodules
- **DNET**
  - Almost all in patients < 20 years
  - Chronic epilepsy
  - "Bubbly" appearing, cortically based mass
  - "Ring" sign on FLAIR
- **Craniopharyngioma**
  - Nearly half of pediatric suprasellar masses
  - 90% Ca++/cystic/enhance

Helpful Clues for Less Common Diagnoses
- **Germinoma**
  - Suprasellar + pineal masses together best clue
  - Early ependymal infiltration

BRAIN TUMOR IN CHILD > 1 YEAR

- **Choroid Plexus Papilloma**
  - Densely enhancing
  - Cotyledon- or frond-like surface
- **Neurofibromatosis Type 2**
  - If multiple schwannomas, think NF2+
  - Look for "hidden," dural-based meningiomas with C+
- **Pineoblastoma**
  - Restricts on DWI
  - Look for CSF spread (ventricles, ependyma)
- **Pleomorphic Xanthoastrocytoma**
  - Cortically based tumor (temporal lobe most common site)
  - Dural reaction ("tail") common
  - Enhancing ill-defined mass plus cyst
- **Anaplastic Astrocytoma**
  - Diffusely infiltrating
  - Classic do not enhance
- **Glioblastoma Multiforme**
  - Typically arises from lower grade astrocytoma
- **Gliomatosis Cerebri**
  - Less likely to enhance
  - More likely bilateral
  - More likely to spread across callosal tracts
- **Supratentorial PNET**
  - Infant with large, bulky, complex hemispheric mass
  - Ca++, hemorrhage, necrosis common
  - Peritumoral edema sparse/absent
- **Teratoma**
  - Neonate with large bulky midline mass
  - Ca++, soft tissue, cysts, fat

Helpful Clues for Rare Diagnoses

- **Astroblastoma**
  - Large, hemispheric
  - Well-circumscribed
  - "Bubbly" solid and cystic
- **Choroid Plexus Carcinoma**
  - Similar to CPP
    - Invades ependymal surface and brain
    - Less homogeneous than CPP
- **Atypical Teratoid-Rhabdoid Tumor**
  - Heterogeneous intracranial mass in infant
  - 50% infratentorial, early CSF spread
- **Metastases**
  - Pial, leptomeningeal
    - PNET
    - Ependymoma
    - Anaplastic astrocytoma
    - Germinoma
    - Choroid plexus carcinoma
  - Falx
    - Leukemia involves both sides of falx
  - Bone and dura: Neuroblastoma > leukemia
    - CT: Bone spiculation, "hair on end"
    - MR: Bone expanded and marrow replaced
- **Central Neurocytoma**
  - "Bubbly" lobulated mass in body of lateral ventricle
- **Dysplastic Cerebellar Gangliocytoma**
  - Look for evidence of Cowden disease
  - Striated cerebellum
    - Enlarged low signal cerebellar folia

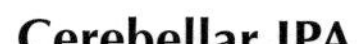

Cerebellar JPA

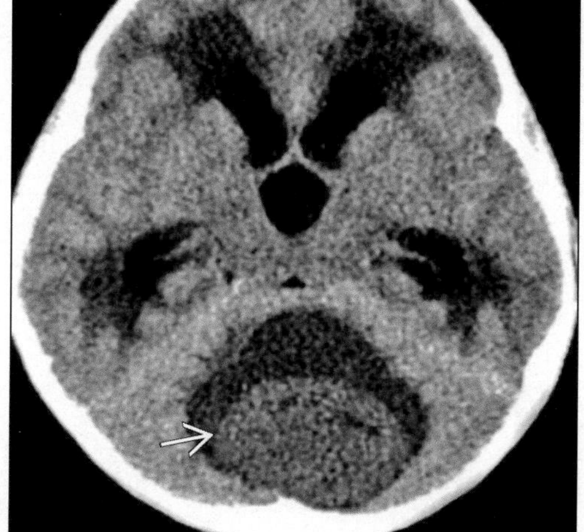

Axial NECT shows a typical midline cystic tumor with a large low-density mural nodule ➔. There is hydrocephalus with interstitial edema.

Cerebellar JPA

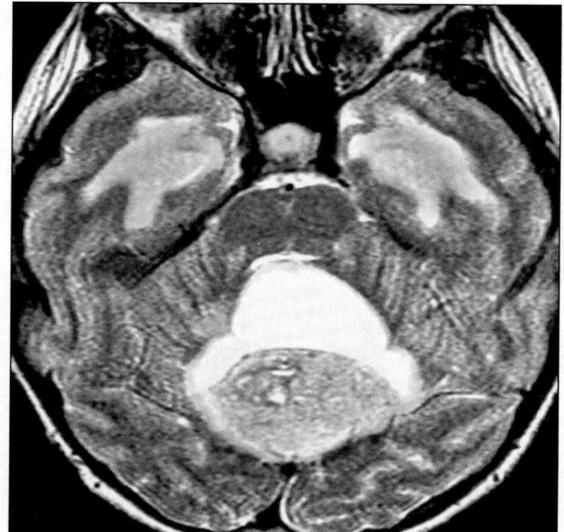

Axial T2WI MR shows the nodule to be high signal intensity, a clue to the high nuclear-to-cytoplasm ratio in cerebellar JPA tumors.

BRAIN TUMOR IN CHILD > 1 YEAR

(Left) *Axial T2WI MR shows poorly marginated hyperintensity ➡ that extends posteriorly from the optic chiasm/hypothalamus along both optic radiations.* **(Right)** *Axial T2WI MR shows a large, hyperintense, well-circumscribed mass. It arises from the hypothalamic region and demonstrates no edema of adjacent structures.*

Optic Pathway Glioma

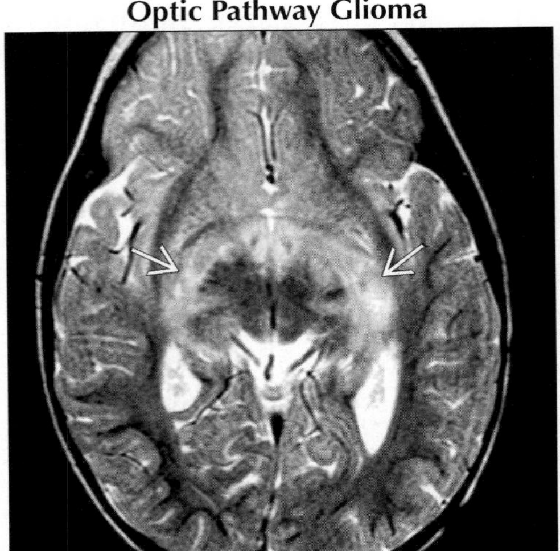

Pilomyxoid Astrocytoma (Rare)

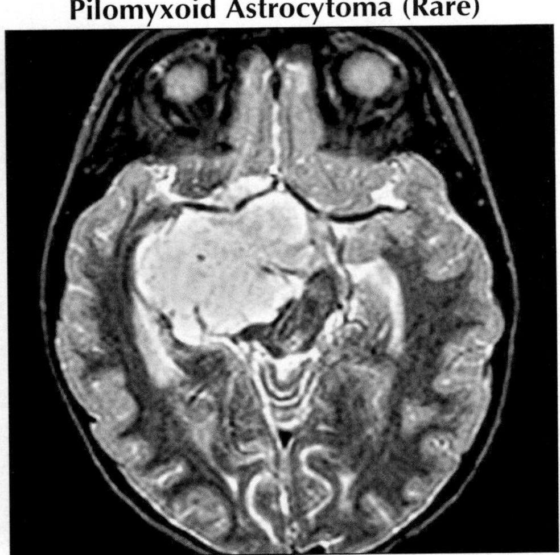

(Left) *Axial T2WI MR shows a low signal midline tumor. There is an associated cyst ➡.* **(Right)** *Axial DWI MR shows diffusion restriction within the tumor nodule, an excellent clue to the aggressive nature of the lesion.*

Medulloblastoma (PNET-MB)

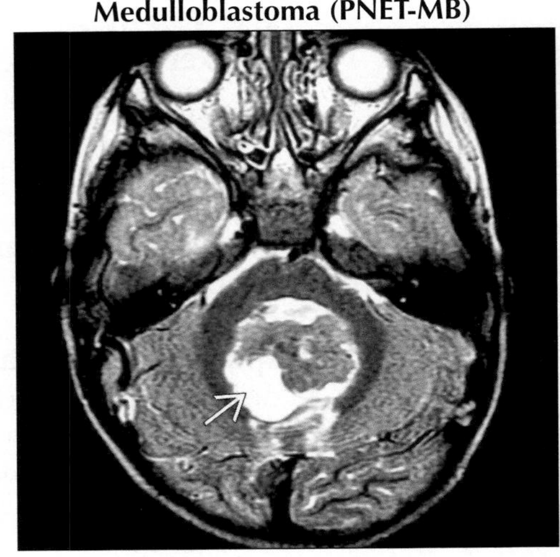

Medulloblastoma (PNET-MB)

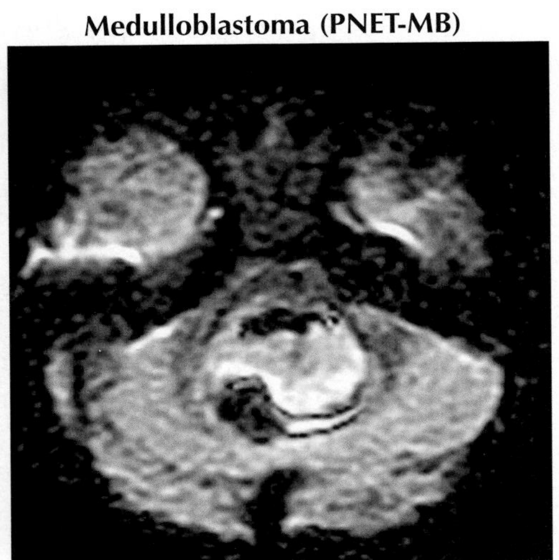

(Left) *Sagittal T2WI MR shows a large, heterogeneous, low signal mass that widens the tegmento-cerebellar angle and extends through the inferior recesses of the 4th ventricle. There is extension into the upper cervical spinal canal ➡.* **(Right)** *Sagittal T2WI MR shows diffuse expansion of the pons and medulla due to an infiltrating glioma.*

Ependymoma

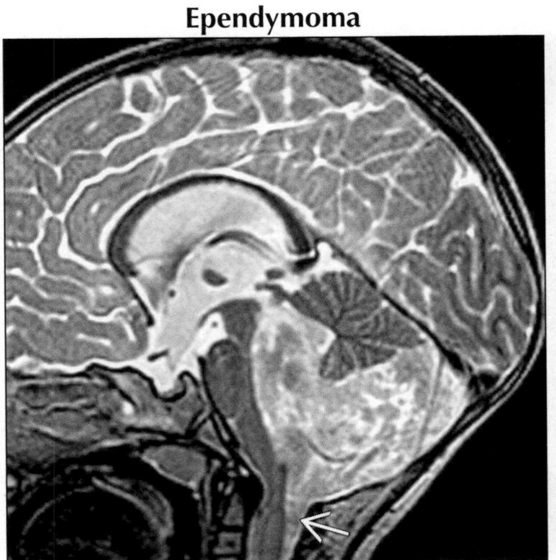

Pediatric Brainstem Glioma

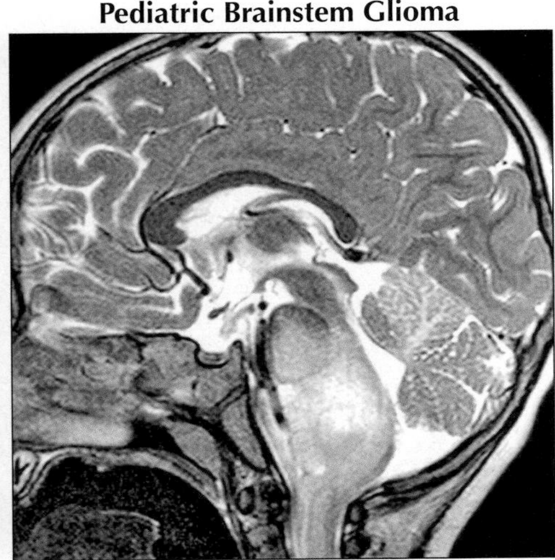

BRAIN TUMOR IN CHILD > 1 YEAR

Subependymal Giant Cell Astrocytoma

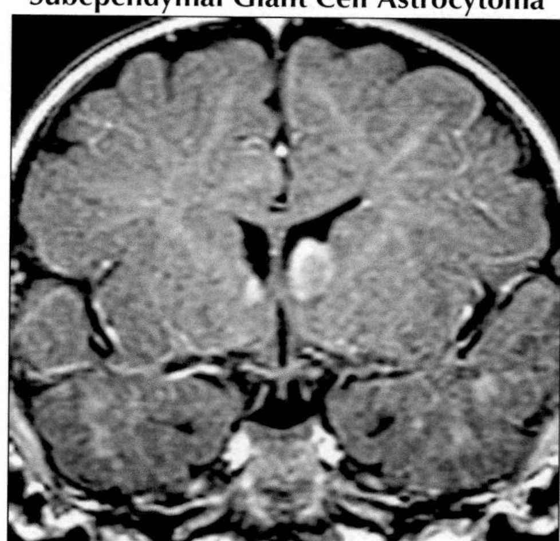

DNET

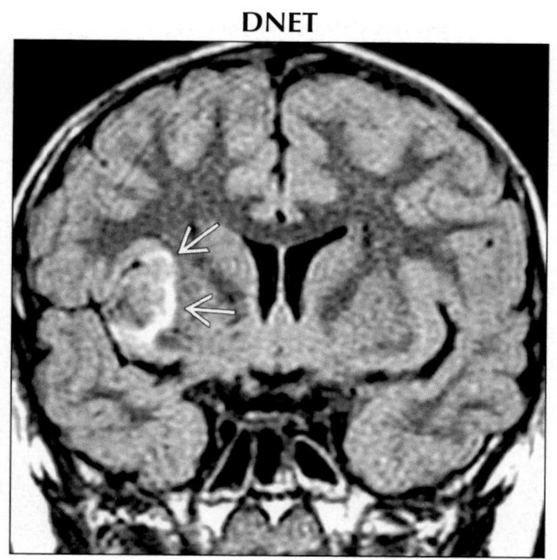

(Left) Coronal T1 C+ MR shows bilateral, asymmetric enhancing lesions at the foramina of Monro. The location is characteristic for subependymal giant cell astrocytoma. The child also had skin and other brain lesions typical of tuberous sclerosis. *(Right)* Coronal FLAIR MR in a child with seizures shows an insular-based lesion with a partial bright ring ➡, the DNET FLAIR "ring" sign.

Craniopharyngioma

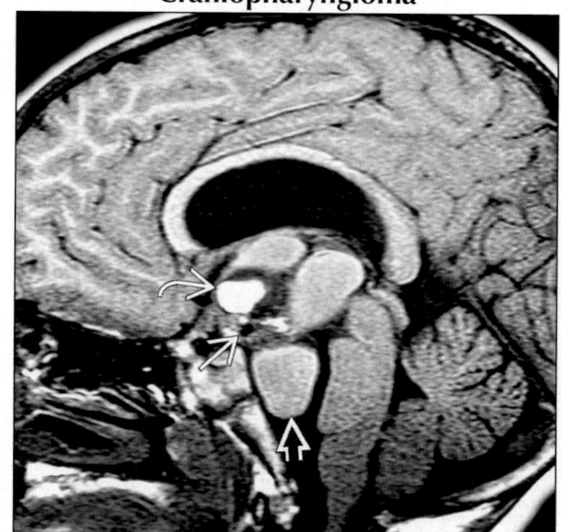

Germinoma

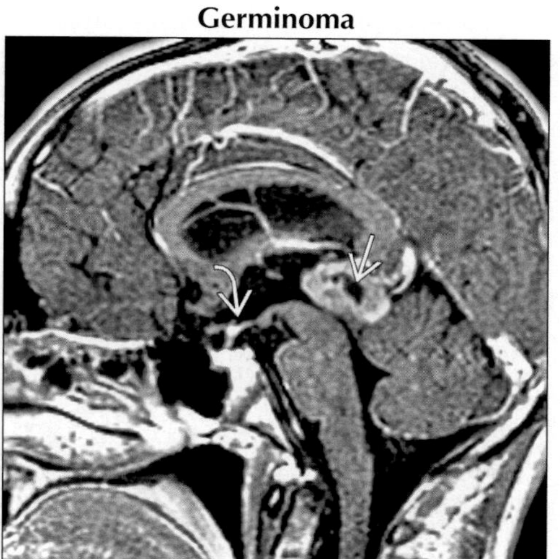

(Left) Sagittal T1WI MR shows a suprasellar collection of cysts of many signal intensities. One ➡ is very high signal intensity, likely due to protein; another extends behind the clivus ➡; and the remainder herniate into 3rd ventricle. Calcification ➡ is noted in the solid component above the dorsum sella. *(Right)* Sagittal T1WI C+ MR shows a medium-sized pineal mass with central necrosis ➡. Note the very small enhancing mass in the infundibular recess ➡.

Choroid Plexus Papilloma

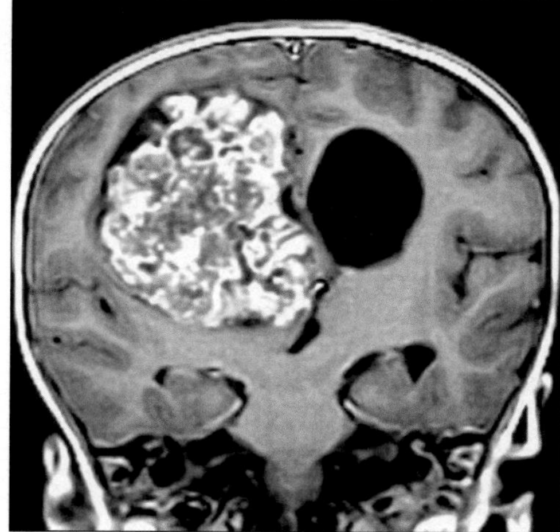

Ganglioglioma

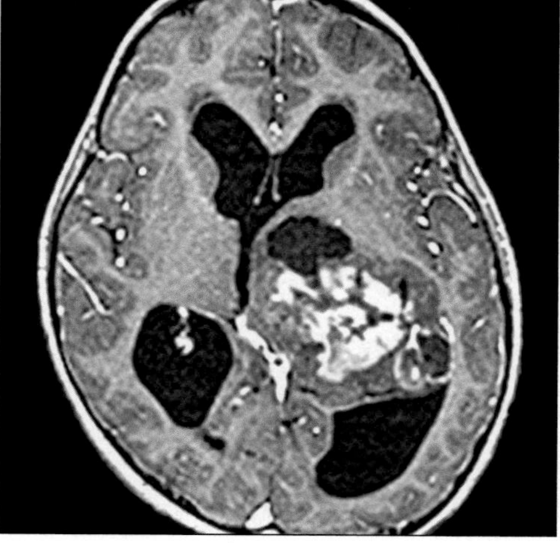

(Left) Coronal T1 C+ MR shows a large enhancing mass within the right lateral ventricle. The surface is frond-like, and there is no brain invasion. The appearance is typical for a choroid plexus papilloma. *(Right)* Axial T1 C+ MR shows a cystic and solid thalamic mass. This lesion was heavily calcified on NECT (not shown).

BRAIN TUMOR IN CHILD > 1 YEAR

(Left) *Coronal T2WI MR shows multiple dural-based meningiomas ➡ at the vertex. There are also bilateral, asymmetric, vestibular schwannomas ➡ in this teen with NF2.* **(Right)** *Sagittal T2WI MR shows a low signal pineal mass that obstructs the aqueduct. This lesion was dense on NECT and restricted on DWI.*

Neurofibromatosis Type 2

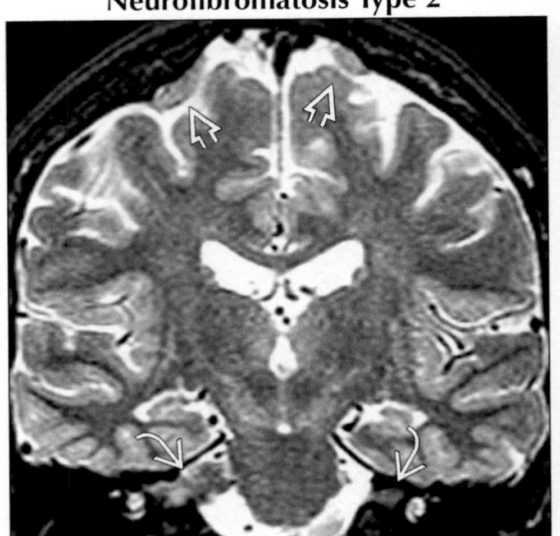

Pineoblastoma

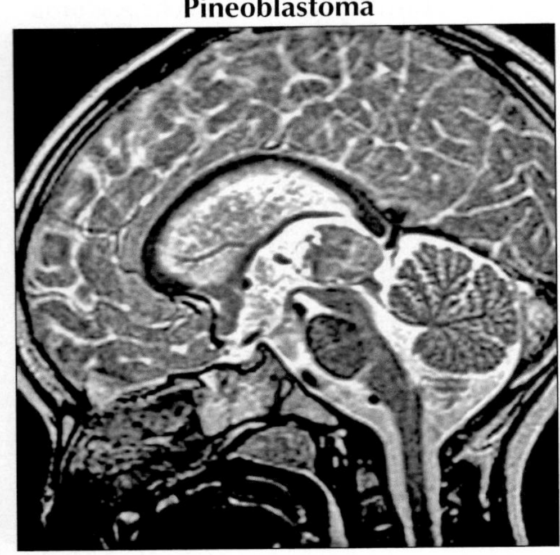

(Left) *Coronal T1 C+ MR shows a cortically based temporal lobe tumor. It is ill-defined, invades adjacent brain tissue, enhances, and contains a rim-enhancing cyst ➡.* **(Right)** *Axial T2WI MR shows bithalamic involvement by homogeneous tumor, which did not enhance on T1 C+ image (not shown).*

Pleomorphic Xanthoastrocytoma

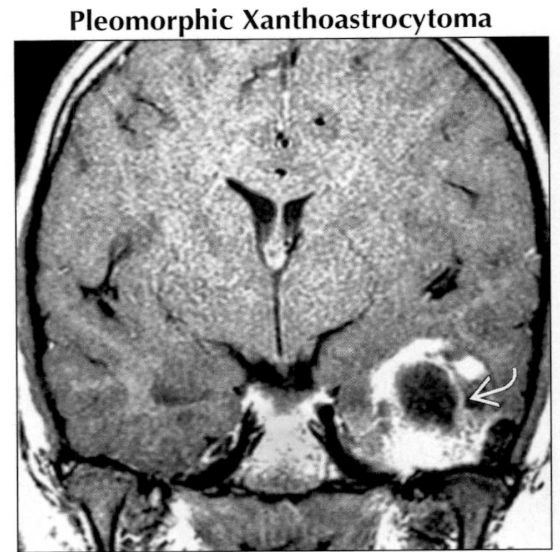

Glioblastoma Multiforme

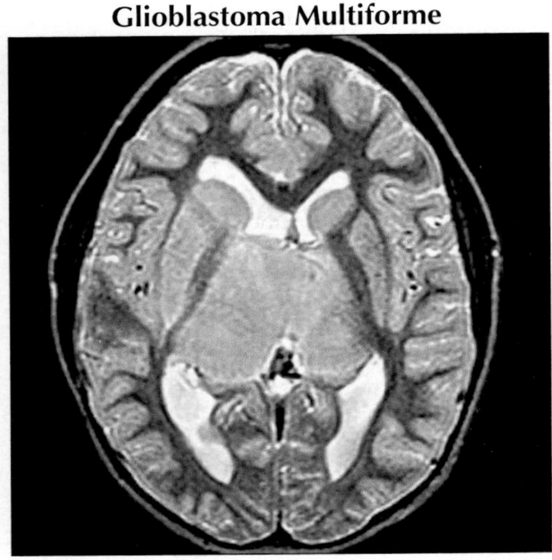

(Left) *Coronal T1WI MR shows marked expansion of the left temporal lobe by a hemorrhagic ➡ mass.* **(Right)** *Sagittal T2WI MR shows a mixed solid, cystic, and calcified pineal region mass ➡ that obstructs the aqueduct of Sylvius. This teenaged patient presented with Parinaud phenomenon. There is acute edema involving the septal-callosal interface ➡.*

Supratentorial PNET

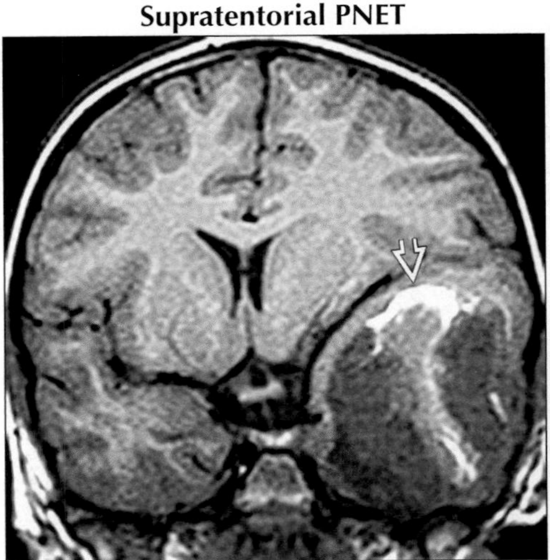

Teratoma

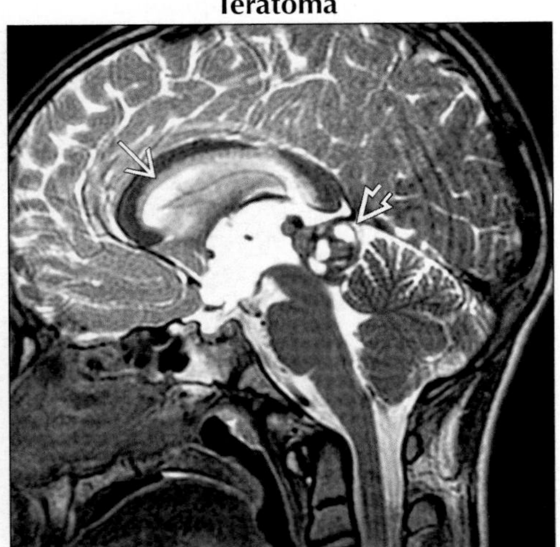

Choroid Plexus Carcinoma

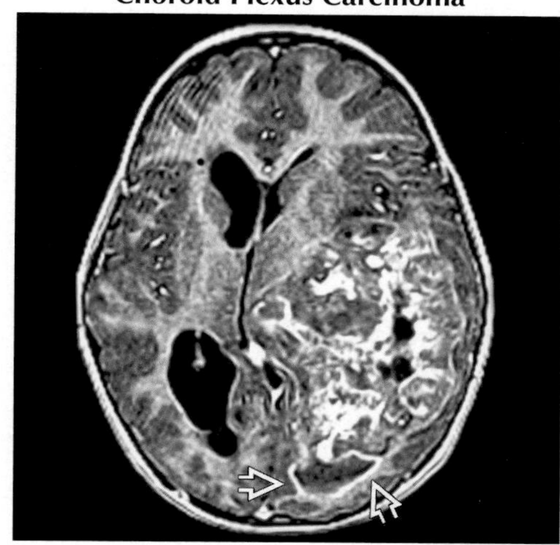

Atypical Teratoid-Rhabdoid Tumor

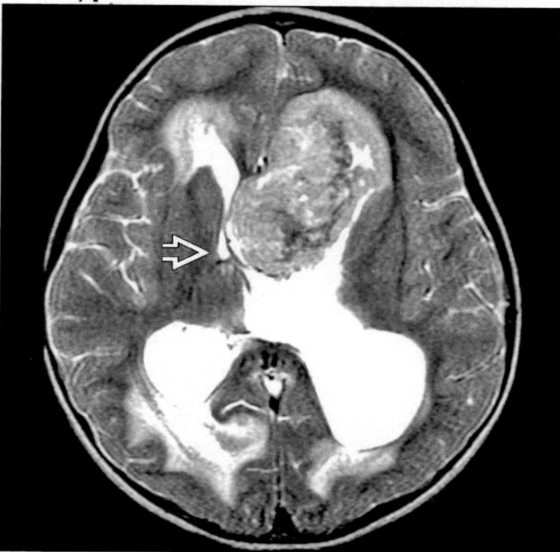

*(**Left**) Axial T1 C+ MR shows a large heterogeneously enhancing trigonal mass with brain invasion and ependymal spread ➡. (**Right**) Axial T2WI MR shows a mixed signal mass obstructing both the right ➡ and left foramina of Monro.*

Atypical Teratoid-Rhabdoid Tumor

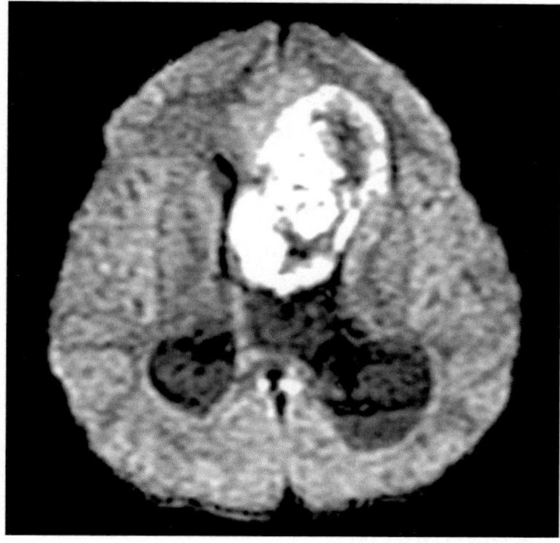

Skull and Meningeal Metastases

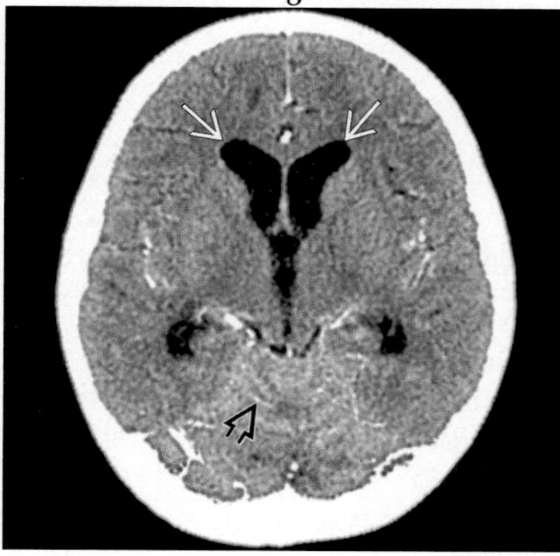

*(**Left**) Axial DWI MR in the same patient shows extensive diffusion restriction in the left frontal ATRT. (**Right**) Axial CECT in this patient with metastatic PNET-MB shows comb-like enhancement of the interfoliate sulci ➡. Note the moderately enlarged lateral ventricles ➡, caused by extraventricular obstructive hydrocephalus from diffuse cisternal metastases.*

Leukemia

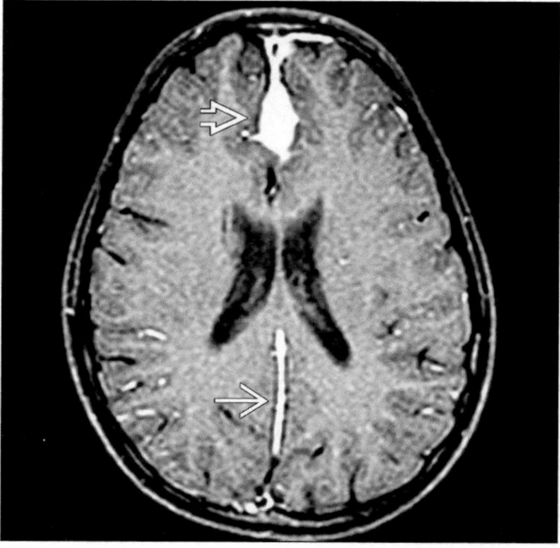

Metastatic Neuroblastoma

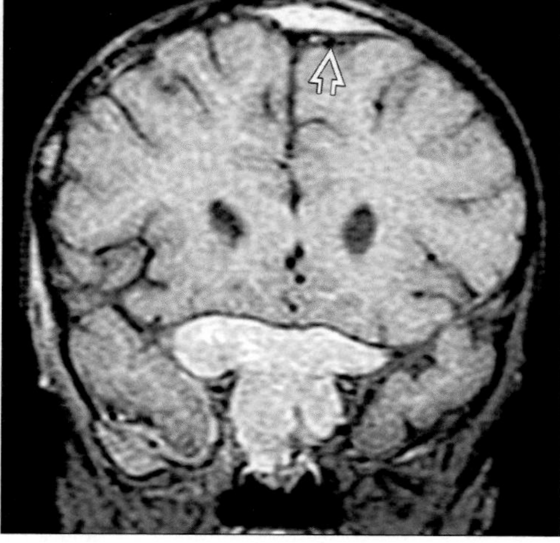

*(**Left**) Axial T1 C+ FS MR in a child with ALL shows involvement of the posterior ➡ and anterior ➡ falx by densely enhancing tissue. Both sides of the falx are involved ventrally. (**Right**) Coronal FLAIR MR shows expansion of the lesser wing of sphenoid by neuroblastoma. There is an additional calvarial and dural-based focus at the vertex ➡.*

RING-ENHANCING LESIONS

DIFFERENTIAL DIAGNOSIS

Common
- Abscess
- Pilocytic Astrocytoma
- Neurocysticercosis

Less Common
- Demyelinating Disease
  - ADEM
  - Multiple Sclerosis
- Ganglioglioma

Rare but Important
- Aneurysm (Thrombosed)
- Other Infections
  - Tuberculosis
  - Fungal Diseases
  - Acquired Toxoplasmosis
  - Lyme Disease
- Other Neoplasms
  - Parenchymal Metastases
  - Lymphoma, Primary CNS
  - Glioblastoma Multiforme
- Subacute Cerebral Infarction
- Subacute Intracerebral Hematoma

ESSENTIAL INFORMATION

Key Differential Diagnosis Issues
- Solitary ring-enhancing lesions most often tumor, infection, or demyelination
- Metastatic lesions typically subcortical; primary tumors more often deep
- Smooth, thin rim of enhancement typical of organizing abscess
- Thick, irregular rim of enhancement suggests necrotic neoplasm

Helpful Clues for Common Diagnoses
- **Abscess**
  - Pyogenic, fungal, granulomatous, or parasitic
  - Single or multiple
  - Thin, smooth rim contrast enhancement (CE)
  - Thin T2 hypointense rim
  - Restricted diffusion central cavity
  - MRS: ↑ amino acids (0.9 ppm), succinate (2.4 ppm), and acetate (1.92 ppm)
  - Early capsule stage: Moderate vasogenic edema and mass effect
  - Late capsule stage: Edema & mass effect ↓
  - ± ventriculitis &/or meningitis
  - ± sinusitis or mastoiditis as a cause
- **Pilocytic Astrocytoma**
  - Cerebellum > optic nerve/chiasm > adjacent to 3rd ventricle > brainstem
  - Peak: 5-15 years of age
  - Variable appearance
    - Nonenhancing cyst + CE mural nodule
    - CE cyst wall + CE mural nodule
    - Solid with necrotic center + heterogeneous CE
    - Solid + homogeneous CE
  - Cyst may accumulate contrast on delayed imaging
  - "Aggressive" metabolite spectrum on MRS: ↑ choline, ↓ NAA; however, clinical behavior frequently benign
- **Neurocysticercosis**
  - Pork tapeworm, *Taenia solium*
  - 5-20 mm cyst
  - ± 1-4 mm eccentric scolex
  - Single or multiple
  - Cisterns > parenchyma > intraventricular
  - Appearance depends on developmental stage and host response
    - Simple cyst ± enhancement → complicated cyst + thick enhancing wall
  - ± surrounding edema
  - ± calcification in healed stage

Helpful Clues for Less Common Diagnoses
- **Demyelinating Disease**
  - **ADEM**
    - Autoimmune-mediated demyelination: Brain and spinal cord
    - Typically monophasic, 10-14 days after viral infection or vaccination
    - "Multiphasic" or "relapsing" ADEM may be same entity as MS
    - Multifocal hyperintense T2 and FLAIR signal WM and BG > GM; cerebrum > cerebellum and brainstem
    - Bilateral common, but asymmetric
    - Punctate or ring-like enhancement (complete or incomplete)
    - MRS: ↓ NAA, ± ↑ lactate and choline in acute lesions
  - **Multiple Sclerosis**
    - Probably autoimmune-mediated demyelination in genetically susceptible individuals
    - Relapsing-remitting course

- Imaging may be identical to ADEM
- Multifocal lesions PVWM, subcortical U-fibers, brachium pontis, brainstem, and spinal cord
- Infratentorial: Children > adults
- Perivenular extension along path of deep medullary veins = "Dawson fingers"
- T1WI: Hypointense lesions = axonal destruction ("black holes")
- T2 and FLAIR: Hyperintense linear foci radiating from ventricles
- Nodular or ring enhancement, occasionally semilunar CE or large tumefactive enhancing rings
- MRS: ↓ NAA, ↑ choline, ↑ myoinositol

- **Ganglioglioma**
  - Temporal > parietal > frontal > occipital > BG/thalamus, hypothalamus/optic pathway, cerebellum
  - Solid, cystic, or mixed; usually cortical-based lesion, without surrounding edema
  - Ca++ common
  - Larger and more cystic lesions in children
  - Variable degree of CE: Diffuse or ring-like
  - Marked meningeal enhancement in desmoplastic infantile ganglioglioma
  - Rarely poorly defined, infiltrating lesion

Helpful Clues for Rare Diagnoses

- **Aneurysm (Thrombosed)**
  - Partially or completely thrombosed
  - Laminated appearance of thrombus
  - ± pulsation artifact on MR
- **Other Infections**
  - **Tuberculosis:** *Mycobacterium tuberculosis* infection
    - CNS TB usually with pulmonary TB
    - Thick basilar meningitis
    - ± dural-based tuberculomas
    - ± parenchymal tuberculomas
    - Multiple > solitary tuberculomas
    - Solid CE or necrotic center
  - **Fungal Diseases**: Rare, usually in immunocompromised patients
    - Nocardia, blastomycosis, candidiasis, coccidiomycosis, histoplasmosis
    - Multiple > single
  - **Acquired Toxoplasmosis**: Single or multiple; nodular or ring CE; immunocompromised patients, esp. HIV+
  - **Lyme Disease**: Multifocal PVWM lesions ± CE; cranial nerve CE common; rash and flu-like symptoms
- **Other Neoplasms**
  - Primary neoplasms usually solitary; metastasis: multiple > single; gray-white junction; + vasogenic edema
  - GBM: Central necrosis and rim CE
  - Primary CNS lymphoma: Ring-enhancing in immunocompromised patients
- **Subacute Cerebral Infarction**
  - Common, but rarely image with contrast
  - Edema in vascular territory; gyriform > ring-like CE
- **Subacute Intracerebral Hematoma**
  - History of trauma or coagulopathy; common, but rarely image with contrast

Abscess

Axial T1 C+ MR shows 2 large, rim-enhancing cerebellar abscesses ➡, mass effect, and surrounding edema ➡, typical of early capsule stage, in a child with mastoiditis.

Abscess

Axial CECT shows 2 rim-enhancing frontal lobe abscesses ➡ secondary to sinusitis. Thin rim enhancement is typical of the early and late capsular stage of abscess formation.

RING-ENHANCING LESIONS

(Left) Axial T1 C+ MR shows a typical nonenhancing cyst ➡ with an intensely enhancing mural nodule ➡ in a child with juvenile pilocytic astrocytoma. *(Right)* Axial T1 C+ MR shows a different child with an enhancing nodule with central necrosis ➡ resulting in the ring-enhancing appearance of right temporal lobe pilocytic astrocytoma.

Pilocytic Astrocytoma

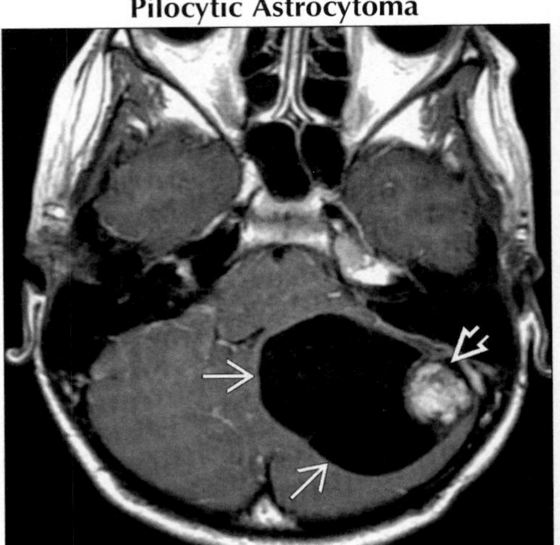

Pilocytic Astrocytoma

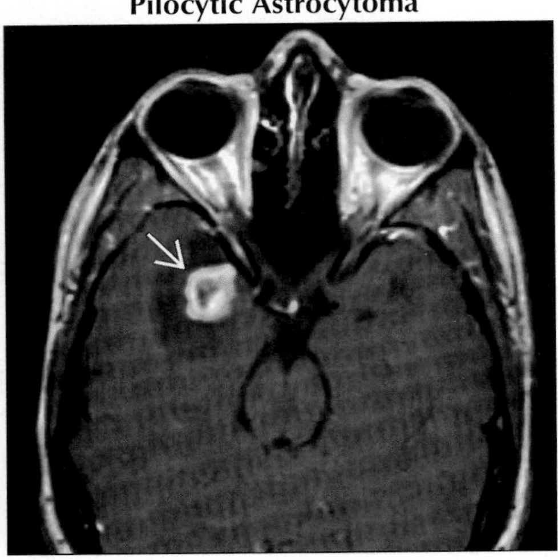

(Left) Sagittal T1 C+ MR shows a less common appearance of pilocytic astrocytoma with an intensely enhancing mural nodule ➡ and rim-enhancing cystic component ➡ in the medulla. *(Right)* Axial T1 C+ MR shows a small rim-enhancing left frontoparietal lesion ➡ with moderate surrounding edema ➡ and possible peripheral scolex in the posteromedial margin of the cavity.

Pilocytic Astrocytoma

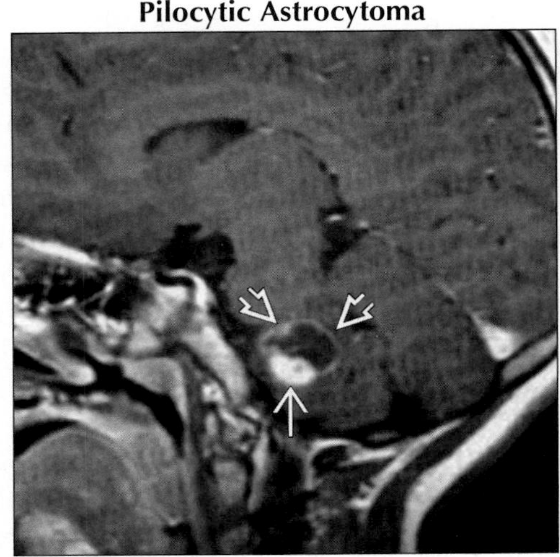

Neurocysticercosis

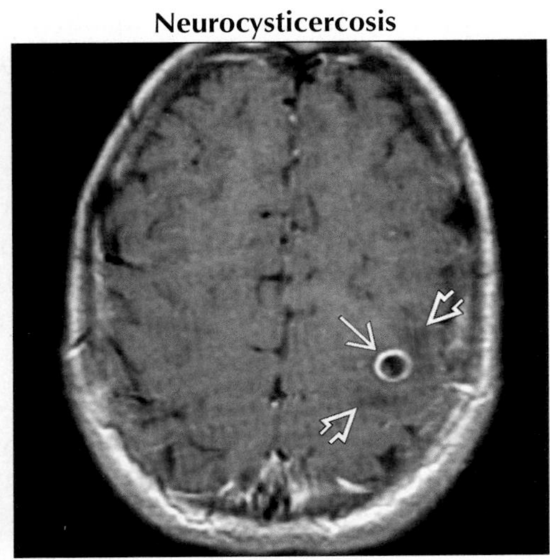

(Left) Axial T1WI C+ MR shows an incomplete ring of peripheral enhancement ➡ at the site of demyelination in a child with ADEM. *(Right)* Axial T1WI C+ MR shows a hypodense mass in the left frontoparietal junction with an incomplete rim of peripheral enhancement ➡. The nonenhancing part of the mass is adjacent to the cortex. This finding is classic for "tumefactive" demyelinating disease, most commonly multiple sclerosis.

ADEM

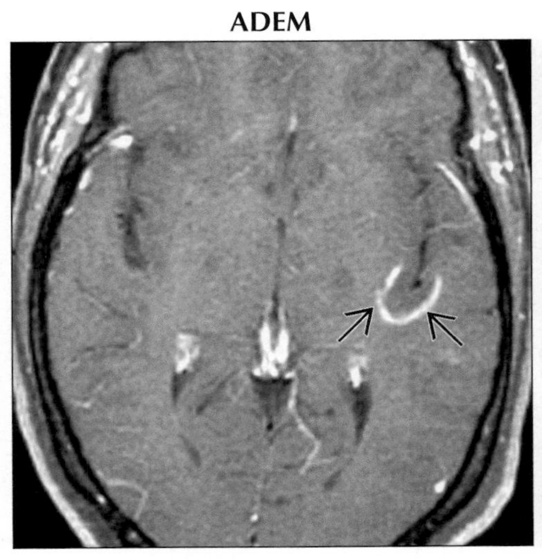

Multiple Sclerosis

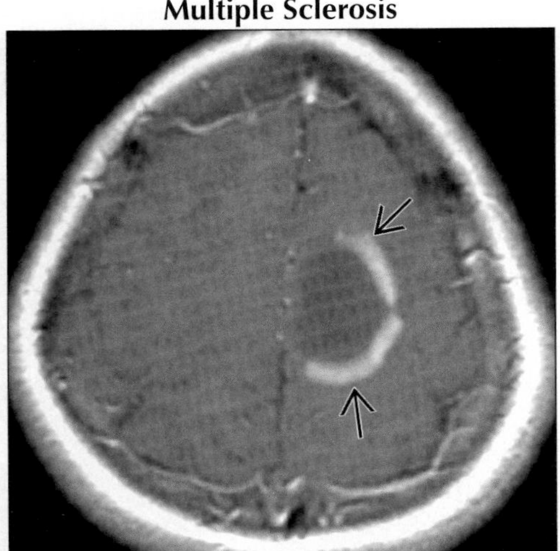

Multiple Sclerosis

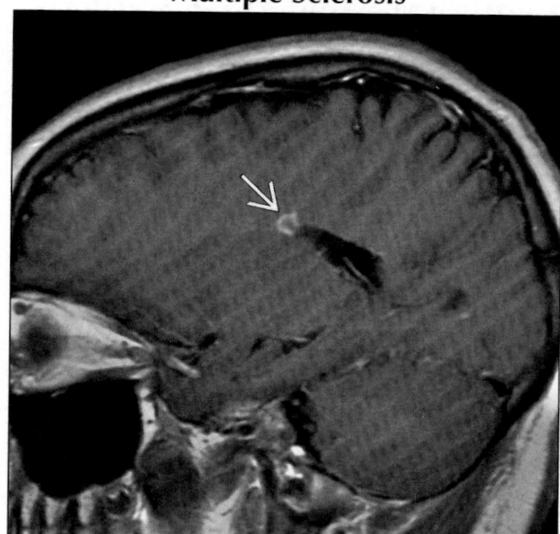

Ganglioglioma

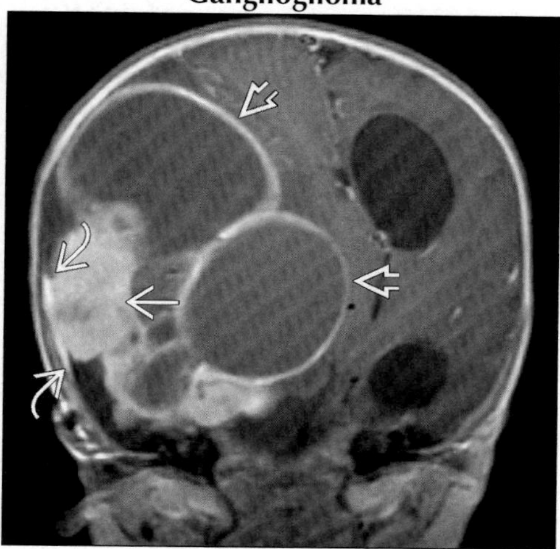

(Left) *Sagittal T1WI C+ MR shows a small ring-enhancing periventricular lesion ➡ in a teenager with multiple sclerosis.* ***(Right)*** *Coronal T1WI C+ MR shows typical MR findings of desmoplastic infantile ganglioglioma: A large lesion in the right cerebral hemisphere with an enhancing nodular peripheral component ➡, multiple deep cystic components ➡, and dural enhancement ➡.*

Aneurysm (Thrombosed)

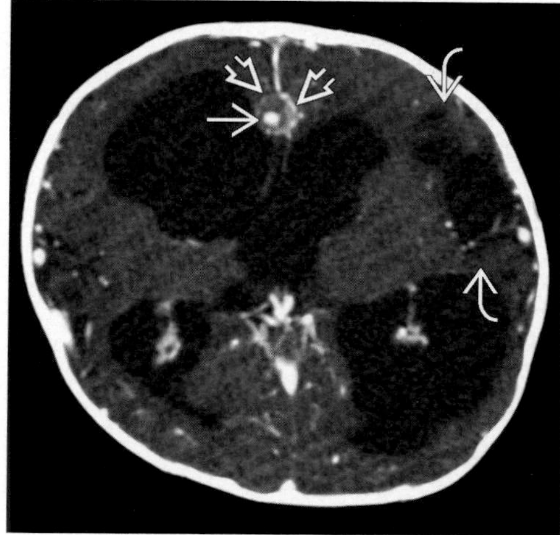

Parenchymal Metastases

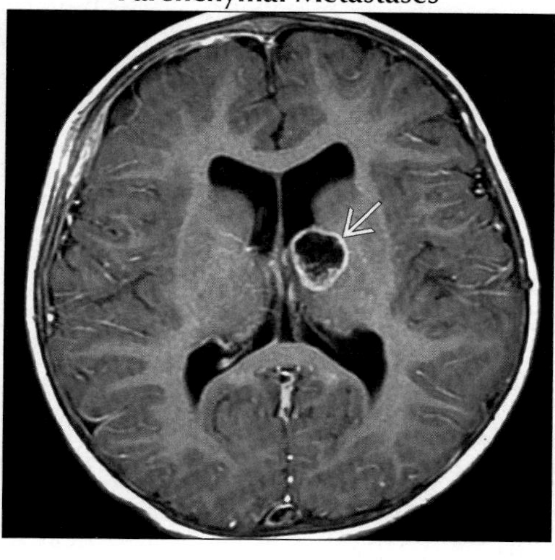

(Left) *Axial CECT shows eccentric enhancement ➡ in the patent lumen of a partially thrombosed pseudoaneurysm ➡, secondary to nonaccidental trauma. Note the remote left MCA infarction ➡ and ventriculomegaly.* ***(Right)*** *Axial T1WI C+ MR shows an irregular rim of enhancement in a solitary focus of metastatic neuroblastoma ➡. In the absence of known extracranial primary neoplasm, primary CNS neoplasm would be a principal consideration.*

Glioblastoma Multiforme

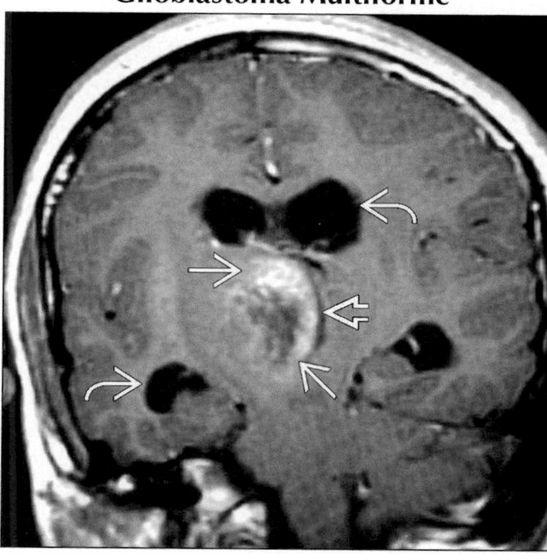

Subacute Cerebral Infarction

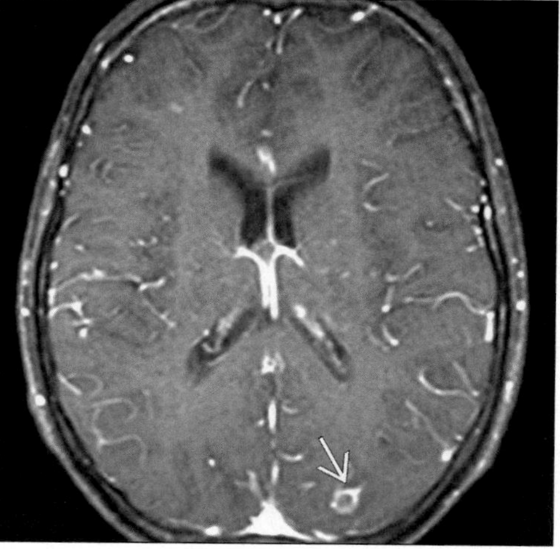

(Left) *Coronal T1 C+ MR shows partial rim enhancement of a large heterogeneous thalamic GBM ➡ with near complete obliteration of the 3rd ventricle ➡ secondary to mass effect and resultant early obstructive hydrocephalus ➡.* ***(Right)*** *Axial T1 C+ FS MR shows a subacute ring-enhancing infarct ➡ 8 days after ictus.*

THICK CORTEX

DIFFERENTIAL DIAGNOSIS

Common
- Encephalitis
- Herpes Encephalitis

Less Common
- Hypomyelination (Pseudo Thick Cortex)
- Tuberous Sclerosis Complex
- Taylor Cortical Dysplasia
- Pachygyria-Polymicrogyria
- Hemimegalencephaly
- Lissencephaly Type 1

Rare but Important
- Neoplasms Associated with Cortical Dysplasia
  - DNET
  - Ganglioglioma
  - Dysplastic Cerebellar Gangliocytoma
- Glioblastoma Multiforme
- Gliomatosis Cerebri
- Meningioangiomatosis
- Congenital Muscular Dystrophy

ESSENTIAL INFORMATION

Key Differential Diagnosis Issues
- EXCLUDES transient (e.g., MELAS, cortical edema from stroke/seizure, etc.)
- Is cortex thick on both T1 and T2W sequences?
- Does cortex follow gray matter signal intensity (malformations)? or is it hyperintense (infection, neoplasm)?
- Is thickened cortex very focal (think neoplasm)? or more generalized (malformation)?

Helpful Clues for Common Diagnoses
- **Encephalitis**
  - Commonly identified agents: *Enterovirus, HSV1, Mycoplasma pneumonia*, Epstein-Barr, HHV-6, influenza
  - Etiology not found in ≈ 50%
  - Hyperintense on T2WI, FLAIR
  - Thickened, hyperintense temporal lobe/insular cortex
- **Herpes Encephalitis**
  - Often bilateral, asymmetric
  - Look for cingulate gyrus, subfrontal cortex involvement
  - Restricts strongly on DWI
  - Enhancement, hemorrhage follow

Helpful Clues for Less Common Diagnoses
- **Hypomyelination (Pseudo Thick Cortex)**
  - Diminished/absent white matter (WM) myelination for age
    - Lacks peripheral "arborization" of white matter
  - Can be primary or secondary
    - Primary hypomyelination (e.g., Pelizaeus-Merzbacher)
    - Secondary (prematurity, malnutrition)
  - Imaging
    - "Pseudo" thick cortex appearance
    - Poor gray-white differentiation on T1WI in children > 1 year
    - Poor gray-white differentiation on T2WI in children > 2 years
    - Small brain with thin corpus callosum
- **Tuberous Sclerosis Complex**
  - Flattened, thickened gyri with "blurred" GM/WM border
  - Can be calcified, involve entire mantle
  - Look for subcortical WM hyperintensities, subependymal nodules
- **Taylor Cortical Dysplasia**
  - Also known as focal cortical dysplasia (FCD) type 2A/B
  - "Balloon cell" dysplasia
  - Malformation of cortical development
  - Refractory focal epilepsy
  - Thickened cortex with T1 hyperintensity, T2 hypointensity in infancy
    - Rare Ca++
  - Lesion conspicuity decreases with WM maturation
- **Pachygyria-Polymicrogyria**
  - Polymicrogyria → excessively small, prominent convolutions ("gyri on gyri")
  - Pachygyria (sometimes called incomplete lissencephaly) → thickened, dysplastic cortex
  - Both cause appearance of "thick cortex" on imaging
  - Density/signal intensity of affected cortex same as normal gray matter
- **Hemimegalencephaly**
  - Hamartomatous overgrowth of part/all of a hemisphere
  - Enlarged hemisphere with thickened, often dysplastic cortex

- Ipsilateral ventricle often enlarged, abnormally shaped
- White matter often overgrows, is hypermyelinated

- **Lissencephaly Type 1**
  - Most severe type (complete agyria) is Miller-Dieker syndrome
  - Thick, multilayered cortex
  - "Hour glass" configuration with shallow sylvian fissures in severe cases

Helpful Clues for Rare Diagnoses

- **DNET**
  - Young patient, longstanding seizures
  - Well-demarcated "bubbly" intracortical mass
  - Often associated with adjacent cortical dysplasia
- **Ganglioglioma**
  - Child/young adult, seizures
  - Superficial hemispheres, temporal lobe
  - Cyst with nodule, ± Ca++, enhancement typical
  - Solid ganglioglioma can resemble Taylor cortical dysplasia (TCD does not enhance)
- **Dysplastic Cerebellar Gangliocytoma**
  - Thickening, overgrowth of cerebellar folia
  - Gyriform "layered" or "striated" pattern
  - Can cause significant mass effect
  - Cowden-Lhermitte-Duclos (COLD) syndrome is considered new phakomatosis
    - Multiple hamartoma-neoplasia syndrome
    - Long-term cancer screening (breast, thyroid)
- **Glioblastoma Multiforme**
  - White matter > > gray matter
  - Tumor infiltration of cortex, subpial extension may occur late
  - Hemorrhage, enhancement common
  - Primary GBM (older patient) 95% necrotic with thick irregular enhancing rim
  - Secondary GBM (younger patient) shows enhancing focus within lower grade tumor
- **Gliomatosis Cerebri**
  - Tumor infiltrates but preserves underlying brain architecture
  - 2 or more lobes affected
  - T2 hyperintense infiltrating mass enlarges cortex, basal ganglia
  - MRS shows elevated myoinositol (mI)
  - Most are WHO grade II or III diffusely infiltrating astrocytoma
- **Meningioangiomatosis**
  - Cortical mass with variable Ca++
  - Linear &/or gyriform enhancement
  - Perivascular proliferation of vessels in meninges, cortex
  - May infiltrate along perivascular spaces, cause mass effect
- **Congenital Muscular Dystrophy**
  - Cobblestone lissencephaly (overmigration)
  - Z-shaped brainstem
  - Hypoplastic rotated cerebellum (similar to Dandy-Walker continuum)

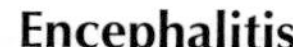

Encephalitis

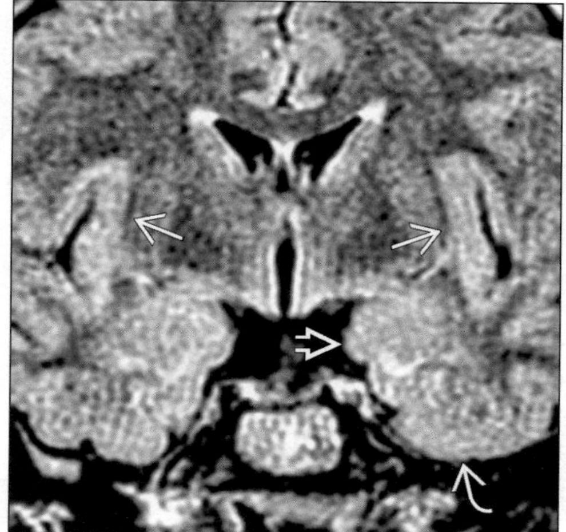

Coronal FLAIR MR shows subtle, bilateral signal increase and swelling in the hippocampus ➔, temporal lobe cortex ➔, and insular cortex ➔ in a child with proven Mycoplasma encephalitis.

Herpes Encephalitis

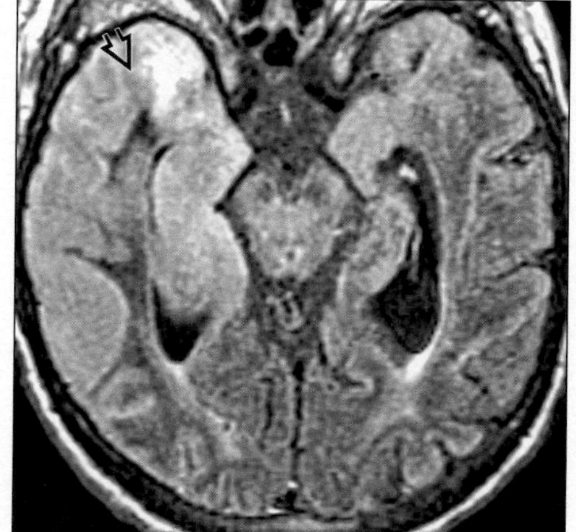

Coronal FLAIR MR shows swollen, hyperintense temporal lobe cortex ➔ with relative sparing of the underlying white matter. DWI (not shown) revealed restricted diffusion in the insular cortex & cingulate gyri.

THICK CORTEX

(**Left**) *Axial NECT in a 4 month old with hypomyelination ➡ shows decreased volume and white matter density. The thin arbors of white matter give a false impression that the cortex, especially in the occipital poles, is thickened ➡.* (**Right**) *Coronal T2WI MR in an 18 month old with Pelizaeus-Merzbacher disease (PMD) shows white matter hypomyelination in the occipital lobes ➡ and cerebellum ➡, giving the appearance of prominent thick cortex.*

Hypomyelination (Pseudo Thick Cortex)

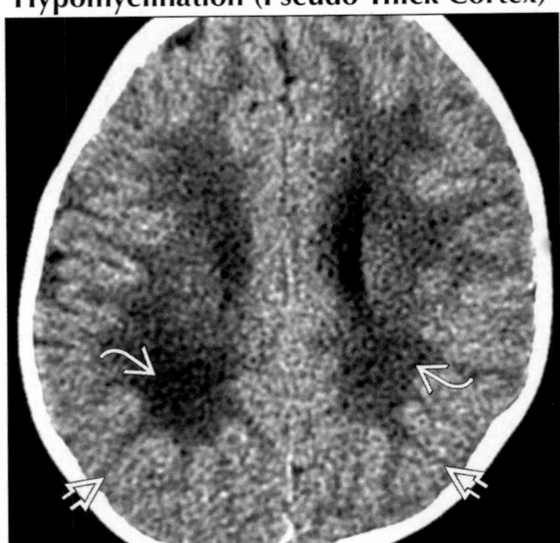

Hypomyelination (Pseudo Thick Cortex)

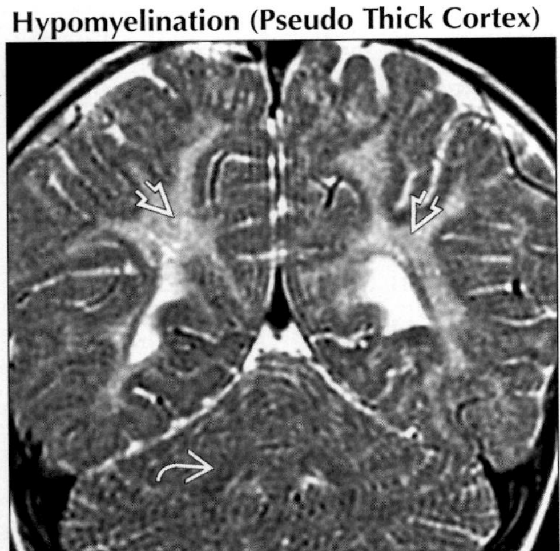

(**Left**) *Axial FLAIR MR shows multiple large, flat, thickened gyri with classic subcortical hyperintensities ➡, characteristic for cortical tubers.* (**Right**) *Axial T2WI MR in an 8 month old shows 2 manifestations of tuberous sclerosis complex: Densely calcified, thickened transmantle hamartoma ➡ in the right parietal lobe and characteristic "tubers" ➡ in the left. Note the multiple subependymal nodules ➡.*

Tuberous Sclerosis Complex

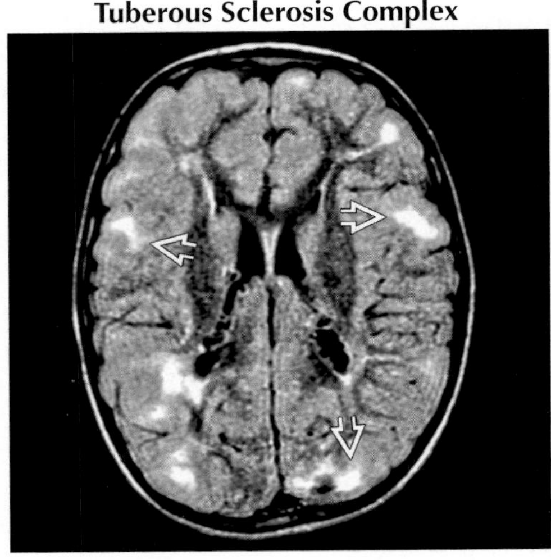

Tuberous Sclerosis Complex

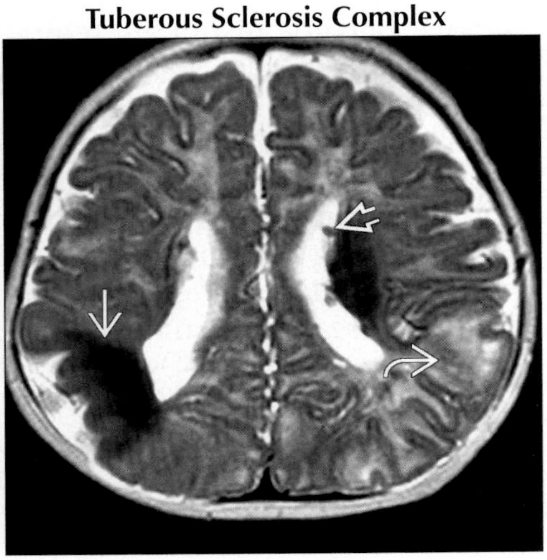

(**Left**) *Coronal PD FSE MR shows focal cortical thickening with high signal of the expanded gyrus ➡.* (**Right**) *Axial CECT in the same child shows a focal-low density, noncalcified cortical/subcortical mass ➡. There is no enhancement, and there are neither subependymal nodules nor a foramen of Monro giant cell astrocytoma.*

Taylor Cortical Dysplasia

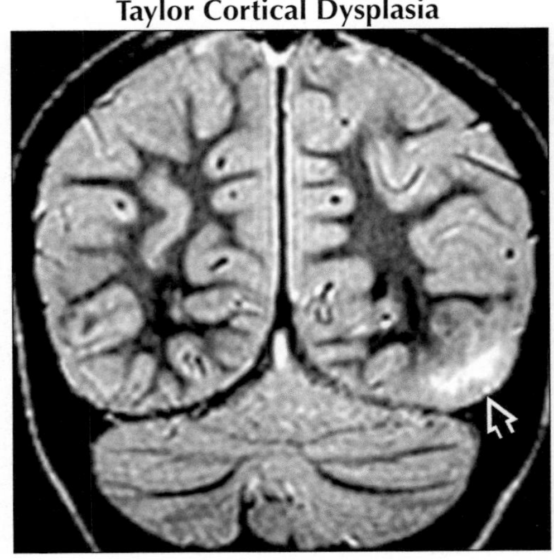

Taylor Cortical Dysplasia

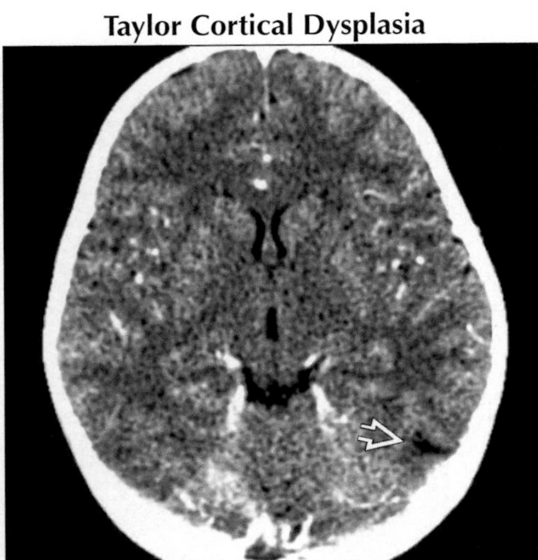

Pachygyria-Polymicrogyria

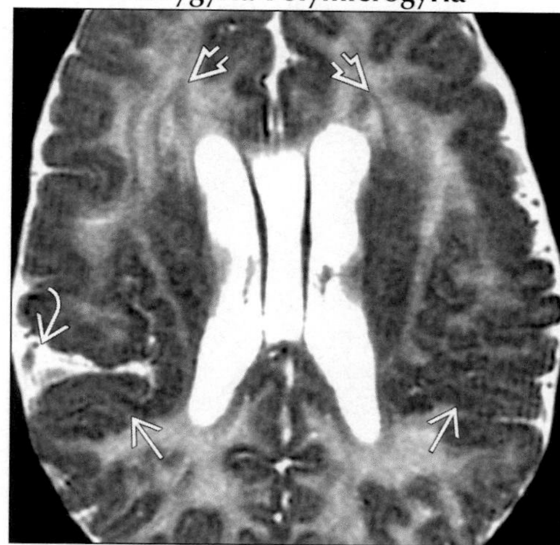

Pachygyria-Polymicrogyria

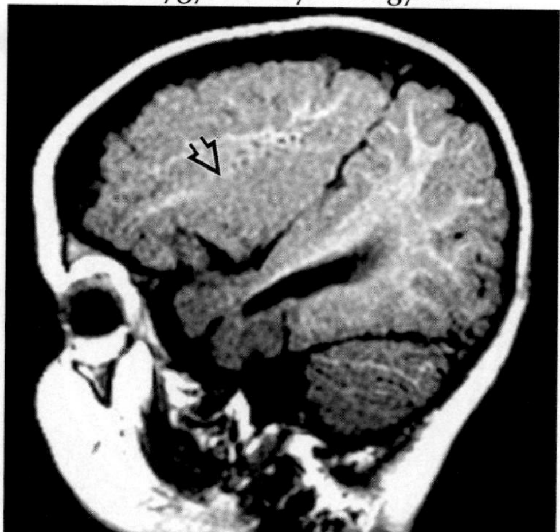

*(**Left**) Axial T2WI MR in a 10 month old with refractory seizures shows bilateral perisylvian foci of polymicrogyria ➡, giving the appearance of thick cortex. Note the abnormal veins ➡ and subtle laminar heterotopia ➡. (**Right**) Sagittal T1WI MR shows a thick cortex ⇨ lining the sylvian fissure in another child with bilateral primitive sylvian fissures and perisylvian polymicrogyria.*

Pachygyria-Polymicrogyria

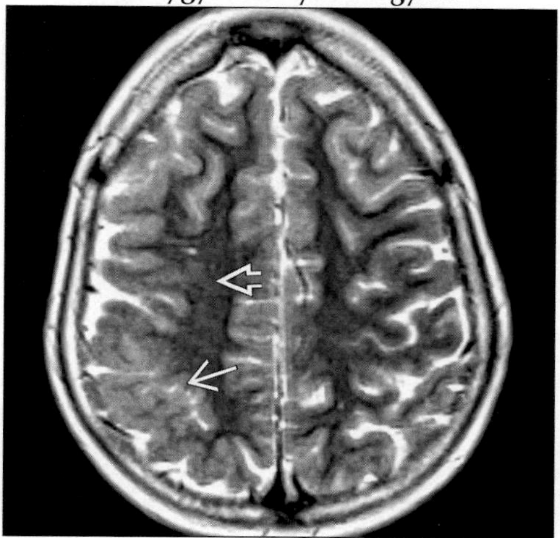

Pachygyria-Polymicrogyria

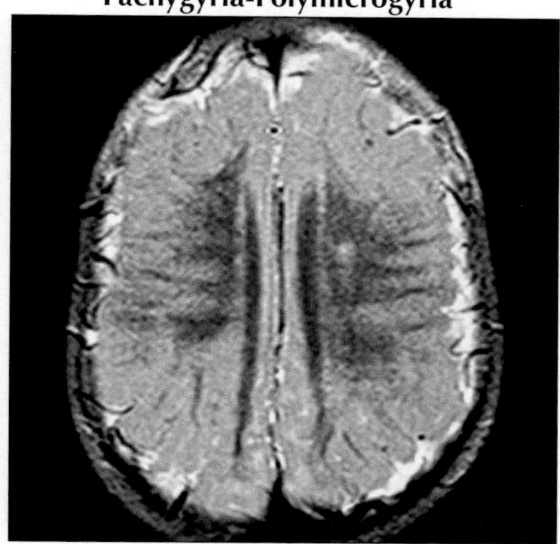

*(**Left**) Axial T2WI MR shows unilateral frontoparietal polymicrogyria with blurring of the gray-white junction ➡ and a nodular appearance ➡. (**Right**) Axial T2WI MR in a different child shows a much more extensively involved brain. Both hemispheres have a diffusely thickened, striated cortex due to polymicrogyria.*

Hemimegalencephaly

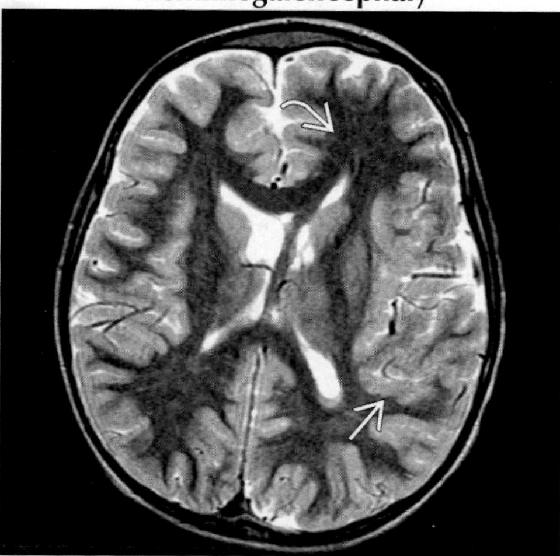

Hemimegalencephaly

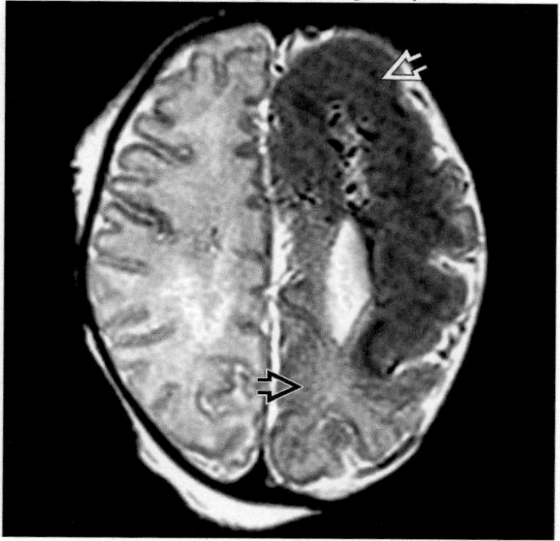

*(**Left**) Axial T2WI MR shows expanded left hemisphere with diffuse overgrowth of white matter ➡ and some gray matter as well ➡. (**Right**) Axial T2WI MR shows a diffusely thickened, partially calcified left frontal cortex ➡. The remainder of the left hemisphere has decreased signal intensity throughout gray and white matter ⇨.*

THICK CORTEX

(**Left**) *Axial T1WI MR in a 2 week old shows the layered appearance of the cortex with a thick inner band of gray matter ➡ and thin outer layer ➡. In between is the "cell sparse" white matter zone ➡.* (**Right**) *Coronal T1WI MR shows a thickened "cobblestone" cortex ➡ and a hypoplastic cerebellum. The 4th ventricle ➡ is opened inferiorly due to vermian hypoplasia and cephalad rotation.*

Lissencephaly Type 1

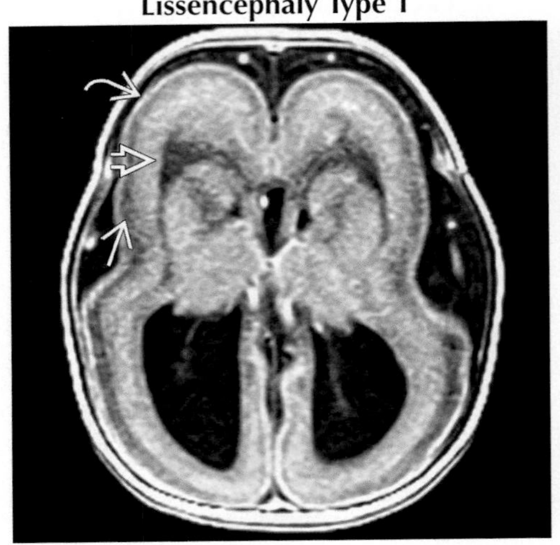

Congenital Muscular Dystrophy

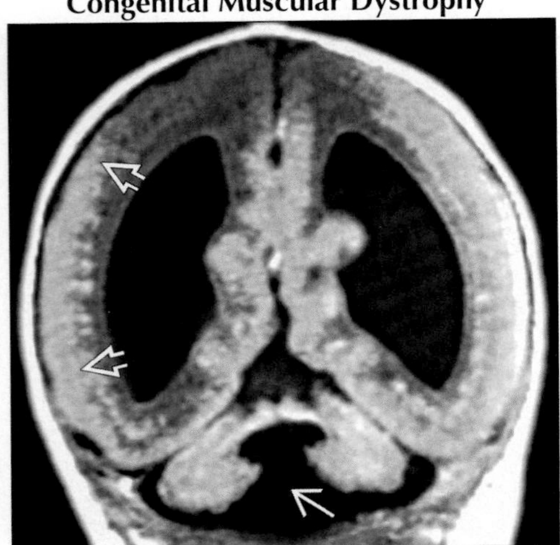

(**Left**) *Axial FLAIR MR shows a thickened, hyperintense, cortically based mass with a "rim" sign of hyperintensity on FLAIR ➡. Lack of edema also is characteristic for DNET.* (**Right**) *Axial T1WI MR shows typical multinodular low signal intensity mass ➡ focally expanding the cortical mantle and remodeling the inner cortex ➡ of the calvarium.*

DNET

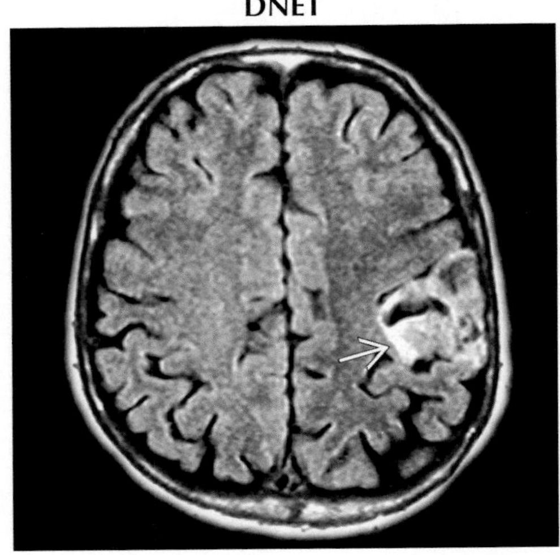

DNET

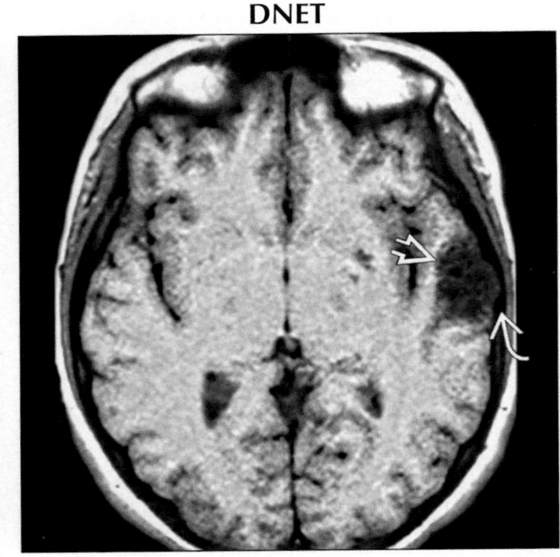

(**Left**) *Axial PD FSE MR shows a thickened, hyperintense cortex ➡ in a 5 year old with epilepsy. Without contrast-enhanced scan, this image would be indistinguishable from Taylor cortical dysplasia.* (**Right**) *Axial T1WI C+ MR in the same patient shows several small enhancing foci ➡. Ganglioglioma was found at surgery.*

Ganglioglioma

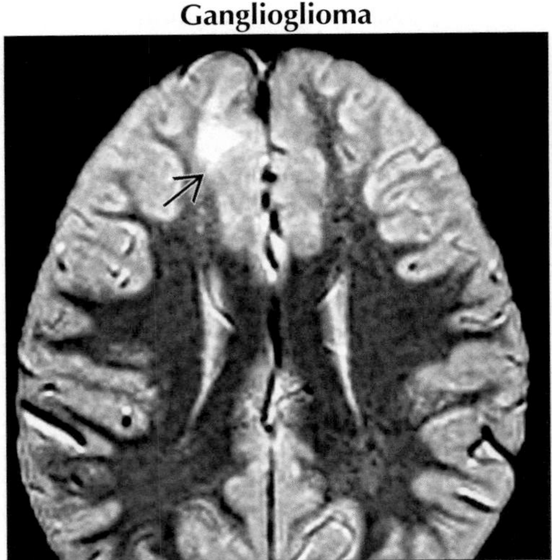

Ganglioglioma

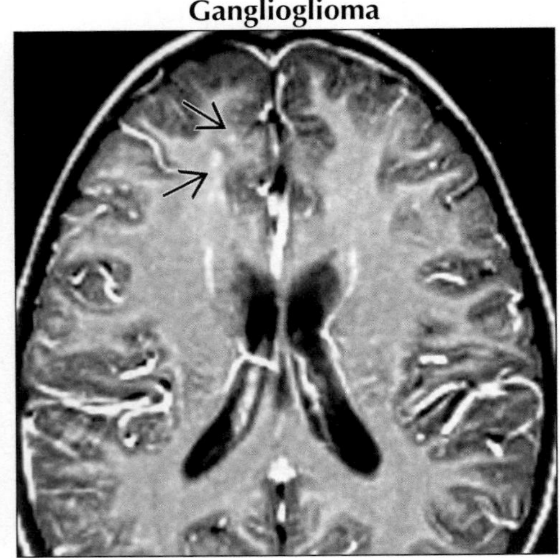

THICK CORTEX

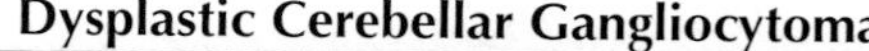

Dysplastic Cerebellar Gangliocytoma

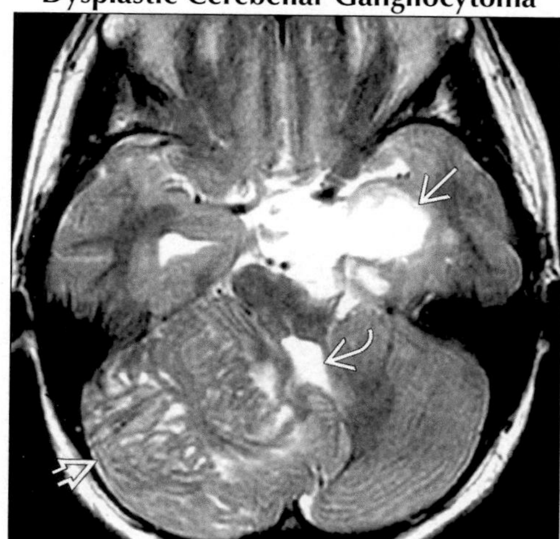

Dysplastic Cerebellar Gangliocytoma

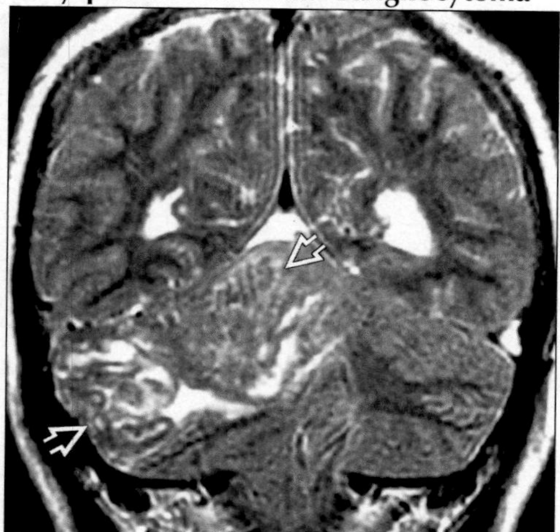

(Left) *Axial T2WI MR shows a striated iso- and hypointense posterior fossa mass that displaces the 4th ventricle. There is an additional epidermoid cyst.* ***(Right)*** *Coronal T2WI MR shows thickened, striated-appearing cerebellar folia in a patient with Lhermitte-Duclos disease. In this case, there was no association with Cowden syndrome.*

Glioblastoma Multiforme

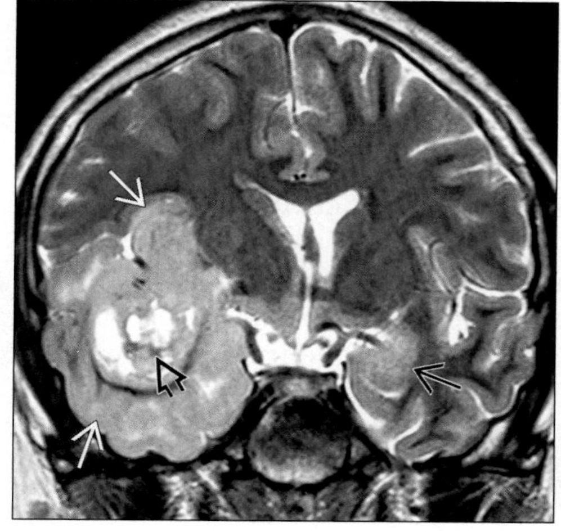

Meningioangiomatosis

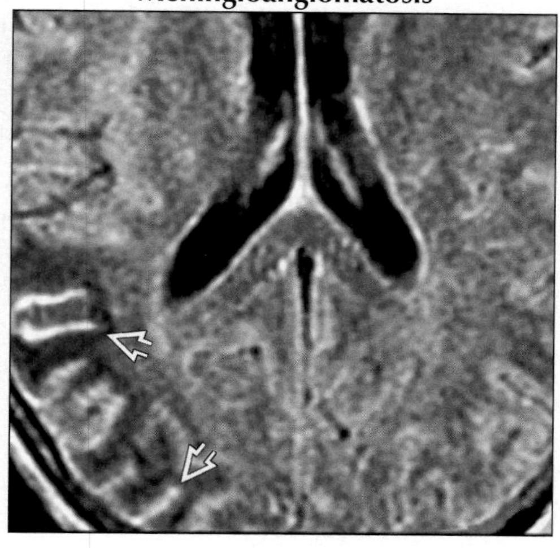

(Left) *Coronal T2WI MR in a 14 year old shows an iso- & hyperintense right temporal lobe & insular mass involving both gray & white matter. Note necrosis, focal hemorrhage. Tumor spread across anterior commissure thickens the left temporal lobe cortex.* ***(Right)*** *Axial FLAIR MR shows a typical case of meningioangiomatosis, most commonly found in NF2. Fine gyriform increased density was present on NECT. FLAIR MR shows linear increased signal.*

Gliomatosis Cerebri

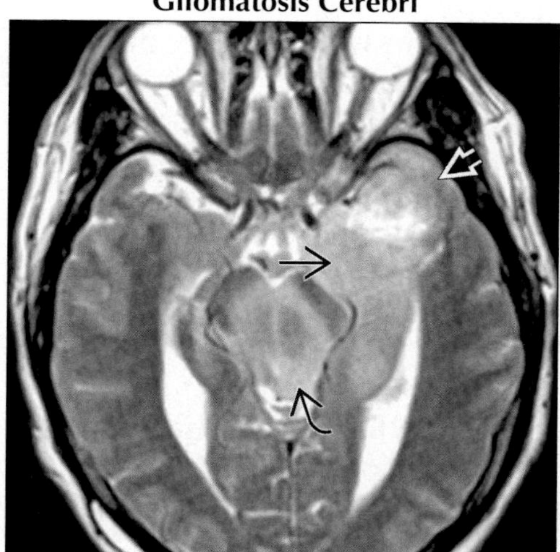

Gliomatosis Cerebri

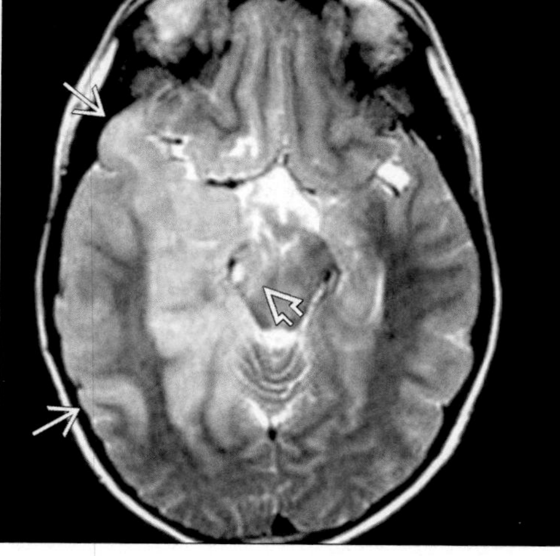

(Left) *Axial T2WI MR in an adult shows involvement of the temporal pole cortex, hippocampus, and mesencephalon. Involvement of more than 1 lobe or region is typical of gliomatosis cerebri.* ***(Right)*** *Axial T2WI FS MR in a 12 year old shows hyperintense, swollen gyri with involvement of the midbrain related to gliomatosis cerebri. WHO grade III diffusely infiltrating astrocytoma was found. (Courtesy M. Warmuth-Metz, MD.)*

METABOLIC DISORDERS AFFECTING PRIMARILY WHITE MATTER

DIFFERENTIAL DIAGNOSIS

Common
- Leukodystrophies
  - X-Linked Adrenoleukodystrophy (X-ALD)
  - Canavan Disease
  - Metachromatic Leukodystrophy (MLD)
  - Krabbe Disease (GLD)
  - Hypomyelination
  - Alexander Disease
  - Vanishing White Matter Disease

Less Common
- Mucopolysaccharidoses

Rare but Important
- Megaloencephalic Leukoencephalopathy with Cysts (MLC)
- Merosin Deficient Congenital Muscular Dystrophy
- Maple Syrup Urine Disease
- Nonketotic Hyperglycinemia
- Urea Cycle Disorders
- Giant Axonal Neuropathy
- Trichothiodystrophies
- Oculocerebrorenal (Lowe) Syndrome
- Hyperhomocysteinemia (Homocystinuria)

ESSENTIAL INFORMATION

Key Differential Diagnosis Issues
- Leukodystrophy
  - Inborn errors of metabolism → abnormal growth or development of myelin sheath → progressive degeneration of WM
  - Symmetric subcortical or deep WM ± GM
- Macrocephaly: Canavan, Alexander, & MLC
- Initial PVWM involvement: MLD, Globoid-cell leukodystrophy (GLD), X-linked ALD
- Initial subcortical WM involvement: MLC, vanishing white matter
- Many → diffuse WM disease and atrophy
- MRS: Majority → ↓ NAA; Canavan → ↑ NAA

Helpful Clues for Common Diagnoses
- **X-Linked Adrenoleukodystrophy (X-ALD)**
  - Most common in males 5-12 years old
  - Immune-mediated inflammation at active zones of demyelination → enhancement
    - 80% splenium ⇒ peritrigonal WM ⇒ corticospinal tracts/fornix/commisural fibers/visual and auditory pathways
    - 15% frontal pattern, genu, anterior/genu internal capsule ± cerebellar (CB) WM
  - Spares subcortical U-fibers
  - ± Ca++
- **Canavan Disease**
  - Macrocephaly
  - ↑ T2 subcortical U-fibers, thalami, and globi pallidi
  - MRS: ↑ NAA
- **Metachromatic Leukodystrophy (MLD)**
  - Most common form is late infantile variant; presents in 2nd year of life
  - Frontal and posterior WM
  - Symmetric, confluent, nonenhancing ↑ T2 PVWM in "butterfly" pattern
  - ± radial stripes (relative sparing of myelin in perivenular regions)
  - Atrophy, subcortical U-fibers involved late
- **Krabbe Disease (GLD)**
  - Globoid-cell leukodystrophy (GLD)
  - CT: Symmetric, bilateral high attenuation in thalami on early CT (3-6 months old)
  - ↑ T2: Thalami, basal ganglia, CB nuclei, PVWM, corticospinal and pyramidal tracts
  - ± optic nerve enlargement
  - ± enhancement at junction of normal and abnormal WM
  - ± lumbar nerve root enhancement
- **Hypomyelination**
  - T2 hypointensity of myelin normally lags behind T1 hyperintensity by 4-8 months
  - Myelination on T2WI should be complete by 3 years, usually by 2 years of age
  - Primary hypomyelination syndromes 2° to chromosome deletions and mutations
    - Pelizaeus-Merzbacher disease (PMD)
    - Spastic paraplegia type 2 (SPG2)
    - Hypomyelination with atrophy of basal ganglia and cerebellum (H-ABC)
    - 18q-syndrome
    - Jacobsen syndrome (11q-)
    - Hypomyelination with congenital cataracts (*DRCTNNB1A*)
    - Hypomyelination + trichothiodystrophy
- **Alexander disease**
  - Macrocephaly
  - Infantile form most common
  - ↑ T2 in bifrontal WM; caudate heads > putamina, thalami
  - Enhancement in periventricular frontal lobe white matter in infantile form

- Enhancement in cerebellum and medulla in juvenile form
- ± enhancement in thalami, brainstem, dentate nuclei, cerebellar cortex, optic chiasm, fornix
- ± obstructive hydrocephalus 2° to periaqueductal disease

• **Vanishing White Matter Disease**
- Childhood ataxia with diffuse CNS hypomyelination, childhood ataxia with central hypomyelination (CASH)
- WM ultimately becomes isointense to CSF, begins in central cerebral WM

Helpful Clues for Less Common Diagnoses

• **Mucopolysaccharidoses**
- Hunter & Hurler syndrome most common
- Enlarged Virchow-Robin spaces, filled with glycosaminoglycans
- Mild PVWM disease

Helpful Clues for Rare Diagnoses

• **Megaloencephalic Leukoencephalopathy with Cysts (MLC)**
- a.k.a. van der Knaap disease
- Macrocephaly
- Peripheral WM swollen with enlarged gyri
- Less severe involvement of CB WM
- Subcortical cysts in posterior frontal and anterior temporal lobes

• **Merosin Deficient Congenital Muscular Dystrophy**
- Hypomyelination of central cerebral WM
- ± CB vermis and pontine hypoplasia

• **Maple Syrup Urine Disease**
- Acute phase: Edema and restricted diffusion in areas where normal neonatal WM should be myelinated
  - Deep CB and perirolandic WM, dorsal brainstem, cerebral peduncles, posterior limb internal capsule ± globi pallidi

• **Nonketotic Hyperglycinemia**
- Delayed myelination and edema in frontal cortex and subcortical WM
- Long-echo MRS: Abnormal peak at 3.56 ppm probably represents glycine

• **Urea Cycle Disorders**
- Multiple different enzyme deficiencies
- Severe edema in cortex, subcortical WM, and basal ganglia

• **Giant Axonal Neuropathy**
- ↑ T2 in cerebral and cerebellar WM, spares subcortical U-fibers

• **Trichothiodystrophies**
- Galactosemia: Delayed myelination in subcortical WM on T2WI, normal on T1WI; ± cerebral and CB atrophy
- Cockayne syndrome: ↑ T2 periventricular WM, basal ganglia, CB dentate nuclei

• **Oculocerebrorenal (Lowe) Syndrome**
- X-linked recessive
- Multiple CSF cysts in subcortical WM
- Confluent areas of ↑ T2 in WM, sparing subcortical U-fibers

• **Hyperhomocysteinemia (Homocystinuria)**
- Myelin destruction and ↓ volume deep cerebral WM, sparing internal capsule, peripheral WM, and subcortical U-fibers

X-Linked Adrenoleukodystrophy (X-ALD)

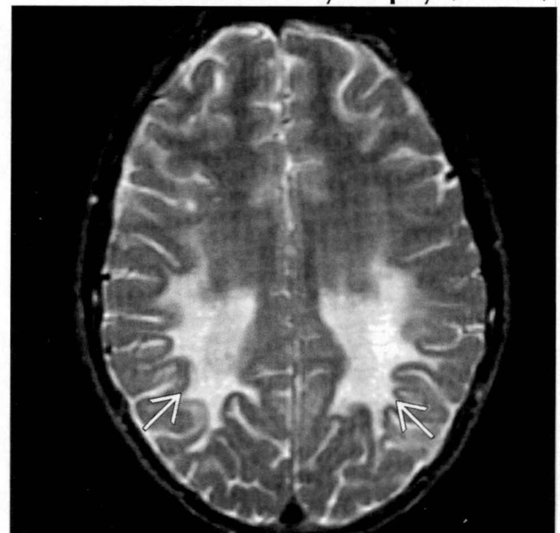

Axial T2WI MR in a 15-year-old male shows symmetric, bilateral confluent areas of hyperintense signal abnormality ➔ in the posterior parietal lobe white matter.

Canavan Disease

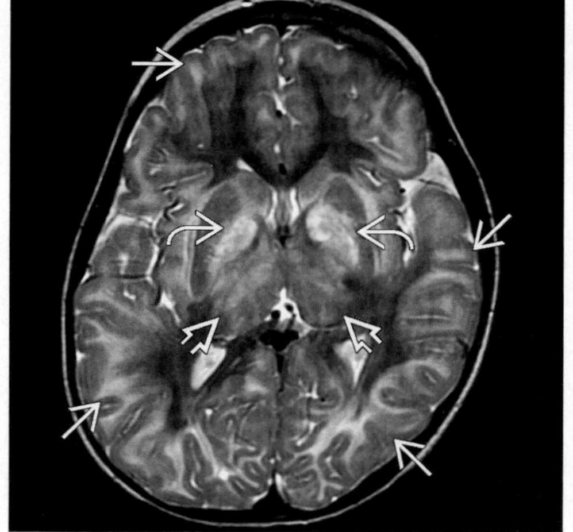

Axial T2WI MR shows symmetric, bilateral, abnormal hyperintense signal in the subcortical U-fibers ➔, the thalami ➔, and the globi pallidi ➔ in a macrocephalic 3 year old.

METABOLIC DISORDERS AFFECTING PRIMARILY WHITE MATTER

(Left) Axial T2WI MR shows bilateral, symmetric hyperintense signal in the parietal and frontal lobe deep white matter ➔, sparing the subcortical U-fibers ➔. (Right) Axial T2WI MR shows typical "radial stripes" of relatively spared myelin ➔ in the perivenular regions.

Metachromatic Leukodystrophy (MLD)

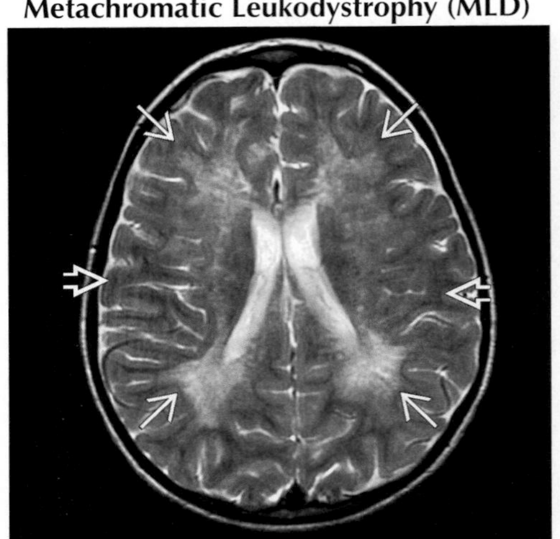

Metachromatic Leukodystrophy (MLD)

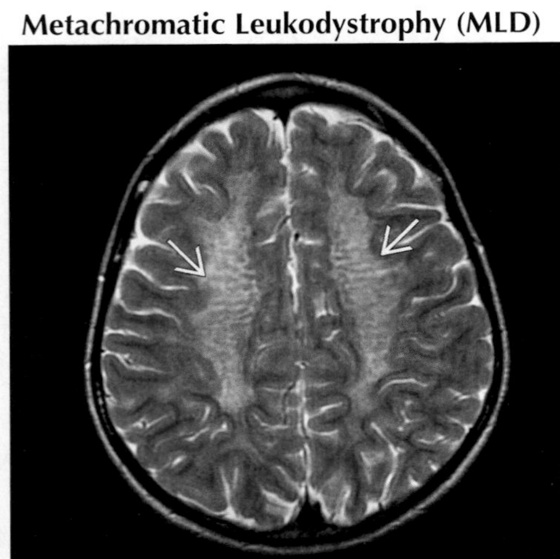

(Left) Axial NECT shows hyperdense foci ➔ in the thalami. The CT findings of hyperdensity may precede abnormalities on MR in patients with Krabbe disease. (Right) Axial T2WI MR shows symmetric, bilateral increased signal in the periventricular white matter ➔ and corticospinal tracts ➔.

Krabbe Disease (GLD)

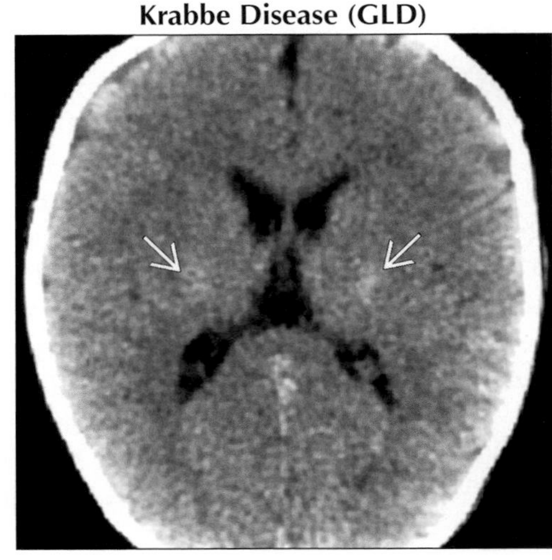

Krabbe Disease (GLD)

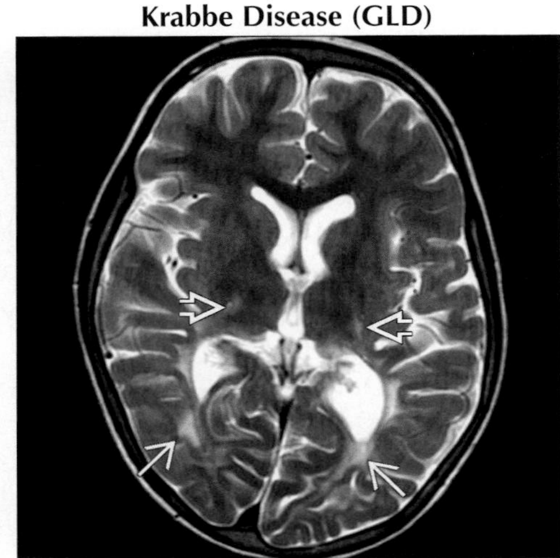

(Left) Axial T2WI MR in a 2 year old shows diffuse lack of T2-hypointense myelin in the deep white matter of both cerebral hemispheres ➔, the corpus callosum ➔, and the internal capsules ➔. Nearly all of the WM structures should be myelinated (hypointense on T2WI) at this age. (Right) Axial T1 C+ MR shows abnormal, symmetric, bilateral hypointensity in the frontal lobe white matter ➔, as well as periventricular contrast enhancement ➔.

Hypomyelination

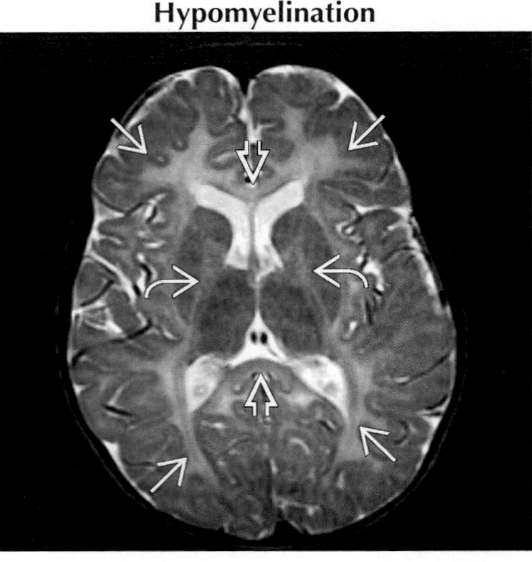

Alexander Disease

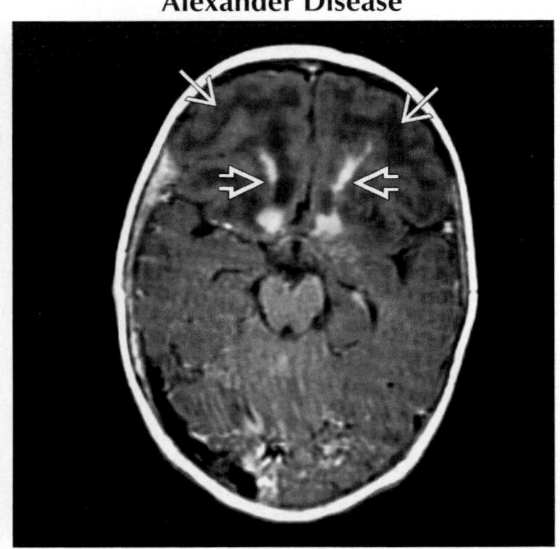

Vanishing White Matter Disease

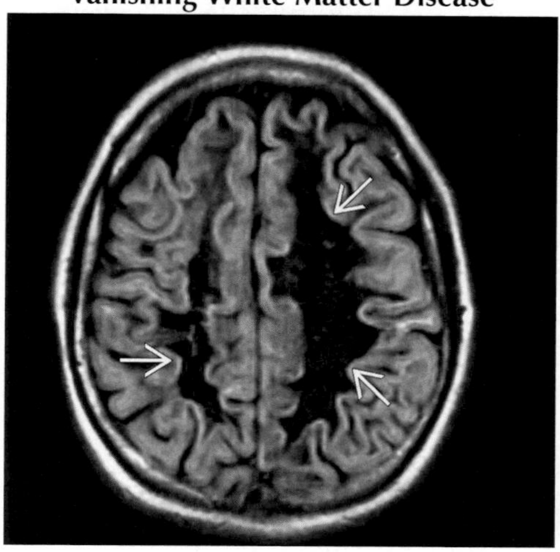

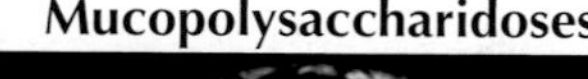

Mucopolysaccharidoses

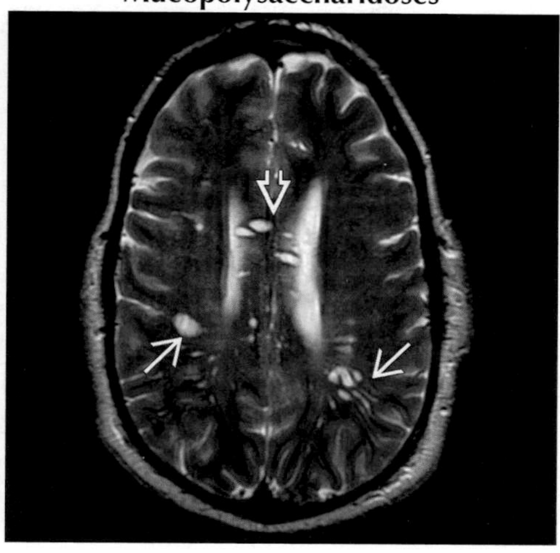

(Left) *Axial FLAIR MR shows symmetric, bilateral, isointense to CSF central white matter* → *in a child with vanishing white matter disease, also known as childhood ataxia with diffuse CNS hypomyelination (CASH).* ***(Right)*** *Axial T2WI FSE MR shows large Virchow-Robin perivascular spaces in the parietal lobe white matter* → *and the corpus callosum* ⇨ *in a child with Hunter syndrome. The enlarged spaces are thought to be filled with glycosaminoglycans.*

Megaloencephalic Leukoencephalopathy with Cysts (MLC)

Megaloencephalic Leukoencephalopathy with Cysts (MLC)

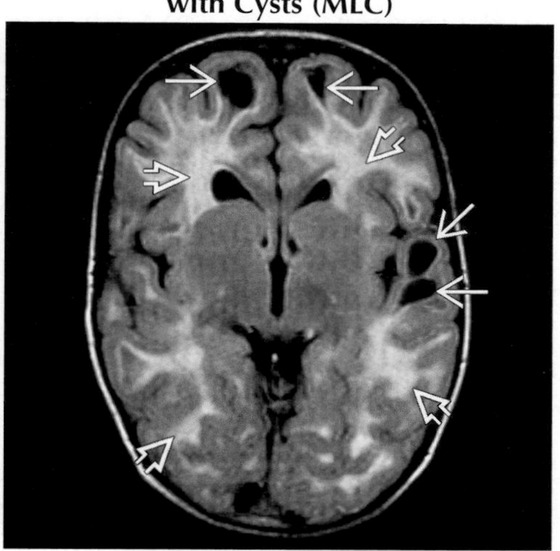

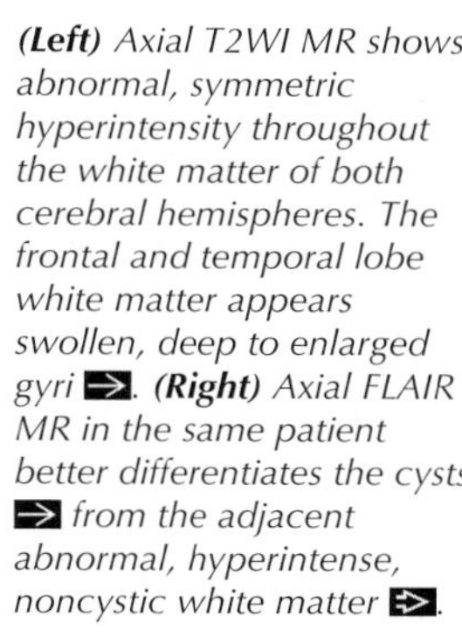

(Left) *Axial T2WI MR shows abnormal, symmetric hyperintensity throughout the white matter of both cerebral hemispheres. The frontal and temporal lobe white matter appears swollen, deep to enlarged gyri* →. ***(Right)*** *Axial FLAIR MR in the same patient better differentiates the cysts* → *from the adjacent abnormal, hyperintense, noncystic white matter* ⇨.

Merosin Deficient Congenital Muscular Dystrophy

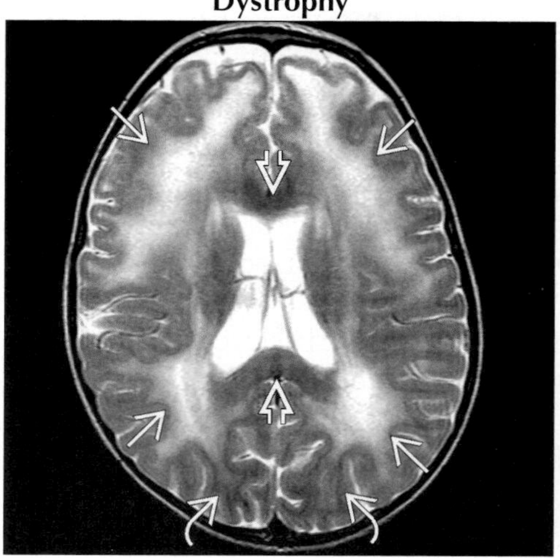

Maple Syrup Urine Disease

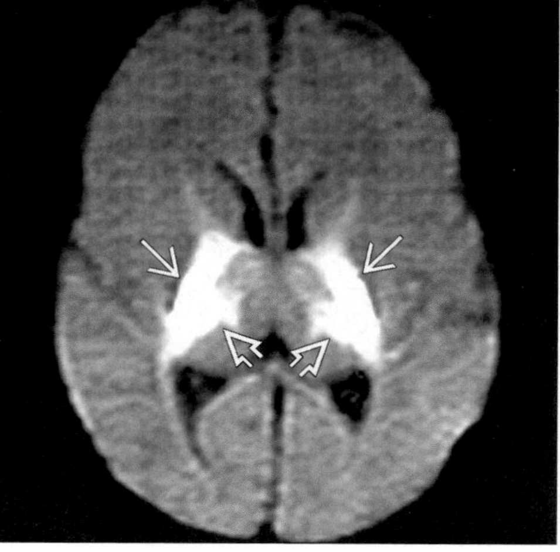

(Left) *Axial T2WI MR shows diffusely abnormal, hyperintense white matter* → *throughout both cerebral hemispheres. The corpus callosum is spared* ⇨*, and the subcortical U-fibers are partially spared* ↷. ***(Right)*** *Axial DWI MR shows marked diffusion restriction in the posterior limb of the internal capsules* → *and lateral thalami* ⇨. *DWI during crisis is helpful in confirming involvement during the acute phases.*

POSTERIOR FOSSA NEOPLASM

DIFFERENTIAL DIAGNOSIS

Common
- Pilocytic Astrocytoma
- Medulloblastoma (PNET-MB)
- Ependymoma
- Brainstem Glioma

Less Common
- Ganglioglioma
- Schwannoma
- Meningioma, CPA-IAC
- Hemangioblastoma
- Choroid Plexus Papilloma

Rare but Important
- Anaplastic Astrocytoma
- Atypical Teratoid-Rhabdoid Tumor
- Choroid Plexus Carcinoma
- Medulloblastoma Variants
- Medulloepithelioma
- Dysplastic Cerebellar Gangliocytoma

ESSENTIAL INFORMATION

Key Differential Diagnosis Issues
- Most common pediatric posterior fossa (PF) tumors
  - Medulloblastoma (PNET-MB)
  - Astrocytomas
    - Pilocytic astrocytoma (PA)
    - Infiltrating "glioma" (astrocytoma, WHO grade II)
  - Ependymoma
- Imaging
  - Findings on conventional MR overlap
  - Location helpful in differential diagnosis
    - Tectum, cerebellum: PA
    - Pons: Diffusely infiltrating astrocytomas
    - Midline (vermis, 4th ventricle): PNET-MB, PA
    - 4th ventricle + lateral recess/CPA mass: Ependymoma
  - DWI, MRS (normalized to water)
    - Can discriminate between pediatric PF tumors
    - PNET-MB, atypical teratoid-rhabdoid tumor (ATRT) show DWI restriction
  - Examine ENTIRE neuraxis in child with PF tumor prior to surgery!
    - T1 C+ essential (look for CSF spread)
- History, PE (e.g., cutaneous markers) important

Helpful Clues for Common Diagnoses
- **Pilocytic Astrocytoma**
  - Child with cystic cerebellar mass + mural nodule
  - Solid component low density NECT, high signal T2
- **Medulloblastoma (PNET-MB)**
  - Early childhood: Solid vermis mass extends into, fills, &/or obstructs 4th ventricle
  - Later onset: Lateral cerebellar mass
  - Hypercellular: ↑ density on NECT, ↓ T2
  - DWI: Restricts
  - 2-5% have nevoid basal cell carcinoma (Gorlin) syndrome (BCCS)
    - Typically seen with desmoplastic variant
    - Look for jaw cysts, bifid ribs, etc.
    - XRT can lead to induced basal cell carcinomas, other intracranial neoplasms within irradiated field
- **Ependymoma**
  - Extrudes through 4th ventricle outlet foramina into cisterns
  - Coarse calcifications
  - Diffusion restriction uncommon, may predict anaplastic behavior
- **Brainstem Glioma**
  - Tectal plate glioma
    - NECT: Increased density progresses to Ca++
    - CECT/MR: Faint or no enhancement
  - Pontine glioma
    - Enlarged pons engulfs basilar artery
    - Enhances late in course, rarely at diagnosis
  - Dorsal exophytic glioma
    - Tumor protrudes into 4th ventricle
    - If large, may be difficult to differentiate from pilocytic astrocytoma
    - Look for FLAIR signal change in dorsal brainstem or peduncles

Helpful Clues for Less Common Diagnoses
- **Ganglioglioma**
  - Brainstem most common posterior fossa site
  - Look for expansion of nucleus cuneatus/gracilis
- **Schwannoma**
  - Vestibular schwannoma (ICA/CPA) looks like "ice cream on cone"
  - T2 hyperintensity helps differentiate from meningioma

- Multiple in NF2
- **Meningioma, CPA-IAC**
  - Broad dural base, covers IAC
  - Variable signal, but T2 hypointensity common
  - Hyperostosis, tumoral calcifications
  - May have intra- or juxtatumoral cyst(s)
- **Hemangioblastoma**
  - Late teen or adult
  - Intraaxial (cerebellum > medulla, cord)
    - Cyst + nodule > solid
    - Solid component shows flow voids, enhances avidly
    - Multiple lesions diagnostic of von Hippel-Lindau (VHL)
  - Avidly enhancing mural nodule abuts pia
  - Look for visceral markers of VHL in any child/young adult with hemangioblastoma
- **Choroid Plexus Papilloma**
  - Frond-like 4th ventricle or CPA tumor
  - Avidly enhancing
  - Hydrocephalus common

Helpful Clues for Rare Diagnoses

- **Anaplastic Astrocytoma**
  - Infiltrating mass involves predominantly white matter
  - Enhancement: None to sparse or patchy
  - Ring enhancement suggests progression to GBM
- **Atypical Teratoid-Rhabdoid Tumor**
  - Imaging similar to PNET-MB plus
    - ATRT patients generally younger
    - Cysts, hemorrhages more common
    - CPA involvement more common
    - Frequent metastases at diagnosis
  - Both ATRT, PNET-MB show diffusion restriction
- **Choroid Plexus Carcinoma**
  - Similar to choroid plexus papilloma plus
    - Cysts, necrosis, bleeds
    - CSF/ependymal/parenchymal spread
- **Medulloblastoma Variants**
  - Desmoplastic medulloblastoma (MB)
    - 5-25% of all medulloblastomas
    - 55-60% of PNET-MBs in children < 3
    - PNET-MB in older children, young adults often also desmoplastic variant
    - Desmoplastic subtype of MB in children < 2 is major diagnostic criterion for basal cell nevus syndrome (Gorlin syndrome)
    - Nodular collections of neurocytic cells bounded by desmoplastic zones
    - Lateral (cerebellar) location
  - MB with extensive nodularity (MBEN)
    - Formerly called "cerebellar neuroblastoma"
    - Usually occurs in infants
    - Gyriform or grape-like appearance
    - May mature → better prognosis
- **Medulloepithelioma**
  - Rare embryonal brain &/or ocular tumor
  - Inhomogeneous signal, enhancement
- **Dysplastic Cerebellar Gangliocytoma**
  - Diffuse or focal hemispheric mass
  - Thick cerebellar folia with "striated" appearance
  - Evaluate for Cowden syndrome

Pilocytic Astrocytoma

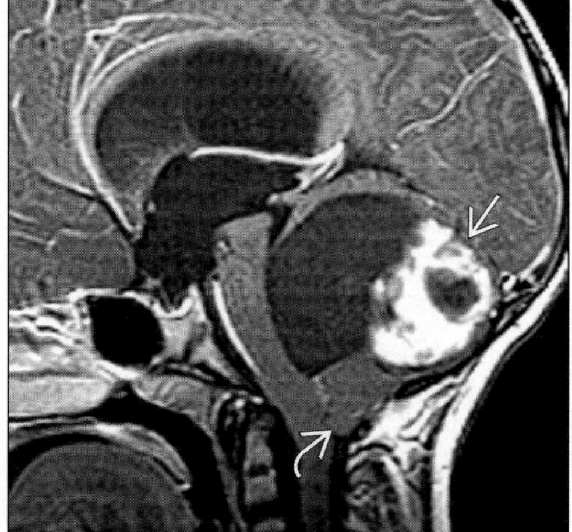

Sagittal T1WI C+ MR shows a typical tumor cyst with an enhancing mural nodule ➔. There is hydrocephalus and protrusion of the cerebellar tonsils ➔ through the foramen magnum (acquired Chiari 1).

Pilocytic Astrocytoma

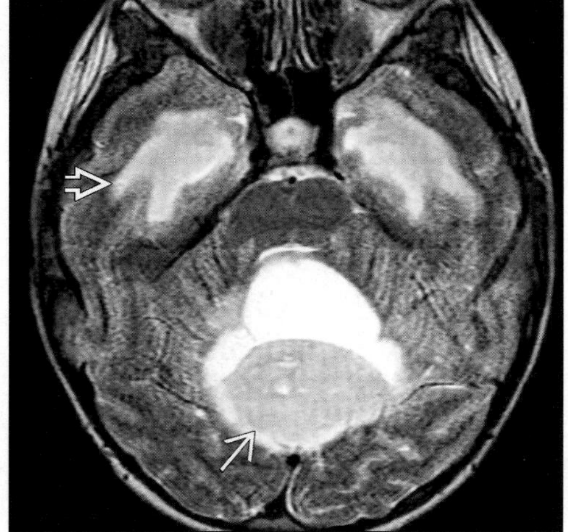

Axial T2WI MR shows increased signal of the solid component ➔ of the mass. Interstitial edema ➔ is present in the temporal lobes.

POSTERIOR FOSSA NEOPLASM

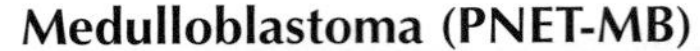

Medulloblastoma (PNET-MB)

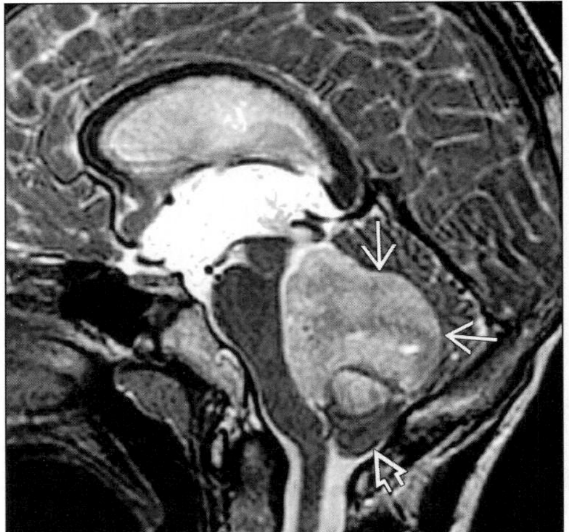

Medulloblastoma (PNET-MB)

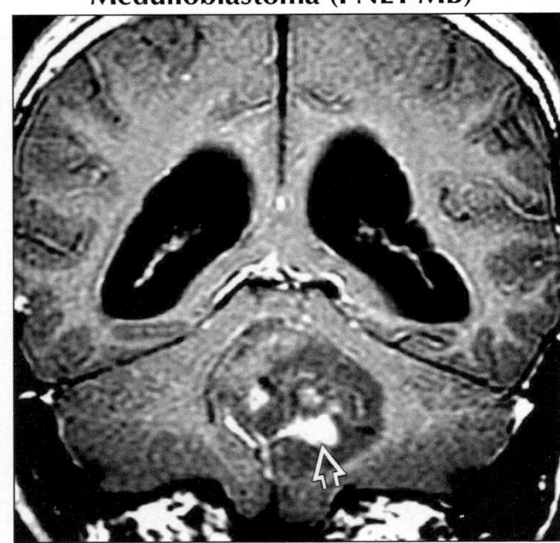

(Left) *Sagittal T2WI MR shows a low signal mass lesion filling and expanding the 4th ventricle. The tumor does not extend through the 4th ventricular outlet foramina. There is hydrocephalus with acquired tonsillar herniation.* ***(Right)*** *Coronal T1 C+ MR shows heterogeneous enhancement of the 4th ventricular PNET-MB.*

Ependymoma

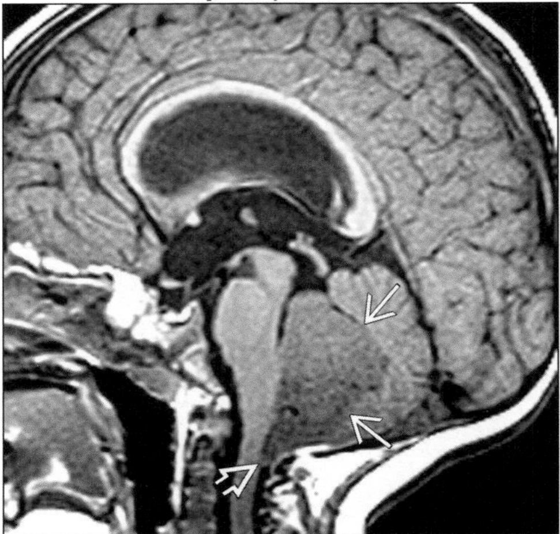

Ependymoma

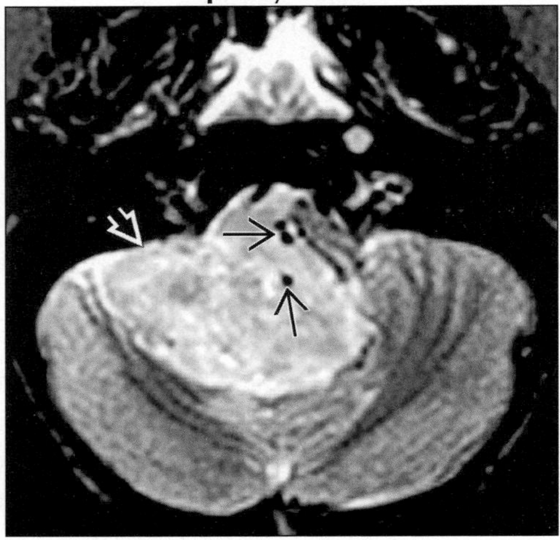

(Left) *Sagittal T1WI MR shows a large tumor filling the 4th ventricle and extruding through the obex into the upper spinal canal.* ***(Right)*** *Axial T2WI MR shows a heterogeneous tumor expanding and extruding through the right foramen of Luschka. There are a few coarse calcific foci within the tumor.*

Brainstem Glioma

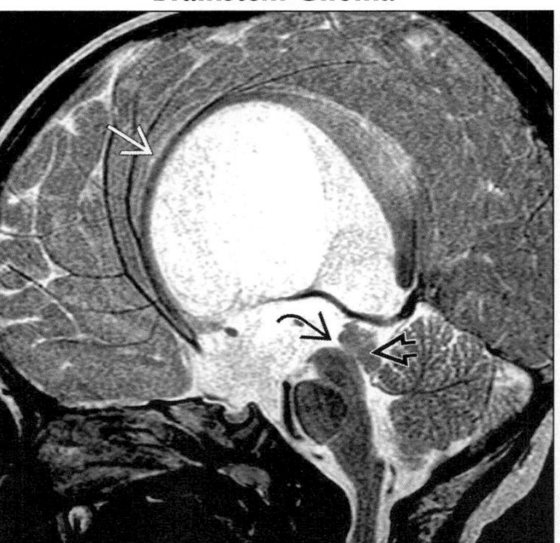

Brainstem Glioma

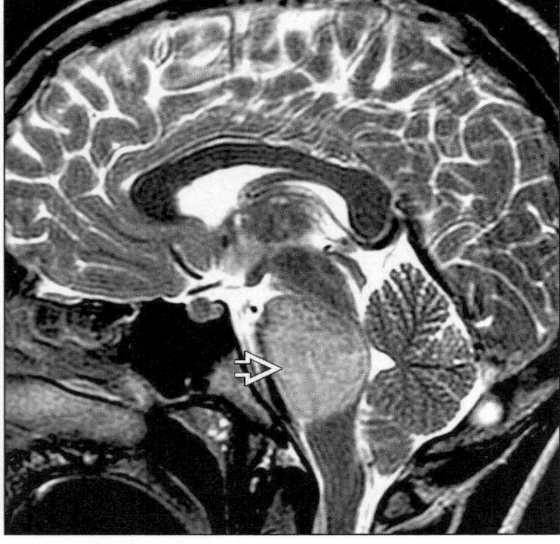

(Left) *Sagittal T2WI MR in an infant with a tectal plate glioma shows marked hydrocephalus involving the 3rd and lateral ventricles. The corpus callosum is stretched thin. The tectal plate is bulbous and slightly increased in signal intensity. The aqueduct of Sylvius is obstructed.* ***(Right)*** *Sagittal T2WI MR in this child with a diffusely infiltrating pontine glioma shows homogeneous signal intensity of the expanded pons.*

Brainstem Glioma

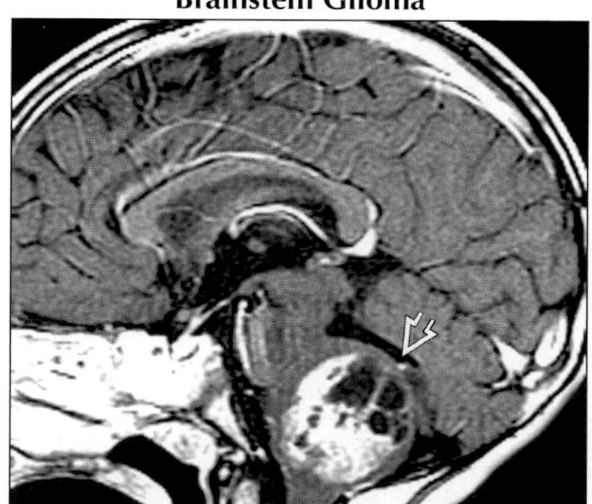

Ganglioglioma

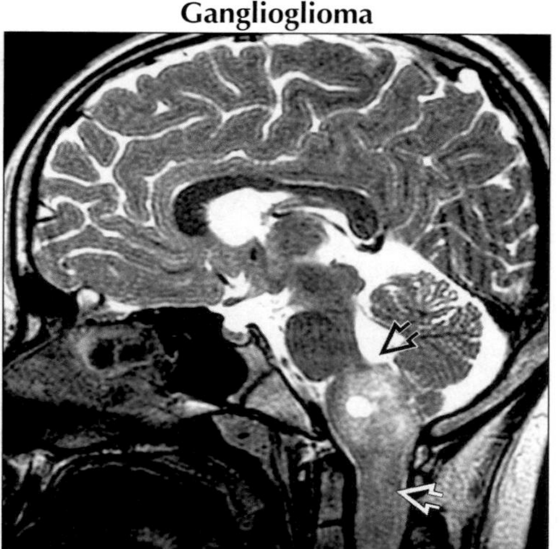

(Left) Sagittal T1 C+ MR shows marked expansion of the medulla ➡ by a complex mass with intralesional cystic areas and avid, but heterogeneous, enhancement in this child with dorsal exophytic brainstem glioma. The inferior 4th ventricle is deformed by the protruding mass. (Right) Sagittal T2WI MR shows marked expansion of the medulla and upper cervical spinal cord ➡. The inferior 4th ventricle is deformed ➡ by the dorsally protruding mass.

Schwannoma

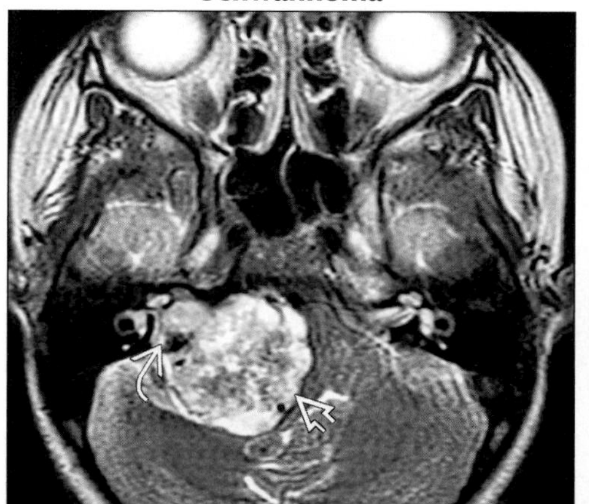

Schwannoma

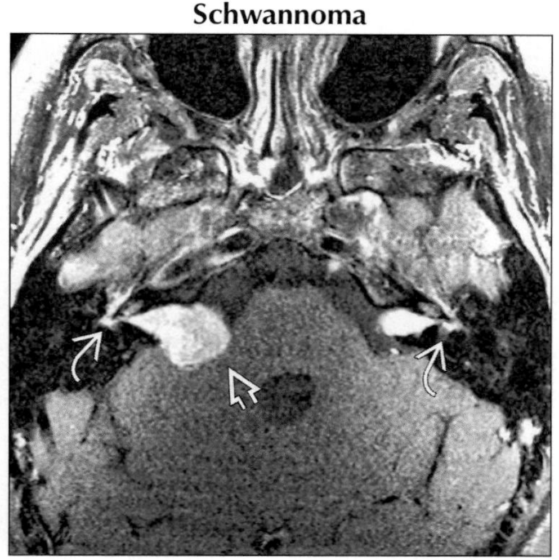

(Left) Axial T2WI MR shows a bulky heterogeneous right cerebellopontine angle mass ➡, which crosses the midline. There is also extensive remodeling of the right internal auditory canal ➡ by this schwannoma. (Right) Axial T1WI C+ MR in another child shows small bilateral vestibular schwannomas. The right lesion ➡ assumes the appearance of "ice cream on a cone." Both demonstrate intralabyrinthine extension ➡.

Meningioma, CPA-IAC

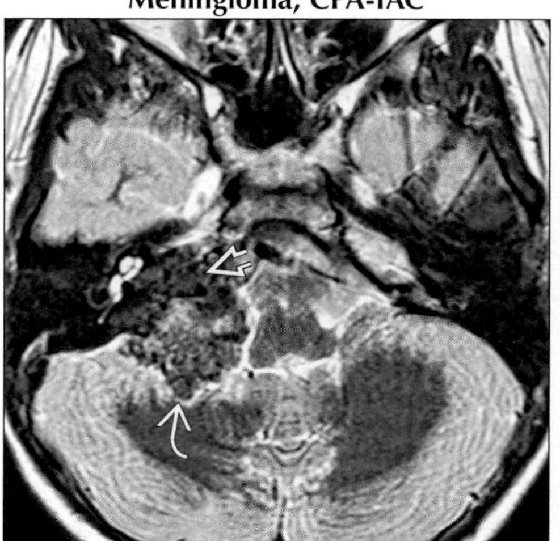

Meningioma, CPA-IAC

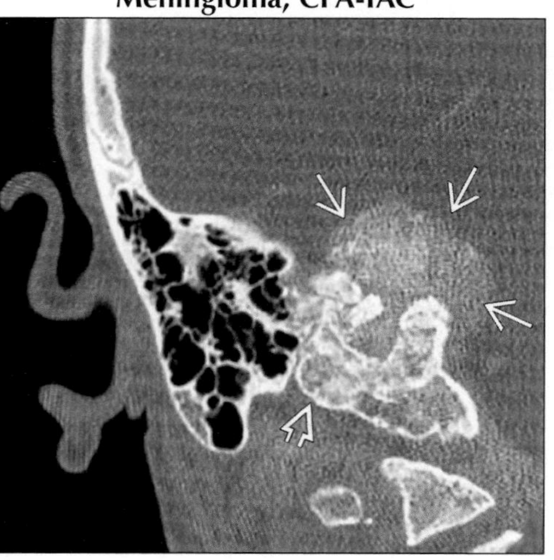

(Left) Axial T2WI MR shows a low signal, lobular, cerebellopontine angle mass ➡ with hyperostosis ➡ of the adjacent petrous apex. There is mild rotation of the medulla due to mass effect. (Right) Coronal NECT shows diffuse hyperostosis ➡ adjacent to the meningioma ➡.

(Left) *Sagittal T2WI MR shows a solid component with multiple flow voids ⊳, a cyst →, and edema of the medulla and upper cervical cord ⊳. **(Right)** Sagittal T1 C+ MR shows the cyst ⊳ to better advantage than the prior T2WI image. Here, the cyst's contents have slightly increased signal.*

Hemangioblastoma

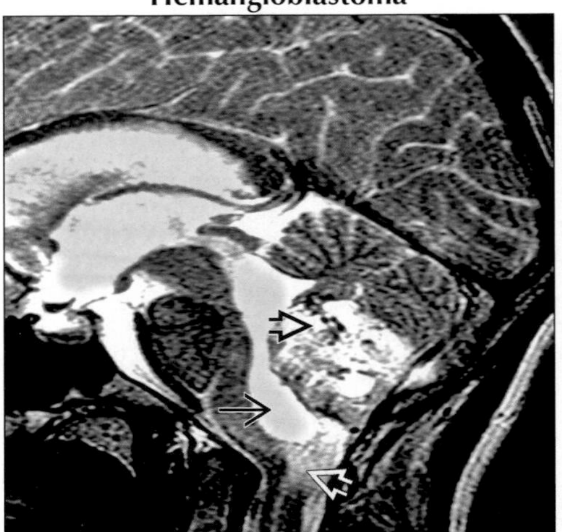

Hemangioblastoma

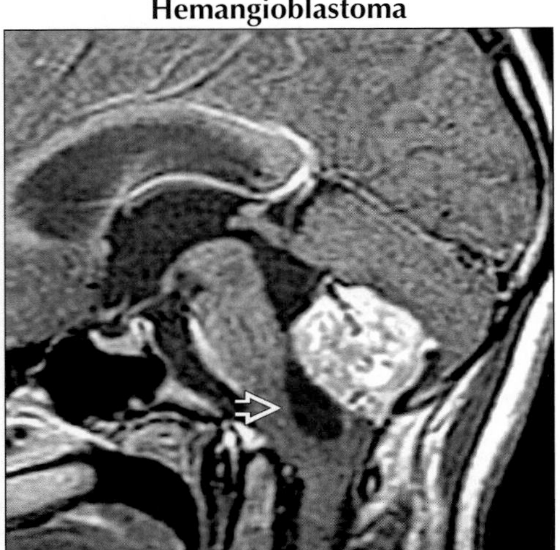

(Left) *Axial T2WI MR shows multiple foci of abnormal signal intensity in the peripheral right cerebellar hemisphere and in the cerebellar white matter ⊳ adjacent to the lateral recess of the 4th ventricle. **(Right)** Axial T1 C+ MR shows enhancement ⊳ following gadolinium administration. The lesion adjacent to the 4th ventricle lateral recess has ill-defined margins.*

Anaplastic Astrocytoma

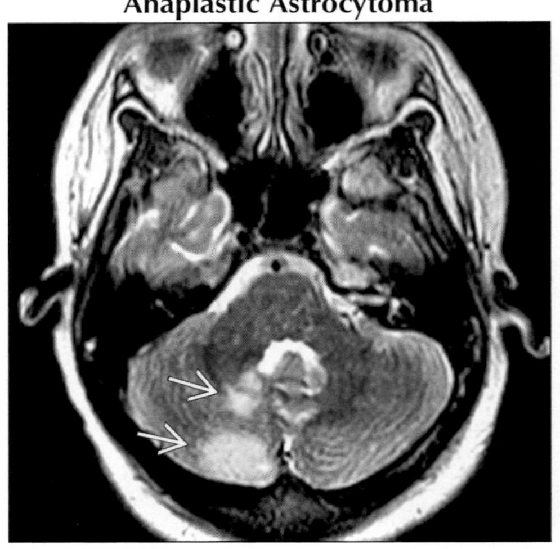

Anaplastic Astrocytoma

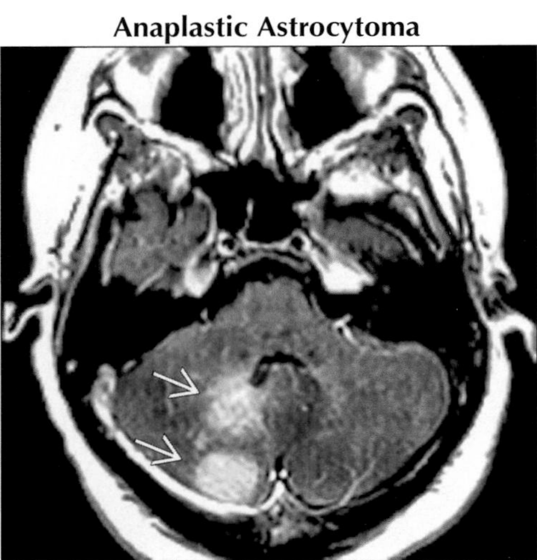

(Left) *Sagittal T2WI MR shows extensive posterior fossa ⊳, pineal region →, and intraventricular ⊳ low signal intensity masses. Multifocal deposits of tumor at diagnosis are strongly suggestive of an atypical teratoid-rhabdoid tumor. **(Right)** Sagittal T1 C+ MR shows quite variable enhancement of the posterior fossa ⊳, pineal region ⊳, and intraventricular ⊳ tumor deposits. There is marked hydrocephalus.*

Atypical Teratoid-Rhabdoid Tumor

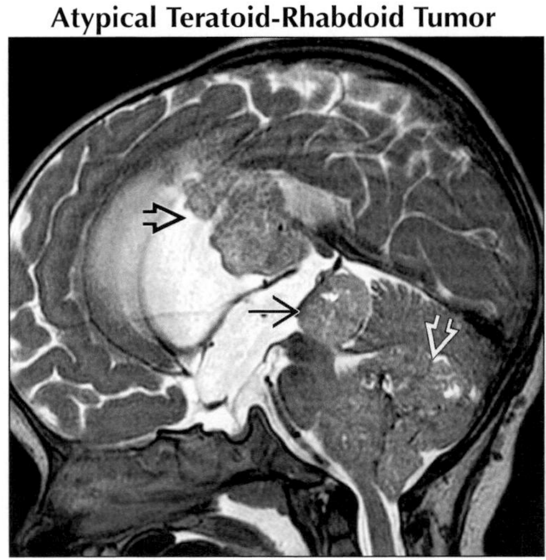

Atypical Teratoid-Rhabdoid Tumor

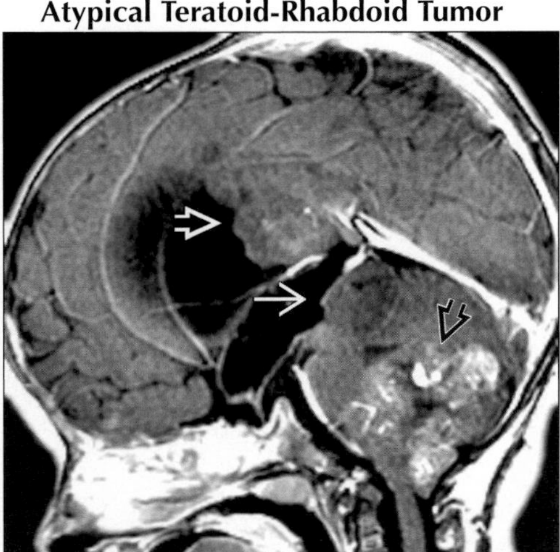

Choroid Plexus Carcinoma

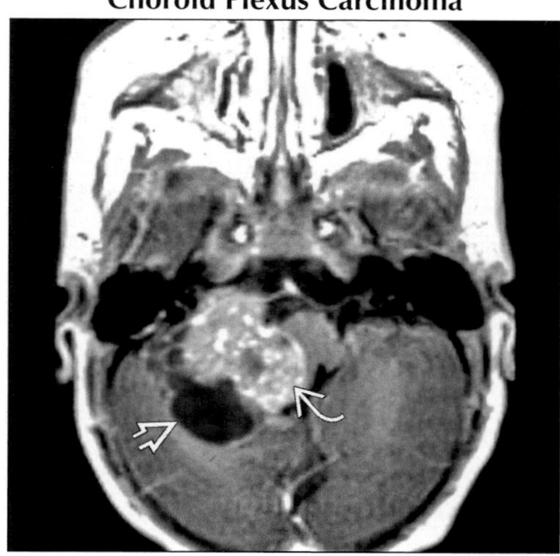

Choroid Plexus Carcinoma

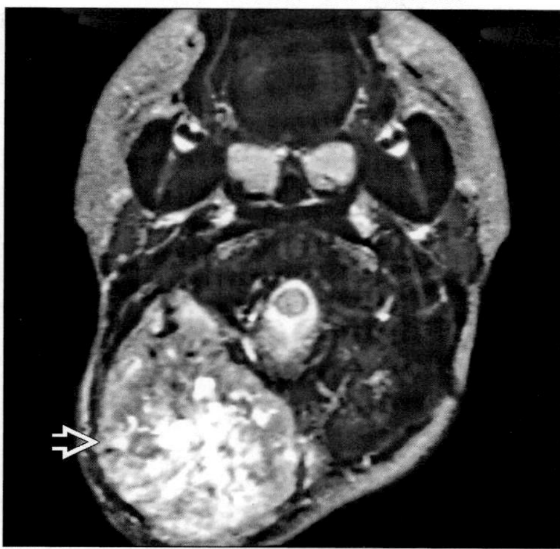

*(**Left**) Axial T1 C+ MR shows a slightly heterogeneous, but avidly enhancing, mass within the right foramen of Luschka. There is an associated cyst. (**Right**) Axial T2WI MR in a different child undergoing treatment for choroid plexus carcinoma shows a large skull base metastatic deposit.*

Medulloepithelioma

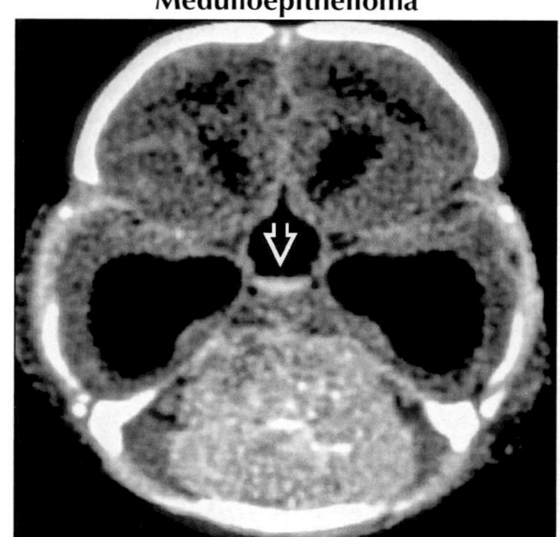

Medulloepithelioma

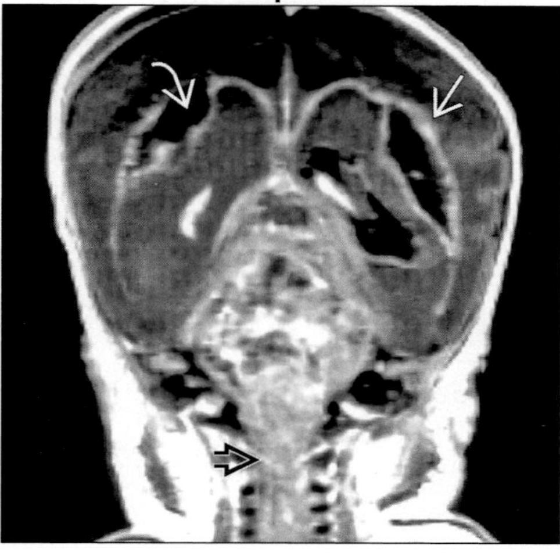

*(**Left**) Axial NECT in a 1-day-old infant shows a dense, lobular mass filling the posterior fossa. Foci of increased density superimposed in the mass are due to hemorrhage. Note the blood-CSF level in the dilated infundibular recess. (**Right**) Coronal T1 C+ MR in the same infant following biopsy shows extension into the spinal canal. Gas in the ventricular system follows neurosurgical intervention. There is extensive ependymal seeding.*

Dysplastic Cerebellar Gangliocytoma

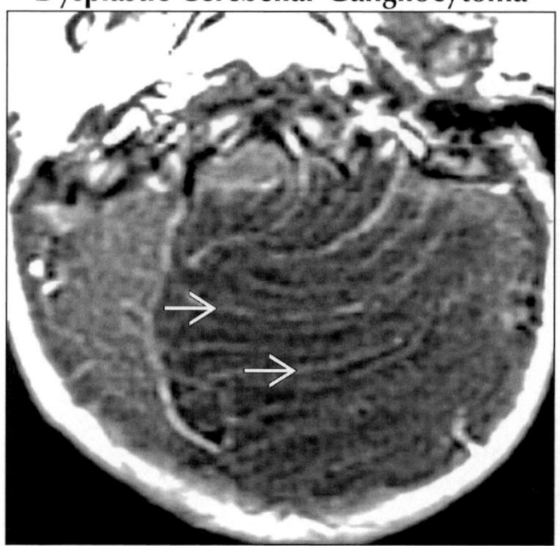

Dysplastic Cerebellar Gangliocytoma

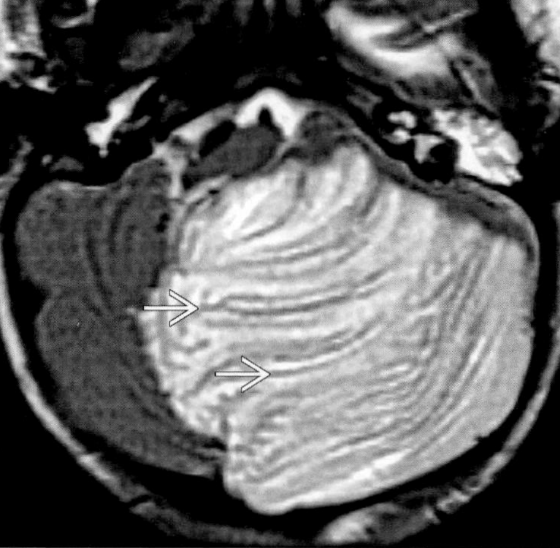

*(**Left**) Axial T1 C+ MR shows a large nonenhancing mass involving the left cerebellar hemisphere. Preservation of the cerebellar folia pattern, or "striated cerebellum", is characteristic for dysplastic cerebellar gangliocytoma (Lhermitte-Duclos). This disease has a strong association with Cowden syndrome. (**Right**) Axial T2WI MR again shows the pattern of a "striated cerebellum".*

CYSTIC-APPEARING POSTERIOR FOSSA LESION

DIFFERENTIAL DIAGNOSIS

Common
- Mega Cisterna Magna
- Arachnoid Cyst
- Dandy-Walker Continuum
- Pilocytic Astrocytoma
- Encephaloceles
- Obstructive Hydrocephalus

Less Common
- Epidermoid Cyst
- Dermoid Cyst
- Neuroglial Cyst
- Ependymal Cyst
- Hemangioblastoma
- Schwannoma (Cystic)
- Abscess
- Enlarged Perivascular Spaces

Rare but Important
- Syringobulbia
- Neurenteric Cyst
- Atypical Teratoid-Rhabdoid Tumor
- Other Intracranial Metastases
- Neurocysticercosis
- Chordoma
- Congenital Muscular Dystrophy

ESSENTIAL INFORMATION

Key Differential Diagnosis Issues
- Cystic-appearing lesion EXACTLY like CSF on all sequences?
  - Mega cisterna magna (MCM), arachnoid cyst (AC), Dandy-Walker Continuum (DW)
  - Trapped 4th ventricle, enlarged perivascular spaces (↑ PVSs), neuroglial or ependymal cyst
- Cystic-appearing lesion NOT exactly like CSF?
  - Congenital inclusion cyst (dermoid, epidermoid, neurenteric cysts)
  - Infection such as abscess, neurocysticercosis (NCC)
  - Neoplasm (pilocytic astrocytoma, hemangioblastoma, metastasis, chordoma)
- Is cyst intra- or extraaxial?
- Intraaxial
  - Trapped 4th ventricle (4th V), ↑ PVSs
  - Neoplasm (e.g., pilocytic astrocytoma), infection (abscess, NCC)
  - Inclusion cyst in 4th V (epidermoid)
- Extraaxial
  - MCM, AC, DW, neurenteric cyst, NCC, neoplasm (schwannoma)
- DWI, T1 C+ scans helpful additions

Helpful Clues for Common Diagnoses
- **Mega Cisterna Magna**
  - Communicates freely with all CSF spaces
  - Normal tegmento-vermian angle (< 5-10°)
- **Arachnoid Cyst**
  - Mass effect on vermis
  - ± Hydrocephalus
  - Use FLAIR, DWI to exclude epidermoid
- **Dandy-Walker Continuum**
  - "Classic" Dandy-Walker malformation
    - Cystic dilatation 4th V ⇒ ↑ posterior fossa (PF), torcular-lambdoid inversion
    - Hypoplastic vermis
    - Vermian remnant rotated anterosuperiorly over cyst
  - Blake pouch cyst (BPC)
    - Embryonic BPC doesn't regress
    - Enlarged PF, 4th V open inferiorly
    - Vermis anatomically complete
- **Pilocytic Astrocytoma**
  - Cystic cerebellar mass
  - Enhancing mural nodule
- **Encephaloceles**
  - Isolated encephalocele: Lacks Chiari 2
  - Chiari 3 = Chiari 2 PLUS
    - Occipital or cervical encephalocele containing cerebellum
  - Syndromic occipital encephalocele
    - Klippel-Feil, Meckel-Gruber, etc.
- **Obstructive Hydrocephalus**
  - Outlets obstructed→ 4th ventricle ↑ ↑
  - Maintains "kidney bean" configuration
  - 3rd V, shunted lateral ventricles small

Helpful Clues for Less Common Diagnoses
- **Epidermoid Cyst**
  - Cerebellopontine angle > 4th V > diploic
  - Frond-like, cystic (CSF-like)
  - Doesn't suppress completely on FLAIR
  - Restricts on DWI
- **Dermoid Cyst**
  - Midline "fatty" mass
    - "Droplets" in CSF if ruptured
    - Look for dermal sinus, midline vertebral/skull base anomalies
- **Neuroglial Cyst**
  - CSF-like parenchymal cyst
  - No enhancement, DWI restriction

CYSTIC-APPEARING POSTERIOR FOSSA LESION

- **Ependymal Cyst**
  - CSF-like
  - Intra- > paraventricular
- **Hemangioblastoma**
  - Posterior fossa mass with cyst, enhancing mural nodule that abuts pia
  - ± Arterial feeders, flow-voids
  - Look for markers of von Hippel-Lindau (VHL)
    - Visceral cysts, renal clear cell carcinoma
  - Adult > > older teen (unless VHL)
    - Check family history!
- **Schwannoma (Cystic)**
  - Vestibular schwannoma (VS) looks like "ice cream on cone"
  - Cysts can be intratumoral or VS-associated (arachnoid)
  - Solid component enhances
- **Abscess**
  - T2 hypointense rim with surrounding edema
  - Ring-enhancing
  - Hyperintense on DWI, hypointense on ADC
- **Enlarged Perivascular Spaces**
  - CSF-like, nonenhancing, nonrestricting
  - Most common PF site = dentate nuclei
  - Less common = cerebellum, pons

Helpful Clues for Rare Diagnoses

- **Syringobulbia**
  - Chiari 1 or 2, holocord syrinx common
  - May rarely extend to syringocephaly
- **Neurenteric Cyst**
  - Slightly hyperintense extraaxial cystic mass, nonenhancing
  - Anterior pontomedullary, CPA cisterns
- **Atypical Teratoid-Rhabdoid Tumor**
  - 50% infratentorial (usually off-midline)
  - Intratumoral cysts, hemorrhage common
  - Gross macrocysts less common
- **Other Intracranial Metastases**
  - Myriad of nonenhancing interfoliate cysts
    - Low- or high-grade brain or spine primary
    - Also reported with breast primary
  - Choroid plexus papilloma cysts can be entirely extra-axial, nonenhancing
- **Neurocysticercosis**
  - Cyst with "dot" (scolex) inside
  - Subarachnoid spaces, sulcal depths most common
  - Intraventricular cysts often isolated
    - 4th ventricle most common
- **Chordoma**
  - High signal on T2
  - Moderate to marked enhancement unless necrotic, mucinous
  - High-attenuation foci (CT) may be occult on MR
- **Congenital Muscular Dystrophy**
  - Best diagnostic clues
    - Severely "floppy" infant
    - Z-shaped or cleft pons
    - Multiple small CSF-like cerebellar cysts (may be PVSs or trapped CSF from overmigration of neurons)

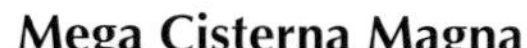

Mega Cisterna Magna

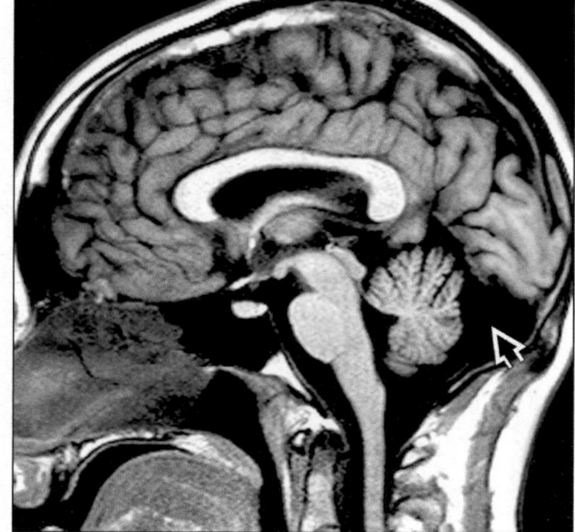

Sagittal T1WI MR shows a mega cisterna magna ➔. The tentorium is normally located, and the posterior fossa is mildly prominent. There is no mass effect upon the vermis.

Arachnoid Cyst

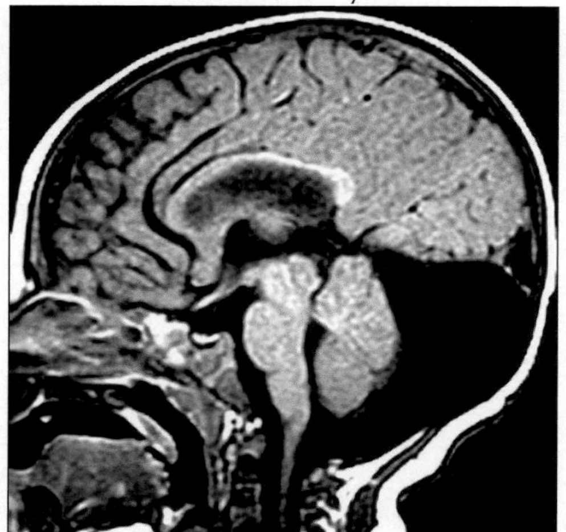

Sagittal T1WI MR shows a retrocerebellar arachnoid cyst. There is enlargement of the posterior fossa, elevation of the tent, and mild compression of the vermis.

CYSTIC-APPEARING POSTERIOR FOSSA LESION

(Left) *Sagittal T1WI MR shows typical enlarged posterior fossa, upward rotation of the small vermian remnant, elevation of the tentorium, and mass effect upon the brainstem in "classic" Dandy-Walker malformation.* ***(Right)*** *Sagittal T2WI MR shows enlargement of the inferior 4th ventricle ➙, which communicates with an enlarged cisterna magna in this infant with a Blake pouch cyst.*

Dandy-Walker Continuum

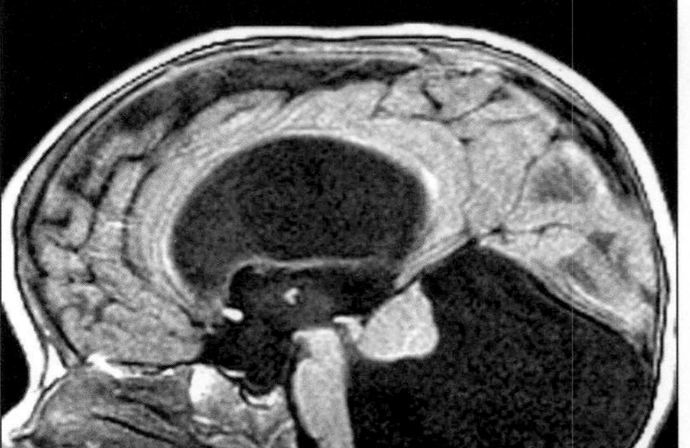

Dandy-Walker Continuum

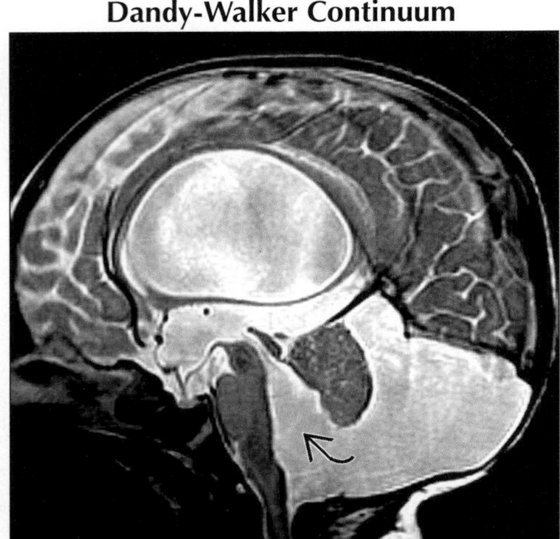

(Left) *Sagittal T1WI C+ MR shows a large cystic neoplasm of the vermis. There is compression of the brainstem and 4th ventricle ➙ by the rim-enhancing mass. Nodular thickening ➙ is present in the caudal aspect of this cerebellar "juvenile" pilocytic astrocytoma (JPA).* ***(Right)*** *Axial T2WI MR shows the very high signal of the cystic component. The solid rim of the JPA is thick ➙ and brighter than gray matter.*

Pilocytic Astrocytoma

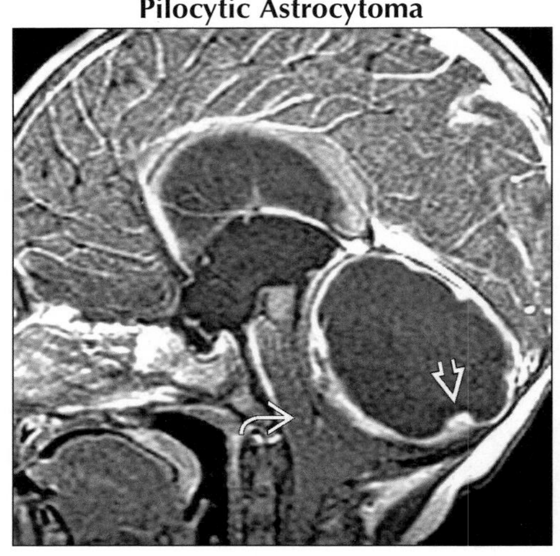

Pilocytic Astrocytoma

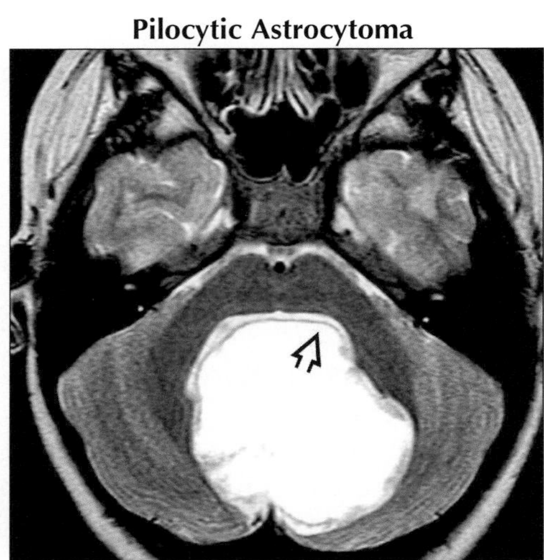

(Left) *Sagittal PD FSE MR shows a classic Chiari 3 malformation with extension of infratentorial tissue and also the venous system ➙ into the large occipital encephalocele.* ***(Right)*** *Axial T2WI MR shows cerebellar tissue ➙ protruding into the encephalocele sac.*

Encephaloceles

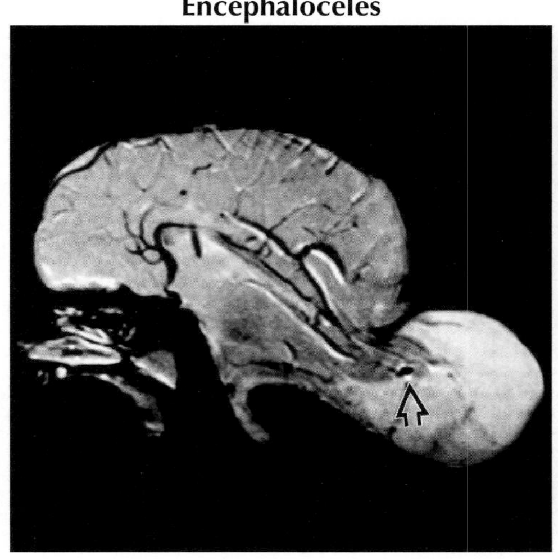

Encephaloceles

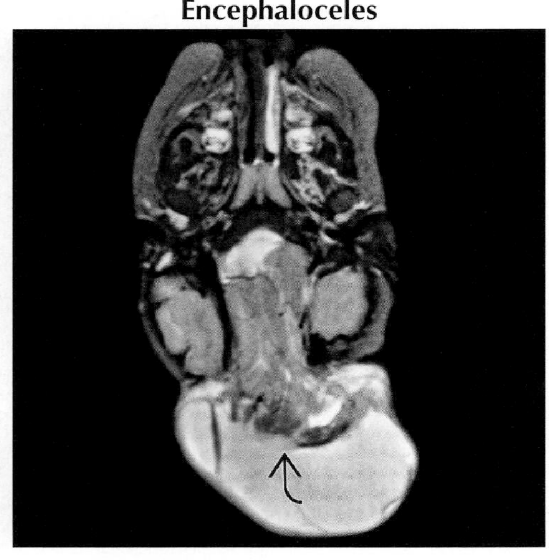

Obstructive Hydrocephalus

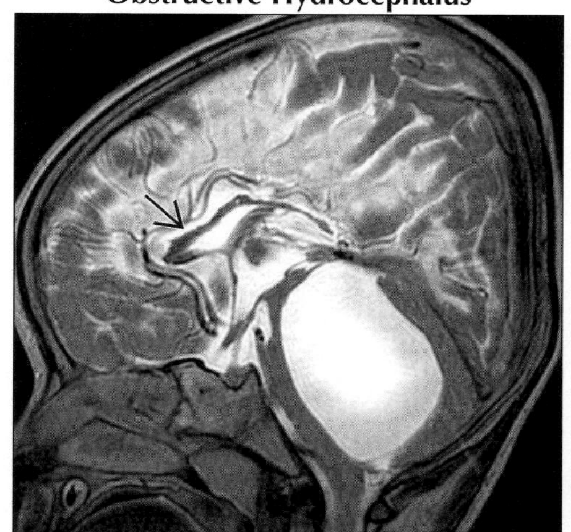

Syringobulbia

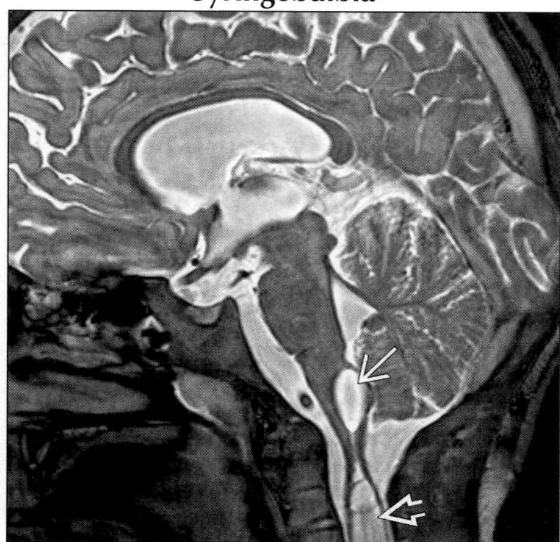

(Left) *Sagittal T2WI MR shows a dilated trapped 4th ventricle in a child with a history of hydrocephalus due to intraventricular hemorrhage as a premature infant. Note the corpus callosum ➔, thinned due to periventricular leukomalacia. The 3rd ventricle, unlike the 4th ventricle, is normal in size.* ***(Right)*** *Sagittal T2WI MR in a child with mild ventriculomegaly and holocord syrinx ➔ demonstrates extension of the syrinx into the medulla ➔.*

Epidermoid Cyst

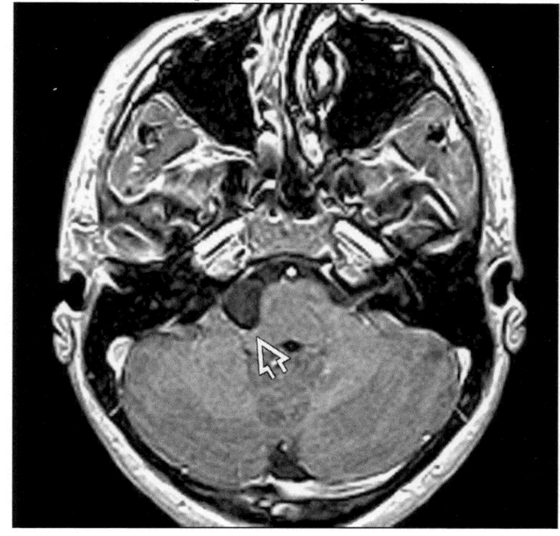

Epidermoid Cyst

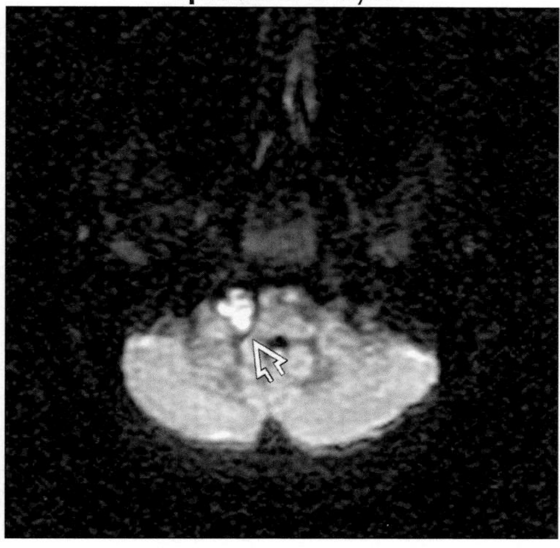

(Left) *Axial T1 C+ MR shows a small, CSF-like cyst ➔ deforming the right cerebellopontine angle.* ***(Right)*** *Axial DWI MR shows diffusion restriction of the lobular mass ➔, confirming the presence of an epidermoid tumor. An arachnoid cyst would not restrict diffusion.*

Dermoid Cyst

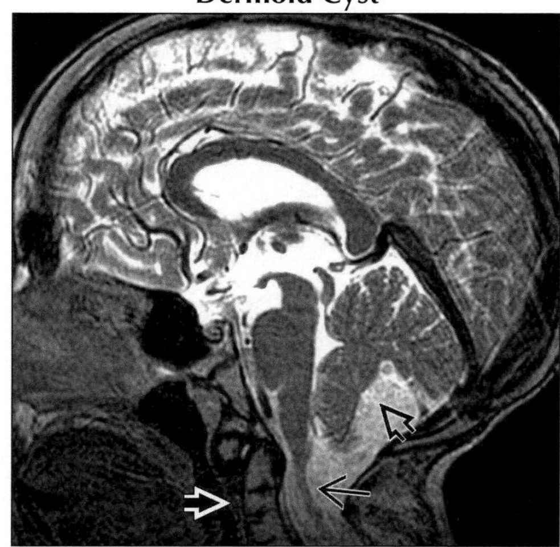

Dermoid Cyst

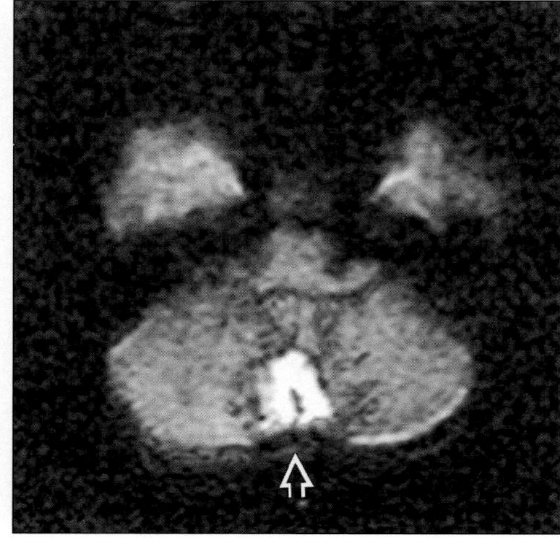

(Left) *Sagittal T2WI MR shows a cystic structure ➔ indenting the inferior vermis. Note also the segmentation anomalies of C2 ➔ and the midline sagittal clefting ➔ of the upper cervical cord in this child with Klippel-Feil anomaly.* ***(Right)*** *Axial DWI MR in the same child shows diffusion restriction ➔. The dermoid was subjacent to a dermal sinus.*

CYSTIC-APPEARING POSTERIOR FOSSA LESION

(Left) Sagittal T2WI MR shows a large CSF intensity cyst ➡ filling the pineal/quadrigeminal region. With the rim of brain parenchyma stretched around the mass, it is intraaxial and most likely represents a neuroglial cyst. (Right) Sagittal T1 C+ MR shows a small, well-delineated CSF-filled cyst ➡ in the inferior 4th ventricle. Cyst displaces the enhancing choroid plexus ➡, which is draped over it.

Neuroglial Cyst

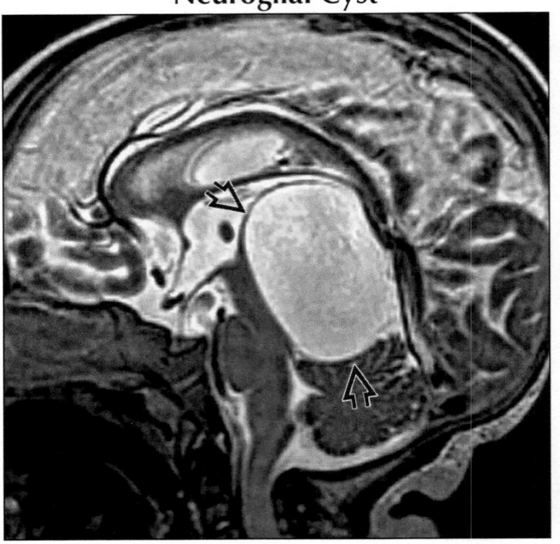

Ependymal Cyst

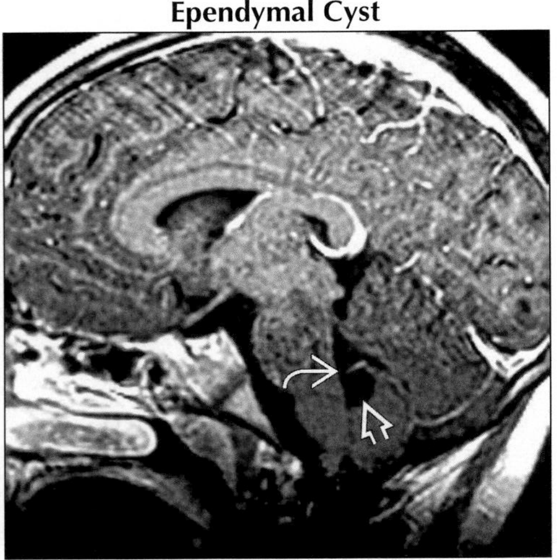

(Left) Sagittal T2WI MR in a teenager with von Hippel-Lindau shows a large tumor-associated cyst ➡ in the medulla. There are flow voids ➡ within the adjacent soft tissue mass. Typical upper cervical cord edema ➡ is present. (Right) Coronal T1 C+ MR in the same patient shows enhancement of the soft tissue nodule ➡. This is classic hemangioblastoma with tumor nodule, cyst wall composed of nonneoplastic tissue (compressed cerebellum).

Hemangioblastoma

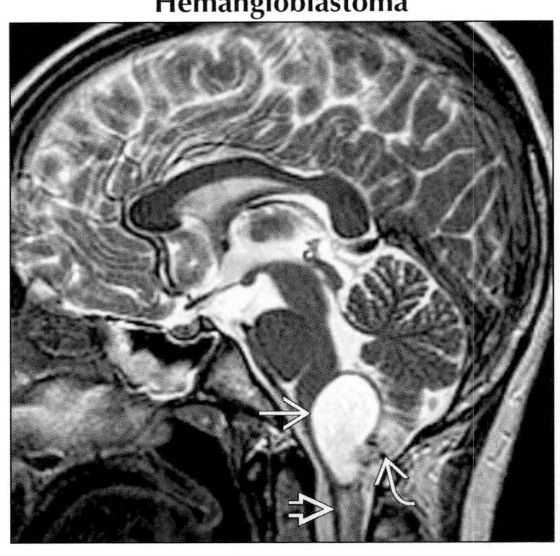

Hemangioblastoma

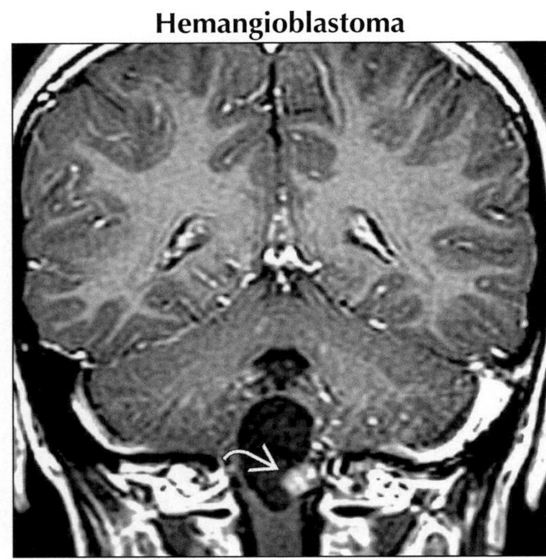

(Left) Axial T1WI C+ MR shows a large cyst that is associated with an IAC-CPA mass. Note the classic "ice cream on a cone" ➡ enhancement, typical for vestibulocochlear schwannoma. Associated cysts are uncommon. (Right) Axial T2WI MR shows typical low signal intensity rim of the abscess cavity ➡ surrounded by edema. There is mastoiditis ➡, the underlying etiology of the abscess in this child.

Schwannoma (Cystic)

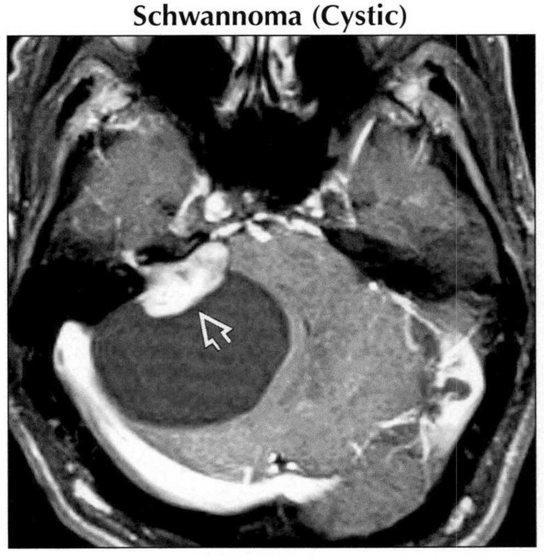

Abscess

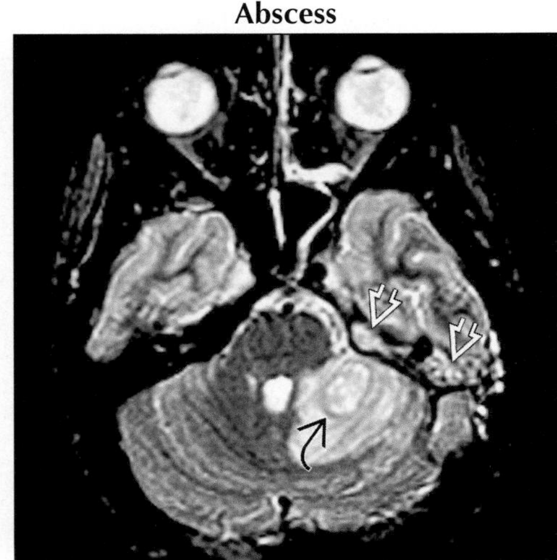

Enlarged Perivascular Spaces

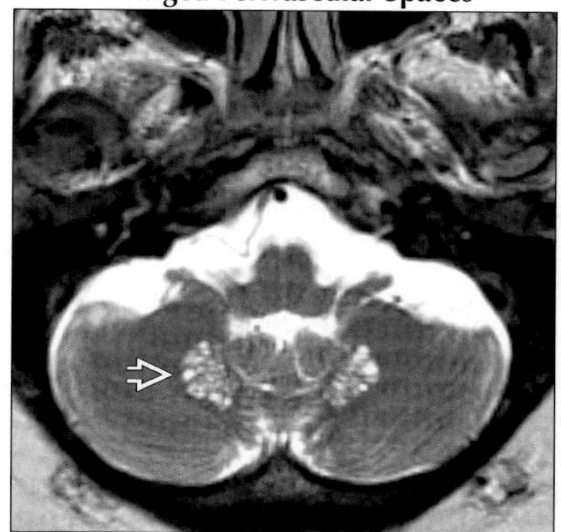

Neurenteric Cyst

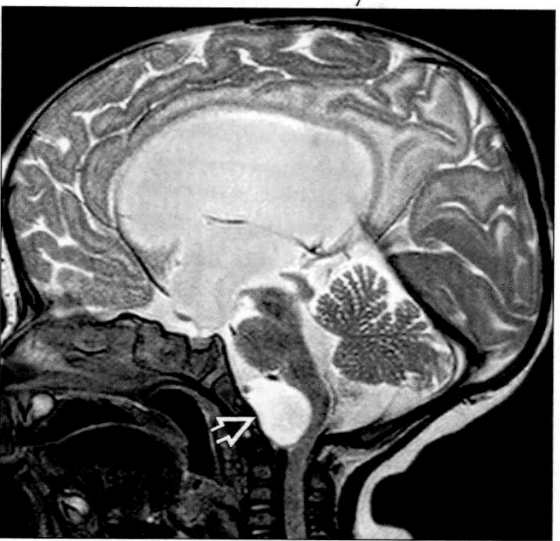

(Left) *Axial T2WI MR shows clusters of multiple tiny hyperintense cystic areas in dentate nuclei ➡. The cystic "lesions" are clusters of enlarged perivascular spaces. This is considered a normal variant and typically does not cause symptoms.* ***(Right)*** *Sagittal T2WI MR shows a high signal cystic mass ➡ that indents the anterior aspect of the medulla.*

Atypical Teratoid-Rhabdoid Tumor

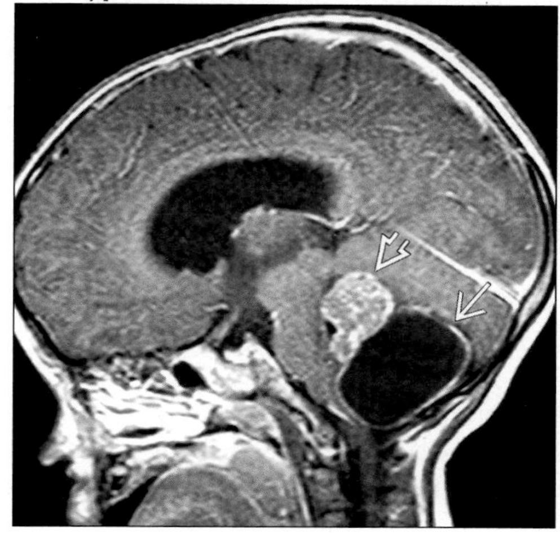

Other Intracranial Metastases

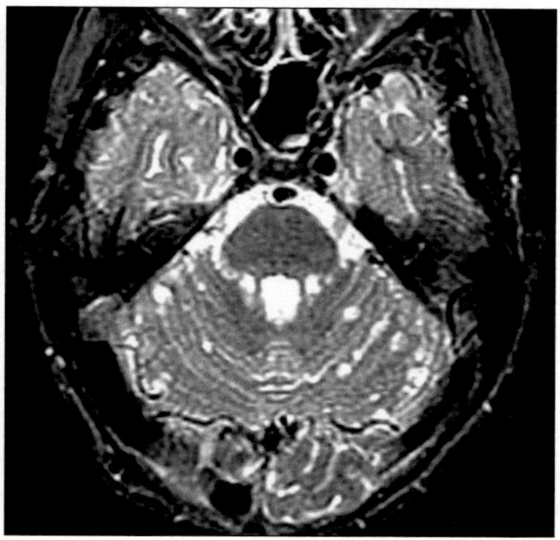

(Left) *Sagittal T1 C+ MR shows a superior 4th ventricle mass ➡ and a large rim-enhancing ➡ cyst. Cysts are more common with posterior fossa atypical teratoid-rhabdoid tumor than PNET-MB.* ***(Right)*** *Axial T2WI MR shows extensive interfoliate cystic metastases associated with high-grade spinal astrocytoma.*

Neurocysticercosis

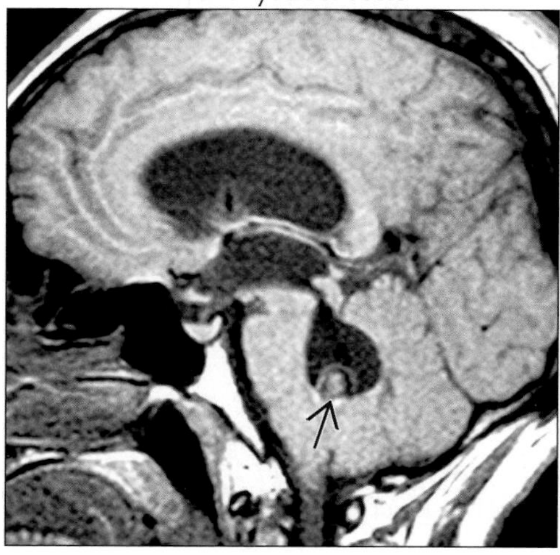

Congenital Muscular Dystrophy

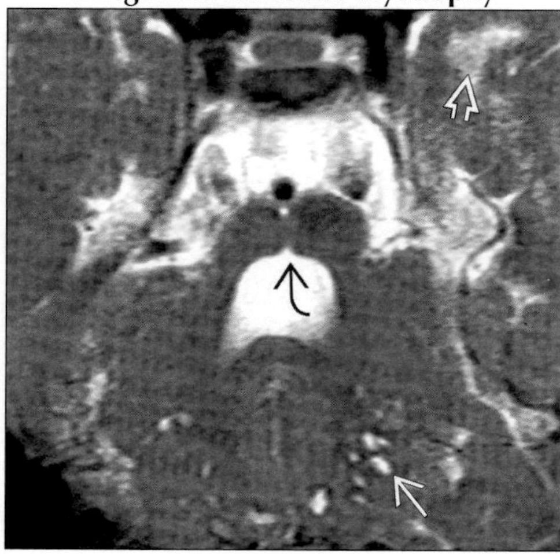

(Left) *Sagittal T1WI MR shows a cyst with a nodule inside the 4th ventricle →. Neurocysticercosis cyst was confirmed pathologically. The protoscolex is the viable larva within the smooth, thin-walled cyst.* ***(Right)*** *Axial T2WI MR shows multiple small cystic lesions in the dysplastic cerebellum ➡. The pons is hypoplastic with dorsal clefting →. Hypomyelination of the temporal lobes is present ➡.*

CONGENITAL CEREBELLAR MALFORMATION

DIFFERENTIAL DIAGNOSIS

Common
- Chiari 1 Malformation
- Chiari 2 Malformation

Less Common
- Cerebellar Hypoplasia
- Cerebellar Dysplasias (Unclassified)
- Dandy-Walker Spectrum

Rare but Important
- Rhombencephalosynapsis
- Molar Tooth Malformations (Joubert)
- Chiari 3 Malformation

ESSENTIAL INFORMATION

Helpful Clues for Common Diagnoses
- **Chiari 1 Malformation**
  - Key facts: Caudal protrusion of pointed cerebellar (CB) tonsils, below foramen magnum (FM)
    - Normal CB tonsils rounded
    - CB position below "opisthion-basion line": 1st decade (6 mm), 2nd-3rd decade (5 mm), 4th-8th decade (4 mm), and 9th decade (3 mm)
    - Underdeveloped bony posterior fossa → downward hindbrain herniation
  - Imaging
    - CB tonsils low and pointed; CSF at foramen magnum effaced; small bony posterior fossa
    - Cine MR: Motion of CB tonsils
    - ± syrinx, presyrinx edema, or ventriculomegaly
    - ± short clivus, dorsal tilt of dens, craniovertebral anomalies
    - Rarely develop over time; rarely resolve without treatment
- **Chiari 2 Malformation**
  - Key facts
    - ~ 100% associated with open neural tube defect, usually myelomeningocele
    - ↓ incidence with ↑ in folate replacement
  - Imaging
    - Small posterior fossa, large FM
    - Large funnel-shaped foramen magnum
    - "Cascade" or "waterfall" herniation of tissue downward, behind medulla
    - "Peg" = uvula/nodulus/pyramid of vermis
    - Cervicomedullary "kink"
    - "Towering" cerebellum through incisura → compressed "beaked" tectum
    - 4th ventricle elongated, without fastigium (posterior point)
    - Low insertion of tentorium/torcular
    - ± syringohydromyelia (20-90%)
    - ± corpus callosum dysgenesis (90%)
    - ± posterior arch C1 anomalies, diastematomyelia, Klippel-Feil syndrome
    - ± aqueduct stenosis, GM heterotopia, absent septum pellucidum/fused forniceal columns, stenogyria

Helpful Clues for Less Common Diagnoses
- **Cerebellar Hypoplasia**
  - Key facts: Inherited or acquired, isolated or syndromic
  - Imaging
    - Isolated small CB hemisphere(s) with normal fissures and interfoliate sulci
    - + brainstem hypoplasia = pontocerebellar hypoplasia
    - ± vermian hypoplasia, abnormal CB fissures, cortical dysplasia
    - ± Dandy-Walker spectrum, molar tooth syndromes, rhombencephalosynapsis
    - Presence of gliosis suggests atrophy rather than congenital hypoplasia
- **Cerebellar Dysplasias (Unclassified)**
  - Key facts: Developmental abnormality
  - Imaging
    - CB hemispheres &/or vermis; abnormal orientation of fissures and lobules
    - Affected structure usually small
    - Focal or diffuse, single or multiple, unilateral or bilateral
    - Diffuse usually associated with supratentorial anomalies: Congenital muscular dystrophies, lissencephalies, polymicrogyria
- **Dandy-Walker Spectrum**
  - Key facts: Continuum = "classic" Dandy-Walker malformation (DWM) → CB vermian hypoplasia → Blake pouch cyst (BPC) → mega cisterna magna (MCM)
    - Intelligence normal in up to 50% of "classic" DWM cases
  - Imaging
    - "Classic" DWM: Cystic dilatation of 4th ventricle → large posterior fossa, torcular-lambdoid inversion, superiorly rotated hypoplastic vermis

- CB vermian hypoplasia: Vermis hypoplasia ± upward rotation; normal-sized posterior fossa and brainstem
- BPC: Herniation of inferior 4th ventricle through foramen of Magendie into vallecula and retrovermian cistern; enhancing choroid plexus in cyst wall
- MCM: Enlarged pericerebellar cisterns communicate with basal subarachnoid spaces; normal vermis/4th ventricle; cistern crossed by falx cerebelli
- Imaging cannot precisely distinguish between mild DWM, BPC, and MCM
- ± associated callosal anomalies, cortical dysplasia, heterotopia

Helpful Clues for Rare Diagnoses

- **Rhombencephalosynapsis**
  - Key facts
    - Fusion of CB hemispheres, dentate nuclei, and superior CB peduncles
  - Imaging: Complete or partial fusion CB hemispheres
    - Absent primary fissure on sagittal; transverse folia on axial and coronal; keyhole-shaped 4th ventricle on axial
    - Fused horseshoe-shaped dentate nuclei
    - Absent posterior CB notch and vallecula
    - Absent or severely hypoplastic vermis
    - ± absent septum pellucidum, olivary hypoplasia, anomalies of limbic system, multiple cranial suture synostoses
    - ± corpus callosum dysgenesis, aqueductal stenosis, cortical dysplasia
- **Molar Tooth Malformations (Joubert)**
  - Key facts: Joubert anomaly is prototype
    - Joubert patients present with episodic hyperpnea, abnormal eye movements, ataxia, and mental retardation
    - Identical imaging findings in some patients without classic Joubert syndrome symptoms; some with renal or ocular anomalies, hepatic fibrosis/cysts, hypothalamic anomalies
  - Imaging: "Molar tooth" = large superior CB peduncles (do not decussate in dorsal midbrain) on axial images
    - Sagittal: Small, high CB vermis
    - Coronal: "Split vermis"
    - Axial: Small dysplastic vermis → triangular-shaped mid 4th ventricle and bat wing-shaped superior 4th ventricle
- **Chiari 3 Malformation**
  - Key facts: Extremely rare; Chiari 2 malformation + high- to mid-cervical cephalocele, which contains cerebellum
    - Controversy: May actually be high cervical myelocystocele rather than Chiari malformation
  - Imaging
    - CCJ or high cervical cephalocele: Meninges, cerebellum ± brainstem, cisterns, 4th ventricle, or dural sinuses
    - ± hydrocephalus
    - ± intracranial Chiari 2 findings

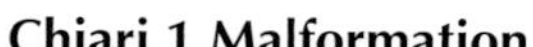

Chiari 1 Malformation

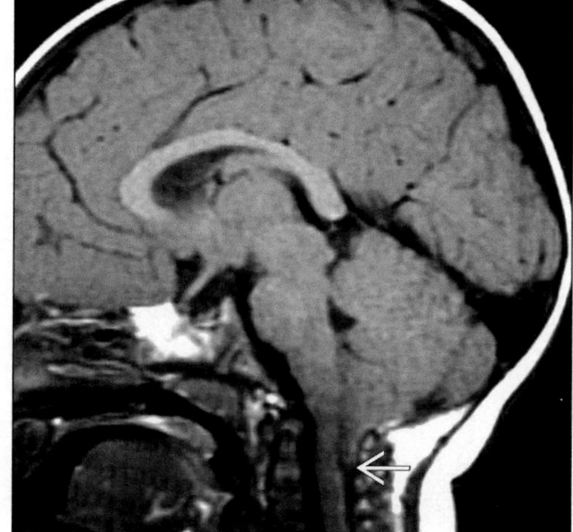

Sagittal T1WI MR shows a pointed cerebellar tonsil, extending well below the basion-opisthion line, effacement of CSF, and mass effect on the dorsal aspect of the cervical cord.

Chiari 1 Malformation

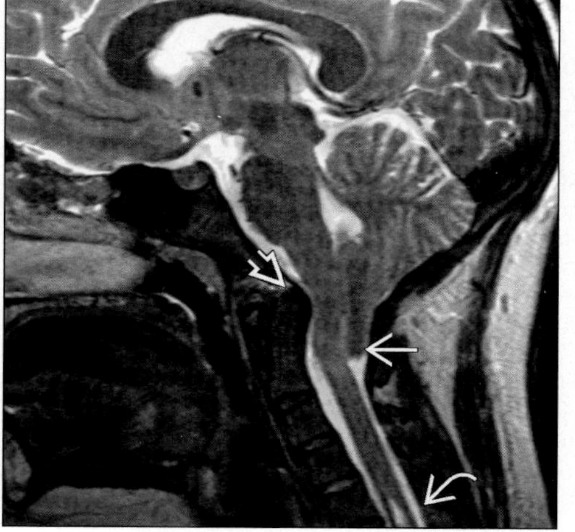

Sagittal T2WI FSE MR shows a pointed, low-lying cerebellar tonsil, effacement of CSF at the foramen magnum, dorsally tilted dens, small posterior fossa, and small lower cervical syrinx.

CONGENITAL CEREBELLAR MALFORMATION

Chiari 2 Malformation | **Chiari 2 Malformation**

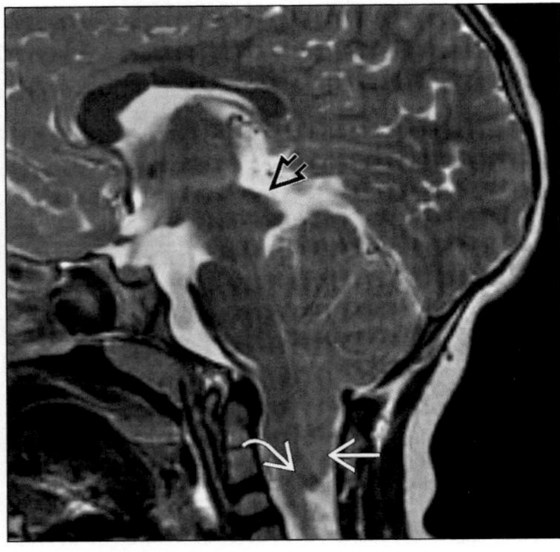

(Left) *Sagittal T1WI MR shows typical features of a Chiari 2 malformation: Small posterior fossa, low cerebellar "peg" → and cervicomedullary junction, tectal "beaking" →, and large massa intermedia →.* ***(Right)*** *Sagittal T2WI FSE MR shows a low-lying cerebellar "peg" →, "beaked" tectum →, cervicomedullary "kink" →, small posterior fossa with low tentorial insertion, and dysplastic corpus callosum.*

Cerebellar Hypoplasia | **Cerebellar Hypoplasia**

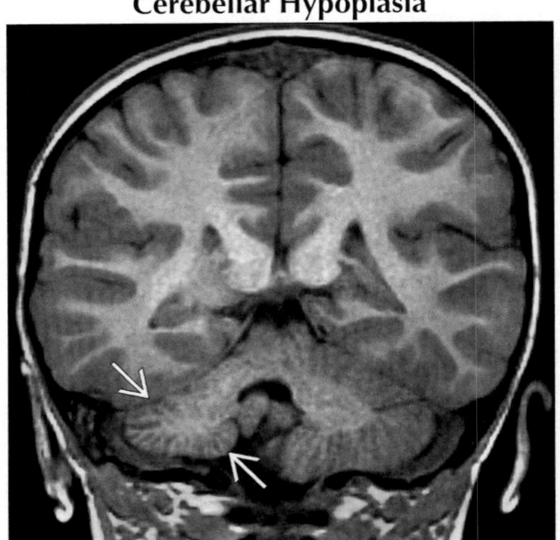

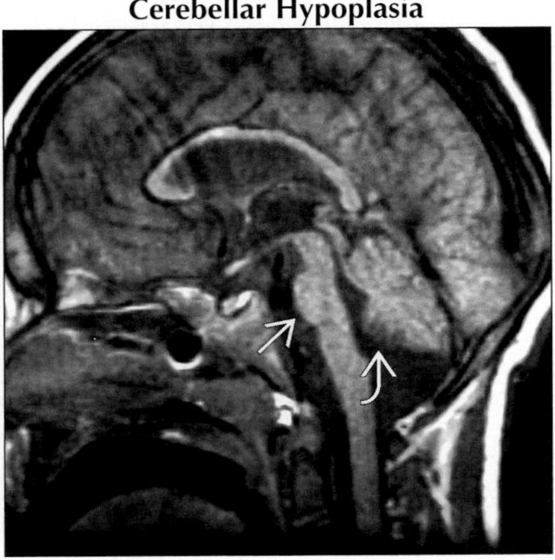

(Left) *Coronal T1WI MR shows a small right cerebellar hemisphere → secondary to congenital hypoplasia.* ***(Right)*** *Sagittal T1WI MR shows deficient inferior cerebellar vermis → and prominent associated hypoplasia of the pons → in a child with pontocerebellar hypoplasia.*

Cerebellar Dysplasias (Unclassified) | **Dandy-Walker Spectrum**

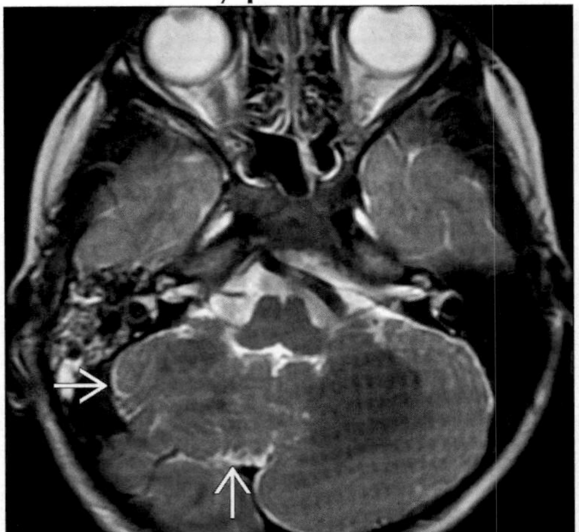

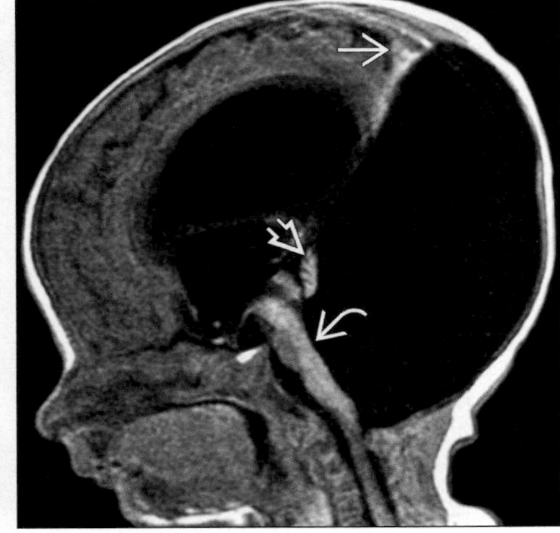

(Left) *Axial T2WI FSE MR shows a hypoplastic and dysplastic right cerebellar hemisphere → with abnormal orientation of the cerebellar folia and irregular gray-white junction* ***(Right)*** *Sagittal T1WI MR shows cystic dilatation of the 4th ventricle, very large posterior fossa, torcular/lambdoid inversion →, and severely hypoplastic, superiorly rotated cerebellar vermis →. The brainstem → is compressed.*

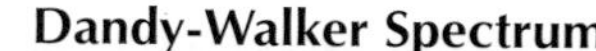

Dandy-Walker Spectrum

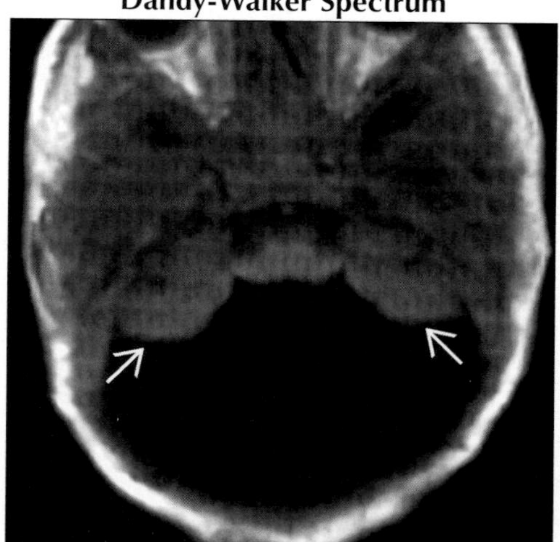

Dandy-Walker Spectrum

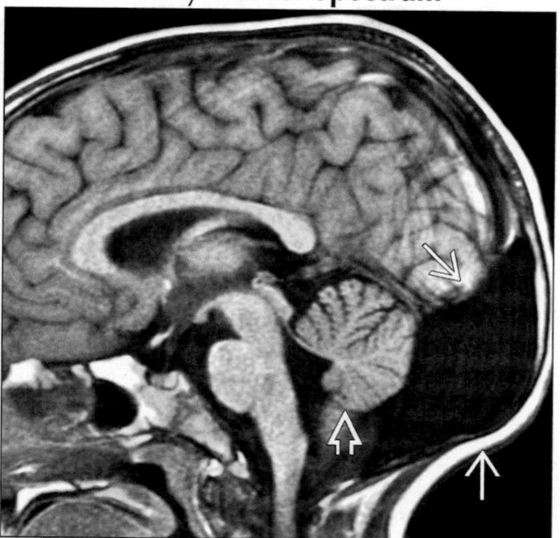

*(**Left**) Sagittal T1WI MR in the same patient shows continuity of the cyst with the 4th ventricle, hypoplastic cerebellar hemispheres ➡ pushed superiorly and laterally by the cyst. (**Right**) Sagittal T1WI MR shows prominent retrocerebellar CSF ➡ dorsal to a normal vermis ➡ and mild enlargement of the posterior fossa = mega cisterna magna vs. arachnoid cyst. Subsequent cisternogram (not shown) demonstrated rapid communication, consistent with MCM.*

Rhombencephalosynapsis

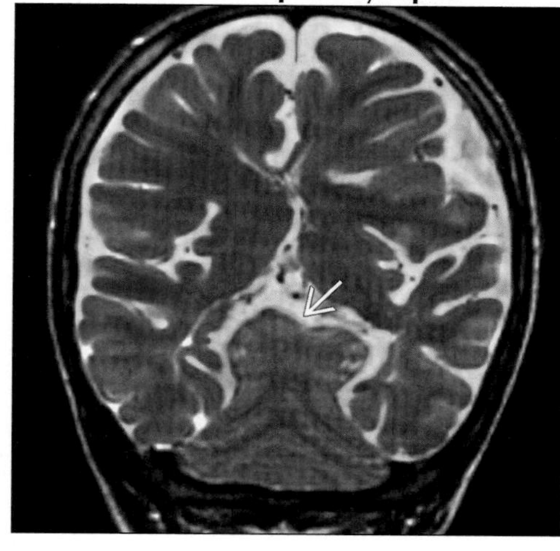

Rhombencephalosynapsis

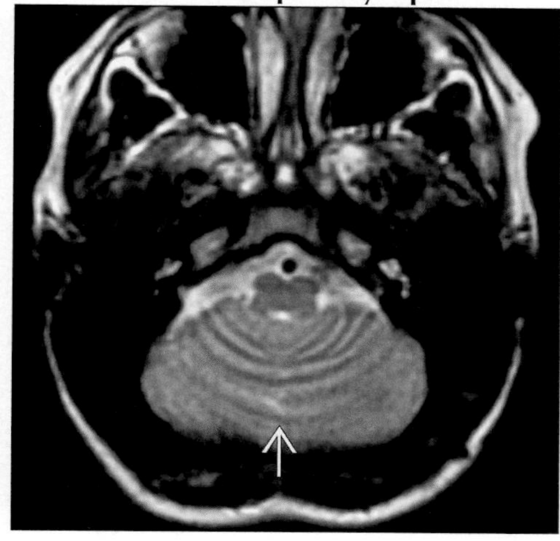

*(**Left**) Coronal T2WI FSE MR shows fusion of the cerebellar tonsils ➡ without intervening midline vermis. (**Right**) Axial T2WI FSE MR shows fusion of the cerebellar hemispheres ➡ without intervening vermis.*

Molar Tooth Malformations (Joubert)

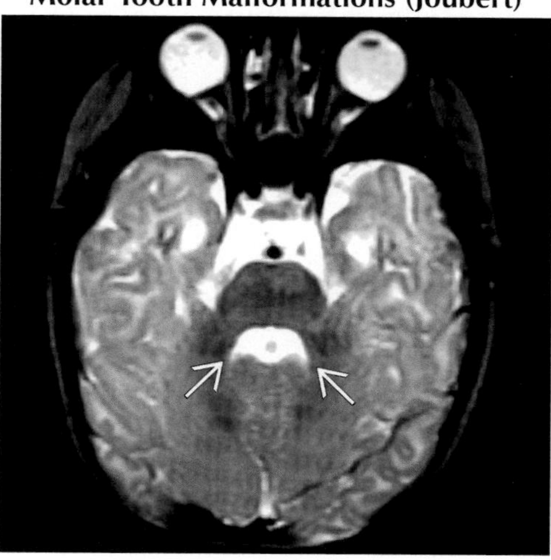

Molar Tooth Malformations (Joubert)

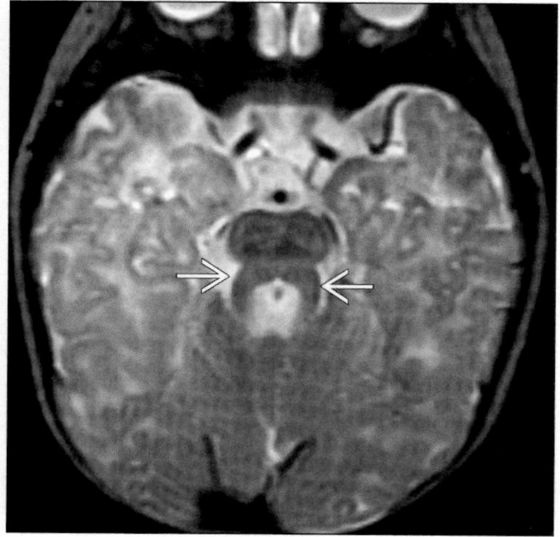

*(**Left**) Axial T2WI FSE MR shows a "bat wing" configuration of the upper 4th ventricle ➡. (**Right**) Axial T2WI FSE MR shows the "molar tooth" appearance of the midbrain secondary to the large superior cerebellar peduncles ➡.*

SECTION 7
Spine

INTRAMEDULLARY SPINAL CORD LESION

DIFFERENTIAL DIAGNOSIS

Common
- Syringomyelia
- ADEM
- Idiopathic Acute Transverse Myelitis
- Acute Transverse Myelopathy

Less Common
- Contusion-Hematoma
- Multiple Sclerosis
- Astrocytoma
- Cellular Ependymoma
- Abscess

Rare but Important
- Dermoid and Epidermoid Tumors
- Cavernous Malformation
- Infarction
- Hemangioblastoma

ESSENTIAL INFORMATION

Key Differential Diagnosis Issues
- Tumor vs. demyelinating disease
  - Tumors tend to be ovoid in shape, frequently enlarge cord ± cyst
  - Demyelinating disease tends to be flame-shaped without cord enlargement or cyst
  - Differentiation may require follow-up
- Adult vs. child spinal cord tumors
  - Intramedullary tumors tend to be more rostral in children than adults; 50% are cervical or cervicothoracic in children
  - Astrocytoma is most common spinal cord tumor in children; ependymoma is most common spinal cord tumor in adults
- Hemorrhage: Ependymoma, cavernoma, hemangioblastoma, cord contusion

Helpful Clues for Common Diagnoses
- **Syringomyelia**
  - Key facts
    - Hydromyelia = cystic central canal
    - Syringomyelia = cystic cord cavity, not contiguous with central canal
    - Syringohydromyelia = features of both syringomyelia and hydromyelia
  - Imaging findings: Expanded cord + nonenhancing cyst or dilated central canal
    - Tubular, beaded, or sacculated
    - ± widened canal, vertebral scalloping
    - ± hydrocephalus, Chiari 1, Chiari 2, dysraphism, tethered cord, or scoliosis
- **ADEM**
  - Key facts: Self-limiting, para-/postinfectious or postimmunization illness
    - Typically monophasic
    - Brain > spinal cord involvement
  - Imaging findings: ↑ T2 SI ± enhancement
- **Idiopathic Acute Transverse Myelitis**
  - Key facts: No etiology found
  - Imaging findings: Normal in up to 50%
    - ↑ T2 SI with variable enhancement
    - Mild fusiform cord enlargement
    - Usually central in location, > 2/3 cross-sectional area of cord
    - Usually 3-4 vertebral segments in length
    - Lacks associated intracranial lesions
- **Acute Transverse Myelopathy**
  - Key facts: Secondary to collagen vascular disease, viral infection, post-vaccination or post-irradiation, paraneoplastic syndrome; chronic ischemia/venous stasis secondary to AVM
  - Imaging findings: Same as idiopathic ATM

Helpful Clues for Less Common Diagnoses
- **Contusion-Hematoma**
  - Key facts: Post-traumatic
  - Imaging findings
    - Acute contusion = edema or hematoma
    - Transection: Best identified on T1WI
    - Chronic: Gliosis, atrophy ± cyst, hemosiderin scar
    - ± associated fracture, subluxation, traumatic disc herniation
- **Multiple Sclerosis**
  - Key facts: Multiphasic demyelinating disease of central nervous system
  - Imaging findings
    - ↑ T2 SI ± patchy or confluent CE
    - Multiple lesions of variable enhancement
    - Cervical cord most common site
    - Usually < 2 vertebral segments in length; < 1/2 cross-sectional area of spinal cord
    - Cord enlargement uncommon
    - Majority of patients have associated brain lesions: Periventricular, subcallosal, brain stem, or cerebellar white matter
- **Astrocytoma**
  - Key facts: Most common spinal cord tumor in children (60%)

- Tumor margins frequently extend beyond enhancing tissue
  - Imaging findings
    - Fusiform enlargement of cord, infiltrative margins of T2 hyperintensity
    - More eccentric and less enhancing than ependymomas
    - Peritumoral cysts in up to 40%
    - ± expansion of canal, scoliosis
- **Cellular Ependymoma**
  - Key facts: 2nd most common cord tumor in children (30%)
    - Tumor margins usually = margin of enhancing tissue
  - Imaging findings: Circumscribed and enhancing, usually central in cord
    - Peritumoral cysts in up to 80%
    - Hemosiderin ("cap" sign) at superior and inferior borders, present in 20%
    - ± widened canal, scoliosis, scalloping
- **Abscess**
  - Key facts: Direct extension from dysraphism in children; idiopathic or hematogenous spread in adults
  - Imaging findings: Irregular ring enhancement + cord expansion; ± restricted diffusion

Helpful Clues for Rare Diagnoses

- **Dermoid and Epidermoid Tumors**
  - Key facts: Benign tumor
    - Intramedullary (40%), extramedullary (60%), extradural (rare)
    - From cells that produce skin, hair follicles, sweat, and sebaceous glands
  - Imaging findings
    - Similar to CSF on T1 and T2WI ± hyperintense T1 fat in dermoid
    - Epidermoid may be hyperintense on DWI, slightly hyperintense on FLAIR
    - ± mild ring enhancement
    - ↑ ↑ enhancement, suspect infection
- **Cavernous Malformation**
  - Key facts: 3-5% in spinal cord
    - Thoracic > cervical > > conus
  - Imaging findings: Heterogeneous 2° to varying ages of blood products
    - Absent or minimal CE
    - Edema if recent hemorrhage
    - ± speckled or "popcorn" appearance
- **Infarction**
  - Key facts: Sudden onset of symptoms; rare in children
  - Imaging findings
    - Hyperintense T2WI/DWI, ± cord expansion, ± patchy enhancement in subacute phase
    - Length usually > 1 vertebral body
    - ± hemorrhagic conversion
- **Hemangioblastoma**
  - Key facts: Extremely rare in children
  - Imaging findings: Cyst with enhancing nodule in dorsal cord
    - Multiple lesions common (including posterior fossa)

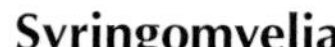

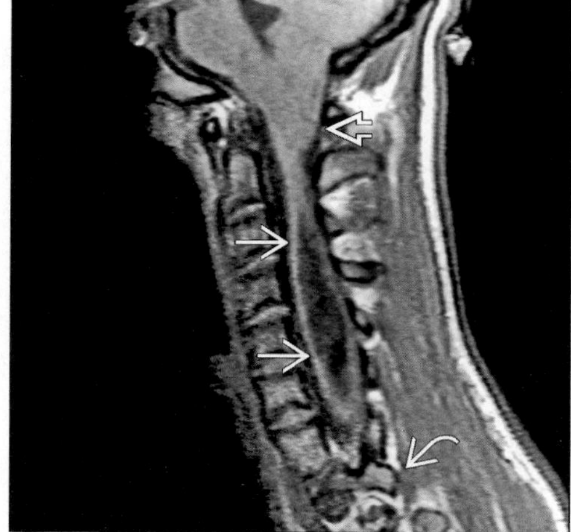

Sagittal T1WI MR shows a large cervical syrinx ➡ in a patient with Chiari 1 ➡ and scoliosis ➡.

ADEM

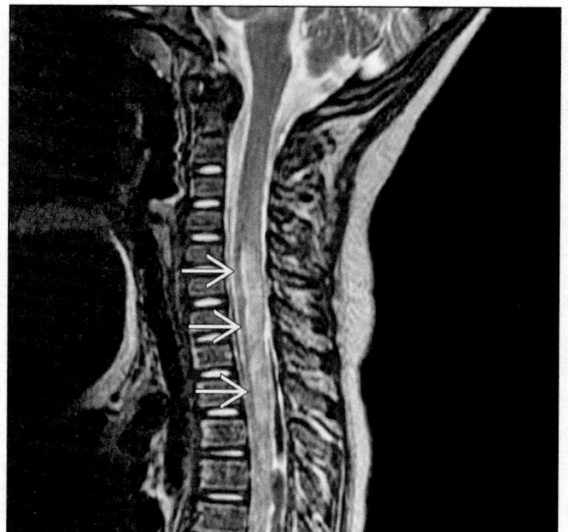

Sagittal T2WI FSE MR shows a long segment of hyperintense T2 signal abnormality ➡ in the mid and dorsal cervicothoracic cord in a child with multiple intracranial lesions (not shown).

INTRAMEDULLARY SPINAL CORD LESION

(Left) *Sagittal T2WI FSE MR shows fusiform cervical cord enlargement and diffuse ill-defined hyperintense T2 signal abnormality in the cervicomedullary junction and the cervical and thoracic cord.* ***(Right)*** *Axial GRE MR demonstrates 2 focal areas of intramedullary hemorrhage → in a child who suffered cervical vertebral body → and lamina → fractures in a diving accident.*

Idiopathic Acute Transverse Myelitis

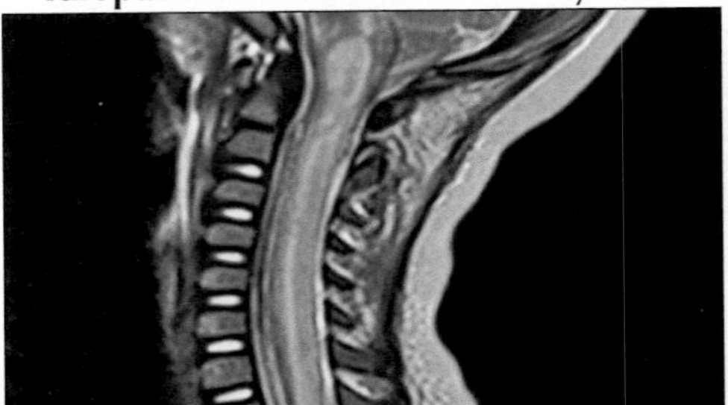

Contusion-Hematoma

(Left) *Sagittal T2WI MR shows multiple hyperintense intramedullary lesions →, typical of multiple sclerosis.* ***(Right)*** *Sagittal T2WI FSE MR shows a single focus of demyelination → in the cervical cord without cord enlargement.*

Multiple Sclerosis

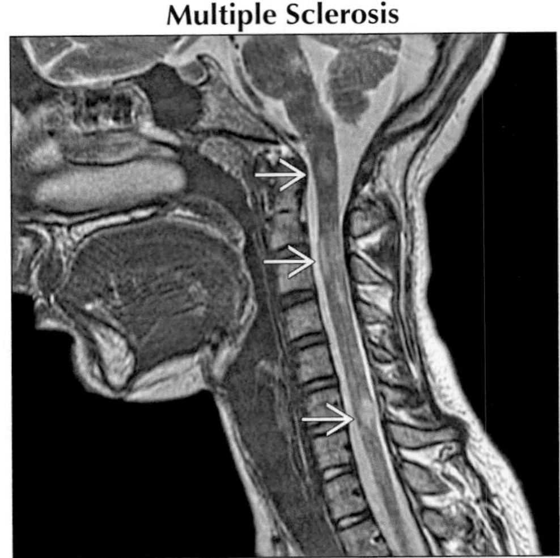

Multiple Sclerosis

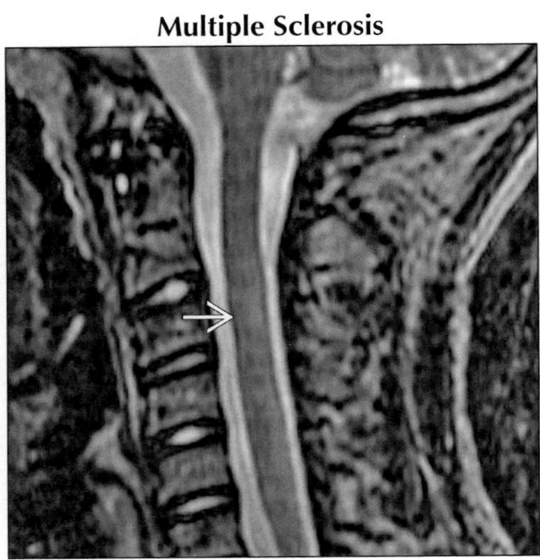

(Left) *Sagittal T1WI C+ MR shows patchy, subtle contrast enhancement within a portion → of cervicothoracic cord neoplasm. Note that the total extent of signal abnormality → is greater than the area of enhancement.* ***(Right)*** *Sagittal T1 C+ MR shows cord enlargement with a solid enhancing portion of tumor → capped by nonenhancing cysts →.*

Astrocytoma

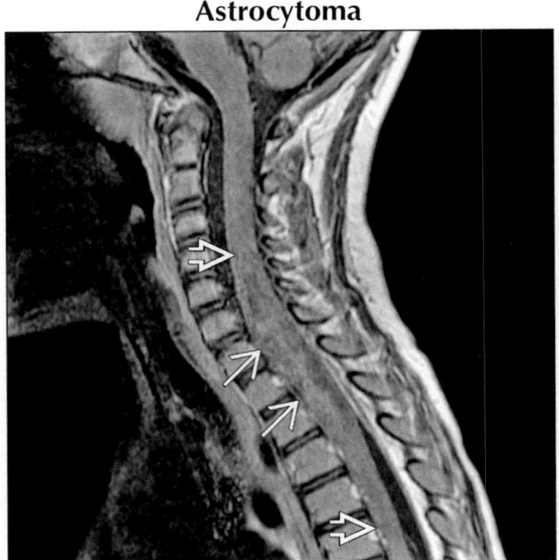

Cellular Ependymoma

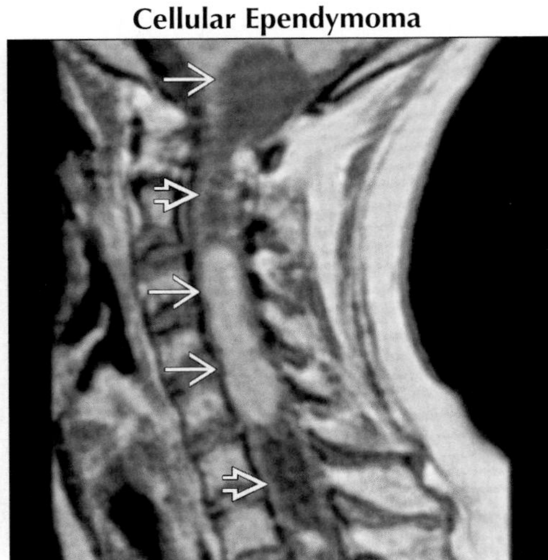

Abscess

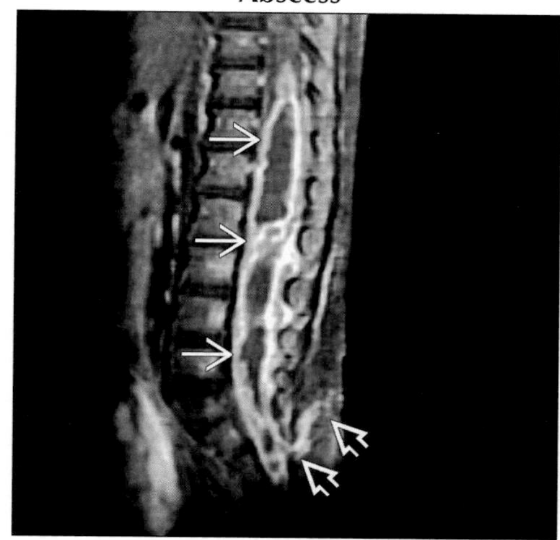

Dermoid and Epidermoid Tumors

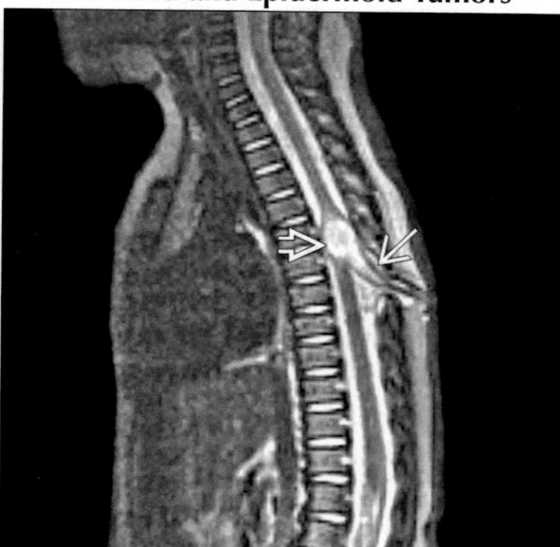

*(**Left**) Sagittal T1WI C+ FS MR shows a large peripherally enhancing intramedullary abscess ➡ within a tethered cord and enhancement of the dorsal dermal sinus ➡ connecting the skin surface to the tethered cord. (**Right**) Sagittal T2WI MR shows a hyperintense intramedullary dermoid tumor ➡ contiguous with an extramedullary component following a dermal sinus tract ➡ to the skin surface.*

Cavernous Malformation

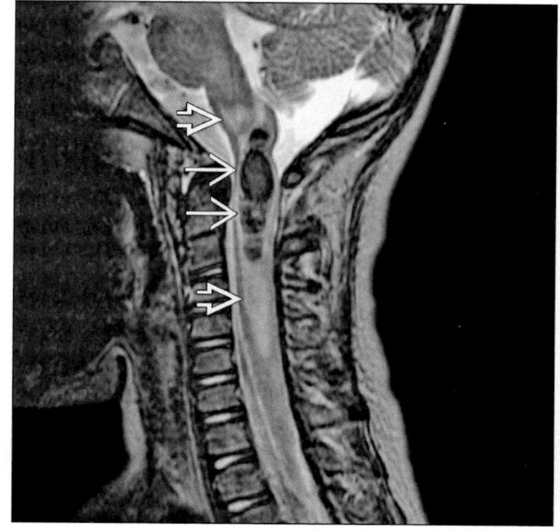

Cavernous Malformation

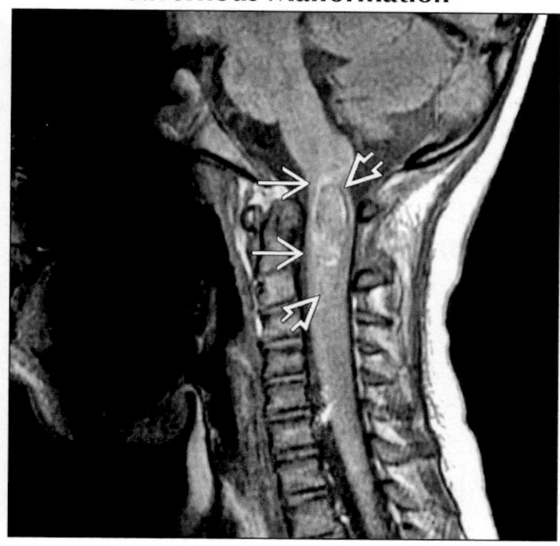

*(**Left**) Sagittal T2WI FSE MR shows hypointense hemorrhage within the cervicomedullary junction ➡ with significant edema ➡ proximal and distal to the intramedullary hemorrhage. (**Right**) Sagittal T1WI MR in the same patient shows ill-defined hyperintense signal consistent with subacute hemorrhage ➡ at the periphery and in the center of the fairly well-defined cervicomedullary cavernoma ➡.*

Infarction

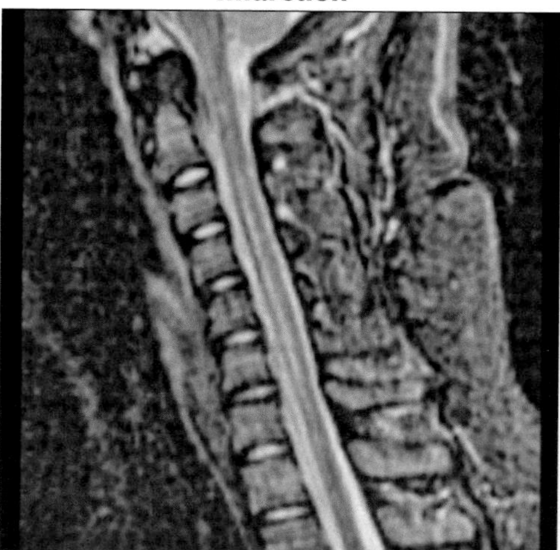

Infarction

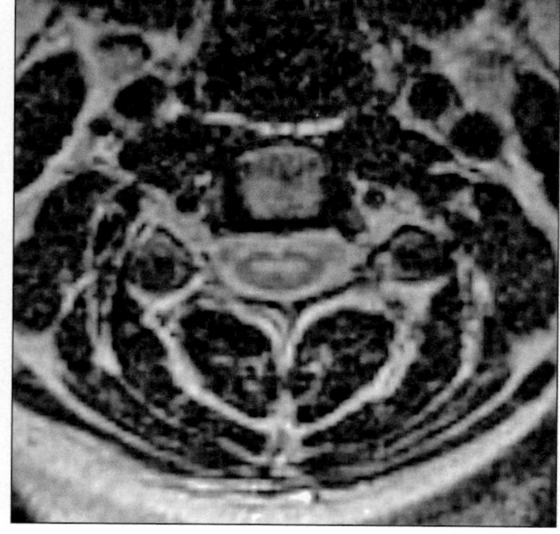

*(**Left**) Sagittal T2WI FSE MR shows long segment central hyperintense cord signal abnormality in a teenager who developed progressive quadriplegia after a back massage (which included another person walking on the patient's back). (**Right**) Axial T2WI FSE MR shows central gray matter hyperintensity in the same patient.*

SCOLIOSIS

DIFFERENTIAL DIAGNOSIS

Common

- Idiopathic Scoliosis
- Degenerative Scoliosis
- Trauma
  - Lateral Compression Fracture, Lumbar
  - Lateral Compression Fracture, Thoracic
  - Lateral Flexion Injury, Cervical
- Neuromuscular Scoliosis
  - Cerebral Palsy
  - Muscular Dystrophy
  - Friedrich Ataxia
  - Poliomyelitis
  - Hemiparesis/Hemiplegia
  - Paraparesis/Paraplegia
- Congenital Scoliosis and Kyphosis
  - Partial Vertebral Duplication
  - Failure of Vertebral Formation
  - Klippel-Feil Spectrum
  - VACTERL Association
- Infection
  - Paraspinal Abscess
  - Pyogenic Osteomyelitis
  - Granulomatous Osteomyelitis
- Failed Back Surgery Syndrome
- Neurogenic (Charcot) Arthropathy
- Limb Length Inequality
- Chest Wall Abnormality
  - Rib Anomaly
  - Sprengel Deformity

Less Common

- Pleural or Pulmonary Abnormality
  - Empyema
  - Pneumonectomy
  - Fibrothorax
- Tumor
  - Pathologic Vertebral Fracture
  - Osteoblastoma
  - Osteoid Osteoma
- Congenital Syndromes with Normal Segmentation
  - Connective Tissue Disorders
  - Neurofibromatosis Type 1
  - Osteogenesis Imperfecta
  - Mucopolysaccharidoses
  - Fibrous Dysplasia
  - Fetal Alcohol Syndrome
  - Proteus Syndrome
  - Tethered Spinal Cord
- Radiation Therapy in Childhood

ESSENTIAL INFORMATION

Helpful Clues for Common Diagnoses

- Painful scoliosis
  - Trauma, tumor, infection
- Short-curve scoliosis
  - Congenital anomaly, tumor, infection, trauma, degenerative, postoperative
- Balanced S-curve scoliosis
  - Idiopathic, connective tissue disorders
- C-curve scoliosis
  - Neuromuscular, osteogenesis imperfecta

Idiopathic Scoliosis

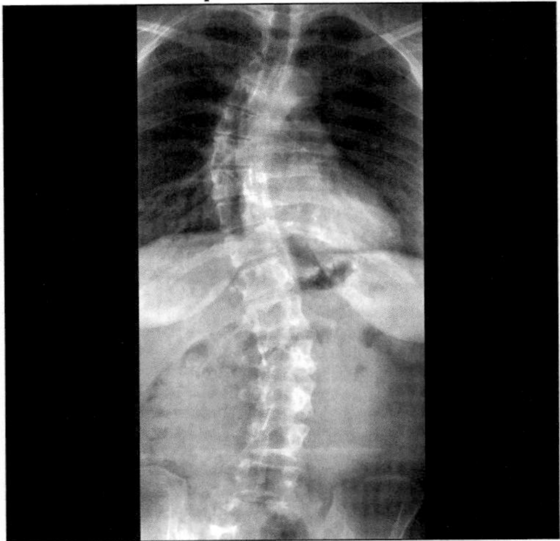

Anteroposterior radiograph shows a classic, balanced, S-shaped curve, convex to right in thoracic spine. There is often minimal wedging of vertebrae on concave side of scoliosis.

Trauma

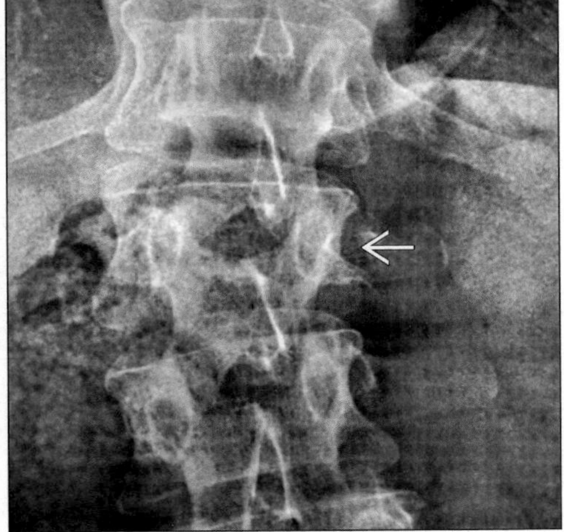

Anteroposterior radiograph shows lateral compression fracture of L1 ➔ resulting in short-curve scoliosis.

Neuromuscular Scoliosis

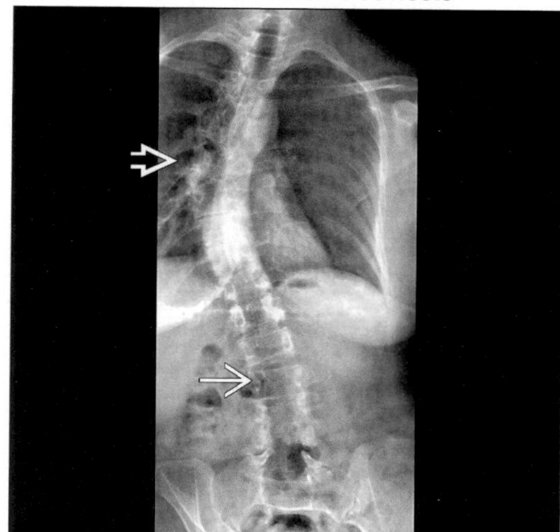

Neuromuscular Scoliosis

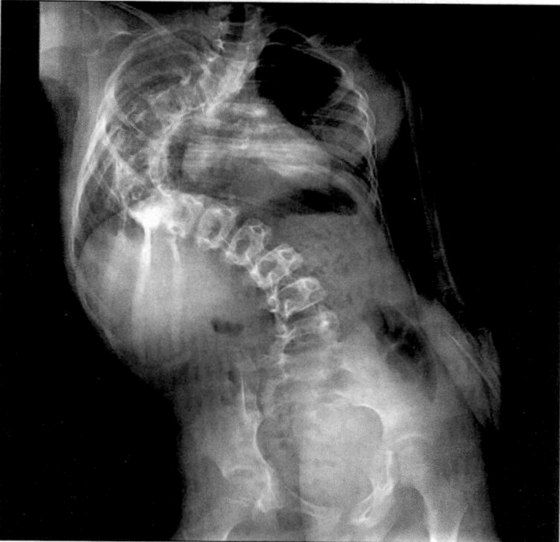

*(**Left**) Anteroposterior radiograph shows C-shaped curve ➡ characteristic of neuromuscular scoliosis. Failure of fusion of the posterior elements ➡ is seen in the lumbar spine. (**Right**) Anteroposterior radiograph shows a more severe, unbalanced C-shaped scoliosis. Neuromuscular scoliosis sometimes yields "hairpin" curve.*

Congenital Scoliosis and Kyphosis

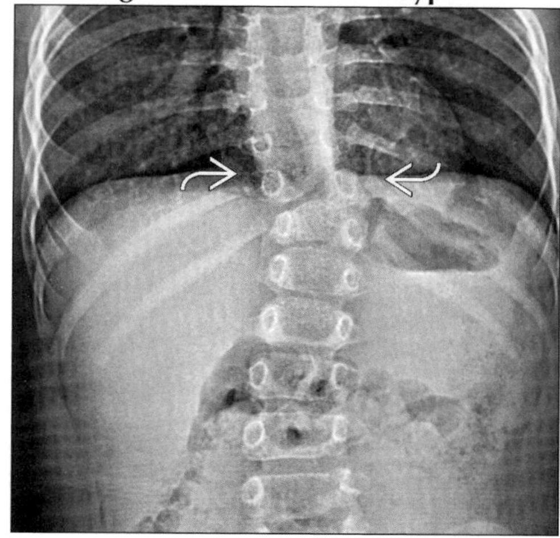

Rib Anomaly

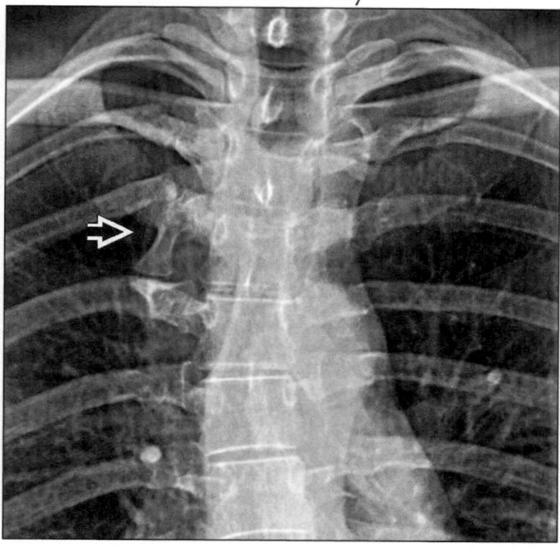

*(**Left**) Anteroposterior radiograph shows left T11 hemivertebra ➡ fused to T12, and right T11 hemivertebra fused to T10. (**Right**) Anteroposterior radiograph shows dextroscoliosis related to the rib anomaly ➡ that has caused separation of the right 4th and 5th ribs.*

Osteoid Osteoma

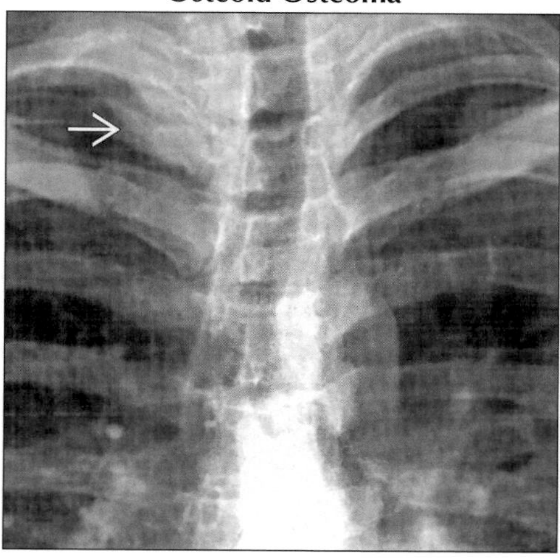

Osteogenesis Imperfecta

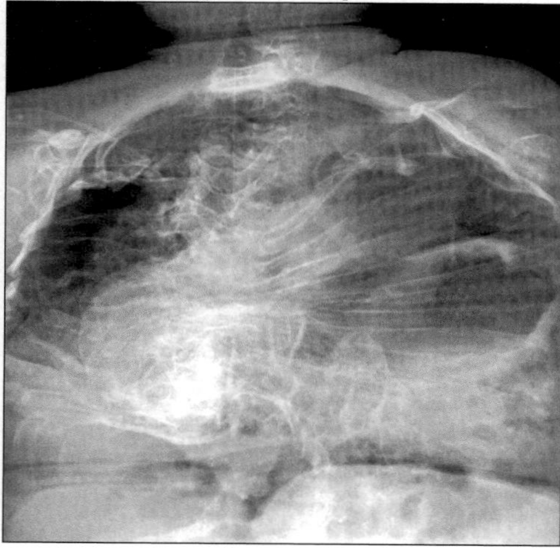

*(**Left**) Anteroposterior radiograph shows short-curve scoliosis and pleural thickening ➡ in a patient with focal pain. Because of these findings, a CT scan was performed; it revealed osteoid osteoma. (**Right**) Anteroposterior radiograph shows extreme scoliosis leading to shortening of the trunk in this patient with osteogenesis imperfecta. Multiple rib fractures are also present.*

KYPHOSCOLIOSIS

DIFFERENTIAL DIAGNOSIS

Common
- Traumatic
  - Burst Thoracolumbar Fracture
  - Lateral Compression Fracture, Lumbar
  - Lateral Compression Fracture, Thoracic
  - Lateral Flexion Injury, Cervical
  - Chance Fracture, Thoracic
- Congenital
  - Congenital Scoliosis and Kyphosis
  - Failure of Vertebral Formation
  - Klippel-Feil Spectrum
  - Partial Vertebral Duplication
  - Tethered Spinal Cord
  - Caudal Regression Syndrome
- Idiopathic Scoliosis,
- Scheuermann Disease
- Neuromuscular Scoliosis
- Juvenile Idiopathic Arthritis
- Idiopathic Kyphosis
- Kyphosis Normal in Infants

Less Common
- Infection
  - Pyogenic Osteomyelitis
  - Granulomatous Osteomyelitis
  - Prevertebral Abscess
  - Postoperative Infection
- Tumor
  - Osteoid Osteoma
  - Osteoblastoma
  - Aneurysmal Bone Cyst
  - Ewing Sarcoma
  - Langerhans Cell Histiocytosis
- Syringomyelia
- Neurofibromatosis Type 1
- Connective Tissue Disorders
- Postoperative Spinal Complications
- Diastematomyelia

Rare but Important
- Post-Radiation

ESSENTIAL INFORMATION

Key Differential Diagnosis Issues
- MR may be useful in certain cases
  - Painful scoliosis: Tumor, infection
  - Atypical curve: Often have underlying bony or neural abnormalities
  - Congenital scoliosis: Assess full extent of bony abnormalities
- CT useful to characterize congenital scoliosis

Helpful Clues for Common Diagnoses
- Congenital curve may progress rapidly, especially if it includes unfused hemivertebrae
- Scheuermann kyphosis presents in adolescence, may be misdiagnosed as fracture
  - Involves multiple levels, look for Schmorl nodes or undulation of endplates without angular deformity
- Lumbar kyphosis normal in infants
  - Lumbar lordosis develops after infant begins to sit upright

Traumatic

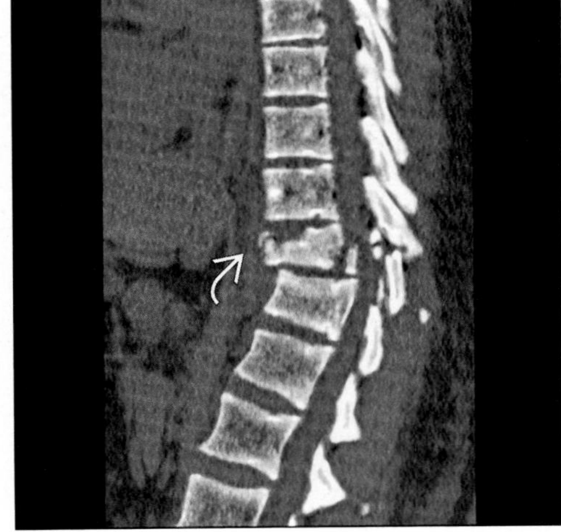

Sagittal bone CT shows kyphotic deformity ➔ in this patient with a flexion-distraction type injury. Kyphosis also seen due to burst or compression fracture.

Congenital

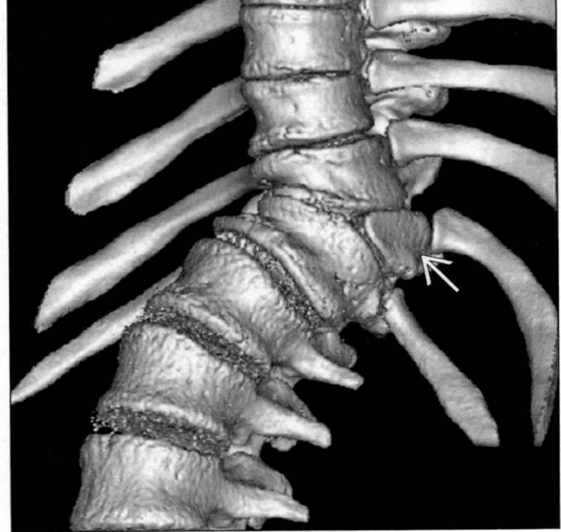

Anteroposterior bone CT 3D reformation shows left T11 hemivertebra ➔. Short-curve, unbalanced kyphoscoliosis is typical of congenital kyphoscoliosis.

KYPHOSCOLIOSIS

Congenital

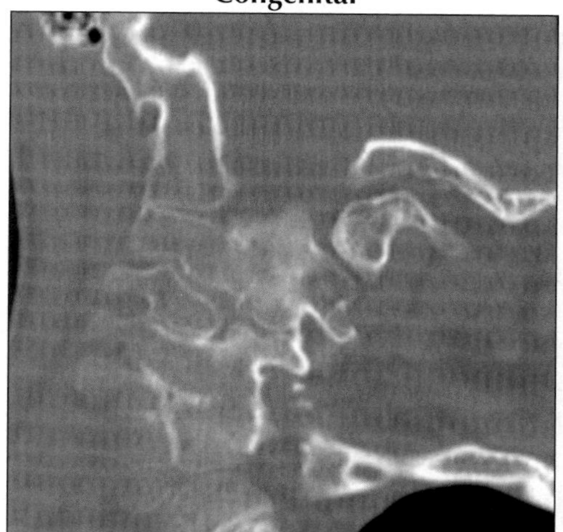

Scheuermann Disease

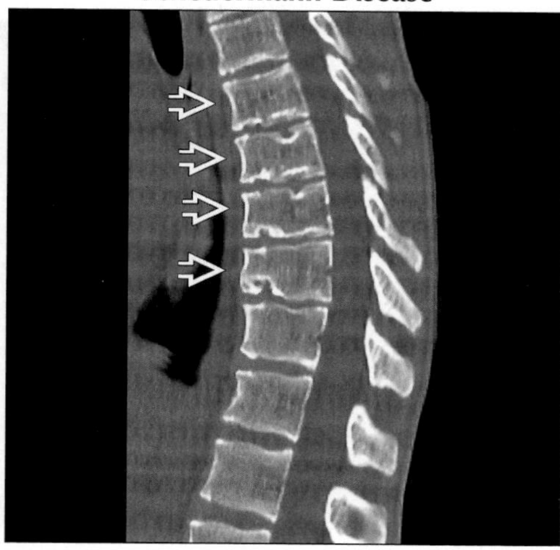

(Left) *Coronal bone CT shows a patient with Klippel-Feil spectrum, including extensive fusion anomalies of the cervical spine and dextroscoliosis. Kyphosis was also present.* ***(Right)*** *Sagittal bone CT shows kyphosis due to vertebral wedging ➡. Note the undulating endplates and Schmorl nodes at 4 contiguous levels. Scoliosis is seen in 15% of Scheuermann cases.*

Neuromuscular Scoliosis

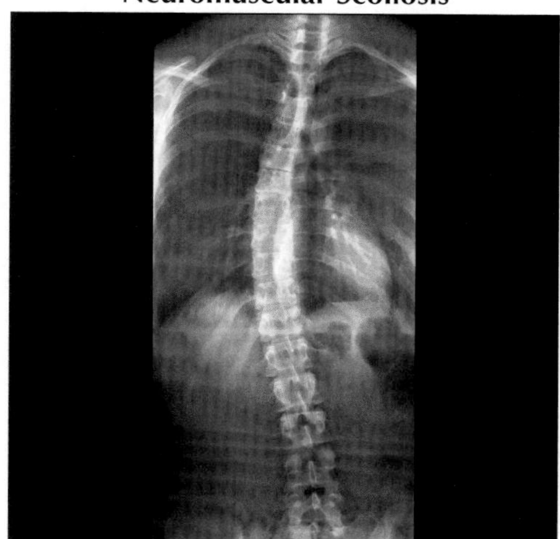

Juvenile Idiopathic Arthritis

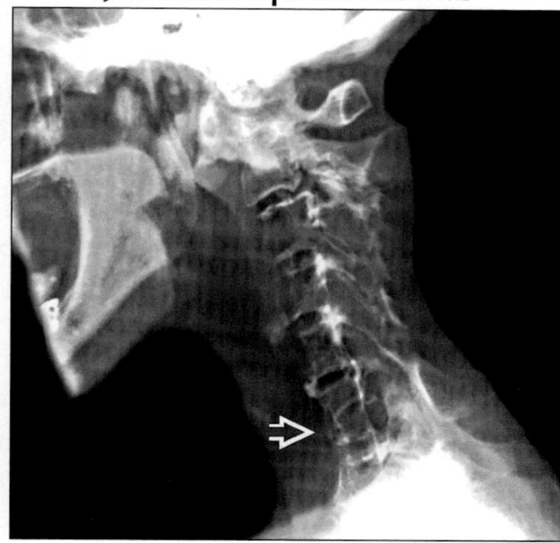

(Left) *Anteroposterior radiograph shows C-shaped scoliosis typical of neuromuscular scoliosis. There is also often persistence of infantile kyphosis in neuromuscular disease.* ***(Right)*** *Lateral radiograph shows mild kyphosis due to cervical fusions ➡. Kyphosis due to juvenile chronic (idiopathic) arthritis is usually not severe.*

Infection

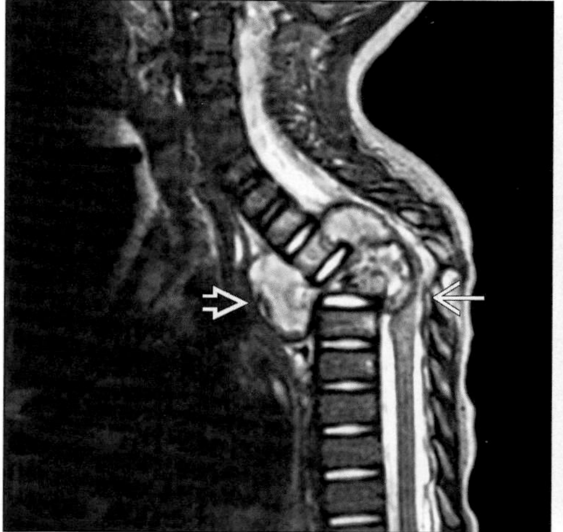

Tumor

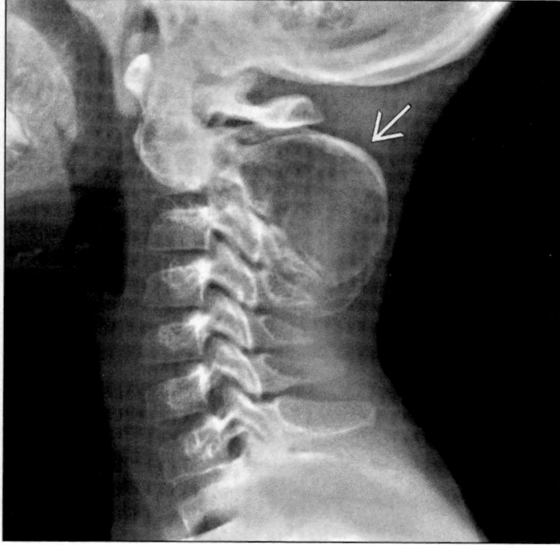

(Left) *Sagittal T2WI MR shows infantile tuberculosis causing kyphotic deformity, epidural abscess ➡, and prevertebral abscess ➡. Spinal TB can be present without pulmonary abnormalities.* ***(Right)*** *Lateral radiograph shows a large expansile mass ➡, an aneurysmal bone cyst in this case, involving posterior elements and causing kyphotic deformity at the C2-3 level.*

BULLET-SHAPED VERTEBRA/ANTERIOR VERTEBRAL BODY BEAKING

DIFFERENTIAL DIAGNOSIS

Common
- Achondroplasia
- Down Syndrome (Trisomy 21)

Less Common
- Radiation-Induced Growth Deformities
- Hypothyroidism (Congenital)
- Pseudoachondroplasia

Rare but Important
- Morquio Syndrome
- Hurler Syndrome

ESSENTIAL INFORMATION

Key Differential Diagnosis Issues
- Bullet shape: Down, achondroplasia, pseudoachondroplasia, hypothyroidism, Hurler, Morquio
- Anterior beaking: Achondroplasia, radiation-induced, Hurler, Morquio

Helpful Clues for Common Diagnoses
- **Achondroplasia**
  - Rhizomelic dwarf
  - Exaggerated lumbar lordosis, posterior vertebral scalloping, narrow foramen magnum, congenital spinal stenosis, decreased interpediculate distance
  - Squared iliac wings, narrow sciatic notch, horizontal acetabular roof
  - Trident hand, flared anterior ribs
- **Down Syndrome (Trisomy 21)**
  - Congenital heart disease, GI abnormalities
  - Brachycephaly, abnormal facies
  - Short stature, atlantoaxial instability, developmental hip dysplasia

Helpful Clues for Less Common Diagnoses
- **Radiation-Induced Growth Deformities**
  - Regional osteoporosis ± scoliosis
- **Hypothyroidism (Congenital)**
  - Mental retardation, delayed growth, short stature, stippled epiphyses
  - Abnormal skull and face with thick protruding tongue, delayed dentition
- **Pseudoachondroplasia**
  - Rhizomelic dwarf
  - C1-2 subluxation, accentuated lumbar lordosis, early osteoarthritis
  - Short thick tubular bones especially in hands and feet, metaphyseal excrescences

Helpful Clues for Rare Diagnoses
- **Morquio Syndrome**
  - Short stature, macrocephaly, coarse facial features, widely spaced teeth
  - Odontoid hypoplasia, increased lumbar lordosis, bell chest, & paddle-shaped ribs
  - Flared iliac wings, inferior tapering iliac bones, steep acetabuli, coxa valga
- **Hurler Syndrome**
  - Mental retardation, short stature
  - Coarse facial features, macrocephaly, and other craniovertebral anomalies including J-shaped sella
  - Small iliac bones with inferior tapering, steep acetabuli, abnormal femoral heads
  - Thickened tubular bones, contractures

Achondroplasia

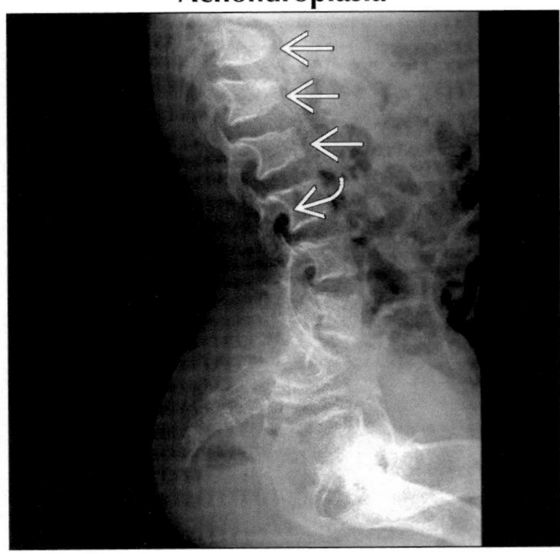

Lateral radiograph shows bullet-shaped vertebrae at the lumbosacral junction ➡ and scalloping of the posterior vertebral cortices ➡, findings commonly seen in patients with achondroplasia.

Achondroplasia

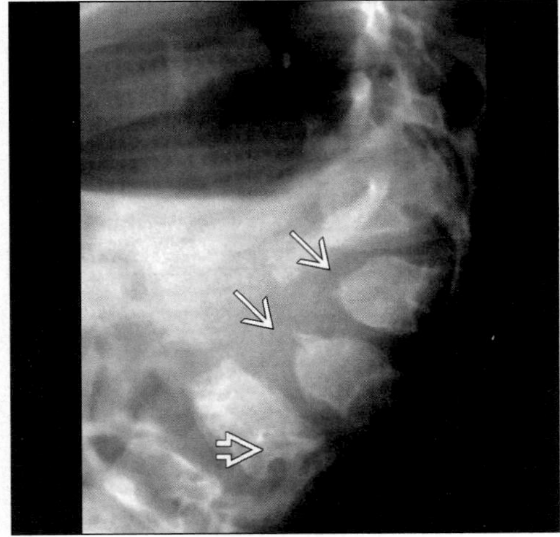

Lateral radiograph shows posterior vertebral scalloping ➡, hypoplasia of L1 and L2, and anterior beaking ➡ with focal kyphosis in this patient with achondroplasia.

Radiation-Induced Growth Deformities

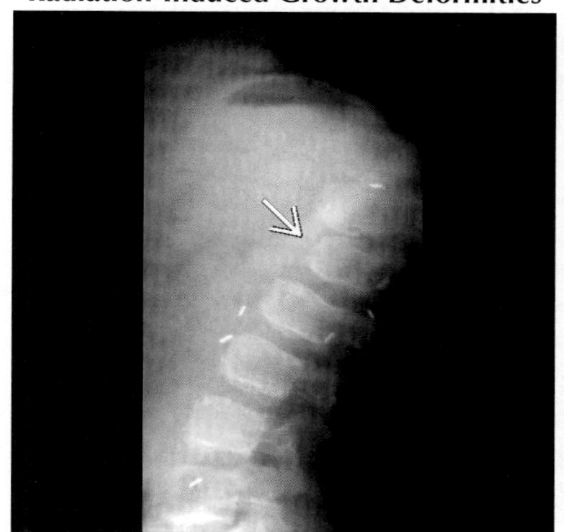

Pseudoachondroplasia

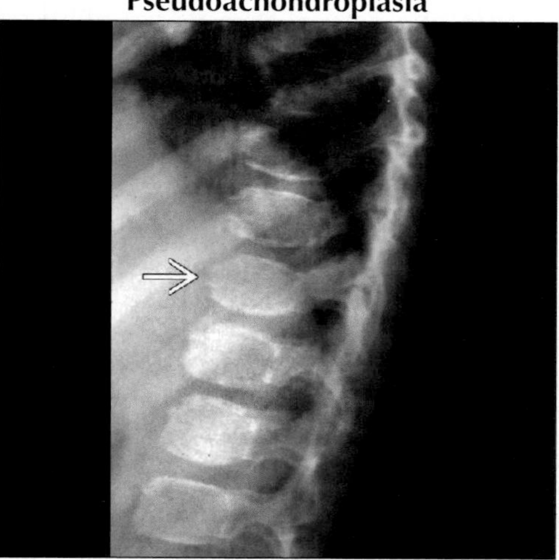

*(**Left**) Lateral radiograph shows a hypoplastic, almost bullet-shaped L1 ➡ in a child who was radiated 1 year earlier for Wilms tumor. Radiation of growing bone slows or stops growth due to vascular damage. (**Right**) Lateral radiograph shows very mild platyspondyly with mild anterior beaking ➡ in a patient with pseudoachondroplasia.*

Morquio Syndrome

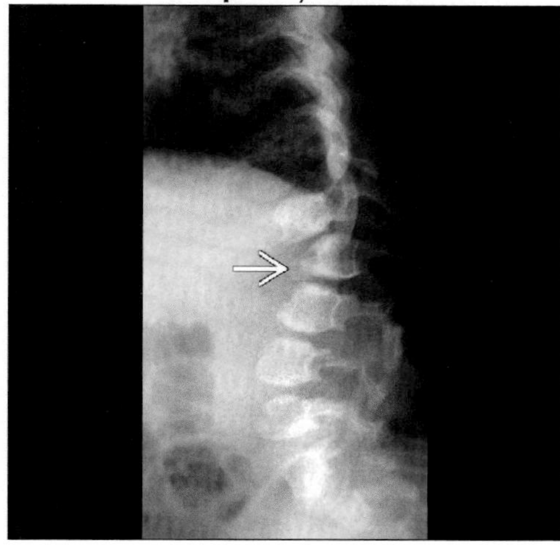

Morquio Syndrome

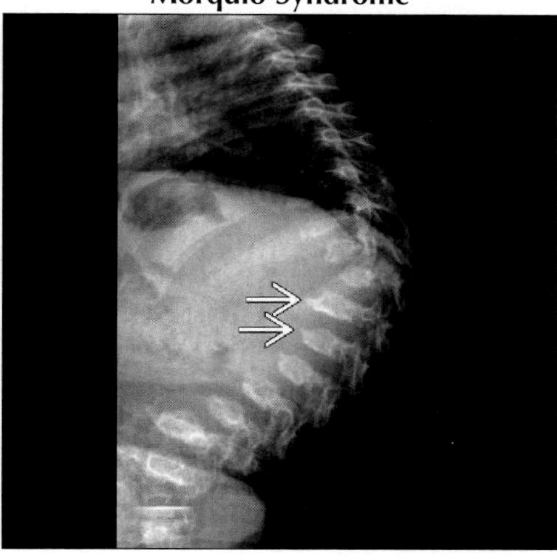

*(**Left**) Lateral radiograph shows a thoracolumbar kyphosis, with a hypoplastic oval L1 and central anterior beaking ➡, in this patient with Morquio syndrome. (**Right**) Lateral radiograph shows a classic example of Morquio syndrome, including dorsolumbar gibbus with vertebral beaking ➡.*

Hurler Syndrome

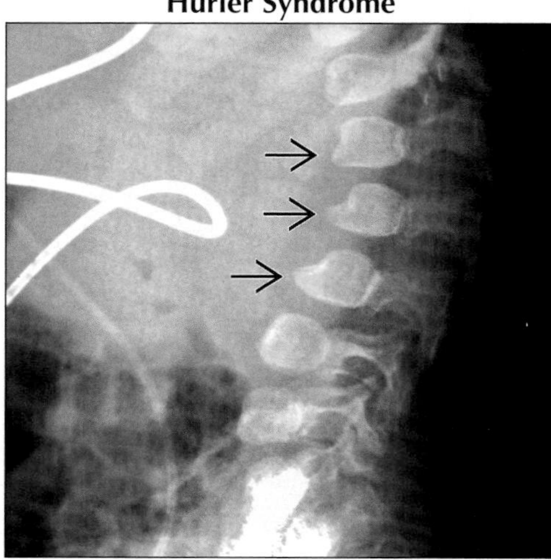

Hurler Syndrome

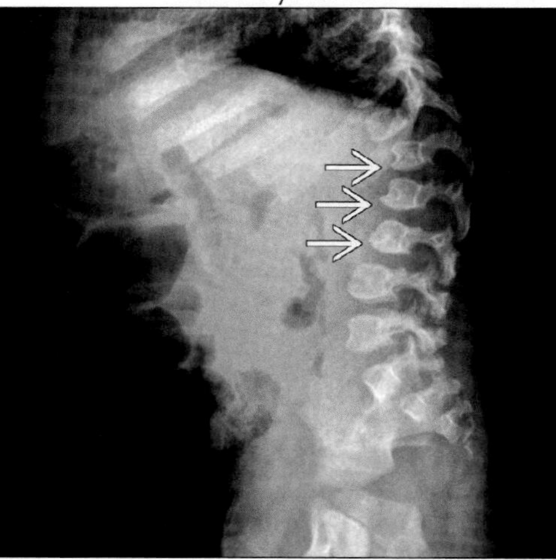

*(**Left**) Lateral radiograph shows inferior beaking ➡ of 3 vertebral bodies in this patient with many classic findings of Hurler syndrome. (**Right**) Lateral radiograph shows the typical skeletal findings of dysostosis multiplex, including vertebral body beaking ➡, in this patient with Hurler syndrome.*

SCALLOPED VERTEBRAL BODIES

DIFFERENTIAL DIAGNOSIS

Common
- Vertebral Segmentation Failure
- Spinal Dysraphism

Less Common
- Achondroplasia
- Mucopolysaccharidoses
- Dural Dysplasia

Rare but Important
- Syringomyelia
- Intraspinal Mass

ESSENTIAL INFORMATION

Helpful Clues for Common Diagnoses
- **Vertebral Segmentation Failure**
  - Single or multiple levels, widened or narrow canal ± dorsal scalloping
- **Spinal Dysraphism**
  - Myelomeningocele: Open neural tube defect, wide osseous dysraphism ± diastematomyelia, syrinx, congenital or developmental kyphoscoliosis
    - ≈ 100% have Chiari 2 malformation
  - Lipomyelocele or lipomyelomeningocele: Skin covered; neural placode/lipoma complex contiguous with SQ fat through osseous dysraphic defect
  - Diastematomyelia ± fibrous, osteocartilaginous, or osseous spur, intersegmental vertebral fusion, thick filum, or tethered cord

Helpful Clues for Less Common Diagnoses
- **Achondroplasia**
  - Flat or bullet-shaped vertebra + short pedicles + posterior scalloping
  - Spinal stenosis secondary to degenerative disease + congenital short pedicles
  - Lumbar hyperlordosis, thoracolumbar kyphoscoliosis
  - ± costochondral junction stenosis, rarely C1-2 instability
- **Mucopolysaccharidoses**
  - Inherited lysosomal storage disorders, Hurler syndrome (MPS I-H) most common
  - Vertebral beaking, thoracolumbar gibbus ± spinal stenosis, dorsal vertebral scalloping
  - Narrow foramen magnum, short posterior C1 arch, odontoid hypoplasia
- **Dural Dysplasia**
  - Patulous sac + dorsal vertebral scalloping
    - ± neurofibromas or other spinal neoplasms in neurofibromatosis type 1
    - ± arterial dissection or aneurysm in Marfan and Ehlers-Danlos syndrome
    - Osteoporosis in homocystinuria

Helpful Clues for Rare Diagnoses
- **Syringomyelia**
  - ± wide canal, spinal dysraphism, Chiari 1, or neoplasm
- **Intraspinal Mass**
  - Intramedullary or extramedullary mass ⇒ enlargement of canal &/or vertebral scalloping

Vertebral Segmentation Failure

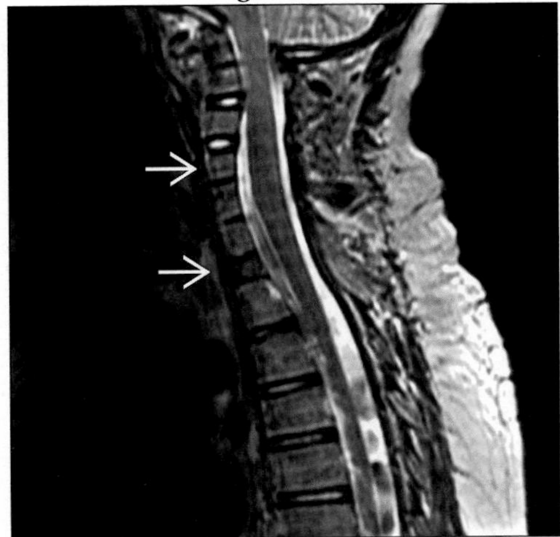

Sagittal T2WI FSE MR shows C4-7 partial block vertebrae ➡, with decreased AP dimension of each vertebral body, narrowed disc spaces, smooth dorsal concavity, and widening of the cervical canal.

Spinal Dysraphism

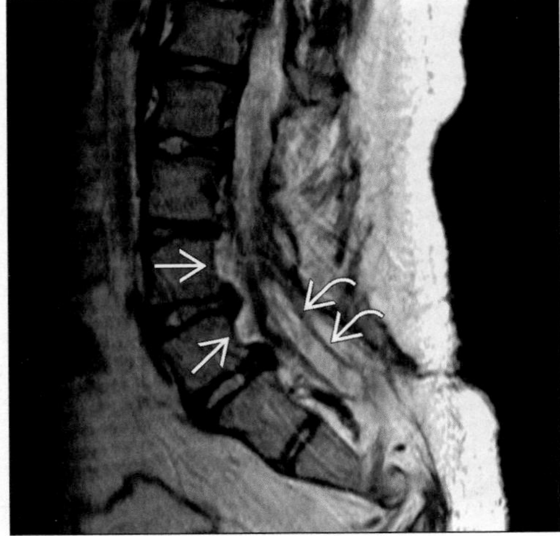

Sagittal T2WI FSE MR shows dorsal vertebral body scalloping ➡ and syrinx involving the distal neural placode ➡ in a child with a prior myelomeningocele repair.

SCALLOPED VERTEBRAL BODIES

Achondroplasia

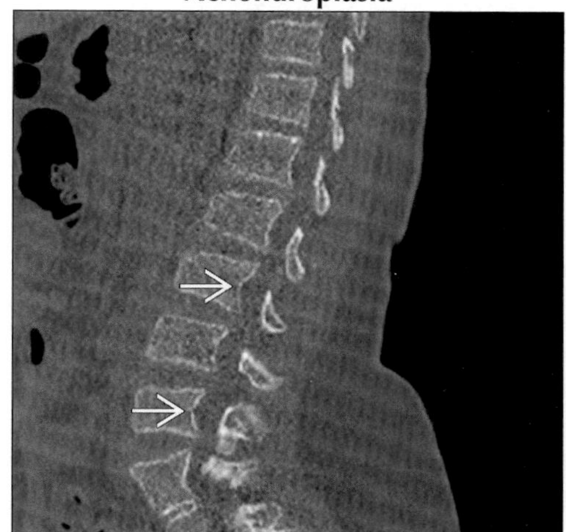

Achondroplasia

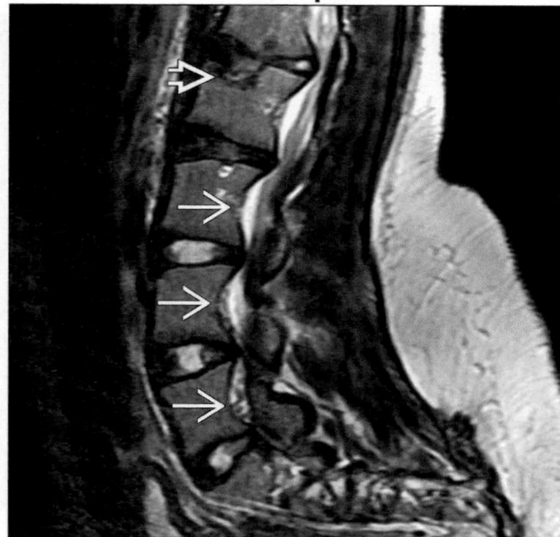

(Left) Sagittal reformat NECT demonstrates multilevel vertebral body scalloping ➔ and severe spinal stenosis in a child with achondroplasia. (Right) Sagittal T2WI FSE MR shows dorsal vertebral body scalloping ➔, severe spinal stenosis, and endplate disc herniation ⇨ in a child with achondroplasia.

Mucopolysaccharidoses

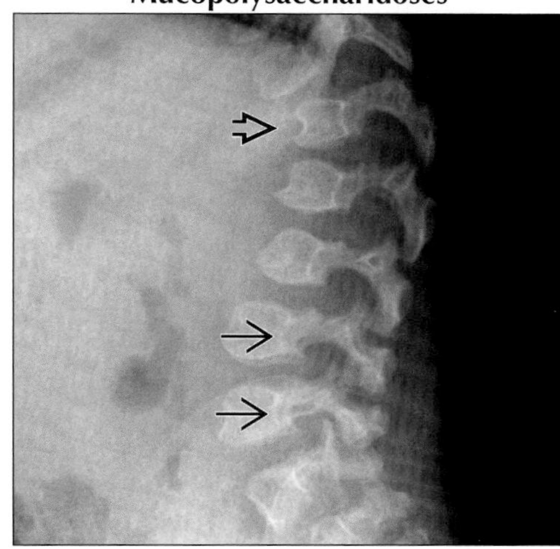

Dural Dysplasia

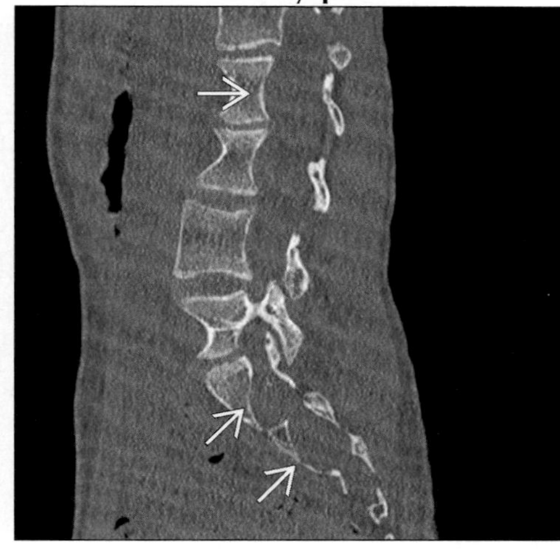

(Left) Sagittal radiograph shows widening of the lumbar canal, scalloping of the vertebral bodies →, and gibbus deformity at the thoracolumbar junction, secondary to abnormal, bullet-shaped upper lumbar vertebrae ⇨. (Right) Sagittal reformat NECT clearly defines vertebral scalloping and neural foraminal enlargement ➔ secondary to diffuse lumbosacral dural dysplasia in a teenager with Marfan syndrome.

Syringomyelia

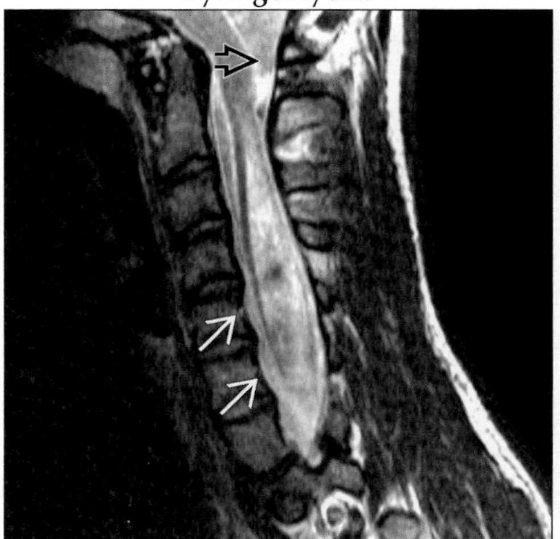

Intraspinal Mass

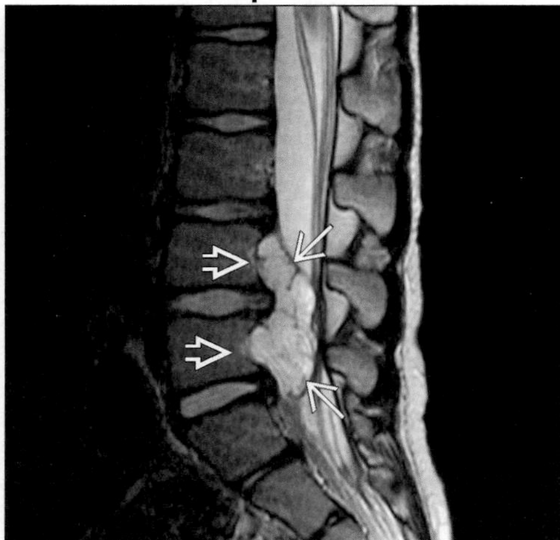

(Left) Sagittal T2WI FSE MR shows enlargement of the cervical canal, dorsal vertebral body scalloping ➔, and syrinx in a child with Chiari 1 ⇨. (Right) Sagittal T2WI FSE MR depicts a mildly heterogeneous intraspinal chordoma ➔ as the cause of smooth dorsal vertebral body scalloping ⇨ in a child who presented with back pain.

DYSMORPHIC VERTEBRAL BODY

DIFFERENTIAL DIAGNOSIS

Common

- Single Vertebral Body
  - Post-Traumatic Deformity
  - Schmorl Node
  - Limbus Vertebra
  - Lytic Osseous Metastases
- Multiple but not all Vertebral Bodies
  - Abnormal Segmentation
    - Partial Vertebral Duplication
    - Vertebral Segmentation Failure
    - Klippel-Feil Spectrum
  - Scheuermann Disease
  - Scoliosis
  - Lytic Osseous Metastases
  - Juvenile Idiopathic Arthritis
  - Neurogenic (Charcot) Arthropathy
  - Post-Radiation Changes
- Diffusely Abnormal Vertebral Bodies
  - Sickle Cell
  - Osteogenesis Imperfecta
  - Achondroplasia

Less Common

- Single Vertebral Body
  - Kümmell Disease
  - Osteochondroma
  - Ewing Sarcoma
  - Langerhans Cell Histiocytosis
- Multiple Vertebral Bodies
  - Pyogenic Osteomyelitis
  - Granulomatous Osteomyelitis
- Diffusely Abnormal Vertebral Bodies
  - Thanatophoric Dwarfism
  - Mucopolysaccharidoses

ESSENTIAL INFORMATION

Key Differential Diagnosis Issues

- Single vertebrae with abnormal appearance usually post-traumatic
- 2 or more adjacent vertebrae with abnormal appearance usually segmentation anomaly

Helpful Clues for Common Diagnoses

- Scheuermann disease causes undulating appearance of vertebral endplates
- Cushing disease causes cupping deformity of vertebral endplates
- Infection and neurogenic arthropathy are centered on intervertebral disc and show endplate erosions
- Juvenile idiopathic arthritis results in vertebral bodies that are tall relative to anteroposterior diameter
- Kümmell disease distinguished by gas in vertebral body
- Sickle cell causes "Lincoln Log" deformity
- Mucopolysaccharidoses and achondroplasia cause "bullet vertebrae" with anterior portion of body small
- Vertebral bodies near apex of a scoliosis often mildly misshapen
- Tumors involving only part of vertebral body may cause a dysmorphic appearance due to partial collapse

Schmorl Node

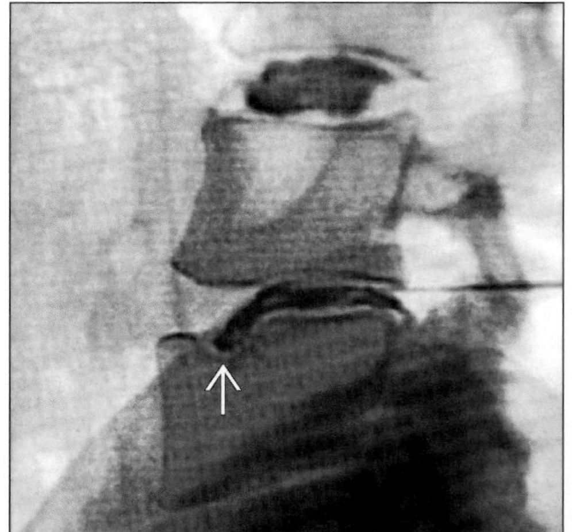

Lateral fluoroscopy shows discographic contrast extending into Schmorl node ➡. Schmorl nodes are caused by disc intravasation into vertebral body.

Limbus Vertebra

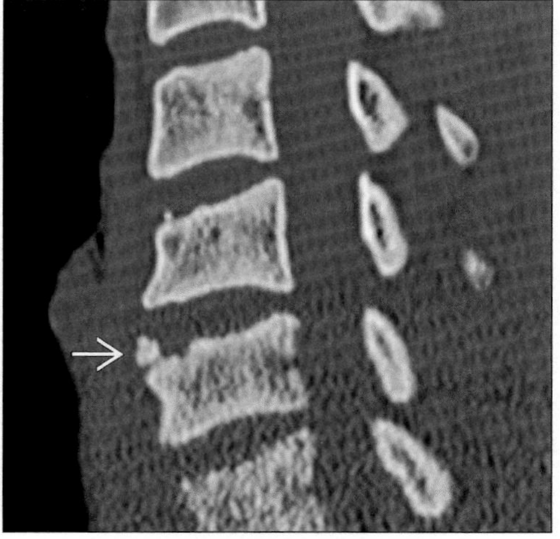

Sagittal bone CT shows a well-marginated ossicle ➡ at the anterior corner of a vertebral body. Limbus vertebra is due to disc herniating between vertebral body and ring apophysis, preventing normal fusion.

Vertebral Segmentation Failure

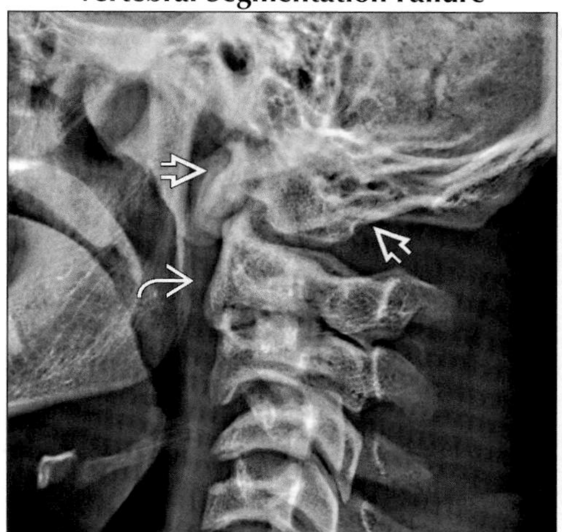

Scheuermann Disease

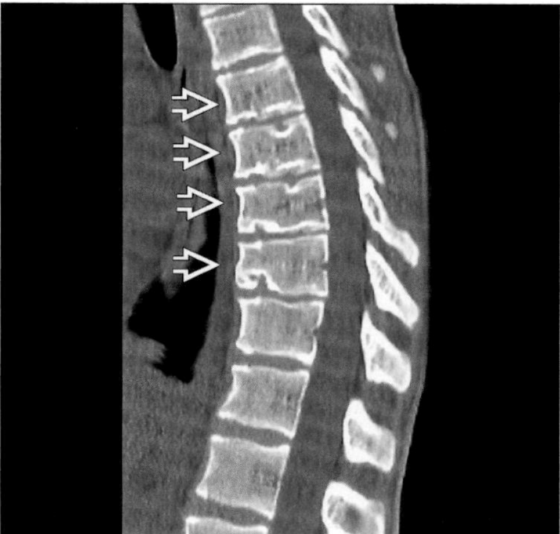

(Left) *Lateral radiograph shows congenital fusion of occiput and C1, with resultant abnormal motion causing a dysmorphic appearance of C2. C4 and C5 are flatter than normal, without definite fusion anomaly.* ***(Right)*** *Sagittal bone CT shows mild anterior wedging and irregular vertebral endplates due to multiple Schmorl nodes, characteristic of Scheuermann kyphosis.*

Juvenile Idiopathic Arthritis

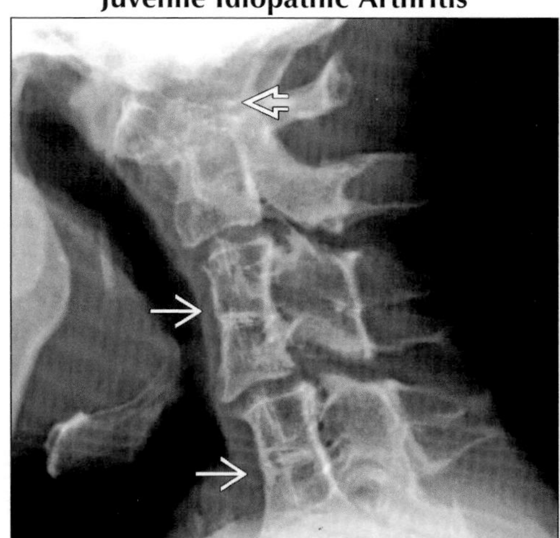

Sickle Cell

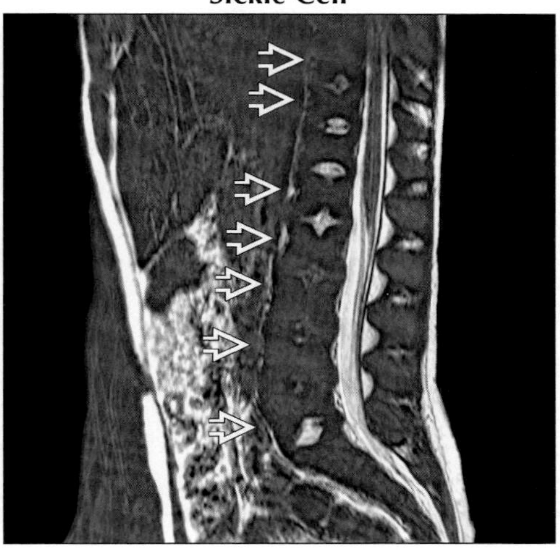

(Left) *Lateral radiograph shows fused vertebrae with narrow AP diameter due to growth failure. Erosion of dens is a clue to the diagnosis.* ***(Right)*** *Sagittal T2WI MR shows "Lincoln Log" appearance of almost all the included vertebrae, with preserved peripheral body height and central flattening reflecting bone infarcts.*

Osteochondroma

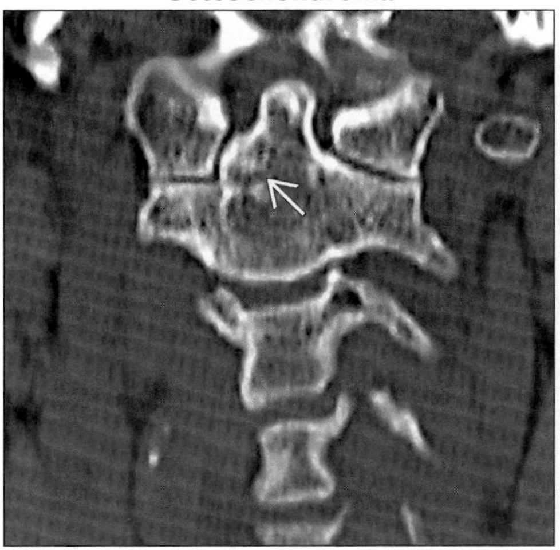

Granulomatous Osteomyelitis

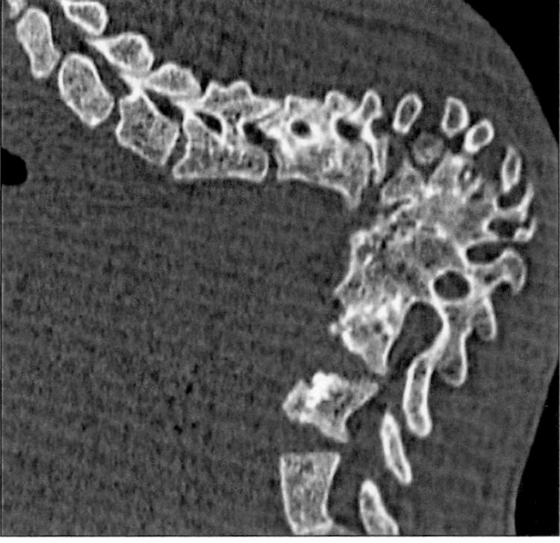

(Left) *Coronal bone CT shows an osteochondroma of C2, causing deformity of both the C2 and C1. Osteochondromas of the spine are very rare, even in patients with multiple hereditary exostoses.* ***(Right)*** *Sagittal bone CT shows multiple, fused, misshapen vertebrae and kyphosis due to tuberculosis.*

SPINAL DYSRAPHIC LESION

DIFFERENTIAL DIAGNOSIS

Common
- Incomplete Fusion, Posterior Element
- Myelomeningocele
- Lipomyelomeningocele (LMM)
- Lipomyelocele (LM)

Less Common
- Diastematomyelia
- Dorsal Dermal Sinus

Rare but Important
- Meningocele, Dorsal Spinal
- Terminal Myelocystocele
- Segmental Spinal Dysgenesis

ESSENTIAL INFORMATION

Key Differential Diagnosis Issues
- Spina bifida: Incomplete closure of posterior bony elements
- Spina bifida aperta = spina bifida cystica: Protrusion of spinal canal elements through posterior bony defect
  - Simple meningocele: Dura and arachnoid, no neural elements
  - Myelocele: Midline plaque of neural tissue exposed, flush with skin surface
  - Myelomeningocele: Myelocele protrudes above skin surface + expansion of subarachnoid space posterior to placode
- Occult spinal dysraphisms develop beneath intact skin surface
  - Meningocele, diastematomyelia, split notochord syndrome, dorsal dermal sinus, fibrolipoma of filum terminale, spinal lipoma, lumbosacral hypogenesis, segmental spinal dysgenesis, myelocystocele

Helpful Clues for Common Diagnoses
- **Incomplete Fusion, Posterior Element**
  - Key facts: Spina bifida occulta
  - Imaging
    - Incomplete fusion of spinous process/lamina without underlying neural or dural abnormality
  - Lumbosacral > cervical > thoracic
- **Myelomeningocele**
  - Key facts: Open neural tube defect, lacks skin coverage
    - Level of dysraphism determines neurological deficit
    - Rarely image spine preoperatively
    - Postoperative spinal imaging if neurological decline despite adequate treatment of hydrocephalus or if neurologic exam suggests additional underlying lesions
  - Imaging
    - CSF sac and neural elements protrude through wide osseous dysraphism
    - Fetal elongation of low-lying cord, usually in dorsal aspect of canal deep to skin-covered postoperative repair
  - Associated abnormalities
    - Chiari 2 malformation (≈ 100%)
    - Hydrocephalus, kyphoscoliosis, segmentation anomalies, diastematomyelia and dermal sinus, syrinx, intraspinal dermoid/epidermoid, orthopedic abnormalities
- **Lipomyelomeningocele (LMM)/Lipomyelocele (LM)**
  - Key facts: Cutaneous stigmata in up to 50%; hemangioma, dimple, dermal sinus, skin tag, or hairy patch
  - Imaging
    - LMM = spinal subarachnoid space expanded ventrally → placode, tethered cord, subarachnoid space, and dura extend dorsally through spina bifida
    - LM = tethered cord and junction between placode and lipoma within spinal canal, lipoma through bony defect
    - Lipoma attached to dorsal aspect of neural placode and contiguous with SQ fat
    - Dorsal and ventral nerve roots exit from ventral surface of placode
    - ± segmentation anomalies, sacral anomalies, syrinx, diastematomyelia, anorectal and GU abnormalities
- **Diastematomyelia**
  - Key facts: Majority between T9 and S1
  - Imaging
    - Split cord malformation (SCM) = sagittal split into 2 hemicords ± fibrous, osteocartilaginous, or osseous spur
    - Pang type 1 SCM = separate dural sac, arachnoid space around each hemicord, separated by fibrous/osseous spur

- Pang type 2 SCM = single dural sac and arachnoid space without spur ± adherent fibrous bands tethering cord
- Nearly all reunite below split
- ± thick filum, tethered cord, syringohydromyelia in 1 or both hemicords, myelocele, or MM
- ± intersegmental laminar fusion ≈ pathognomonic for diastematomyelia

Helpful Clues for Less Common Diagnoses

- **Dorsal Dermal Sinus**
  - Key facts
    - Midline or rarely paramedian dimple or pinpoint ostium ± pigmented patch, hairy nevus, or cutaneous hemangioma
    - Differentiate from simple sacral dimple (< 2.5 cm from anus, extends inferiorly toward coccyx) and pilonidal sinus (low ostium, does not enter spine)
    - High suspicion if dimple above intergluteal fold
  - Imaging
    - ↓ curvilinear tract through ↑ SQ fat
    - May end in SQ tissue or extend into canal, terminating in conus medullaris, subarachnoid space, filum terminale, nerve root, fibrous nodule on surface of cord, or dermoid/epidermoid cyst
    - Dural "tenting" at dural penetration
    - LS > occipital > T > C spine
    - ± varying degrees of dysraphism; incomplete posterior element fusion → multilevel dysraphism
    - ± dermoid/epidermoid, abscess, or arachnoiditis
    - ± cord tethering in lumbosacral lesions

Helpful Clues for Rare Diagnoses

- **Meningocele, Dorsal Spinal**
  - Key facts: Skin covered
  - Imaging
    - Meninges protrude through dysraphism into SQ fat
    - Cord tethering and syrinx rare
- **Terminal Myelocystocele**
  - Key facts: Large skin-covered mass, usually sacral/coccygeal
  - Imaging
    - Hydromyelic tethered cord traverses dorsal meningocele, terminates in dilated terminal ventricle
- **Segmental Spinal Dysgenesis**
  - Key facts: Focal dysmorphic/hypoplastic vertebrae, meninges, and spinal cord with normal spine above and below
  - Imaging
    - Dysplastic vertebrae → severe focal kyphosis
    - Thecal sac narrows and then terminates; spinal cord narrows and disappears rostral to thecal sac
    - Thecal sac reappears below dysplastic segments
    - Spinal cord reappears below reappearance of thecal sac

Incomplete Fusion, Posterior Element

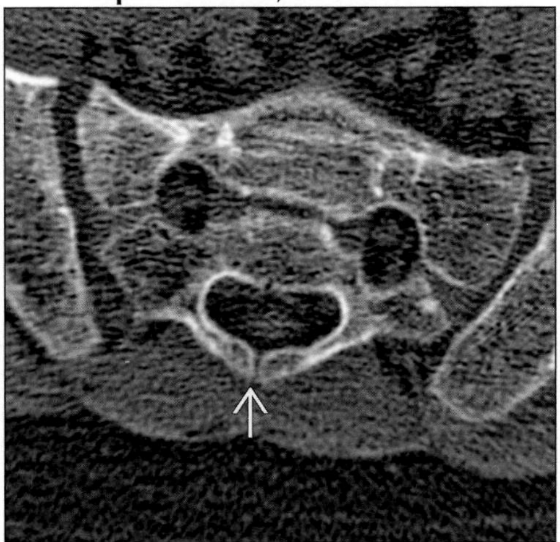

Axial NECT shows incomplete midline fusion of the S2 spinous process ➔.

Myelomeningocele

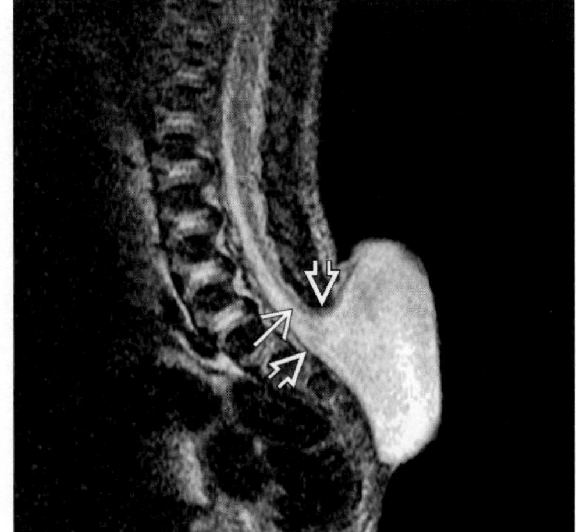

Sagittal T2WI FSE MR shows the low spinal cord ➔ coursing through the dysraphic defect in the upper sacrum ➔, with expansion of the CSF sac, in this infant with open neural tube defect.

(Left) *Sagittal FSE STIR MR shows dysraphic defect and a myelomeningocele sac on a prenatal MR.* ***(Right)*** *Sagittal T1WI MR shows fetal elongation of the cord extending to the level of the postoperative/posterior dysraphic defect in a patient with prior repair of sacral myelomeningocele.*

Myelomeningocele

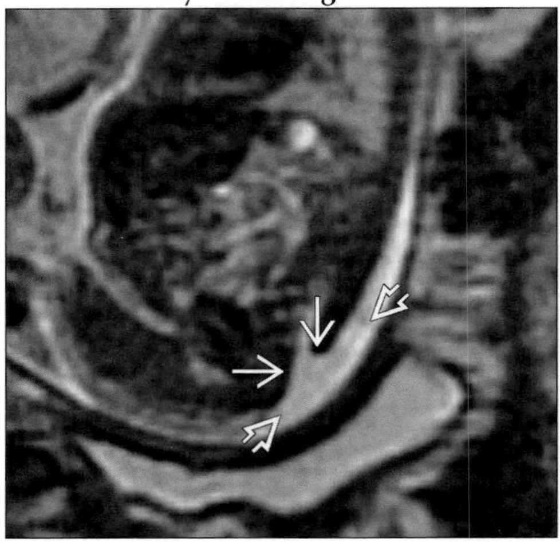

Myelomeningocele

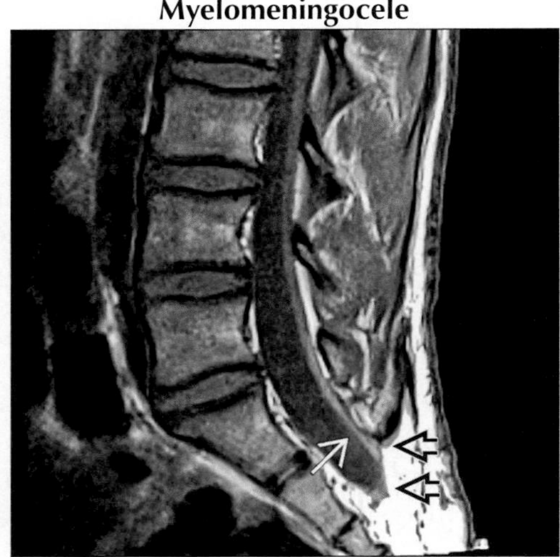

(Left) *Sagittal T1WI MR shows the low-lying cord with neural elements and intraspinal lipoma extending through a lumbar dysraphic defect, with a small CSF sac within the subcutaneous lipomatous mass. Note that the intraspinal lipoma is contiguous with the subcutaneous fat.* ***(Right)*** *Axial T1WI MR shows contiguity of the intraspinal lipoma with the subcutaneous fat and extension of neural tissue through the bony defect.*

Lipomyelomeningocele (LMM)

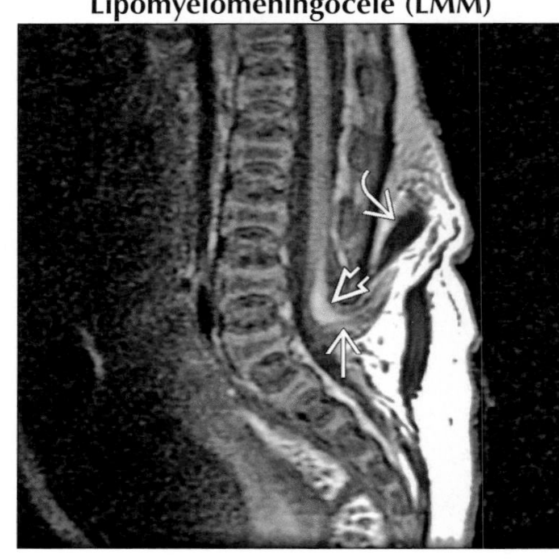

Lipomyelomeningocele (LMM)

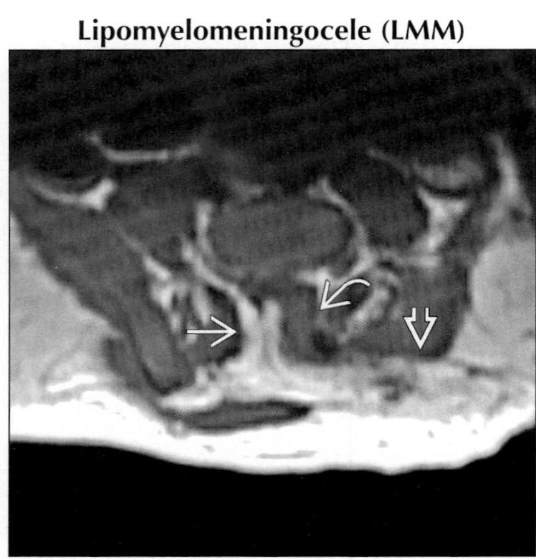

(Left) *Sagittal T1WI MR shows a tethered cord and intraspinal lipoma extending through bony defect, contiguous with subcutaneous fat, without enlargement and extension of CSF sac.* ***(Right)*** *Axial T1WI MR shows split cord malformation with the 2 hemicords separated by a bony spur, indicating Pang type 1 SCM. Note the intraspinal lipoma associated with the left hemicord.*

Lipomyelocele (LM)

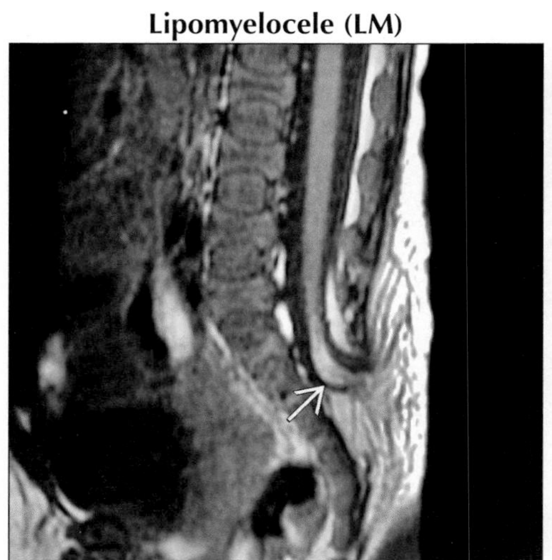

Diastematomyelia

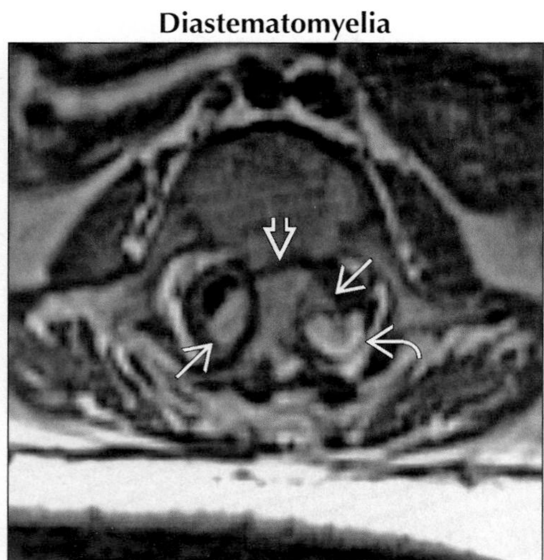

Diastematomyelia

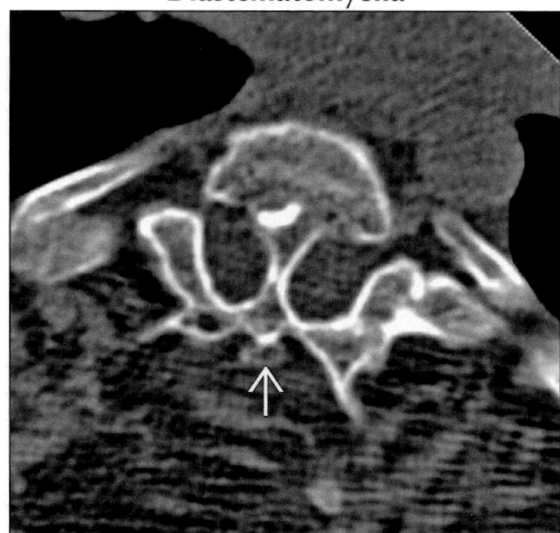

Dorsal Dermal Sinus

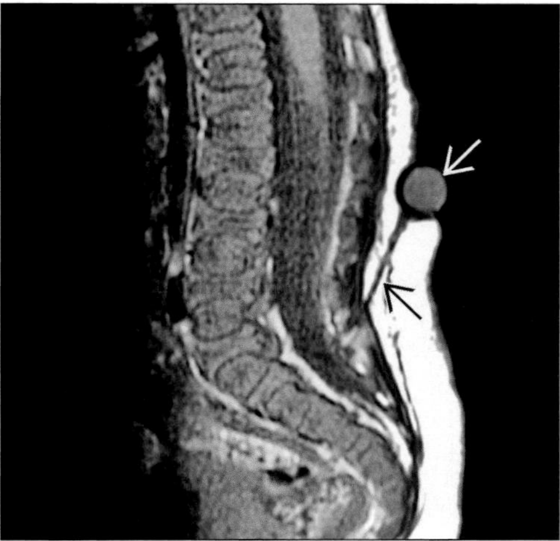

__(Left)__ Axial NECT shows a dense bony spur → separating 2 thecal sacs in this patient with diastematomyelia. __(Right)__ Sagittal T1WI MR shows a dorsal dermal sinus without cord tethering. A small vitamin E capsule marks the level of the dermal sinus opening at the skin surface →. The hypointense dermal sinus descends through the subcutaneous fat → to the interspinous space at the lumbosacral junction, without intraspinal abnormality.

Dorsal Dermal Sinus

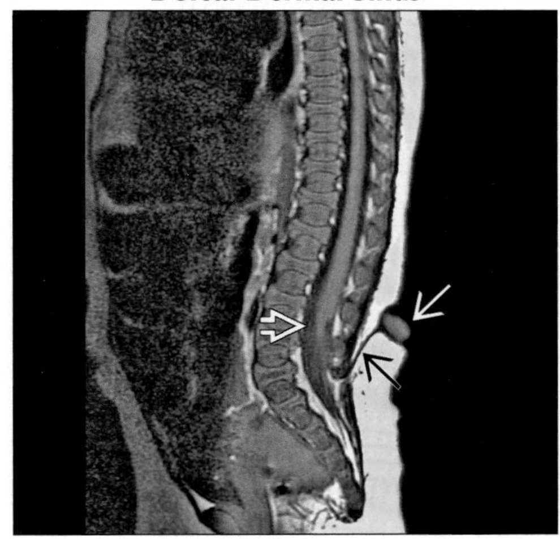

Dorsal Dermal Sinus

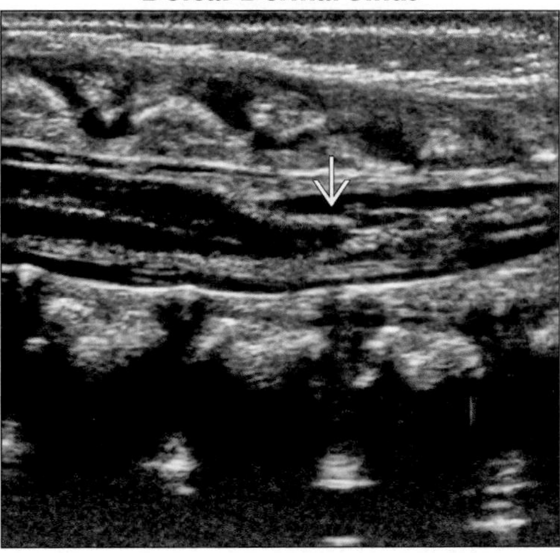

__(Left)__ Sagittal T1WI MR shows a vitamin E capsule marking the opening of a dermal sinus at the skin surface →. The dermal sinus → traverses the subcutaneous fat and enters the dorsal canal at the lumbosacral junction. Note the associated tethering of the spinal cord →. __(Right)__ Longitudinal ultrasound in the same patient shows low conus → at the upper aspect of L5, without adequate visualization of the dorsal dermal sinus.

Meningocele, Dorsal Spinal

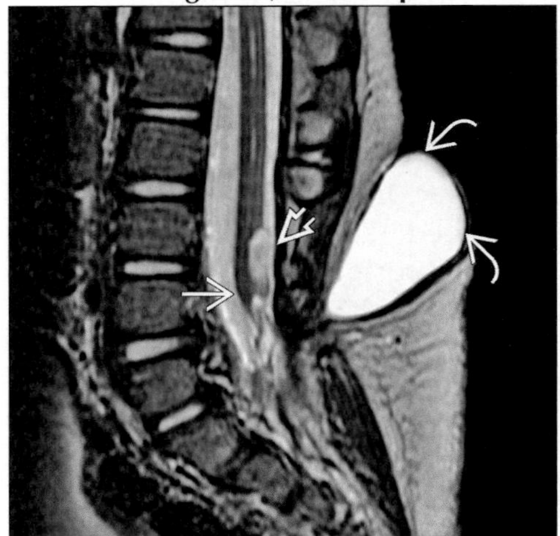

Terminal Myelocystocele

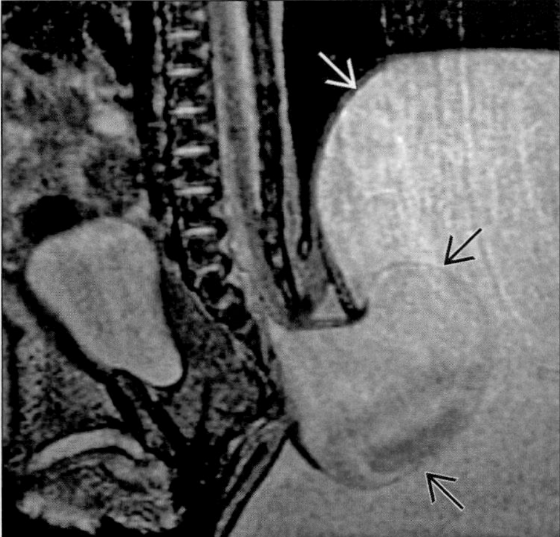

__(Left)__ Sagittal T2WI FSE MR shows a tethered cord →, intraspinal epidermoid →, and meningocele → without neural elements protruding through dysraphic defect. __(Right)__ Sagittal T2WI FSE MR shows terminal myelocystocele → and adjacent meningocele →.

CONGENITAL AND ACQUIRED CHILDHOOD PLATYSPONDYLY

DIFFERENTIAL DIAGNOSIS

Common
- Trauma
- Langerhans Cell Histiocytosis
- Leukemia
- Metastatic Disease
- Ewing Sarcoma

Less Common
- Achondroplasia (Homozygous)
- Osteogenesis Imperfecta
- Pseudoachondroplasia
- Mucopolysaccharidoses
- Radiation-Induced
- Spondyloepiphyseal Dysplasia

Rare but Important
- Homocystinuria
- Idiopathic Juvenile Osteoporosis
- Cushing Disease
- Thanatophoric Dwarfism
- Metatropic Dwarfism
- Kniest Dysplasia
- Short Rib Polydactyly
- Hypophosphatasia

ESSENTIAL INFORMATION

Key Differential Diagnosis Issues
- Platyspondyly: Generalized vertebral collapse maintaining relatively parallel endplates
- Differentiating features: Congenital presentation vs. childhood onset; diffuse collapse vs. solitary or multifocal collapse

Helpful Clues for Common Diagnoses
- **Trauma**
  - Solitary or multifocal, history diagnostic
  - Any age
- **Langerhans Cell Histiocytosis**
  - Childhood; thoracic spine main site
  - Solitary or few vertebra involved
  - May reconstitute during healing
- **Leukemia**
  - Age 2-5 years
  - Variable presentations
    - Generalized osteoporosis, diffuse collapse
    - Focal lesion(s) with permeative destruction, periostitis, soft tissue mass; collapse solitary or multifocal
  - Metaphyseal bands (lucent, dense, or alternating), may involve vertebra
- **Metastatic Disease**
  - Neuroblastoma, retinoblastoma, Wilms
  - ± soft tissue mass, skeletal imaging nonspecific
- **Ewing Sarcoma**
  - Teens, young adults
  - Solitary lesion
  - Permeative destruction, soft tissue mass

Helpful Clues for Less Common Diagnoses
- **Achondroplasia (Homozygous)**
  - Radiographically and clinically mimics thanatophoric dwarfism
  - Both parents have achondroplasia
  - Diffuse collapse
  - Congenital presentation
- **Osteogenesis Imperfecta**
  - Generalized osteoporosis
  - Solitary, multiple, or diffuse vertebra involved
    - Depends on severity of disease
    - Younger patients at presentation have more extensive disease
    - May be congenital
  - Multiple fractures axial and appendicular skeleton
  - Congenital platyspondyly type 2A
  - Micromelia, short ribs
- **Pseudoachondroplasia**
  - Rhizomelic dwarf
  - Normal infancy, manifests by age 2-3 years
  - As child develops, mimics spondyloepiphyseal dysplasia
  - Diffuse collapse develops during childhood
- **Mucopolysaccharidoses**
  - Short stature, diffuse skeletal dysplasia
  - Coarse facial features
  - Diffuse collapse
  - Congenital presentation
  - Morquio, Hunter best known
    - Mental retardation with Hunter
- **Radiation-Induced**
  - Regional osteoporosis
  - May affect only 1 side of vertebra
    - ± scoliosis
  - May induce osteochondroma formation
- **Spondyloepiphyseal Dysplasia**
  - Truncal dwarfism
  - Diffuse spine deformities
  - Delayed ossification long bone epiphyses

- Coxa vara consistent feature of variable severity
- Congenita: Congenital presentation
- Tarda: Develops around puberty
  - Spine changes are not dominant feature

Helpful Clues for Rare Diagnoses

- **Homocystinuria**
  - Nonspecific osteoporosis
  - Scoliosis
  - Diffuse collapse develops in childhood
  - Body habitus mimics Marfan
  - Mental retardation
- **Idiopathic Juvenile Osteoporosis**
  - Typically > 2 years
  - Axial and appendicular osteoporosis
    - Complicated by fractures
    - Spine involvement solitary, multifocal, diffuse
  - May mimic osteogenesis imperfecta tarda
- **Cushing Disease**
  - Rare in children
  - Produces generalized osteoporosis
    - Solitary or multifocal collapse, especially thoracic and lumbar spine
  - May develop osteonecrosis
- **Thanatophoric Dwarfism**
  - Most common lethal bone dysplasia
    - Occurs in 1:10,000 births
    - Fatal within hours to days after birth from respiratory failure
  - Rhizomelic dwarf
    - Micromelia, short ribs
  - Diffuse collapse
    - Excessive intervertebral disc space heights
  - Congenital presentation
  - Telephone receiver femurs (bowing, metaphyseal flaring)
- **Metatropic Dwarfism**
  - Metatropic: Changing
    - Early life short limb, normal trunk
    - Later life short trunk with severe kyphoscoliosis
  - Characteristic short long bones with dramatic metaphyseal flaring
  - Diffuse collapse
  - Congenital presentation
- **Kniest Dysplasia**
  - Short trunk, short limb, large joints
  - Diffuse collapse develops in childhood
- **Short Rib Polydactyly**
  - Lethal dwarfism
  - Short ribs, micromelia, polydactyly
  - Diffuse changes
  - Congenital presentation
  - Includes asphyxiating thoracic dystrophy (Jeune) and Ellis-van Creveld
- **Hypophosphatasia**
  - Varying degrees of poor bone mineralization
  - Congenital (lethal)
    - Diffuse collapse
  - Variable degree and number collapsed vertebra with later presentations

Langerhans Cell Histiocytosis

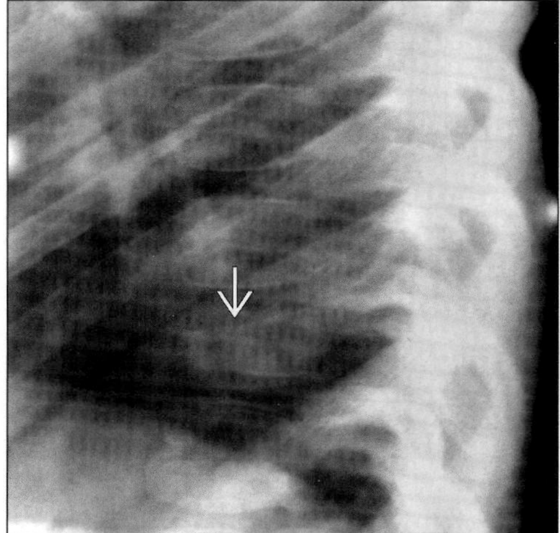

Lateral radiograph shows partial collapse of thoracic vertebral body ➔. The endplates are intact as are the disc spaces and posterior elements. The appearance is common in Langerhans cell histiocytosis.

Langerhans Cell Histiocytosis

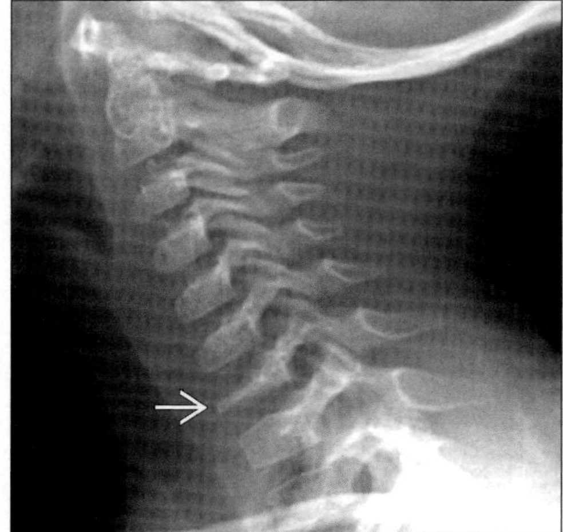

Lateral radiograph shows typical presentation of Langerhans cell histiocytosis with vertebra plana at C7 ➔. Following treatment, this body partially reconstituted its height.

CONGENITAL AND ACQUIRED CHILDHOOD PLATYSPONDYLY

Leukemia

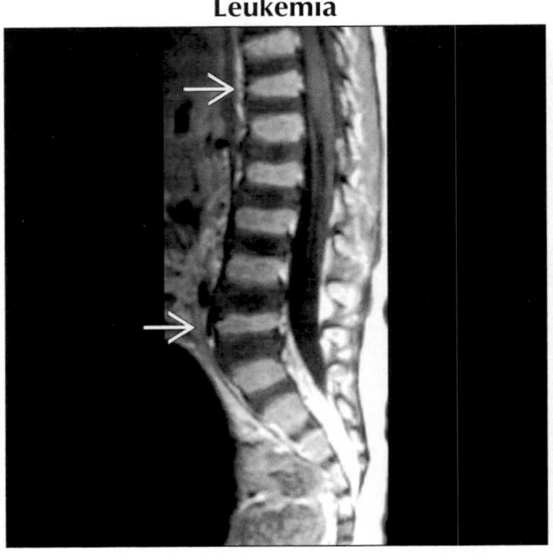

Leukemia

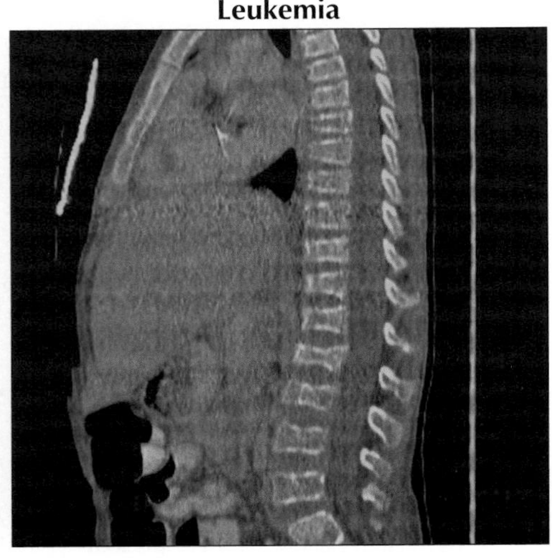

(Left) *Sagittal T1WI C+ MR shows the typical appearance of leukemic marrow infiltration with height loss of varying degrees involving all vertebral bodies ➔. Notice the contrast enhancement of all the vertebral bodies in this child.* ***(Right)*** *Sagittal reformat CECT shows severe osteopenia and diffuse vertebral compressions. This child presented with these compression fractures and proximal femoral metaphyseal bands.*

Ewing Sarcoma

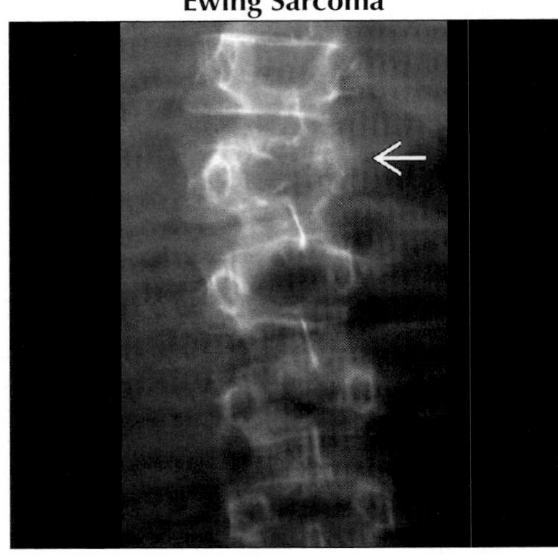

Osteogenesis Imperfecta

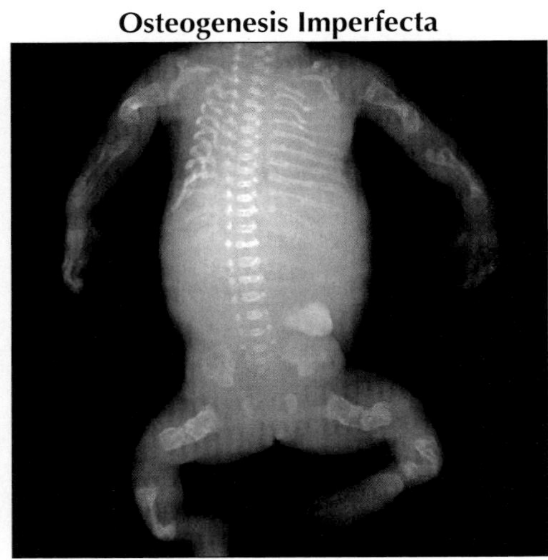

(Left) *Anteroposterior radiograph shows asymmetric platyspondyly ➔ with destruction of the left pedicle in a 12 year old. This proved to be early destruction in Ewing sarcoma.* ***(Right)*** *Anteroposterior radiograph shows multiple rib, vertebral, and long bone fractures in this fetus with osteogenesis imperfecta, type II. The arms and legs are short due to angulation and deformity resulting from the fractures.*

Pseudoachondroplasia

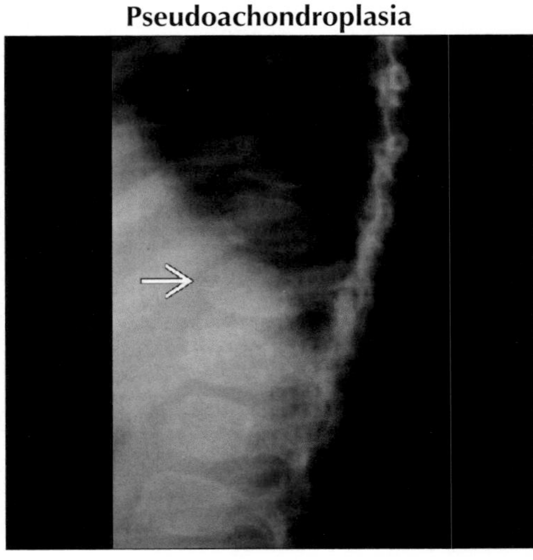

Mucopolysaccharidoses

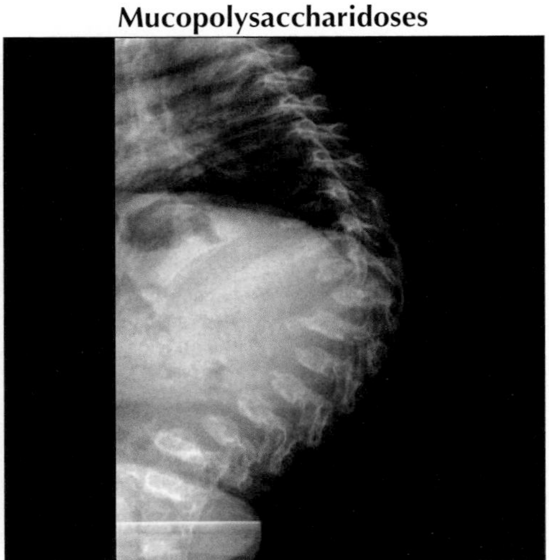

(Left) *Lateral radiograph shows very mild platyspondyly ➔ with mild anterior beaking in this patient with pseudoachondroplasia.* ***(Right)*** *Lateral radiograph shows a classic example of Morquio syndrome, with diffuse vertebral body collapse, dorsolumbar gibbus, and vertebral beaking.*

Radiation-Induced

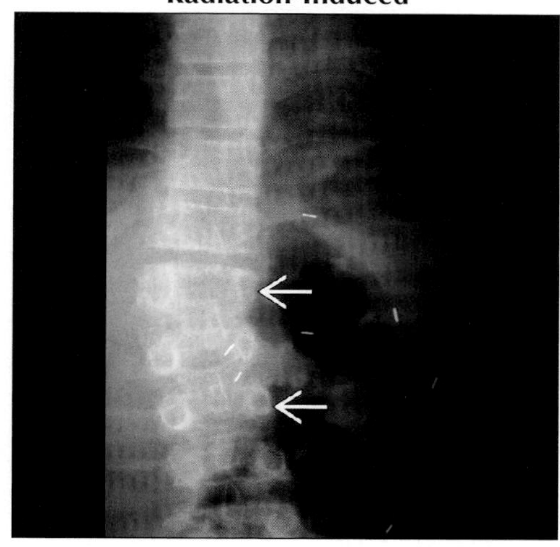

Spondyloepiphyseal Dysplasia

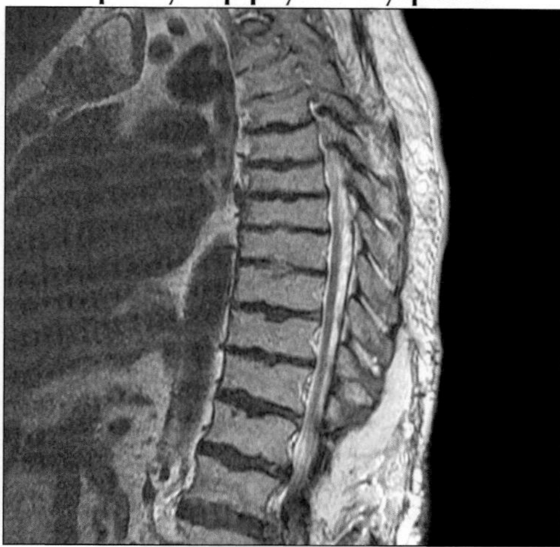

*(**Left**) AP radiograph shows relative hypoplasia of the left side of the T12, L1, L2, and L3 vertebral bodies ➡, creating an asymmetric platyspondyly due to radiation of a left Wilms tumor. Note the clips from the left nephrectomy. (**Right**) Sagittal T2WI MR shows endplate irregularity and diffuse platyspondyly with rectangular-shaped vertebral bodies. There is a generous bony spinal canal dimension. This is the adult appearance of spondyloepiphyseal dysplasia.*

Homocystinuria

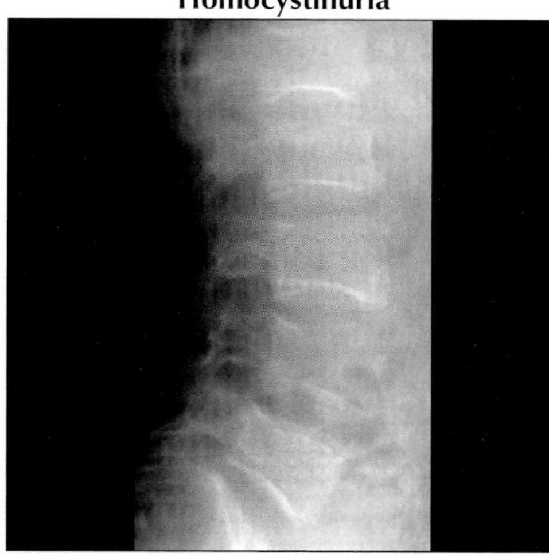

Cushing Disease

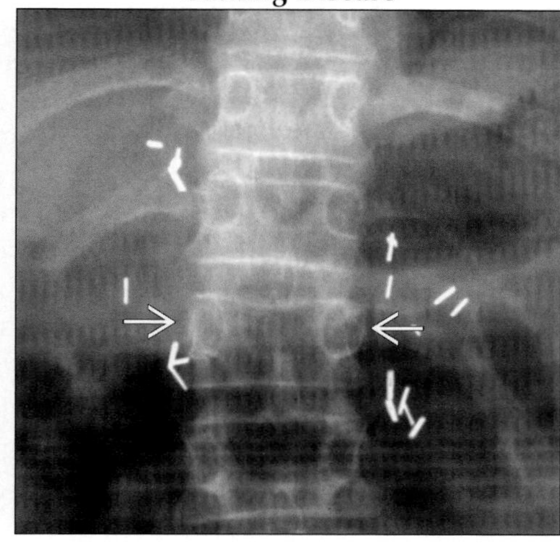

*(**Left**) Lateral radiograph shows diffuse osteopenia and mild generalized platyspondyly. The findings are nonspecific and, in this case, due to homocystinuria. (**Right**) Anteroposterior radiograph shows minimal platyspondyly of T12 ➡. The 11th ribs have been resected as a surgical approach for adrenalectomy in this patient with Cushing disease.*

Thanatophoric Dwarfism

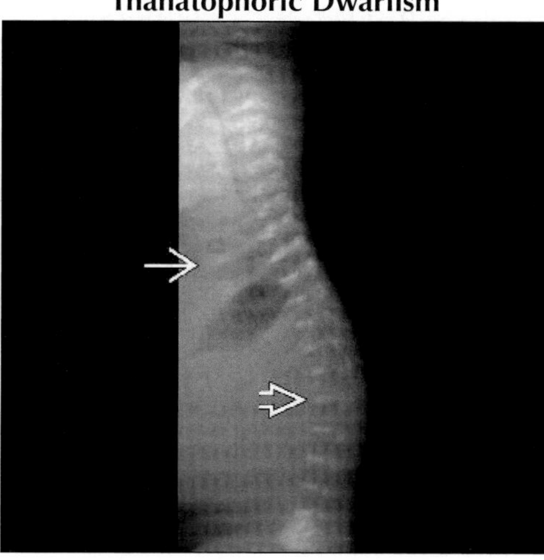

Hypophosphatasia

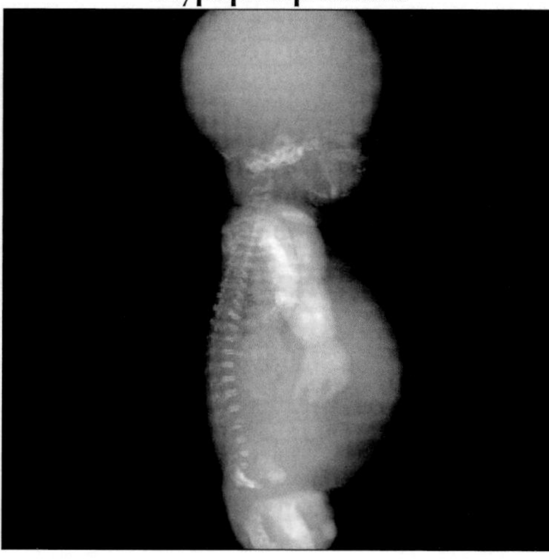

*(**Left**) Lateral radiograph shows short ribs ➡ and classic platyspondyly ⇨, with the widened intervertebral disc spaces associated with many dwarfisms, including thanatophoric dwarfism. (**Right**) Lateral radiograph shows a severe deficit in bone formation. Diffuse platyspondyly is present. The cranium is particularly notable for having no ossification, except at the base of skull, a clue to the diagnosis of hypophosphatasia.*

BACK PAIN

DIFFERENTIAL DIAGNOSIS

Common

- Scoliosis
  - Idiopathic Scoliosis
  - Neuromuscular Scoliosis
  - Congenital Scoliosis
- Trauma
  - Fracture
  - Traumatic Spinal Muscle Injury
- Syringomyelia
- Spondylolysis
- Scheuermann Disease

Less Common

- Congenital Spinal Stenosis
- Guillain-Barré Syndrome
- Neoplasm
  - Lymphoma
  - Neuroblastic Tumor
  - Ewing Sarcoma
  - Myxopapillary Ependymoma, Spinal Cord
  - CSF Disseminated Metastases
  - Hematogenous Metastases
  - Osteoid Osteoma
  - Langerhans Cell Histiocytosis
- Osteomyelitis
  - Granulomatous Osteomyelitis
  - Pyogenic Osteomyelitis

Rare but Important

- Intervertebral Disc Herniation
- Idiopathic Acute Transverse Myelitis
- Secondary Acute Transverse Myelitis

ESSENTIAL INFORMATION

Key Differential Diagnosis Issues

- Clinical history, physical examination, and appropriate laboratory investigations constrain differential considerations

Helpful Clues for Common Diagnoses

- **Scoliosis**
  - **Idiopathic Scoliosis**
    - Usually sigmoid S-shaped
    - Pelvic tilt ⇒ limb-length discrepancy
    - No vertebral segmentation anomalies
  - **Neuromuscular Scoliosis**
    - C-shaped curvature common
    - Baclofen infusion device clue if present
  - **Congenital Scoliosis**
    - Vertebral segmentation and formation anomalies
    - Rib fusions, pedicular bars ⇒ more likely progressive curvature
- **Trauma**
  - **Fracture**
    - Similar criteria to adults
  - **Traumatic Spinal Muscle Injury**
    - MR or CT best for diagnosis
    - T2WI FS MR or STIR MR most helpful for diagnosis, determining extent
- **Syringomyelia**
  - Chiari 1 malformation common association in pediatric patients
  - Always consider traumatic, neoplastic causes
    - Administer contrast if tumor suspected or nodularity detected
- **Spondylolysis**
  - Unilateral or bilateral; may not see osseous break (stress reaction)
  - Oblique plain radiographs, MR show osseous defects well
  - Bone scintigraphy sensitive for detecting stress reaction prior to pars fracture
- **Scheuermann Disease**
  - Most common in adolescent age group
  - Diagnostic criteria include anterior wedging, kyphosis, endplate irregularity
  - May see significant kyphosis ± scoliosis

Helpful Clues for Less Common Diagnoses

- **Congenital Spinal Stenosis**
  - Reduced AP diameter of central spinal canal
  - Pedicles are short, thick, and more laterally angled
  - Predisposes to symptomatic degenerative spine disease at younger age
- **Guillain-Barré Syndrome**
  - Smooth, linear enhancement of cauda equina and conus pia diagnostic in correct clinical context
  - If nodular enhancement, consider tumor or granulomatous infection
- **Neoplasm**
  - **Lymphoma**
    - Hodgkin disease usually seen in adolescents
    - Consider NHL in younger patients
  - **Neuroblastic Tumor**
    - Often diagnosed in younger patients

- Spinal invasion through neural foramina affects surgical treatment planning; MR best for detection
- ○ **Ewing Sarcoma**
  - Usually adolescent age group
  - Aggressive destructive or permeative lesion, cellular MR signal characteristics
- ○ **Myxopapillary Ependymoma, Spinal Cord**
  - May present with chronic or longstanding back pain
  - May have extensive intradural metastases at time of diagnosis
- ○ **CSF Disseminated Metastases**
  - Consider choroid plexus, pineal region, suprasellar, posterior fossa tumors, glial neoplasms, leukemia/lymphoma
  - Most commonly seen in brain tumors with intimate CSF contact
- ○ **Hematogenous Metastases**
  - Relatively rare
  - Consider neuroblastoma, lymphoma, and tumors with bone to bone metastatic patterns (Ewing sarcoma, osteosarcoma)
- ○ **Osteoid Osteoma**
  - Pain classically worst at night
  - Symptoms alleviated with aspirin
- ○ **Langerhans Cell Histiocytosis**
  - May mimic neoplasm symptoms, imaging appearance (small, round blue cell tumor)
  - Classic etiology of severe vertebra plana
  - Vertebral height often makes surprising recovery after treatment

- **Osteomyelitis**
  - ○ **Granulomatous Osteomyelitis**
    - May be centered at disc space; TB tends to spare disc space until late in disease process
    - Look for paravertebral masses with TB
  - ○ **Pyogenic Osteomyelitis**
    - Frequently centered in intervertebral disc space
    - Abnormal marrow signal intensity, paraspinal inflammatory mass

Helpful Clues for Rare Diagnoses

- **Intervertebral Disc Herniation**
  - ○ Diagnostic criteria identical to adults
- **Idiopathic Acute Transverse Myelitis**
  - ○ Idiopathic inflammatory spinal cord disorder ⇒ bilateral motor, sensory, and autonomic dysfunction
  - ○ Central cord lesion extends > 2 vertebral segments (often 3-4 segments), eccentric enhancement
  - ○ Thoracic > cervical cord (10%)
- **Secondary Acute Transverse Myelitis**
  - ○ Inflammatory disorder of spinal cord associated with many etiologies
  - ○ Hyperintense lesion on T2WI with mild cord expansion without significant enhancement
  - ○ Thoracic > cervical > conus medullaris

Idiopathic Scoliosis

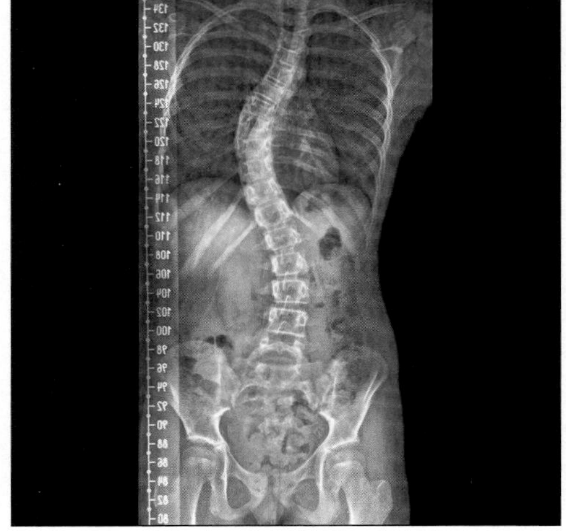

Anteroposterior radiograph in a female adolescent patient shows substantial S-shaped idiopathic thoracic dextroscoliotic curvature with lumbar levoscoliosis.

Neuromuscular Scoliosis

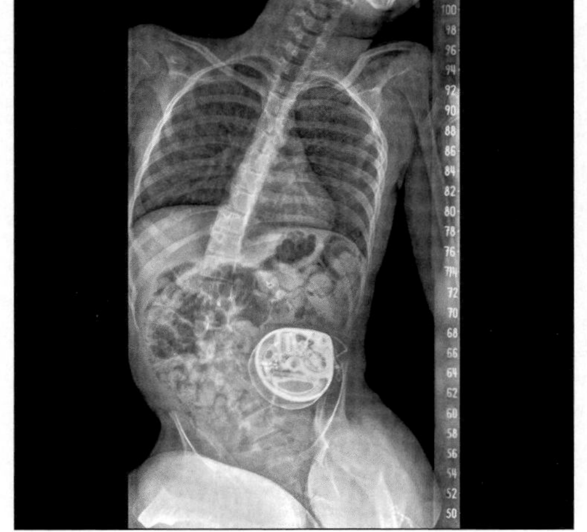

Anteroposterior radiograph in a cerebral palsy patient with spasticity shows convex right C-shaped neuromuscular scoliosis. Note the baclofen infusion system for spasticity treatment.

BACK PAIN

(Left) *Coronal bone CT 3D reformats in a VACTERL patient with convex right spinal curvature demonstrates multiple rib fusions on the left, upper thoracic block vertebra, T7 and T12 hemivertebra ➔, and T9 butterfly vertebra ➔.* ***(Right)*** *Sagittal T1WI MR in a patient with Chiari 1 malformation shows a large cervical syrinx. Despite this sacculated appearance, the syrinx fluid compartments are in contiguity and would likely respond to a single catheter drain.*

Congenital Scoliosis

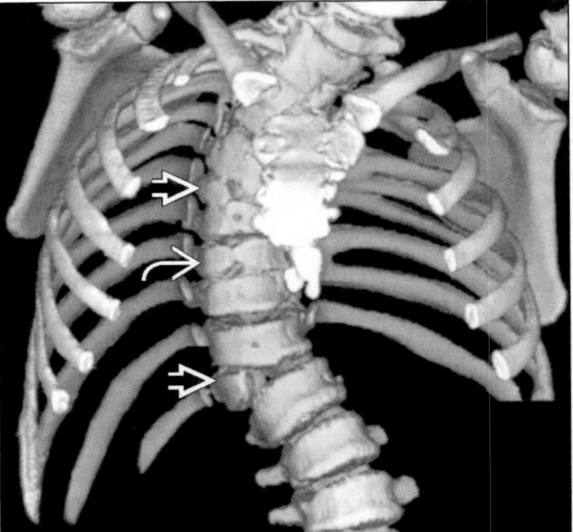

Syringomyelia

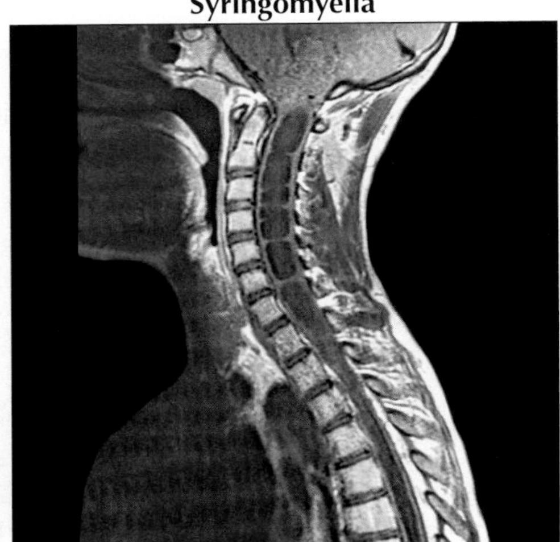

(Left) *Sagittal bone CT in a pediatric patient with back pain reveals an L5 pars defect ➔ with minimal anterior subluxation of L5 on S1.* ***(Right)*** *Sagittal bone CT in an adolescent patient depicts multilevel anterior wedging with endplate irregularities of Scheuermann disease producing rounded kyphotic thoracic deformity.*

Spondylolysis

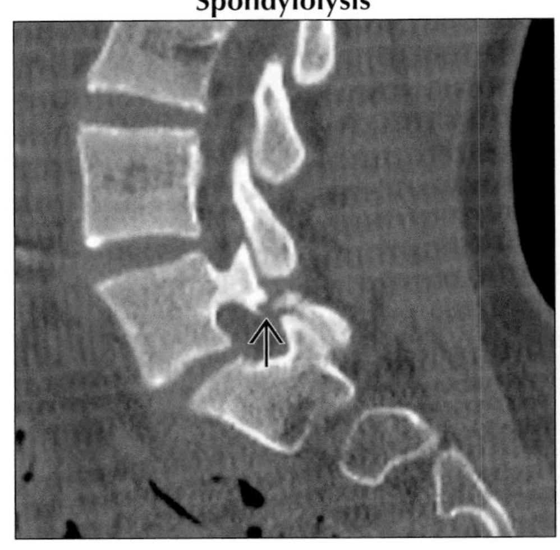

Scheuermann Disease

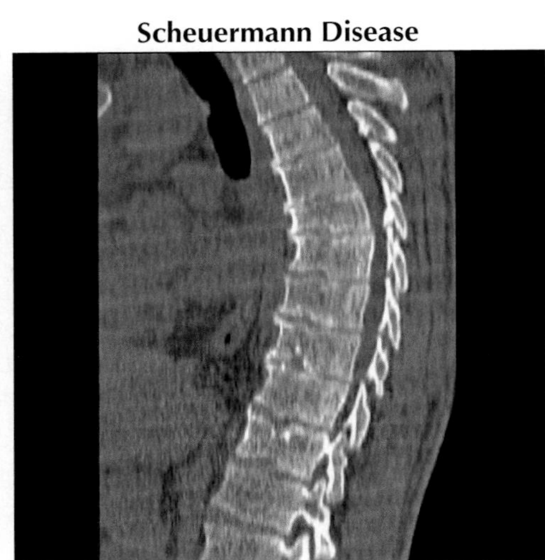

(Left) *Sagittal T2WI MR demonstrates marked narrowing of the lumbar spinal canal anteroposterior diameter. Anteroposterior canal diameter should normally increase rather than decrease in the lower lumbar spine.* ***(Right)*** *Sagittal T1WI C+ MR in a patient with ascending paralysis demonstrates the avid, smooth, linear enhancement of the ventral conus pia and cauda equina.*

Congenital Spinal Stenosis

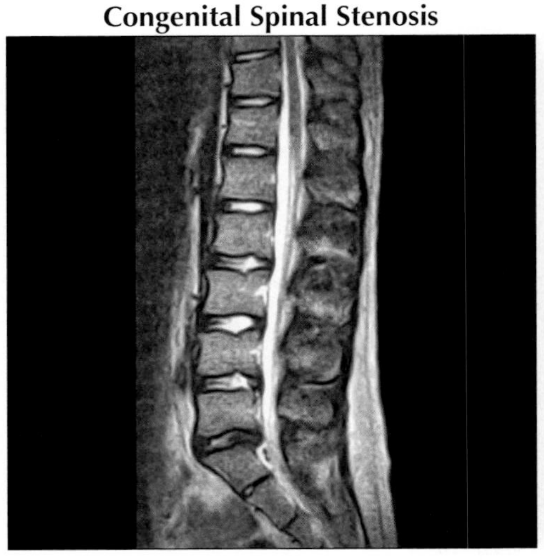

Guillain-Barré Syndrome

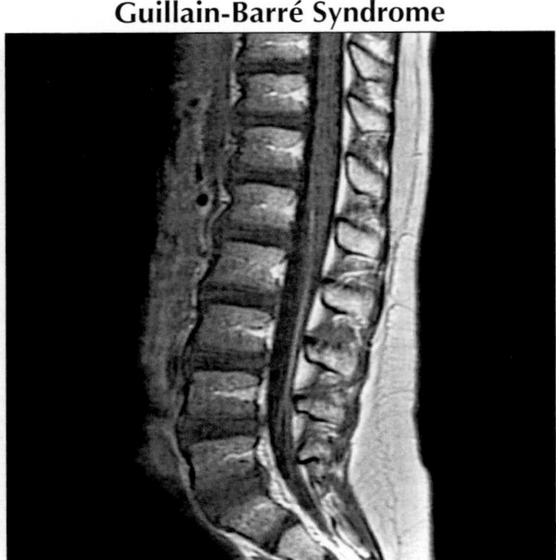

Lymphoma

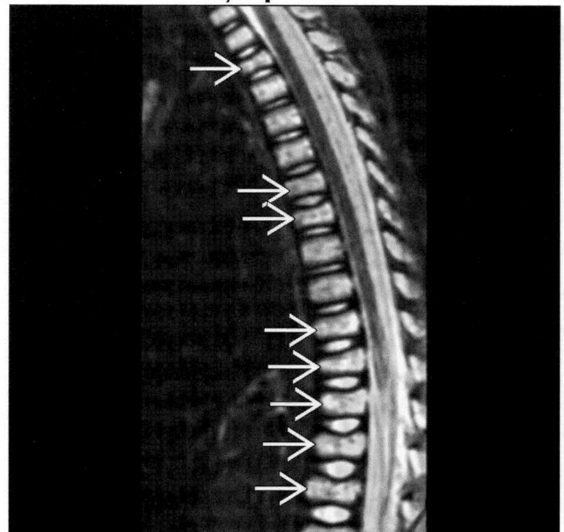

Myxopapillary Ependymoma, Spinal Cord

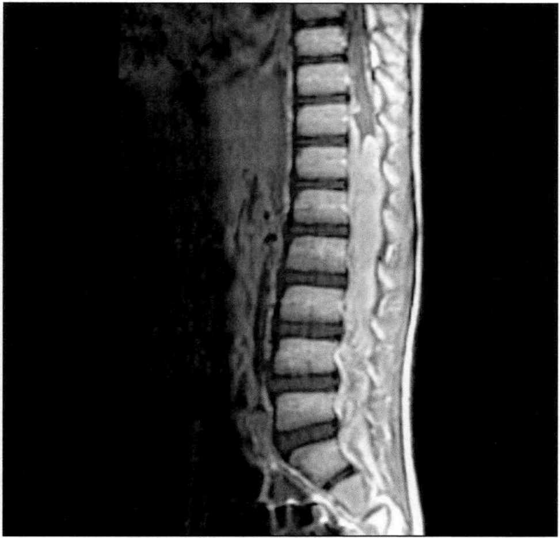

(Left) *Sagittal STIR MR in a newly diagnosed patient reveals abnormal hyperintense marrow signal and numerous vertebral compression fractures* ➡. ***(Right)*** *Sagittal T1 C+ MR reveals diffuse abnormal intradural enhancement within thecal sac, obscuring conus termination and cauda equina and distorting normal conus and cauda equina.*

CSF Disseminated Metastases

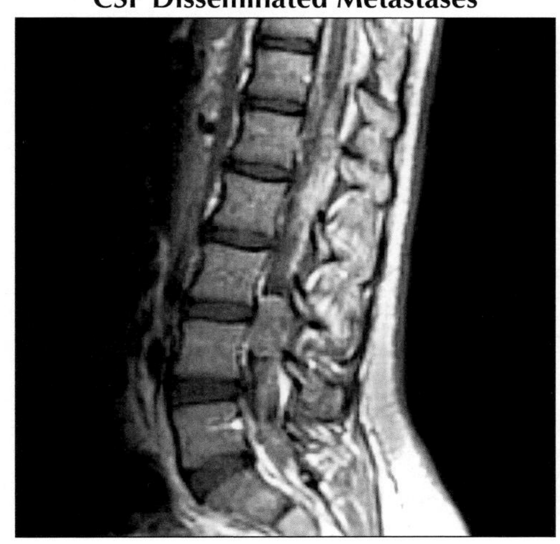

Osteoid Osteoma

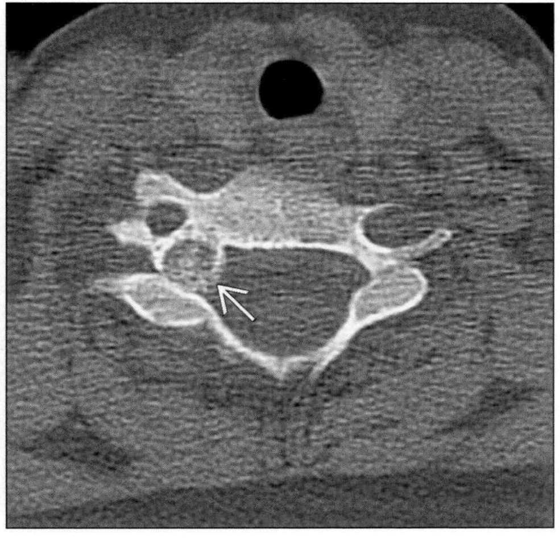

(Left) *Sagittal T1WI C+ MR spinal surveillance imaging in a pediatric patient with a malignant brain glial neoplasm shows extensive smooth and nodular enhancing intradural drop metastases.* ***(Right)*** *Axial bone CT of the cervical spine demonstrates a well-circumscribed lytic lesion in the expanded right pedicle* ➡ *with dense central nidus.*

Pyogenic Osteomyelitis

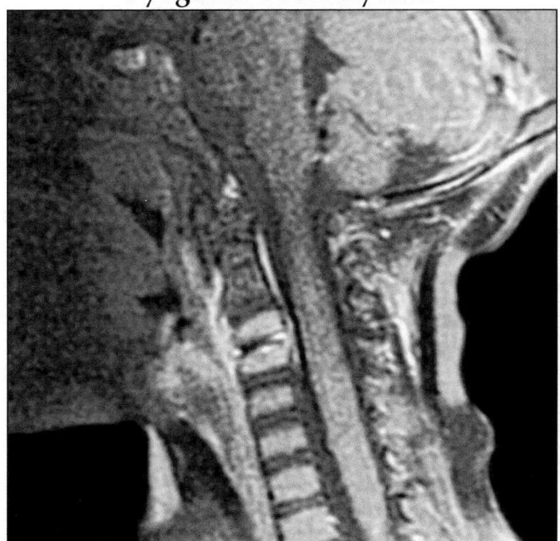

Secondary Acute Transverse Myelitis

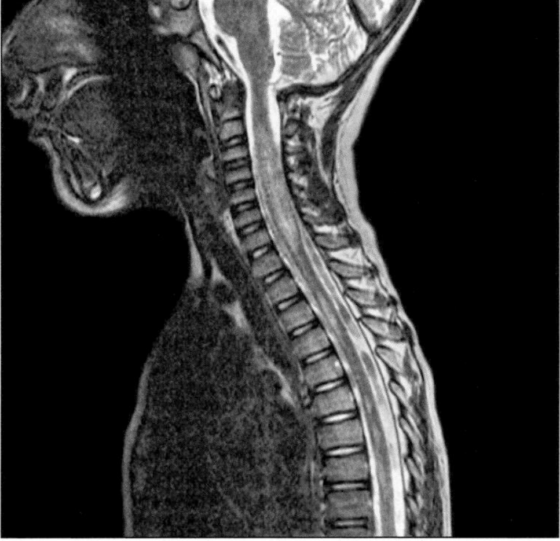

(Left) *Sagittal T1WI C+ FS MR shows C 3/4 disc space height loss with fluid signal intensity and abnormal marrow and epidural enhancement adjacent to disc space indicating discitis with osteomyelitis. No spinal cord compression is present.* ***(Right)*** *Sagittal T2WI MR demonstrates abnormal intramedullary T2 hyperintensity extending to the conus level (not shown). The areas of abnormality are patchy rather than contiguous.*

LUMBAR SOFT TISSUE MASS

DIFFERENTIAL DIAGNOSIS

Common
- Lipomyelomeningocele
- Myelomeningocele
- Spinal Lipoma
- Traumatic Spinal Muscle Injury
- Scoliosis

Less Common
- Plexiform Neurofibroma
- Ewing Sarcoma
- Lymphoma
- Venous Vascular Malformation
- Lymphatic Malformation
- Paraspinal Abscess

Rare but Important
- Lytic Osseous Metastases
- Hemangiopericytoma
- Dorsal Spinal Meningocele
- Pseudomeningocele

ESSENTIAL INFORMATION

Key Differential Diagnosis Issues
- Appearance of overlying skin, pertinent clinical information helps limit differential list

Helpful Clues for Common Diagnoses
- **Lipomyelomeningocele**
  - Lipomyelocele = neural placode-lipoma complex contiguous with subcutaneous fat through dysraphic defect, attaching to and tethering spinal cord
  - Lipomyelomeningocele = lipomyelocele + meningocele, enlargement of subarachnoid space, displacement of neural placode outside of spinal canal
- **Myelomeningocele**
  - Posterior spinal defect lacking skin covering ⇒ neural tissue, CSF, and meninges exposed to air
  - Lumbosacral (44%) > thoracolumbar (32%) > lumbar (22%) > thoracic (2%)
  - Low-lying cord on postoperative MR imaging does not always = clinical tethering
- **Spinal Lipoma**
  - Arise from premature separation (dysjunction) of cutaneous ectoderm from neuroectoderm during neurulation
  - Profound hypodensity on CT and T1WI hyperintensity characteristic of fat
  - Use chemical fat saturation or inversion recovery MR techniques to confirm fat content
- **Traumatic Spinal Muscle Injury**
  - Paraspinal muscle fiber disruption from indirect forces ⇒ abnormal muscle T2 hyperintensity and swelling
  - Most commonly from MVA; also athletic injuries, blow from falling objects, direct injury
- **Scoliosis**
  - General term for any lateral curvature of spine
    - Dextroscoliosis: Curve convex to right
    - Levoscoliosis: Curve convex to left
    - Kyphoscoliosis: Scoliosis with component of kyphosis
    - Rotoscoliosis: Scoliosis which includes rotation of vertebrae
  - Short-curve scoliosis usually has underlying abnormalities; consider congenital, neoplasm, or inflammation

Helpful Clues for Less Common Diagnoses
- **Plexiform Neurofibroma**
  - Long, bulky, multinodular nerve enlargement is pathognomonic for NF1
  - Often affects sacral or brachial plexi
- **Ewing Sarcoma**
  - 5% of all Ewing tumors in spine (sacrum > rest of spine)
  - Usually in adolescents or younger adults
  - Permeative lytic lesion of vertebral body or sacrum involving vertebral body before neural arch
    - Contiguous spread along peripheral nerves from spine or sacral primary but may originate in soft tissues
- **Lymphoma**
  - Lymphoreticular neoplasms with wide variety of specific diseases and cellular differentiation
  - Multiple types demonstrate variable imaging manifestations
- **Venous Vascular Malformation**
  - Congenital trans-spatial vascular malformation of venous channels present from birth

- May be mass-like, frequently enhances moderately (less than soft tissue hemangioma)
- No arterial vessels within lesion, venous channels may be large
- Look for phleboliths to make specific diagnosis

- **Lymphatic Malformation**
  - Congenital trans-spatial vascular malformation of lymphatic channels present from birth
  - Typically minimal to no enhancement, although septations may enhance, especially if previously inflamed
  - Fluid-fluid levels strongly suggest diagnosis
  - May grow rapidly if hemorrhage or concurrent viral infection
- **Paraspinal Abscess**
  - Suppuration of paraspinal soft tissue from direct extension or hematogenous dissemination of pathogens
  - Identification of calcified psoas abscesses suggests tuberculous paraspinal abscess

Helpful Clues for Rare Diagnoses

- **Lytic Osseous Metastases**
  - Osteolytic metastases of primary tumor to spine; bone destruction exceeds bone production ⇒ lytic rather than blastic
  - Lesion usually destroys posterior cortex, pedicle first
- **Hemangiopericytoma**
  - Vividly enhancing hypervascular neoplasm arising from pericytes expanding/eroding spinal canal with large soft tissue component
  - Dural-based if primary, epicenter in bone if metastatic
  - Previously called angioblastic meningioma but probably different tumors
- **Dorsal Spinal Meningocele**
  - Skin-covered dorsal dural sac containing arachnoid, CSF protruding thorough posterior osseous defect into subcutaneous tissues
    - Always skin-covered; skin may be dysplastic or ulcerated
  - Lumbosacral junction, sacrum > > cervical, thoracic
    - Mild cases may show only absent spinous process or localized spina bifida
    - More severe cases show multisegmental spina bifida, spinal canal enlargement
- **Pseudomeningocele**
  - CSF-filled spinal axis cyst with supportive postoperative or post-traumatic ancillary findings
  - Cyst contiguous with thecal sac, not lined by meninges
  - Fat-saturated T2WI best sequence to demonstrate pseudomeningocele and localize dural communication

Lipomyelomeningocele

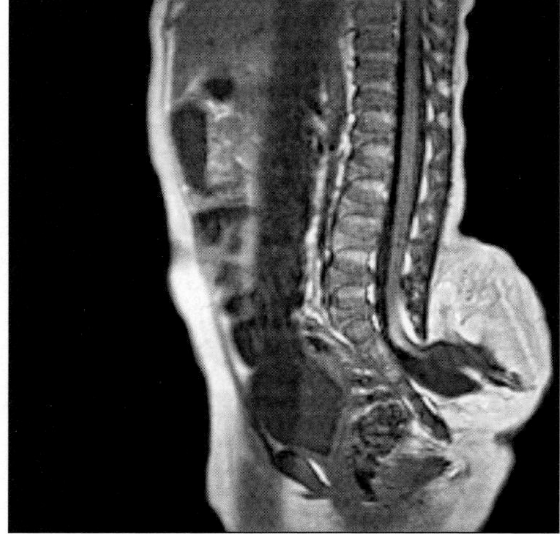

Sagittal T1WI MR demonstrates a low-lying spinal cord inserting into a large lipomatous malformation that is contiguous with subcutaneous fat extending through a posterior dysraphic defect.

Myelomeningocele

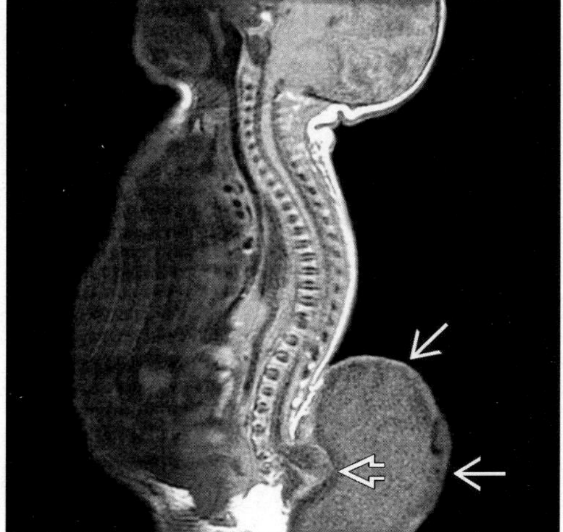

Sagittal T1WI MR shows a large unrepaired myelomeningocele sac ➔. Neural elements are seen protruding into the sac ⇨, which was not skin covered, confirming diagnosis of myelomeningocele.

LUMBAR SOFT TISSUE MASS

Spinal Lipoma

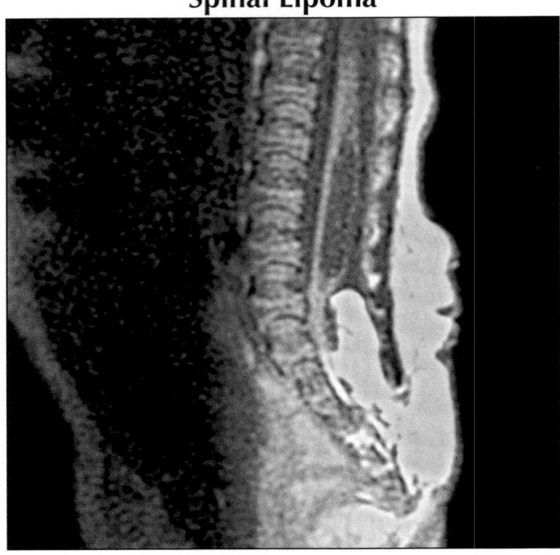

Traumatic Spinal Muscle Injury

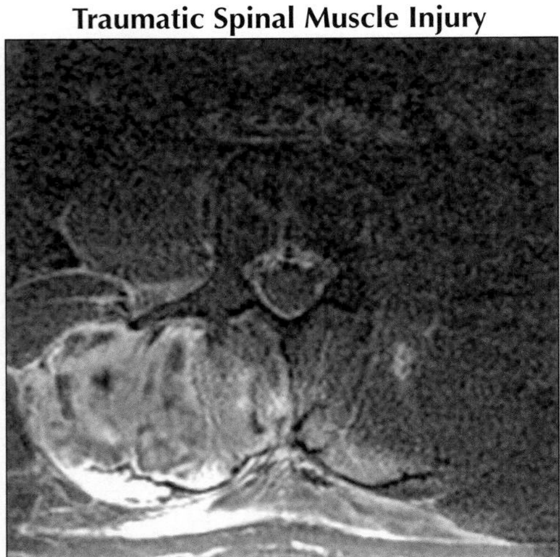

(Left) *Sagittal T1WI MR demonstrates a large terminal lipoma adherent to the distal spinal cord contiguous with subcutaneous fat in a patient clinically presenting with a palpable lumbar mass.* ***(Right)*** *Axial T2WI FS MR in a trauma patient with back pain and swelling reveals characteristic diffuse soft tissue edema in the right paraspinal muscles and subcutaneous tissues.*

Scoliosis

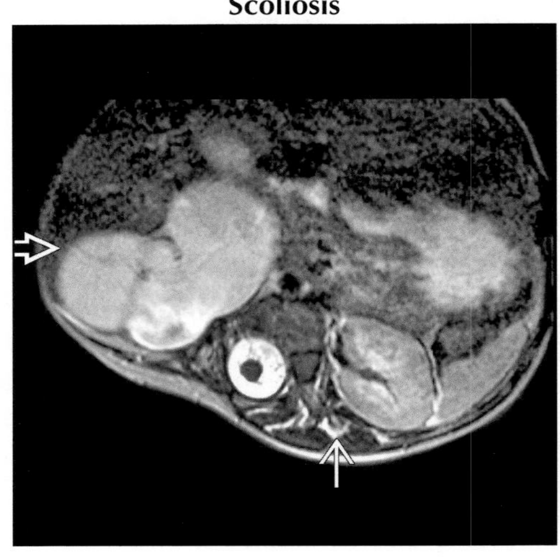

Plexiform Neurofibroma

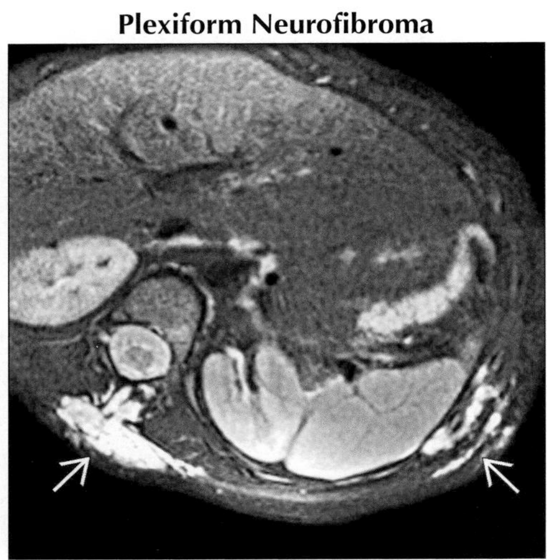

(Left) *Axial T2WI FS MR in a patient with VACTERL demonstrates protrusion of the left paraspinal soft tissues ➔ due to congenital scoliosis, explaining palpable area of clinical concern. Note also the dysplastic right kidney ➔.* ***(Right)*** *Axial STIR MR in this patient with neurofibromatosis type 1 reveals 2 palpable, T2 hyperintense, soft tissue plexiform neurofibromas ➔.*

Ewing Sarcoma

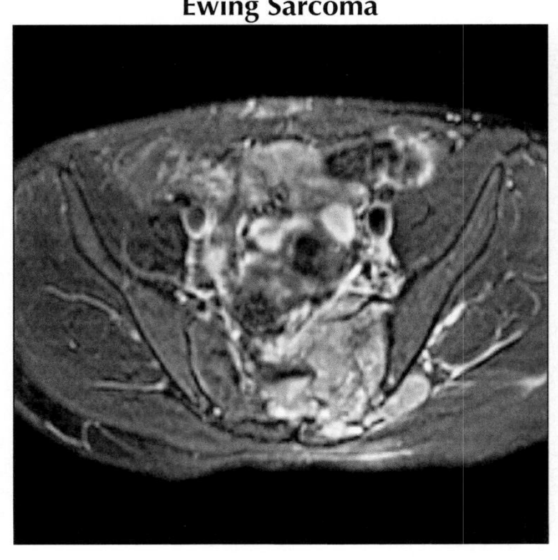

Lymphoma

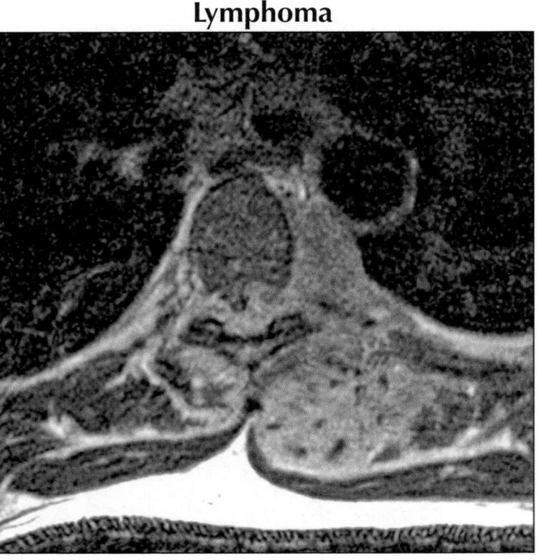

(Left) *Axial T2WI FS MR depicts a large pelvic Ewing sarcoma with tumor extension into the lumbosacral soft tissues, producing pain and a clinically palpable mass.* ***(Right)*** *Axial T1WI C+ MR demonstrates a large enhancing thoracolumbar epidural mass at the site of palpable concern, extending into the paraspinal muscles and epidural space.*

LUMBAR SOFT TISSUE MASS

Venous Vascular Malformation

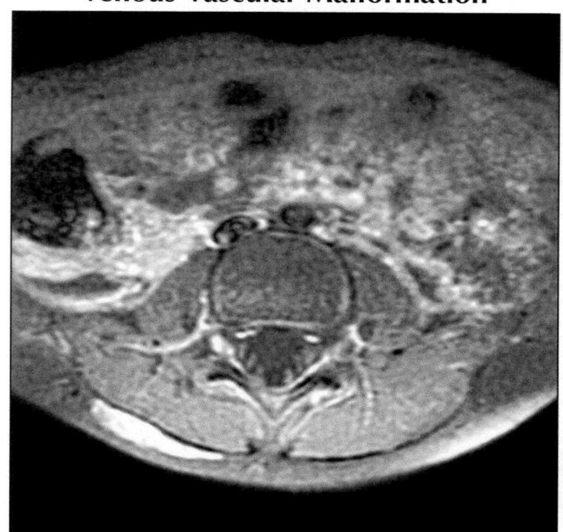

Lymphatic Malformation

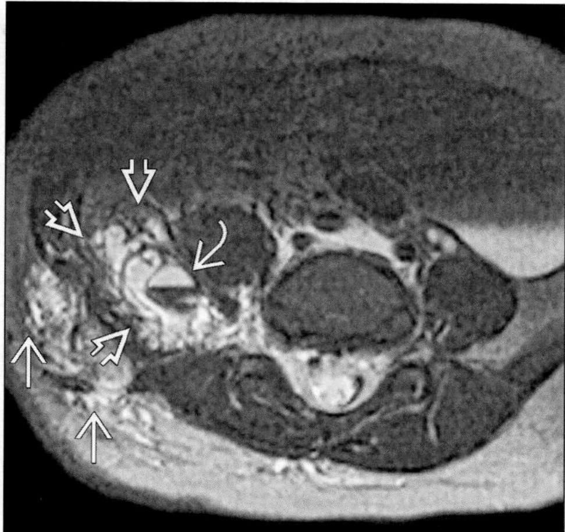

***(Left)** Axial T1WI C+ FS MR shows homogeneous enhancement within a subcutaneous dorsal soft tissue mass. The size of this clinically palpable mass changed with position and onset of crying. **(Right)** Axial T2WI FS MR reveals a large abdominal ➔ lymphatic malformation with trans-spatial extension into the right lumbar flank soft tissues ➔ of this patient with Proteus syndrome. Note the characteristic fluid-fluid level ➔.*

Paraspinal Abscess

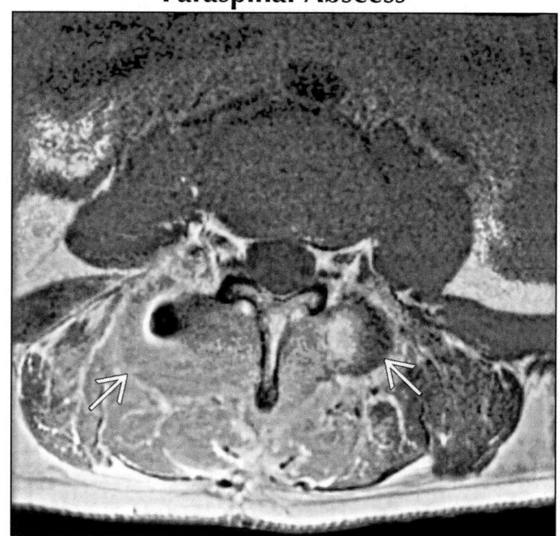

Hemangiopericytoma

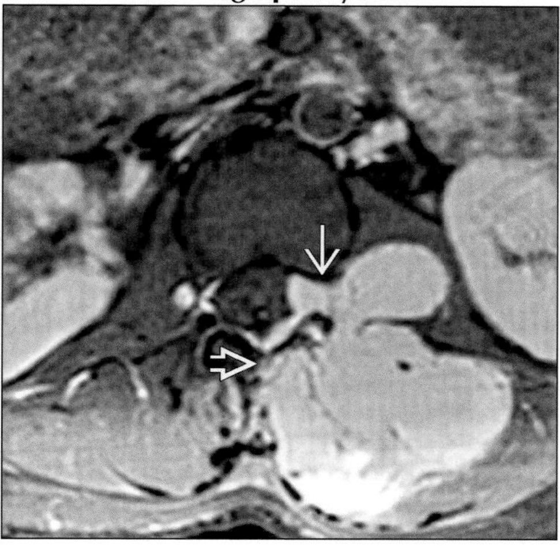

***(Left)** Axial T1WI C+ MR following posterior spinal fusion reveals a large rim-enhancing fluid collection ➔ that surrounds the hardware with marginal inflammation in the dorsal paraspinal soft tissues. **(Right)** Axial T1WI C+ MR shows a large, lobulated, paravertebral enhancing mass that involves the left dorsal elements ➔. Note the extension along the dural margin into the left neural foramen ➔.*

Dorsal Spinal Meningocele

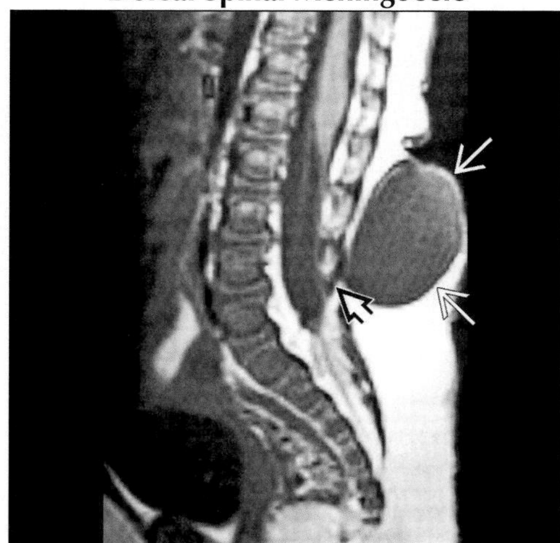

Pseudomeningocele

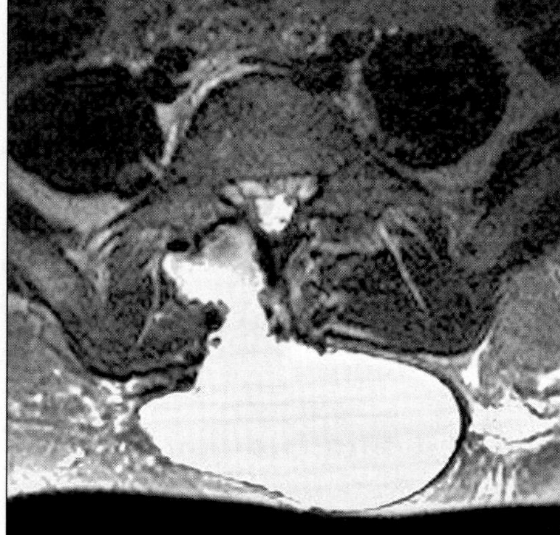

***(Left)** Sagittal T1WI MR shows a mildly low-lying conus at L2 and a large, skin-covered, dorsal CSF signal mass ➔ communicating with the thecal sac via a very thin, fluid signal pedicle traversing the posterior elements ➔. **(Right)** Axial T2WI MR shows a large CSF signal fluid collection in the dorsal lumbar soft tissues, extending from the right hemilaminectomy site into subcutaneous tissues. There is no displacement or mass effect upon the thecal sac.*

SACROCOCCYGEAL MASS

DIFFERENTIAL DIAGNOSIS

Common
- Sacrococcygeal Teratoma
- Presacral Abscess

Less Common
- Neuroblastic Tumor
- Plexiform Neurofibroma
- Lymphoma
- Chondrosarcoma
- Ewing Sarcoma

Rare but Important
- Rhabdomyosarcoma
- Osteosarcoma
- Dermoid and Epidermoid Tumors
- Myxopapillary Ependymoma
- Anterior Sacral Meningocele
- Terminal Myelocystocele
- Enteric Cyst

ESSENTIAL INFORMATION

Key Differential Diagnosis Issues
- Myriad pathologies produce sacrococcygeal masses
  - Clinical data directs differential list
- Fever, elevated inflammatory markers prompt search for infection source
- Identification of tumor matrix narrows differential considerations
- Location and relationship of mass to important regional structures impacts tumor resectability
- Look for osseous invasion or epidural extension, which may alter surgical planning

Helpful Clues for Common Diagnoses
- **Sacrococcygeal Teratoma**
  - Very heterogeneous density/signal intensity, enhancement of solid tumor portions
  - AAP grade based on proportion of external and internal tumor
  - Worse outcome portended by
    - Male sex
    - Large proportion of internal tumor
    - Older age at diagnosis
  - Often detected on routine obstetrical ultrasound ⇒ elective cesarean section
    - Fetal MR valuable for confirmation of diagnosis, AAP grading
  - Sacrum and coccyx usually spared, even when tumor spreads into spinal canal via sacral hiatus
  - Coccyx must be resected or recurrence risk high
- **Presacral Abscess**
  - Fever, serum inflammatory markers usually elevated, prompting clinical consideration of diagnosis
  - Regional soft tissue inflammation, discitis, epidural abscess, or vertebral osteomyelitis
  - Rim enhancement and diffusion restriction on DWI MR characteristic

Helpful Clues for Less Common Diagnoses
- **Neuroblastic Tumor**
  - Paraspinal location along sympathetic chain (neural crest derivatives)
  - Benign (ganglioneuroma) → intermediate grade (ganglioneuroblastoma) → highly malignant (neuroblastoma)
  - Frequently calcified, encircles vessels and regional structures
  - Important upstaging findings affecting surgical management include bilaterality and epidural extension
    - MR best imaging modality for detecting tumor extension into spinal canal through neural foramen
- **Plexiform Neurofibroma**
  - Neurofibromatosis type 1
  - Grape-like or botryoid morphology with characteristic distribution along nerves (major or minor peripheral nerves/plexi)
  - Hyperintense on STIR MR, T2WI MR
    - "Target" appearance
- **Lymphoma**
  - Protean imaging appearances
  - Often large at diagnosis
  - May be focal or diffuse
  - Relatively low signal intensity on T2WI MR ± mild diffusion restriction reflects high tumor cellularity
- **Ewing Sarcoma**
  - Usually older child/adolescent presentation age
  - Aggressive or permeative bone destruction
  - Cellular signal intensity (relatively low signal intensity on T2WI MR)

Helpful Clues for Rare Diagnoses

- **Rhabdomyosarcoma**
  - Aggressive soft tissue mass with frequent bone invasion
  - Rarely arises primarily in sacrum
    - Usually regional extension from prostate or uterus primary tumor
  - Signal characteristics variable
    - Frequently shows cellular characteristics with lower signal intensity on T2WI MR
- **Osteosarcoma**
  - Destructive lesion with frank bone destruction and large soft tissue mass
  - May arise in preexisting lesion (aneurysmal bone cyst, fibrous dysplasia)
  - Osteoid matrix makes diagnosis
- **Dermoid and Epidermoid Tumors**
  - Consider previous lumbar puncture with nonstyletted needle, congenital dermal sinus tract
  - Contains fat &/or squamous debris
  - Epidermoid component ⇒ diffusion restriction
- **Myxopapillary Ependymoma**
  - Very uncommon sacral and presacral ependymomas have been described
  - Most myxopapillary ependymomas arise near conus or filum (may be confined entirely to filum terminale)
  - CSF-disseminated intradural metastases common
- **Anterior Sacral Meningocele**
  - Cyst contiguity with thecal sac through enlarged neural foramen is diagnostic
  - Most anterior sacral meningoceles are simple CSF signal cysts
    - May also have lipomatous component (complex anterior sacral meningocele)
- **Terminal Myelocystocele**
  - Spinal cord termination always low
  - Cystic dilatation of distal spinal cord central canal (myelocystocele) extending through dilated subarachnoid fluid collection (meningocele)
- **Enteric Cyst**
  - Fortuitous adjacent location to sacrum in isolated mesenteric or intestinal duplication cyst
  - Split notochord malformations (neurenteric cysts)

Other Essential Information

- Patient age and signal characteristics on MR imaging are most helpful criteria to narrow pertinent differential diagnosis list
- Currarino syndrome or triad
  - Sacral agenesis
  - Anorectal malformations
  - Presacral mass
    - Anterior meningocele, teratoma, lipoma, dermoid cyst, enteric cyst
  - Look for associated urogenital and limb anomalies

Sacrococcygeal Teratoma

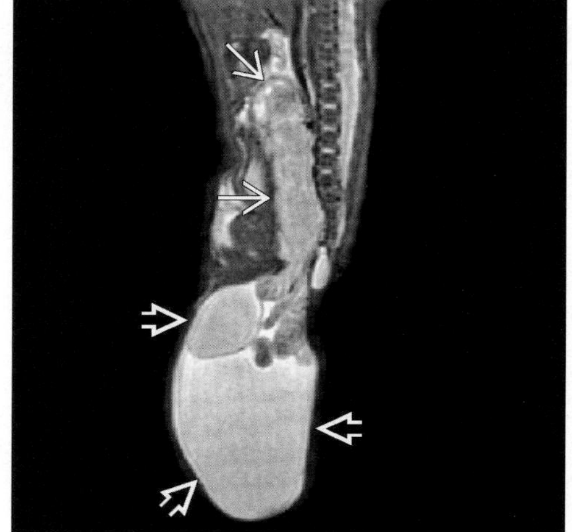

Sagittal T2WI MR shows typical case of large AAP type 2 SCT with mixed cystic and solid mass. The internal portion is predominately solid ➡ and the external portion ➡ is more cystic.

Sacrococcygeal Teratoma

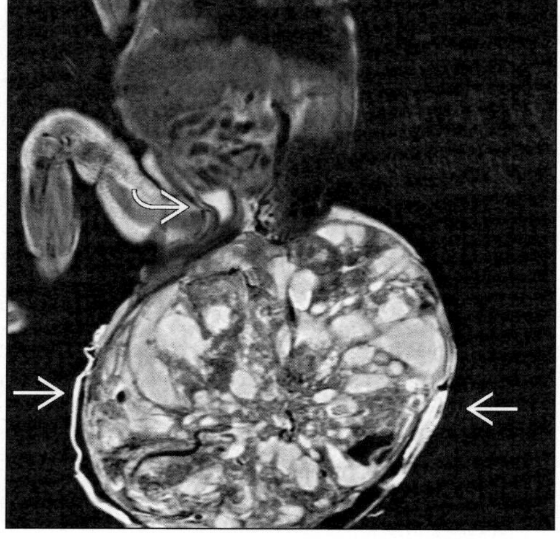

Sagittal T2WI FS MR shows a very large pedunculated mass ➡, predominantly external. Notice the displacement of the urinary bladder ➡ anteriorly.

SACROCOCCYGEAL MASS

(***Left***) *Sagittal STIR MR shows intervertebral disc space infection at L5-S1 level with extensive prevertebral T2 hyperintensity representing a presacral abscess.* (***Right***) *Sagittal T2WI MR demonstrates a large presacral soft tissue mass ➡ with sacral vertebral bone involvement as well as epidural extension ⇨ through the neural foramina.*

Presacral Abscess

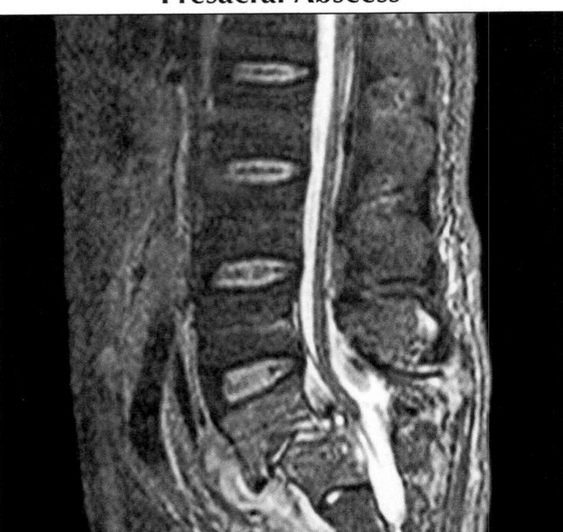

Neuroblastic Tumor

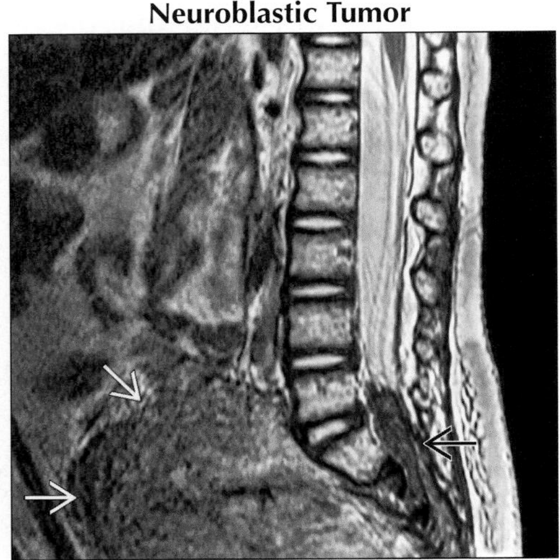

(***Left***) *Coronal STIR MR in a patient with NF1 reveals multilevel, bilateral, T2 hyperintense plexiform neurofibromas involving the spinal and pelvic nerves and relevant plexuses.* (***Right***) *Axial T1 C+ FS MR shows a large destructive sacral mass with avid enhancement spreading into the dorsal soft tissues.*

Plexiform Neurofibroma

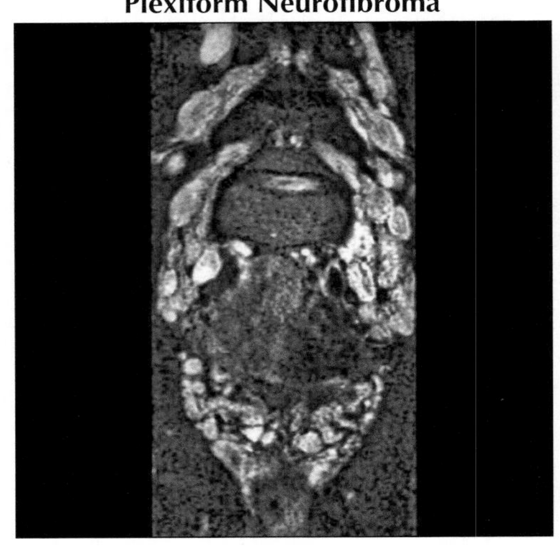

Lymphoma

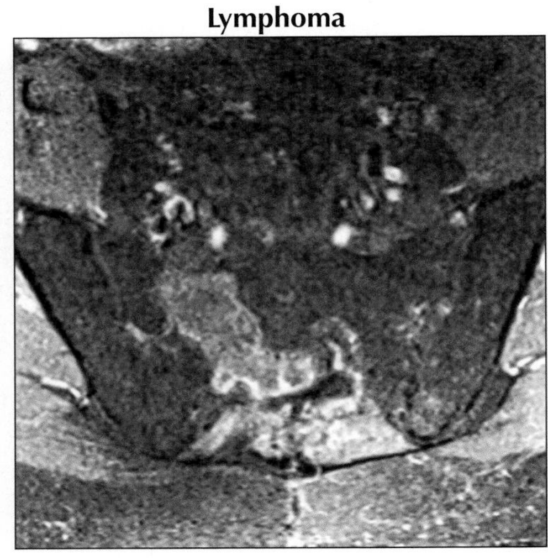

(***Left***) *Axial T2WI FS MR shows a large sacral Ewing sarcoma with bone destruction and extension into the dorsal lumbosacral soft tissues.* (***Right***) *Sagittal T2WI MR demonstrates a large exophytic sacral mass engulfing the lower sacral vertebra and extending into the central spinal canal ➡ through the sacral hiatus ⇨.*

Ewing Sarcoma

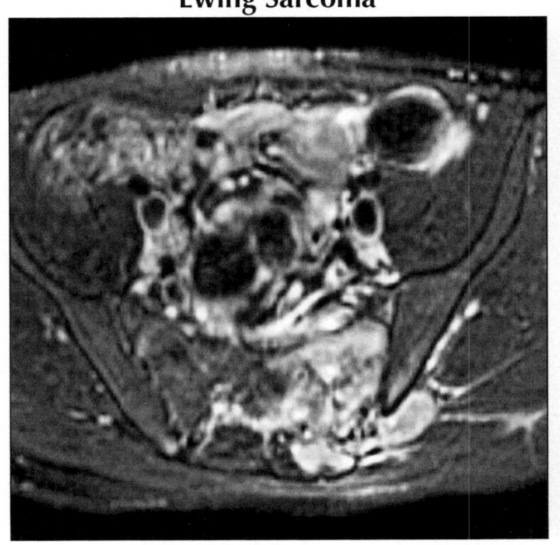

Rhabdomyosarcoma

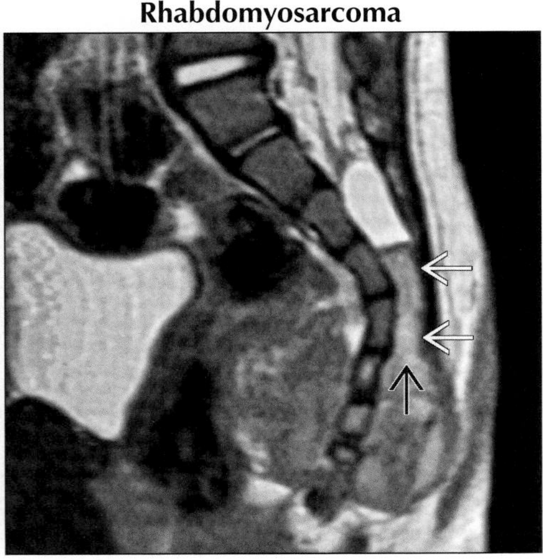

SACROCOCCYGEAL MASS

Osteosarcoma

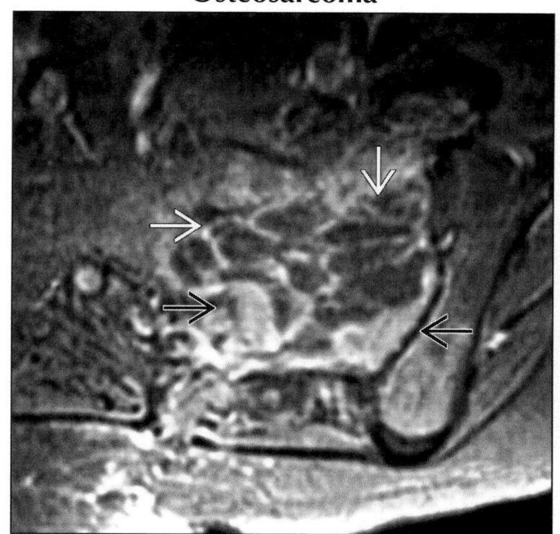

Dermoid and Epidermoid Tumors

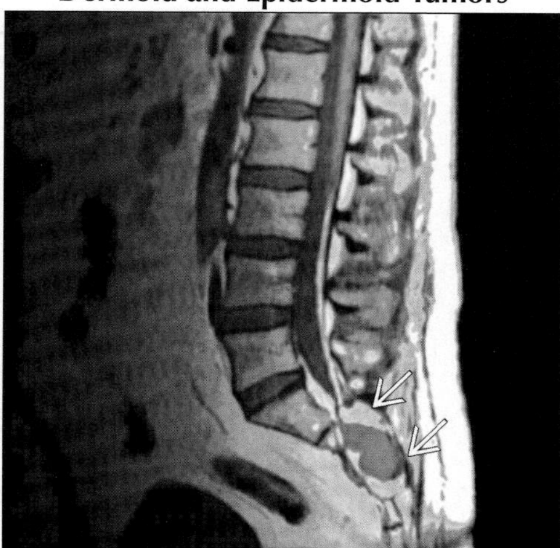

(Left) *Axial T1 C+ FS MR demonstrates a destructive pelvic mass with multiple enhancing areas of solid tumor ⇨ as well as fluid-filled, nonenhancing necrotic regions ➔.* ***(Right)*** *Sagittal T1WI MR depicts a mixed signal intensity expansile extradural sacral mass ➔. Additional findings include low-lying spinal cord and fatty filum infiltration.*

Myxopapillary Ependymoma

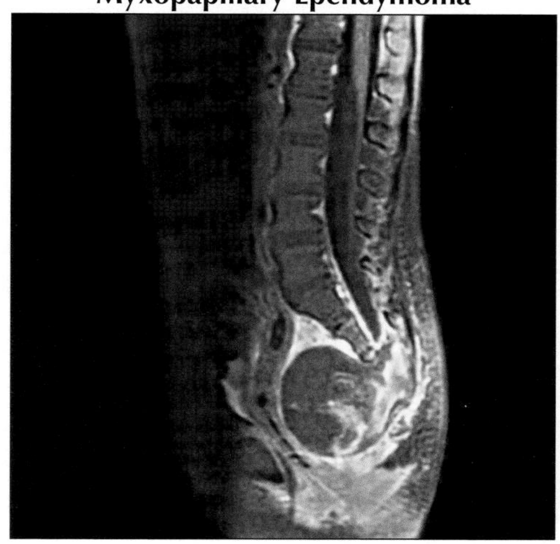

Anterior Sacral Meningocele

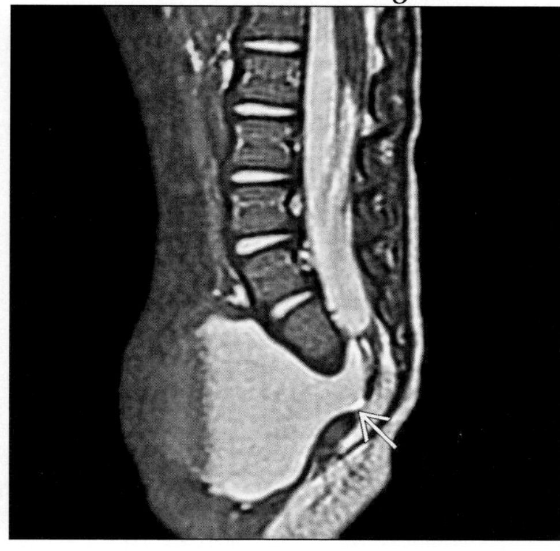

(Left) *Sagittal T1 C+ FS MR reveals a heterogeneous presacral mass with osseous destruction and spinal extension. Conus is low lying. Exact pathological diagnosis of this rare lesion has been debated but shows many features of sacral ependymoma.* ***(Right)*** *Sagittal T2WI MR demonstrates a large CSF signal intensity presacral cyst that is contiguous with the thecal sac through an enlarged sacral foramen ➔.*

Anterior Sacral Meningocele

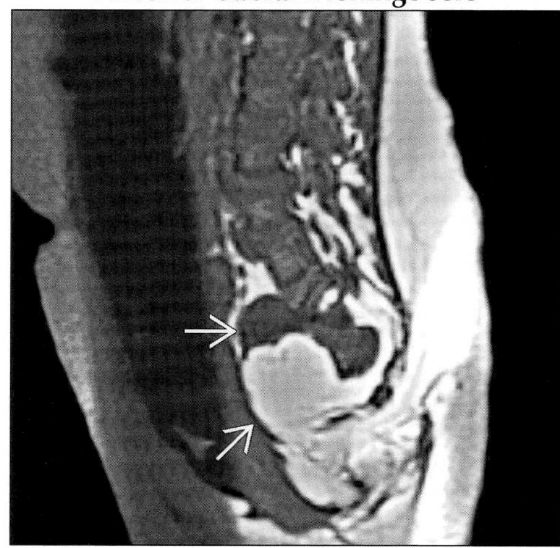

Terminal Myelocystocele

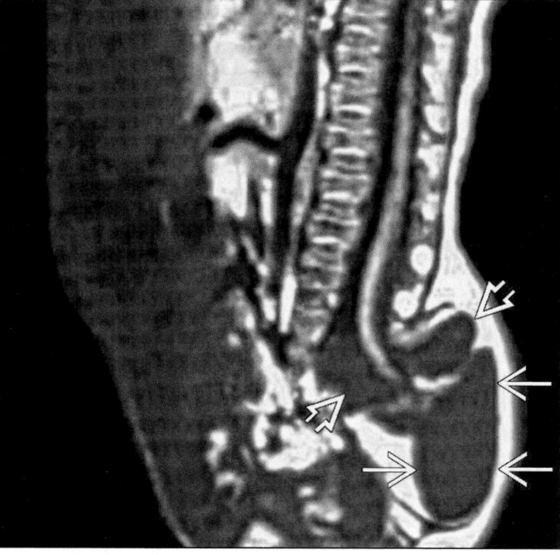

(Left) *Sagittal T1WI MR in a patient with caudal regression depicts a variant complex ASM with both cyst and lipoma components ➔ extending through the sacral foramina to produce a sacral mass.* ***(Right)*** *Sagittal T1WI MR shows the classic appearance of terminal myelocystocele, with a low-lying tethered spinal cord and distal hydromyelia ➔ traversing a meningocele ⇨.*

INDEX

A

INDEX

INDEX

INDEX

B

INDEX

C

INDEX

INDEX

INDEX

D

INDEX

E

INDEX

INDEX

INDEX

H

INDEX

INDEX

INDEX

I

J

INDEX

K

INDEX

L

INDEX

INDEX

M

INDEX

INDEX

INDEX

O

INDEX

INDEX

INDEX

R

INDEX

INDEX

INDEX

INDEX

T

INDEX

U

INDEX

V